Current Tumor Diagnosis:
Applications
Clinical Relevance
Research – Trends

Cancer of the Lung
State and Trends in Diagnosis and Therapy

**7th Symposium on Tumor Markers
Hamburg
December 5. – 8. 1993**

Scientific Advisory Board:

Prof. Dr. U. Büll, Aachen
Prof. Dr. H. Caffier, Würzburg
Prof. Dr. J. F. Chatal, Nantes
Prof. Dr. N. Dahlmann, Hamburg
Dr. A. van Dalen, Gouda
Prof. Dr. M. Dietel, Kiel
Prof. Dr. A. Encke, Frankfurt
Dr. A. A. Epenetos, London
Prof. Dr. D. Gonnermann, Hamburg
Priv.-Doz. Dr. J. R. Izbicki, Hamburg
Prof. Dr. A. Khalifa, Cairo
Prof. Dr. R. Kreienberg, Ulm
Prof. Dr. R. Lamerz, München
Dr. M. Lüthgens, Stuttgart
Prof. Dr. H. Maass, Hamburg
Prof. Dr. K. Marlicz, Stettin
Prof. Dr. W. Müller-Ruchholtz, Kiel
Prof. Dr. P. Pour, Omaha
Prof. Dr. L. Schmid, Oberstaufen
Prof. Dr. H. J. Weh, Hamburg

7th Symposium on Tumor Markers, Hamburg 1993

Current Tumor Diagnosis:
Applications
Clinical Relevance
Research – Trends

Satellite Symposium

Cancer of the Lung
State and Trends in Diagnosis and Therapy

Edited by
R. Klapdor

W. Zuckschwerdt Verlag München · Bern · Wien · New York

The Editor:

Prof. Dr. R. Klapdor
Medical Clinic
University of Hamburg
Martinistraβe 52
D-20251 Hamburg

Distributors:

Germany:	Switzerland:	Austria:	USA:
Brockhaus Kommission	Hans Huber Verlag	Maudrich Verlag	Scholium International Inc.
Verlagsauslieferung	Längassstrasse 76	Spitalgasse 21a	14 Vanderventer Ave
Kreidlerstrasse 9	CH-3000 Bern	A-1097 Wien	Port Washington
D-70806 Kornwestheim			11050 NewYork

Die Deutsche Bibliothek – CIP-Einheitsaufnahme:

Current tumor diagnosis : applications, clinical relevance, research, trends / 7th Symposium on Tumor Markers, Hamburg 1993 ; Satellite Symposium Cancer of the Lung – State and Trends in Diagnosis and Therapy. Ed. by R. Klapdor. – München ; Bern ; Wien ; New York : Zuckschwerdt, 1994
ISBN 3-88603-509-3
NE: Klapdor, Rainer [Hrsg.]; Hamburger Symposium über Tumormarker <7, 1993>; Satellite Symposium Cancer of the Lung – State and Trends in Diagnosis and Therapy <1993, Hamburg>

Insofar as this book mentions any dosage or application, readers may rest assured that the authors, editors and publishers have made every effort to ensure that such references are strictly in accordance with the state of knowledge at the time of production of the book. Nevertheless, every user is requested to carefully examine the manufacturer's leaflets accompanying each drug to check on his own responsibility whether the dosage schedules recommended therein or the contraindications stated by the manufacturers differ from the statements made in the present book. Such examination is particularly important with drugs that are either rarely used or have been newly released on the market.

Trade-mark protection will not always be marked. The absence of a reference does not indicate an unprotected trade-mark.

The opinions expressed in this presentation are those of the panelists and are not attributable to the sponsor of the publisher or the editor.

All rights reserved. No part of this publication may be produced, stored in a retrieval system, or transmitted in any form or by any means, electronic, mechanical, photocopying, recording or otherwise, without prior permission from the publisher.

© 1994 by W. Zuckschwerdt Verlag GmbH, Kronwinkler Strasse 24, D-81245 München (Germany). Printed in Germany by Presse-Druck Augsburg.

ISBN 3-88603-509-3

Contents

Preface XV

In Vitro Diagnosis
Gastroenterology

Friedrich R.E., Plambeck K., Hellner D., Thoms V.W., Bahlo M., Klapdor R. (Hamburg):
Initial values of tumor associated antigens (TAA) in the sera of patients with primary oral
squamous cell carcinomas 3

Friedrich R.E., Krüll A., Plambeck K., Hellner D., Thoms V., Bahlo M., Klapdor R. (Hamburg):
Tumor-associated antigens (SCC, CEA, TPA) in patients with squamous cell carcinomas of the
head and neck before and after preoperative percutaneous irradiation. A preliminary report . 7

Friedrich R.E., Plambeck K., Hellner D., Thoms V., Bahlo M., Klapdor R. (Hamburg):
Determination of tumor-associated antigens (TAA) in sera of patients with carcinomas
of the salivary glands in the head and neck (diagnosis and follow-up) 10

Reiter W., Stieber P., Reuter C., Cramer C., Fateh-Moghadam A. (Munich): CA 72-4, CEA, CA 19-9
in diagnosis of relapse and metastases and in prognosis of stomach cancer patients 13

Gärtner U., Scheulen M.E., Aghabi E., Wiefelspütz J., Delbrück H. (Wuppertal, Bad Gandersheim,
Essen): Determination of CA 72-4 by IRMA or ELISA in the follow-up of gastric cancer patients 17

Safi F., Kuhns V., Beger H.G. (Ulm): Tumor markers in gastric cancer 20

Oremek G.M., Kirsten D., Lorenz M., Kirsten R., Nelson K., Seiffert U.B. (Frankfurt/M):
Phospholipids and tumor markers in the differential diagnosis and therapy of gastric cancer . 28

Lamerz R., Mann K., Segura E., Spöttl G., Brandt A. (Munich): Use of AFP and its LCA-differentiation
for the detection, monitoring, and differential diagnosis of hepatocellular carcinoma 30

Cichoż-Lach H., Celiński K., Slomka M., Pokora J. (Lublin): Levels of alpha-fetoprotein in
chronic liver diseases 34

Lundin J., Roberts P.J., Kuusela P., Haglund C. (Helsinki): The prognostic value of preoperative
serum levels of CA 19-9, CA 242 and CEA in patients with pancreatic cancer 37

Friess H., Hammer K., Auerbach B., Müller M., Büchler M.W. (Bern, Marburg):
CA 494: High sensitivity and specificity in pancreatic cancer 41

Plebani M., Basso D., Panozzo M.P., Navaglia F., D'Angeli F., Del Giudice G., Battistel M.,
Del Favero G. (Padova): CA 242 – A real new tumor marker of pancreatic carcinoma? 46

Wiklund B., Silén Å., Nilsson S., Andersson E.L. (Borlänge, Uppsala, Lund): Monoclonal TPAcyk
assays quantifying human cytokeratin 8 and 18 fragments in serum of cancer patients 50

Pohlmann G., Klapdor R., Bahlo M., Gross E. (Hamburg): Preliminary data on the influence of
octreotidacetat (S 100) on the parameters amylase, lipase as well as CA 19-9, CA 125 and
TPS in the course of pancreatic surgery 55

Carpelan-Holmström M., Haglund C., Kuusela P., Järvinen H., Roberts P.J. (Helsinki):
Preoperative CA 242 and CEA serum levels in patients with colorectal cancer 57

Gebauer G., Müller-Ruchholtz W. (Kiel): Quantitative measurement of the tumor markers CEA,
CA 19-9, CA 15-3, CA 125, AFP, β-HCG and SCC in tumor tissue, healthy colonic mucosa and
serum of patients with colorectal cancer 61

Paul M.A., Visser J.J., van Kamp G.J., Mulder C., Meijer S. (Amsterdam): Biliary CEA levels in
patients with liver metastases of colorectal cancer 66

Riedl S., Bodenmüller H., Schlag P., Faissner A. (Heidelberg, Tutzing, Berlin): Clinical significance
of tenascin serum levels in colorectal carcinomas 70

Khalifa A., Eissa S., Zaki S., Khalid M., El-Ghor H., Abdalla A., El-Banna M. (Cairo): Correlation
between cell cycle kinetics and serum markers: CEA and CA19-9 in colorectal cancer 72

Jaunalksne I., Donina S., Zakenfelds G., Januskevics V., Svarcbergs A. (Riga): Comparison of the
tumor markers CA 19-9 and CEA for follow-up of patients with gastrointestinal cancer 77

Meyer-Pannwitt U., Dorß V.A., Fröschle G., Klapdor R., Schreiber H.W. (Hamburg): Significance
of neuron-specific enolase (NSE) as a tumor marker in the diagnosis and follow-up of surgical
patients with abdominal neuroendocrine tumors 80

Plebani M., Navaglia F., Basso D., De Paoli M., Bortolotti L., Cipriani A. (Padova): CYFRA 21-1 serum determination: Which utility in the diagnosis of gastrointestinal tumors? 87

Hansson L.-O. (Stockholm): Comparison of two assays (TPA and TPS) for cytokeratin polypeptides in serum using three different patient groups and in healthy subjects 90

Hryniewiecki L., Klincewicz K., Breborowicz D. (Poznań): Tumor markers in ascitic fluid. Efficacy of the method as a tool for screening studies and differential diagnosis 93

Nägele H., Gebhardt A., Niendorf A., Sandersfeld F., Klapdor R., Daerr W., Meyer-Pannwitt U. (Hamburg): Tumor markers and cholesterol metabolism in patients with gastrointestinal cancer 97

Gynecology

Sturm G., Schmidt-Rhode P., Chari S., Bauer T. (Marburg): Evaluation of cancer associated serum antigen (CASA) as an additional tumor marker in ovarian carcinoma 105

Ward B.G., McGuckin M.A. (Herston): Practical uses of CASA and CA 125 estimation in the management of ovarian cancer 108

Kristen P., Dörffler P., Caffier H. (Würzburg): Clinical value of CASA versus CA 125 in ovarian cancer 111

Meisel M., Weise J., Straube W. (Greifswald): Time course of tumor markers CASA and CA 125 in patients with ovarian carcinoma 115

Hasholzner U., Baumgartner L., Stieber P., Meier W., Hofmann K., Fateh-Moghadam A. (Munich): Significance of the tumor markers CA 125 II, CA 72-4, CASA and CYFRA 21-1 in ovarian carcinomas 119

Malm A.M., Costa S.D., Huober J., Roth H.J., Diel I.J., Bastert G. (Heidelberg): Comparison of the cancer-associated serum antigen (CASA) with CA 125 – Specificity and sensitivity in benign and malignant disorders 123

Kenemans P., Verstraeten A.A., van Kamp G.J., Hilgers J. (Amsterdam): Tumor markers in gynecology 125

Nilsson O., Karlsson B., Lindholm L., Pettersson A. (Gothenburg): Development of assays for determination of MUC-1 breast cancer antigen 130

Torre G.C., Barbetti V., Paganuzzi M., Mazzei C., Onetto M., Bobbio B., Bruzzone M., Lucchese V., Boccardo F., Gaffuri M., Rembado R. (Pietra Ligure, Genova): Tissue polypeptide specific (TPS) antigen in benign and malignant gynecological diseases 134

Walker R.P., Crebbin V., Stern J., Brown J., Scudder S., Schwartz P. (Alameda, San Francisco, Davis, New Haven): Urinary gonadotropin peptide (UGP) as a marker for gynecologic malignancies . . . 138

Gaarenstroom K.N., Bonfrer J.M.G., Korse C.M., Van Huizen M.E., Helmerhorst Th.J.M. (Leiden, Amsterdam): Prognostic value of serum fragments of cytokeratin 19 in patients with cervical cancer 143

Oremek G.M., Vering A., Stegmüller M., Seiffert U.B. (Frankfurt): Clinical value of mammary serum antigen (MSA) as a tumor marker for breast carcinoma 146

Meisel M., Straube W., Versümer C. (Greifswald): Time course of tumor markers MSA, CA 15-3 and CA 549 in patients with breast cancer 149

Heilenkötter U., Jagella P., Bahlo M., Klapdor R. (Geesthacht, Hamburg): TPS compared to CA 15-3 and CEA in primary diagnosis of breast cancer 152

Spitz J., Benz P., Ewald L., Rink Th., Berle P. (Wiesbaden): The diagnostic efficiency of the tumor marker CA 15-3 155

Essmann-Seboth D., Fuchs I., Jakesz R., Reiner G., Zekert F., Zekert M. (Wien): CA 15-3 in the postoperative follow-up of breast cancer patients 158

Alter G., Mende T. (Halle): The diagnostic value of the serum tumor markers CEA and CA 549 in patients with scintigraphically verified skeletal metastases of mammary carcinomas 160

Drahovsky M., Greiner-Mai E., Lentfer D. (Dietzenbach): Follow-up of breast cancer using CA 15-3 immunoluminometric determination 163

Krämer S., Katalinic A., Jäger W. (Erlangen): Survival time in breast cancer patients with osseous metastases after increase of CEA compared to CA 15-3 167

Jäger W., Kissing A., Cilaci S., Palapelas V., Lang N. (Erlangen): Is an increase of CA 125 in breast cancer patients an indicator of pleural metastases? 170

Schelp C., Wege S., Pfleiderer P., Boßlet K., Madry N. (Marburg): A new chemiluminescence immunoassay for the detection of PEM in breast cancer sera 174

Van Dalen A., Blusse van OudAlblas A., Heering K.J., vd Linde D.L. (Gouda): Are tumor marker changes in breast cancer reliable? 178

Krämer S., Reinhardt G., Jäger W. (Erlangen): Is there still a relevance for measuring CEA during follow-up in breast cancer patients? 181

Bach F., Söletormos G., Bjerregaard B., Bach F.W., Horn Th. (Herlev, Copenhagen): Cerebrospinal fluid TPA and CK-BB in comparison with cytology in diagnosing central nervous system metastases secondary to breast cancer 184

Beck E., Moldenhauer A., Kiesewetter F., Jäger W., Wildt L., Lang N. (Erlangen): In vitro analysis of CA 125 production and release by ovarian cancer cells 187

Möbus V.J., Kieback D.G., Grill H.-J., Kreienberg R. (Ulm): Detection of the tumor-associated antigens CA 125, TPS, CA 72-4 and CASA in the supernatant of 25 human ovarian cancer cell lines 192

Lung

Ebert W., Dienemann H., Fateh-Moghadam A., Müller Ch., Scheulen M.E., Konietzko N., Schleich Th., Bombardieri E., Banauch D., Mühlhofer W. (Heidelberg, Munich, Essen, Nuremberg, Milano, Mannheim): Enzymun-test CYFRA 21-1: Results of the clinical phase 1 multicenter study in bronchogenic carcinoma 199

Scheulen M.E., Klanig H., Wiefelspütz J.K., Kämper P., Wagner B., Konietzko N., Seeber S. (Essen): Radioimmunoassay of CYFRA 21-1 in 240 patients with untreated lung cancer 204

Van der Gaast A., Schoenmaker C., Kok T.C., Blijenberg B.G., Splinter T.A.W. (Rotterdam-Dijkzigt): Clinical applications of CYFRA 21-1 in patients with non-small cell lung cancer 207

Rastel D. (Gif-sur-Yvette): CYFRA 21-1, a non-small cell lung cancer tumor marker. Report of the first multicenter evaluation 210

Bonfrer J.M.G., Korse C.M., Baas P. (Amsterdam): CYFRA 21-1, a new marker tested during follow-up of patients treated for adenocarcinoma of the lung 215

Van der Gaast A., Schoenmaker C., Kok T.C., Blijenberg B.G., Splinter T.A.W. (Rotterdam-Dijkzigt): Prognostic significance of TPS in patients with non-small cell lung cancer 218

Gittermann G., Klapdor R., Bahlo M., Kaukel E., Beuerlein I., Dahlmann N., Jaworrek D. (Harburg, Hamburg, Tutzing): Cyfra 21-1, TPA, TPAcyk and TPS versus CEA, CA 19-9, SCC and NSE in lung cancer 220

Lüdtke B., Bahlmann G., Wood W.G. (Stralsund): Can CYFRA 21-1 replace tissue polypeptide antigen (TPA)? Studies on different patient groups including those with renal insufficiency 227

Bodenmüller H., Ofenloch B., Lane B., Banauch D., Dessauer A. (Tutzing, Dundee): Biochemical characterization of CYFRA 21-1, a serum marker for monitoring of lung cancer 231

Rameken M., Bahlo M., Hassanein A., Klapdor R., von Osten A., Niendorf A. (Hamburg): Secretion of CYFRA 21-1, TPS and TPA as well as CEA in relation to growth kinetics – Studies in nude mice bearing xenografts of human lung and pancreatic carcinomas 234

Auerbach B., Takamatsu K., Lang N., Gerardy-Schahn R., Jaques G., Madry N. (Marburg, Frankfurt, Hannover, Yokohama): Embryonic NCAM isoform as a serum tumor marker in small cell lung cancer. Biochemical characterization and methods for detection 239

Ebert W., Brömmer H., Schapöhler B., Muley Th. (Heidelberg): Elevated serum levels of ICTP do not prove bone metastases in small cell lung cancer 242

Brenner W., Zimmermann J., Bohuslavizki K.H., Eberhardt J.-U., Clausen M., Henze E. (Kiel): Clinical value of the tumor marker TPS versus TPA in different malignancies 246

Oremek G.M., Seiffert U.B., Jonas D. (Frankfurt): Determination of the tissue polypeptide antigen (TPA/TPS) with different commercially available assays. A methodological comparison 249

Khalifa A., Mady E.A., Tag El-Din M.A., El-Dessouki H.M. (Cairo): Tumor markers profile in broncho-alveolar lavage in lung cancer 252

Urogenital Tract

Schambeck C., Stieber P., Hell H., Hasholzner U., Hofmann K., Schmeller N., Fateh-Moghadam A. (Munich): Significance of the tumor markers TATI, NSE, CYFRA 21-1 and TPAcyk in carcinomas of the kidney 257

El-Ahmady O., Gamal El-Din A., Eissa S., Helal Th., Khalaf I. (Cairo): Comparison between TPA and CA 50 expression in Egyptian bladder cancer patients 260

Katzenwadel A., Schultze-Seemann W., Struve I., Sommerkamp H. (Freiburg): Plasma SCC (squamous cell carcinoma related antigen) levels in patients with bladder cancer 267

Schultze-Seemann W., Katzenwadel A., Struve I., Sommerkamp H. (Freiburg):
SCC (squamous cell carcinoma related antigen) in urine - A possible tumor marker
in patients with transitional cell carcinoma 270
Rohde D., Küsters D., Sikora R., Jakse G. (Aachen): sICAM-1 level in urine of bladder
cancer patients 274
Soloway M.S., Freiha F.S., DeVere White R.W., Graham S.D., Lamm D.L., Feygin M., Fischer L.N.
(Miami, Stanford, Sacramento, Atlanta, Morgantown, Stratford, Bromma): Tissue polypeptide
antigen (TPA) immunoradiometric assay (IRMA) in regional and systemic staging of transitional
cell carcinoma (TCC) of the urinary tract 281
Blottner S., Blottner A., Hingst O., Schadow D. (Berlin): Use of TPS as a proliferation marker
in studies of mammalian spermatogenesis 285
Nilsson O., Dahlen U., Grundström B., Karlsson B., Nilsson K. (Gothenburg): Development of
immunoassays specific for the different serological forms of PSA 289
Bluestein B., Tewari P., Zhou A., Caldwell G., Larsen F. (East Walpole): Clinical significance of free
und complexed forms of PSA in prostate cancer 297
Huber P.R., Strittmatter B., Maurer A., Schmid H.-P. (Basel): Free PSA analyzed by
chromatofocusing, molecular sieving and immunological methods 302
Spitz J., Benz P., Köllermann M. (Wiesbaden): Combined estimation of free and complexed PSA –
First clinical results 305
Huland E., Hübner D., Haese A., Huland H. (Hamburg): Early diagnosis of recurrent prostate
cancer after radical prostatectomy by a new and simple ultrasensitive PSA-detection 309
Donn F., Kondziella P., Becker H., Hannemann-Pohl K. (Hamburg): Prostate specific antigen as
a screening test for prostate cancer 313
Donn F., Kondziella P., Becker H., Hannemann-Pohl K. (Hamburg): Clinical use of serum prostate
specific antigen (PSA) 317
*Darte C., Southwick P.C., Catalona W.J., Richie J.P., Ahmann F.R., Hudson M.A., Scardino P.T.,
Flanigan R.C., deKernion J.B., Ratliff T.L., Kavoussi L.R., Dalkin B.L., Waters W.B.,
MacFarlane M.T.* (Liege, San Diego, St. Louis, Boston, Tucson, Houston, Chicago, Los Angeles):
Evaluation of prostate specific antigen (PSA) and digital rectal examination (DRE) for early
detection of prostate cancer. Results of a multicenter study of 6630 men 321
Spitz J., Benz P., Bickert Th., Köllermann M. (Wiesbaden): Clinical relevance of PSA values in urine   323
Silén Å., Nilsson S., Wiklund B., Lennartsson L. (Borlänge, Uppsala): Cytokeratin fragments –
A release product from growing prostate cancer cells? 326
Cooper E.H., Purves D.A., Yerna M-J. (Leeds, Liège): Tandem®Ostase™ – An IRMA for bone
alkaline phosphatase evaluated in breast and prostate cancer 330
Semjonow A., Adomeit H.J., Rathert P. (Münster, Düren): Skeletal alkaline phosphatase and
total alkaline phosphatase as serum markers for bone metastases 334
Saller B., Hoermann R., Reichel G., Spoettl G., Grossmann M., Mann K. (Essen, Munich):
HCG and free hCGβ as markers in trophoblastic and non-trophoblastic tumors ... 337
Otto T., Fuhrmann C., Goepel M., Krege S., Rübben H. (Essen): Tumor marker in the supernatant
of primary germ cell culture - A new test system for detection of vital tumor cells 341

Varia

Kaiser U., Jaques G., Auerbach B., Havemann K. (Marburg): Serum NCAM: A potential
new prognostic marker for multiple myeloma 347
Schambeck C., Fateh-Moghadam A., Bartl R., Lamerz R., Wick M. (Munich): Clinical significance
of the labeling index in multiple myeloma compared with beta-2-microglobulin, thymidine
kinase and bone marrow histology 350
Micke O., Schäfer U., Wilken Ch., Prott F.J., Wörmann B., Hiddemann W. (Münster, Göttingen): Soluble
interleukin-2 receptors, serum thymidine kinase and beta-2-microglobulin as tumor markers in
therapy monitoring and follow-up of patients with high-grade non-Hodgkin's lymphoma 354
Kowalzick L., Köhler I., Meißner K. (Hamburg): Serum level of soluble interleukin-2 receptor
is a marker for disease activity in cutaneous T-cell lymphoma (CTCL) 358
Gerding H., Cremer-Bartels G., Krause K., Busse H. (Münster): Neopterin is an indicator of
metastatic disease in patients with choroidal melanoma 362
*Scheefers-Borchel U., Scheefers H., Michel A., Will H., Fischer G., Basenau D., Dahlmann N., Laumen
R., Mazurek S.,. Eigenbrodt E.* (Wettenberg, Göttingen, Hamburg-Harburg, Gießen): Quantitative
determination (ELISA) of pyruvate kinase type tumor M2 – A new tumor marker 365

New Assays

Henne V., Jung S., Schmutz M. (Basel): Cobas® Core CA 72-4 EIA: Analytical performance of a fast and automated determination for TAG-72 antigen on the Cobas® Core immunochemistry analyzer 371

Lentfer D., Greiner-Mai E., Drahovsky M. (Dietzenbach): CA 72-4 in gastrointestinal malignancies – Experience with a new assay 376

Heinze T., Theunissen R., Greiner-Mai E., Lentfer D. (Berlin, Dietzenbach): Immunoluminometric determination of CA 72-4 in the follow-up of gynecological tumors 380

Uhl W., Denk B. (Penzberg): Improved CA 125 determinations using two different monoclonal antibodies 384

Hasholzner U., Stieber P., Baumgartner L., Pahl H., Meier W., Fateh-Moghadam A. (Munich): CA 125 mechanized microparticle enzyme immunoassay (MEIA). A clinical and methodical evaluation 389

Bonfrer J.M.G., Jansen E., de Feij-de Graaf H.M., Korse C.M. (Amsterdam): Evaluation of a new CA 125 assay: The LIA-mat CA 125 II 392

Nustad K., Nilsson O., Kierulf B., Varaas T., Thrane-Steen K., Paus E., Okkenhaug C., Olsen K.H., Børmer O.P. (Oslo, Gothenburg): Immunoassays for the CA 125-related antigen using new monoclonal antibodies 397

Nilsson O., Jansson E.-L., Dahlen U., Nilsson K., Nustad K., Högberg T., Lindholm L. (Gothenburg, Oslo, Lund): New monoclonal antibodies for determination of the ovarian cancer associated antigen CA 125 401

Meyer M., Darte C., Wilmet M., Sokoloff R.L., Rittenhouse H.G., Wolfert R.L. (Liège, San Diego): Consistency of Tandem® PSA dual-monoclonal assay and its clinical importance 406

Drahovsky M., Fritsch U., Schlett R., Mack M., Oed M., Reum L. (Dietzenbach): Automated chemiluminescence immunoassay for prostate specific antigen (PSA) 410

Blijenberg B. G., Greiner-Mai E. (Rotterdam -Dijkzigt, Dietzenbach): Evaluation of the LIA-mat® PSA assay 415

Huber P.R., Schmid H.P., Stremmel C., Gallati H., Maurer A., Thein M. (Basel): Tumor necrosis factor p55 and p75 measured in sera of prostatic cancer patients using Cobas® Core 419

Correale M., Arnberg H., Blockx P., Bombardieri E., Castelli M., Encabo G., Gion M., Klapdor R., Nilsson S., Reutgen H., Ruggeri G., Safi F., Stegmuller M., Vering A. (Bari, Uppsala, Edegem, Milano, Roma, Barcelona, Venezia, Hamburg, Berlin, Brescia, Ulm, Frankfurt): A new monoclonal antibody based immunoassay for tissue polypeptide antigen. Preliminary clinical results 423

Fischer L.N., Carbin B.E., Bäcklander M., Lanneskog A.C., Sundström B. (Bromma, Stockholm): A standardized protocol for determination of TPA in urine by a monoclonal assay and its clinical significance 426

Ayanoglu G., Chen D., Sverlow K. (Alameda): Serum cytokeratin antigen (CKA): An enzyme immunoassay for quantitative measurement of serum cytokeratins in carcinoma 431

Bonfrèr J.M.G., Lodewijks R., Jansen E., Lentfer D. (Amsterdam, Dietzenbach): Evaluation of a new AFP assay 435

Dahlen U., Karlsson B., Lindholm L., Nilsson O. (Gothenburg): Development of an enzyme immunoassay for determination of the tumor-associated antigen CA 242 438

Drahovsky M., Lentfer D., Völcker P. (Dietzenbach): Monitoring of oncological patients with an automated luminescence-labeled immunoassay for ferritin 442

Kessler A.-Ch. (Tutzing): Technical and clinical evaluation of seven tumor marker assays based on ELISA technology – Results of a multicenter study 446

Pfleiderer P., Giradin Ph., Henne V., Maurer A. (Basel): Performance of tumor marker assays on the true Random Access Immunochemistry Analyzer Cobas® Core 449

Poley S., Fateh-Moghadam A., Nüssler V., Pahl H. (Munich): β2-Microglobulin enzyme immunoassay (Cobas® Core) – A methodical and clinical evaluation 452

Round Table:
Quality Control and Standardization

Maurer A. (Basel): Quality control and standardization of tumor marker assays 457

Jansen H.-M., Stieber P., Fateh-Moghadam A. (Munich): Sensitivity profiles and normalized dot plots. Tools for the clinical evaluation of new methods and comparison of methods 461

Scheurlen H., Fateh-Moghadam A., Fiedler H., Klapdor A., Kreienberg R., Möbus V., Spitzer R., Stieber P., Diziol P., Ziergöbel R., Spanuth E. (Heidelberg, Munich, Suhl, Hamburg, Ulm, Mannheim): The analysis of variance as a statistical procedure for assessing tumor marker tests 464
Lamerz R., Brandt A., Segura E. (Munich): Long-term quality control exemplified by laboratory radioimmunoassays for AFP and CEA 472
Dahlmann N. (Hamburg): Long-term standardization of tumor marker tests 477
Zwirner M., Risse Th., Benz R., Birkmeyer G.D., Buchterkirche W., Baum U., Brandt B., van Dalen A., Förster R., Hubl W., Kapp S., Klapdor R., Spitz J., Wieser N. (Tübingen, Ulm, Wien, Bremen, Frankfurt, Münster, Gouda, Essen, Mainz, Hamburg, Wiesbaden, Ingelheim): Determination of CA 19-9 with various commercial assays. Results of an international proficiency study 481
Haglund C. (Helsinki): Quality control and standardization of tumor marker tests in Finland 487
Zucchelli G.C., Pilo A., Cohen R., Cianetti A., Torre G.C. (Pisa, Lyon, Roma, Pietra Ligure): Tumor markers: Quality control and standardization in Italy 488
Fischer L.N. (Bromma): Tumor marker determinations: How should they be reported? 492
Nap M., Wilhelm W.W. (Leeuwarden, Utrecht): Quality control in immunohistology: Evaluation of the interpretation instead of technique and reagents 494

Oncogenes – Receptors – Cytokines

Meden H., Marx D., Fattahi A., Rath W., Krohn M., Wuttke W., Schauer A., Kuhn W. (Göttingen): Serum levels of a c-erbB-2 oncogene product in ovarian cancer patients 501
Kynast B., Isola J., Binder L., Teramoto Y., Marx D., Oellerich M., Bokemeyer C., Poliwoda H., Schmoll H.-J., Schauer A. (Hannover, Tampere, Göttingen, Alameda): Detection of p185^{HER-2} fragments in sera of breast cancer patients – A new prognostic factor and tumor marker? 505
Sampson E., Teramoto Y. (Alameda): Quantitation of c-erbB-2 oncoprotein in human breast tissue 510
Teramoto Y., Konrad K. (Alameda): Measurement of the extracellular domain of the c-erbB-2 oncoprotein in sera of breast cancer patients 516
Beckmann M.W., Scharl A., Tutschek B., Göhring U.J., Schenko G., Beckmann A., Niederacher D., Schnürch H.G. (Düsseldorf, Köln): Comparison of the epidermal growth factor receptor (EGF-R) and of Her-2/neu protein (p$^{185/Her2}$) expression in breast cancer 521
Nekarda H., Nakamura T., Hoelscher A.H., Becker K., Bollschweiler E., Siewert J.R. (Munich, Tokyo): Prognostic impact of c-erbB-2 oncoprotein overexpression in adenocarcinoma of the esophagus 526
Harvey J., Crebbin V., Gorrin G., Hammond S., Mauceri J., Teramoto Y., Walker R. (Alameda): An enzyme immunoassay for the detection of epidermal growth factor receptor in tissue extracts of breast cancer specimens 533
Suciu E.-M., Sing S., Stocking C., Meybohm I., Goedde H.W. (Hamburg): Expression and function of GM-CSF receptors in solid tumor cell lines 538
Minguillon C., Judith D., Heinze T., Schäfer A., Köppen B., Lichtenegger W. (Berlin, Hamburg): Interleukin-6 (IL-6) expression in breast cancer and correlation with pathological prognostic factors 542
Vainas I., Dimitriadis K., Pasaitu K., Stergiou I., Tsirintanis I., Kapetanos D., Zakapas E., Delopoulos D. (Thessaloniki): Steroid hormone receptors (SR) in normal (NTT) and pathological (PTT) thyroid tissue samples – New tumor markers? 545
Müller W., Borchard F. (Düsseldorf): Expression of p53 in gastric cancer 548
Biermann C.W., de Riese W., Ulbright T.M., Orazi O., Hinkel A., Foster R.S., Senge Th. (Herne, Indianapolis): Immunohistochemical p53 protein expression and its correlation with proliferative activity in clinical stage I non-seminomatous germ cell tumors of the testis (NSGCT) 551
Kuczyk M.A., Serth J., Allhoff E.P., Höfner K., Thon W.F., Jonas U. (Hannover, Würselen): p53 immunohistochemistry as a new prognostic factor for bladder cancer 554
Minguillon C., Schönborn I. Friedmann W., Judith D., Bartel U., Lichtenegger W. (Berlin): Expression of the nuclear oncogene p53 in human breast cancer in relation to prognostic factors 559
Galle P.R., Müller M., Zentgraf H., Volkmann M. (Heidelberg): Detection of p53-antibodies by immunoblot and ELISA in various human malignancies - A new serological test? 562

Immunohistochemistry

Hagedorn H., Schreiner M., Wiest I., Schleicher E., Nerlich A. (Munich): Basement membrane expression as a marker for the differentation of squamous cell carcinomas of the larynx 567

Friedrich R.E., Hellner D., Arps H. (Hamburg, Fulda): Detection of keratins in microvascularized jejunal autografts to the oral cavity and adjacent oral mucosa 571

Friedrich R.E., Bartel-Friedrich S., Niedobitek G., Herbst H., Lobeck H. (Hamburg, Berlin): Undifferentiated carcinomas of the nasopharyngeal type (UCNT) – Correlation of EBV-genome detection by ^{35}S-labeled plasmids and detection of keratin, vimentin and EMA 575

Friedrich R.E., Bartel-Friedrich S., Lobeck H. (Hamburg, Berlin): Detection of keratins in lymph node metastases of poorly differentiated carcinomas in the head and neck region. Comparison of patterns of expression to primary sites of lesions 579

Friedrich R.E., Bartel-Friedrich S., Lobeck H., Friedrich K.H., Hellner D. (Hamburg, Berlin): Correlation of the immunocytochemical demonstration of keratin phenotypes in undifferentiated carcinomas of the nasopharyngeal type (UCNT) to the hypotheses of its histogenesis 582

Broll R., Kayser K., Vollmer G., Bruch H.-P. (Lübeck): Expression of tenascin in gastric carcinoma – An immunohistochemical investigation 586

Dippe B., Lorenz M., Petrowsky H., Engels F., Krüger S., Schneider M. (Frankfurt, Lübeck): Different growth patterns in primary colorectal carcinomas and their lymph node metastases 590

Basso D., Plebani M., Del Giudice G., Panozzo M.P., Venturini R., Meggiato T., Carbone M.D., Del Favero G., Del Mistro A., Burlina A. (Padova): Concanavalin A affinity pattern of CA 19-9. An in vitro and in vivo study 594

Göhring U.-J., Scharl A., Stoffl M., Thelen U., Crombach G. (Köln): A high fraction of proliferating cell nuclear antigen (PCNA) in breast cancer indicates poor prognosis 598

Beckmann M.W., Tutschek B., Göhring U.J., Scharl A., Loaiciga K., Bracht M., Beinlich A., Schnürch H.G. (Düsseldorf, Cologne): Immunohistochemical detection of cathepsin D (Cath D) in formalin-fixed, paraffin-embedded breast cancer samples 602

Weitz S., Khabbaz N., Carne L., Harvey J. (Alameda): Cathepsin D tissue cytosol enzyme immunoassay (EIA) and immunohistochemical (IHC) reagent in breast cancer prognosis 606

Paganuzzi M., Onetto M., Marroni P., Bruzzone M., Alama A., Catsafados E., Reggiardo G., Ragni N., Torre G.C., Boccardo F. (Genoa, Pietra Ligure): Relationship between tumor labeling index, serum markers of cell proliferation and CA 125 609

Willemse F., Nap M., Foekens J.A., Henzen-Logmans S.C. (Groningen, Leeuwarden, Rotterdam): Epithelial percentage in breast cancer sections obtained by true color image analysis – Correction factor for quantitative data on cytosolic tumor extracts? 612

Fernö M., Borg Å., Killander D., Hirschberg L., Brundell J. (Lund, Bromma): Prognostic significance of elevated levels of urokinase in breast cancer cytosols – A novel quantitative luminometric assay applicable on steroid receptor cytosols 617

Abdel Salam A., Mangoud A., Ramadan M., Khalifa A., El-Ahmady O. (Zagazik, Cairo): OKT9 as a tumor marker in endometrial and uterine cervical carcinoma 621

Abdel Salam A., Mangoud A., Ramadan M., Khalifa A., El-Ahmady O. (Zagazik, Cairo): Epithelial antigens in normal ovary and ovarian mixed mesodermal tumors 625

Ardoino S., Durante P., Ferro M.A., Li Causi F., Parodi C., Puppo P., Sanguineti G., Vitali A. (Pietra Ligure): Immunohistochemistry in prostatic pathology – Diagnostic value of PSA, PSAP and high molecular weight cytokeratin. Evaluation of 650 fine needle biopsies 630

Götze S., Caselitz J. (Hamburg): DNA cytophotometry of human bladder carcinomas – A comparative study of scanning cytophotometry and flow cytophotometry 634

El-Ahmady O., El-Din A.G., Eissa S., Helal T., Khalaf I. (Cairo): Expression of CEA in normal and malignant tissue of Egyptian bladder cancer patients 636

Otto T., Heider K.-H., Goepel M., Noll F., Raz A., Rübben H. (Essen, Karlsruhe, Detroit): The role of motility, adhesion- and migration factors in bladder carcinomas 640

De Riese W., Biermann C.W., Crabtree W.N., Ulbright T.M., Hinkel A., Allhoff E.P., Senge Th. (Herne, Indianapolis, Würselen): Ki-67 immunostaining as a new prognosticator in non-metastatic renal cell carcinoma 643

Makovitzky J., Gyürüs P. (Halle, Pecs): Comparative immunohistochemical examinations on the corpora amylacea in the brain, lung and prostatic gland 647

Latif M.S. (Cairo): DNA synthesis in human osteosarcoma (HOS) cells treated with lead chromate 650

Holzhausen H.-J., Knolle J., Bahn H., Rath F.-W., Gabius H.-J. (Halle, Munich): Expression of endogenous sugar-binding proteins (endogenous lectins) in tumors of peripheral nerves in correlation to the growth pattern 655

Knolle J., Bahn H., Holzhausen H.-J., Rath F.-W., Gabius H.-J. (Halle, Munich): Patterns of endogenous sugar-binding proteins in benign and malignant soft tissue tumors 659

Nerlich A., Berndt R., Wiest I., Schleicher E. (Munich, Worms): Immunohistochemical analysis of various basement membrane components in dermal cylindromas 662

Egert Sylvia, Senekowitsch Reingard (Munich): Characterization of LDL receptor-binding and LDL internalization with various human cell lines 665

Immunoscintigraphy

Fritsche L., Grünert B., Heissler E., Barzen G., Cordes M., Felix R. (Berlin): Radioimmunoscintigraphy of head and neck squamous cell cancer with 99mTc-labeled antibody SQ174 – First results in 10 patients 671

Behr Th., Pavel M., Becker W., Hensen J., Wolf F. (Erlangen): Urine 5-HIAA excretion alone or in combination with ^{123}I-MIBG scintigraphy in patients with carcinoids? 675

Platz D., Gratz K.F., Luebeck M. (Hamburg): Clinical value of ^{111}In-pentetreotide SPECT in the assessment of gastro-entero-pancreatic (GEP) tumors and medullary thyroid cancer (MTC) .. 678

Scheidhauer K., Hildebrandt G., Luyken C., Schomäcker K., Klug N., Schicha H. (Cologne): Somatostatin receptor imaging of intracranial tumors 681

Scharl A., Göhring U.-J., Scheidhauer K., Schomäcker K. (Cologne): Visualization of peptide hormone receptor complexes using [^{111}In]octreotide in breast cancer in vivo 684

Franke W.-G., Wiener S., Weiß S., Siegert E., Koehler K. (Dresden): Detection and delineation of rhabdo- and leiomyosarcomas using ^{111}In labeled antimyosin-antibodies (Fab) as a hopeful tool in oncology 688

Bockisch A., Mörschel M., Hach A., Schmitz A. (Mainz): Immunoscintigraphy with the B72.3 antibody in presurgical patients with suspected colorectal cancer 694

Oehr P., Germer U., Liu Q. (Bonn): Application of anti-TPS antibodies for in vivo diagnostics and therapy 698

Richter H., Reinsberg J., Wagner U., Biersack H.J. (Bonn): Formation of anti-idiotype antibodies and the induction of cellular immunity after in vivo administration of the monoclonal antibody OC 125 701

Popp A., Bahlo M., Klapdor R., Platz D. (Hamburg): Biodistribution and tumor visualization with ^{111}In labeled B72.3 antibodies. Studies in nude mice bearing xenografts of human pancreatic carcinomas 707

Therapy

Riva P., Arista A., Sturiale C., Franceschi G., Riva N., Spinelli A., Casi M., Moscatelli G., Campori F., Gentile R. (Cesena): Intratumoral radioimmunotherapy in glioblastomas by means of ^{131}I radiolabeled monoclonal antibodies 713

Bosslet K., Czech J., Hoffmann D. (Marburg): Fusion protein mediated tumor-selective prodrug activation 717

Pantel K., Schlimok G., Fackler-Schwalbe I., Oberneder R., Hofstetter A., Loibner H., Riethmüller G. (Augsburg, Munich, Vienna): Immunocytological monitoring of antibody-mediated reduction of individual disseminated breast cancer cells 724

Gast B., Reinsberg J. (Bonn): Determination and characterization of human antibodies after application of the monoclonal antibody B72.3 729

Schwaibold H., Huland E., Heinzer H., Huland H. (Hamburg): Toxicity of local continuous and cyclic, high-dose bladder perfusion with recombinant and natural interleukin-2 in advanced cancer of the urinary bladder 733

Heinzer H., Huland E., Falk B., Huland H. (Hamburg): Inhalative natural interleukin-2 (IL-2) in combination with low dose systemic IL-2 and interferon-α (IFNa). Longterm follow-up and toxicity of patients with pulmonary metastasis of renal cell carcinoma 737

Eggermont A.M.M., Goey S.H., Slingerland R., Punt C.J.A., Gratama J.W., Oosterom R., Bolhuis R.L.H., Stoter G. (Rotterdam): Intrapleural administration of interleukin-2 in malignant pleural mesothelioma. A phase I-II study 740

Eggermont A.M.M., Lienard D., Schraffordt Koops H., Kroon B.B.R., Rosenkaimer F., Lejeune F.J. (Rotterdam, Lausanne, Groningen, Amsterdam, Ingelheim): High dose TNFα, gamma-interferon and melphalan in isolated limb perfusion for stage III melanoma and irresectable soft tissue sarcomas of the extremities – A highly effective regimen 744

Mansour M., Stenke L., El-Ahmady O., Lindgren J.A. (Cairo, Stockholm): Formation and proliferative effects of leukotrienes and lipoxins in human bone marrow cells 748

Wiegel T., Baumann M., Bressel M., Arps H. (Hamburg, Fulda): Immediate adjuvant hormonal therapy and radiotherapy following radical prostatectomy for stage D1 adenocarcinoma of the prostate 752

Wiegel T., Schmidt R., Steiner P., Arps H., Göckel-Beining B. (Hamburg, Fulda, Steinheim): Three-dimensional treatment planning for radiotherapy of prostate cancer: Technique and acute toxicity 756

Carl U.M., Bahnsen J., Fröschle G., Wiegel T. (Hamburg, Düsseldorf): Para-aortic radiation treatment in FIGO stage III ovarian carcinomas – A sensible complementary approach in connection with cytotoxic drugs? 760

Friedrich R.E., Krüll A., Hellner D., Plambeck K., Schwarz R. (Hamburg): Local tumor control in patients with advanced stages of squamous cell carcinomas of the oral cavity: Interstitial brachytherapy with iridium-192 764

Friedrich R.E., Donath K., Hellner D. (Hamburg): A caseous-tuberculoid reaction in lymph node metastases following radiochemotherapy of undifferentiated nasopharyngeal carcinoma 767

Falk B., Huland E., Hübner D., Huland H. (Hamburg): Longterm continuous release and bioactivity of interleukin-2 depot preparations in human tumor bearing nude mice 770

Adams S., Baum R.P., Schnürch H.G., Stegmüller M., Bender H.G., Hör G. (Frankfurt): Successful labeling of the murine monoclonal anti-EGF-receptor-antibody MAb[425] with technetium-99m. First experimental results 772

Nußbaumer J., Gunsenheimer B., Haunschild J., Steiner K., Senekowitsch R. (Munich): Anti-EGF-receptor MAb 425 has a growth-inhibiting influence on tumor cells and leads to a differentiation of multicell tumor spheroids 776

Friedrich R.E., Mestmacher P., Hellner D. Arps H. (Hamburg, Fulda): Evidence of a growth inhibition effect of high levels of recombinant human erythropoietins on sarcoma cell lines in vitro 780

Friedrich R.E., Mestmacher P., Hellner D., Reymann A., Arps H. (Hamburg, Fulda): Tumor cell growth stimulation by stable PGE_1 and PGI_2 derivatives on human sarcoma cell lines in vitro 784

Friedrich R.E., Mestmacher P., Hellner D., Arps H. (Hamburg, Fulda): Lack of tumor cell growth stimulating activity of recombinant human erythropoietins (Erypo 4000™, Recormon 1000™) on sarcoma cell lines in vitro 788

Mattes J., Matzen K., Truckenbrodt R., Senekowitsch R. (Munich): In vitro studies to assess the response of human adenocarcinoma cell spheroids to radiotherapy using fluorodeoxyglucose and thymidine 791

Matzen K., Mattes J., Truckenbrodt R., Senekowitsch R. (Munich): Autoradiographical studies to evaluate C14-FDG uptake by human tumor cell spheroids as response to radiotherapy 795

Workshop 1
10 Years CA 19-9 and CA 125

Klapdor R. (Hamburg): CA 19-9 and CA 125 – 10 years Hamburg Symposia on Tumor Markers . . . 801

Haglund C., Lundin J., Roberts P.J. (Helsinki): 10 years experience of CA 19-9 in patients with pancreatic cancer 803

Makovitzky J. (Halle): The occurrence of the carbohydrate antigen 19-9 in the organism of man 808

Meier W., Stieber P., Baumgartner L., Hasholzner U., Fateh-Moghadam A. (Munich): 10 years experience with the tumor marker CA 125 in ovarian cancer. A critical review 811

Chatal J.F., Peltier P., Chetanneau A., Resche I. (Nantes): Current status of immunoscintigraphy after ten years of clinical experience 816

Syrigos K.N., Epenetos A.A. (London): Achievements, failings and promises of radioimmunotherapy 818

Noujaim A.A., Baum R.P., Sykes T.R., Madiyalakan R., Sykes C.J., Hertel A., Niesen A., Hör G. (Alberta, Frankfurt): Monoclonal antibody B43.13 for immunoscintigraphy and immunotherapy of ovarian cancer 823

Sommer K., Crone-Münzebrock W. (Hamburg): Evolution of CT and MRI in oncologic diagnosis and their current value 830

Workshop 2
Gene Technology in Diagnosis and Therapy

Blum H.E. (Zurich). Recombinant DNA technology: Diagnostic and therapeutic aspects 835
Shipman R. (Basel): Applications of the polymerase chain reaction to tumor analysis
and diagnosis 839
Frisch J., Schulz G., Nemunaitis J., Steward W.P., Verweij J., Brugger W., Kanz L., Mertelsmann R.
(Marburg, Dallas, Glasgow, Rotterdam, Freiburg): Adjuvant therapy with recombinant CSFs
in patients with solid tumors 846
Huland E., Heinzer H., Falk B., Schwaibold H., Hübner D., Huland H. (Hamburg): Modification
of local and systemic host response by topical cytokine application in malignant disease.
Experimental and clinical experiences 851

Workshop 3
Immunosuppression, -deficiency (Transplantation/AIDS) and Cancer

Brunkhorst R., Lang H., Behrendt M., Frei U. (Hannover): De novo cancers in renal
transplant recipients 855
*Rogiers X., Langwieler T.E., Malagó M., Kuhlencordt R., Knoefel W.T., Fischer L., Sterneck M.,
Broelsch C.E.* (Hamburg): Limiting factors of liver transplantation in patients with liver tumors 859
Nägele H., Klapdor R., Bahlo M., Kalmar P., Rödiger W. (Hamburg):
Determination of tumor markers after heart transplantation 861
Gallati H., Pracht I., Bock A., Thiel G. (Basel): Serum level of tumor necrosis factor receptor
p55 and p75 in patients with kidney transplantations 866
Hauser H.-P., Gürtler L., Knapp S., Eberle J., von Brunn A., Kaptue L. (Marburg, Munich, Youndé):
Genetic variability of HIV – A new HIV subtype from Cameroon 869
Markus B.H. (Frankfurt): Immunological phenomenons and problems after
organ transplantation 871

Satellite Symposium:
Cancer of the Lung – State and Trends in Diagnosis and Therapy

Amthor M. (Rotenburg): Histopathologic diagnosis of lung cancer –
Classification, problems, pitfalls 877
Steiner P. (Hamburg): Clinical staging of primary lung cancer 880
Stieber P., Dienemann H., Hasholzner U., Zimmermann A., Hofmann K., Fateh-Moghadam A.
(Munich): Tumor markers in lung cancer 886
Schirren J., Trainer S., Richter W., Schneider P., Bülzebruck H., Vogt-Moykopf I. (Heidelberg):
Stage related surgery of bronchial carcinoma 892
Heckmayr M., Gatzemeier U. (Hamburg-Großhansdorf): Chemotherapeutic treatment of
bronchial carcinoma 895
*Koch K., Broll I., Frank W., Hartmann H., Kaiser D., Krumhaar D., Loddenkemper R.,
Matthiessen W., Neusetzer H.* (Potsdam): Radiotherapy for lung cancer 898
Eggermont A.M.M., Stoter G. (Rotterdam): Intrapleural administration of cytokines for
malignant pleural effusions 903

Sponsors 907

Preface

The present book contains the contributions presented at the 7th Hamburg Symposium on Tumor Markers, December 5-8, 1993.

More than 250 presentations given by participants from all over the world reflect the increasing national and international interest in these Hamburg Symposia, in 1993 it extended to a four days meeting.

As in the preceeding Symposium major topics were again: *In Vitro Diagnosis,* including subjects like *New Assays, Oncogenes, Receptors, Cytokines,* as well as *Immunohistochemistry, Immunoscintigraphy and Therapy.*

The discussions on the topic *Quality Control and Standardization* were continued in two scientific sessions and within the *6th Meeting of the Working Group Quality Control and Standardization* established during the Hamburg Symposium in 1991.

These Proceedings also include the lectures of the *Satellite Symposium* which in 1993 had the title *Cancer of the Lung – State and Trends in Diagnosis and Therapy* under the chairmenship of *Prof. Branscheid* and *Prof. Kaukel.*

The discussion of new aspects/trends in oncology as a main focus was intended by two workshops: *Gentechnology in Diagnosis and Therapy* and *Immunosuppression/Deficiency (Transplantation/AIDS) and Cancer.*

A third workshop *10 Years CA 19-9 and CA 125* preceeding the scientific programm on December 5 was dedicated to the developments in the field of tumor marker oncology during the past decade, since the clinical introduction of the two monoclonal antibody defined tumor associated antigens CA 19-9 and CA 125 – and since the 1st Hamburg Symposium with about 15 contributions and 20 participants.

Finally, I would like to take the opportunity to thank once again all the assistants and coworkers for their help in preparing and organizing this 7th Symposium on Tumor Marker.

The authors, too, deserve our thanks for their rapid submission of manuscripts, the sponsors of the meeting for their generous financial support, and again *W. Zuckschwerdt* and his coworkers for their advice and rapid puclication of the Proceedings – a new comprehensive documentation of the efforts undertaken all over the world to evaluate and improve the usefulness of tumor markers for in vivo diagnosis, for prognosis, for monitoring therapy and possibly even for therapy – that means for the benefit of all our patients.

R. Klapdor
Hamburg, October 1994

In Vitro Diagnosis

Gastroenterology

Initial values of tumor associated antigens (TAA) in the sera of patients with primary oral squamous cell carcinomas

R. E. Friedrich[a], K. Plambeck[a], D. Hellner[a], V.W. Thoms[a], M. Bahlo[b], R. Klapdor[b]

[a]Department of Oral and Maxillofacial Surgery, [b]Department of Internal Medicine, Eppendorf University Hospital, University of Hamburg, Germany

Introduction

There are still no screening methods available indicating or excluding the presence of squamous cell carcinoma of the oral cavity or oropharynx by serological assays. The clinical inspection is the most important tool of initial diagnosis and follow-up. Several reports deal about the clinical application of serological assays of tumor associated antigens (TAA) in the diagnosis and follow-up of oral and oropharyngeal carcinomas (OSCC) indicating that the additional evaluation of TAA levels give further information about the staging, recurrence, and clinical outcome of this entity (1–4). To get a better estimation of the clinical value of so-called "tumor markers" in carcinomas of the oral cavity, we determined a panel of TAA at the time of the first diagnosis (primary tumors).

Material and methods

From 1991 to 1993 the TAA levels of up to 112 patients with oral and oropharyngeal squamous cell carcinomas were measured. Excepting one female with a clinical recurrence of local and distant metastases of a breast carcinoma at the time of the initial diagnosis of the OSCC in all patients only one tumor was present (C2).
The analysis of serum levels of oral and oropharyngeal carcinoma patients included: squamous cell carcinoma antigen (abbreviated: SCC), carcino-embryonic antigen (CEA), tissue polypeptide antigen (TPA), ferritin, TAG-72 and CA 19-9. According to instructions of the suppliers the cut-off levels of the antigens are as follows: SCC: 1.5 ng/ml; CEA: 3 ng/ml; CA 19-9: 35 U/ml; ferritin 220 µg/l (females) and 330 µg/l (males); TPA: 95 U/l; TAG-72: 3.5 U/ml. Up to 112 patients (for TAG-72:106, for SCC: 95; for TPA: 84) with oral squamous cell carcinomas were investigated. Patients with local recurrences were excluded.
For detection of antigens the products of several suppliers were used (SCC: Microparticle Immunoassay (MEIA), (IMX SCC assay, Abbott, Wiesbaden, Germany); TPA: LIA-mat® Immunoassay, Byk-Sangtec, Dietzenbach, Germany; CA 19-9: Cobas®Core CA 19-9 EIA, Roche, Basel, Switzerland; TAG-72 Immunoradiometric assay, Sorin Biomedica, Saluggia, Italy; CEA: Enzymun-Test®, Boehringer Mannheim, Germany).

Results

In the majority of cases the values were in the physiological range of healthy volunteers (below cut-off values).
SCC: SCC values within the physiological range were determined in 77 of 111 patients (69.4%); 27 patients with values > 1.5 ng/ml of a total of 34 are T4 carcinomas (figures 1, 2).
TPA: TPA values within the cut-off levels were determined in 67 of 85 patients (78.8%), TPA values > 150 U/l are rare: n = 3, (figure 4).
CEA: CEA values within the physiological range were determined in 77 of 112 patients (68.75%), CEA values > 5ng/ ml: n = 8, (figure 3).
CA 19-9: CA 19-9 values within the PR were determined in 95 of 110 (86.3%), (CA 19-9 values > 100 U/ml: n = 4).
Ferritin: 1. Adult women (n = 35): physiological values of ferritin values were determined in 26 patients, ferritin values > 400 µg/ml: 6 and > 800

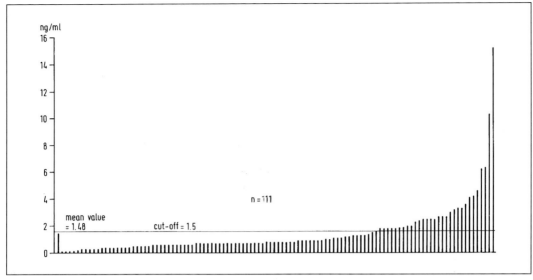

Figure 1. Variation of SCC values in OSCC patients at the time of diagnosis.

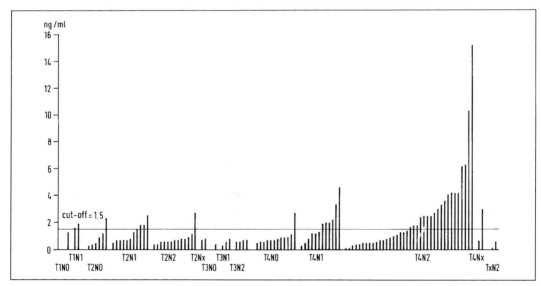

Figure 2. Correlation of SCC values and TNM stages in 111 patients with OSCC (initial values, primary tumors).

µg/ml: n = 3. 2. Adult men (n = 73): ferritin values > 330 µg/ml were found in 15 patients (20.5%) including 3 patients with levels > 800 µg/ml.
TAG-72: TAG-72 values within the PR were determined in 90 of 108 patients (84.06%), TAG-72 of > 8 U/ml: n = 4.
Emphasizing on the application of SCC the correlation of these values and TNM stages is demonstrated in figure 2.

Discussion

Up to the knowledge of the authors so far this is the first study presenting the results of a broad panel of serological TAA in patients with oral and oropharyngeal squamous cell carcinomas at the time of the initial diagnosis.
Interestingly, TAA indicated for the follow-up of carcinomas of the stomach (TAG-72) but not used

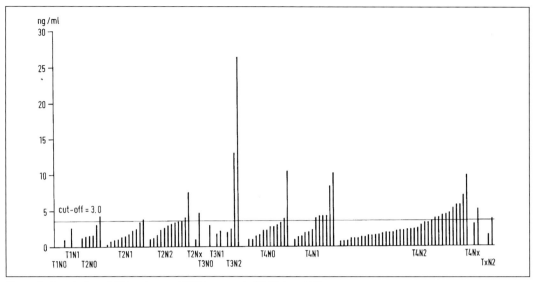

Figure 3. Correlation of CEA values and TNM stages in OSCC (n = 112).

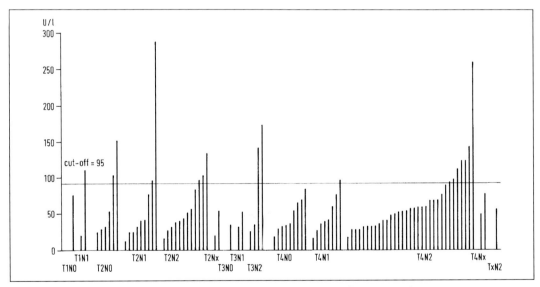

Figure 4. Variation of TPA values in 94 patients with OSCC (initial values, primary tumors).

for application in carcinomas of the oral cavity were in the physiological range in the vast majority of cases. So, although an abuse of alcohol and nicotine in more than 90% of our patients was documented and there is a risk of second malignancies of the respiratory and alimentary tract in these patients, the marker is not affected by the presence of oral and oropharyngeal carcinomas even in advanced stages. Standard x-rays or CT scans of thorax and abdominal ultrasound are part of our routine staging in oral cancer.

The application of CA 19-9 is in the domain of diagnosis and follow-up of cancers of the gastrointestinal tract but elevated values also can be found in other diseases, e.g. chronic pancreatic inflammations. So, chronic abuse of alcohol and nicotine without evidence of a malignancy of the exocrine pancreas, colon, stomach and gall bladder does not interfere with normal serological values of this gastrointestinal cancer antigen.

CEA is supposed to be the serological marker of first choice in head and neck cancer but it seemed to be less sensitive than SCC regarding squamous cell carcinomas of the oral cavity (1).

The distribution of TPA in tissues is similar to the one identified for subsets of intermediate filaments and currently it is suggested TPA to represent keratins No. 8, 18 and 19 (simple type epithelia kertatins) or to be of an origin related to keratin proteins. Obviously these keratins are hardly secreted to the blood stream and in up to 4 of 5 patients with advanced stages of oral squamous cell carcinomas the TPA levels are in the accepted physiological range.

SCC antigen was first described in 1977 by *Kato* and *Torigoe* (5) and applied in patients with cervix or lung cancers (sensitivity: 40–54%, (5, 6, 7)). In contrast, the sensitivity of SCC in oral squamous cell carcinomas was lower: 24–43% (1, 8, 9, 10), in this range are our own results.

However, neither SCC nor CEA are sensitive enough for detecting small primary tumors of the oral cavity which are successfully resected in a lot of cases.

Positive evidence is much higher in clinical inspection than in SCC serum levels due to the good accessibility of the oral cavity. Indeed, even in advanced stages of OSCC in a lot of patients the secreted amounts of SCC are within the physiological range. Vice versa, in the majority of $T_{3-4}N_{1-2}$ oral squamous cell carcinoma patients neither the malignant tumor nor the known abuse of alcohol and nicotine leads to an elevation of SCC levels.

It is concluded that the serological tumor associated antigens tested so far give further information of the stage and follow-up of the disease only in a subgroup of patients which presently is poorly defined. Regarding the rationale of surgical therapy with respect to oral squamous cell carcinoma the markers are not sensitive enough in the majority of cases. They are not recommended for screening tests. On the other hand, initial values of TAA are useful for estimation of follow-up in some cases, especially in patients with pathological values at the time of diagnosis which might be altered during therapy (irradiation, ablative surgery). So, in some cases with elevated titers of TAA, e.g. SCC, TPA or CEA, the use of these markers for follow-up might be helpful.

References

1. Hellner D, Klapdor R, Schmelzle R (1990) SCC and CEA in maxillofacial surgery. In: Klapdor R (ed) Recent results in tumor diagnosis and therapy. Zuckschwerdt, München, pp 3–7
2. Kurokawa H, Tsuru S, Okada M, Nakamura T, Kajiyama M (1993) Evaluation of tumor markers in patients with squamous cell carcinoma in the oral cavity. Int J Oral Maxillofac Surg 22: 35–38
3. Söderholm A-L, Lindqvist C, Haglund C (1992) Tumor markers and radiological examinations in the follow-up of patients with oral cancer. J Cran Max Fac Surg 20:211–215
4. Tsuji T, Sasaki K, Shinozaki F (1989) An expression of squamous cell carcinoma-related antigen in oral cancers. Int J Oral Maxillofac Surg 18:241–243
5. Kato H, Torigoe T. (1977) Radioimmunoassay for tumor antigen of human cervical squamous cell carcinoma. Cancer 40:1621–1628
6. Kato H, Miyauchi F, Morioka H, Fujino T, Torigoe T (1979) Tumor antigen of human cervical squamous cell carcinoma. Cancer 43:585–590
7. Mino N, Lio A, Hamamoto K (1991) Availability of tumor antigen 4 as a marker of squamous cell carcinoma of the lung and other organs. Cancer 55:302–308
8. Fischbach W, Rink C (1988) SCC-Antigen: ein sensitiver und spezifischer Tumormarker für Plattenepithelcarcinome? Dtsch med Wschr 113:289–293
9. Hellner D, Klapdor R, Gundlach KKH, Schmelzle R (1989) Erfahrungen mit dem SCC-Antigen beim Plattenepithelcarcinom der Mundhöhle. Dtsch Z Mund-Kiefer Gesichts Chir 13:286–290
10. Yoshimura Y, Harada T, Oka M, Sugihara T, Kishimoto H (1988) Squamous cell carcinoma antigen in the serum of oromaxillary cancer. Int J Oral Maxillofac Surg 17:49–53

Address for correspondence:
Dr. med. Dr. med. dent. R. E. Friedrich
Klinik für Mund-, Kiefer- und Gesichtschirurgie
(Nordwestdeutsche Kieferklinik)
Martinistraße 52
D-20246 Hamburg, Germany

Tumor-associated antigens (SCC, CEA, TPA) in patients with squamous cell carcinomas of the head and neck before and after preoperative percutaneous irradiation

A preliminary report

R.E. Friedrich[a], A. Krüll[b], K. Plambeck[a], D. Hellner[a], V. Thoms[a], M. Bahlo[c], R. Klapdor[c]

[a]Department of Oral and Maxillofacial Surgery, [b]Department of Radiotherapy, [c]Department of Internal Medicine, Eppendorf University Hospital, University of Hamburg, Germany

Introduction

Until now no markers are available indicating the response of carcinoma cells to a preoperative percutaneous irradiation in patients with advanced stages of squamous cell carcinomas of the head and neck. On the other hand control of therapy efficiency by means of squameous cell carcinoma antigen SCC values has been reported. Permanently elevated SCC levels in squamous cell carcinomas after intervention are suspected for relapses or failure of therapy (1).

The pattern of proteins detected by tissue polipeptide antigen (TPA) and tissue polypeptide specific antigen (TPS) in sera was correlated to the patterns of expression of keratins (simple epithelia) and identified as keratins no. 8, 18 and 19 (5). In solid carcinomas, e.g. squamous cell carcinomas of the upper aerodigestive tract, a de novo expression of simple type of epithelia characterizing keratins is well known; for review see (4).

Both the release of tumor associated antigens (TAA) in irradiated patients as a result of epithelial damage (keratin fragments) and tumor necrosis on the one hand and the impaired differentiation of oral epithelia in an irradiation field on the other might lead to an alteration of TAA comparing pre- to post-values.

Alterations of SCC values in the beginning of irradiation of squamous cell carcinomas in the head and neck region have to be considered in estimating therapy response by means of this marker. So, in a preliminary study pre- and post values of tumor associated antigens in patients with a primary head and neck cancer were measured.

Material and methods

In a pilot study we determined the initial values of several serological antigens (SCC, CEA, TPA) in patients with advanced stages (T_{2-4}, N_{1-2}, M_0) of carcinomas of the head and neck region (n = 14). Blood samples were collected at the time of diagnosis and about three month after irradiation ((RT) exception: pat. no. 12 (one week after RT). The cut-off levels are defined: SCC = 1.5 ng/ml (IMX, Abbott), CEA = 3.0 ng/ml (Enzymun, BM), TPA = 95 U/l (LIA-mat, Byk-Sangtec). The TNM staging and localization of primaries are presented in table I.

Results and discussion

Summarizing all pre- and post-values a decline of serological levels was restricted to SCC. On the other hand even in large tumors the majority of patients had normal SCC values. TPA values are hardly affected neither by the disease nor RT and in no case levels higher than 95 U/l were found in patients with normal pretreatment values. CEA levels are not altered by RT substantially. Due to a higher subgroup of elevated CEA levels using a cut-off level 3 ng/ml there is no patient with elevated pretreatment values gaining this margin after RT. In individuals were differences of serum levels related to irradiation, e.g. in some patients was a short increase of SCC levels (even within the physiological range) but others were not altered at all and in three cases was a constant decline of SCC. Based on the present preliminary data it is concluded that serological markers like SCC, CEA, and TPA might be useful for selecting the response to irradiation in a subgroup of patients with head and neck cancer. The criteria of these patients have to be clarified in further studies.

Table I. Clinical and serological data of patients with squamous cell carcinomas of the head and neck. In all patients prior to ablative surgery a percutaneous irradiation (60–75.5 Gy) was applied. The sera were investigated before and after irradiation.

Patient	TNM	Localization	SCC pre-	post	CEA pre-	post	TPA pre-	post
1	T2N1M0	floor of the mouth	0.8	1	1.5	2.1	n.d.	n.d.
2	T4N1M0	alveolar process	0.1	0.9	4.5	4.3	92.4	113
3	T3N1M0[a]	floor of the mouth	4.6	1.1	10.2	6.7	76.8	54.4
4	T4N2M0[b]	floor of the mouth	4.1	1.5	5.8	5.0	144	29.1
5	T4N0M0	maxillary sinus/orbit	0.6	0.8	1.8	1.2	24.6	30.6
6	T4N0M0	maxillary sinus/orbit	0.7	1.2	3.9	3.1	36.9	50.8
7	T4N2M0	floor of the mouth	2.4	1.8	1.1	0.8	40.9	37.3
8	T3N0M0	intermaxillary	0.4	0.2	3	3.5	n.d.	n.d.
9	T4N2M0	base of the tongue	1.1	1.8	10.3	8.3	156	114
10	T2N2M0	intermaxillary	0.6	1.2	3.3	4.9	113	43.2
11	T4N1M0	base of the tongue	3.3	1.4	5.4	4.7	101	97.4
12	T2N2M0[c]	intermaxillary/bucc.	30.5	2.1	42	44.8	535	422
13	T4N2M0	tonsills	0.1	0.8	0.9	1	69.5	30
14	T4N2M0	floor of the mouth	3	0.3	2.4	3.2	n.d.	n.d.
15	T4N2M0	floor of the mouth	0.5	0.5	4.2	4.5	n.d.	n.d.

[a] Six years before a laryngeal carcinoma had been resected, reduced general condition; at autopsy a second carcinoma of the lower esophagus was found.
[b] Patient died half a year later due to multiple pulmonary metastases, which were not detectable on chest x-ray/CT at the first staging.
[c] Synchronous relapse of an adenocarcinoma of the breast with multiple bone metastases during therapy, palliative intended irradiation of head and neck region.
n.d. = not determined.

Table II. Comparison of TAA values in patients with advanced stages of squamous cell carcinomas of the head and neck. The TAA values are subgrouped according to pretreatment cut-off values ($\leq$ or $\geq$ cut-off levels, 95% specifity) and follow-up values are collected for each subgroup separately.

Pre-values		After RT	
		$\leq$ cut-off	> cut-off
SCC $\leq$ cut-off = 9		8	1
SCC > cut-off = 6		4	2
	total:	12	3
CEA $\leq$ cut-off = 6		4	2
CEA > cut-off = 9		0	9
	total:	4	11
TPA $\leq$ cut-off = 5		5	0
TPA > cut-off = 6		2	4
	total:	7	4

References

1. Fateh-Moghadam A, Stieber P (1993) Tumormarker und ihr sinnvoller Einsatz. 2. Auflage, Hartmann Verlag, Marloffstein-Rathsberg, p 63–64
2. Fischbach W, Meyer Th, Barthel K (1990) Squamous cell carcinoma antigen in the diagnosis and treatment follow-up of oral and facial squamous cell-carcinoma. Cancer 65:1321–1324
3. Hellner D, Klapdor R, Schmelzle R (1990) SCC and CEA in maxillofacial surgery. In: Klapdor R (ed) Recent results in tumor diagnosis and therapy, 5th Symposium on tumor markers. Hamburg, Zuckschwerdt, München, pp 3–7
4. Lobeck H (1991) Orthologie und Pathologie der Zytokeratine. Habilitationsschrift, Freie Universität Berlin
5. Moll R, Franke WW, Schiller DL, Geiger R, Krepler R (1982) The catalogue of human cytokeratins. Patterns of expression in normal epithelia, tumors and cultured cells. Cell 31:11–24

Address for correspondence:
Dr. med. Dr. med. dent. R. E. Friedrich
Klinik für Mund-, Kiefer- und Gesichtschirurgie
(Nordwestdeutsche Kieferklinik)
Martinistraße 52
D-20246 Hamburg, Germany

Determination of tumor-associated antigens (TAA) in sera of patients with carcinomas of the salivary glands in the head and neck (diagnosis and follow-up)

R.E. Friedrich[a], K. Plambeck[a], D. Hellner[a], V. Thoms[a], M. Bahlo[b], R. Klapdor[b]

[a]Department of Oral and Maxillofacial Surgery, [b]Department of Internal Medicine, Eppendorf University Hospital University of Hamburg, Germany

Introduction

Due to local recurrences and distant metastases even decades after surgical treatment it is necessary to establish a long-terme follow-up in adenocarcinomas of the salivary glands in the head and neck region (2, 3). The clinical value of determination of tumor associated antigens (TAA) is yet not well established in these entities. In addition, there are in a lot of cases no tumor specific clinical symptoms complained and its not a rare situation to be surprised by the histological diagnosis of a malignant disease originating from the salivary glands despite an almost unaffected oral tissue (2). To add some more information on the excretory activity of salivary gland tumors, a panel of TAA was investigated in sera of patients with a history of salivary gland carcinomas of the head and neck region.

Material and methods

We investigated the levels of tumor-associated antigens (TAA) in 13 patients with different salivary gland carcinomas of the head and neck region (adenoid-cystic carcinomas (n = 3) (ACC), mucoepidermoid carcinomas (n = 10) (MEC), epithelial-myoepithelial carcinoma (n = 1) (EMC)). Ablative surgery in patients with MEC was done six month up to 20 years before and during the recall of the patients. In none but one female there was a recurrence suspected (restaging). Three patients with large ACC were used to study the value of TAA in patients which are clinically suspected to have a fatal outcome of their disease. Cut-off levels are defined: SCC = 1.5 ng/ml (IMx, Abbott), CA 19-9 = 37 U/ml (EIA Roche), CEA = 3 ng/ml (Enzymun, BM), TPA = 95 U/l (L/A-mat, Byk-Sangtec), TAG 72 = 3.5 U/ml (IRMA, Sorin).

Results

In the majority of MEC patients tested the serological levels of the tumor-associated antigens were in the physiological range. In three patients of this rare entity, initial values were available. In two of these cases SCC levels were elevated, but there is obviously no correlation to tumor size.
Indeed, in the third patient with normal initial SCC values and a large primary tumor destroying the entire left maxilla initially only CEA levels were elevated and immediately decreased after surgery. Up to now during follow-up there are neither signs of local recurrence nor distant metastases and CEA values are still in the physiological range.
In the patient suffering from epithelial-myoepithelial carcinoma the TAA used in this study hardly give any information about the progress of the disease. Excepting the tendency of CA 125 values coming up to the cut-off level all TAA tested are not affected neither by large pulmonary metastases nor by the metastases infiltrating soft and hard tissues of the left foot.
In ACC in one patient the elevated CEA value (15 ng/ml) did not decrease substantially (from 15 to 12 ng/ml) after a subtotal resection and irradiation of the parotid tumor infiltrating the pharynx and skull base. An increase of CEA (from 23 to 32 ng/ml) was noticed about six month before scintigraphy detected the multifocal distant metastases. On the other hand, in patients treated with curative

Gastroenterology   11

Table I. Comparison of TAA with [1]history, sex and primary staging of patients with mucoepidermoid carcinomas ([a]initial values; [b]after local resection, residual tumor; [c]status after resection of pulmonary metastases; n.d. = not determined).

Patient	Sex	Years[1]	T-staging	SCC (ng/ml)	TPA (U/l)	CEA (ng/ml)
1	m	5	T1	3.5[a]	33	< 0.1[a]
2	m	0.6	T1	2.0[b]	42.7	2.6
3	m	24	T2	0.4	47.6	1.7
4	m	23	T2[a]	n.d.	n.d.	2.4
5	f	28	T1	0.9	27.6	1.8
6	f	9	T2[a]	0.6	21.0	1.2
7	m	5	T1[a]	2.1[a]	95	0.5
8	f	0.75	T4	0.3[a]	73.7[a]	3.9[a]
9	m	22	T1	0.4	23.8	3.3[c]
10	m	19	T2[a]	0.8	35.0	1.2
11	f	5	T1	0.5	28.6	1.4
12	m	12	T1	1.0	70.7	3.5
13	m	11	T1[a]	0.9	39.9	3.7
14	f	10	T4	0.8	22.3	1.1

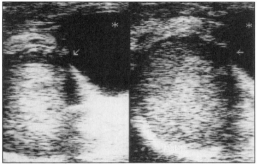

1.a.

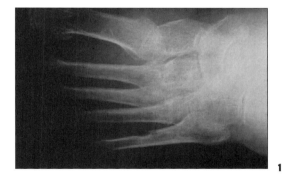

1.c.

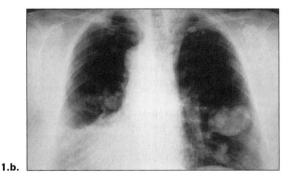

1.b.

Figure 1. Epithelial-myoepithelial carcinoma presumed to originate from the right parotid gland about 18 years ago. The tumor invades the orbit and infiltrates into the right eye (ultrasound imaging: asterix = bulbus oculi, arrow indicating invasion of the tumor (left) (1.a.)), the pulmonary tumors are known for more than three years (1.b.). About 8 month ago the patient complained on a small tumor of the left foot which was resected. Soon occured a local recurrence infiltrating the bone (1.c.). During local treatment to save the right eye (left side: congenital strabism) and follow-up the TAA applied were in the physiological range.

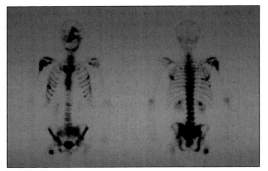

Figure 2. Scintigraphy of a patient with adenoid-cystic carcinoma of the left parotid gland infiltrating the pharynx and skull base. One year after surgery and irradiation multiple bone metastases were detected. CEA levels (≥12 ng/ml) slightly decreased after surgery and irradiation. Several months before the time of diagnosis of distant metastases (bones, brain) CEA levels markedly increased (23-32 ng/ml).

intention for several times but still suffering from local recurrences the marker is not indicative (n = 2). These data need confirmation in a larger series of patients. Further TAA investigated are not affected by the diseases.

Discussion

In large ACC CEA levels might be elevated. Tumor reduction can be associated by a slight decrease of CEA levels and during a percutaneous irradiation of the tumor region there is a further decrease. CEA levels never became normal and about 12 month after combined surgery and radiotherapy multifocal distant metastases appeared. Thus, elevated CEA levels can indicate an activity of the tumor in ACC.

In the patient with an EMC there is a history of the malignant disease of 18 years and during the palliative treatment of the local recurrences of the tumor invading the orbit for a long time a very slow progress of lung metastases was known. TAA constantly were in the physiological range (SCC, CEA, CA 19-9, TAG-72, NSE, TK, CA 15-3) and not altered by palliatively intended local resections. CA 125 levels were increasing from 26 to 34 U/ml (cut-off level 35 U/ml) which might be correlated to a progression of the disease (fast local recurrence in the right maxillary and orbital region; distant metastases of the left foot), but this correlation needs confirmation during follow-up and is not helpful in clinical management.

Elevated CEA, CA-50 and CA 19-9 values (CEA > 5 U/ml, CA-50 > 17 U/ml, CA 19-9 > 37 U/ml) were found in histogenetically different head and neck neoplasms including tumors of the salivary glands (malignant salivary gland tumors: CEA 4/18, CA-50 6/18, CA 19-9 4/18; benign salivary gland tumors: CEA 3/21, CA-50 1/21, CA 19-9 0/21) (1). Comparing benign and malignant salivary gland tumors there seems to be no difference regarding CEA sensitivity.

It is concluded that TAA might not be applied for screening of patients with a history of a MEC of the salivary glands and no clinical suspicion of a tumor recurrence. There are no serological markers to control patients with EMC but CA 125 might give some additional information about the progress of the disease. CEA can be used for the follow-up of ACC.

References

1. Gustafsson H, Franzén L, Grankvist, Anniko M, Henriksson R (1988) Glycoprotein tumor markers in head and neck neoplasms – a consecutive study on CA-50, CA 19-9, and CEA. J Cancer Res Clin Oncol 114: 394-398
2. Lentrodt J (1977) Mukoepidermoidtumoren. HNO-Praxis 3/2: 190-193
3. Seifert G (1992) Histopathology of malignant salivary gland tumours. Oral Oncol Eur J Cancer 28B (1): 49-56

Address for correspondence:
Dr. med. Dr. med. dent. R. E. Friedrich
Klinik für Mund-, Kiefer- und Gesichtschirurgie
(Nordwestdeutsche Kieferklinik)
Martinistraße 52
D-20246 Hamburg, Germany

CA 72-4, CEA, CA 19-9 in diagnosis of relapse and metastases and in prognosis of stomach cancer patients

W. Reiter[a], Petra Stieber[a], C. Reuter[b], C. Cramer[b], A. Fateh-Moghadam†[a]

[a]Institute of Clinical Chemistry, [b]Chirurgical Clinic and Poliklinic, Klinikum Großhadern, Ludwig-Maximilians-University, Munich, Germany

Introduction

Stomach cancer is beside breast, lung, colon and prostatic cancer the most frequent cause of cancer death in the FRG.
The aim of the study was to investigate the relevance of CA 72-4 in stomach cancer in comparison to the established but not satisfying markers CEA and CA 19-9.
We focused our interest on the question of prognostic significance of these markers in stomach cancer.

Patients and methods

The present retrospective study was done using frozen sera (stored at $-70°$ C) of 216 patients. All sera were collected at an active stage of disease pretherapeutically. The patient group included sera of 146 patients with histologically proven stomach cancer: 112 at the time of primary diagnosis, 18 with distant metastases and 16 patients with local relapse. As a clinically relevant reference group we investigated the CA 72-4, CEA and CA 19-9-levels in 70 patients with benign disorders of the gastrointestinal tract (cholelithiasis, cirrhosis of liver, hepatitis, M. Crohn, colitis ulcerosa, prim. bil. cirrhosis).
We determined the CA 72-4 concentrations by a solid phase radioimmunoassay (Centocor, Isotopen Diagnostik) (1–7). CEA (MEIA, Abbott, IMx) and CA 19-9 concentrations (EnzymunR, Boehringer Mannheim, ES 700) were determined by automized assays each of them based on the sandwich principle.
Life table analysis was calculated according to Kaplan-Meyer. The patients were divided into two groups, respectively, according to the preoperative marker levels. Two cut-off levels (which discriminate best) were used: < 3 U/ml versus ≥ 3 U/ml for CA 72-4, < 4 ng/ml versus ≥ 4 ng/ml for CEA and < 60 U/ml versus ≥ 60 U/ml for CA 19-9. The statistical significance between the survival curves was calculated using chi-square (log-rank)-test.

Results

Specificity

Postulating a specificity of 95% for all three markers investigated versus benign gastrointestinal diseases (12) the cut-off value of CA 72-4 was 3.9 U/ml, of CEA 7.2 ng/ml and of CA 19-9 166 U/ml. This fact is very important as well for differential diagnostic decisions at the time of primary diagnosis as during follow-up care and for control of therapy efficacy in stomach cancer.

Sensitivity

Using the above mentioned cut-off values at a specificity of 95% CA 72-4 showed the highest overall sensitivity in stomach cancer with 40% in comparison to CEA (17%) and CA 19-9 (21%). At the time of primary diagnosis, the sensitivity was 36% for CA 72-4, 14% for CEA, and 20% for CA 19-9. There was a significant increase of true positive test results in recurrent disease: At the time of local relapse respectively distant metastases the sensitivity of CA 72-4 was 56% (56%), of CEA 19% (33%), and of CA 19-9 18% (28%).

Table I. Sensitivity (%) of CA 72-4, CEA, CA 19-9 and simultaneous determinations in stomach cancer at the time of primary diagnosis, metastatic gastric carcinoma and relapse. Specificity = 95% versus benign gastrointestinal diseases.

Marker	Cut-off	n = 146	Prim. diag. n = 112	Metastases n = 18	Relapse n = 16
CA 72-4	3.9 U/ml	40	36	56	56
CEA	7.2 ng/ml	17	14	33	19
CA 19-9	166 U/ml	21	20	28	19
CA 72-4 or CEA		48	43	72	56
CA 72-4 or CA 19-9		41	37	56	56
CEA or CA 19-9		24	20	60	23

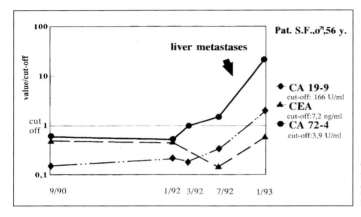

Figure 1. Long-term follow-up of a 56-years-old patient with stomach cancer.

Marker combinations

For the calculations of marker combinations both markers had to fulfill a specificity of 95% versus benign gastrointestinal diseases and at least one of the two markers had to show a true positive test result. As far as the different marker combinations are concerned, the simultaneous determination of CA 72-4 and CEA showed the highest additive sensitivity. Overall sensitivity in stomach cancer was 48% in comparison to CA 72-4/CA 19-9 (41%) and CEA/CA 19-9 (24%). At the time of primary diagnosis, the sensitivity was 43% for CA 72-4/CEA, 37% for CA 72-4/CA 19-9, and 20% for CEA/CA 19-9; at the time of local relapse 56% for CA 72-4/CEA, 56% for CA 72-4/CA 19-9 and 23% for CEA/CA 19-9. There was a significant increase of sensitivities in metastatic stomach cancer: CA 72-4/CEA = 72%, CA 72-4/CA 19-9 = 56%, and CEA/CA19-9 = 60%. The combination of all three markers did not increase sensitivity significantly.

Prognosis

Patients with a preoperative CA 19-9 concentration $\geq$ 60 U/ml (CEA: $\geq$ 4 ng/ml) have a significant shorter survival time than those with lower values. The survival rates in the group of patients with serum concentrations $\geq$ 60 U/ml for CA 19-9 were in 81% of the cases < 2 years versus 19% $\geq$ 2 years (CEA: $\geq$ 4 ng/ml in 79% < 2 years versus 21% $\geq$ 2 years/ CA 72-4: $\geq$ 3 U/ml in 67% < 2 years versus 33% $\geq$ 2 years). The preoperative value of CA 19-9 (log-rank = 13.8) represents the best prognostic factor beside CEA (log-rank = 12.2). CA 72-4 shows a log-rank of 6.9.

Conclusions

CA 72-4 is a sensible marker in stomach cancer. The simultanous determination of CA 72-4 and CEA in sera of patients with stomach cancer is recommended because of the best specificity /

Table II. The distribution of patients with stomach cancer according to preoperative CA 72-4-, CEA- and CA 19-9 levels. Cut-off: CEA = 4 ng/ml, CA 72-4 = 3 U/ml, CA 19-9 = 60 U/ml.

Survival time	Marker					
	CEA < 4	CA 72-4 < 3	CA 19-9 < 60	CEA ≥ 4	CA 72-4 ≥ 3	CEA 19-9 ≥ 60
≥ 2 Years	57	59	57	21	33	19
< 2 Years	43	41	43	79	67	81

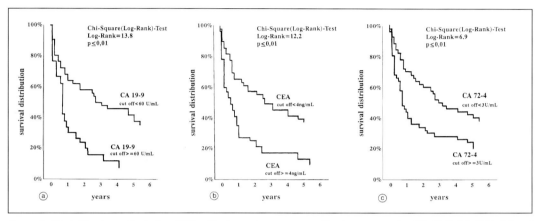

Figure 2. Life-tables for patients (n = 103) with stomach cancer according to preoperative CA 19-9- (a), CEA- (b) and 72-4 (c) levels. When a cut-off of 60 U/ml for CA 19-9, 4 ng/ml for CEA and 3 U/ml for CA 72-4 was used the prognosis was significantly better in patients with serum concentrations below this cut-off.

sensitivity-profile in recurrency, the importance of prognostic significance, and also from an economic point of view.

If one of the two markers becomes clearly positive during follow-up care this "leading" marker is sufficient as a single determination for control of therapy efficacy.

References

1. Nuti M, Teramoto YA, Mariani-Costantini R, Horan Hand P, Colcher D Schlom J (1982) A monoclonal antibody (B 72.3) defines patterns of distribution of a novel tumor-associated antigen in a human mammary carcinoma cell population. Int J Cancer 29:539–545
2. Johnson, VG, Schlom J, Paterson AJ, Bennett J, Magnani JL, Colcher D (1986) Analysis of a human tumor-associated glycoprotein (TAG 72) identified by monoclonal antibody B 72.3. Cancer Res 46:850–857
3. Thor A, Ohuchi N, Szak A, Johnston WW, Schlom L (1986) Distribution of oncofetal antigen tumor-associated glycoprotein-72 defined by monoclonal antibody B 72.3. Cancer Res 46:3118–3124
4. Fateh-Moghadam A, Stieber P, Bayerl B, Brandl R, Knedel M (1988) Klinische Einsatzmöglichkeiten des neuen Tumormarkers CA 72-4. Aktuell (Isotopen Diagnostik CIS) 10,3
5. Stieber P, Fateh-Moghadam A, Wädlich H (1989) CA 72-4: Ein neuer Tumormarker beim Magenkarzinom. J Clin Chem Clin Biochem 27:767–768
6. Stieber P, Fateh-Moghadam A, Wädlich H, Nagel D, Lamerz R, Denecke H (1990) CA 72-4: A new marker for stomach cancer. In: Klapdor R (ed) Recent results in tumor diagnosis and therapy. Zuckschwerdt, München, pp 23–26
7. Stieber P, Fateh-Moghadam A (1991) Klinische Wertigkeit von CA 72-4. mta 6:3–5
8. Reiter W, Stieber P, Denecke H, Lamerz R, Fateh-Moghadam A (1993) CA 72-4: Ein sinnvoller Tumormarker beim Magenkarzinom (Wertigkeit im Vergleich mit CEA und CA 19-9). Lab med 17:239
9. Stieber P, Reiter W, Denecke H, Fateh-Moghadam A (1993) CA 72-4: a sensible tumor marker in gastric carcinoma. Lab med 17:441–444

10 Reiter W, Stieber P, Denecke H, Fateh-Moghadam A (1993) Klinische Wertigkeit des CA 72-4 bei Patienten mit Magenkarzinom. Abstracta, XXI. Kongreß der Gesellschaft für Gastroenterologie in Bayern: 32

11 Reiter W, Stieber P, Reuter C, Cramer C, Fateh-Moghadam A (1993) CA 72-4 in der Diagnostik von Rezidiven und Metastasierung bei Patienten mit Magenkarzinom. In: Klapdor R (Hrsg) Aktuelle Tumordiagnostik: Möglichkeiten, Klinische Relevanz, Forschung–Perspektiven. Kurzfassungen/Abstracts. 7. Hamburger Symposium über Tumormarker. Zuckschwerdt, München, pp 5

12 Arbeitsgruppe Qualitätskontrolle und Standardisierung von Tumormarkertests im Rahmen der Hamburger Symposien über Tumormarker (1992). Tumordiagnose und Therapie 13, XIX–XXII, Thieme, Stuttgart

Address for correspondence:
Dr. med. Petra Stieber
Institut für Klinische Chemie
Klinikum Großhadern
Marchioninistraße 15
D-81377 München, Germany

Determination of CA 72-4 by IRMA or ELISA in the follow-up of gastric cancer patients

U. Gärtner[b], M. E. Scheulen[c], E. Aghabi[a], J. Wiefelspütz[c], H. Delbrück[a]

[a]Clinic Bergisch-Land, Wuppertal, [b]Paracelsus-Clinic, Bad Gandersheim, [c]University Hospital of Internal Medicine (Tumor Research), Tumor Center of West Germany, Essen, Germany

Introduction

The CA 72-4 assay determines the human tumor-associated glycoprotein TAG-72 and is defined by the monoclonal antibodies B 72.3 and CC 49 (3, 7). It is expressed by a variety of carcinomas with highest sensitivities in gastric and ovarian cancer (2, 8, 10, 11).
The aim of this study was to find out whether CA 72-4 either determined by IRMA or ELISA is of higher value than the commonly used tests for CEA and CA 19-9 in the follow-up of gastric cancer patients or may advantageously add to the cumulative sensitivity when used in combination (1, 4, 5, 6, 9).

Patients and methods

Patients

Determinations of the tumor markers CA 72-4 by IRMA or ELISA, CEA and CA 19-9 were performed in a prospective study in the sera of 243 patients in two hospitals. All patients had undergone gastrectomy because of histologically confirmed cancer of the stomach in curative intention one to 48 months before (median four months). Seventy patients (29%) had a partial and 173 patients (71%) a total gastrectomy, respectively. Beside tumor marker determinations common clinical investigations such as ultrasound of the abdomen, endoscopy and x-ray were done at the two hospitals where the patients were admitted during the follow-up after tumor gastrectomy. In case of the suspicion of a tumor relapse computertomography was performed. A relapse had to be proven by histological examination. Sensitivity and specificity of each single tumor marker and various combinations were calculated.

CA 72-4 IRMA

Altogether, 201 sera were analyzed with the Centocor® CA 72-4™ IRMA (Centocor Inc., Malvern, Penn., USA), a two-step solid-phase sandwich radio-immunometric assay. A cut-off value of 3.8 U/ml was used.

CA 72-4 ELISA

CA 72-4 was automatically analyzed in 157 sera with the ES 300 using the Enzymun-Test® CA 72-4 (Boehringer Mannheim GmbH, Mannheim, Germany), a new one-step solid phase sandwich enzyme linked immunosorbant assay with streptavidin-biotin technology. A cut-off value of 6.8 U/ml was used.

CEA and CA 19-9 ELISA

For the determination of CEA in 240 and CA 19-9 in 234 sera the Enzymun-Test® (Boehringer Mannheim GmbH, Mannheim, Germany) were used with the cut-off values 5.0 ng/ml and 37.0 U/ml, respectively.

Results

Out of the 243 gastric cancer patients of the study 56 patients (23%) had relapses during follow-up after gastrectomy including 27 with

Table I. Sensitivity and specificity of the tumor markers.

Marker	Number of patients	Sensitivity	Specificity
CA 72-4 (IRMA)	201	49% (24/49)	92% (140/152)
CA 72-4 (ELISA)	157	31% (12/39)	93% (110/118)
CA 19-9	234	51% (28/55)	86% (154/179)
CEA	240	27% (15/56)	89% (164/184)
CA 72-4 (IRMA)/CA 19-9	193	75% (36/48)	77% (112/145)
CA 19-9/CEA	238	62% (34/55)	78% (142/183)
CA 72-4 (IRMA)/CA 19-9/CEA	192	84% (38/45)	68% (100/147)

local progression of disease (48%), 12 with liver metastases (22%), and 17 with metastatic disease in other locations (30%) such as lung, kidney, scrotum, bone and peritoneum, respectively.

CA 72-4 was determined in 201 patients with the IRMA and in 157 patients with the ELISA in comparison to CA 19-9 in 234 patients and CEA in 240 patients, respectively.

The sensitivities and specificities of the tumor markers are listed in table I according to a calculation based on the cut-off values determined in a population of healthy blood donors (95%-confidence limit).

Accordingly, sensitivites were higher for CA 72-4 IRMA with 49% and CA 19-9 with 51% in comparison to CA 72-4 ELISA with 31% and CEA with 27%. The corresponding specificities were 92% for CA 72-4 IRMA, 93% for CA 72-4 ELISA, 86% for CA 19-9 and 89% for CEA, respectively.

When two or three tumor markers were combined the calculation of cumulative sensitivities led to higher figures of 75% for CA 72-4 IRMA and CA 19-9, 62% for CA 19-9 and CEA and 84% for CA 72-4 IRMA, CA 19-9 and CEA with a corresponding decrease in specificity to values of 77, 78 and 68%, respectively.

Discussion

With respect to specificity, in our population of patients with gastric cancer CA 72-4 IRMA proved to be the marker with the highest sensitivity during follow-up after gastrectomy comparable to CA 19-9 and can be recommended as the tumor marker of first choice in this malignant disease.

By combination of CA 72-4 with CA 19-9 or even with CA 19-9 and CEA the sensitivity can be further increased to 75 or 84%, respectively. However, this increase in sensitivity is accompanied by a marked decrease in specificity to only 77 or 68%. Thus, the combined determination of tumor markers results in a substantially high proportion of patients with false positive results and may induce unjustified physical and psychic stress as well as diagnostic expenses as long as the results of salvage therapy are only palliative in the majority of relapsing patients (9).

In agreement with other investigations (2, 6, 8, 10, 11) CA 72-4 is the tumor marker of first choice in the follow-up of patients with gastric cancer. However, the benefit of an early detection of relapses is questionable as long as there is no curative salvage treatment for most of the patients with this disease (9).

References

1 Borlinghaus P, Lamerz R (1991) Zirkulierende Tumormarker bei gastrointestinalen Tumoren. Leber-Magen-Darm 5: 199-205

2 Byrne DJ, Browning MCK, Cuschieri A (1990) CA 72-4: a new tumor marker for gastric cancer. Br J Surg 77: 1010-1013

3 Colcher D, Horan Hand P, Nuti M, Schlom J (1981) A spectrum of monoclonal antibodies reactive with human mammary tumor cells. Proc Natl Acad Sci USA 78: 3199-3202

4 Delbrück H (1988) Magenkarzinom. In: Delbrück H (Hrsg) Tumornachsorge. Thieme, Stuttgart, pp 352-361

5 Klug TL, Sattler MA, Colcher D, Schlom J (1986) Monoclonal antibody in immunoradiometric assay for an antigenic determinant (CA 72) on a novel pancarcinoma antigen (TAG 72). Int J Cancer 38: 661-669

6 Heptner G, Domschke S, Domschke W (1989) Comparison of CA 72-4 with CA 19-9 and carcino-

embryonic antigen in the serodiagnostic of gastrointestinal malignancies. Scand J Gastroenterol 24: 745

7 Paterson AJ, Schlom J, Sears HF, Bennett J, Colcher D (1986) A radioimmunoassay for the detection of a human tumor-associated glycoprotein (TAG-72) using monoclonal antibody B 72.3. Int J Cancer 37: 659–666

8 Patzke B, Klapdor R, Meyer-Pannwitt U, Weh P, Schreiber HW (1990) TAG 72 in comparison with CA 19-9, CEA, and CA 125 in diagnosis and follow-up of stomach cancer. In: Klapdor R (ed) Recent results in tumor diagnosis and therapy. Zuckschwerdt, München, pp 31–36

9 Scheulen ME (1990) Welche Tumormarker sind für die Krebsnachsorge von praktischer Bedeutung? Münch med Wschr 132: 240–245

10 Scheulen ME, Klapdor R, Delbrück H, Milewski A, Bahlo M, Kämper P, Wiefelspütz J, Klenner D, Jaworek D (1992) Determination of CA 724 in serum with a new one-step enzyme-immunoassay: technical evaluation and first clinical results in patients with gastric cancer and other malignancies. In: Klapdor R (ed) Tumor associated antigens, oncogenes, receptors, cytokines in tumor diagnosis and therapy at the beginning of the nineties. Zuckschwerdt, München, pp 237–241

11 Schmid L, Bauer R, Rauthe G, Langhammer HR, Bryxi V (1990) The use of TAG 72 in oncological follow-up. Comparison with CEA and CA 19-9 in gastric carcinoma and with CA 125 and CEA in ovarian cancer. In: Klapdor R (ed) Recent results in tumor diagnosis and therapy. Zuckschwerdt, München, pp 94–99

Address for correspondence:
Prof. Dr. med. H. Delbrück
Klinik Bergisch-Land
Im Saalscheid 5
D-42369 Wuppertal, Germany

Tumor markers in gastric cancer

F. Safi, V. Kuhns, H. G. Beger
Department of General Surgery, University of Ulm, Germany

Introduction

Recent advances in hybrid technology and the discovery of new tumor-associated antigens have created new possibilities for serological diagnosis and tumor follow-up. The tumor marker CA 19-9 has an important place in the diagnosis and follow-up of patients with pancreatic carcinoma (1). One of the most widely used of the serum tumor markers is the 180-kD glycoprotein, carcinoembryonic antigen (2,3). Recently a high molecular weight mucin-like protein, termed tumor-associated glycoprotein-72 (TAG-72), has been identified and characterized using monoclonal antibody (MoAb) B72.3 and a panel of second generation MoAb that include CC49 and CC83 (4,5). Elevated serum CA 72-4 levels are found in a high proportion of patients with gastrointestinal malignancies, ovary, endometrium and breast cancer (6). Expression of the antigen was found rarely in most normal adult human tissues, with the exception of secretory phase endometrium, apocrine metaplasia of the breast and transitional colonic mucosa (6–11).

The present prospective study was designed to compare the tumor markers CA 72-4, CEA and CA 19-9 with regard to their sensitivity and specificity in the diagnosis of different stages of gastric cancer, and in the detection of recurrences during the follow-up of gastric cancer patients after curative surgical therapy.

Patients and methods

Patients

Serum samples for the determination of tumor marker concentrations were collected from patients admitted to the Department of Surgery, University Hospital of Ulm. Sera were examined prospectively. Pre-operative serum samples were obtained from the following groups of patients admitted to our surgical department for the following reasons:

1. Gastric cancer (n = 115), age 38-85 years, median age 66 years, 77 males and 38 females. The patients were classified by the TNM system (12) after surgery and histological examination of operative specimen. Stage I: n = 26; stage II: n = 27; stage III: n = 28; stage IV: n = 34.

2. Sera from 167 patients with malignancies not involving the stomach were analysed for CA 72-4: 91 males, age 49–87 years, median age 64 years; 76 females, age 24–90 years, median age 69 years.

3. Benign disorders: 266 males, age 17–83 years, median age 53 years; 210 females, age 16–86 years, median age 51 years. The diagnoses are based on clinical, labaratory, histological and/or operative findings. None of the patients in the control benign group has yet developed a carcinoma.

The diagnoses of gastric cancer and other malignancies were ascertained histologically after the appropriate surgical measure.

CA 72-4, CEA and CA 19-9 were measured simultaneously in 59 patients who had undergone surgery for gastric cancer and had no post-operative evidence of metastasis. These patients were refered to our follow-up clinic. These patients are first seen in our follow-up clinic four months after surgery, then at regular four months intervals thereafter. At each appointment, the patients were examined and blood samples taken for the determination of liver parameters and the tumor markers CA 72-4, CEA and CA 19-9. Abdominal sonography and endoscopy of the upper GI-tract are performed every eight months, upper gastrointestinal series of a new stomach, chest X-ray (a.p. and lateral) annually, and CT of the upper abdomen every 16 months. If a tumor marker continues to rise during the follow-up period, an intensive metastasis search through imaging procedures is started, independently of the follow-up program. During the follow-up period (range 4–71 months; median 13 months) recurrences of gastric cancer intra-abdominally were detected in 29 of 59 patients by imaging procedures.

Methods

Early morning fasting blood samples were obtained from those patients in hospital for treatment. Blood samples were centrifuged and the sera assayed during the same day.
The tumor marker CA 72-4 was determined by radioenzymassay (RIA technique; Centocor Company). The intra-assay coefficient of variability was 9–13% as determined in 20 measurements of five patients and standard sera, with the concentrations ranging between 2.5 to 100 U/ml. The inter-assay coefficient of variability established in 20 determinations was 11.5%. The normal value of CEA is ≤ 3 ng/ml. Carcinoembryonic antigen (CEA) and tumor-associated antigen (CA 19-9) were assayed with the Isotope Diagnostic Enzymimmunoassays Testkit (Dreieich, FRG). The sensitivity of the test is established by the percentage of true-positive values in patients with cancer: TP/(TP + FN) x 100 (TP = true positive, FN = false negative). The specificity is the percentage of the true negative values in patients with benign diseases TN/(TN + FP) x 100 (TN = true negative, FN = false positive). Fisher's test was used for statistical evaluation. The difference betweeen CA 72-4 serum levels in the different groups was calculated with the Kruskal-Wallis-Test (13). Patients with adeno-carcinoma of the stomach were separated in various groups depending on histological type of Laurén and degree of differentation (14).

Table I. Distribution of CA 72-4 levels in patients with gastric cancer and three control groups.

CA 72-4 (U/ml)	Group I gastric cancer		Group II colorectal cancer		Group III other malignancies		Group IV benign diseases	
	n	%	n	%	n	%	n	%
≤ 2.5	45	39	43	55	65	73	438	92
> 2.5	70	61	35	41	24	27	38	8
> 10	30	26	20	25	6	7	2	0.4
Total number of patients	115		78		89		476	

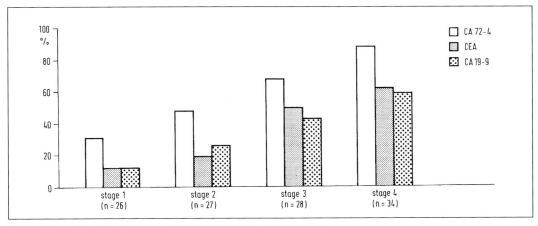

Figure 1. Sensivity of the tumor markers in dependence on tumor stage.

Table II. CA 72-4 concentration depending on histological type of Laurén and grading.

	n	CA 72-4 (U/ml)			
		≤ 2.5		> 2.5	
		n	%	n	%
Histological type					
intestinal	51	17	33	34	67
diffuse	54	25	46	29	54
Histological grading					
G1	3	2	67	1	33
G2	31	16	52	15	48
G3	45	14	31	31	69
G4	29	12	41	17	59

Table III. Sensitivity of the tumor markers CA 72-4, CEA and CA 19-9 in gastric cancer depending on the estimation of one marker or more and on tumor stage.

Tumor marker	Sensitivity (%)				
	stage I	stage II	stage III	stage IV	total
Only CA 72-4	31	48	68	88	61
Only CEA	12	19	50	62	37
Only CA 19-9	12	26	43	59	37
CA 72-4/CEA	35	52	75	88	64
CA 72-4/CA 19-9	35	56	79	91	67
CA 72-4/CEA/CA 19-9	38	63	82	91	70
CEA/CA 19-9	15	30	54	68	43

Results

Pre-operative CA 72-4 serum levels

Table I shows the CA 72-4 determination in the gastric cancer group and in three control groups. Of all gastric cancer patients (group I), 61% had pathological values above 2.5 U/ml, and 26% were above 10 U/ml. The latter were patients with advanced tumor stage III and IV. The median CA 72-4 values were 2.8 U/ml (range 0.8–1730) for gastric cancer patients, 2.3 U/ml for colorectal carcinoma patients (range 0.8–2739), 1.7 U/ml for patients with other malignancies (range 0.8–144) and 1.5 U/ml for patients with benign diseases (range 0.8–25). The differences in the findings between group I and II ($p < 0.06$) were not significant between group I and III, and group I and IV were statistically significant ($p < 0.0001$). The frequency of elevated serum levels of CA 72-4, CEA and CA 19-9 in gastric cancer is shown in figure I. The more advanced the tumor stage, the higher the percentage of patients with pathological CA 72-4, CEA and CA 19-9 concentrations before surgery. CA 72-4 was more sensitive than CEA and CA 19-9 in all stages. The differences in the sensitivity of CA 72-4 and CEA or CA 19-9 for stage II and IV ($p < 0.02, 0.004$) were significant, for stage I and III not significant.

Histological grading of the gastric cancer was documented in 108 patients and histological type of Laurén in 105 patients. The CA 72-4 serum concentration was independent on differentiation of the carcinoma and on histological type of Laurén (table II).

Table III summarizes the sensitivity of one tumor marker or of two or more estimated markers in gastric cancer depending on tumor stage. In fact, the analysis of the patients' sera for the presence of CA 72-4 and/or CEA and/or CA 19-9 and CA 72-4 and/or CEA/CA 19-9 increased the percentage positive from 61 to 70%.

Table IV. Sensitivity of CA 72-4 and CEA in colorectal cancer and other malignancies.

Location of the carinoma	n	Sensitivity of			
		CA 72-4 (%)		CEA (%)	
		≤ 2.5 U/ml	> 2.5	≤ 3 ng/ml	> 3
Colorectal	78	55	41	40	60
Pancreas	33	67	33	41	59
Esophageal	18	94	6	67	33
Lung	14	50	50	21	79
Breast	9	100	0	44	56
Others	15	66	34	87	13

Table V. CA 72-4 and CEA determination in patients with benign surgical diseases.

Disease	n	CA 72-4 > 2.5 U/ml		CEA > 3 ng/ml		Median value (range)	
		n	%	n	%	CA 72-4	CEA
Gastritis/ulcus	30	2	7	4	13	1.6 (0.8–9.4)	1.9 (1.9–6.9)
Colorectal polyps	77	4	5	5	6	1.5 (0.8–6.1)	1.9 (1.9–7.9)
Gastroenteritis	11	1	9	2	18	1.3 (0.8–3.2)	1.9 (1.9–6.6)
Hepatitis/ liver cirrhosis	30	3	10	14	47	1.3 (0.8–10.9)	2.2 (1.9–12.5)
Cholecystolithiasis	61	5	8	13	21	1.4 (0.8–9.3)	1.9 (1.9–9.9)
Pancreatitis	52	4	8	15	29	1.3 (0.8–3.4)	1.9 (1.9–9.7)
Cardio-vascular disease	62	6	10	15	24	1.5 (0.8–4.8)	1.9 (1.9–9.3)
Benign disease of the thyroid gland	69	6	9	5	7	1.6 (0.8–3.7)	1.9 (1.9–19.5)
Others	84	7	8	14	17	1.6 (0.8–25)	1.9 (1.9–7.5)
Total	476	38	8	87	18	1.6 (0.8–25)	1.9 (1.9–19.5)

The important control groups II and III (patients with other malignancies) is analyzed separately with regard to the specificity of the marker to the stomach. Table IV shows the results in these groups. CA 72-4 values were above 2.5 U/ml in 0–50% of patients with colorectal, pancreas, esophageal, lung and breast carcinoma. Values of more than 10 U/ml were found in only 0–21% of the same patients groups.

CEA was more sensitive in every group of patients and high values of CEA (> 10 ng/ml) were frequently observed (0–43%) of the patients.

CA 72-4 levels in patients with benign disease

All benign diseases caused a moderate elevation of serum CA 72-4 levels, between 2.5–10 U/ml, and only 0.4% of the patients had CA 72-4 above 10 U/ml. Elevated levels of CEA were found in 18% of this group of patients (table V). If we assume the normal value of CA 72-4 to be below 2.5 U/ml, then the sensitivity of this marker is 61%, its specificity 92%, and its total accuracy 82%. Using other cut-off values (2, 3, 4, 5, and 10 U/ml) a total accuracy of 79%, 80%, 79%, 80% and 77% can be estimated, respectively.

Table VI. CA 72-4, CEA and CA 19-9 in follow-up patients.

Tumor marker	Patients with recurrences n = 29		Patients without recurrences n = 30	
	n	%	n	%
CA 72-4 >2.5 U/ml	27	93	2	7
CEA > 3 ng/ml	17	35	11	37
CA 19-9 > 37 U/ml	10	25	1	3

Gastric cancer recurrences and follow-up with CA 72-4, CEA and CA 19-9 (table VI)

A total of 59 patients were regularly followed-up in our cancer clinic. Recurrences were found in 29 patients at a median follow-up time of 13 months (range 4-71 months) by imaging techniques. CA 72-4 was more sensitive than CEA and CA 19-9. The pathological values of CA 72-4 were observed in median five months (range 1-15) before recurrences diagnosed via radiological examinations.

Of patients (n = 30) with no metastases detected during the course of the median observation time of 21 months (range 5-152 months), 93% had normal CA 72-4 concentrations, and 7% moderately elevated levels with a median value of 2.1 U/ml (range 0.6-2.9). If these patients in the follow-up clinic are considered as a control group, then the sensitivity for CA 72-4 in recognizing recurrences was 93% versus 35% for CEA and 25% for CA 19-9, the specificity of CA 72-4 was also 93%.

Discussion

Various serological markers have been credited with diagnostic importance in the case of carcinoma of the stomach. In clinical studies the accuracy of the carcinoembryonic antigen (CEA) and carbohydrate antigen (CA 19-9) have been evaluated in the diagnosis and follow-up of gastric cancer (15, 16). None of the markers mentioned above have so far proved to be specific to gastric carcinoma (16). In the present study, CA 72-4 levels were elevated in 61% of patients with gastric cancer, in the literature sensitivity varied between 38% by *Patzke* (17) and *Piantino* (18) and 66% by *Stieber* (19).

The difference in sensitivity is due to a) different cut-off values in the literature, ranging from 2.2 U/ml (*Motoo*) (20) to 6 U/ml (*Piatino*) (18), and b) the fact that the gastric cancer colletives of the various authors are different in regard to tumor stages (a patient collective with more patients in an advanced tumor stage shows a higher sensitivity than a colleictve with more patients in an early stage). Therefore we advocate an internationally uniform cut-off value; furthermore, sensitivity should be given as related to the tumor stage.

Like CEA, the best investigated tumor marker in gastric cancer and CA 19-9 (16), CA 72-4 is not suitable for diagnosing gastric cancer in early stage, i.e., for use as a screening test (17, 21). Only 31% of the CA 72-4 values were above normal for stage I. In our study, therefore, not even one in three of those with early gastric cancer would have been recognized by elevated CA 72-4 levels. As a whole, the marker concentration shows a good correlation to the tumor stage, as described by other authors (22, 23). The more advanced the cancer and the larger the tumor mass present, the higher the percentage of pathological values, i.e., the amount of freely circulating antigen. The results obtained from this study showed 88% sensitivity of the marker in stage IV patients, suggesting that CA 72-4 may be considered as a marker for advanced diseases.

No correlation between sex of patients with gastric cancer, or between degree of differentiation or between histological type of Laurén and the serum concentration of CA 72-4 was found. *Motoo* et al. (20) confirmed the same results. A correlation between degree of differentiation and serum concentration of CA 72-4, a higher sensitivity of CA 72-4 in patients with intestinal tumor type than in those with diffuse type were shown by *Brandt* et al. (22). Quantitatively, CA 72-4 thus seems superior to CEA and CA 19-9 in the whole collective of patients with gastric cancer and in every tumor stage. In contrast to our results *Lorenz* and *Schmid* (21, 24) found that CEA and CA 19-9 were more sensitive than CA 72-4. Both authors used the cut-off value of 4 U/ml. Using our cut-off value of 2.5 U/ml we found the best total accuracy of the marker (84%). The simultaneous estimation of CA 72-4, CEA and CA 19-9 increase the sensitivity in diagnosing gastric cancer from 61% (by using CA 72-4 alone) to 70% (by using CA 72-4, CEA and CA 19-9). This increase in the sensitivity up to 9% is in our opinion very low. We decide to use only CA 72-4 in patients with gastric cancer.

To evaluate the specificity of CA 72-4, the serum antigen levels were determined on a series of patients with benign and malignant diseases. We found antigen concentrations above 2.5 U/ml in 8% of patients with benign diseases. The specificity of the marker distinction between patients with benign and malignant diseases was 92%. In the literature the specificity varied between 88 and 100% (11, 22, 25-27).

In our group with malignant disease not originating in the stomach, we found pathological CA 72-4 values of over 2.5 U/ml in 35% of the cases. In all subgroups of patients with malignancies, not involving the stomach, CEA was more sensitive than CA 72-4 (28, 29), particularly for tumors of the colorectum and pancreatic carcinoma. The highest percentages of pathological marker levels were found for ovarian cancer with 58 to 69% of cases having pathological values (11, 30–32).

Since pathological CA 72-4 values were found both in patients with gastric cancer and in patients with malignant primary manifestations other than of the stomach, we must assume that this tumor-associated antigen is not able to distinguish between neoplasms of the stomach and those of other organs. As a consequence, CA 72-4 does not constitute a specific marker for gastric cancer.

Previous studies have demonstrated that a sustained post-operative rise of CEA and CA 19-9 in patients with GI-adenocarcinoma points to the possibility of local recurrence of metastases (16, 33). In agreement with the current literature, our study shows that metastasizing gastric cancer was associated with increased CA 72-4 levels (21, 24). The recurrences of gastric cancer mainly were located intra-abdominally. A continuous increase in CA 72-4 during tumor follow-up is frequently the first indication of recurring tumor growth and precedes the diagnosis of recurrences by a median time of five months (range 1–16 months). The determination of CA 72-4 levels at four months intervals enabled us to detect cancer metastases in 93% of the follow-up patients with recurrences. CA 72-4 was more sensitive than CEA and CA 19-9 in the recognition of recurrences. The difference in the sensitivity was highly significant ($p < 0.0001$). A comparison of the tumor marker determinations either in the diagnosis or the follow-up period confirms the conclusion that CA 72-4 is of greater clinical relevance than CEA and CA 19-9 in gastric cancer patients. However, it is questionable whether the diagnosis of metastases is important for increasing survival time of these affected patients. An effective systemic therapy for the treatment of patients with recurred adenocarcinoma of the stomach is not available.

With the simple method of measuring the serum levels of the tumor marker CA 72-4, we obtained the diagnosis of metastases. Another question will be the therapy of these metastases.

Conclusions

CA 72-4 represents the most sensitive tumor marker for gastric cancer. CA 72-4 was above the normal limits of 2.5 U/ml in 61% of the patients with gastric cancer, in 35% of patients with other malignancies, and in 7% in patients with benign diseases. CEA and CA 19-9 were elevated in 37% of patients with gastric cancer (> 3 ng/ml for CEA and > 37 U/ml for CA 19-9). CA 72-4 levels were above 10 U/ml in 26% of the gastric cancer patients, in 15% of patients with other malignancies, and in 0.4% of the patients with benign diseases. There was a good correlation between CA 72-4 level and tumor stage in gastric cancer. CA 72-4 serum levels were more than 2.5 U/ml, respectively, 31%, 48%, 68% and 88% of the patients with stages I, II, III and IV.

CA 72-4 was found to be more sensitive than CEA and CA 19-9 in detecting recurrences of gastric cancer. In the post-operative care period, carcinoma recurred in 29 patients. Of these 93% had CA 72-4 concentrations above 2.5 U/ml, whereas only 59% and 35% had pathological CEA and CA 19-9 serum levels ($p < 0.002$, $p < 0.0001$). Although neither CA 72-4 nor CEA and CA 19-9 are sensitive enough for screening and diagnosis of early gastric cancer, CA 72-4 is superior to CEA and CA 19-9 in the detection of gastric cancer recurrences.

References

1. Safi F, Beger HG, Bittner R, Büchler M, Krautzberger W (1986) CA 19-9 and pancreatic adenocarcinoma. Cancer 57:779–783
2. Fletcher RH (1986) Carcinoembryonic antigen. Ann Intern Med 104:66–73.
3. Sikorska H, Shuster J, Gold P (1988) Clinical applications of carcinoembryonic antigen. Cancer Detect Prev 12:321–355
4. Johnson VG, Schlom J, Paterson AJ, Bennett J, Magnani JL, Colcher D (1986) Analysis of a human tumor-associated glycoprotein (TAG-72) identified by monoclonal antibody B72.3. Cancer Res 46:850–857
5. Muraro R, Kuroki M, Wunderlich D (1988) Generation and characterization of B72.3 second genera-

tion monoclonal antibodies reactive with the tumor-associated glycoprotein-72 antigen. Cancer Res 48:4588–4596
6. Thor A, Ohuchi N, Szpak CA, Johnson WW, Schlom J (1986) Distribution of oncofetal antigen tumor-associated glycoprotein 72 defined by monoclonal antibody B72.3.Cancer Res 46:3118–3124
7. Thor A, Viglione MJ, Muraro R, Ohuchi N, Schlom J, Gorstein F (1987) Monoclonal antibody B72.3 reactivity with human endometrium: A study of normal and malignant tissues. Int J Gynecol Pathol 6:235–247
8. Gastagna M, Nuti M, Squartini F (1987) Mammary cancer antigen recognized by monoclonal antibody B72.3 in apocrine metaplasia of the human breast. Cancer Res 47:902–906
9. Stramignoni D, Bowen R, Atkinson B, Schlom J (1983) Differential reactivity of monoclonal antibodies with human colon adenocarcinomas and adenomas. Int J Cancer 31:543–552
10. Wolf BC, D'Emilice JC, Salem RR (1989) Detection of the tumor-associated glycoprotein antigen (TAG-72) in premalignant lesions of the colon. J Natl Cancer Inst 81:1913–1917
11. Klug TL, Sattler MA, Colcher D, Schlom J (1986) Monoclonal antibody immunoradiometric assay for an antigenic determinant (CA 72) on a novel pancarcinoma antigen (TAG-72). Int J Cancer 38:661–669
12. Hermanek P, Scheibe O, Spiessl B, Wagner G (1987) TNM-Klassifikation maligner Tumoren. Springer, Berlin
13. Weber E (1972) Grundriß der Biologischen Statistik. Fischer, Stuttgart
14. Laurén P (1965) The two histological main types of gastric carcinoma: diffuse and so-called intestinal-type carcinoma. Acta Path Microbiol Scand 64:31–49
15. Quentmeier A, Schlag P, Schmidt-Gayk H, Herfarth Ch (1983) CA 19-9 and CEA in gastric cancer detection, staging, follow-up. Advances in cancer research. Int Soc Oncodevelop Biol Medicine (abstract)
16. Safi F, Bittner R, Poos R, Roscher R, Beger HG (1985) CA 19-9 in der Diagnose des Magen- und Kolorektalkarzinoms. Med Klin 80:676–679
17. Patzke B, Klapdor R, Meyer-Pannwitt U, Weh P, Schreiber HW (1990) TAG 72 in comparison with CA 19-9, CEA and CA 125 in diagnosis and follow-up of stomach cancer. In: Klapdor R (ed) Recent results in tumor-diagnosis and therapy. Zuckschwerdt, München, pp 31–36
18. Piantino P, Ranadone A, Fusari A, Cerchier A, Daziano E (1990) CA 72-4, CA 125 and CA 19-9 as diagnostic aid in gastric carcinoma. J Nucl Med Allied Sci 34:103–106
19. Stieber R, Fateh-Moghadam A, Wädlich H, Nagel D, Lamerz R, Denecke H (1990) Ca 72-4: A new tumor marker for stomach cancer. In: Klapdor R (ed) Recent results in tumor diagnosis and therapy. Zuckschwerdt, München, pp 23–26
20. Motoo Y, Satomura Y, Kawwakami H, Watanabe H, Ohta H, Okai T, Sawabu N (1990) Serum-levels of tumor-associated glycoprotein (TAG-72) in digestive cancers. Oncology 47:456–462
21. Lorenz M, Weber T, Baum RP, Runge U, Hertel A, Hottenrott C (1990) Clinical experience with CA 72-4 in comparison with CA 19-9 and CEA RIMES in gastrointestinal tumors and benign diseases. In: Klapdor R (ed) Recent results in tumor diagnosis and therapy. Zuckschwerdt, München, pp 64–68
22. Brandt B, Liffers E, Sasse W, Assmann G (1988) CA 72-4: Marker 1. Wahl für das Magenkarzinom. In: Klapdor R (ed). Tumorassoziierte Antigene, Onkogene, Rezeptoren, Zytokine in Tumordiagnostik und -therapie zu Beginn der 90er Jahre. Zuckschwerdt, München
23. Buda F, Aragona P, Giani G, Sisto R, Di Nardo G, Binotto F, Gangemi P, De Zerbi T, Gentile G, Papadia A. (1989) Pretreatment evaluation of CA 72-4 in patients with carcinoma of the stomach versus CEA, TPA, CA 19-9, FER. G Ital Oncol 9:67–72
24. Schmid L, Bauer R, Rauthe G, Langhammer HR, Bryxi V. The use of TAG-72 in oncological follow-up. In: Klapdor R (ed) Recent results in tumor diagnosis and therapy. Zuckschwerdt, München, pp 94–99
25. Gero EJ, Colcher D, Ferroni P, Melsheimer R, Giani S, Schlom J, Kaplan P (1989) The CA 72-4 radio-immunoassay for the detection of the TAG-72 carcinoma associated antigen in serum of patients. J Clin Lab Anal 3:360–369
26. Heptner G, Domschke S, Schneider MU, Domschke W (1988) Der neue Tumormarker CA 72-4 im Vergleich zu CA 19-9 und CEA bei gastrointestinalen Erkrankungen. Nuc compact 19:132–134
27. Klapdor R, Patzke B, Bahlo M, Strüven D, Hirschmann M. Serum (1988) Tag-72 bei benignen und malignen Erkrankungen des Magen-Darm-Traktes. Z Gastroenterol 26:611
28. Gamisch R, Senekowitsch R, Schaibold H, Schelling M, Pabst W (1990) Diagnostic value of the new tumor marker CA 72-4 for malignancies of the gastrointestinal tract compared to CEA and CA 19-9. In: Klapdor R (ed) Recent results in tumor diagnosis and therapy. Zuckschwerdt, München, pp 27–30
29. Heptner G, Domschke S, Domschke W (1989) Comparison of CA 72-4 with CA 19-9 and carcinoembryonic antigen in the serodiagnostics of gastrointestinal malignancies. Scand J Gastroenterol 24:745–750
30. Bayerl B, Meier W, Stieber P, Albiez M, Eiermann W, Fateh-Moghadam A (1990) Significance of CA 72-4

in the diagnosis of ovarian cancer. In: Klapdor R (ed) Recent results in tumor diagnosis and therapy. Zuckschwerdt, München, pp 111–112

31 Gadducci A, Ferdeghini M, Ceccarini T, Prontera C, Facchini V, Bianchi R, Fioretti P (1989) The serum concentrations of TAG-72 antigen measured with CA 72-4 IRMA in patients with ovarian carcinoma. Preliminary data. J Nucl Med Allied Sci 1989; 33:32–36

32 Hettenbach A, Hofmann I, Schleich HG, Schmidt R (1989) CA 125, CA 72-4 and SRA bei Patienten mit Ovarialkarzinomen, gutartigen Ovarialtumoren und Kontrollen. Aktuell 11:11–16

33 Guadagni F, Roselli M, Amato T, Cosimelli M, Mannella E, Perri P, Abbolito MR, Cavaliere R, Colcher D, Greiner JW, Schlom J (1991) Tumor-associated glycoprotein-72 serum levels complement carcinoembryonic antigen levels in monitoring patients with gastrointestinal carcinoma. Cancer 68:2443–2450

Address for correspondence:
Priv.-Doz. Dr. med. F. Safi
Abteilung für Allgemeinchirurgie der Universität Ulm
Steinhövelstraβe 9
D-89075 Ulm, Germany

Phospholipids and tumor markers in the differential diagnosis and therapy of gastric cancer

G.M. Oremek[a], D. Kirsten[b], M. Lorenz[b], R. Kirsten[c], K. Nelson[c], U.B. Seiffert[a]

[a]Central Laboratory, Department of Internal Medicine, [b]Department of Surgery, [c]Department of Pharmacology, University Hospital Frankfurt/Main, Germany

Introduction

Gastric cancer is on rank three regarding letal outcome of tumor desease in Germany. Even more effective diagnostic procedures and early therapy onset has not altered much the poor prognosis in the past (1). Many attempts were done to find out more sensitive and more specific markers for the early detection of gastric tumors. The aim of this study was to evaluate the clinical usefullness of phospholipids and tumor markers CEA, CA 72-4, CA 19-9, and CA 50 in patients with gastric carcinoma (2). Tumor markers CEA, CA 19-9 and CA 50 are already helpfull in monitoring patients with gastric carcinoma (2). Little is known about phospholipids in these patients. Phospholipids as lysophosphatidylcholine, phosphatidylethanolamine, phosphatidylinositol, phosphatidylserin and sphingomyelin are essential for a well functionating transport mechanism in the cell membrane. In healthy persons the amount of phospholipids required and synthesized is kept in balance. During some desease or exercise the allover concentration of the decomposed phospholipids might be higher than that of the new synthesized one (3). Concentration lowering of some parts of phospholipids and elevation of the others have been observed. It is supposed, that phospholipids will show some change in their pattern in patients with malignoma or inflammation.

Patients and methods

We measured tumor marker and phospholipid concentration in 92 patients and 50 healthy volunteers. 40 patients suffered from a gastric carcinoma (22 primary gastric carcinoma, ten with organ metastasis and eight with a relaps), 40 patients had a gastric ulcer an 12 an acute pancreatitis. We used the enzym analyzer ES 700 (Boehringer Mannheim) to determine the concentrations of CEA, CA 19-9 and CA 72-4. CA 50 concentration was measured by Delfia fluorescence test (Fluorometer 1230 Arcus, Pharmacia). The phospholipids were determined by HPLC method as described by *Folch* (4).

Results

The results of tumor markers are shown in table I. Primary gastric cancer without organ metastasis: The sensitivity of the tumor markers CEA, CA 19-9, CA 50 and CA 72-4 is very low in early stages of gastric cancer. The best result was obtained by CA 72-4 with a sensitivity of 48%. Using a combination of CEA and CA 72-4 the sensitivity will increase to 54%. Other combinations are less effective: CA 72-4/CA 19-9 = 43%; CA 72-4/CA 50 = 38%.
Gastric carcinoma with metastasis: In this group CA 72-4 has a sensitivity of 67%. A simultaneous determination of CA 72-4 with CEA shows the highest sensitivity of 78%.
Relaps: Patients with a relaps were best detected by CA 72-4 with a sensitivity of 53%. Other tumor markers were not reliable with sensitivities between 19 and 28%.
Benign gastric desease: In persons with benign gastric desease we saw false positive results in CA 72-4 (7%), CA 19-9 (12%), CA 50 (13%) and CEA (15%).
Phospholipid concentration: In healthy volunteers (n = 50, 18–65 years) concentration was between 2.5 and 3.5 mmol/l ($\bar{x}$ = 3.08 mmol/l). In patients with benign gastric desease phospholipid

Table I. Percent of elevated tumor marker serum concentrations in patients with benign and malignant gastric diseases and healthy controls.

	CEA > 5 ng/ml	CA 19-9 > 37 U/ml	CA 50 > 25 U/ml	CA 72-4 > 3 U/ml
Primary gastric cancer	17	25	18.2	48
Gastric cancer with metastases	36.4	32	29	67
Relaps	20	28	19	53
Benign gastric desease	15	12	13.8	7
Controls	7.5	9.8	10.5	3

concentration was similar with $\bar{x}$ = 2.95 mmol/l (2.5 – 3.46 mmol/l). Patients with gastric carcinoma show a lower allover concentration of phospholipids with $\bar{x}$ = 2.7 mmol/l (0.9 – 2.9 mmol/l). Phosphatidylinositol, one part of the entire phospholipid group showes even a reduction of 46%, phosphatidylcholine of 10% and phosphatidylethanolamine an elevation of 15%. A change in the allover phospholipid concentration and composition is also described in patients with hepatocellular carcinoma and colon cancer (5, 6). In patients with hepatocellular carcinoma there is a reduction of phosphatidylinositol, in patients with colon cancer a reduction of phosphatidylcholine.

Conclusions

The prognosis of patients with gastric carcinoma is so much the better the earlier the diagnosis is found out (7, 8). Therefore one needs reliable tests to confirm the diagnosis. None of the available tests fullfill the demand for a high sensitive and specific test. Nevertheless we could show in our investigations that CA 72-4 is superior to other tumor markers. CA 19-9 and CA 50 are apperantly comparable. Simultaneous determination of CA 72-4 and CEA allows a better detection of patients with gastric carcinoma than using parameters as single test. Alterations of the phospholipid composition especially of phosphatidylcholine and phosphatodylinositol and changes of the allover concentration are already notable in patients with gastric carcinoma without metastasis. Determination of phospholipids, CA 72-4 and CEA are helpfull and favorable in monitoring patients with gastric carcinoma.

References

1. Delbrück H, Severin M (1990) Aspekte der Lebensqualität und des Leistungsvermögens potentiell kurativ operierter Magenkarzinompatienten. Tumordiagn Ther 11:116–119
2. Lamerz R (1989) Tumormarker – Prinzipien und Klinik. Dtsch Ärztebl 86:678–682
3. Eibel HJ (1984) Phospholipide als funktionelle Bausteine biologischer Membranen. Angew Chem 96:247–261
4. Folch J, Lees M, Stanley GH (1957) A simple method for isolation and purification of total lipides from animal tissues. J Biol Chem 226:497–509
5. Eggens I, Bäckmann L, Jakobsson A, Voltersson C (1988) The lipid composition of highly differentiated human hepatomas, with special reference to fatty acids. Brit J Exp Path 69:671–683
6. Kasimos JW, Merchant TE, Gierke L, Glonek T (1990) 31P magnetic resonance spectroscopy of human colon cancer. Cancer Res 57:143–171
7. Stieber P, Reiter W, Denecke H, Fateh Mogahdam A (1993) CA 72-4: ein sinnvoller Tumormarker bei Magenkarzinom. Lab Med 17:441–444
8. Stieber P, Fateh-Moghadam A (1989) Ein neuer Tumormarker beim Magenkarzinom. J Clin Chem Clin Biochem 27:767–768

Address for correspondence:
Dr. med. G. M. Oremek
Zentrum der Inneren Medizin
Zentrallabor
Universitätskliniken
Theodor-Stern-Kai 7
D-60590 Frankfurt/Main, Germany

Use of AFP and its LCA-differentiation for the detection, monitoring, and differential diagnosis of hepatocellular carcinoma

R. Lamerz, K. Mann, E. Segura, G. Spöttl, A. Brandt
Medical Department II, Klinikum Großhadern, University of Munich, Germany

Introduction

Since its detection alpha-fetoprotein (AFP) is regarded as an essential tumor marker of hepatocellular carcinoma (HCC) (1,2). Nevertheless, its tumor specificity is limited in general by its increase in benign liver diseases (hepatitis, liver cirrhosis). Moreover its tumor organ specificity remains limited as other tumors such as germ cell tumors with sinusoidal tissue elements and less frequently other cancers (lung, pancreatic, stomach, biliary carcinomas) are also able to produce this marker (3). While AFP kinetics in follow-up are important for the differentiation between benign and malignant AFP elevations in serum (transitory versus constant often exponential increase), the lectin binding of its carbohydrate side chains (about 5%) is of value for the differentiation of AFP from different sources (4). Besides the well known determination of concanavalin A binding of AFP for differentiation of yolk sac tumor AFP (non-binding) from liver AFP (binding) with less clinical relevance, lens culinaris agglutinin (LCA) binding for AFP differentiation in benign (less binding) and malignant liver diseases (binding) has reached clinical interest and more significance (5) by means of a commercially available test kit (L-kit, Wako Chemicals, Neuss) for better discrimination between benign liver diseases and malignant HCC. Here we report on our preliminary experiences with the LCA differentiation kit in comparison with conventionally determined AFP and CEA serum levels.

Material and methods

AFP was determined in serum of 249 patients aged between 1 and 88 years (86% between 40 and 80 years, 72 females, 183 males) with histologically proven or clinically highly probable HCC (elevated AFP, liver tumor detected by ultrasound or CT, pre-existing liver disease, exclusion of other primary tumors) in comparison with 246 patients with benign liver diseases and 148 (AFP)/252 (CEA) patients with secondary liver tumors (colorectal, pancreatic, lung, breast, gynecologic carcinomas). LCA differentiation was investigated in sera of 35 patients with HCC and 11 patients with chronic liver disease without clinical or ultrasound/CT evidence for HCC but a serum AFP elevation of ≥ 30 ng/ml.

AFP and CEA were determined using conventional double antibody tests developed by our laboratory (sensitivity 2–3 ng/ml; intra-/inter-assay variation < 5%/15%) (8, 9). AFP-LCA differentiation was performed by means of a commercially available L-differentiation kit (Wako Neuss/Osaka, Japan) described in detail elsewhere (LCA agarose gel electrophoresis and AFP antibody affinity blotting on prelabeled NC membranes, immunoreaction and enzymatic staining according to the tetrazolium method) (6). The test detects a fucosyl-group inserted at the asparagin-N-acetyl-glucosamin-anchoring of the carbohydrate chain which is incorporated in HCC and other tumor AFP by means of a tumor fucosyl-transferase not present in benign liver diseases. The test was performed according to the prescription of the manufacturer using an electrophoresis equipment of LKB/Pharmacia and an immunoblotting chamber developed by our

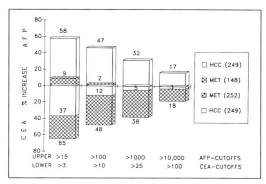

Figure 1. Sensitivity rates according to different increasing cut-offs of AFP (upper line) and CEA (lower line) in patients with hepatocellular cancer (n = 249) and other primaries with liver involvement (AFP: n = 148; CEA: n = 252).

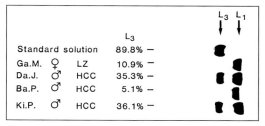

Figure 2. AFP-LCA lectin electrophoresis of standard solution and sera of one patient with liver cirrhosis and three patients with HCC (working AFP concentration about 100 ng/ml). Anode to the right. LCA binding rates (L3) indicated.

laboratory. Finally, the intensities of stained formazan bands were evaluated by computer-directed scanner densitometry and quantified as percent of total intensity.

Results and discussion

Normal serum AFP concentrations ≤ 15 ng/ml were found in 42% of HCC patients, elevated levels > 15 ng/ml in 58%, > 100 ng/ml in 47%, > 1000 ng/ml in 32% and > 10.000 ng/ml in 17% (10th/50th/90th percentiles 3/81/30970 ng/ml) (figure1). Non-correlating (r = 0.01, n.s.) CEA serum concentrations ≤ 3 ng/ml were observed in 63% of patients, elevations > 3 ng/ml in 37%, > 10 ng/ml in 12%, > 25 ng/ml in 5% and > 100 ng/ml in 3% (10th/50th/90th perc. 2/2/13 ng/ml). By comparison patients with other primary tumors and liver metastases showed elevated serum AFP levels (n = 148) only in 9% of cases with concentrations mostly < 100 ng/ml and in 2% up to 350 ng/ml. In contrast more striking serum CEA elevations (n = 252) were encountered > 3 ng/ml in 65%, > 10 ng/ml in 48%, > 25 ng/ml in 38% and in 18% > 100 ng/ml (colorectal cancer: 84%, 67%, 53%, 38%). In spite of an increase of HCC cases with normal serum AFP concentrations due to a more frequent detection of smaller liver foci in contrast to our former investigations, there is still a remarkable discrimination between primary (HCC) and secondary liver tumors by means of AFP and CEA serum determination (figure 1). The combination of an elevated serum AFP level and a normal or only slightly elevated CEA level is highly suspicious of HCC, in contrast to the combination of an elevated CEA and normal AFP level which is highly suspicious of a secondary liver tumor (10).

In contrast to HCC patients, patients with benign chronic liver diseases showed transitory or constantly lower pathologic serum AFP elevations mostly < 500 ng/ml in 22% of patients with chronic hepatitis (n = 39) and in 15% of patients with liver cirrhosis (n = 207) mostly < 100 ng/ml and only in four cases elevations up to 500 ng/ml consistent with other investigators (11).

In the follow-up (n = 47) 16 HCC patients showed always normal, 14 showed increased and further increasing AFP serum levels. Following operation or liver transplantation (LTX) or during chemotherapy seven patients developed a serum AFP decrease to normal values, two patients with recurrence an AFP elevation from the normal range, whereas seven further patients after operation or LTX experienced a decrease and re-increase of serum AFP and a further patient following operation a re-increase and later normalization following LTX. From 32 patients following LTX, meanwhile 18 (56%) patients have deceased, 13 (41%) of them in the first, four cases (12%) in the second and one in the third post-transplant year. Actually alive are three patients in the first, two in the second, five in the third, one in the fourth, two in the fifth and one patient in the eighth year following LTX.

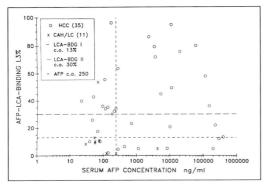
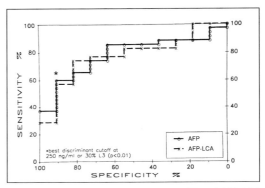

Figure 3. Total serum AFP concentrations and AFP-LCA binding values (L3 %) in patients with benign liver disease (n = 11) and hepatocellular carcinoma (n = 35) discriminated by one AFP cut-off (250 ng/ml) and two AFP-LCA cut-offs (I = 13%, II = 30%).

Figure 4. ROC analysis of total serum AFP and AFP-LCA binding rates in patients with benign liver disease (n = 11) and with hepatocellular carcinoma (n = 35). Best discriminating cut-offs at 250 ng/ml (AFP) or 30% (AFP-LCA) (p < 0.01).

According to our preliminary results of AFP-LCA differentiation in 35 HCC and eleven patients with chronic hepatitis or liver cirrhosis with AFP serum values ≥ 30 ng/ml, all cases depicted stained bands in the L1- (non-binding) and L3- (binding) position (figure 2). Following relative intensity determination the L3-values (%) were ≤ 13% in 9/11 CAH/LC cases or ≤ 30% in 10/11 cases with total AFP values ≤ 100 ng/ml in 8/11 or ≤ 250 in all cases (figure 3). In contrast L3-values >13% were detected in 25/35 (71%) or > 30% in 20/35 (57%) HCC patients with total AFP values >100 in 28/35 (80%) and > 250 ng/ml in 21/35 (60%) cases (p < 0.01). According to ROC analysis (figure 4) the best discriminant cut-off for total serum AFP discrimination between benign/malignant liver AFP was found at 250 ng/ml (prev. = 76%; s = 60%, sp = 91%, pv+ = 96%, pv- = 42%, p < 0.01) and for AFP-LCA discrimination at 30% (prev. = 76%; s = 57%, sp = 91%, pv+ = 95%, pv- = 40%; p < 0.01) slightly higher than indicated by other investigators (10–20%) (7, 12, 13).

According to the basic investigations of *Aoyagi* et al. (5) the well known concanavalin A binding of AFP can be used for discrimination between yolk sac or generally non-liver-tumor AFP (non-binding) and liver tumor AFP (binding). The Con A non-binding of AFP is caused by steric blocking by an additional N-acetyl-glucosamine group at the branching mannose residue of the biantennary AFP carbohydrate chain. According to *Aoyagi* this non-binding of Con A is termed glucosaminylization index which thus is high for yolk sac AFP and low for benign or malignant liver AFP (5). In contrast lentil culinaris lectin (LCA) binding is effectuated by an additionally inserted fucosyl-group by means of a tumor activated fucosyl-transferase and allows a discrimination between benign liver AFP (low binding) and malignant liver AFP (>10-20% binding in 80% of cases). Yet the fucosylation index is found still more regularly elevated in other primaries than the liver (e.g. germ cell tumors). Therefore the method does not discriminate between primary or secondary liver tumors (5). A further lectin differentiation of interest in primary liver tumors is the use of erythro-agglutinin-phytohemagglutinin differentiation with high binding for HCC-AFP, the values of which are partially overlapping with the results of AFP-LCA differentiation (6, 7).

Further investigations showed no correlation between AFP-LCA binding and total serum AFP values, but a correlation between AFP-LCA values and the size of liver HCC tumors (12). A further important finding was reported preliminarily by a long-term follow-up of eight patients with liver cirrhosis and elevated serum AFP values in whom the measurement of fucosylation index showed that all patients with low LCA binding in spite of increasing AFP values during an observation period of three to nine years did not develop HCC tumors, whereas this was observed in three patients with high LCA binding (32–62%)

following nine months or two and four years, respectively (13). Only one of our cases with serum AFP values ≥ 30 ng/ml and benign chronic liver diseases who had liver cirrhosis and a L3–value of 65% with constantly rising AFP values in the follow-up, developed a HCC that was proven two years later and operated by partial hepatectomy.

Conclusions

AFP is still the most interesting tumor marker of first choice in HCC (> 250 ng/ml: s = 60%, sp = 91%) and may be supplemented by AFP-LCA binding determination for detecting patients with chronic liver disease and an elevated risk for HCC (> 13%: s = 71%; > 30%: s = 57%) who should be monitored more strictly and frequently.

References

1. Regan LS (1989) Screening for hepatocellular carcinoma in high-risk individuals. Arch Int Med 149:1741–1744
2. Tremolda F, Benevegnu L, Drage C, Casarin C, Cechetto A, Realdi A, Realdi G, Ruol A (1989) Early detection of hepatocellular carcinoma in patients with cirrhosis by alpha-fetoprotein, ultrasound and fine-needle biopsy. Hepato-Gastroenterol 36:519–521
3. Lamerz R (1992) Alpha-Fetoprotein. In: Thomas L (ed) Labor und Diagnose. Medizinische Verlagsgesellschaft, pp 1153–1162
4. Taketa K, Sekiya C, Namiki M, Akamatsu K, Ohta Y, Endo Y, Kosaka K (1990) Lectin-reactive profiles of alpha-fetoprotein characterizing hepatocellular carcinoma and related conditions. Gastroenterol 99:508–518
5. Aoyagi Y, Suzuki Y, Igarashi K, Saitoh A, Oguro M, Yokota T, Mori S, Nomoto M, Isemura M, Asakura H (1991) The usefulness of simultaneous determinations of glycosaminylation and fucosylation indices of alpha-fetoprotein in the differential diagnosis of neoplastic diseases of the liver. Cancer 67:2390–2394
6. Shimizu K, Taniichi T, Satomura S, Matsuura S, Tage H, Taketa K (1993) Establishment of assay kits for the determination of microheterogeneities of alpha-fetoprotein using lectin-affinity electrophoresis. Clin Chim Acta 214:2–12
7. Sato Y, Nakata K. Kato Y, Shima M, Ishii N, Koji T, Taketa K, Endo Y, Nagataki S (1993) Early recognition of hepatocellular carcinoma based on altered profiles of alpha-fetoprotein. N Engl J Med 328:1802–1806
8. Lamerz R, Rjosk H, Schmalhorst U, Fateh-Moghadam A (1976) Alpha-Fetoprotein: Methodik und klinische Erfahrungen mit einem neuen Radioimmunoassay. Z Anal Chem 279:120
9. Lamerz R, Ruider H (1976) Bestimmungen von karzinoembryonalem Antigen bei Patienten mit Dickdarmtumoren. Erfahrungen mit einem neuen Radioimmunoassay. Münch med Wschr 118:377–380
10. Lamerz R, Stieber P, Borlinghaus P, Fateh-Moghadam A (1991) Tumor markers in cancer of the liver. Diagn Oncol 1:363–372
11. Lamerz R (1980) Die klinische Bedeutung von Alpha-Fetoprotein bei Lebererkrankungen. Bayer Internist 2:19–23
12. Kuromatsu R, Tanaka M, Tanikawa K (1993) Serum alpha-fetoprotein and lens culinaris agglutinin-reactive fraction of alpha-fetoprotein in patients with hepatocellular carcinoma. Liver 13:177–182
13. Aoyagi Y, Saitoh A, Suzuki Y, Igarashi K. Oguro M, Yokota T, Mori S, Suda T, Isemura M, Asakura H (1993) Fucosylation index of alpha-fetoprotein, a possible aid in the early recognition of hepatocellular carcinoma in patients with cirrhosis. Hepatology 17:50–52

Address for correspondence:
Prof. Dr. med. R. Lamerz
Medizinische Klinik II, Klinikum Großhadern
Marchioninistraße 15
D-81377 München, Germany

Levels of alpha-fetoprotein in chronic liver diseases

Halina Cichoż-Lach, K. Celiński, Maria Słomka, J. Pokora
Department of Gastroenterology, Medical Academy, Lublin, Poland

Introduction

Alpha-fetoprotein, a biological tumor marker, is a glycoprotein consisting of 590 aminoacids, which is not synthesized in healthy adults (2, 4). Its role in detection of primary liver cancer is emphasized during the last time. There are many studies relating to AFP serum levels in chronic liver diseases particularly in cirrhosis and in hepatocellular carcinoma (3, 9)
This paper presents the results of investigations on alpha-fetoptrotein (AFP) serum levels in patients with chronic liver diseases.

Material and methods

115 patients were admitted to our study: 38 with chronic active hepatitis (CAH), 70 with hepatic cirrhosis (HC) (20 active and 50 inactive) and seven with primary liver cancer (PLC). There were 73 males and 42 females aged 21 to 74 years, mean age 45 years. Diagnosis was documented by clinical, biochemical and histological abnormalities.
It was recognized that each patient had been HBV infected, because each was HBsAg serum positive. The other serological markers of HBV were examined too. They were HBeAg, anti-HBs, anti-HBe, anti-HBc and anti-HBc IgM. Radioimmunoassay (Abbott Laboratories) was used to assay serological markers.
Hepatitis B DNA-polymerase activity was not assayed in all patients, only in six cases with CAH. Table I shows occurrence of HBV serological markers in the examined patients. 14 patients with CAH, nine with HC and none with PLC were HBeAg positive. Measurement of AFP serum level was done by radioimmunoassay (7). Our own norm is 3 + 0.5 ng/ml (IU/ml).

Results

AFP serum levels in chronic liver diseases are shown in table II. In the group with CAH the mean value of AFP levels was 12.7 ng/ml (range 1–40), with HC it was 6.9 ng/ml (range 0.5–13), and with PLC it was significantly higher, 348 ng/ml (range 250–420). The differences were statistically highly significant ($p < 0.001$). Statistical analysis was calculated using Student's test by Statgraph version 2.
In all HBeAg positive patients (and high HBV DNA-polymerase activity in all six cases, 1720 cpm), both in the CAH and the HC group, higher AFP levels than in anti-HBe positive patients were observed. In the group with CAH the mean value was 18.2 + 4.7 ng/ml, with HC it was 8.8 + 2.4 ng/ml whereas in anti-HBe positive patients it was 8.4 + 2.0 ng/ml and 5.2 + 2.1 ng/ml, respectively. The differences were highly significant ($p < 0.001$) (figure 1).
Similarly higher AFP serum levels were observed in patients with active hepatic cirrhosis than in inactive. The mean value in the active cirrhosis group was 8.0 + 2.2 ng/ml as opposed to 4.8 + 1.7 ng/ml and in the inactive group.
In four of PLC patients three measurements of AFP levels were performed once every two months. The levels were decreasing systematically, in the first patient from 294 ng/ml to 220 after two months and to 102 after additional two months, in the second 400-210-156 ng/ml, in the third 382-256-210 ng/ml, in the fourth 356-198-124 ng/ml, as shown in the figure 2. This study will be continued and results will be presented in the near future.

Table I. Occurrence of HBV serological markers in examined patients.

	HBsAg	HBeAg	anti-HBs	anti-HBe	anti-HBc	anti-HBc IgM
CAH	38	14	0	24	38	4
HC	70	9	0	61	0	70
PLC	7	0	0	7	7	0

Table II. Levels of AFP in examined patients in ng/ml (IU/ml).

	Range	Mean	+ SE	p-Value[a]
Own norm		3.0	0.5	$p < 0.001$ CAH/PLC
CAH	1–4	12.7	4.0	
HC	0.5–13	6.9	2.1	$p < 0.001$ HC/PLC
PLC	250–240	348	56	

[a] The differences between CAH, HC, PLC and controls were highly significant ($p < 0.001$)

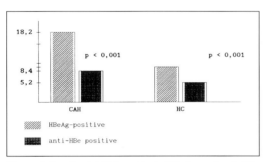

Figure 1. Levels of AFP in patients HBeAg and anti-HBe positive in ng/ml (IU/ml).

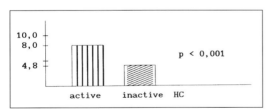

Figure 2. Levels of AFP in active and inactive hepatic cirrhosis.

Discussion

The highest AFP serum levels were observed in primary liver cancer. This is in agreement with other authors (9, 14). Significantly lower AFP levels were noticed in chronically active hepatitis and cirrhosis but still they exceeded the norm (1).

In HBsAg, HBeAg and DNA-polymerase positive chronic liver disease patients (suggesting HBV replication) AFP serum levels are usually higher than in anti-HBe positive patients (15).
In our study, in four patients decreasing AFP levels were observed during progressive liver neoplasmatic process. Zhou et al. and Iwamura have shown, that the AFP levels decline in the terminal stage of hepatocellulare (6, 16). This problem still remains difficult to explain.

Conclusions

We found, that the AFP serum level is the best marker in early detection of primary liver cancer and its clinical value has been thoroughly assessed (11).
Consequently, the long-term follow-up study of AFP levels in patients with chronic liver diseases, particularly with cirrhosis, can be useful in early detection of hepatocellular cancer which develops on their base. Therefore monitoring AFP serum levels is important in patients with chronic liver diseases (3, 5, 8, 9, 10, 12, 13, 14).

References

1 Collazos J, Genolla J, Ruibal A (1992) Preliminary study of alpha-fetoprotein in nonmalignant liver diseases. A clinico-biochemical evaluation. Int J Biol Markers 7(2):97–102

2. Deugnier Y, Auffret P, Lehry D, Brissot P, Bourel M (1987) Marqueurs bilogiques du carcinome hepatocellulaire. Gastroenterol Clin Bioll 11:648–657
3. Di Bisceglie AM, Hoofnagle JH (1989) Elevations in serum alpha-fetoprotein levels in patients with chronic hepatitis. B Cancer 64(10):2117–2120
4. Dumas O, Barthelemy C, Audigier JC (1990) Faut-il depister les carcinomes hepatocellulaires sur cirrhose? Gastroenterol Clin Biol 14:715–726
5. Imberti D, Fornari F, Sbolli G, Buscarini E, Squassante L, Buscarini L (1993) Hepatocellular carcinoma in liver cirrhosis. A prospective study. Scand J Gastroenterol 28(6):540–544
6. Iwamura K (1985) Investigations of a screening test for early diagnosis of hepatocellular carcinoma. Mat Med Pol 4(56):232–239
7. Johnson PJ, Portmann B, Williams R (1978) Alpha-fetoprotein concentrations measured by radioimmunoassay in diagnosing and excluding hepatocellular carcinoma. Br Med J 2:661–663
8. Leandro G, Basso D, Fabris C, Zizzari S, Elba S, Del-FaveroG, Di-Mario F, Meggiato T, Angonese C, Naccarato R (1989) Alpha-fetoprotein, tissue polypeptide antigen and ferritin in diagnosing primary hepatocellular carcinoma in patients with liver cirrhosis. J Cancer Res Clin Oncol 115(3):276–278
9. Li GH, Li JQ (1989) Subclinical primary liver carcinoma. J Surg Oncol 42(3):181–183
10. Lok AS, Lai CL (1989) Alpha-Fetoprotein monitoring in Chinese patients with chronic hepatitis B virus infection: role in the early detection of hepatocellular carcinoma (see comments). Hepatology 9 (1):110–115
11. Maussier ML, Valenza V, Schinco G, Galli G (1990) AFP, CEA, CA 19-9 and TPA in hepatocellular carcinoma. Int J Biol Markers, 5(3):121–126
12. Okazaki N, Yoshino M, Yoshida T, Takayasu K, Moriyama N, Makuuchi M, Yamazaki S, Hasegawa H, Noguchi M, Hirohashi S (1990) Early diagnosis of hepatocellular carcinoma. Hepatogastroenterol 37(5):480–483
13. Tang Z.Y, Yu YQ, Zhou X.D, Yang B.H, Ma Z.C, Lin ZY (1993) Subclinical hepatocellular carcinoma: an analysis of 391 patients. J Surg Oncol Suppl 3:55–58
14. Tremolda F, Benevegnu L, Drago C, Casarin C, Cechetto A, Realdi G, Ruol A (1989) Early detection of hepatocellular carcinoma in patients with cirrhosis by alphafetoprotein, ultrasound and fine-needle biopsy. Hepatogastroenterol 36(6):519–521
15. Vajro P, Fontanella A, De-Vincenzo A, Lettera P, Greco L, Coppa A, D'Armiento M (1991) Monitoring of serum alpha-fetoprotein levels in children with chronic hepatitis B virus infection. J Pediatr Gastroenterol Nutr 12(1):27–32
16. Zhou XD, Tang ZY, Yu YQ, Hou Z (1991) Current management of hepatocellular carcinoma. Hepato-Gastroenterol 38:46–55

Address for correspondence:
Dr. Halina Cichoż-Lach
Department of Gastroenterology
Medical Academy
ul Jaczewskiego 8
PL-20-950 Lublin, Poland

The prognostic value of preoperative serum levels of CA 19-9, CA 242 and CEA in patients with pancreatic cancer

J. Lundin[a], P.J. Roberts[a], P. Kuusela[b], C. Haglund[b]
[a] IV. Department of Surgery, [b] Department of Bacteriology and Immunology,
University of Helsinki, Helsinki, Finland

Introduction

The overall prognosis of pancreatic cancer is poor, the 5-year survival rate being 0.2–3.4 per cent (3). Even after surgery for cure the 5-year survival in a meta-analysis was only 3.4 per cent (3). The effect of chemotherapy in different studies has so far been limited. However, if patients are selected for adjuvant therapy, knowledge of factors having influence on prognosis would be of great importance. Clinical stage is known to correlate with prognosis (1). When comparing patients within the same stage of pancreatic cancer, very few prognostic factors are known.

The aim of this study was to evaluate the prognostic value of the preoperative serum levels of CA 19-9, CA 242 and CEA in different stages of pancreatic cancer. CA 242 is a novel tumor marker that is related, although not identical, to the antigenic epitope of CA 19-9 (6).

Patients and methods

Patients

Serum samples were taken from 128 patients with pancreatic cancer. Patients were classified according to TNM-stage and divided into three groups. Group I consisted of 23 patients with resectable disease (16 stage I patients, six stage II patients and one stage III patient). Group II consisted of 37 patients with locally non-resectable disease (17 stage II patients and 20 stage III patients). Group III consisted of 68 patients with advanced disease, that is stage IV patients. In group I and II, patients who died within 30 days from operation were excluded. In group III, all patients were evaluated, since the mean survival was extremely short and many patients did not undergo surgery at all.

Assays

The serum concentrations of CA 19-9, CEA and CA 242 were determined by commercially available assays (Centocor, Malvern, PA; Abbott, Wiesbahn, Germany; Wallac Oy, Turku, Finland).

Statistical analysis

Life-tables were calculated according to *Kaplan-Meier*. Patients were divided into groups having a preoperative tumor marker value above or below a certain cut-off level and their survival was compared. The statistical significance of the difference in survival of the groups was calculated using the log-rank test. By gradually raising the cut-off level, every achieved marker value was tested as cut-off point. The lowest cut-off level that discriminated the patients significantly according to prognosis was considered optimal for prognostic evaluation (5).

Results

The optimal cut-off levels for evaluation of prognosis

In group II, a significant difference in survival between patients with marker values below versus above a certain cut-off level was reached at the preoperative CA 19-9 value of 370 U/ml ($p < 0.05$). Since no significant difference in survival was seen for the other groups, 370 U/ml was

Table I. The median and mean survival times of patients with pancreatic cancer divided according to stage and preoperative serum-CA 19-9 and serum-CA 242 level.

		Serum-CA 19-9		Serum-CA 242	
		< 370 U/ml	> 370 U/ml	< 200 U/ml	> 200 U/ml
Group I (n = 23)	no. of patients	14	9	17	6
	median (months)	20.4	12.2	21.4	10.5
	mean (months)	27.8	14.4	26.8	10.7
Group II (n = 37)	no. of patients	18	19	21	16
	median (months)	10	5.1	11.4	5.1
	mean (months)	12.4	6.2	13.2	6.4
Group III (n = 68)	no. of patients	26	42	31	37
	median (months)	2.5	1.3	2.3	1.6
	mean (months)	5	3.3	4.9	3.1
All patients (n = 128)	no. of patients	58	70	69	59
	median (months)	9.6	3.8	9.5	3.1
	mean (months)	13.1	5	12.6	4.7

chosen as cut-off level in all groups when evaluating CA 19-9 as a prognostic factor.

Using CA 242, a difference in survival was seen in all groups and the lowest cut-off level that discriminated the patients with non-resectable disease significantly according to survival was 200 U/ml.

The analysis of CEA showed a significant difference in survival only in group III, where patients with a preoperative value below 15 ng/ml had a slightly longer survival than those with a value above this level.

Survival according to stage

In group I, the median survival was 16.6 months, in group II 6.6 months and in group III two months. The corresponding mean survival was 22.6 months, 9.7 months and four months respectively. The differences between the survival curves of the stage groups were highly significant ($p < 0.001$).

CA 19-9

When analysing all patients, there was a significant difference in survival between those with a preoperative CA 19-9 level below 370 U/ml (58 patients) and those whose level was above 370 U/ml (70 patients) ($p < 0.01$). In group I and III, the difference in survival between patients

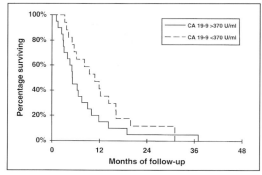

Figure 1. Life-tables for patients with non-resectable pancreatic cancer (Group II) and preoperative CA 19-9 lower respectively higher than 370 U/ml. Patients with a preoperative CA 19-9 level lower than 370 U/ml had significantly better prognosis than patients with CA 19-9 higher than 370 U/ml.

with a preoperative CA 19-9 level below versus above 370 U/ml was not significant ($p > 0.05$). Only in group II, a statistically significant difference between the survival curves was seen ($p < 0.05$) (figure 1). Median and mean survival of patients in different groups are shown in table I.

CA 242

A significant difference in survival was seen between patients with a preoperative CA 242 level below 200 U/ml and those whose level was

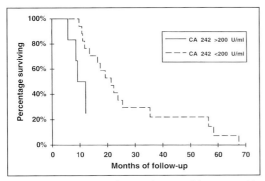

Figure 2. Life-tables for patients with resectable pancreatic cancer and preoperative CA 242 lower respectively higher than 200 U/ml. Patients with a preoperative CA 242 level lower than 200 U/ml had significantly better prognosis than patients with CA 242 higher than 200 U/ml (p < 0.01).

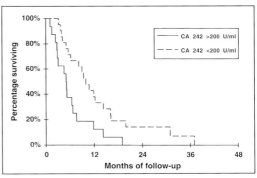

Figure 3. Life-tables for patients with non-resectable pancreatic cancer and preoperative CA 242 lower respectively higher than 200 U/ml. Patients with a preoperative CA 242 level lower than 200 U/ml had significantly better prognosis than patients with CA 242 higher than 200 U/ml (p < 0.05).

above 200 U/ml when analysing all patients and also analysing group I–III separately. For all patients the p-value was 0.001. For group I, group II and group III the p-values were 0.01, 0.05 and 0.05 respectively. Median and mean survival of patients in different groups are shown in table I.

CEA

When analysing all patients, there was a significant difference in survival between those with a preoperative CEA level below (97 patients) versus above 15 ng/ml (31 patients) (p < 0.001). In group I and II the difference was not significant and only in group III a significant difference was seen (p < 0.01).

Discussion

The CEA and CA 19-9 levels have previously been shown to correlate with prognosis in patients with pancreatic cancer (2, 4). However, in these studies stage of disease has not been taken into account. The prognostic value of CA 242 has not been reported previously. We decided to evaluate whether high or low preoperative CA 19-9, CA 242 and CEA levels also might predict prognosis within stage.

By testing several cut-off levels we found that those recommended for diagnostic purposes were not optimal for prognostic evaluation. For final analyses we therefore determined the lowest cut-off level that divided the patients into groups with significant differences in survival (5). These cut-off values were 370 U/ml, 200 U/ml and 15 ng/ml for CA 19-9, CA 242 and CEA respectively, that is much higher than the corresponding cut-off levels recommended for diagnostic use (37 U/ml, 20 U/ml and 5 ng/ml respectively).

Also in this study there was a significant difference in survival between patients with a low versus high preoperative tumor marker level when patients were analysed as one group. When divided according to stage a difference in survival was still seen for CA 242 in all groups and for CA 19-9 in group II. This might reflect a difference in biological behavior between tumors associated with a low respectively high serum level of the tumor markers. On the other hand, it might reflect differences in tumor burden and spread of disease within stage.

Theoretically, one might have expected the correlation between survival and the preoperative tumor marker levels in serum to be more pronounced. A weak or lacking correlation in some stage groups might be explained by the fact that the serum level of a tumor marker is not a reflection of the ability of the tumor tissue to synthesise the antigen, but rather a consequence of many other factors affecting the amount of circulating antigen. Among these factors are incretion of produced antigen into the blood stream, metabolism and excretion of the antigen and occurrence of liver metastases. These factors are difficult to measure and the mechanisms are partly unknown.

Conclusions

When predicting prognosis of patients with pancreatic cancer, the preoperative serum levels of CA 242 and CA 19-9 seems to be of limited value in patients with resectable disease. They might, however, be of some clinical value in patients with non-resectable tumors, in whom spread of disease may be difficult to assess even at surgery. CA 242 seems, in an univariate analysis, to be a stronger prognostic factor and predict prognosis within stage more clearly than CA 19-9 and CEA.

References

1 Andren-Sandberg A, Ihse I (1983) Factors influencing survival after total pancreatectomy in patients with pancreatic cancer. Ann Surg 198:605–10

2 Bottger T, Zech J, Weber W, Sorger K, Junginger T (1990) Relevant factors in the prognosis of ductal pancreatic carcinoma. Acta Chir Scand 156:781–8

3 Gudjonsson B (1987) Cancer of the pancreas. 50 years of surgery. Cancer 60:2284–303

4 Kalser MH, Barkin JS, Redlhammer D, Heal A (1978) Circulating carcinoembryonic antigen in pancreatic carcinoma. Cancer 42:1468–1471.

5 Lundin J, Roberts PJ, Kuusela P, Haglund C (1994) The prognostic value of preoperative serum levels of CA 19-9 and CEA in patients with pancreatic cancer. Br J Cancer 69:515–519

6 Nilsson O, Johansson C, Glimelius B, Persson B, Norgaard PB, Andren SA, Lindholm L (1992) Sensitivity and specificity of CA242 in gastrointestinal cancer. A comparison with CEA, CA50 and CA 19-9. Br J Cancer 65:215–21

Address for correspondence:
C. Haglund, M.D.
IV. Department of Surgery
Helsinki University Central Hospital
Kasarmikatu 11–13
SF-00130 Helsinki, Finland

CA 494: High sensitivity and specificity in pancreatic cancer

H. Friess[a], K. Hammer[a], B. Auerbach[b], M. Müller[a], M.W. Büchler[a]
[a]Department of Visceral and Transplantation Surgery, University of Berne, Switzerland,
[b]Research Laboratories, Behringwerke AG, Marburg, Germany

Introduction

The incidence of pancreatic cancer still increases in industrialized Western countries (10). The only way to improve the infaust prognosis of pancreatic cancer is the early diagnosis of the tumor followed by a possibly curative resection. So far only 10% –20% of the patients have resectable tumor at the time of diagnosis (4).

Tumor markers defined by monoclonal antibodies (MAB) seemed to be a non-invasive, simple diagnostic tool in cancer diseases. But due to low sensitivity and specificity they are mainly used to follow up cancer patients and to provide information about the efficiency of a therapeutical strategy (3, 9, 11). In pancreatic cancer, CA 19-9 is the reference tumor marker which is widely used in clinical practice (7, 8).

The monoclonal antibody BW 494/32 has been shown to have a high binding capacity to pancreatic cancer cells in vitro and in vivo and has been used for passive immunotherapy in patients with ductal pancreatic cancer (2, 6). It was isolated from BALB/c mice which were immunized with a human colon cancer cell line (1). This antibody has been used to establish an assay which detects its antigen CA 494 in serum.

In the present study CA 494 serum levels were measured in pancreatic and non-pancreatic disorders and compared with the reference tumor markers CA 19-9 and carcino-embryonic antigen (CEA).

Methods and patients

Patients

Overall 494 patients were included in this study. 59 patients had a histologically confirmed pancreatic adeno-carcinoma. Six patients were diagnosed in tumor stage I, six in stage II, 33 in stage III and 14 patients in tumor stage IV. Non-pancreatic gastrointestinal cancers were confirmed histologically in 97 patients. 51 patients had a colorectal cancer, 46 patients a cancer of the stomach. 100 patients with chronic pancreatitis as the most important benign differential diagnosis to pancreatic cancer were included. In addition, 124 patients with benign non-pancreatic gastrointestinal diseases, for example, gastric ulcer (24), benign jaundice (19), cholecystolithiasis (15), hemorrhoids (14), irritable bowel disease (11), liver cirrhosis (10), and 114 healthy volunteers served as controls.

All blood samples were taken preoperatively and the sera were stored at −80 °C immediately.

Methods

The enzyme immunoassay established to measure the antigen CA 494 is described in figure 1. 20 µl of each serum sample or control and 100 µl phosphate-buffered incubation medium (pH 6.8) incubated in the wells of microtiter plates coated with the MAB BW 494 for 2 h at 37 °C. After having been washed 3 times a 100 µl-solution of the tracer antibody was filled into each well (2 h, 37 °C). It was impossible to bind radioactivity or an enzyme to the MAB BW 494 without inducing a great loss of the binding activity to its epitope. Thus we used the MAB C50 (IgM; Pharmacia, Uppsala, Sweden) conjugated to horseradish peroxidase as the tracer antibody. Finally, the bound enzymatic activity was determined photometrically at 450 nm using the peroxidase-dependent reaction of hydrogen peroxide and 3, 3', 5, 5' tetramethylbenzidine (TMB).

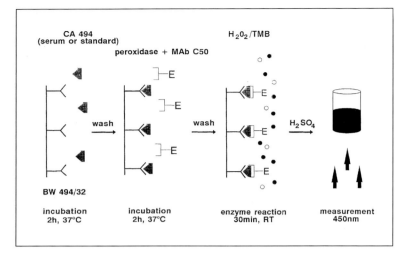

Figure 1. Measurement of CA 494 in serum by ELISA technique.

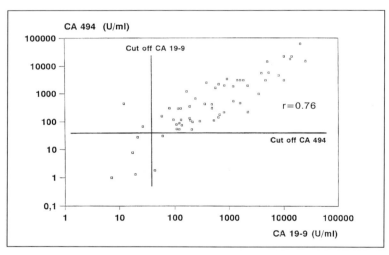

Figure 2. Correlation of CA 19-9 (U/ml) and CA 494 (U/ml) in 59 patients with pancreatic cancer. The cut-off level was 37 U/ml for CA 19-9 and 40 U/ml for CA 494. Correlation coefficient r = 0.76; p < 0.001. The horizontal line represents the cut-off of CA 494 (40 U/ml), the vertical line the cut-off of CA 19-9 (37 U/ml).

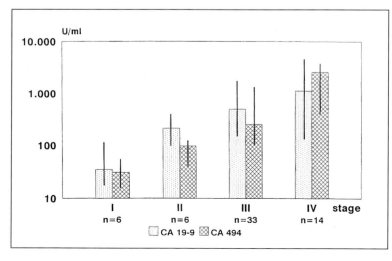

Figure 3. CA 19-9 (U/ml) and CA 494 (U/ml) in dependence on the tumor stages in 59 patients with pancreatic cancer. Values are medians ± upper and lower quartiles.

Table I. Sensitivity of CA 19-9, CEA, CA 494 in patients with pancreatic cancer, colorectal cancer and gastric cancer.

	CA 19-9 > 37 U/ml	CEA > 3 ng/ml	CA 494 > 40 U/ml
Pancreatic cancer	53/59 (90%)	26/59 (44%)	53/59 (90%)
Colorectal cancer	20/51 (39%)	28/51 (55%)	9/51 (18%)
Gastric cancer	16/46 (35%)	17/46 (37%)	19/46 (41%)

Table II. Specificity of CA 19-9, CEA, CA 494 in patients with chronic pancreatitis, benign non-pancreatic gastrointestinal diseases (GI-dis.) and healthy volunteers.

	CA 19-9 < 37 U/ml	CEA < 3 ng/ml	CA 494 < 40 U/ml
Chronic pancreatitis	86/100 (86%)	74/100 (74%)	94/100 (94%)
Benign non-pancreatic GI-dis.	112/124 (90%)	95/124 (77%)	118/124 (95%)
benign jaundice	19/19 (100%)	19/19 (100%)	19/19 (100%)
liver cirrhosis	8/10 (80%)	3/10 (30%)	9/10 (90%)
others	85/95 (89%)	73/95 (77%)	90/95 (95%)
Healthy volunteers	108/114 (95%)	98/114 (86%)	113/114 (99%)
Total	306/338 (91%)	267/338 (79%)	325/338 (96%)

The absorbance values of the CA 494 ELISA correlated directly with the concentration (0–300 U/ml) of the CA 494 antigen in the sample. The analytical sensitivity, measuring an analyte free sample + 2 standard deviation (S0 + 2SD), was determined as < 4 U/ml. The intra-assay coefficient of variation (CV, n = 15) of various serum specimens (32–223 U CA 494/ml) was in the range of 6%–13%; the interassay CV (n = 21) of two control sera were found to be 9.9% (41.9 U/ml) and 6.1% (77.1 U/ml), respectively. The range of the assay was between 1 and 300 U/ml. Linearity and recovery studies produced results between ±15% of the expected concentrations. Hemolysis did not interfere with the assay.

The upper cut-off level of the CA 494 assay was set at 40 U/ml. Using this cut-off the specificity in a group of 251 (median age: 46 years; range: 26–65 years) healthy volunteers was 99%. The mean CA 494 serum concentration was 6.8 ±9.9 (mean ± standard deviation).

To compare this new assay for CA 494 we used two commercially available tumor marker assays: A CA 19-9 – immunoradiometric assay (EISA CA 19-9, CIS, Dreieich, Germany) and an enzyme immunoassay for CEA (EIA CEA, CIS, Dreieich, Germany). As recommended by the manufacturer, the cut-offs were set at 37 U/ml for CA 19-9 and 3 ng/ml for CEA.

Results

In patients with pancreatic cancer the sensitivitiy for CA 19-9, CEA and CA 494 was 90% (53/59), 44% (26/59) and 90% (53/59), respectively. Linear regression analysis indicated that there was a positive correlation (r = 0.76, p < 0.001) between the serum concentration of CA 19-9 and CA 494 in pancreatic cancer patients (figure 2). Due to the high correlation between these markers a combined determination was not advantageous compared with the single determination of CA 494 or CA 19-9. The slight increase in the sensitivity from 90% to 93% (55/59) implied a loss of about 10% in specificity. The median serum levels of CA 19-9 and CA 494 increased with the tumor stage (I to IV according to the UICC) in which the patients have been diagnosed. There has been no difference in sensitivity between the tumor markers CA 19-9 and CA 494 in the various tumor stages (figure 3). The serum level did not depend on the grade of differentiation of the carcinoma.

In patients with non-pancreatic gastrointestinal cancer the sensitivity of the tumor markers was low compared to pancreatic cancer. In gastric cancer there was no difference between CA 19-9, CEA and CA 494 with 35% (16/46), 37% (17/46) and 41% (19/46). In the group of patients with colorectal cancer CEA proved its value with 55% (28/51) serum levels above the cut-off. The values for CA 19-9 and CA 494 in this group were 39% (20/51) and 18% (9/51), respectively.

The specificity of CA 19-9, CEA and CA 494 in patients with chronic pancreatitis, as the most important benign control group to pancreatic cancer, was 86% (86/100), 74% (74/100) and 94% (94/100), respectively. The specificity of CA 19-9, CEA and CA 494 in patients with benign non-pancreatic disorders was 90% (112/124), 77% (95/124) and 95% (118/124). In a subgroup of 19 patients with benign jaundice we did not find elevated serum levels, neither for CA 494 nor for CA 19-9.

The specificity in the group of healthy volunteers was 99% for the new tumor marker CA 494, 95% and 86% for CA 19-9 and CEA, respectively. In total, we found a significant difference in specificity between CA 494 (96%) and CA 19-9 (91%, $p < 0.05$) and CA 494 and CEA (79%, $p < 0.001$).

Discussion

The accurate and early diagnosis (tumor stage I, II) of pancreatic cancer is a clinical challenge and the only way to improve the poor prognosis. So far no convincing conservative treatment regime exists that provides better surviving rates or a higher quality of life (4).

Tumor markers are simple, non-invasive and comparably cheap tools that provide information about the efficiency of a therapeutical strategy and prognosis or recurrency after tumor resection (3, 9, 11).

The serum tumor marker CA 19-9 is accepted as the reference tumor marker in pancreatic cancer (7, 8). The sensitivity of CA 19-9 in pancreatic cancer is reported to be between 71% and 87% (5, 8). In the present study, we have confirmed this value with 90%. The new tumor marker CA 494 showed an identical sensitivity in pancreatic cancer.

Only six patients with tumor stage I and six patients with stage II could be included in this study. Due to this fact we can not describe the new marker CA 494 as a helpful tool in detecting early stages of pancreatic cancer. This must be cleared up in further examinations. But our results indicate that the higher specificity of this new marker allows a better discrimination between pancreatic cancer and benign disorders. One hypothetical explanation for the higher specificity of CA 494 compared with CA 19-9 could be the use of two antibodies in one assay. Thus we only measure a subgroup of mucins that bear both, the epitope for MAB BW 494 and the epitope for MAB C50.

Conclusion

We described a hopeful new tumor marker CA 494 that seems to combine a better specificity than that of the reference marker CA 19-9 with its high sensitivity in pancreatic cancer.

References

1 Bosslet K, Kern HF, Kanzy EJ, Steinstraesser A, Schwarz A, Lüben G, Schorlemmer HV, Sedlacek HH (1986) A monoclonal antibody with binding and inhibitory activity on human pancreatic carcinoma cells. Cancer Immunol Immunother 23:185–191

2 Büchler M, Friess H, Schultheiss K-H, Gebhardt C, Kübel R, Muhrer KH, Winkelmann M, Wagener T, Klapdor R, Kaul M (1991) A randomized controlled trial of adjuvant immunotherapy (murine monoclonal antibody 494/32) in resectable pancreatic cancer. Cancer 68 (7):1507–1512

3 Glenn J, Steinberg WM, Kurtzman SH, Steinberg SM, Sindelar WF (1988) Evaluation of the utility of a radioimmunoassay for serum CA 19-9 levels in patients before and after treatment of carcinoma of the pancreas. J Clin Oncol 6 (3):462–468

4 Gudjonsson B (1987) Cancer of the pancreas. 50 years of surgery. Cancer 60: 2284–2303

5 Haglund C, Roberts PJ, Kuusela P, Scheinin TM, Mäkelä O, Jalanko H (1986) Evaluation of CA 19-9 as a serum tumour marker in pancreatic cancer. Br J Cancer 53:197–202

6 Kübel R, Büchler M, Bosslet K, Baczako K, Beger HG (1987) Immunohistochemical analysis of new monoclonal antibodies for pancreatic carcinoma associated antigens. In: Klapdor R (ed) New tumour markers and their monoclonal antibodies. Thieme, Stuttgart, New York pp 354–358

7 Pleskow DK, Berger HJ, Gyves J, Allen E, McLean A, Podolsky K (1989) Evaluation of a serologic marker, CA 19-9, in the diagnosis of pancreatic cancer. Ann Intern Med, 110:704–709

8 Safi F, Beger HG, Bittner R, Büchler M, Krautzberger W (1986) CA 19-9 and pancreatic adenocarcinoma. Cancer 57: 779–783

9 Safi F, Roscher R, Bittner R, Beger HG (1988) The clinical relevance of tumor marker CEA, CA 19-9 in regional chemotherapy of hepatic metastases of colorectal carcinoma. Int J Biol Mark 3 (2):101–106
10 Silverberg E, Lubera JA (1989) Cancer statistics 1989. Cancer J Clinicians 3:3–39
11 Staab HJ (1987) The combined use of CA 19-9 and carcino-embryonic antigen (CEA) in malignancies of the gastrointestinal tract. Acta Gastro-ent Belg 46:29–35

Address for correspondence:
Prof. Dr. med. M.W. Büchler
Abteilung für Viszeral- und Transplantationschirurgie
Universität Bern (Inselspital)
Murtenstraβe 35
CH-3010 Bern, Switzerland

CA 242 – A real new tumor marker of pancreatic carcinoma?

M. Plebani[a], D. Basso[a], M.P. Panozzo[a], F. Navaglia[a], F. D'Angeli[b],
G. Del Giudice[a], M. Bottistel[a], G. Del Favero[b]

[a]Department of Laboratory Medicine, [b]Department of Gastroenterology,
University Hospital of Padova, Italy

Introduction

In the last decades the determination of several tumor markers in serum has been proposed to provide clinical help in the diagnosis of pancreatic cancer (1–4).

Various epitopes are now suitable for their detection in biological fluids (CA 19-9, CA 50, CAR-3, DU-PAN-2 and others) (1, 3, 5–7). They are all borne on glycoprotein macromolecules and in some cases the same macromolecule bears two or more epitopes (8, 9).

To date, the best serological indicator of pancreatic adenocarcinoma is CA 19-9, an epitope of a mucin-type glycoprotein identical to the sialylated Lewis a antigen, and recognized by the antibody 1116 NS 19-9 (7, 10). However, CA 19-9 determination has demonstrated some limits in pancreatic cancer diagnosis: a) It is not sensitive enough to suggest the presence of a tumor in an early stage (11), b) its circulating levels are influenced by any liver dysfunction, and jaundice in particular (4, 12, 13).

To overcome these limits, new tumor markers have been proposed. Among them one of the more recently introduced is CA 242, which has been claimed as useful not only for pancreatic cancer, but also for colon cancer diagnosis (14,15); in addition, it seems to offer some advantages in the follow-up of pancreatic cancer (16). This epitope is a sialylated carbohydrate structure related to the type I chain and situated on the same macromolecule as CA 50, though it is completely different from the latter (15).

The aims of the present study were: 1. to assess the behavior of serum CA 242 by comparison with that of CA 19-9 in patients with pancreatic cancer, 2. to verify any relationship between these two markers and tumor dimensions and spread or patient survival, 3. to assess the role of liver dysfunction in influencing the results, 4. to verify whether CA 242 serum determination can improve findings obtained with CA 19-9.

Materials and methods

We studied a total of 259 patients. Fifty-nine were control subjects (34 males, 25 females, age range 18-65), i.e. healthy members of the medical staff or blood donors. Twenty-seven (17 males, 10 females, age range 39-81) were patients affected by pancreatic cancer of duct cell origin, histologically confirmed on surgical or autoptic specimens. Fifteen of them had liver metastases and ten were followed up from two to eleven months (median = three months) after serum sampling. Twelve patients (nine males, three females, age range 37–67) were affected by chronic pancreatitis, diagnosed on the basis of at least two of the following: plain abdomen x-ray for pancreatic stones, pancreatic ultrasonography, computed axial tomography and endoscopic retrograde pancreatography. Twenty-six patients (16 males, 10 females, age range 40–80) were affected by gastric cancer and sixty-seven (40 males, 26 females, age range 30–82) had colon cancer. Five patients with colon cancer had liver metastases and 30 had lymph node involvement; none of the gastric cancer cases had metastatic liver involvement, while twelve had lymph node invasion. Fourteen patients (eleven males, three females, age range 22–90) had other gastrointestinal malignancies (gastric lymphoma: seven cases; hepatocellular carcinoma: four cases; adenocarcinoma of the papilla of Vater: three cases). Thirty patients (15 males, 15 females, age range 38–73) had benign hepato-biliary diseases (liver cirrhosis: 20 cases; bile duct stones: eight cases; primary biliary cirrhosis: one case; liver steatosis: one case). Twenty-four patients (12 males, 12 females, age range 28–66) had benign gastrointestinal diseases (peptic ulcer: 15 cases; ulcerative cholitis: three cases; Crohn's disease: six cases).

CA 19-9 and CA 242 were assayed in fasting serum by means of ILMA and IFMA procedures (Byk Sangtec and Pharmacia, respectively).

Statistical analysis was performed using analysis of variance (ANOVA one-way), Bonferroni's test for pairwise comparisons, Student's t-test, receiver operating characteristic (ROC) curves and Fisher's exact test.

Results

Figure 1 shows the individual serum levels of CA 242. CA 242 was significantly higher in pancreatic cancer patients than in any other group (ANOVA one-way: F = 9.36, p < 0.001). CA 19-9 increased in all patient groups as compared to controls, in pancreatic cancer as compared to all the other groups and in patients with hepato-biliary diseases as compared to patients with benign gastrointestinal pathologies (F = 18.73, p < 0.001). In pancreatic cancer neither CA 242 nor CA 19-9 were related to the presence of liver metastases (t = 1.09, p:ns and t = 1.61, p:ns respectively) or tumor size (above or below 4 cm; t = 0.93, p:ns and t = 0.68, p:ns respectively).

Figure 2 reports the results of the ROC curves of CA 242 and CA 19-9 in distinguishing pancreatic cancer from the remaining patients. The best diagnostic accuracy was obtained using a cut-off value of 60 U/ml (86%) for CA 242 and 80 U/ml (84%) for CA 19-9.

Pancreatic cancer patients with pathological CA 242 or CA 19-9 (> 30 U/ml and 37 U/ml respectively) had a shorter survival than those with normal CA 242 or CA 19-9 serum levels (Fisher's exact test: p < 0.05 for CA 242 and p < 0.005 for CA 19-9).

Considering the patients all together, CA 242 and CA 19-9 were correlated (r = 0.962, p < 0.001); this correlation was confirmed when pancreatic cancer patients were evaluated singly (r = 0.880, p < 0.001).

Considering the patients overall, CA 242 and CA 19-9 correlated with total bilirubin (r = 0.274, p < 0.001 and r = 0.362, p < 0.001), with ALP

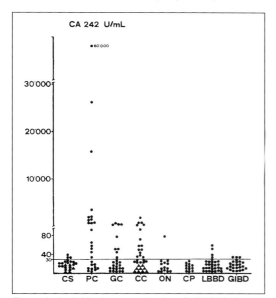

Figure 1. Individual serum levels of CA 242 in our material. The continuous line represents the upper normal limit (mean + 2 SD of our controls). CS = control subjects; PC = pancreatic cancer; GC = gastric cancer; CC = colon cancer; ON = other gastrointestinal neoplasias; CP = chronic pancreatitis; LBBD = liver-biliary benign diseases; GIBD = gastro-intestinal benign diseases. Each triangle represents the values from five subjects.

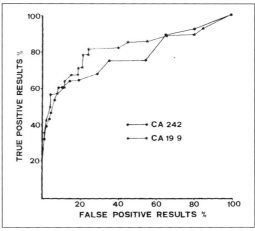

Figure 2. Receiver operating characteristic (ROC) curves of CA 242 and CA 19-9 in distinguishing pancreatic cancer from the remaining patients.

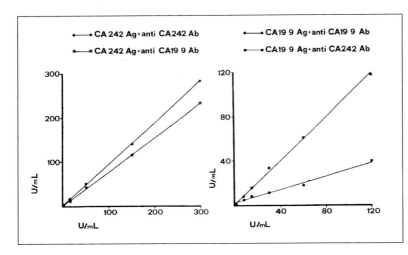

Figure 3. Dilution curves obtained using standard CA 242 and CA 19-9 materials. Ag = antigen; Ab = antibody.

($r = 0.281$, $p < 0.001$ and $r = 0.407$, $p < 0.001$) and with GGT ($r = 0.206$, $p < 0.01$ and $r = 0.352$, $p < 0.001$).
Figure 3 reports the dilution curves obtained with standard CA 242 and CA 19-9 antigens and antibodies.

Discussion

CA 242 antibody was first isolated in 1985 by *Lindholm* et al. after the immunization of mice with the human adenocarcinoma cell line COLO 205 and fusion with the Sp 2/0 mouse myeloma cell line (17). The epitope, a sialylated carbohydrate structure, is detectable in serum.
Mean CA 242 serum levels were significantly higher in pancreatic cancer patients than in control subjects or in patients with other benign or malignant gastrointestinal diseases. A similar pattern was observed for CA 19-9, though some patients with benign hepato-biliary diseases had higher mean values than those with no liver or biliary involvement. The sensitivity of these tumor markers in diagnosing pancreatic cancer was 63% for CA 242 and 69% for CA 19-9 when 30 U/ml (mean + 2 SD of our controls) and 37 U/ml (according to *Del Villano*) (18) were used as cut-off limits; the corresponding specificities were 85% and 89%. The similarity in sensitivity and specificity between these two markers was also confirmed by the ROC curves for different cut-off values and the best accuracy (84%) was obtained considering 80 U/ml for CA 19-9 and 60 U/ml for CA 242.
No relationship was found between tumor marker levels and tumor spread or tumor size in our patients with pancreatic cancer. Firstly, tumor spread and tumor size do not necessarily reflect the number of neoplastic cells; in fact neoplastic cells, vessels, connective tissue and necrotic tissue coexist inside the tumor. Secondly, the circulating levels of a tumor marker might increase because of an enhanced tumor production, but also due to a reduced metabolism. The latter event has to be considered particularly for glycoprotein tumor markers in pancreatic cancer, since an altered liver function is a frequent finding in pancreatic cancer and it may greatly interfere with glycoprotein metabolism (19). The correlation found cholestasis indices and both CA 242 and CA 19-9 further supports the above considerations for both markers.
Though CA 242 and CA 19-9 serum determination may be of little help in pancreatic cancer staging, it could provide some useful information on prognosis. In fact high levels of these markers were associated with a shorter survival.
The very similar behavior of CA 19-9 and CA 242 and the highly significant correlation found between these two markers induced us to question whether CA 242 is really a new tumor marker. So we performed the following experiment: standard CA 242 antigen was made to

react with standard CA 19-9 antibody and vice versa. The results allow us to claim that the antibodies raised against CA 19-9 or CA 242 react with both antigens, so the different nature of these two antigens is open to doubt. In any case, for clinical purposes, CA 242 offers no significant advantages over CA 19-9 in pancreatic cancer diagnosis.

References

1 Satake K, Kanazawa G, Kho I, Chung Y-s, Umeyama K (1985) Evaluation of serum pancreatic enzymes, carbohydrate antigen 19-9, and carcinoembryonic antigen in various pancreatic diseases. Am J Gastroenterol 80:630–636
2 Del Favero G, Fabris C, Plebani M, Panucci A, Piccoli A, Perobelli L, Pedrazzoli S, Baccaglini U, Burlina, A, Naccarato R (1986) CA 19-9 and carcinoembryonic antigen in pancreatic cancer diagnosis. Cancer 57:1576–1579
3 Sakamoto K, Haga Y, Yoshimura R, Egami H, Yokoyama Y, Akagi M. (1987) Comparative effectiveness of the tumor diagnostics, CA 19-9, CA 125 and carcinoembryonic antigen in patients with diseases of the digestive system. Gut 28:323–329
4 Basso D, Fabris C, Del Favero G, Panucci A, Plebani M, Angonese C, Leandro G, Dodi G, Burlina A, Naccarato R (1988) Combined determination of serum CA 199 and tissue polypeptide antigen: why no improvement in pancreatic cancer diagnosis? Oncol 45:24–29.
5 Basso D, Panozzo M.P, Fabris C, Meggiato T, Faggian D, Fogar P, Scalon P, Del Favero G, Plebani M, Burlina A, Naccarato R (1991) Does serum CAR-3 play a role in pancreatic cancer diagnosis? Oncol 48:22–25
6 Fabris C, Malesci A, Basso D, Bonato C, Del Favero G, Tacconi M, Meggiato T, Fogar P, Panozzo MP, Ferrara C, Scalon P, Naccarato R (1991) Serum DU-PAN-2 in the differential diagnosis of pancreatic cancer: influence of jaundice and liver dysfunction. Br J Cancer 63:451–453
7 Magnani JL, Steplewski Z, Korpowsiki H, Ginsburg V (1983) Identification of the gastrointestinal and pancreatic cancer-associated antigen detected by monoclonal antibody 19-9 in the sera of patients as a mucin. Cancer Res 43:5489–5492
8 Lam MS, Bast RC, Colnaghi MI, Knapp RC, Colcher D, Schlom J, Metzger S (1987) Co-expression of human cancer-associated epitopes on mucin molecules. Int J Cancer 39:68–72
9 Kawa S, Kato M, Oguchi H, Kobayashi T, Furuta S, Kanai M (1991) Preparation of pancreatic cancer-associated mucin expressing CA 19-9, CA 50, Span-I, Sialyl SSEA-I, and Dupan-2. Scand J Gastroenterol 26:981–992
10 Uhlenbruck G, Holler U, Heising J, Van Mill A, Dienst C. (1985) Sialylated Lea blood group substances detected by the monoclonal antibody CA 19-9 in human seminal plasma and other organs Urol Res 13:223–226
11 Frebourg T, Bercoff E, Manchon N, Senant J, Basuyau J-P, Breton P, Janvresse A, Brunelle P, Bourreille J (1988) The evaluation of CA 19-9 antigen level in the early detection of pancreatic cancer. A prospective study of 866 patients. Cancer 62: 2287–2290.
12 Albert MB, Steinberg WM, Henry JP (1988) Elevated serum levels of tumor marker CA 19-9 in acute cholangitis. Dig Dis Sci 33:1223–1225
13 Basso D, Meggiato T, Fabris C, Plebani M, Fogar P, Panozzo MP, Del Favero G (1992) Extra-hepatic cholestasis determines a reversible increase of glycoproteic tumor markers in benign and malignant diseases. Eur J Clin Invest 22:800–804
14 Nilsson O, Johansson C, Grimelius B, Persson B, Norgaard-Pedersen B, Andren-Sandberg A, Lindholm L (1992) Sensitivity and specificity of CA242 in gastrointestinal cancer. A comparison with CEA, CA50 and CA 19-9. Br J Cancer 65:215–221
15 Rothlin MA, Joller H, Largiader F (1993) CA 242 is a new tumor marker for pancreatic cancer. Cancer 1993 71:701–707
16 Banfi G, Zerbi A, Pastori S, Parolini D, Di Carlo V, Bonini P (1993) Behaviour of tumor markers CA 19.9, CA 195, CAM43, CA242, and TPS in the diagnosis and follow-up of pancreatic cancer. Clin Chem 39:420–423
17 Lindholm L, Johansson C, Jansson E-L, Hallberg C, Nilsson O (1985). An immunoradiometric assay (IRMA) for the CA-50 antigen. In: Holmgren J (ed) Tumor marker antigen. p123. Studentliteratur: Lund, Sweden
18 Del Villano B-C, Brennan S, Brock P, Bucher C, Liu V, McClure M, Rake B, Space S, Westrick B, Schoemaker H, Zurawski VR (1983) Radioimmunometric assay for a monoclonal antibody-defined tumor marker, CA 19-9. Clin Chem 29:54–552
19 Thomas P (1980) Studies on the mechanisms of biliary excretion of circulating glycoproteins. Biochem J 192:837–843

Address for correspondence:
Dr. M. Plebani
Istituto di Medicina di Laboratorio
c/o Laboratorio Centrale
Via Giustiniani 2
I-35128 Padova, Italy

Monoclonal TPAcyk assays quantifying human cytokeratin 8 and 18 fragments in serum of cancer patients

B. Wiklund[a], A. Silén[a], S. Nilsson[b], E.L. Andersson[c]

[a]AB IDL, Borlänge, [b]Oncology Department, University Hospital, University of Uppsala, Uppsala
[c]Cell Biology Department, University Hospital, University of Lund, Lund, Sweden

Introduction

The cytokeratins, of which 20 have been analyzed from different epithelial tissues, can be further subdivided into type I (cytokeratins 9–19 and perhaps 20) and type II (cytokeratins 1–8) (4, 5, 10, 15, 16). It is now widely accepted that, for a normal formation of intermediate filaments, two different cytokeratins are necessary, one type I and one type II, which form a pair. Cytokeratins appear in different combinations in different epithelial tissue, and in each cell type there is one or more cytokeratin pair (9, 13).

Cytokeratin expression remains throughout almost all stages of epithelial malignancy. The smallest cytokeratin pair, 8 and 18, is found in large quantities in simple, ductal and glandular epithelium, pseudostratified epithelium, transitional epithelium and carcinomas arising therefrom (9, 13).

Cells in growing tumors and metastases release growth factors which stimulate the endothelial cells in blood vessels to produce new blood vessels. The increased vascularization in the tumor results in further cell growth in parts of the tumor and an increased release of substances related to cell growth. This increased growth results in a blocking of blood vessels, cell death and cell lysis and release of proteolytic enzymes. Proteolysis of cell material releases solubilized fragments of cytokeratins which can leak out into the circulation. It can also be postulated that cytokines endogenously produced as a result of cell division in growing tumors can affect epithelial cells. This could cause not only a restructuring of the cytoskeleton but also a significant release of cytokeratin fragments into the circulation.

TPA (tissue polypeptide antigen) first described in 1957 (3) as a tumor associated antigen is present in a variety of malignant tumors. Numerous clinical investigations during the last decades have shown that elevated levels of TPA in serum are found in a high frequence among patients with tumor progression. An even more increased frequency of elevated values are found among patients with distant metastases.

A relation between TPA and (cyto)keratins 8, 18 and 19 has been previously demonstrated (7, 17). Sequence identity between major fragments of TPA and cytokeratin 8 has been established as well as a high degree of homology (72%) between sequences of a TPA fragments and cytokeratin 18 (2, 6, 14).

It has been shown that monoclonal antibodies against pertinant epitopes of cytokeratins 8, 18 and 19 could replace, individually or in pairs, the polyclonal TPA antibody used in a TPA IRMA kit on the market (8). An increased concentration of cytokeratin fragments in serum correlates with tumor progression.

In this study, we have made a technical and clinical evaluation of two new monoclonal assays (TPAcyk ELISA and IRMA, AB IDL, Sweden) and compared them with two other TPA assays available on the market.

Material and methods

Human cytokeratins 8 and 18, were purified through preparative SDS-PAGE, and have been proved pure (95%) by analytical electrophoresis. The cytokeratins were fragmentised by enzymatical degradation to a size of 10-50 kD. These fragments have been used as immunogen and antigen material in different assays.

Monoclonal antibodies were developed against purified human solubilised cytokeratins 8 and 18.

The reactivity of the monoclonals against cytokeratin fragments were shown in SDS-PAGE/blotting.
A TPAcyk ELISA method was developed as a sandwich assay, with a one-step primary incubation in microtiter plates (strips 12 x 8 wells), coated with two monoclonal antibodies against cytokeratin 8 and 18, respectively. The HRP-tracer antibody was an affinity purified polyclonal antibody.
A TPAcyk IRMA method was developed as a sandwich assay, with a one-step incubation in tubes with a plastic bead, coated with two monoclonal antibodies against cytokeratin 8 and 18, respectively. The tracer antibody was an affinity purified polyclonal antibody, labelled with iodine-125. A polyclonal TPA IRMA test from Byk-Sangtec, Germany was used for correlation studies of patient sera.
A monoclonal TPS IRMA test, Hermann Biermann GmbH (Beki Diagnostics, Sweden), was used for correlation studies of patient sera and for immunochemical studies.
Blood samples of patients with metastatic pancreatic cancer were collected at the University Hospital of Lund, Sweden. After separation the sera were kept at −20 °C. An evaluation of the TPAcyk tests and the TPS IRMA test on 101 cancer patient sera with different epithelial tumor diagnoses has been performed at a major German hospital (1300 beds), linked to a university clinic. "Diluent": 5% BSA in PBS pH 7.5.

Results and discussion

The TPAcyk ELISA and IRMA assays were evaluated technically in parallell and both assays revealed essentially the same characteristics.

Precision, detection limit and hook effect

The intra-assay precision was calculated from ten replicates of different concentrations (1–30 ng/ml) and resulted in CVs of 1–5%. The inter-assay between-kit precision was determined by repeated testings of control sera over a period of 300 days, resulting in a CV of 7.3% (n = 34) for a value of 1.29 ng/ml and a CV of 5.5% (n = 34) for a value of 3.86 ng/ml.
The detection limits of the assays were calculated as the average + 3 SD from 30 replicates of the standard 0 and resulted in a value of ≤ 0.1 ng/ml.

The hook effect was demonstrated to occur above a dose of > 500 ng/ml. Most patient sera show a value of 0–30 ng/ml, with some few values up to 100 ng/ml.

Reference range and specificity

The reference range was determined by testing of sera from several hundreds of blood donors. The cumulative frequence of 95% of the apparently healthy population was found to be 0.95 ng/ml in both assays, giving a "cut-off" of 0.95 ng/ml (at 95% specificity). Very high dose-responses were shown in both assays for solubilised cytokeratins 8 and 18, respectively, verifying the specificity of the catching mononclonal antibodies in SDS-PAGE/blotting.

Dose-response

The TPAcyk ELISA has a dose-response of 0–2.0 absorbance units at 490 nm for the concentration range of 0–15 ng/ml of TPAcyk. The TPAcyk IRMA has a dose-response of 0–70,000 CPM for the concentration range of 0–30 ng/ml of TPAcyk.

Correlation to other TPA assays

The correlation between the TPAcyk ELISA and IRMA was found to be > 0.95.

Polyclonal TPA

When testing patient sera (n = 321) with different cancer diagnoses (e.g. bladder, prostate, lung, kidney) a correlation between the TPAcyk ELISA/IRMA and the polyclonal TPA IRMA was found to be in the order of 0.9. The factor of 100 between ng/ml and U/l TPA was established from the cut-off value in the TPAcyk tests of 0.95 ng/ml and the polyclonal TPA kit (cut-off = 95 U/l).
These results coincide with the previously published data, that TPA and cytokeratins 8, 18 and 19 were related (7, 17). Later it was found that sequences from antigenically active fragments of TPA were identical to cytokeratin 8 sequences (56 amino acid residues) (6, 14). In the same paper it was shown that several shorter sequences were

52 In Vitro Diagnosis

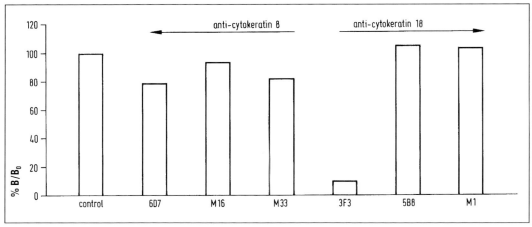

Figure 1. The TPS tracer showed a high reactivity to cytokeratin 8 and 18, coated on the beads (27.5% B/T). A significant inhibition (90% B/Bo) of the TPS tracer was revealed by the monoclonal 3F3 (anti-cytokeratin 18) as well as a less inhibition (20% B/Bo) by the monoclonals 6D7 and M33 (both anti-cytokeratin 8). These results confirm the strong relation between the TPA M3 epitope and the cytokeratins 18 and 8 (less). Control = solvent; other bars refer to the different antibody clones.

similar to cytokeratin 18. It was shown that monoclonal antibodies against pertinant epitopes of cytokeratins 8, 18 and 19 could replace, individually or in pairs, the polyclonal TPA antibody used in a TPA IRMA kit on the market (8).

TPA M3 epitope

One study of 41 patient sera tested in the TPAcyk tests and TPS IRMA (TPA M3 epitope) test, showed a correlation of 0.95 with a 40% higher values of samples in the TPAcyk test. The patient sera were from different diagnoses, e.g. breast, lung, bladder.

In a second study, in cooperation with a German laboratory, of 101 patients' sera with both the TPAcyk test and the TPS IRMA (TPA M3 epitope) test, we found a very high correlation of 0.97 with 45% higher values in the TPAcyk test. The patient sera were from many different diagnoses (n = 25), e.g. rectum, colon, breast, thyroid, bronchial, etc. The high correlations between the TPAcyk tests and the TPS IRMA test, with higher sensitivity for the TPAcyk tests, are in coincidence to a previous report from another German laboratory (1).

The high correlation between the TPAcyk tests and the TPS IRMA (TPA M3 epitope) test, with many different diagnoses, is indicating a strong relation between the human cytokeratin 8/18 and the TPA M3 epitope, supporting previous reports that the TPS (TPA M3 epitope) test showed high dose-response to cytokeratin 18 and 8, with a response-ratio between cytokeratins 18 and 8 of 10:1 in one study (11) and of 70:1 in another study (12).

To further investigate the immunochemical specificity of the TPA M3 epitope, we tested different concentrations of the solubilised human cytokeratin 8 and 18 in the TPS IRMA test revealing a very high response (67 U/l TPS per 1 ng/ml) to purified cytokeratin 8 and 18 (1:1 mixture). The response-ratio between cytokeratin 18 and 8, respectively was 15:1.

In another experiment, monoclonal antibodies against cytokeratin 8 (clones: 6D7, M16, M33), cytokeratin 18 (clones: 3F3, 5B8, M1) and the monoclonal TPS IRMA tracer (TPA M3 epitope) were reacted against beads, coated with cytokeratin 8:18 (1:1), in a simultaneous competition test as follows:

- 100 µl TPS tracer+100 µl diluent (= control, defined as 100% B/Bo) + 1 bead
- 100 µl TPS tracer + 100 µl 6D7 antibody, 10 µg/ml + 1 bead
- 100 µl TPS tracer + 100 µl M16 antibody, 10 µg/ml + 1 bead

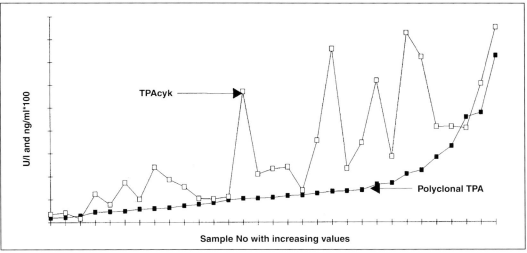

Figure 2. A higher dose-response for a majority of the sera of patients with metastatic pancreatic disease was found with the TPAcyk assay compared to the polyclonal TPA IRMA. All sera, elevated in the polyclonal TPA test, were also elevated in the TPAcyk tests.

- 100 µl TPS tracer + 100 µl M33 antibody, 10 µg/ml + 1 bead
- 100 µl TPS tracer + 100 µl 3F3 antibody, 10 µg/ml + 1 bead
- 100 µl TPS tracer + 100 µl 5B8 antibody, 10 µg/ml + 1 bead
- 100 µl TPS tracer + 100 µl M1 antibody, 10 µg/ml + 1 bead

After an incubation of 17 hours at 22 °C, the total CPM was measured, the beads were washed in 3 x 3 ml saline and the bound CPM was measured. The B/T was calculated and the control with TPS tracer and only diluent (= no inhibition) showed a binding of 27.5%. To compare the other series, with different monoclonal antibodies in simultaneous competition with the TPS tracer, we defined the control as 100% B/Bo. The B/Bo values of the other series is shown in figure 1.

Clinical study of samples from patients with pancreatic metastatic disease

High sensitivities for local (83%) and metastatic (94%) pancreatic cancer disease were found at 95% specificity for the TPAcyk assays when testing patient sera from these groups. The relation between the TPAcyk tests and the polyclonal TPA IRMA for the metastatic pancreatic patient sera is shown in figure 2.

Conclusions

The TPAcyk ELISA and IRMA tests are specific for cytokeratins 8 and 18 fragments, in the size of 10–50 kD. They show high correlations (> 0.95) to the TPA M3 epitope. The TPA M3 epitope is strongly related to human cytokeratin 18 and 8 with a response-ratio of 15:1 between the cytokeratins. The TPAcyk tests show a correlation in the order of 0.9 to the polyclonal TPA IRMA test for different diagnoses, e.g. prostate, colon, bladder, kidney. The TPAcyk tests show high sensitivity (94%) for patient sera of metastatic pancreatic cancer, where TPAcyk (in parallell with CA19-9) could be a good signal of metastatic disease.

References

1 Bahlo M, Strüven D, Klapdor R (1993) TPAcyk ELISA zur quantitativen Bestimmung des Tissue Polypeptide Antigen im Serum. GIT Labor Medizin 1-2/93:24–26
2 Bahr J, Carlsson K, Lüning B (1988) An epitope in Coil 2B of cytokeratin 8. Acta Chem Scand B42: 442–447
3 Björklund B, Björklund V (1957) Antigenicity of pooled human malignant and normal tissues by cyto-immunological technique: Presence of an insoluble heat-labile tumor antigen. Int Arch Allergy 10:153–184

4. Lazarides E (1980) Intermediate filaments as mechanical integrators of cellular space. Nature 282:249–256
5. Lazarides E (1982) Intermediate filaments: a chemically heterogenous developmentally regulated class of proteins. Ann Rev Biochem 51:219–250
6. Leube RE, Bosch FX, Romano V, Zimbelman R, Höfler H, Franke WW (1986) Cytokeratin expression in simple epithelia. III Detection of mRNAs encoding human cytokeratins nos. 8 and 18 in normal and tumor cells by hydridization with cDNA sequences in vitro and in situ. Differentiation 33:69–85
7. Lüning B, Nilsson U (1983) Sequence homology between TPA and intermediate filament proteins. Acta Chem Scand B37:731–753
8. Mellerick DM, Osborn M, Weber K (1990) On the nature of serological TPA; monoclonal keratin 8, 18 and 19 antibodies react differently with TPA prepared from human cultured cells and TPA in human serum. Oncogene 5:1007–1017
9. Moll R, Franke WW, Schiller DL (1982) The catalog of human cytokeratins: Patterns of expression in normal epithelia, tumors and cultured cells. Cell 31:11–24
10. Moll R, Schiller DL, Franke WW (1990) Identification of protein IT of the intestinal cytoskelton as a novel type I cytokeratin with unusual properties and expression patterns. J Cell Biol 111:567–580
11. Oehr P, Lüthgens ML, Liu Q (1992) Tissue polypeptide antigen and specific TPA. In: Sell S (ed) Serological cancer markers. Humana Press Inc, Totowa, New Jersey, pp 193–206
12. Oehr P, Liu Q, Jin HY, Halim AB, El Ahmady O, Nap M, Lackner, Schultes B, Ota Y (1992) TPS: Biology and clinical value. In: Klapdor R (ed) 6th Symposium on tumor markers. Zuckschwerdt, München, Bern, Wien, New York, pp 213–218
13. Quinlan RA, Schiller DL, Hatzfeld M, Achtstätter T, Moll R, Jorcano JL, Magin TM, Franke WW (1985) Patterns of expression and organization of cytokeratin intermediate filaments. In: Wang E, Fishman D, Liem RRH, Sun TT (eds) Intermediate filaments. Ann NY Acad Sci 455:282–306
14. Redelius P, Lüning B, Björklund B (1980) Chemical studies of Tissue Polypeptide Antigen (TPA). II. Partial amino acid sequence of cyanogen bromide fragments of TPA subunit B1. Acta Chem Scand B34:265–273
15. Steinart PM, Steven AC, Roop DR (1985) The molecular biology of intermediate filaments. Cell 42:411–419
16. Weber K, Geisler N (1984) Intermediate filaments – from wool-keratins to neurofilament. A structural overview. In: Levine AJ, van de Woulde GF, Topp WC, Watson JD (eds) Cancer cell, the transformed phenotype. Cold Spring Harbor Laboratory, New York, pp 153–159
17. Weber K, Osborn M, Moll R, Wiklund B, Lüning B (1984) Tissue polypeptide antigen (TPA) is related to the non-epidermal keratins 8, 18 and 19 typical of simple and non-squamous epithelia: Re-evaluation of a human tumor marker. EMBO J 3:2707–2714

Address for correspondence:
Dr. Ph. B. Wiklund
AB IDL
P.O. Box 426
S-19124 Sollentuna, Sweden

Preliminary data on the influence of octreotidacetat (S 100) on the parameters amylase, lipase as well as CA 19-9, CA 125 and TPS in the course of pancreatic surgery

G. Pohlmann[a], R. Klapdor[b], M. Bahlo[b], E. Gross[a]

[a] I. Department of Surgery, [b] General Hospital Barmbek,
Department of Medicine, University Hospital, Hamburg, Germany

Introduction

Basing on previous studies demonstrating a significant increase of TPS during pancreatic surgery in contrast to a decrease of the tumor associated antigens CA 19-9 and CA 125 (2, 3) we recently started to study the effects of pancreatic surgery on the parameters amylase, lipase, CA 19-9, CA 125 and TPS without and with simultaneous subcutaneous treatment with octreotidacetat (1, 4) (Sandostatin 100).

Material and methods

In eleven patients, nine females and two males, mean age 61 years, range 43-75 years, suffering from exocrine pancreatic carcinoma (6), chronic pancreatitis (2), carcinoid (1) and papillomas (2) the parameters amylase, lipase, CA 19-9 (Cobas Core EIA Roche), CA 125 (Enzymun EIA BM) and TPS (IRMA Beki) were measured by commercially available test systems before, during and after resective or palliative pancreatic surgery (before and at the end of the surgical procedure as well as 4, 8, 12, 24, 48, 72 hours and 5, 8, 14, 21 and 28 days after operation).
In six patients Sandostatin was applied s.c., 0.1 mg three times a day, starting 24 hours preoperatively and continued up to day 5 after surgery.

Results and discussion

1. In the preoperative period elevated levels of amylase and lipase were found in 36% of the patiens (maximal levels 358 U/l and 2620 U/l). CA 125 was found to be elevated (> 35 U/ml) in one patient, CA 19-9 (> 37 U/ml) in three patients and TPS (>100 U/l) in five patients. No correlation was found between the serum concentrations of the parameters amylase/lipase and the tumor markers CA 125/CA 19-9 and TPS.

2. Intra- and postoperatively the serum concentrations of the tumor associated antigens CA 19-9 and CA 125 showed a significant long lasting or temporary decrease, as could be expected from previous studies.
In contrast, serum concentrations of TPS showed an increase with maximal values at the end of the surgical procedure (mean increase for TPS 430% in relation to the preoperative levels). A remarkable increase of more than 1000% was found in two patients after pancreatico-duodenectomy and left resection, respectively.
In some patients serum amylase and lipase also showed a temporary increase (mean 497 and 562 %), however, in contrast to TPS peak values were found 24–48 hours after operation.

3. In the course of the postoperative period the serum concentrations of amylase and lipase decreased into normal ranges in 8/11 pateints within 100 hours.
In contrast, for TPS there was found a second temporary increase in 6/9 patients with a peak value between 10 and 14 days (mean increase 370% compared to the preoperative levels).
Interestingly also CA 125 showed a significant temporary increase up to a mean of 99 U/ml, beginning 4–5 days after surgery and with maximal values between 8 and 15 days (figure 1).

4. In this non-randomized preliminary study s.c. injection of Sandostatin did not show a significant effect on the serum concentrations of the measured parameters (figure 1).

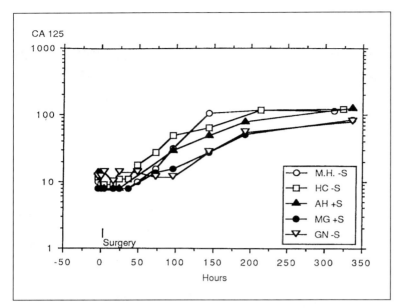

Figure 1. Typical examples for postoperative transient increases of serum CA 125 in patients after pancreatic surgery over a postoperative period up to 14 days.

References

1. Büchler M (1992) Role of octreotide in the prevention of postoperative complications following pancreatic resection. Amer J Surg 163:125–131
2. Klapdor R, Pohlmann G, Gross E, Bahlo M (1992) Influence of pancreatic surgery on behaviour of serum levels of the TAA CA 19-9, CEA, CA 125, TK and TPS in the pre- and postoperative period. Intern J Pancreatol 12:100
3. Pohlmann G, Gross E, Biermann CW, Klapdor R (1992) Intra- and postoperative serum levels of TPS and CA 125 in pancreatic surgery. Digestion 52:114
4. William ST, Woltering EA, O'Dorisio TM, Flechter WS (1989) Effect of octreotidacetat on pancreatic exocrine function. Amer J Surg 157:459–462

Address for correspondence:
Dr. med. G. Pohlmann
Abteilung für Chirurgie
Allgem. Krankenhaus Barmbek
Rübenkamp 148
D-22307 Hamburg, Germany

Preoperative CA 242 and CEA serum levels in patients with colorectal cancer

M. Carpelan-Holmström[a], C. Haglund[a], P. Kuusela[b], H. Järvinen[c], P.J. Roberts[a]

[a] IV. Department of Surgery, Helsinki University Central Hospital,
[b] Department of Bacteriology and Immunology, University of Helsinki,
[c] Second Department of Surgery, Helsinki University Central Hospital, Helsinki, Finland

Introduction

CEA is the most commonly used tumor marker for colorectal cancer. However, CEA is seldom elevated in tumors limited to the bowel wall, and therefore, CEA is not clinically useful in the early diagnosis of this disease.

CA 242 is a new tumor marker defined by the monoclonal antibody C 242, which was obtained by immunizating mice with a human colorectal carcinoma cell line COLO· 205 (4). CA 242 is a sialylated carbohydrate epitope present on the same mucinous type of antigen as CA 19-9 and CA 50. This antigen can be found in various carcinomas (1, 2, 5). The CA 242 epitope can be detected in serum by a DELFIA assay (1, 5).

The CA 242 levels are low in healthy subjects and in patients with benign diseases, while elevated levels may be found in patients with gastrointestinal cancer (3, 5).

The aim of this present study was to investigate the preoperative serum expression of CA 242 in patients with colorectal cancer and to compare the results with the preoperative serum levels of CEA.

Patients and methods

Patients

260 patients with colorectal cancer were included in the study (39 patients with Dukes' A, 100 patients with Dukes' B, 60 patients with Dukes' C and 61 patients with Dukes' D colorectal cancer), representing the incidence of different stages of colorectal cancer in Finland. 153 patients had colonic cancer (16 patients with Dukes' A, 63 patients with Dukes' B, 36 patients with Dukes' C and 38 patients with Dukes' D) and 107 patients had rectal cancer (23 patients with Dukes' A, 37 patients with Dukes' B, 24 patients with Dukes' C and 23 patients with Dukes' D).

Sera from 29 patients with benign colorectal diseases (ulcerative colitis, polyposis coli, diverticulitis and Crohns disease) were used as controls.

Methods

Serum samples were taken preoperatively and stored at −20 °C for further evaluation. The serum levels of CEA were determined by a commercially available solid phase radioimmunoassay (Abbot-Diagnostics, Chicago, IL, USA). The serum levels of CA 242 were measured by a dissociation enhanced lanthanide fluoroimmunoassay (DELFIA) (Pharmacia Wallac Oy, Turku, Finland). Both CEA and CA 242 were quantitated from the same serum samples.

The cut-off levels recommended by the manufacturers were 5 ng/ml for CEA and 20 U/ml for CA 242. The correlation between CA 242 and CEA were calculated by linear regression.

Results

CEA

Using the recommended cut-off level of 5 ng/ml, the overall sensitivity of the CEA-test was 43% and the specificity 86% (table I). The preoperative CEA level was elevated in 26% of patients with Dukes' A, 32% of patients with Dukes' B, 38% of patients with Dukes' C and 77% of patients with Dukes' D colorectal cancer (table I).

Table I. Sensitivities of CEA and CA 242 for colorectal cancer according to Dukes' stage, using the cut-off value of 5 ng/ml for CEA and 20 U/ml for CA 242.

Sensitivity	Dukes' A	Dukes' B	Dukes' C	Dukes' D	All
CEA	26%	32%	38%	77%	43%
CA 242	26%	26%	40%	67%	39%

Table II. Sensitivity and specificity of CEA and CA 242 for colorectal cancer at different cut-off levels.

CEA	> 5 ng/ml	>10 ng/ml	> 50 ng/ml	> 100 ng/ml
Sensitivity	43%	28%	15%	10%
Specificity	86%	93%	100%	100%

CA 242	> 20 ng/ml	>40 ng/ml	> 200 ng/ml	> 400 ng/ml
Sensitivity	39%	24%	12%	9%
Specificity	90%	97%	100%	100%

When the two-fold, ten-fold and twenty-fold cut-off values of 10 ng/ml, 50 ng/ml and 100 ng/ml, respectively, were used, the overall sensitivity decreased to 28%, 15% and 10%, while the specificity increased to 93%, 100% and 100%, respectively (table II).
The highest CEA-level found in Dukes' A colorectal cancer was 11 ng/ml, in Dukes' B 1453 ng/ml, in Dukes' C 297 ng/ml, in Dukes' D 9000 ng/ml and in the control group 14 ng/ml. The median values were all below 3 ng/ml except in Dukes' D colorectal cancer, where it was 54 ng/ml.
The sensitivity for Dukes' A, B, C and D colonic cancer was 19%, 32%, 31% and 71%, while the sensitivity for rectal cancer was 30%, 32%, 50% and 83%, respectively (table III). The overall sensitivity was higher in rectal cancer (47%) than in colonic cancer (40%) (table III).

CA 242

Using the recommended cut-off level of 20 U/ml, the overall sensitivity of the CA 242-test was 39% and the specificity 90% (table I). CA 242 was elevated preoperatively in 26% of patients with Dukes' A, 26% of patients with Dukes' B, 40% of patients with Dukes' C and 67% of patients with Dukes' D colorectal cancer (table I).
The highest CA 242 level in Dukes' A colorectal cancer was 144 U/ml, in Dukes' B 1000 U/ml, in Dukes' C 265 U/ml, in Dukes' D 20 000 U/ml and in the control group 41 U/ml. The median values were 8 U/ml, 9 U/ml, 7,5 U/ml and 105 U/ml for Dukes' A, B, C and D colorectal cancer, respectively, and for the control group 5 U/ml.
When the two-fold, ten-fold and twenty-fold cut-off values of 40 U/ml, 200 U/ml and 400 U/ml, respectively were used, the overall sensitivity decreased to 24%, 12% and 9%, while the specificity increased to 97%, 100% and 100%, respectively (table II).
The sensitivity for Dukes' A, B, C and D colonic cancer was 31%, 27%, 36% and 63%, respectively, while the sensitivity for rectal cancer was 22%, 24%, 21% and 74% respectively (table III). The overall sensitivity was higher in colonic cancer (39%) than in rectal cancer (34%) (table III).

Comparison of CEA and CA 242

If either CEA or CA 242 was required elevated for a positive test, the overall sensitivity was 58% and the specificity of the combination was 80%. The correlation between CEA and CA 242 serum levels was low (r^2-value = 0.335).
In Dukes' A colorectal cancer 46% of the patients had an elevated CEA and/or an elevated CA 242 serum level, in this group only 5% had both markers elevated (table IV). In Dukes' B cancer 46% had an elevated CEA and/or an elevated CA

Table III. Sensitivity of CEA, CA 242 and of the combination of the markers in patients with colonic and rectal cancer, using the cut-off level of 5 ng/ml for CEA and 20 U/ml for CA 242. The number of patients (elevated/total) in the different groups are found in brackets.

Colonic cancer	Dukes' A	Dukes' B	Dukes' C	Dukes' D	All
CEA+	19% (3/16)	32% (20/63)	31% (11/36)	71% (27/38)	43% (61/153)
CA 242+	31% (5/16)	27% (17/63)	36% (13/36)	63% (24/38)	39% (59/153)
CEA+ and CA 242+	16% (2/16)	13% (8/63)	11% (19/36)	50% (19/38)	22% (33/153)
CEA+ and/or CA 242+	38% (6/16)	46% (29/63)	53% (19/36)	74% (32/38)	56% (86/153)

Rectal cancer	Dukes' A	Dukes' B	Dukes' C	Dukes' D	All
CEA+	30% (7/23)	32% (12/37)	50% (12/24)	83% (19/23)	47% (50/107)
CA 242+	22% (5/23)	24% (9/37)	36% (11/24)	74% (17/23)	39% (42/107)
CEA+ and CA 242+	0% (0/23)	11% (4/37)	25% (6/24)	70% (16/23)	24% (26/107)
CEA+ and/or CA 242+	52% (12/23)	46% (17/37)	71% (17/24)	87% (20/23)	62% (66/107)

Table IV. Proportion of different combinations of elevated CEA and CA 242 serum levels in patients with Dukes A, B, C and D colorectal cancer, respectively, using the cut-off value of 5 ng/ml for CEA and 20 U/ml for CA 242.

	Dukes' A	Dukes' B	Dukes' C	Dukes' D	All
CEA- CA 242-	53%	54%	40%	15%	42%
CEA+ and/or CA 242+	47%	46%	60%	85%	58%
CEA+ CA 242+	5%	12%	18%	59%	23%
CEA+ CA 242-	21%	20%	20%	18%	20%
CEA- CA 242+	21%	14%	22%	8%	15%

242 serum level, of which 12% had both markers elevated (table IV).
In Dukes' C cancer 60% had an elevated CEA and/or an elevated CA 242 serum level, of which 18% had both markers elevated (table IV). In Dukes' D cancer 85% had an elevated CEA and/or an elevated CA 242 serum level and 59% had both markers elevated (table IV).
The correlation between CEA and CA 242 serum levels were low in all stages of colorectal cancer (r^2-value: 0.016; 0.092; 0.002 and 0.334 in Dukes' A, B, C and D colorectal cancer, respectively).
An elevated CEA level and/or an elevated CA 242 serum level was found in 38%, 46%, 53% and 74% of the patients with Dukes' A, B, C and D colonic cancer, respectively, whereas elevated CEA and/or CA 242 levels were found in 52%, 46%, 71% and 87% in rectal cancer patients, respectively (table III). Thus 56% of the patients with colonic cancer and 62% of the patients with rectal cancer had either or both of the tumor markers elevated (table III).

Discussion

CEA has a low sensitivity, especially in early stages of colorectal cancer, i.e. Dukes' A and B tumors (3, 5, 6). In Dukes' C and D tumors the sensitivity increases, but an elevation of the CEA level does not always precede clinical diagnosis.
In our material a combination of CEA and CA 242 increased the sensitvity for colorectal cancer by 21% in Dukes' A, by 14% in Dukes' B, by 22% in Dukes' C and by 8% in Dukes' D colorectal cancer. The overall sensitivity increased by 15%. When both or either of the markers was required to be elevated, the sensitivity increased to 46%, 46%, 60% and 80% in Dukes' A, B, C and D colorectal cancer, respectively. Other studies have shown corresponding results (3, 5, 7). The fact that a combination of CEA and CA 242 increased the sensitivity also in Dukes' A and B colorectal cancer might be of clinical value.
There was a low correlation between the serum levels of CEA and CA 242, which also has been notified by other authors (3, 5, 7), indicating that

CEA and CA 242 are expressed independently. Interestingly, only 5–12% of the patients with local colorectal cancer (Dukes' A-B) had an elevated serum level of both CEA and CA 242. A combination of CEA and CA 242 increased the sensitivity in all stages of colorectal cancer.

This study strongly supports the use of both CEA and CA 242 in the preoperative diagnosis of patients with colorectal cancer.

CEA showed higher sensitivities for rectal cancer than for colonic cancer, while the opposite was true for CA 242. A combination of CEA and/or CA 242 resulted in a higher sensitivity for both rectal and colonic cancer, but the sensitivity was more increased in patients with rectal cancer.

The control group of this report was very small but has later been enlarged to 92 patients with benign colorectal diseases. Preliminary results indicate that the assay parameters remain similar compared to those reported in this paper.

The main clinical use of CEA is monitoring operated patients with colorectal cancer for early detection of recurrence. A study analysing the value of the new marker CA 242 and the combination of it with CEA in follow-up is in progress. Furthermore, the prognostic value of the preoperative serum levels of CEA and CA 242 will be investigated.

References:

1 Johansson C, NO, Lindholm L (1991a) Comparison of serological expression of different epitopes on the CA50 carrying antigen CanAg. Int J Cancer 48:757–763

2 Johansson C, NO, Bäckström D, Jansson E-L, Lindholm L (1991b) Novel epitopes on the CA50-carrying antigen: Chemical and immunochemical studies. Tumor Biol 12:159–179

3 Kuusela P, Haglund C, Roberts PJ (1991) Comparison of a new tumor marker CA 242 with CA 19-9, CA 50 and carcinoembryonic antigen (CEA) in digestive tract diseases. Br J Cancer 63:636–640

4 Lindholm L, JC, Jansson E-L, Hallberg C, Nilsson O (1985) An immunometric assay (IRMA) for the CA 50 antigen. In: Holmgren J (ed) Tumor marker antigens. Lund, Studentlitteratur, pp 122–133

5 Nilsson O, JC, Glimelius B, Persson B, Norgaard-Pedersen B, Andrén-Sandberg A, Lindholm L (1992) Sensitivity and specificity of CA242 in gastrointestinal cancer. A comparison with CEA, CA50 and CA19-9. Br J Cancer 65:215–221

6 Roberts PJ (1988) Tumor markers in colorectal cancer. Scand J Gastroenterol 23:50–58

7 Roberts PJ, Kuusela P, Carpelan-Holmström M, Haglund C (1991) Value of different tumor markers in colorectal cancer. In: Klapdor R (ed) Tumor Associated antigens, oncogens, receptors, cytokines in tumor diagnosis and therapy at the beginning of the nineties. Zuckschwerdt, München, pp 30–32

Address for correspondence:
P.J. Roberts, M.D.
IV. Department of Surgery
Helsinki University Central Hospital
Kasarmikatu 11–13
SF-00130 Helsinki, Finland

Quantitative measurement of the tumor markers CEA, CA 19-9, CA 15-3, CA 125, AFP, β-HCG and SCC in tumor tissue, healthy colonic mucosa and serum of patients with colorectal cancer

G. Gebauer, W. Müller-Ruchholtz
Department of Immunology, University of Kiel, Germany

Introduction

The examination of tumor-associated molecules in serum is a useful method for tumor monitoring in cancer follow-up (1). But to what extent serum concentrations describe the marker expression in tumor tissue itself and especially the enhancement of its production compared with healthy tissue is not known. Several qualitative studies claimed that stromal parts of cancerous tissues and healthy mucosa do not contain any markers in immunohistochemically detectable quantities at all (2, 3, 4, 5). In cancerous tissues the tumor markers were described in carcinoma cells whereas in the adjacent normal mucosa epithelial cells the immunohistochemical staining of tumor markers was either weak or not possible (2, 3, 4, 6, 7). Stromal parts of tissue samples vary extremely between different carcinoma specimens. Therefore a comparison of tumor marker concentrations between several tumors and specimens without considering the variety of stromal parts of tissue samples is not possible with sufficient accuracy. Taking this into consideration in our study tumor antigen concentrations in tumor samples were only calculated for the part of tumor cells.

The aims of our study were:
1. Definition of tissue cut-offs of tumor markers for colorectal mucosa.
2. Comparison of the sensitivity of tumor markers in serum and tumor tissue in colorectal cancer patients.
3. Examination of the distribution of individual ratio between cancerous and healthy colorectal tissues.
4. Examination of the correlation between marker content in tissue and serum.
5. Study on the correlation between tumor marker concentrations and grading and staging of the tumor.

Material and methods

The tumor markers CEA, CA 19-9, CA 15-3, CA 125, AFP, β-HCG, and SCC were measured quantitatively in tumor tissue, healthy colonic mucosa and serum of 56 patients with colorectal adenocarcinomas. Blood samples for serum analysis were taken preoperatively, the tissue specimens immediately after surgery and put to storage at −80° C until marker extraction. For preparation of the tissue extracts the KCl extraction method (8) was used. Tissue samples at a weight of 25–50 mg were incubated for 16 hours at + 6° C with 3 molar potassium chloride solution in PBS (phosphate buffered saline, pH 7.4). After adding of 300 µl of the dilution standard of the testkits and centrifugation at 12000 g for three minutes, the supernatant was tested with Abbott monoclonal in vitro EIA testkits for CEA, CA 19-9, CA 125, AFP, β-HCG and SCC and with the Centocor monoclonal in vitro RIA testkit for CA 15-3. For getting a better comparability of different tissue samples, stromal and carcinoma cell parts in the cancer tissue specimens were determined in representative histological sections and the tumor marker concentrations were calculated accordingly.

To establish a tumor-immunological classification of the cases under study, the 95th percentile of the distribution of marker concentrations in

normal colonic mucosa was defined as normal tissue cut-off value.
For a comparison of marker concentrations in serum, mucosa and tumor tissues the Wilcoxen-Rank-Test was used for statistical analysis. The Mann-Whitney-U-Test was used for comparing the differences in marker concentrations between tumors of different grading or staging.

Results

In the vast majority of the tissue samples – in carcinomas as well as in normal mucosa – all markers were detectable. Except for AFP and CA 15-3 concentrations in normal mucosa were significantly higher than those in serum. The AFP content of mucosa was similar to that of serum. CA 15-3 was detected in higher concentrations in serum than in healthy tissue. Compared with normal mucosa and serum the marker concentrations in tumor tissue were significantly elevated for all markers. The marker concentrations are listed in the tables I, II and III, the levels of significance of the Wilcoxen-Rank-Test in table V.
Tissue cut-offs of CEA, CA 19-9, CA 125, β-HCG and SCC – defined as the 95th percentile of the distribution of marker concentrations in histologically normal mucosa – were much higher than those used for serum examination whereas those for CA 15-3 and AFP were below serum cut-offs (tables I and II).
In tumor tissue the sensitivity of all markers was considerably higher than in serum. The highest sensitivity could be demonstrated for CA 15-3 (87%) followed by CEA (83%) and β-HCG (64%), whereas only 57% of all tumors were CA 19-9 positive (table III). The sensitivities of the markers CA 15-3, CEA, β-HCG and CA 19-9 in serum were only 6%, 41%, 2% and 17% (table I). Obviously tumor markers established for serum analysis of patients with colorectal cancer are not necessarily the markers of highest sensitivity for tissue examination.
For individual comparison of marker concentrations in the two tissue types, the ratio of the concentrations in tumor tissue and healthy mucosa was calculated for each patient. The concentrations were assessed as different, when the tissue contents differed from each other more than twofold. Only few patients had lower concentrations in the tumor than in their healthy mucosa. In most cases the tumor concentrations were higher than those of the corresponding mucosa. In several cases the marker concentrations were elevated in the tumor tissue more than hundred, in a few cases even more than 1000 times (table IV). Especially the contents of CEA, CA 15-3 and CA 19-9 in cancer tissues were much higher than those of the adjacent normal mucosa (table IV). For all other markers similar high differences in marker content could only be demonstrated in some cases.
A correlation of tumor tissue and serum concentration was not observed for any marker by using the Spearmen-Rank-Correlation. All of the CA 15-3, CA 125, AFP and β-HCG serum-positive patients as well as 19 of the 21 CEA and seven of the eight CA 19-9 serum-positive patients were also marker positive in the tumor tissue. In contrast to this elevated marker concentrations in the tissues were associated in a considerable lower number of cases with simultaneous serum positivity.

Table I. Tumor marker concentrations and sensitivities in serum of patients with colorectal carcinomas.

	CEA ng/ml	CA 19-9 E/ml	CA 15-3 E/ml	CA 125 E/ml	AFP ng/ml	β-HCG miu/ml	SCC ng/ml
Sample size	54	54	54	50	54	53	52
Maximum	11120.0	7843.0	49.5	206.5	66.3	5.7	4.0
Upper quartile	6.2	30.2	17.6	11.3	3.2	2.3	1.3
Median	2.0	11.4	14.2	8.4	2.2	0.8	0.8
Lower quartile	1.0	5.3	9.0	6.2	1.4	0.1	0.5
Minimum	0.0	0.0	4.9	2.3	0.0	0.0	0.0
Average	355.4	242.7	14.2	15.7	3.7	1.4	1.0
Cut-off	2.5	40.0	24.0	35.0	20.0	5.0	2.5
Sensitivity	41%	17%	6%	6%	2%	2%	8%

Table II. Tumor marker concentrations in healthy colorectal mucosa of patients with colorectal carcinomas.

	CEA ng/g	CA 19-9 E/g	CA 15-3 E/g	CA 125 E/g	AFP ng/g	β-HCG miu/g	SCC ng/g
Sample size	55	55	55	55	55	55	55
Maximum	42948.8	16377.9	32.8	1252.5	30.5	251.2	1211.5
Upper quartile	4330.9	1002.4	5.3	80.4	5.9	49.6	13.4
Median	2172.2	234.4	2.6	45.0	3.5	30.1	6.2
Lower quartile	939.5	76.7	1.0	0.1	0.1	20.2	2.3
Minimum	158.8	0.1	0.1	0.1	0.1	0.1	0.1
Average	3964.8	1000.7	3.7	90.6	3.7	44.3	36.5
Cut-off	14968.0	4373.0	8.8	488.0	12.5	189.6	153.0

Table III. Tumor marker concentrations and sensitivities in tissue of colorectal carcinomas.

	CEA ng/g	CA 19-9 E/g	CA 15-3 E/g	CA 125 E/g	AFP ng/g	β-HCG miu/g	SCC ng/g
Sample size	52	52	52	52	52	52	52
Maximum	1170662.4	2128658.5	663.7	7104.4	99.3	1142.2	1958360.4
Upper quartile	156854.0	23962.4	76.8	390.2	15.5	263.5	101.8
Median	73141.3	8553.8	30.4	151.5	2.3	153.4	22.5
Lower quartile	19507.5	1081.9	16.2	45.4	0.1	80.2	10.2
Minimum	915.7	0.0	0.0	0.0	0.0	24.1	0.0
Average	1127450.0	147917.2	72.2	638.4	12.5	2177	38094.6
Sensitivity	83%	57%	87%	19%	20%	64%	13%

Table IV. Relative frequencies of individual ratios between tumor marker concentrations in tumor tissue and healthy mucosa in percent.

	CEA	CA 19-9	CA 15-3	CA 125	AFP	β-HCG	SCC
Sample size	51	51	51	51	51	51	51
Ratio ≤ 0.49	0	2	2	4	2	2	4
Ratio 0.5–2	4	12	6	39	45	18	29
Ratio 2.1–10	18	27	37	41	45	63	49
Ratio 10.1–100	55	29	47	14	8	18	12
Ratio ≥ 100	24	31	8	2	0	0	6

Table V. Values of probability of the Wilcoxen-Rank-Test; comparison of serum, tumor tissue and mucosa concentrations.

	CEA	CA 19-9	CA 15-3	CA 125	AFP	β-HCG	SCC
Serum/mucosa	$5 \cdot 10^{-8}$	$5 \cdot 10^{-7}$	$5 \cdot 10^{-9}$	$5 \cdot 10^{-4}$	n.s.	$5 \cdot 10^{-9}$	$1 \cdot 10^{-9}$
Serum/tumor	$1 \cdot 10^{-9}$	$5 \cdot 10^{-8}$	$5 \cdot 10^{-7}$	$5 \cdot 10^{-8}$	$5 \cdot 10^{-2}$	$5 \cdot 10^{-9}$	$5 \cdot 10^{-9}$
Mucosa/tumor	$1 \cdot 10^{-9}$	$5 \cdot 10^{-8}$	$5 \cdot 10^{-9}$	$1 \cdot 10^{-5}$	$1 \cdot 10^{-2}$	$5 \cdot 10^{-9}$	$5 \cdot 10^{-7}$

Furthermore, it was found that six of the seven CA 15-3 tissue-negative patients had no metastases, neither in lymphnodes nor in other organs. Staging data of the 7th patient were not known. For CA 125 too, the concentrations of locally restricted tumors were much lower than of carcinomas associated with metastases (p < 0.001).

A correlation between tumor grading and marker concentration in carcinoma tissues could not be observed for any marker. However, even the highest concentrations of CEA, CA 15-3 and AFP in undifferentiated tumors were found below the lower quartile of the other carcinomas.

Discussion

In several studies tumor markers were measured quantitatively in colorectal tissues (9, 10 11, 12, 13, 14). But in none of them it was taken into consideration that the proportion of the tumor cells and stroma in a cancer tissue sample may differ strongly from case to case. So it is to say that no calculation of the tumor marker content of the truely cancerous cells was attempted in any of these studies. The lack of such correction is obviously one of the most important reasons for the controversial results of different studies, not only according to concentrations in cancerous tissues but also to the correlation between tumor marker content of carcinomas and histological grading (4, 10, 12). Another reason for variable results of quantitative marker measurement in tissues may be seen in different extraction techniques. But because of the heterogenicity of tumor cells themselves (7) a calculation of marker concentrations based on the marker producing parts of tissue samples does not allow a description of marker concentration on the level of a single cell.

By defining tumor marker cut-offs for tissues an assessment of the results of quantitative tumor marker measurement similar to the evaluation of serum values is possible. The decision which tumor-associated molecule is of highest sensitivity is only valid on the basis of tissue cut-offs. Until now such cut-offs were not established for any gastrointestinal tissue. Therefore a comparison of different tumor markers in respect of their qualification for tissue analysis was not possible.

Previous studies on sensitivities of tumor-associated molecules in any gastrointestinal carcinoma tissue are not known. Therefore an integrative discussion of the data presented in this study is not possible. Similar investigations about tumor marker content of carcinomas of the mammary gland claimed lower sensitivities for CEA and CA 15-3 (15, 16, 17) than those presented in this study for colorectal cancer. This is surprising especially for CA 15-3, a tumor marker of first choice for cancer of the mammary gland but without any importance at all for serum analysis in patients with gastrointestinal cancers. Obviously markers established in serum follow-up of patients with malignant diseases are not necessarily qualified markers for tissue examination as well.

The different patterns of tumor marker concentrations in serum and tumor tissues show that the analysis of serum is not predictive for marker expression in the tumor itself. All markers were produced in the tumor cells in higher quantities compared with the healthy mucosa, but only CEA and in several cases CA 19-9 were released into the serum in amounts high enough to cause serum positivity. Thus, not only the enhanced expression of tumor-associated molecules in carcinoma cells but also the mechanism of marker release is important for the elevation of the serum concentration.

Until now the prognostic value of tumor marker examinations in cancerous tissues is not known. Qualitative immunohistochemical studies on CEA in colorectal and stomach cancer reported significantly higher survival rates of patients with CEA-negative carcinomas (4, 18, 19). However, long-term quantitative studies have not been published so far. Preliminary studies on CA 19-9 and CA 125 tumor marker concentrations in colorectal tumors appear to indicate a considerable prognostic relevance especially for CA 125 (13). In this context our finding of higher CA 15-3 and CA 125 tumor marker concentrations in patients with metastases may be an indication that some markers could be used as a sign for biological aggressiveness of carcinomas. Long-term monitoring of these patients would allow to study the prognostic relevance of quantitative tumor marker examinations in cancer tissues.

For immunoscintigraphic approaches the selective accumulation of antibodies is necessary. Quantitative studies on tumor marker expression in tissues will allow better specification of the conditions for their successful utilisation. Antibodies against CEA, CA 15-3, CA 19-9 and in some cases CA 125 and SCC as well could be useful for such purposes because these tumor-associated molecules often fulfill the characteristic of extremely enhanced expression in malignant tissues. But the quantitative analysis presented above is not able to describe the localization of markers in tumor cells especially their expression on the cell surface. Therefore additional immunocytochemical investigations should be conducted to complement the results of quantitative studies.

References

1. Barillari P, Sammartino P, Cardi M, Ricci M, Gozzo P, Cesareo S, Cesari A (1990) Gastrointestinal cancer follow-up: The effectiveness of sequential CEA, TPA, and CA 19-9 evaluation in the early diagnosis of recurrences. Aust N Z J Surg 61:675–680
2. Mori M, Shimono R, Adachi Y, Matsuda H, Kuwano H, Sugimachi K, Ikeda M, Saku M (1990) Transitional mucosa in human colorectal lesions. Dis Colon Rectum 33:498–501
3. Savoie SC, Sikorska HM (1991) Immunohistochemical charracterization of a new anticarcinoembryonic antigen monoclonal antibody. Anticancer Res 11:1–12
4. Cunningham L, Stocking B, Halter SA, Kalemeris G (1986) Immunoperoxidase staining of carcinoembryonic antigen as a prognostic indicator in colorectal carcinoma. Dis Colon Rectum 29:111–116
5. Mc Manus LM, Naughton MA, Martinez-Hernandez A (1976) Human chorionic gonadotropin in human neoplastic cells. Cancer Res 36:3476–3481
6. Martin F, Martin MS (1972) Radioimmunoassay of carcinoembryonic antigen in extracts of human colon and stomach. Int J Cancer 9:641–647
7. Dietel M, Arps H, Klapdor R, Müller-Hagen S, Sieck M, Niendorf A, Hoffmann L (1986) Comperative studies of the tumor markers CA 125, CA 19-9, CEA, 17-1A, and CA 50 in tissue sections and sera of patients with ovarian tumors. In: Greten H, Klapdor R (ed) Clinical relevance of new monoclonal antibodies. Thieme, Stuttgart, pp 296–304
8. Meltzer MS, Leonard EI, Rapp HJ, Borsos T (1971) Tumor-specific antigen solubilized by hypertonic potassium chloride. J Nat Cancer Inst 47:703–709
9. Casale V, Castelli M, Coloni F, Sega E, Sega FM, Sciarretta F (1983) The biological and clinical significance of tumor markers in tissue extracts. Cancer Detect Prev 6:61–66
10. Quentmeier A, Möller P, Schwarz V, Abel U, Schlag P (1987) Carcinoembryonic antigen, CA 19-9, and CA 125 in normal and carcinomatous human colorectal tissue. Cancer 60:2261–2266
11. Wagener C, Müller-Wallraf R, Nissen S, Gröner J, Breuer H (1981) Localization and concentration of carcinoembryonic antigen (CEA) in gastrointestinal tumors: Correlation with CEA levels in plasma. JNCI 67:539–547
12. Rosandic-Pilas M, Hadzic N, Stavljenic A, Juricic M, Scukanec-Spoljar M (1990) Relationship between tissue and serum concentrations of carcinoembryonic antigen (CEA) in gastric and colonic carcinomas. Acta Med Austriaca 17:89–93
13. Quentmeier A, Schwarz V, Schlag P (1990) Relevance of cell surface markers for the prognosis of colorectal cancer. In: Klapdor R (ed) Recent results in tumor diagnosis and therapy. Zuckschwerdt, München, pp 335–338
14. Porciani S, Becciolini A, Lanini A, Bandettini L, Bechi P, Benucci A, Tommasi M (1990) Tissue CEA concentration in colorectal carcinoma and in the proximal mucosa. J Nucl Med Allied Sci 34 (4 suppl): 301–304
15. Gent H-J (1990) Quantitative zellbiologische und immunbiologische Parameter beim Mammakazinom. Thieme, Stuttgart, p 92–93
16. Gent H-J, Rodewald G, Mecke H, Harpprecht J, Müller-Ruchholtz W (1990) Quantitative analysis of carcinoembryonie antigen in fresh specimens of the mammary gland. In: Klapdor R (ed) Recent results in tumor diagnosis and therapy. Zuckschwerdt, München, pp 366–370
17. Gent H-J, Dietrich H, Grillo M, Müller-Ruchholtz W, Quantitative analysis of CA15-3 in fresh specimens of the mammary gland. In: Klapdor R (ed) Recent results in tumor diagnosis and therapy. Zuckschwerdt, München, pp 357–361
18. Shousha, S, Lyssiotis T, Godfrey VM, Scheuer PJ, Carcinoembryonic antigen in breast-cancer tissue: A useful prognostic indicator. Br Med J 1:777–779
19. Jessup JM, Giavazzi R, Campbell D, Cleary KR, Morikawa K, Hostetter R, Atkinson EN, Fidler IJ (1989) Metastatic potential of human colorectal carcinomas implanted into nude mice: Prediction of clinical outcome in patients operated upon for cure. Cancer Res 49:6906–6910

Address for correspondence:
Prof. Dr. Dr. h. c. W. Müller-Ruchholtz
Institut für Immunologie im
Klinikum der Universität zu Kiel
Brunswikerstraße 4
D-24105 Kiel, Germany

Biliary CEA levels in patients with liver metastases of colorectal cancer

M.A. Paul[a], J.J. Visser[a], G.J. van Kamp[b], C. Mulder[b], S. Meijer[a]

Departments of [a]Surgery and [b]Clinical Chemistry, Free University Hospital, Amsterdam, The Netherlands

Introduction

Occult liver metastases, which escape detection at the time of initial surgery, are present in 20 to 30 percent of curatively resected colorectal cancer patients. Improved imaging techniques, such as intra-operative ultrasonography, may have decreased this percentage, but accurate detection of early liver metastases still remains a significant clinical problem. Because patients with occult metastases may benefit from chemotherapy, adjuvant treatment is given to most patients with advanced stage (Astler-Coller B2 and C) colorectal cancer. Consequently, many patients are overtreated and more sensitive tests to identify patients at risk for developing liver metastases are urgently needed.

Recently *Yeatman* and coworkers (1) suggested that the biliary level of carcinoembryonic antigen (CEA) might be a proper marker for early liver metastasis. This novel hypothesis was based on the following rationales: CEA derived from the liver metastases may be transported not only to the blood but also to the bile. The volume of bile is smaller than the volume of blood, and, moreover, bile becomes concentrated ten- to twelve-fold in the gallbladder. A detectable level of CEA, therefore, might be found at an earlier stage in gallbladder bile than in serum. Support for this hypothesis was found in *Yeatman's* study, which showed that high levels of CEA occurred in gallbladder bile in all patients with liver metastases. Based on regression analysis of estimated tumor volume versus biliary CEA, this study demonstrated that even very small metastases with a volume of 1 ml or less might be detectable by an elevation in the biliary CEA level.

These findings suggest that accurate determination of CEA levels in gallbladder bile could become a significant improvement in the early detection of colorectal liver metastases (1, 2). To study the usefulness of this new test we measured serum and biliary CEA levels in patients who had developed liver metastases during follow-up after resection of a colorectal carcinoma.

Materials and methods

Serum and gallbladder bile samples were obtained from thirty patients with metachronous liver metastases of colorectal cancer who underwent exploratory laparotomy for tumor resection or hepatic artery perfusion. Patients with prior cholecystectomy or concomitant gallstone disease and patients who were found to have extrahepatic spread of tumor were excluded from the study.

The group comprised eighteen males and twelve females, aged 37 to 73 years, with a mean age of 59 years. Serum samples were obtained by peripheral vein puncture. Bile samples were obtained by transhepatic gallbladder puncture, prior to manipulation of the tumor.

In patients who underwent partial liver resection (n = 16), the diameter of the tumor was measured in the surgical specimen and tumor volume ($4/3\pi r^3$) and surface area ($4\pi r^2$) were calculated. Neither central necrosis, which may be present in large tumors, nor irregularities in the shape of the tumors were considered. When more than one tumor was present, the sum of the values was taken. All tumors were positive for CEA on immunohistochemical staining. A non-parametric statistical method was applied and the correlations between a) the CEA level in serum and bile and b) the tumor volume or surface and the biliary CEA level were examined using Spearman's rank coefficient and linear regression analysis. Bile-to-serum ratios of CEA levels were calculated to measure the extent of CEA accumulation in bile.

CEA was measured with a commercially available immunoassay (Enzymun-Test CEA, Boehringer Mannheim GmbH). Bile samples were pretreated by extraction with perchloric acid. CEA was precipitated from this extract with phosphotungstic acid, washed with ethanol and redissolved in CEA-free serum. The recovery of the extraction procedure was 86.8 + 4.7% (mean + SD). The within-run and between-run coefficients of variation of the CEA assay in bile were < 10% and < 15%, respectively. A cut-off value of 5 ng/ml was used for CEA in serum, whereas for bile a cut-off value of 10 ng/ml, as recommended by *Yeatman* et al., was taken.

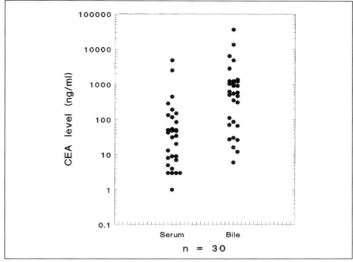

Figure 1. CEA levels in serum and gallbladder bile. Biliary levels are significantly higher than corresponding serum levels (p > 0.001).

Results

Serum and biliary CEA levels of the study group are shown in figure 1. CEA varied from 1–4800 (mean 315) ng/ml in serum and from 6–35.760 (mean 2523) ng/ml in gallbladder bile. Biliary CEA levels were significantly higher than the corresponding serum levels (p < 0.001). The bile-to-serum ratio varied from 0.3–203 (mean 43.7, median 12.3). In only two of the patients did the serum level exceed the biliary level. These two patients had gross involvement of one liver lobe which probably reduced the production of bile in that lobe.

There was a significant correlation between the levels of CEA in serum and in bile (r = 0.68, p < 0.001, figure 2).

Serum CEA was elevated above the cut-off level of 5 ng/ml in 23 (77%) of the patients, whereas

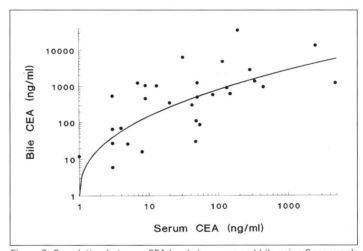

Figure 2. Correlation between CEA levels in serum and bile using Spearman's rank correlation (r = 0.68, n = 30, p < 0,001).

biliary CEA was elevated above the cut-off level of 10 ng/ml in 29 (97%).

In the 16 patients in whom the tumor was resected, a significant correlation was found between biliary CEA and a) tumor volume (r = 0.82, p < 0.001, figure 3) and b) tumor surface area (r = 0.81, p < 0.001, figure 4). Using a linear regression analysis, the cut-off level of 10 ng/ml was shown to correspond with a tumor volume of less than 4 ml and a tumor surface area of less than 6 cm^2.

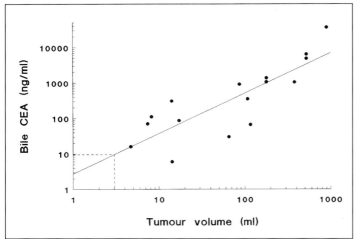

Figure 3. Relation between the biliary CEA level and the tumor volume. Using a linear regression analysis (r = 0.82, n = 16, p < 0.001), the cut-off value of 10 ng/ml corresponds with a volume of less than 4 ml.

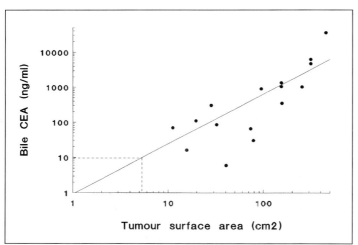

Figure 4. Relation between the biliary CEA level and the tumor surface area. Using a linear regression analysis (r = 0.81, n = 16, p < 0.001), the cut-off value of 10 ng/ml corresponds with a surface area of less than 6 cm^2.

Discussion

Our results, which are generally in agreement with those previously reported by Yeatman et al. (1), indicate that determination of CEA in gallbladder bile may well be a new and useful adjunct to the early detection of liver metastasis. Biliary CEA levels were found to be significantly elevated in 97% of our patients, all of whom had histologically proven liver metastases. Moreover, there was a strong positive correlation between biliary CEA and tumor volume. Regression analysis showed that at a cut-off level of 10 ng/ml a single metastasis with a diameter of 2 cm could potentially produce an elevation in biliary CEA. This finding indicates that relatively small metastases could be detected by this test.

However, before the implementation of this test in clinical practice as a screening method for occult liver metastases three main problems remain. The first is the optimal cut-off value for biliary CEA. Control bile samples for determination of normal CEA levels are mostly obtained during surgery in patients with biliary tract pathology. In patients with asymptomatic cholelithiasis, however, levels above 20 ng/ml occur, while markedly elevated levels up to 200 ng/ml are found in patients with acute cholecystitis and in patients with malignant or benign biliary obstruction (1, 3). These elevations may be due at least partly to the presence of cross-reacting glycoproteins (4). In patients without any biliary tract pathology gallbladder bile CEA levels are usually less than 3 ng/ml (own observations, reference 1, 3). More bile samples of patients without biliary tract pathology have to be studied to determine the optimal cut-off level, but these samples are hard to obtain. In our study group the sensitivity of biliary CEA in detecting liver metastases was 97% at the cut-off level of 10 ng/ml recommended by Yeatman et al. (1) and 90% at the cut-off level of 22 ng/ml used by Lamerz et al. (3).

The second problem is also related to the fact that biliary tract pathology may give rise to falsely elevated CEA levels. This implies that the test will only be a reliable marker for liver metastases in the absence of gallbladder pathology and biliary tract obstruction other than by the liver metastases themselves. Benign biliary tract pathology occurs frequently. In our series of 70 colorectal cancer patients with curative resection, twenty-seven percent had had cholecystectomy or were found to have concomitant gallstone disease.

The third issue is the optimal moment at which gallbladder bile should be sampled. Gallbladder bile is most easily obtained during laparotomy for primary tumor resection. If the assumption that most or all of the CEA in bile is indeed derived from liver metastases and not from the primary tumor holds true, then any elevation in biliary CEA should be indicative for the presence of liver metastases. This assumption is supported by experimental evidence in rats and monkeys which indicated that only a minor amount of intravenously injected CEA is recovered in bile (5). However, human studies on biliary excretion of circulating CEA are lacking. Furthermore, in the animal studies CEA was given by single injection, a situation which differs from the continuous secretion of CEA in the bloodstream by the primary tumor. It is possible that an elevation in biliary CEA may occur in the absence of liver metastases due to 'spill-over' of primary tumor CEA into the bile. A possible indication for this 'spill-over' is the discovery of a low biliary CEA level (< 3 ng/ml) in one of our patients who had had an elevated level at the time of primary tumor resection two months before. To avoid false positive biliary CEA levels it may be advisable to sample gallbladder bile some time after resection of the primary tumor. Any elevation in biliary CEA would then indicate the presence of recurrence, either in the liver or elsewhere in the abdomen. A study which compares patients sampled during primary tumor resection with patients who are sampled some time after the resection, is needed to establish the best time of sampling. If the 'spill-over' of CEA occurs, all curatively resected patients should have their bile sampled not during surgery, but later on. Bile can be obtained by percutaneous transhepatic, ultrasonography guided, puncture of the gallbladder, or by a naso-biliary drain. Both procedures are invasive, but should be considered, because of the important therapeutical implications of the result.

Conclusion

CEA in gallbladder bile is a sensitive marker for colorectal liver metastases. Further studies to determine the usefulness of this test in the screening and follow-up of patients with colorectal cancer are now in progress.

References

1. Yeatman TJ, Bland KI, Copeland EM, Hollenbeck JI, Souba WW, Vogel SB, Kimura AK (1989) Relationship between colorectal liver metastases and CEA levels in gallbladder bile. Ann Surg 210:505–512
2. Yeatman TJ, Komura AK, Copeland EM, Bland KI (1991). Rapid analysis of carcinoembryonic antigen levels in gallbladder bile-identification of patients at high risk of colorectal liver metastases. Ann Surg 213:113–117
3. Lamerz R, Meijer G, Heiss M, Brandt A, Vogel S, Jauch KW (1992). Gallbladder and serum CEA in cholecystolithiasis and malignant gastrointestinal diseases. In: Klapdor R (ed) Tumor associated antigens, oncogenes, receptors, cytokines in tumor diagnosis and therapy at the beginning of the nineties. Cancer of the breast – state and trends in diagnosis and therapy. Zuckschwerdt, München, pp 23–27
4. Svenberg T, Hammarström S, Hedin A (1979) Purification and properties of biliary glycoprotein I (BGP I). Immunochemical relationship to carcinoembryonic antigen. Mol Immunol 16: 245–252
5. Thomas P (1980). Studies on the mechanisms of biliary excretion of circulating glycoproteins. Biochem J 192:837–843

Address for correspondence:
M.A. Paul, M.D.
Department of Surgery
Free University Hospital
P.O. Box 7057
NL-1007 MB Amsterdam, The Netherlands

Clinical significance of tenascin serum levels in colorectal carcinomas

S. Riedl[a], H. Bodenmüller[b], P. Schlag[c], A. Faissner[d]

[a]Surgical Clinic of the University, Heidelberg, [b]Boehringer Mannheim GmbH, Research Center Tutzing, [c]Klinikum Robert Virchow of the FU, Berlin, [d]Institute of Neurobiology of the University, Heidelberg, Germany

Introduction

Tenascin is a hexameric glycoprotein of the extracellular matrix. Different isoforms ranging from 180 kD to 300 kD are produced by alternative RNA-splicing. An increased tenascin tissue content is observed during benign and neopastic proliferation. In embryologic development tenascin occurs primarily in sites of epithelial-mesenchymal interaction but also in mesenchymal organs such as liver, brain, muscle and bone. In addult tissue tenascin is present in very restricted locations and in low concentration. In the murine small intestine tenascin was found only in the basal lamina of the villous tips but not in the crypts. It has been suggested that tenascin is involved in physiological cell shedding (7). Our studies confirm the site restricted occurence of tenascin in human colorectal mucosa (8). Reparative and hyperproliferative processes such as wound healing of the epidermis for example result in an increased tenascin content of the tissue. The termination of these processes lead to a complete remission of tenascin upregulation (4, 5, 9). Increased tenascin concentrations correlate well with cell diferentation, cell migration and mitogenic activity (1, 3).

A strong neoexpression of tenascin exists in the extracellular matrix of different tumors, especially carcinomas, such as cancer of the ovary, colorectum, thyroid, stomach, urinary bladder, parotid, lung, and some sarcomas of the soft tissue (2, 6). The aim of our study was to investigate wether alterations of tissue content of tenascin cause elevated serum levels in patients with colorectal carcinomas.

Material and methods

118 patients with primary colorectal carcinomas (70 male, 48 female from 30 to 87 years of age, median age 64 years) and 51 healthy volunteers (33 male, 18 female from 24 to 90 years of age, median age 47 years) were investigated. After surgical tumor therapy the TNM-classification (UICC) was used. There were 14 patients with stage I, 29 patients stage II, 36 patients stage III with lymph node metastases and 32 patients stage IV with synchronous distant metastases. In ten cases the histological T-category could not be defined. Three patients without distant metastases and six patients with distant metastases had an unclear histological N-category. The tumor grading was GI in two cases, GII in 73 cases, GIII in 31 cases and GIV in three cases (in consideration of the lowest grading of the tumor). Prior to surgery blood samples were obtained. Serum was produced by centrifugation and stored at −70 °C in plastic tubes. A three step sandwich assay with the steptavidin-biotin technology was used. The concentration was calculated from a standard curve, for which we used a preparation of purified tenascin (purity > 90%) from human fibroblast cultures as standard material. Statistical analysis was carried out by Wilcoxon-test, Kruskal-Wallis-test and Jonckheere-test.

Results

Patients with colorectal carcinomas (n = 118) show a significantly higher tenascin serum level of 5.0 ± 4.2 µg/ml ($\bar{x} \pm s$), range 0.9 to 26.9 µg/ml,

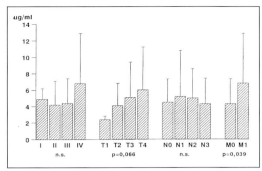

Figure 1. Tenascin serum levels in relation to tumor stage and categories of TNM classification (UICC) ($\bar{x}$;s).

compared to healthy voluteers with a tenascin level of 3.2 ± 1.7 µg/ml ($\bar{x}$ ± s), range 0.9 to 7.1 µg/ml (p = 0.007). Assuming a specifity of 95% a sensitivity of 25% for colorectal carcinomas results. Different tumor stages do not show significant differences of tenascin levels. But stage IV with synchronous distant metastases had the highest level compared to other stages. In increasing T-categories a trend of higher tenascin levels was found (p = 0.066). The N-categories representing presence and number of lymph node metastases had no influence on tenascin serum levels. In patients with synchronous distant metastases a significantly higher tenascin serum level was observed as compared to those without distant metastases (p = 0.039) (figure 1).

Discussion

The neoplastic increase of tenascin found by immunohistological examinations in colorectal carcinomas causes a significant elevation of tenascin serum levels in patients with primary carcinomas. The diagnostic relevance of the tenascin serum level in patients with primary colorectal carcinomas is low on account of a low sensitivity. The altitude of the tenascin serum level possibly correlates with the total tumor mass.

Therefore, tenascin could be a valuable parameter in the follow-up of colorectal cancer patients during therapy. The correlation of tenascin serum levels and distant metastases needs further investigations to study the prognostic significance of tenascin.

References

1. End P, Panayotou G, Entwistle A, Waterfield MD, Chiquet M (1992) Tenascin: a modulator of cell growth. Eur J Biochem 209:1041–1051
2. Erickson HP (1989) Tenascin: an extracellular matrix protein prominent in specialised embryonic tissues and tumors. Annu Rev Cell Biol 5:71–92
3. Faissner A, Kruse J (1990) Tenascin is a repulsive substrate for central nervous system neurons. Neuron 5:627–637
4. Howeedy AA, Virtanen I, Laitinen L, Gould NS, Koukoulis GK, Gould VE (1990) Differential distribution of Tenascin in the normal, hyperplastic, and neoplasic breast. Lab Invest 63:798–806
5. Mackie EJ, Halfter W, Liverani D (1988) Induction of Tenascin in healing wounds. J Cell Biol 107:2757–2767
6. Natali PG, Nicotra MR, Bigotti A, Botti C, Castellani P, Risso AM, Zardi L (1991) Comparative analysis of the expression of the extracellular matrix protein Tenascin in normal human fetal, adult and tumor tissues. Int J Cancer 47:811–816
7. Probstmeier R, Martini R, Schachner M (1990) Expression of Jl/Tenascin in the crypt-villus unit of adult mouse small intestine: Implications for its role in epithelial cell shedding. Development 109:313–321
8. Riedl SE, Faissner A, Schlag P, von Herbay A, Koretz K, Müller P (1992) Altered content and distribution of Tenascin in colitis, colon adenoma, and colorectal carcinoma. Gastroenterol 103:400–406

Address for correspondence:
Dr. med. S. Riedl
Chirurgische Universitätsklinik
Kirschnerstraße 1
D-69120 Heidelberg, Germany

Correlation between cell cycle kinetics and serum markers: CEA and CA 19-9 in colorectal cancer

A. Khalifa[a], Sanaa Eissa[a], S. Zaki[b], M. Khalid[b], H. El-Ghor[b], A. Abdalla[b], M. El-Banna[b]

[a]Oncology Diagnostic Unit (Biochemistry Department),
[b]Surgical Department, Ain-Shams Faculty of Medicine, Abbassia, Cairo, Egypt

Introduction

Accurate clinical and pathological staging of patients with colorectal cancer is of great importance in taking the decision of the surgical procedure. It assists in the selection of patients for adjuvant therapy and in the choice of the most useful among the alternative treatment options available. It also helps in predicting the prognosis (1). The pathological classification of colorectal cancer has remained essentially the same for 50 years. Preoperative staging is not accurate enough and the data offered by pathologic staging are not available preoperatively. It has been shown that it is possible to divide patients with primary colorectal cancer into prognostic groups before surgery on the basis of the preoperative serum levels of tumor markers (1). By supplementing microscopic morphology with FCM and DNA testing, it is possible 1. to improve the sensitivity and specificity of the detection of malignant cells, 2. to achieve more biologically meaningful tumor subclassification, and 3. to obtain information that can facilitate the prediction of individual patient tumor therapy responses (2, 3).

In order to clarify the significance of recent parameters, DNA ploidy, CEA and CA 19-9, a group of patients with colorectal cancer has been studied.

Material and methods

Twenty eight patients with resectable colorectal adenocarcinomatous tumors were the subjects of this study, 39.3% were females and 60.7% were males. TNM staging revealed 57.1% in stage II and 42.9% in stage III. When Dukes' classification was applied 21.4% were Dukes' A, 35.7% Dukes' B and 42.9% Dukes' C.

Operative specimens were sent for histological examination and one cubic centimetre samples representative of the tumor, were excised from the operative specimen preserved in RPMI media, either processed freshly or stored at $-70\ °C$ till time of FCM analysis. Blood samples were preoperatively collected from patients and controls. Sera obtained by centrifugation were divided into aliquots and stored at $-20\ °C$ until assayed.

Flow cytometric (FCM) DNA analysis

Preparation of single cell suspension

The presence of representative tumor tissue was confirmed on a hematoxylin and eosin section. Tissue specimens in RPMI media were dispersed mechanically by scrapping the cut surface of the tumor with a scalpel to release cells into the media. Cell suspension was filtered through 45 μm nylon mesh. The filtrate was gently centrifuged at 500 g for five minutes (min) and washed in PBS (10 mM phosphate buffered saline, pH 7.4). The cells were counted using Coulter T660 cell counter and adjusted to a concentration of $3-10 \cdot 10^5$/ml using PBS.

DNA staining (4, 5, 6)

Cells were stained using Coulter procedure. At first cells were lysed and permeabilized to PI using 100 μl of lysing permeabilizing reagent (LPR) (< 0.01% potassium cyanide, < 0.1% sodium azide, non-ionic detergent in saline). Then cells were treated with 1 ml staining solution which is composed of propidium iodide (PI = 50 μg/ml) and RNase (type III, bovine pancreas, 4 ku/ml). Propidium iodide (PI) binds by intercalation to the double stranded DNA and RNA. In combination with ribonuclease digestion, PI can be used as a DNA specific cytochemical probe. When measured by flow cytometry, the intensity of integrated red fluorescence of PI is directly proportional to the amount of DNA bound by the dye. By comparing the intensity of each cell to the intensity of cells containing diploid amounts of DNA (stromal cells in the tumor) the relative quantity of DNA in the cells of interest can be determined. The quantity is defined as the DNA index. Bit map gating on integrated versus peak red fluorescence is used to minimize doublets included in the histogram.

Sample running

Chicken RBCs (Coulter, France) were used as an internal DNA standard. This DNA standard was added to one of two duplicate specimens. This allowed quality control of staining variability. After setting the bit map gate 20,000 events were collected using Coulter Profile II flow cytometer. Peak channel numbers and corresponding CVs were recorded for the G0/G1 and G2/M peaks, and the ratio of the G2/M peak channel to G0/G1 channel was recorded. Single parameter histograms were used to evaluate the cell cycle.

Interpretation of DNA histograms

Cell cycle evaluation of the DNA histogram was performed by m-cycle computer soft developed by *Peter S. Rabinovitch* (Phoenix Flow Systems, San Diego, CA). Histograms with CVs less than five were accepted for evaluation. Tumors were classified into two groups based on the ploidy status: diploid, when they had a DNA index of 0.99 –1.1, or aneuploid tumor when 10% of the total cell population had a DNA index = 0.99 –1.1. Tumors are considered tetraploid, if >15 % cells had their DNA index = 2 or termed multiploid, if they had multiple aneuploid populations. The cell cycle events were analyzed to determine the synthetic phase fraction (SPF). CA 19-9 was measured by immunoradiometric assay (Centocor, France) [7]; CEA was measured by EIA method (Eurogenetics, USA) [8].

Results

Cut-off values were selected as 5 ng for CEA, 37 U/ml for CA 19-9, 10% and 20% for SPF. In the control group, CEA ranged from 1.2 – 5 ng/ml with a mean value of 1.8 ± 0.1 ng/ml and CA 19-9 ranged from 1.7 – 39.5 U/ml with a mean value of 13.4 ± 2.7 U/ml. In the colorectal cancer patients CEA ranged from 0.5 – 83 ng/ml with a mean

Table I. The relation between studied parameters and TNM staging.

Parameter	TNM stage (n)	
	II (16)	III (12)
CA 19-9 (U/ml)		
mean ± SE[a]	11.3 ± 5	166.6 ± 20.9
positivity[a] (no.)	0% (0)	66.7% (8)
CEA (ng/ml)		
mean ± SE[a]	3.7 ± 0.4	29 ± 5.8
positivity[a] (no.)	25% (4)	75% (9)
CEA + CA 19-9		
positivity (no.)	25% (4)	91.7% (11)
DNA aneuploidy (no.)[a]	43.7% (7)	83.3% (10)
SPF		
> 10% (no.)	50% (8)	75.0% (9)
> 20% (no.)	25% (4)	58.3% (7)

[a] Significant difference between stage II and III at $p < 0.05$

Table II. Relations between venous invasion of the tumor and parameters studied.

Parameter	Venous invasion (n)	
	present (11)	absent (17)
CA 19-9 (U/ml)		
mean ± SE[a]	94.8 ± 20	66.6 ± 13.3
positivity (no.)[a]	63.6% (7)	5.9% (1)
CEA (ng/ml)		
mean ± SE[a]	34.3 ± 6.7	3.7 ± 0.49
positivity (no.)[a]	81.8% (9)	23.5% (4)
CEA + CA 19-9		
positivity (no.)		
DNA aneuploidy	72.7% (8)	52.9% (9)
SPF		
mean ± SE		
> 10 % (no)	72.7% (8)	52.9% (9)
> 20 % (no)[a]	63.6% (7)	23.5% (4)

[a] Significant difference between the two groups at $p < 0.05$

Table III. The relation between Dukes' stage of the tumor and parameters studied.

Parameter	Dukes' stage (n)		
	A (6)	B (10)	C (12)
CA 19-9 (U/ml)			
mean ± SE[a]	4.9 ± 2.50	14.7 ± 1.6	166.6 ± 58.7
positivity (no.)[a]	0% (0)	0% (0)	66.7% (8)
CEA (ng/ml)			
mean ± SE[a]	2.5 ± 0.28	4.4 ± 0.5	29 ± 6.6
positivity (no.)[a]	0 % (0)	40 % (4)	75.0% (9)
CEA + CA 19-9			
positivity (no.)	0 % (0)	40% (4)	91.7% (11)
DNA aneuploidy[a]	33.3 % (2)	50% (5)	83.3% (10)
SPF			
> 10 % (no.)	66.7 % (4)	40% (4)	75% (9)
> 20 % (no.)[a]	0% (0)	40% (4)	58.3% (7)

[a] Significant difference between the three Duke's stages at $p < 0.05$

Table IV. Relations between DNA ploidy of the tumor, its SPF, serum CA 19-9 and CEA.

	Diploid (n = 11)	Non-diploid (n = 17)			
		aneuploid	tetraploid	multiploid	total
CA 19-9 (U/ml)					
mean+SE[a]	27.6 + 18.4	138 + 86.2	39.3 + 33.5	65 + 61.1	112 + 26
positivity (no.)	18.2% (2)	27.3%	33.3%	33.3%	35.3% (6)
CEA (ng/ml)					
mean + SE[a]	4.1 + 0.7	7.8 + 3	5.2 + 2.6	55.1 + 25.3	16.3 + 6.5
positivity	36.4% (4)	36.4%	50%	100%	81.8% (9)
CEA + CA 19-9					
positivity	36.4% (4)	55.6%	100%	100%	81.8% (9)
SPF					
mean + SE[a]	9.5 + 1.1	15.8 + 2.3	5.1 + 1.9	32.3 + 7.5	17.5 + 2.8
> 10 (%)	54.5% (6)	63.6%	50%	100%	64.7% (11)
> 20 (%)	27.3% (3)	36.4%	50%	100%	47.1% (8)

[a] Significant difference between diploid and non-diploid tumors at $p < 0.05$

value of 14.6 ± 4.4 ng/ml and CA 19-9 ranged from 1.7 – 962 U/ml with a mean value of 77.7 ± 35.3 U/ml. The difference was significant at $p < 0.05$ between both groups for both markers. No correlation was found between CEA and CA 19-9 values. The relation between studied parameters, TNM, Dukes' staging and venous invasion of the tumor are shown in tables I,II,III. Histological grading of the tumor was not correlated to any of the parameters studied. Only a significant difference was found between Gr I (grade 1) and Gr III for DNA index ($p < 0.05$). Table IV shows DNA pattern of tumors in relation to CEA, CA 19-9 and SPF.

Discussion

The natural history of colorectal cancer is characterized by great variation in clinical behavior. A most important problem in the management of patients is that of predicting the malignant potential of this neoplasm, especially its potential for local and systemic progression. The classical clinico-pathological variables used to predict prognosis for colorectal cancer patients are subjective, irreproducible and non-quantitative. In recent years a number of studies have investigated the significance of new parameters such as tumor markers, DNA, oncogenes in order to refine the clinico-pathological classification of colorectal cancer.

In evaluating the possible adjunctive value of parameters studied, DNA ploidy, cell cycle, serum CA 19-9 and CEA, we evaluate the possible inter-relationships between these parameters and conventional clinico-pathological findings. The specificity/sensitivity analysis demonstrated, that the sensitivity of CEA is superior to that of CA 19-9 at every specificity, confirming other findings (1). However, the combined assay of both markers increases the sensitivity only in stage III tumors, a result supported by *Safi* et al. (9).

Significant correlations were found between tumor stage (TNM Dukes) and either CEA or CA 19-9 serum levels which agrees with other publications (1, 9, 10, 11, 12, 13, 14). What is stated on the tumor stage applies to its lymph node status. Yet, for the primary tumor (T), the relations were different as CEA does not correlate while CA 19-9 significantly does, a finding reported by others (15). This suggests that CA 19-9 is affected by extramural extension of the tumor while CEA is more sensitive to lymph node spread. Serum CEA and CA 19-9 were dependent on Dukes' stage which is consistent with others (1, 9, 12, 13, 14). Venous invasion was found to correlate with serum CEA. This is keeping with *Tabuchi* and his coworkers, who suggested that serum CEA may be hematogenousely drained by the portal system via draining veins of the tumor (16). No significant relations between the histological grade of the tumor, neither CEA nor CA 19-9 were found, that confirm the previous findings (11).

Abnormal DNA content which reflects abnormal chromosomal rearrangements is frequently associated with an aggressive clinical course in colorectal cancer (3,10). The DNA ploidy pattern was significantly correlated to both TNM and Dukes' staging of the tumor which agrees with *Benner* et al. (17) and disagrees with others (18, 19). On this basis *Benner* and his coworkers hypothesized that the measurement of DNA ploidy on biopsy specimens might provide information regarding the likelihood of tumor spread prior to difinitive surgery. The relation between histological grading, and DNA ploidy revealed a tendency of tumors to have a non-diploid pattern as they become more undifferentiated, a finding supported by others (3, 18, 21).

CEA and CA 19-9 mean values were higher in non-diploid versus diploid tumors. This confirms the previous findings concerning CEA, but for CA 19-9 the correlation has not been reported before (22). Tumors were divided into high or low proliferative tumors dependent on cut-off values chosen for SPF as 10% and 20% (23, 24). Non-diploid tumors with SPF > 10% and > 20% were more frequent than diploid tumors. The relation was similar to that found by others (25).

Strong relations were found between SPF and both Dukes' and venous invasion. The relation between SPF and Dukes has been reported by others but its relation with venous invasion has not been mentioned in the reviewed literature and it indicates that highly proliferative tumors invade the circulation more frequently (26).

The preoperative elevation of CEA alone or in combination with CA 19-9 in non-diploid tumors than diploid tumors may provide information in selecting individuals, who are in need for frequent follow-up by CEA and CA 19-9 after a potentially curative colorectal resection.

References

1 Putzki H, Student A, Jablonski M, Heymann H (1987) Comparison of the tumour markers CEA, TPA, and CA 19-9 in colorectal carcinoma. Cancer 11, 59(2):223–6

2 Darzynkiewicz, Z (1988) Flow cytometry in cytopathology. Analyt Quant Cytol Histol 10(6):459–461

3 Jones DJ, Moore M, Schofield PF (1988) Prognostic significance of DNA ploidy in colorectal cancer prospective flow cytometric study. Br J Surg 75:28–33

4 Krishan, A, Ganapathi, RN, Israel, M (1978) Effect of adriamycin and analogs on the nuclear fluorescence of propidium iodide-stained cells. Cancer Res 38:3656–3662

5 Raber, MN, Barlogis, R (1990) DNA flow cytometry of human solid tumors In: Groten H, Klapdor R (eds) Flow cytometry and sorting. Wiley-Liss, New York, pp 745–754

6. Shapiro, HM (1988) Practical flow cytometry: Parameters and probes. Alan Liss, New York, p 133–148, 164
7. Gold, P, Freedman, SO (1965) Demonstration of tumor-specific antigens in human colonic carcinoma by immunologic tolerance and absorption techniques. J Exp Med, 121:439
8. Del Villano BC, Brennan S, Brock P (1983) Radiometric assay for a monoclonal antibody-defined tumor marker, CA 19-9. Clin Chem 29:549–552
9. Safi F, Bittner R, Beger HG (1986) The signifying value of CA 19-9 compared to CEA in gastric and colorectal carcinoma and their follow-up treatement. In: Groten H, Klapdor R (eds) New tumour associated antigens two year clinical experience with monoclonal antibodies. Thieme, Stuttgart, New York, pp 11–18
10. Dallek M, van Ackeren H, Klapdor R, Klapdor U, Bahlo M, Gereten H, Saeger W (1986) Primary diagnosis and follow up of colorectal and stomach cancer with the tumor associated antigens CEA, CA 19-9 and CA 125 in two year clinical experience with monoclonal antibodies. In: Groten H, Klapdor R (eds) Thieme, Stuttgart, New York, pp 35–42
11. Staab HJ, Brummendorf T, Glock S, Hornung A, Rauskaher V, Anderer FA, Kieninger S (1986) CA 19-9 and CEA in the diagnosis and follow-up of gastrointestinal carcinomas. In: Groten H, Klapdor R (eds) New tumour associated antigens. Two year clinical experience with monoclonal antibodies. Thieme, Stuttgart, pp 19–24
12. Gupta MK, Arciaga R, Bocci L, Tubbs R, Bukowski R, Deodhar SD (1985) Measurement of a monoclonal-antibody-defined antigen (CA 19.9) in the sera of patients with malignant and non malignant diseases. Cancer 56:277–283
13. Lewi H, Blumgart LH, Carter DC, Gillis CR, Hole D, Ratcliffe JG, Wood C, McArdle CS (1984) Preoperative carcinoembryonic antigen and survival in patients with colorectal cancer. Br J Surg 71: 206–208
14. Wanebo HJ, Stearns M, Schwartz MK (1978) Use of CEA as a guide to a selected second look procedure in colorectal cancer. Ann Surg 188:481
15. Durdey P, Williams NS, Brown DA (1984) Serum carcinoemhoryonic antigen and acute phase reactant proteins in the preoperative detection of fixation of colorectal tumors. Br J Surg 71(7): 881–884
16. Tabuchi Y, Deguchi H, Imanishi K, Saitoh Y (1987) Comparison of carcinoembryonic antigen levels between portal and peripheral blood in patients with colorectal cancer. Correlation with histopathologic variables. Cancer 59(7):1283–88
17. Benner BF, De La Vega JET, Roseman DL, Coon JS (1985) Should flow cytometric DNA analysis precede definitive surgery for colon cancer? Ann Surg 202:740–744
18. Quirke P, Dyson JED, Dixon MF, Bird CC, Joslin CAF (1985) Heterogeneity of colorectal adenocarcinoms evaluated by flow cytometry and histopathology. Br J Cancer 51:99–106
19. Koha M, Caspersson T, Wikstrom B, Brismar B (1990) Heterogeneity of DNA distribution pattern in colorectal carcinoma: A microspectrophotometric study of fine needle aspirates. Analyt Quant Cytol Histol 12:348–351
20. Remvikos Y, Muleris M, Vieth Ph, Salmon RJ, Dutrillanx B (1988) DNA content and genetic evolution of human colorectal adenocarcinoma. A study by flow cytometry and cytogenetic analysis. Int J Cancer 42:539–543
21. Bauer KD (1993) Colorectal neoplasia. In: Bauer KD, Duque RE, Shankey TV, Williams, Wilkins (eds) Clinical flow cytometry principles and applications. pp 307–316
22. Kouri M, Pyrohonen S, Mecklin JP, Varvinen H, Laasonen A, Franssila K, Kuusela P, Nordling S (1991) Serum carcinoembryonic antigen and DNA ploidy in colorectal carcinoma. A prospective study. Scand J Gastroenterol 26(8):812–8
23. Witzing TE, Loprinzi CL, Gonchoroff NJ (1991) DNA ploidy and cell kinetic measurements as predictors of recurrence and survival in stages B2 and C colorectal adenocarcinoma. Cancer (68):879–88
24. Joennsuu H, Klemi PJ, Eerola E (1988) Flow cytometric DNA analysis combined with fine needle aspiration biopsy in the diagnosis of palpable metastases. Analyt Quant Cytol Histol 1(4):256–260
25. Kallioniemi OP, Blanco G, Alavaikko M, Hietanen T, Mattila J, Lauslahti K, Lehtinen M, Koivula T (1988) Improving the prognostic value of DNA flow cytometry in breast cancer by combining DNA index and s-phase fraction. Cancer (62):2183–2190
26. Temple WJ, Sugarbaker EV, Thomthwaite JT, Henstey GT, Ketcham AS (1980) Correlation of cell cycle analysis with Dukes' staging in colon cancer patients. J Surg Res 28:314–318

Address for correspondence:
Prof. Dr. A. Khalifa
Oncology Diagnostic Unit
Ain-Shams Faculty of Medicine
ET-Abbassia, Cairo, Egypt

Comparison of the tumor markers CA 19-9 and CEA for follow-up of patients with gastrointestinal cancer

I. Jaunalksne, S. Donina, G. Zakenfelds, V. Januskevics, A. Svarcbergs

Institute of Experimental Clinical Medicine, Riga, Latvia

Introduction

Carcinoembrionic antigen (CEA) and carbohydrate antigen (CA 19-9) are generally accepted as tumor markers and have been used to monitor gastrointestinal cancer (1, 2, 4). None of these markers, however, is tumor specific, but not all cancer patients have elevated serum levels of CEA or CA 19-9 (3).

Materials and methods

In order to asses the diagnostic sensitivity of the tumor markers CEA and CA19-9 as well as their combination 200 patients with histologically proven gastrointestinal carcinomas before surgical treatment were investigated: 123 patients with gastric cancer and 77 with colorectal cancer (52 from these 77 with rectal cancer). The investigations were carried out during 1989–1992 in Latvian Oncological Center. Patients were distributed according to TNM classification (5) on the stages of the disease. Gastric cancer patients: 1 stage 14; 2 stage 23; 3 stage 30; 4 stage 56; colorectal cancer patients: 1 stage 18; 2 stage 23; 3 stage 23; 4 stage 13. Follow-up serial determinations were carried out in 103 patients in postoperative period every three months with an average follow-up time of 18 months and the data were correlated with clinical findings.

CEA and CA 19-9 were determined in patient sera by enzyme immuno-assay using kits from Hoffman La Roche, Switzerland. As cut-off values we used for CEA 5 ng/ml, for CA 19-9 35 U/ml.

Results and discussion

The incidence of gastric cancer patients with CEA (above 5 ng/ml) and CA 19-9 (above 35 U/ml) arises as malignant process vasted. The percentage of gastric cancer patients with elevated levels of CEA ranged from 15–52% and with elevated CA 19-9 fluctuated from 15 to 42% (table I).

In CEA negative patients (under 5 ng/ml) the percentage of patients with CA 19-9 above 35 U/ml increases with disease stage, it ranges from 18 to 48% (figure 1). In the patient group with elevated CEA levels (above 5 ng/ml) the incidence of CA 19-9 positive gastric cancer patients increases with stage, it ranged from 20–46% (figure 1). It means that with elevation of CEA level the incidence of CA 19-9 positive gastric cancer patients increases. This is shown in figure 2.

The diagnostic sensitivity of CEA is 36.5% and for CA 19-9 50.6%. When both markers are used the sensitivity increases to 71.4%. Analysis of these data allow to conclude, that elevation of serum CA 19-9 level is a sign of a vasting process and it is the marker of first choice for gastric cancer.

If the gastric cancer patients depending on the stage of disease were CEA positive (> 5 ng/ml) in 15 – 52%, in colorectal cancer patients it ranged from 21 to 62%, especially patients with rectal cancer have CEA levels of 33–63%. The elevated level of CA 19-9 was found in 20–45% colorectal cancer patients depending on the stage of disease (table I).

Nevertheless the colorectal cancer patients with CEA concentrations below the cut-off value have elevated CA 19-9 levels from 18–40%, depending on the stage of disease (figure 3).

Patients with rectal cancer have a higher incidence of pathological values of 28–60%. 25–63% of the patients with CEA values above the cut-off have elevated CA 19-9 serum levels depending on the stage of the disease (figure 3). Concentration of CA 19-9 augments with increasing CEA serum levels. CA 19-9 level may serve as indicator of advanced disease (figure 4).

Table I. Changes of CEA and CA 19-9 concentration of gastric and colorectal cancer patients in dependence of disease stage.

Tumor marker	Tumor localization	Stage I	Stage II	Stage III	Stage IV
CEA ng/ml					
≤5	gastric cancer	85%	78%	68.9%	48.2%
	colorectal cancer	77.9%	65.3%	47.8%	38.4%
>5	gastric cancer	15%	22%	31.1%	51.8%
	colorectal cancer	22.1%	34.7%	52.2%	61.6%
CA 19-9 U/ml					
<10	gastric cancer	69%	45.5%	32%	46.6%
	colorectal cancer	33.4%	23.8%	30%	56%
10-35	gastric cancer	15.5%	40.9%	28%	11.1%
	colorectal cancer	46.6%	38%	25%	0%
>35	gastric cancer	15.5%	13.6%	40%	42.3%
	colorectal cancer	20%	38%	45%	44%

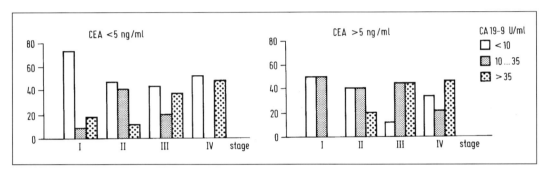

Figure 1. Distribution of serum CA 19-9 values of gastric cancer patients in dependence of disease stage.

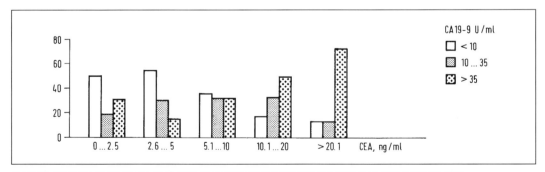

Figure 2. Changes of serum CA 19-9 level of gastric cancer patients depending on CEA concentration.

The diagnostic sensitivity of CEA for colorectal cancer patients was 41.5 % and for CA 19-9 36%. If both markers are used sensitivity increases for colorectal cancer patients up to 81.5%. The analysis of these data allow us to conclude, that CEA is a marker of first choice for colorectal cancer. The complementary assay of CA 19-9 antigen level gives additive information.

Follow-up serial determinations of CEA and CA 19-9 give better chance to choice one elevated marker during the preoperative period for monitoring the course of disease during the postoperative period. Progression of disease in gastric cancer patients is more expressed and connected with CA 19-9 level above 35 > U/ml during the preoperative period as it is in colorec-

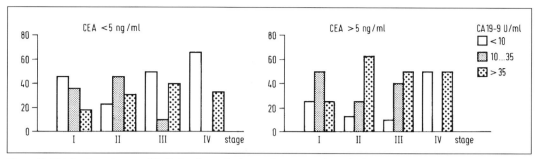

Figure 3. Distribution of serum CA 19-9 values of colorectal cancer patients in dependence of disease stage.

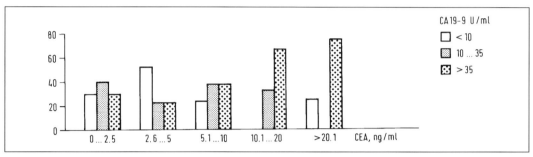

Figure 4. Changes of serum CA 19-9 level of colorectal cancer patients depending on CEA concentration.

tal cancer patients with CEA level above 5 ng/ml. Our conclusions agree with authors, who found CA 19-9 for gastric cancer to reveal a sensitivity comparable or slightly superior to CEA (2). In colorectal cancer CA 19-9 represents a tumor marker comparable to or slightly less relevant than CEA (4). In cases of gastric and colorectal cancer simultaneous determination of CA 19-9 in addition to CEA results in an increase of sensitivity of about 5–10% (3).

Conclusion

CA 19-9 is the marker of first choice for gastric cancer. CEA is the marker for first choice for colorectal cancer. Complementary assay of both raise the diagnostic sensitivity. In patients without elevation of CEA, the elevation of CA 19-9 allows to predict recurrence or metastases. High values of preoperative CA 19-9 levels may serve as indicators of advanced disease.

References

1. Klapdor R (1990) Markers for tumors of the gastrointestinal tract. In: Workshop Report-Enzymun-Test CA19-9. Berlin, April 23rd, 24th p 3–15
2. Klapdor R (1988) Stellenwert der Tumormarker bei der Früherkennung gastrointestinaler Tumoren. Verh Dtsch Ges Inn Med 94:29–40
3. Schelling M, Schmid L, Senekowitsch R et al (1990) First experience with CA195 in gastrointestinal carcinomas compared to CA 19-9 and CEA. In: Klapdor R (ed) Recent results in tumor diagnosis and therapy. Zuckschwerdt, München, Bern, Wien, San Francisco, pp 37–42
4. Staab HI, Hornung A, Anderer FA et al (1984) Klinische Bedeutung des zirkulierenden tumorassoziierten Antigens CA19-9 bei Karzinomen des Verdauungstraktes. Dtsch med Wschr 109: 1141–1147
5. TNM classification of malignant tumors. (1989) Blinova NA (ed) Health Ministry of USSR, Moscow, p 131

Address for correspondence:
Dr. I. Jaunalksne
Institute of Experimental Clinical Medicine
4,0 Vaciesha Str.
LV-1004 Riga, Latvia

Significance of neuron-specific enolase (NSE) as a tumor marker in the diagnosis and follow-up of surgical patients with abdominal neuroendocrine tumors

U. Meyer-Pannwitt[a], V. A. Dorß[a,1], G. Fröschle[a], R. Klapdor[b], H. W. Schreiber[a]

[a]Division of General Surgery, [b]Department of Medicine, University of Hamburg, Germany

Introduction

Abdominal neuroendocrine tumors consist mainly of endocrine pancreatic and gastrointestinal carcinoid tumors. Patients with these relatively rare malignancies often have long and unusual clinical courses that challenge surgeons, internists, and pathologists (1).

Neuron-specific enolase (NSE) is a glycolytic enzyme found in the cytoplasm of both nerve cells and neuroendocrine cells of various organs. Tumors derived from these cells produce large amounts of NSE that can be measured in serum by radioimmunoassay (RIA) (2). In small-cell lung cancer, NSE was found to have a stage-dependent sensitivity of about 40 to 80 percent (3). Most investigators judged serum NSE measurements to be a useful tool for monitoring therapy and predicting survival (4, 5). By contrast, only a few studies of serum NSE in patients with abdominal neuroendocrine tumors have been conducted, with conflicting results (6, 7, 8, 9, 10, 11). Therefore, the significance of NSE serum measurements in the diagnosis and particularly in the long-term follow-up of patients with these tumors demands further investigation.

At our institution, serial serum samples from patients with abdominal neuroendocrine tumors treated for many years were collected and stored frozen. In this study, the disease courses of the patients were analyzed, and NSE was measured in the sera by RIA. The aim of this retrospective study was to compare the clinical courses with the NSE concentrations at the time of diagnosis, during various forms of treatment, and as the disease progressed.

Patients and methods

Patients with endocrine pancreatic and gastrointestinal carcinoid tumors were eligible for this study if their hospital charts could be reviewed and if frozen serum samples were available for NSE measurements.

Serum had been stored at −68 °C and −20 °C. NSE was measured by radioimmunoassay using the Pharmacia NSE-RIA kit (Pharmacia AB, Uppsala, Sweden). Visibly hemolytic serum was not used. Sensitivity calculations were based on a cut-off value of 12.5 µg/l, as stated by the manufacturer and used by most investigators (12, 13).

Results

Patient characteristics and disease course

22 patients with abdominal neuroendocrine tumors were studied retrospectively (12 male, 10 female). At the time of diagnosis, they were 20 to 77 years old (mean: 51.8 years). Table I shows the diagnoses in detail.

At the initial diagnosis, which was made between 1970 and 1989, eleven patients already had lymph node or liver metastases. From seven months to 17 years later (median 19 months), metastatic disease was diagnosed in seven additional patients. The liver was the most frequent site of metastasis (17 cases), followed by mesenteric and paraaortic lymph nodes (eight cases) and peritoneal dissemination (two cases). One patient with multiple endocrine neoplasia (MEN), type I, had Zollinger-Ellison syndrome in

---

[1]Formerly Division of General Surgery, University of Hamburg, now Department of Anesthesiology, General Hospital Barmbek, Hamburg.

Table I. Diagnoses of abdominal neuroendocrine tumors.

Endocrine pancreatic carcinoma	11
not hormone producing	6
hormone producing	5
insulinoma, metastatic	4
glucagonoma, metastatic	1
Carcinoid tumor	10
ileum, metastatic	4
stomach, not metastatic	3
coecum, metastatic	2
duodenal papilla, metastatic	1
Gastrinoma	1
duodenum, metastatic	

addition to multiple gastric carcinoid tumors. The patient with the gastrinoma also had serotonin overproduction and many features of the carcinoid syndrome.

Eight patients required surgical exploration for definitive diagnosis of the tumor. All ten tumor specimens that were analyzed for NSE by immunohistology were strongly positive. Serum assays for other tumor markers were mostly negative throughout the entire disease course: CEA, CA 19-9, CA 125, and AFP were normal in 84, 81, 75, and 72 percent of the patients, respectively. All patients with hormone producing tumors had elevated blood hormone levels that also reflected tumor growth and response to therapy. Largely the same was true of the urinary excretion of 5-hydroxy-indoleacetic acid (5-HIAA) in patients with disseminated carcinoid tumors and the carcinoid syndrome (figure 6).

Treatment was predominantly surgical. Eighteen patients underwent at least one laparotomy and 12 had tumor resections for cure. Palliative operations were also frequent, and five patients were reoperated because of surgical complications. There was one postoperative fatality. Chemotherapy was mostly based on fluorouracil (5-FU) plus streptozocin, among other agents. Seven patients were treated with somatostatin or its long-acting analogue, octreotide. Cytotoxic and hormone therapy resulted in temporary control of symptoms caused by excessive hormone secretion. Eight patients had up to four embolizations each of hepatic metastases, with temporary improvement of symptoms.

Even with metastatic tumors, a large proportion of patients survived for several years (up to 17) with relatively few and mild symptoms.

NSE in the diagnosis and during follow-up

NSE was measured in 217 serum samples drawn at the time of the initial diagnosis or during follow-up from 1982 until 1990. Per patient up to 28 samples collected during up to six years were analyzed. An additional large number of serum samples was analyzed that had been drawn

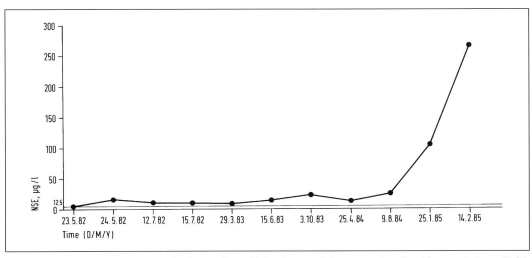

Figure 1. Serial serum NSE concentration in a patient with insulinoma of the pancreatic tail and liver metastases (H.S.). Despite chemotherapy with 5-FU and streptozocin that led to improvement of symptoms, at autopsy the liver was largely replaced by metastases and weighed 12.5 kg. In this case the serum NSE appears to reflect the disease course.

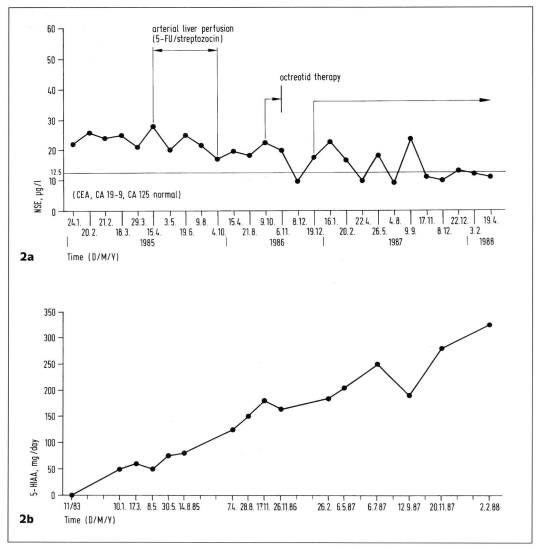

Figure 2a, b. Serum NSE (upper panel) and urinary excretion of 5-HIAA (lower panel) in a patient with metastatic carcinoid tumor of the coecum (H.Mö.). NSE reduction is seen during cytotoxic arterial perfusion of the liver, normalization during octreotide therapy, with relief of symptoms. The urinary excretion of 5-HIAA, however, is continuously rising and reflects the continuously growing liver metastases that finally replace almost the entire liver.

during and shortly after embolizations of liver metastases.
At diagnosis, eight of 16 patients had NSE concentrations above 12.5 µg/l, which equals a sensitivity of 50 percent. Three exceeded 25 µg/l. Five of the eight patients with initial NSE elevations already had metastatic disease. Two additional patients, one of which had undergone high-dose chemo- and radiation therapy for suspected inoperable adenocarcinoma, had borderline NSE concentrations.
During the following clinical course, 14 of 17 patients with metastases (82 percent) had NSE concentrations above 12.5 µg/l, ten patients (59 percent) exceeded 25 µg/l. The percentage numbers of patients with endocrine pancreatic cancer did not differ substantially from those with gastrointestinal carcinoids. All three patients that

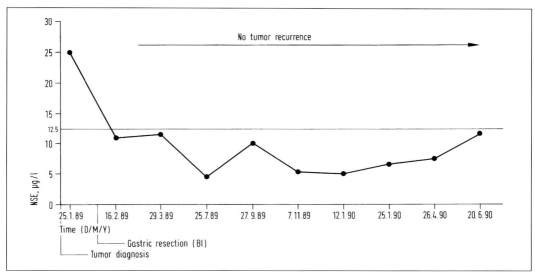

Figure 3. Serum NSE in a patient with a gastric carcinoid tumor before and after gastric resection (H.D.). There is a postoperative normalization that lasts while the patient remains tumor-free.

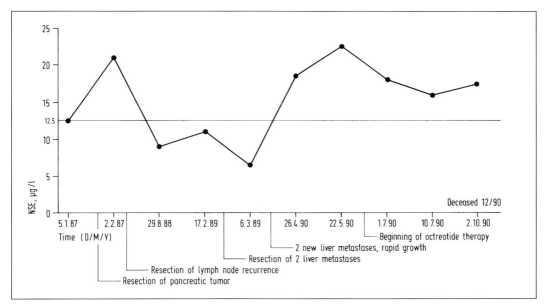

Figure 4. Serum NSE in a patient with metastatic endocrine pancreatic carcinoma without hormone production (H.M.) A lymph node recurrence and – later – two liver metastases are diagnosed and resected while NSE stays normal. Later, newly diagnosed liver metastases that grow rapidly are accompanied by rising serum NSE.

remained tumor-free after therapy had normal posttherapeutic NSE concentrations. NSE was also normal in the patient with MEN type I syndrome. Two patients with the largest metastatic tumor burden reached the highest NSE concentrations (> 200 µg/l; figure 1). In spite of this, there was no clear correlation between the NSE concentration and the tumor size or the extent of metastases as measured by ultrasound, computed tomography, or at autopsy. For instance, in four

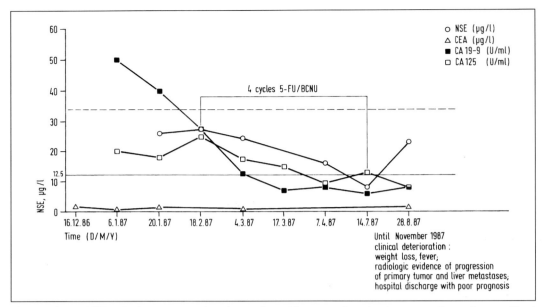

Figure 5. Serum NSE and other tumor markers in a patient with metastatic endocrine pancreatic carcinoma without hormone production undergoing chemotherapy (W.K.). NSE and CA 19-9 are elevated initially and become normal. After conclusion of therapy, there is further tumor progression and clinical deterioration of the patient, while NSE rises again.

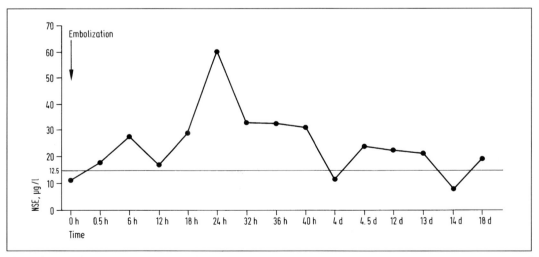

Figure 6a. Transient increase of serum NSE in a patient with metastatic insulinoma (G.W.) following embolization of the left liver lobe. There was improvement of hypoglycemic symptoms.

patients who survived for several years while their liver metastases were growing very slowly or not at all, NSE concentrations in serum decreased intermittently or even normalized (figure 2a,b).

After complete resection of the tumor, three patients with preoperative NSE elevations and one patient with a borderline NSE concentration had normal NSE concentrations or a significant reduction, respectively (figure 3). NSE was again

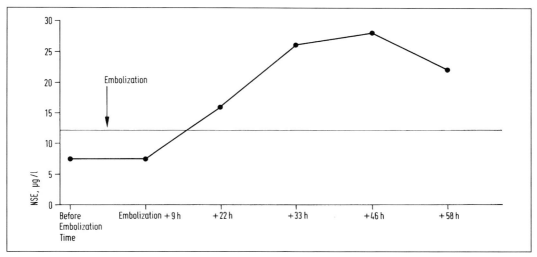

Figure 6b. Serum NSE in a patient with endocrine pancreatic carcinoma without hormone production (E.B.). The course shows a temporarily rising NSE concentration after embolization of liver metastases.

elevated when a tumor recurrence was diagnosed. Increasing serum NSE concentrations were often coincidental with clinical deterioration and rapid tumor growth detected by imaging techniques. Many of these patients succumbed to their disease only weeks or months later (figures 4 and 5). Effective chemotherapy and treatment with octreotide resulted in falling NSE concentrations (figure 2, 4) that rose again after termination of treatment (figures 4).

During 6 chemo-embolizations of liver metastases by interventional radiology, we were able to monitor closely short-term changes of the NSE serum concentration. Six to 48 hours after successful embolization, sharp increases were seen (up to 1500 µg/l), occasionally with multiple peaks (figure 6a, b). Other tumor markers, such as CEA or CA 19-9, did not change significantly. Within a few days, the NSE concentration returned to normal or the pretreatment level, respectively.

Discussion

In this retrospective study, the long-term clinical course of 22 surgical patients with abdominal neuroendocrine tumors was compared with serial serum measurements of the neuroendocrine tumor marker neuron-specific enolase (NSE). Sensitivities of about 50 percent at diagnosis and more than 80 percent during follow-up of patients with metastatic disease were found. Thus, NSE seems to be as sensitive in these tumors as it is in small-cell lung cancer.

There was a clear response to therapy, with complete tumor resection leading to normalization, and chemo- or octreotide treatment resulting in significant reductions or normalizations of the serum level. Rising NSE levels during or shortly after therapy indicated a poor prognosis in individual patients.

There appears to be no reliable correlation between the serum NSE concentration and the amount of tumor present. However, if there is high proliferative activity of tumor cells, such as when new metastases develop or when the primary tumor and its metastases start to grow rapidly, or when tumor tissue becomes necrotic for other reasons, the serum NSE concentration rises.

We conclude that NSE may indeed be a useful serum tumor marker in patients with abdominal neuroendocrine tumors.

Measuring serum NSE may be worthwhile under the following circumstances: 1. a neuroendocrine abdominal tumor is suspected, 2. during follow-up of patients with endocrine pancreatic and gastrointestinal carcinoid tumors, especially if there are no elevated hormone or 5-HIAA levels to monitor, 3. for monitoring cytotoxic and octreotide therapy, and particularly after embolization of liver metastases.

References

1. Moertel CG. (1989) Approach to the management of carcinoid tumors and islet cell cancer. In: Kelley WN (ed) Textbook of Internal Medicine. 1st ed Philadelphia J.B. Li ppincott, pp 1285–1291
2. Tapia EJ, Polak JM, Barbosa AJA, Bloom SR et al (1981) Neuron-specific enolase is produced by neuroendocrine tumours. Lancet 1:808–811
3. Carney DN, Marangos PJ, Ihde DC, Bunn PA, Cohen MH, Minna JD, Gazdar AF (1982) Serum neuron-specific enolase: a marker for disease extent and response to therapy of small cell lung cancer. Lancet 1:583–585
4. Fischbach W, Jany B (1986) Neuron-specific enolase in the diagnosis and therapy monitoring of lung cancer: A comparison with CEA, TPA, ferritin and calcitonin. Int J Biol Markers 3:129–136.
5. Nöu E, Steinholtz L, Bergh J, Nilsson K, Pahlman S (1990) Neuron-specific enolase as a follow-up marker in small cell bronchial carcinoma. A prospective study in an unselected series. Cancer 65(6):1380–1385.
6. Prinz RA, Marangos PJ (1982) Use of neuron-specific enolase as a serum marker for neuroendocrine neoplasms. Surgery 92:887–889.
7. Prinz RA, Bermes EW, Kimmel JR, Marangos PJ (1983) Serum markers for pancreatic islet cell and intestinal carcinoid tumors: a comparison of neuron-specific enolase, β-human chorionic gonadotropin and pancreatic polypeptide. Surgery 94(6):1019–1023.
8. Prinz RA, Marangos PJ (1983) Serum neuron-specific enolase: a serum marker for nonfunctioning pancreatic islet cell carcinoma. Am J Surg 145:77–81.
9. Fischbach W, Jany B, Nelkenstock R (1986) Bedeutung der neuronspezifischen Enolase (NSE) in der Diagnostik von Bronchialkarzinomen und neuroendokrinen Tumoren. Dtsch med Wochenschr 111:1722–1725.
10. Cunningham RT, Johnston CF, Irvine GB, Buchanan KD (1992) Serum neuronespecific enolase levels in patients with neuroendocrine and carcinoid tumours. Clin Chim Acta 212(3):123–131.
11. D'Alessandro M, Mariani P, Lomanto D, Carlei F, Lezoche E, Speranza V (1992) Serum neuron-specific enolase in diagnosis and follow-up of gastrointestinal neuroendocrine tumors. Tumour Biol 13(56):352–357
12. Pharmacia Diagnostics (1988) Instruction manual Pharmacia NSE RIA, Pharmacia Diagnostics AB, Uppsala, Sweden, 3:17–23
13. Cooper EH, Splinter TAW, Brown DA, Muers MF, Peake MD, Pearson SL (1985) Evaluation of a radioimmunoassay for neuron specific enolase in small cell lung cancer. Br J Cancer 52:333–338

Address for correspondence:
Dr. med. U. Meyer-Pannwitt
Chirurgische Universitätsklinik
Martinistraße 52
D-20246 Hamburg, Germany

CYFRA 21-1 serum determination: Which utility in the diagnosis of gastrointestinal tumors?

M. Plebani[a], F. Navaglia[a], D. Basso[a], M. De Paoli[a], L. Bortolotti[b], A. Cipriani[c]

[a]Department of Laboratory Medicine, [b]Department of Surgery,
[c]Department of Pneumology, University-Hospital, Padova, Italy

Introduction

Cytokeratins, biochemically related to intermediate fragments (IF), form an intracellular network of filaments which is belived to provide an important structural role in the integrity of the cell (1). Cytokeratins 8, 18 and 19 are the most abundant cytokeratins in carcinomas (2). They are released into necrotic areas and can be found intratumorally and in the blood, circulating as partially degraded complexes and as such can be used as tumor markers (3). A fragment of cytokeratin 19, refered as CYFRA 21-1, can now be detected in serum by immunological methods (immunoradiometric or enzyme immuno-assays) based on the use of two mouse monoclonal antibodies. This serum determination has been suggested as useful diagnostic and prognostic marker of squamous cell carcinoma of the lung (4).

The aims of this study were therefore: 1. to assess the diagnostic usefulness of CYFRA 21-1 in evaluating gastric and colon cancers in comparison with lung cancers, 2. to ascertain the CYFRA 21-1 discriminatory capacity towards benign conditions which may enter in the differential diagnosis with colon, gastric and lung cancers, and 3. to ascertain whether renal and/or liver function and inflammatory disease may influence circulating CYFRA 21-1 levels in serum.

Materials and methods

We studied a total of 252 subjects, ninety-one (40 males, 51 females, age range 21–82 years) serve as controls; twenty-five (20 males and 5 females, age range 42–75 years) were patients with lung cancer. Of them, 17 had squamous cell carcinoma, six had adenocarcinoma and two had small cell carcinoma. The staging was: stage I = 43%, stage II = 19%, stage III = 14% and stage IV = 24%. Nineteen patients (10 males, 9 females, age range 47–79) had gastric cancer without metastases, twenty patients (10 males, 10 females, age range 38–70 years) had colon cancer. Of these, six had liver metastases and eight had lymph node involvement. 37 patients with benign lung disease (22 males, 15 females, age range 19–73 years), 27 patients with peptic ulcer (17 males, 10 females, age range 19–66 years) and 34 patients with other gastrointestinal disease (17 males, 17 females, age range 21–68 years) were also investigated. A serum sample was obtained from each subject after overnight fasting. The sera were kept at −80 °C for no more than one month until the biochemical determination.

CYFRA 21-1 was assayed using an ELISA method (Boehringer Mannheim, Italia). Results were expressed as mg/l. Statistical analysis was performed using the analysis of variance (ANOVA one-way), Bonferroni's test for pairwise comparison, and receiver operating characteristic (ROC) curves.

Results

Figure 1 illustrates the individual values of CYFRA 21-1 in the material studied. The continuous line represents the cut-off value calculated by means of mean + 2 standard deviation of our controls (1.7 mg/l). The mean value of the patients with lung cancer (5.42, SD 8.74 mg/l) was higher than that of all the other groups.

Figure 2 illustrates the results of ROC curves for CYFRA 21-1 in discriminating patients with lung

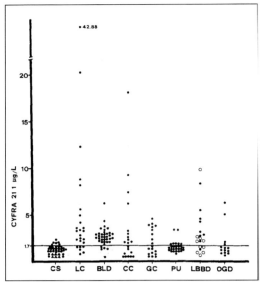

Figure 1. Individual serum values of CYFRA 21-1 in the material studied. CS = control subjects; LC = lung cancer; BLD = benign lung disease; CC = colon cancer; GC = gastric cancer; PU = peptic ulcer; LBBD = liver and biliary (open dots) benign diseases; OGD = other gastrointestinal benign diseases. Each triangle represents 10 CS. The continuous line represents the upper normal limit calculated by mean + 2 standard deviation of our CS (ANOVA: F = 7.78, p < 0.001).

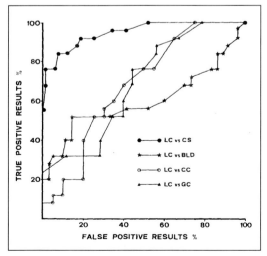

Figure 2. Receiver operating characteristic (ROC) curves in discriminating patients with lung cancer (LC) from control subjects (CS), patients with benign lung diseases (BLD), with colon cancer (CC) and with gastric cancer (GC).

cancer from those with gastric or colon cancer, patients with benign lung diseases and controls. The best discriminant value between lung cancer and controls was 1.7 mg/l, while it was 3.2 mg/l between lung cancer and benign lung disease (sensitivity = 52%, specificity = 86%). Considering the first cut-off, the sensitivity of CYFRA 21-1 in diagnosing colon cancer (CC), gastric cancer (GC) and lung cancer (LC) was 55%, 50% and 76%, respectively. With the same cut-off the specificity towards benign gastrointestinal diseases (BGID) and peptic ulcer (PU) was 80% and 70%, respectively. In patients with CC, GC, and LC, CYFRA 21-1 levels vary neither in relation to tumor stage nor in relation to tumor grading. Considering the patients all together, CYFRA 21-1 levels correlated with serum bilirubin ($r = 0.177$, $p < 0.05$), gamma-glutamyltranspeptidase ($r = 0.593$, $p < 0.001$) and inversely with serum albumin ($r = -0.219$, $p < 0.05$). Moreover, CYFRA 21-1 correlated with circulating C-reactive protein ($r = 0.458$, $p < 0.001$).

Discussion

CYFRA 21-1 is a fragment of cytokeratin 19, which is present in normal epithelial cells as well as in malignant cells of epithelial origin (5). The ELISA technique based on two different monoclonal antibodies is able to detect the serum fragment of cytokeratin subunit 19 with both, sensitivity and specificity (4). Higher levels of CYFRA 21-1 were found in lung cancer than in other pathological conditions, whether benign or malignant. High levels of CYFRA 21-1 were also found in patients with colon cancer and with hepatobiliary diseases, but not in patients with gastric cancer. These results probably reflect the normal tissue distribution of cytokeratin 19, which is well represented in normal lung, colon mucosa and bile duct epithelia, but only weakly in stomach epithelial wall (5). The thresholds of 1.7 and 3.2 mg/l determined using the ROC curve analysis were found to give the maximal accuracy in discriminating lung cancer patients from controls and from patients with benign lung disease, respectively. In particular for lung cancer, when using a cut-off value of 3.2 mg/l instead of 1.7 mg/l, a slight decrease in sensitivity was observed; however, specificities towards benign lung diseases and gastric or colon cancer significantly increased. The limit of 3.2 mg/l may therefore be useful in the assessment of lung cancer patients. The sensitivity of CYFRA 21-1 in diagnosing gastric or colon cancer was invariably too low to consider this marker as useful index in the assessment of these two neoplasias. We found significant correlations between serum levels of CYFRA 21-1 and some indices of cholestasis. We may therefore suggest that CYFRA 21-1 undergoes liver metabolism and that cholestasis may reduce its hepatic clearance and may induce an augmented release of the fragment from ductular epithelial cells. Finally, a relation was found between CYFRA 21-1 and C-reactive protein, suggesting that the presence of inflammation may contribute to favoring cytokeratin fragment release from damaged epithelial cells.

Conclusion

CYFRA 21-1 does not seem to possess a sensitivity and specificity high enough to be proposed for the diagnosis of colon and gastric cancer. Considering a cut-off level of 3.2 mg/l it may be of some utility in discriminating benign from malignant lung diseases. Liver disfunction and cholestasis can influence the serum levels of this substance, probably because it undergoes an altered liver metabolism; moreover, the presence of inflammatory reaction can enhance CYFRA 21-1 circulating levels. Further studies are necessary to evaluate the clinical usefulness of CYFRA 21-1 measurement in monitoring of patients with lung cancer.

References

1 Lazarides E (1980) Intermediate filaments as mechanical integrators of cellular space. Nature 283:249–256
2 Moll R, Franke W, Schiller DL, Geiger B, Krepler R (1982) The catalog of human cytokeratins: patterns of expression in normal epithelia, tumors and cultured cells. Cell 31:11–24
3 Sun T-T, Eichner R, Nelson WG, Tseng SCG, Weiss RA, Jarvinen M, Woodcock-Mitchell J (1983) Keratin classes: molecular markers for different types of epithelial differentiation. J Invest Dermatol 81:109s–115s.
4 Pujol J-L, Grenier J, Daures J-P, Daver A, Pujol H, Michel F-B (1993) Serum fragment of cytokeratin subunit 19 measured by CYFRA 21-1 immunoradiometric assay as a marker of lung cancer. Cancer Res 53:61–66
5 Kasper M, Stosiek P, Typlt H, Karsten U (1987) Histological evaluation of three new monoclonal anti-cytokeratin antibodies. 1. Normal tissues. Eur J Cancer Res Clin Oncol 23:137–147

Address for correspondence:
Dr. med. M. Plebani
Istituto di Medicina di Laboratorio
Laboratorio Centrale
Via Giustiniani
I-2-35128 Padova, Italy

Comparison of two assays (TPA and TPS) for cytokeratin polypeptides in serum using three different patient groups and in healthy subjects

L.-O Hansson

Department of Clinical Chemistry, Karolinska Hospital, Stockholm, Sweden

Introduction

The cytokeratins (CK) belong to the intermediate filaments of cytoplasmatic structural components, a group of 10 nm rope-like polymeric proteins. The cytokeratins are found in epithelial cells. At least 19–20 different but biochemically and immunologically related proteins belong to the cytokeratin-family (figure 1).
The polyclonal antibody used in the TPA Prolifigen IRMA kit (Sangtec) is immunologically related to the type II cytokeratins 8, 18 and 19, while the monoclonal TPS IRMA kit (BEKI) is related only to epitope M3, on the probably – as tumor marker – less important cytokeratin 18 (figure 1: 18), especially in e.g. lung cancer. There seems to be a unique cytokeratin combination, regarding type and amount, in different types of epithelia. These differences are both a challenge and a possibility when using cytokeratins as tumor markers. The most common cytokeratins in tumors are CK 7, 8, 18 and 19.

Methods

We have compared the original polyclonal Prolifigen TPA IRMA kit with the monoclonal TPS kit using serum samples from healthy subjects (50 men and 36 women) and from patients with three different types of tumors (colorectal n = 30, ovarian n = 30, and prostatic n = 43).

Results

When comparing the TPA and TPS kits using samples from healthy subjects we found significantly lower values for TPS compared to TPA even though the range of the values was much wider for the TPS assay, especially for the subjects with the 20% highest values (figure 2 and table II). The wider range (27.6 – 92.3) and larger SD for the TPS results on healthy subjects can eventually cause problems regarding the cut-off between the healthy subjects and patients with cancer.
The results of the different comparisons using samples from patients with different malignant diseases are presented in the following figures

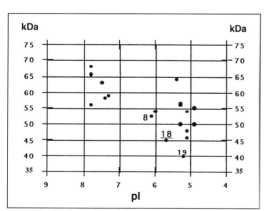

Figure 1. Cytokeratin molecular mass in relation to pl.

Table I. Cytokeratin expression by some epithelial carcinomas.

Epithelia	Cytokeratin					
Breast		7	8		18	19
Colorectal			8		18	19
Lung		7	8		18	19
Ovaries		7	8		18	19
Prostate	5	7	8		18	19
Urinary bladder	5	7	8	13	17	18	19

Table II. Results for TPS and TPA in healthy controls and cancer patients.

	Regression equation	R	TPA, mean ± SD (range) U/l	TPS, mean ± SD (range) U/l	TPA median	TPS median
Healthy subjects	y = 3.09x – 115.8	0.62	47.6 ± 1.7 (45.8 – 58.0)	32.0 ± 10.2 (27.6 – 92.3)	47.2	29.0
Colorectal	y = 1.58x – 36.1	0.89	253.4 ± 255.5 (24.1 – 957)	318.6 ± 406.2 (21.9 – 1367)	179.7	46.3
Ovarian	y = 0.54x + 51.2	0.48	205.5 ± 282.0 (24.6 – 957)	156.9 ± 307.8 (23.6 – 1448)	90.8	28.5
Prostatic	y = 2.64x + 103.5	0.73	169.6 ± 306.7 (21.7 – 1664)	629.9 ± 925.4 (37.3 – 3000)	53.9	218.5

TPS(y) = slope · TPA(x) + intercept

Table III. Inserted TPA and TPS calibrators and control samples assayed with the opposite kit; x = assigned value, y = assayed value.

Samples	Assay used	Regression	r^2
TPA controls	TPS IRMA	y = 0.654x + 489.4	two samples
TPS controls	TPA IRMA	y = 0.480x + 7.7	two samples
TPA calibrators	TPS IRMA	y = 1.57x + 61.57	0.999
TPS IRMA calibrators	TPA IRMA	y = 0.465x + 20.78	1.0

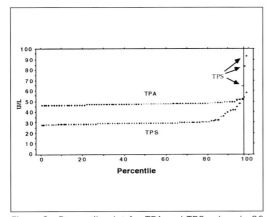

Figure 2. Percentile plot for TPA and TPS values in 86 healthy subjects.

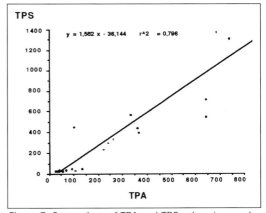

Figure 3. Comparison of TPA and TPS values in samples from patients with colorectal cancer.

(figures 3–5) and summarized in table II. From these figures and the results of the correlation studies with different study groups using the TPA and TPS assays it is evident that there are significant differences concerning the two assays, and that information collected using the TPA assay can not be transformed to clinical evaluations using the TPS kit even, though both tests are related to cytokeratins. The TPA kit generally measures higher values in patients with ovarian cancer while the TPS kit reveales higher values especially in prostatic carcinoma but also in colorectal carcinoma. The discrepancy regarding the mean and median values for TPS in patients with colorectal

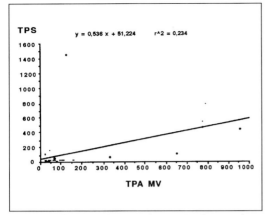

Figure 4. TPA and TPS values in samples from patients with ovarian cancer.

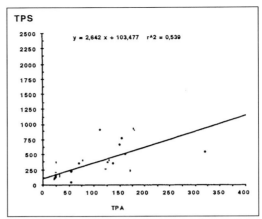

Figure 5. TPA and TPS values in samples from patients with prostatic cancer.

cancer results from the fact that more than 50% of these patients had relatively low TPS values and some patients had very high values. No information concerning the diagnostic value of the two assays can be drawn from the present study.
In this study we have also analyzed the different calibrators and control samples supplied in the respective kit with the opposite kit. These results are summarized in table III.

Conclusions

To be able to explain these obtained differences three important factors have to be considered: 1. the patient-samples investigated, 2. the calibrators, and 3. the antibodies used.
In this study using two different tests reacting with cytokeratins, the differences probably depend on the fact that Prolifigen TPA reacts with both CK 8, 18 and 19 while TPS reacts with only one epitope M3 on CK 18. There seems to be a significant difference in the assigned value of the calibrators used in the two kits. Another important factor is given by the differences in the relative amount and availability of the different epitopes in serum samples from different patient-groups. The expression of cytokeratin can probably also vary as a function of disease progression. Thus it is very important to measure more than just one epitope (cytokeratin) with the assay used. From our short study it is also clear, that the vast historical knowledge collected for the Prolifigen TPA kit can not be transferred when using the TPS assay.

References

1   Moll R, Franke WW, Schiller D, Geiger B, Keppler R (1982) The catalog of human cytokeratins: Pattern of expression in normal epithelia, tumors and cultured cells. Cell 455:282–306
2   Weber K, Osborn M, Moll R, Wiklund B, Lüning B (1984) Tissue polypeptide antigen (TPA) is related to the non-epidermal keratins 8, 18 and 19 typical of simple and non-squamous epithelia: re-evaluation of a human tumor marker. EMBO J 3:2707–2714
3   Mellerick DM, Osborn M, Weber K (1990) On the nature of serological tissue polypeptide antigen (TPA); monoclonal keratin 8, 18 and 19 antibodies react with differently with TPA prepared from human cultured carcinoma cells and TPA in human serum. Oncogene 5:1007–1017

Address for correspondence:
L.-O. Hansson, M.D.
Department of Clincial Chemistry
Karolinska Hospital
S-104 01 Stockholm, Sweden

Tumor markers in ascitic fluid. Efficacy of the method as a tool for screening studies and differential diagnosis

L. Hryniewiecki, K. Klincewicz, D. Breborowicz

Department of Gastroenterology, University School of Medicine, Poznań, Poland

Introduction

Ascites may be a common symptom of chronic liver diseases as well as tumors of GI tract or accompany some kidney or heart diseases. Examination of ascitic fluid could provide valuable information about the origin of the disease and might be a good diagnostic tool especially in differential diagnosis.

The purpose of the present study has been to evaluate the diagnostic value of some tumor markers measured in ascitic fluid: carcinoembrional antigen (CEA), alpha fetoprotein (AFP) and other biochemical paramethers as total cholesterol and total protein for the differentiation of ascites of malignant origin from the one due to chronic liver diseases.

Material and methods

The study was done including 84 patients with ascites, aged from 18 to 81 years, 48 men and 36 women, which were divided into two groups. The first group consisted of 46 patients with malignant ascites. This group consisted of nine patients with liver cancer, ten patients with large bowel cancer, five patients with gastric cancer, 8 patients with pancreatic cancer, ten patients with ovary cancer and four patients with lymphomas. The second group comprised 38 patients with liver cirrhosis.

Diagnosis of all patients was based upon clinical and laboratory examinations as well as imaging techniques (ultrasound and CT examinations) and fine-needle biopsies. Liver disease was confirmed by liver biopsies.

The following tumor markers and biochemical parameters were measured in ascitic fluids of all patients. Carcinoembrionic antigen and alpha fetoprotein concentrations were determined by the double antibody method with the use of radioimmunoassay. Values of 10 ng/ml and 5 ng/dl were considered as discriminative ones for CEA and AFP respectively. Total cholesterol levels were determined by HOD–PAP enzymatic method using commercial test kits (Analco). A value of 50 mg/dl was considered to be discriminative. Total protein was measured by a commercial biuret method (POCH). The discriminative value for this parameter was 3 g/dl.

After classification of all data into four categories (true positive (a), true negative (b), false positive (c) and false negative (d); the sensitivity was calculated as $(a/(a = d)) \times 100$, the specifity as $(b/(b + c)) \times 100$ and the efficiency as $(a + b) / (a + b + c + d)$.

Maan-Whitney and Cochran-Cox tests were used for statistical evaluation of data. A 5% level was considered as statistically significant.

Results

All results are presented on the following figure and table. Figure 1 shows levels of tumor markers and some biochemical parameters in ascitic fluid in patients with tumor disease and liver cirrhosis. The mean CEA concentration in malignant patients was 83.2 ng/ml but only 4.2 ng/l in cirrhotic ones and this difference was statistically significant. In non-malignant patients only 8.6% of all cases showed CEA levels above 10.0 ng/l, which has been considered as discriminative value. Mean AFP concentration in malignant patients amounted to 51.8 ng/ml, being 6.0 ng/ml in cirrhotic ones. This difference was statistically not significant because of very large

Table I. Diagnostic values of some ascitic indices of malignancy for separating ascites of malignant origin from ascites due to chronic liver diseases.

Category	Cholesterol	Total protein	CEA	AFP
Discrimination value	> 50 mg/dl	> 3.0 g/dl	> 10 ng/ml	> 5 ng/ml
Sensitivity	94%	75%	45%	17%
Specifity	79%	84%	88%	74%
Efficiency	87%	81%	61%	38%

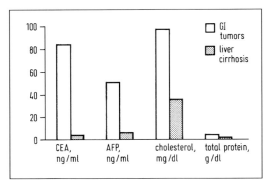

Figure 1. Ascitic tumor markers and some ascitic biochemical parameters in patients with GI tumors and liver cirrhosis.

variation of individual measurements (standard deviation was 216.7 ng/ml). The highest level of AFP in liver cancer exceeded 1000 ng/ml and only 17.6 % of malignant patients had values above the discriminative value, which had been 5.0 nl/ml. On the other hand, also in 26% of cirrhotic patients AFP values were above 5.0 ng/ml. This rather low sensitivity of AFP determination in separation of malignant from non-malignant ascitic fluids was caused by high specifity only for diagnosing liver cancer. In our material only 19% of all tumors were liver cancers.

It has been assumed that differential diagnosis of ascites could be improved by the application of measurements of ascitic cholesterol and ascitic total protein. The mean concentration of cholesterol was 96.2 mg/dl in the group of malignant patients and 36.1 mg/dl in the non-malignant one. The difference was statistically significant. It is noteworthy, that in malignant patients values below the discriminative value of 50 mg/ml were asserted only in 13% of all cases and in cirrhotic ones the values above this level were observed in 13% of all cases too.

The mean total protein level in ascitic fluid was 3.39 g/dl in malignant patients and only 1.87 g/ml in cirrhotic ones. The difference was statistically significant. Nevertheless, 32.6% of the patients of the malignant group showed total protein levels below 3.0 g/dl, which was considered to be the discriminative value.

Cytological examination of ascitic fluids much improves the sensitivity of measurements of these biochemical markes of malignancy. It was possible to confirm malignancy in our material in 90% of all cases.

Table I shows diagnostic values of the studied tumor markers for separating ascites of malignant origin from ascites due to chronic liver diseases, expressed in terms of sensitivity, specifity and efficiency. Applying discriminative values it has been possible to reveal that the diagnostic efficiency ranged from 87% to 38%. The efficiency of 87% for cholesterol, 81% for total protein and only 61% for CEA and 38% for AFP are calculated. These data give evidence that determinations of total cholesterol and total protein in ascitic fluid are better tumor markers for the separation of malignant from non-malignant cases than measurements of CEA and AFP. However, estimation of ascitic cholesterol levels seems to be superior to the determination of ascitic total protein.

In order to establish whether there exists any link between accumulation of cholesterol and total protein in ascitic fluids, regression analysis has been performed. The correlation coefficient calculated was only 0.39, that means rather weak interrelationship. These findings indicate, that there is a different mechanism for accumulation of cholesterol and total protein in ascitic fluids, which up to now is not clearly elucidated.

Discussion

There are many ascitic parameters such as total protein, serum fluid albumin gradient, fibronectin, pH or lipoproteins, which have been investigated for separation of malignant ascites from non-malignant ones, (2, 3, 4, 10, 11, 12, 13, 15) a number of these indices require application of complicated and sometimes very expensive techniques. The purpose of our studies has been to find out a simple but reliable and cost-effective method for quick differential diagnosis of malignant and non-malignant ascites. Estimation of CEA is very useful as it is a specific marker of malignancy. Our study revealed also high specifity of this marker which amounted up to 88% but its sensitivity was only 45%. This was caused by a number of false negative results. Previous studies have shown that CEA concentrations were higher in ascitic fluids than in blood serum (1). Other reports confirmed these findings (8, 11). These data suggest, that only a high concentration of CEA in ascitic fluid could be of reliable diagnostic value for the estimation of malignancy.

Measurements of ascitic AFP are of lower value because of a number of false negative and false positive results. An elevation of AFP levels was observed in 22% of cirrhotic patients. Nevertheless, a high value of this marker may suggest neoplastic metaplasia in cirrhotic liver.

Determination of cholesterol and to a lesser extent of total protein seems to be a very useful diagnostic tool for differential diagnosis of malignancy, in particular due to its simplicity, rapidity and cost-effectiveness (4, 5). Our data revealed high sensitivity and specifity as well as efficiency of these parameters confirming reports of other authors (4, 5). Additional cytological examination of ascitic fluids could improve the diagnostic value of the measurement of cholesterol and total protein accumulation in ascitic fluids.

All data presented have shown, that determination of ascitic cholesterol and total protein could be a good and fast screening test in the diagnosis of malignancy of ascitic patients completing the use of other tumor markers and indicating the necessity of applying more specific tests and examinations for a more thorough estimation of the origin and localisation of the neoplasm.

Conclusions

Measurement of total cholesterol and total protein in ascitic fluid could be a simple and not expensive screening test for separation of ascites of malignant origin from the one due to chronic liver diseases. Lipid accumulation in ascitic fluid seems to have a better diagnostic value for differential diagnosis of malignancy than measurements of total protein level. Determination of ascitic CEA and AFP enables differentiation of some types of GI tract tumors. Additional cytological examination of ascitic fluid might improve the sensitivity and efficiency of the tests applied.

References

1. Brêborowicz D, Klincewicz H, Breborowicz J (1990) Oznaczanie antygenu CEA i AFP w diagnostyce róznicowej plynów wysiekowych. Nowiny Lek 2:49
2. Cacaloglu Y, Okten A, Yalein S (1991) Serum – ascites albumin concentration gradient in the prediction of portal hypertension in ascitic patients. Gastroenterol 100:1484
3. Dirsch OK, Landelt U, Pedio G (1991) Möglichkeiten der Zytodiagnostik in Ascites. Leber Magen Darm 3:108
4. Hoefs JC (1990) Diagnostic paracentesis. A potent diagnostic tool. Gastroenterol 98:230
5. Jüngst D, Gerbes AL, Martin R, Paumgartner G (1986) Value of ascitic lipids in the differentiation between cirrhotic and malignant ascites. Hepatol 8:1104
6. Mc Kenna JM, Chandrashkar AJ, Henkin RE (1980) Diagnostic value of CEA in exsudative pleural effusions. Chest 78:587
7. Mezger J Parmenetter W, Gerbes AL et al (1988) Tumor associated antigens in diagnosis of serum effusions. J Clin Path 41:633
8. Nystrom JS, Dyce B, Wada J et al (1983) CEA titer in effusion fluid. Arch Int Med 137:875
9. Pare P, Talbot J, Hoefs JC (1983) Serum-ascites albumin concentration gradient a physiologic approach to the differential diagnosis of ascites. Gastroenterol 85:240
10. Prieto M, Gomez-Lechon MJ, Melchior H (1988) Diagnosis of malignant ascites. Dig Dis Sci 33:833
11. Rector W, Reynolds T (1984) Superiority of the serum-ascites albumin difference over ascites total protein concentration in separation of "transudative" and "exsudative" ascites. Am J Med 29:16
12. Rieder H, Ramadori G, Mayer zum Büchenfelde KH et al (1991) Genese des Fibronektin im Ascites –

Nachweis von zellurären und Plasma-Fibronektin in portalen und malignen Aszites. Z Gastroenter 29:16
13 Runyan BA, Hoefs JC, Morgan TE (1988) Ascitic fluid analysis in malignancy related ascites. Hepatol 8:1104
14 Sales H, Lauvet H, Zeitoun P, Deltour G (1979) Dosages de l'antigene carcino-embryonaire dans les liquides d'epanchement. La Nouvelle Presse Medicale 8:526
15 Suzuki N, Kawashima S, Degushi K et al (1980) Low density lipoproteins from human ascites plasma J Biochem 87:1253

Address for correspondence:
Prof. Dr. habil. L. Hryniewiecki
Department of Gastroenterology
University School of Medical Sciences of Poznań
ul Przybyszewskiego 49
PL-60-355 Poznań, Poland

Tumor markers and cholesterol metabolism in patients with gastrointestinal cancer

H. Nägele[a], A. Gebhardt[c], A. Niendorf[c], F. Sandersfeld[a], R. Klapdor[b], W. Daerr[b], U. Meyer-Pannwitt[a]

[a]Surgical Clinic, [b]Medical Clinic, [c]Institute of Pathology,
University Hospital Hamburg-Eppendorf, Hamburg, Germany

Introduction

It is well accepted that high cholesterol levels are significantly correlated with the development of atherosclerosis and its complications (6). There are some controversies on the significance of low serum lipids. Epidemiological studies showed an increased mortality in the lowest cholesterol percentile, leading to a "J-shaped curve", mostly due to an increased cancer rate (8). In the "Lipid Research Clinics Program Mortality Follow-Up Study" the relative risk of men to die of colon carcinoma was 5.7, when their total cholesterol was below 187 mg/dl (3). Many other studies described an association between low cholesterol levels and malignant disease, especially gastrointestinal cancer and leukemia (1, 4, 5, 7, 9, 11, 13, 18, 21, 23, 25). It is under discussion whether low serum lipids are a consequence or a cause and possibly a marker of malignancy. Some authors even called in question common recommendations for lowering lipids in cardiovascular prevention (2, 16). Therefore it is necessary to define more precisely the mechanisms of "tumor-associated hypocholesterolemia". To address this issue we conducted a prospective study on the course of serum lipids, tumor markers and cellular lipid metabolism in patients who underwent surgery for gastrointestinal cancer.

Patients and methods

From 1990 to 1992 99 patients with gastrointestinal cancer, who where admitted to the department of surgery, were included in the study. 35 patients who underwent surgery for benign conditions (resection of gall bladder, gastric resection for ulcer disease and others) were included as controls. The localizations of the carcinomas were as follows: esophagus 1, stomach 15, bile duct 6, hepatocellular 3, pancreas 12, colon 13, sigma 4, rectum 12, anus 3. In 15 patients an attempt was made to resect liver metastasis, two patients had sarcomas and seven patients had various other malignancies with abdominal localization (germ cell tumors, melanoma, undifferentiated carcinoma of unknown origin). 18 patients died perioperatively or where lost for follow-up. In six patients the suspected malignancy was not confirmed intra- or postoperatively, these patients were followed in the control group.

At the initial evaluation patients had to give a written consent to be included in the study. Preoperatively, 10 days, 3 and 12 month after the operation the patients status of health was checked, especially the results of imaging techniques were collected to determine, if there was any evidence of tumor progression. After one year of follow-up the patients were divided into three subgroups: curative surgery = 24 patients, relapse or disease progression = 20 patients, tumor death = 31 patients. 18 patients died perioperatively or where lost of follow-up. Therefore only 44 patients (or 47%) were followed over one year. The 15 patients with stomach cancer were analyzed separately because of stable low cholesterol levels independent of the state of disease. These patients had significantly increased HDL cholesterol levels which highlights the special role of the stomach in lipid metabolism (12). At the described time blood was drawn after an overnight fasting for the determination of blood lipids (total-, LDL-, HDL-, VLDL-cholesterol, triglycerides, apolipoproteins B, AI, AII) and the

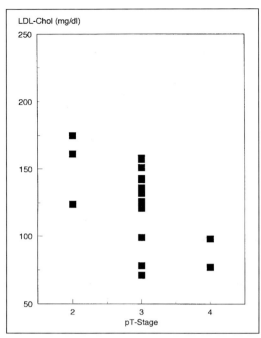

Figure 1. Preoperative LDL cholesterol levels in relation to pathological tumor size (pT stage).

tumor markers carcinoembryonal antigen (CEA Enzymun®, Boehringer Mannheim and CA 19-9 EIA, La Roche) with commercially available kits. Blood was cooled down immediately, centrifuged and the serum/plasma stored at –70 °C in aliquots. Blood of a single patient was analyzed in one assay. When possible, tumor tissue was harvested and cellular cholesterol metabolism was determined (results of this part of the study were described elsewhere (15). Thyroid hormone and blood glucose levels and informations on the medication and the diet were collected to exclude secondary dyslipidemias. At the end of the study laboratory values were correlated in respect to pathologic findings and different prognostic groups.

Results

Preoperatively there was no significant difference in lipid values between cancer patients and controls (data not shown), although some patients had very low total cholesterol levels (below 140 mg/dl). When LDL cholesterol levels of patients with colon cancer were compared to their pT-stage a negative association was observed (figure 1). Nearly all patients and controls showed a significant depression of lipid values at the tenth postoperative day, possibly due to the operation trauma. When control patients reached initial values after three month, the cancer patients showed a heterogeneous response. Four typical patients with low preoperative levels of total- and LDL cholesterol had no signs of relapse at one year of follow-up. These patients showed a marked increase in both total and LDL cholesterol (figure 2). The patient with the deepest preoperative cholesterol value (114 mg/dl preoperatively) had a coecal carcinoma. This observation is in agreement with another study which showed

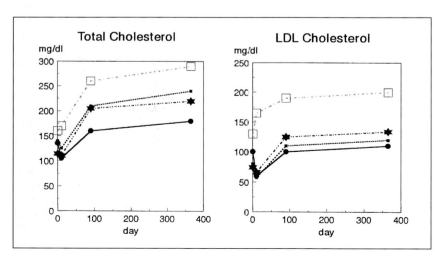

Figure 2. Levels of total and LDL cholesterol (y-axis) in follow-up (days 0, 10, 90 and 365) of four typical patients with curative surgery.

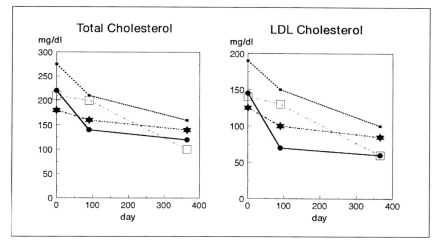

Figure 3. Levels of total and LDL cholesterol (y-axis) in follow-up (days 0, 90 and 365) of four typical patients with non-curative surgery.

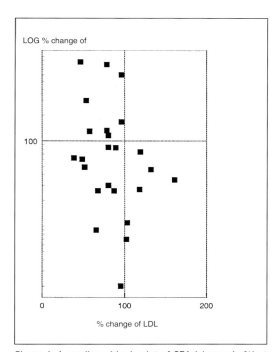

Figure 4. A semilogarithmic plot of CEA (change in %) at month 3 in relation to levels at entry (=100%) against change (%) of LDL cholesterol levels at month 3 versus values at entry (=100%).

Table I. Different prognostic groups in relation to changes in LDL cholesterol levels in follow-up.

LDL cholesterol month 3 (% of pre-OP)		
	≥ 95%	< 95%
Curative	65% (11/17)	35% (6/17)
Non-curative	32% (8/25)	68% (17/25)
LDL cholesterol month 12 (% of pre-OP)		
	≥ 95%	< 95%
Curative	75% (12/16)	25% (4/17)
Non-curative	42% (8/25)	58% (17/25)
LDL cholesterol month 12 (% of month 3)		
	≥ 95%	< 95%
Curative	73% (11/15)	27% (4/15)
Non-curative	35% (5/14)	65% (9/14)

deeper cholesterol values in patients with right-sided colon cancer (14). Four other patients with progression of disease showed an impressive drop of cholesterol levels during observation (figure 3). Although the other patients showed minor changes a comparison of the percentual changes of total and LDL cholesterol levels at month 3 and 12 versus entry showed that most patients with curative surgery had stable or even increased values, whereas patients with relapse or progression tended to have a decrease in lipid levels over time (table I). Changes in the levels of apolipoprotein B are similar to LDL (data not shown). As expected, an analysis of the tumor marker results in gerneral showed higher serum concentrations in patients with disease progression or tumor death, both preoperatively and in follow-up (data not shown). A combination of tumor marker and LDL cholesterol results showed that no patient with an increase in CEA showed an increase in LDL cholesterol (figure 4). Similar results were obtained for CA 19-9 (data not shown).

Discussion

Our data show that in some patients with gastrointestinal cancer the values of total and LDL cholesterol are correlated with the course of disease. When total- or LDL cholesterol levels fell in follow-up of patients after resection of gastrointestinal cancer, disease progression should be suspected and vice versa. In this setting total- and LDL cholesterol levels are additional "tumor markers". The classical tumor markers CEA and CA 19-9 showed comparable changes in follow-up. No patient with tumor progression and tumor marker increase showed a rise in lipid levels. We suggest a careful observation of the often determined cholesterol levels in cancer patients. Further and larger studies should clarify the exact role of this inexpensive "tumor marker" in contrast to the classical markers CEA and CA 19-9.

The changes in blood lipids seem to reflect a secondary response to tumor size and tumor kinetics, because they were seen in follow-up and not initially. The mechanism how the tumor lowers cholesterol levels in cancer patients may be a direct uptake of LDL particles via the LDL receptor pathway to fulfill its enhanced demand in cell surface synthesis. This hypothesis is supported by some in vitro (17) and in vivo (23) data. Another part of our study investigated the cholesterol metabolism of the tumor cells. These results published elsewhere are in agreement with the "hypothesis of consumption" and showed high levels of expression of LDL receptors in the cancer cells which correlated with positive intraindividual shifts of serum cholesterol after surgery (15). The enhanced cholesterol demand of tumor cells may be a new and exciting therapeutic approach either in targeting cytotoxic drugs via the LDL receptor pathway (10) or in inhibition of intracellular cholesterol synthesis by mevinolin or dehydroepiandrosterone to arrest cell division (20).

Conclusion

It can be concluded that the course of total- and LDL cholesterol levels after resection of gastrointestinal cancer has some value in assessing prognosis of these patients. Therefore lipid values in cancer patients should be observed carefully.

Our data are further arguments that tumor-associated hypocholesterolemia is a consequence rather than a cause of malignancy.

References

1 Beaglehole R, Foulkes MA, Prior IA, Eyles EF (1980) Cholesterol and mortality in New Zealand Maoris. Brit Med J 280:285–287
2 Bräuer H, Scheffer K, Schreiber G (1986) Sind niedrige Cholesterinwerte wirklich erstrebenswert? Fortschr Med 104:674–678
3 Cowan LD, Osonnell DL, Ciqui MH, Barrettconner E, Bush TL, Wallace RB (1990) Cancer mortality and lipid and lipoprotein levels – The lipid research clinics program mortality follow-up study. Am J Epidemiol 131:468–482
4 Garcia-Palmieri MR, Sorlie PD, Costas R Jr, Havlik RJ (1981) An apparent inverse relationship between serum cholesterol and cancer mortality in Puerto Rico. Am J Epidemiol 114:29–40
5 Kagan A, Mcgee DL, Yano K, Rhoads GG, Nomura A (1980) Serum cholesterol and mortality in a Japanese-American population: The Honolulu Heart program. Am J Epidemiol 114:11–20
6 Kannel W, Castelli W, Gordon T, McNamara P (1971) Serum cholesterol, lipoproteins and the risk of coronary heart disease. The Framingham study. Ann Intern Med 74:1–12
7 Kark JD, Smith AH, Hames CG (1980) The relationship of serum cholesterol to the incidence of cancer in Evans County, Georgia. J Chronic Dis 33(5): 311–32
8 Levy R (1982) Consideration of cholesterol and non-cardiovascular mortality. Am Heart J 104:324–328
9 Knekt P, Reunannen A, Aromaa A, Heliovaara M, Hakulinen T, Hakarna M (1988) Serum cholesterol and risk of cancer in a cohort of 39,000 men and women. J Clin Epidemiol 41:519–530
10 Masquelier M, Vitols S, Peterson C (1986) Low-density lipoprotein as a carrier of antitumoral drugs: In vivo fate of drug-human low-density lipoprotein complexes in mice. Cancer Res 46:3842–3847
11 Morris DL, Borhani NO, Fitzsimons E, Hardy RJ, Hawkins CM, Kraus JF, Labarthe DR, Mastbaum L, Payne GH (1983) Serum cholesterol and cancer in the hypertension detection and follow-up program. Cancer 52:1754–1759
12 Nägele H, Sandersfeld F, Niendorf A, Kreymann G, Daerr W, Meyer-Panwitt U (1993) Plasma lipid and body composition changes in gastrointestinal cancer. 62nd European Atherosclerosis Society Congress, p 49
13 Neugut A, Johnson C, Fink D (1986) Serum cholesterol levels in adenomatous polyps and cancer of the colon. JAMA 255:365–367

14 Nomura AM, Stemmermann GN, Chyou PH (1991) Prospective study of serum cholesterol levels and large-bowel cancer. J Natl Cancer Inst 83 (19): 1403–1407
15 Niendorf A, Gerding D, Wittke D, Peters A, Nägele H, Meyer-Pannwitt U, Gebhardt A (1993) Tumor associated hypocholesterolemia – high levels of expression of LDL receptors in surgically removed cancer specimen correlate with positive intra-individual shifts of serum cholesterol after surgery. Proceedings of the 84d annual meeting of the American Association for Cancer Research
16 Oliver MF (1991) Might treatment of hypercholesterolemia increase non-cardiac mortality? Lancet 337(8756):1529–1531
17 Peterson C, Vitols S, Rudling M, Blomgren H, Edsmyr F, Skoog L (1985) Hypocholesterolemia in cancer patients may be caused by elevated LDL receptor activities in malignant cells. Med Oncol Tumor Pharmacother 2 :143–147
18 Rose G, Keys A, Taylor HL, Kannell WB, Paul O, Reid DD, Stamler J (1974) Colon cancer and blood-cholesterol. Lancet 1974,I:181–183
19 Schatzkin A, Hoover RN, Taylor PR, Ziegler RG, Carter CL, Albanes D, Larson DB, Licitra LM (1988) Site-specific analysis of total serum cholesterol and incident cancer in the National Health and Nutrition Examination Survey I Epidemiologic Follow-Up Study. Cancer Res 48:452–458
20 Schulz S, Klann RC, Schoenfeld S, Nyce JW (1992) Mechanisms of cell growth inhibition and cell cycle arrest in human colonic adenocarcinoma cells by dehydroepiandrosterone: Role of isoprenoid biosynthesis. Cancer Res 52:1372–1376
21 Toernberg SA, Holm LE, Carstensen JM, Eklund GA (1989) Cancer incidence and cancer mortality in relation to serum cholesterol. J Natl Cancer Inst 81:1917–1921
22 Vitols S, Björnholm M, Gahrton G, Peterson C (1985) Hypocholesterolemia in malignancy due to elevated low-density-lipoprotein-receptor activity in tumour cells: Evidence from studies in patients with leukaemia. Lancet II:1150–1154
23 Wald NJ, Thompson SG, Law MR, Densem JW, Bailey A(1989) Serum cholesterol and subsequent risk of cancer: results from the BUPA study. Brit J Cancer 59:936–938
24 Williams RR, Sorlie PD, Feinleib M, Mcnamara PM, Kannell WB, Dawber (1981) Cancer incidence by levels of cholesterol. JAMA 245:247–252
25 Winawer SJ, Flehinger BJ, Buchhalter J, Herbert E, Shike M (1990) Declining serum cholesterol levels prior to diagnosis of colon cancer. JAMA 263: 2083–2085

Address for corresdondence:
Dr. med. H. Nägele
Chirurgische Klinik
Universitätskrankenhaus Hamburg-Eppendorf
Martinistraβe 52
D-20246 Hamburg, Germany

In Vitro Diagnosis

Gynecology

Evaluation of cancer associated serum antigen (CASA) as an additional tumor marker in ovarian carcinoma

G. Sturm, P. Schmidt-Rhode, S. Chari, T. Bauer,
Department of Gynecology and Obstetrics, University of Marburg, Germany

Introduction

The tumor associated antigen CA 125 has been the most widely used tumor marker for monitoring ovarian cancer. Although it is elevated in 80% of advanced ovarian cancer patients (FIGO stage III/IV;) (1, 2, 3), the marker is not sensitive enough to recognize earlier stages of the tumor. Furthermore, a large number of benign ovarian neoplasms and endometriosis is also associated with elevated levels of CA 125 (4), thus questioning the specificity of the marker. We have studied several other markers such as CEA, TPA and various monoclonal epithelial antigens including CA 72-4. With the exception of the latter, none of the other markers were found to be of any further advantage (5). In an attempt to improve this situation, we have examined the recently developed CASA assay (cancer associated serum antigen). This method employs the two core protein reactive monoclonal antibodies BC2 and BC3 for detection of the MUC-1 antigen (6).

Materials and methods

CA 125 and CA 72-4 were determined by immunoradiometric assay (IRMA: ID-CIS GmbH, Dreieich), the cut-off limit for the two being 65 U/ml and 3.0 U/ml, respectively (3). CASA was determined by solid phase enzyme immunoassay (EIA: medac Diagnostika, Hamburg), the inter- and intra-assay VC being 12.5% and 7.2%, respectively; the cut-off level is set to 4 U/ml. This limit has been obtained by testing 80 serum samples from healthy donors and is in agreement with the manufacturers' data. Further, selected for screening purposes were early- (n = 24), mid- (n = 20) and late pregnancy sera (n = 40), amniotic fluid from normal (n = 20) and pathological (neural tube defects: NTD, anencephaly; n = 20) pregnancies, sera from benign ovarian diseases (ovarian cysts, endometriosis; n = 40), ovarian carcinoma (n = 40) and endometrial cancer (n = 20) (see figure 1).

The sensitivity of different markers was tested in 93 primary sera of ovarian cancer patients. In a retrospective follow-up study we compared CASA with CA 125 and CA 72-4 in 300 sera of 39 patients with ovarian cancinoma of stage III/IV (FIGO).

Results

As shown in figure 1, the CASA levels during early and mid-pregnancy weeks did not significantly differ from the normal range. On the other hand, during late pregnancy, the levels reached lie between 40 – 200 U/ml ($p < 0.001$). The CASA levels in the amniotic fluid of normal pregnancies showed median values of 100 U/ml, whereas in the pathological pregnancies it was in the range of 3–100 U/ml, the median being 12 U/ml. What is of interest is the obvious increase in CASA levels during normal late pregnancy and the significantly lower amounts in amniotic fluid of pathological cases, thus qualifying CASA to be a potential diagnostic tool for screening pregnancy. However, further studies are needed to establish this point. While in benign ovarian diseases the CASA levels were in the normal range, in ovarian cancer patients it ranged from normal up to 700 U/ml. In the collective of 93 primary sera of ovarian cancer patients the sensitivity of CASA was only 57%, whereas that of CA 125 was 78%.

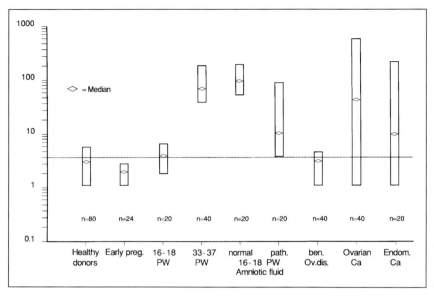

Figure 1.
CASA serum levels in different patient groups.

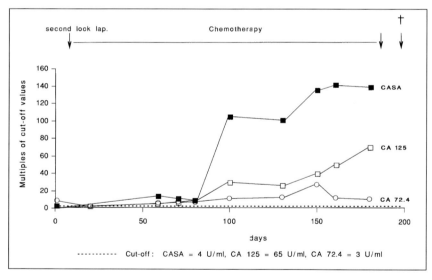

Figure 2.
Follow-up of a patient with endometroidal ovarian carcinoma (pT3 Nx M1 G3).

In advanced endometrial cancer patients, although CASA was elevated in some of them, it did not appear to be better than CA 50 and/or CA 125.

In the follow-up study of 39 patients with ovarian carcinoma two were positive only to CASA, two only to CA 72-4 (histologically identified as mucinous type), and five only to CA 125. Twenty-four were positive not only to CA 125 but also to CASA. In twelve of these 24 cases CASA proved to be an even better marker than CA 125 in terms of expressing the dynamics of tumor growth. This could best be represented by plotting multiples of cut-off values as shown in figure 2.

Discussion

Elevated levels of CA 125 in benign diseases as for e.g. in endometriosis – an observation similar to the reports published (4) – clearly shows the lack of specificity of this marker for ovarian carcinoma. CA 72-4, on the other hand, is a highly sensitive and specific marker for the CA 125 negative mucinous types of ovarian carcinomas and hence here may be used as a primary marker (5). This study also demonstrates that CASA assay can be used to improve the discriminatory ability of CA 125 assay to differentiate between benign gynecological disease and ovarian carcinoma. In nearly one third of the cases studied, CASA was found to be superior to CA 125 in that CASA levels reflected the tumor growth in a more dynamic fashion. In this respect, CASA in combination with CA 125 or CA 72-4 can be regarded as a valuable second marker in ovarian malignomas. Using CASA and CA 125, *Ward* et al.(7) arrived at similar conclusions. Furthermore, on the basis of the above observations, it is worth considering CASA as a possible tool for screening fetal abnormalities in the 16th week of pregnancy (amniotic fluid) and disturbed late pregnancies.

References

1 Schmidt-Rhode P, Sturm G, Künzig HJ, Schulz KD (1986) CA 125 Plasmakonzentrationen und Second Look Operation bei Patientinnen mit Ovarialkarzinom. In: Greten H, Klapdor R (eds) 4. Hamburger Symposium über Tumormarker. Thieme, Stuttgart, New York, pp 110
2 Kaesemann H, Caffier H, Hoffmann FJ, Crombach G, Würz H, Kreienberg R, Möbus V, Schmidt-Rhode P, Sturm G (1986) Untersuchungen zur Sensitivität und Spezifität des Tumormarkers CA 125 beim Ovarialkarzinom - Eine kooperative Studie der GTMG. In: Greten H, Klapdor R (eds) Klinische Relevanz neuer monoklonaler Antikörper. Thieme, Stuttgart, New York, pp 64–72
3 Möbus V, Kreienberg R, Crombach G, Würz H, Caffier H, Hoffmann FJ, Kaufmann M, Schmidt-Rhode P, Sturm G (1988) Evaluation of CA 125 as a prognostic and predictive factor in ovarian cancer. J Tumor Marker Oncol 3:251–258
4 Barbieri RL, Niloff JM, Bast RC, Schätzel E, Kistner RW, Knapp RC (1986) Elevated serum concentrations of CA 125 in patients with advanced endometriosis. Fertil Steril 45:630–634
5 Valet A, Schmidt-Rhode P, Klein A, Sturm G, Schulz KD. (1991) CA 72-4 als Tumormarker für Ovarialkarzinome. Arch Gynecol Obstet 250:186–188
6 McGuckin MA, Layton GT, Bailley MJ, Hurst T, Khoo SK, Ward BG (1990) Evaluation of two new assays for tumor associated antigens, CASA and OSA, found in the serum of patients with epithelial ovarian carcinoma – comparison with CA 125. Gynecol Oncol 37:165–171
7 Ward BG, McGuckin MA, Ramm LE, Coglan M, Sanderson B, Tripcony L, Free KE (1993) The management of ovarian carcinoma is improved by the use of CASA and CA 125 assays. Cancer 71:430–438

Address for correspondence:
Prof. Dr. rer. nat. G. Sturm
Abteilung für Gynäkologie und Geburtshilfe
Universitätsfrauenklinik
Pilgrimstein 3
D-35037 Marburg, Germany

Practical uses of CASA and CA 125 estimation in the management of ovarian cancer

B. G. Ward[a], M. A. McGuckin[b]
[a]Department of Gynecological Oncology,
[b]Department of Obstetrics and Gynecology, University of Queensland, Herston, Australia

Introduction

In the ten years or so since the development of the CA 125 assay, the clinical utility of tumor marker estimations in the management of ovarian cancer has been continuously clarified. The description of the CASA assay in 1990 added a further dimension to tumor marker measurements in that the CASA assay defines an epitope on the MUC-1 polymorphic epithelial mucin, an entirely unrelated protein to OC 125. Measurement of the CASA antigen can correct some of the deficiencies of measurement of CA 125 alone in that the problems of low specificity for ovarian cancer and frequent expression in non-malignant disease suffered by CA 125 are not seen with CASA.

Retrospective studies

Retrospective studies in our department have shown that a combination of CASA and CA 125 achieved a 70% sensitivity for ovarian malignancy at a specificity of 100% when discriminating between benign and malignant ovarian tumors. The tumors which were not detected by the combination of the assays were generally of early stage and were generally easily resectable. The combination of the assays was consistently superior to the use of either CA 125 or CASA alone. CASA consistently was more sensitive than CA 125 for small volume disease whether detecting small volume disease at primary presentation or prior to second look surgery. A combination of these assays on average gave a mean lead time to clinical recurrence of over six months. Finally, postoperative CASA levels were shown to be an independent prognostic factor in women with small volume disease in that women who had normal levels of CASA prior to their chemotherapy had a statistically significantly better chance of survival than women whose levels were abnormal (1, 2).

A study performed in collaboration with the Breast Cancer Screening Clinic at the Royal Women's Hospital of 5,000 healthy women determined the normal range for CASA in this population and demonstrated that CASA levels increased with age and smoking practice. Other studies have demonstrated that CASA is elevated in women with chronic lung disease and those with some lung cancers, and perhaps a common pathway with smokers could be postulated (3).

Prospective study

A prospective study has therefore been underway in our department for three years to confirm these earlier observations. We have concentrated on disease progress monitoring and also on prognostic assessment, as these two areas appear to be the most clinically relevant. One hundred and six patients have been followed with an average follow-up time of some 24 months. Blood from these patients was drawn preoperatively, and then at time points prior to each cycle of chemotherapy. Not all patients had blood drawn at the designated time points and therefore some of the data which follows involves less than the full 106 patients for each of the aspects analysed.

With regard to monitoring of patients, our previous findings have been confirmed in that the combination of CASA (Medical Innovations, Sydney, Australia) and CA 125 (Byk-Sangtec,

Table I. Timing of tumor marker increase versus time of recurrence; percentages in parentheses.

Tumor marker	> 2 Months before rec.	< 2 Months before rec.	After recurrence	No increase
CASA	14 (44)	6 (19)	3 (9)	9 (28)
CA 125	14 (44)	9 (28)	3 (9)	6 (19)
Combined	19 (59)	8 (25)	4 (13)	1 (3)

Table II. Predictive values for death before 24 months.

Pre-chemox cycle	n	CASA		CA 125		Combination	
		PPV	NPV	PPV	NPV	PPV	NPV
1	61	58	74	54	82	54	83
2	63	75	77	94	87	79	90
3	54	69	79	93	85	91	73
4	51	63	72	90	80	69	79

PPV = positive predictive value; NPV = negative predictive value

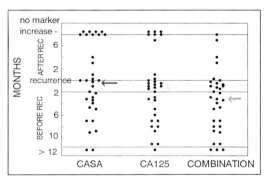

Figure 1. Time of marker increase versus clinical recurrence.

Germany) has an additive effect with 84% of patients having a marker level rise of one or other marker prior to clinical recurrence (table I). Median lead time to recurrence in all patients was three and a half months for the combined assay measurement (figure 1).

When assay levels were analysed with regard to the patient survival, it was found that normalisation of CASA and CA 125 levels prior to the second cycle of chemotherapy was the most statistically significant factor relating to survival. Normal values of both assays prior to the second cycle of chemotherapy have a positive predictive value of 79% for survival of two years, with a negative predictive value of 90%. In other words, if tumor marker levels have normalised by the second cycle of chemotherapy, then the patient has a nearly 80% chance of being alive at two years, whereas if either or both markers have not normalised by this time, the patient has a 10% 2-year survival. These observations are highly significant and may well provide the basis for individualising treatment (table II).

Conclusion

In conclusion, we would suggest that measurement of tumor marker levels have three roles at the present time in the management of women with ovarian cancer. First of all a combination of CASA and CA 125 is very useful in discriminating benign from malignant neoplasms where confusion exists. This may allow relevant streaming of patients towards the relevant gynecological oncology service for management. Secondly, monitoring of women following their treatment with tumor markers allows disease progression to be determined before clinical recurrence in the majority of cases. The difficulty at the present time of course is finding an effective second line treatment. However, the use of intraperitoneal therapy or Taxol may overcome some of these deficiencies. In our institute, the use of tumor marker measurements has taken over from second look operation to determine tumor response. Finally, the measurements of CASA and CA 125 prior to the second cycle of chemotherapy is a highly effective way of determining patient survival and may allow those patients at high risk of recurrence to be treated with less toxic regimens, or alternatively have more intensive treatment regimens to attempt to reverse the situation.

Acknowledgement

Professor Ward acknowledges the assistance of medac GE Diagnostica (Hamburg).

References

1. Ward BG, McGuckin MA, Ramm LE et al (1993) The management of ovarian cancer is improved by the use of cancer associated serum antigen CASA and CA 125 assays. Cancer 71:430–438
2. McGuckin MA, Ramm LE, Joy G, Free K, Ward BG (1992) Preoperative discrimination between ovarian carcinoma and non-ovarian gynecological malignancy and benign gynecological disease using serum levels of CA 125 and the polymorphic epithelium mucin CASA, OSA and MSA. Int J Gynecol Cancer 119–128
3. McGuckin MA, Ramm LE, Joy G, Devine PL, Ward BG (1993) Circulating tumor associated mucin concentrations determined by the CASA assay in healthy women. Clinica Chimica Acta 214:139-151

Address for correspondence:
Prof. Dr. B. G. Ward
Department of Gynecological Oncology
Royal Brisbane Hospital
AUS-Herston, Q 4029, Australia

Clinical value of CASA versus CA 125 in ovarian cancer

P. Kristen, P. Dörffler, H. Caffier
Women's Clinic of the University, Würzburg, Germany

Introduction

Tumor markers are helpful means in monitoring success of therapy and clinical follow-up of malignant disease. In ovarian cancer CA 125 is well established over the last ten years since its first introduction in 1983 (1). It is expressed by epthelian ovarian tumors and serum levels correlate to the extent of surgical treatment and the clinical outcome of patients suffering from ovarian cancer. High serum levels before or after debulking surgery and during clinical follow-up care appear to be of predictive and prognostic significance (2). Besides high sensitivity, CA 125 shows limited specificity, because of often elevated levels in benign gynecological diseases, i.e. in endometriosis. More recently cancer associated serum antigen (CASA) is introduced as a new marker in ovarian malignany (3). The CASA assay uses monoclonal antibodies that bind to an epitope on the polimorphic epithelial mucin. In the following study the clinical position of CASA versus CA 125 is evaluated in patients with ovarian cancer.

Methods

By means of commercially available kits (CA 125: ID CIS Dreieich, CASA: medac, Hamburg) asservated sera of 42 patients with ovarian cancer were tested. All patients had advanced disease of FIGO-stage III and IV. Only patients with histologically confirmed non-mucinous epithelial ovarian carcinomas were enrolled in this retrospective study. Marker determination was done pre- and postoperatively, monthly during chemotherapy and regulary during the clinical follow-up. The cut-off value used for CASA was 4 U/ml, for CA 125 65 U/ml, respectively. So, altogether 467 serum samples of 42 patients were analyzed for both markers.

Results and discussion

As shown in figure 1 there was no direct correlation to be found between the individual serum levels of CASA and CA 125 estimated preoperatively. The same findings could also be observed in the postoperative situation and in the follow-up. Both markers showed strong correlations to the extent of surgical therapy (figure 2). In patients with preoperative low levels of CA 125 and low or negative levels of CASA more often a complete removal of tumor mass was achieved, than in patients with elevated levels of these markers.

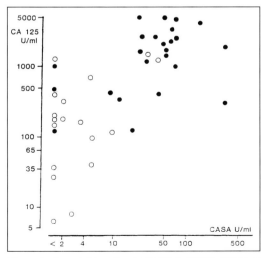

Figure 1. Correlation of preoperative serum levels of CASA versus CA 125. Extent of surgical therapy: ○ complete removal/tumor < 2cm; ● uncomplete removal/tumor > 2cm.

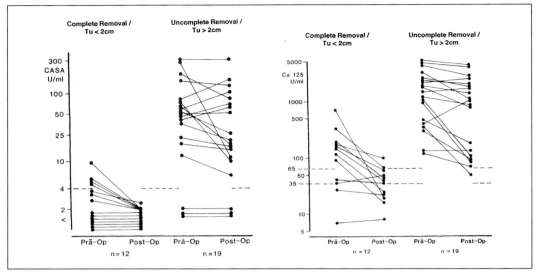

Figure 2. Correlation of CASA and CA 125 to the extent of surgical therapy.

Table I. CASA versus CA 125 in ovarian cancer: serum levels in different clinical situations (cut-off values: CASA = 4 U/ml, CA 125 = 65 U/ml).

Clinical situation	No. pat. = 100%	CASA+ CA 125+	CASA+ CA 125-	CASA- CA 125+	CASA- CA 125-
Prä-op.	42	62%	2%	26%	10%
Post-op. total	39	51%	3%	13%	33%
no tumor/tumor < 2cm	16	13%	–	13%	74%
tumor > 2cm	23	79%	4%	13%	4%
Complete rem./NED	20	6%	6%	–	88%
Three month post-op.	37	41%	8%	8%	43%
Progression	35	66%	7%	19%	17%

Table II. CASA versus CA 125 in ovarian cancer: median serum levels in different clinical situations.

Clinical situation	CASA (U/ml)	CA 125 (U/ml)
Prä-op.	12	40
Post-op. total	6.5	91
no tumor / tumor < 2 cm	<2	37
tumor >2 cm	20	1034
Complete rem./NED	<2	17
Part. rem.	4	70
No change	8	95
Progression	12	346

Table I shows the marker constellation concerning the clinical course of disease. In 62% both markers were positive before therapy in stage III and IV disease. In 2% only CASA and in 26% only CA 125 showed preoperative elevated levels. In 10% of all the patients both of the markers were negative. In the cases with complete remission or no evidence of diesease (NED) both markers were negative in 88%, elevated levels for CASA and CA 125 in this group of patients could be found in 6%, in 6% only CASA was elevated. The median values of the two markers concerning the clinical course of disease are shown in table II. Both markers showed strong correlations in the follow-up of the patients. Figure 3 shows the example of

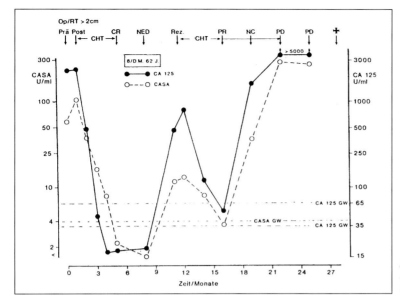

Figure 3. Clinical follow-up of a 62 years old patient with CASA and CA 125.

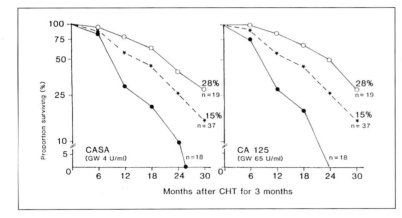

Figure 4. Overall survival in ovarian cancer: serum levels of CASA and CA 125 three month post operation: O—O median survival curve of all patients with negative serum levels; ●—● median survival curve of patients with positive serum levels *—* median survival curve of all patients. Cut-off values: CASA = 4 U/ml; CA 125 = 65 U/ml.

a 62 years old patient with stage IV disease. CASA and CA 125 reflect very strongly the different clinical situations. The level of the two markers three month after therapy is of prognostic relevance as shown in regression analysis (figure 4). When the markers are elevated at this time a significant decrease in median overall survival is found (CASA: 9 versus 31 month; CA 125: 9 versus 27 month)

Summary

The cancer associated antigen (CASA) shows a strong correlation with the extent of surgery as well as the clinical course of patients with ovarian cancer stage FIGO III and IV. In patients with preoperative low or negative values more often a complete removal of the tumor by means of surgery is found than in patients with elevated levels. Concerning the different clinical courses of disease the sensitivity of CASA was about 15% less than sensitivity of CA 125. The prognostic relevance of both markers is comparable and the marker results three month after onset of therapy show a significant correlation with median survival time. To give a statement to the specificity of CASA versus CA 125 the marker levels in benign ovarian tumors have to be examined. It is important to determine CASA in early stage ovarian carcinoma, because CA 125 is elevated in only half of these patients (4). Depending on these further evaluations CASA could become an additional marker in preoperative diagnosis and postoperative monitoring of patients with ovarian malignancy.

References

1. Bast RC, Klug TL, John ES, Niloff J, Lazarus H, Berkowitz RS, Leqvitt T, Griffith CT, Parker L, Zurawski VR, Knapp RC (1983) A radioimmunoassay using a monoclonal antibody to monitor the course of epithelial ovarian cancer. New Engl J Med 309:883–887
2. Kaesemann H, Caffier H, Hoffmann FJ, Crombach G, Wurz H, Kreienberg R, Möbus V, Schmidt-Rhode P, Sturm G (1986) Monoklonale Antikörper in Diagnostik und Verlaufskontrolle des Ovarialkarzinoms. Klin Wochschr 64:781–785
3. Ward BG, McGuckin MA, Ramm LE, Coglan M, Sanderson B, Tripcony L, Free KE (1993) The management of ovarian carcinoma is improved by the use of cancer associated serum antigen and CA 125 assays. Cancer 71:430–438
4. Mogensen O, Mogensen B, Jykobsen A (1989) CA 125 in the diagnosis of pelvic masses. Eur J Cancer Clin Oncol 25:1187–1190

Address for correspondence:
Prof. Dr. med. H. Caffier
Universitätsfrauenklinik
Josef-Schneider-Straße 4
D-97080 Würzburg, Germany

Time course of tumor markers CASA and CA 125 in patients with ovarian carcinoma

M. Meisel, J. Weise, W. Straube

Department of Gynecology and Obstetrics, Ernst-Moritz-Arndt-University, Greifswald, Germany

Introduction

We have used recently developed CASA assay (cancer associated serum antigen), which uses monoclonal antibodies that bind to an epitope on the polymorphic epithelial mucin, for the follow-up during management of ovarian cancer (1).

In addition we have studied the course of CA 125, a tumor marker of the first generation, which is suggested to have a high sensitivity for ovarian carcinoma.

In an attempt to confirm the experience that CASA being a polymorphic epithelial mucin is quite independent of expression of CA 125 (2), we studied the time course of these markers in women suffering from ovarian carcinoma over several months.

Material and methods

Serum samples of 26 patients with ovarian cancer were collected preoperatively and postoperatively throughout several months.

Serum was stored at –20 °C until assay. CASA was determined by an enzymimmunoassay (medac, Hamburg, FRG), the cut-off level being 4 U/ml. CA 125 was determined by Abbott IMX, the cut-off level being 35 U/ml. All samples were tested in duplicate.

All women in our study have had full documentation of surgery and postoperative chemotherapy.

Results

In figure 1 the preoperative expression rate of CASA and CA 125 are related to their respective tumor histology.

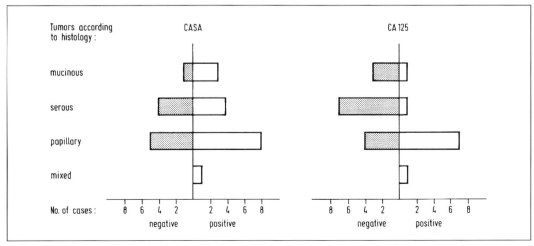

Figure 1. Preoperative tumor marker expression (number of cases) related to the histological type of ovarian tumors.

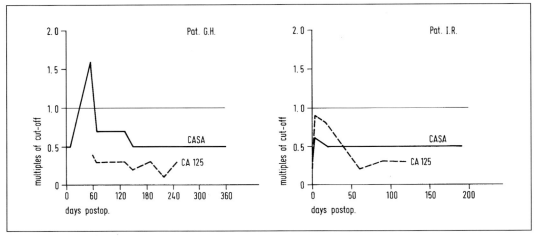

Figure 2. Representative cases of group 1. Pat. G.H. (left): papillary cystadeno carcinoma p(T3NxMo) G2; pat. I.R. (right): serous cystadeno carcinoma p(T3NoMo) G1.

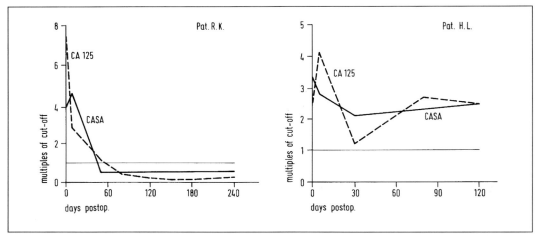

Figure 3. Representative cases of group 2. Pat. R.K. (left): papillary adeno carcinoma p(T3NxMo) G3; pat. H.L. (right): papillary adeno carcinoma p(T2cNxM1) G3.

CASA is shown to recognize all types of ovarian tumors, however, not in every case CASA becomes positive as may be deduced from figures 2 to 5. Only in rare instances it was possible to get nearly the same time courses of CASA and CA 125. So we have tried to group the patients in four representative examples exhibiting a coincident trend in the time course of CASA and CA 125 concentrations.

Group 1: Patients in this group show an identical time course in CASA as well as in CA 125. Levels increase only occasionally beyond the cut-off. In most cases they are below the cut-off in spite of the detected and confirmed tumor. In this group all patients are without complaints (figure 2).

Group 2: Here the expected courses for the tumor markers are shown (figure 3) beginning with pathological figures followed by a considerable decrease postoperative after surgery. As shown, the time course below the cut-off level suggests a favorable prognosis (pat. R.K., left). If there is an initial decline without reaching normal marker concentrations then the prognosis is worse, exitus letalis after a few months (pat. H.L. right).

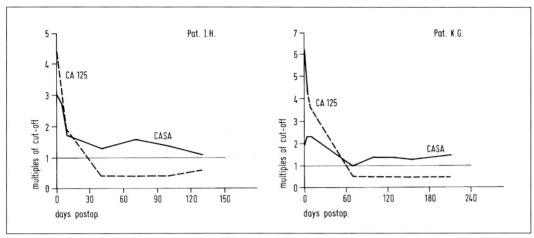

Figure 4. Representative cases of group 3. Pat. I.H. (left): serous cystadeno carcinoma p(T3bNx Mo) G3; pat. K.G. (right): malignant mixed tumor p(T3bNxMo).

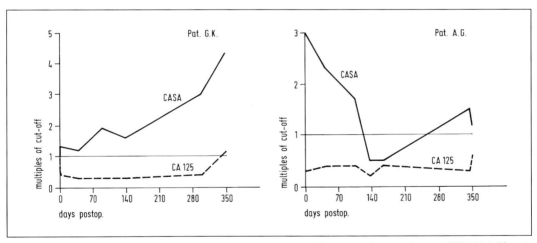

Figure 5. Representative cases of group 4. Pat. G.K. (left): serous papillary cystadeno carcinoma p(T3NxMo) G2; pat. A.G. (right): serous papillary cystadeno carcinoma p(T2aNoMo) G1.

Group 3: Patient with different tumor marker courses in CASA and CA 125 are found, starting with pathological figures of both parameters first and, after chemotherapy, a decrease in CA 125 to normal levels contrasting to CASA which shows values above the cut-off (figure 4). This difference remains unexplained. Six out of 26 patients were considered to belong to this group of time courses. In three cases the patients died some months after surgery.

Group 4: The level of CA 125 remains below the cut-off during the whole observation period (figure 5). In contrast, in these cases CASA levels continue to show advanced values and, obviously, the response to a stimulus leading to further increase is earlier. The patients shown have either a favorable prognosis (pat. A.G., right) or a worse one (pat. G.K., left), exitus letalis.

The latter case shows the additional diagnostic hints which may be given by CASA determinations if CA 125 does not response.

Discussion

High molecular weight mucins, a new class of serum tumor markers, have enormous potential in the detection of ovarian carcinoma, since the use of assays for these markers may overcome many of the problems associated with CA 125.

When used in combination with CA 125, some mucin-based assays have increased the sensitivity and specificity of detection (3). It was shown that two out of ten tumors will be incorrectly classified using CA 125 alone (2).

CASA may be used as second marker for the following reason: CASA may be better suited for differentiating malignant tumors because it reflects the changes in tumor growth during therapy in a more dynamic fashion than CA 125. In another study when CASA determinations were used in addition to the CA 125 assay, the sensitivity for disease was increased from 33 to 62 % (4).

Preoperatively more women had elevated CASA levels than CA 125 ones. In recurrent or persistent disease, CASA levels are elevated more frequently than CA 125 values. This is most likely an indication of the higher sensitivity of CASA over CA 125 for small volume disease (1). We have demonstrated that the CASA assay can be used together with CA 125 to improve the sensitivity for ovarian cancer.

References

1. McGuckin MA, Layton GT, Bailey MJ, Hurst T, Khoo SK, Ward BG (1990) Evaluation of two new assays for tumour associated antigens, CASA and OSA, found in the serum of patients with epithelial ovarian carcinoma: comparison with CA 125. Gynecol Oncol 37:165–171
2. Ward BG (1992) Serum assays in the management of ovarian carcinoma. Int J Gynecol Cancer 1:10-18
3. Devine PL, McGuckin MA, Ward BG (1992) Circulating mucins as tumor markers in ovarian cancer. Anticancer Res 12:707–717
4. Ward BG, McGuckin MA, Ramm LE, Coglan M, Tripcony L, Free KE (1993) The management of ovarian carcinoma is improved by the use of cancer-associated serum antigen and CA 125 assays. Cancer 71:430–438

Address for correspondence:
Prof. Dr. med. W. Straube
Klinikum der Ernst-Moritz-Arndt-Universität
Wollweberstraße 1–3
D-17487 Greifswald, Germany

Significance of the tumor markers CA 125 II, CA 72-4, CASA and CYFRA 21-1 in ovarian carcinomas

Ute Hasholzner[a], L. Baumgartner[b], Petra Stieber[a], W. Meier[b], Karin Hofmann[a], A. Fateh-Moghadam†[a]

[a]Institute for Clinical Chemistry, [b]Gynecological Clinic, Klinikum Großhadern,
Ludwig-Maximilians-University, Munich, Germany

Introduction

Since ten years CA 125 is considered to be a good marker in follow-up care and control of efficacy of therapy in ovarian cancer (1, 2, 3). But also CA 72-4, CASA and CYFRA 21-1 were described as potential markers.
We examined the clinical significance of the tumor marker CA 72-4 (4), the cancer associated serum antigen CASA (5, 6) and CYFRA 21-1 (7) compared with CA 125 II in ovarian carcinomas in order to look for differences of the single tumor markers regarding histology of the ovarian cancer.

Patients and methods

The following investigation was done retrospectively using 262 sera stored at −80 °C. The reference group consisted of 103 sera: 50 sera from healthy women as judged by clinical examination and clinical chemistry and 53 sera from patients with benign gynecological diseases (ovarian cyste, uterus myomatosus, extrauterin gravide, benign ovarian tumors, etc.). 159 sera were from patients with ovarian carcinomas, 72 of them at the time of primary diagnosis (25 serous, 22 mucinous, 25 other histologies) and 87 sera during follow-up care or at a different tumor activity.

We used the following commercially available test kits:
CA 125 II (RIA, Centocor, FRG), CA 72-4 (RIA, Centocor, FRG), CASA (EIA, Medac, FRG) and CYFRA 21-1 (ELISA on ES 700, Boehringer Mannheim, FRG).

Results and discussion

Specificity

Fixing specificity at 95% versus the healthy control group, we found the following cut-off values; CA 125 II: 52 U/ml, CASA: 3.1 U/ml, CA 72-4: 3.0 U/ml and CYFRA 21-1: 1.8 ng/ml. Postulating a specificity of 95% (8) versus the clinically corresponding reference group of benign gynecological diseases we obtained higher cut-off values: 160 U/ml for CA 125 II, 6.5 U/ml for CASA, 6.8 U/ml for CA 72-4 and 2.4 ng/ml for CYFRA 21-1.
These cut-off values (specificity of 95% versus benign gynecological diseases) are taken as basis for dot plots with normalized scales and the calculations of sensitivities. As can be seen in dot plots (figure 1), in serous ovarian carcinomas the same number of values with CA 125 and CASA are elevated, in mucinous ovarian cancer CA 72-4 shows the highest sensitivity. In other histologies consisting of endometroid tumors, dysgerminoma, undifferenciated carcinoma, clearcell carcinoma, germ cell tumor, CA 125, CASA and CA 72-4 were elevated in less than a quarter of cases, CYFRA 21-1 in 12 out of 30 cases.
Most of the elevated cytokeratin-19-levels were from germ cell tumors or embryonal tumors, patients with elevated values of β-HCG or APF at the same time.

Sensitivities

Regarding all ovarian carcinomas (without follow-up) at a specificity of 95% versus benign gynecological diseases, sensitivities of the four markers are lying between 37 and 39%.

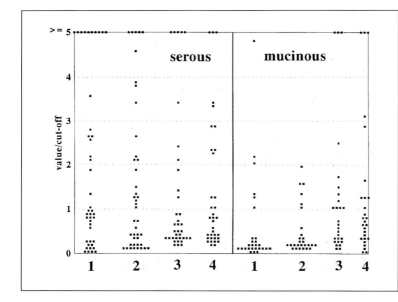

Figure 1. Dotplot: serous ovarian cancer (n = 53) and mucinous ovarian cancer (n = 27); all values are divided through the cut-off value at a specificity of 95% versus benign gynecological diseases. 1= CA 125 II, cut-off = 160 U/ml, 2 = CASA, cut-off = 6.5 U/ml, 3 = CA 72-4, cut-off = 6.8 U/ml, 4 = CYFRA 21-1, cut-off = 2.4 ng/ml

Table I. Sensitivities (%) of CA 125 II, CA 72-4, CASA and CYFRA 21-1 in ovarian cancer at general (n = 110), at time of primary diagnosis (n = 72) and in different histologies: serous (n = 53), mucinous (n = 37), others (n = 30). Specificity is fixed at 95% versus benign gynecological diseases (n = 53) in single marker and in combination of markers.

Marker 1	Marker 2	All	Primary diagnoses	Serous	Mucinous	Others
CA 125 II		38	47	50	21	20
CA 72-4		38	47	36	43	24
CASA		37	31	50	21	22
CYFRA 21-1		39	44	33	36	39
CA 125 II or	CA 72-4	34	58	57	36	28
CA 125 II or	CYFRA 21-1	32	50	54	37	36
CA 125 II or	CASA	30	45	61	26	24
CA 72-4 or	CASA	37	57	57	47	33
CYFRA 21-1 or	CA 72-4	36	50	50	44	39

At the time of primary diagnosis, 47% of the patients have true positive test results with CA 125 II and CA 72-4, 31% with CASA and 44% with CYFRA 21-1. The high positive rate of CA 72-4 in this study is influenced by the high number of mucinous ovarian carcinomas, which are overrepresented in our investigation compared to normal distribution of histological type of ovarian carcinoma.

Regarding sensitivities in relation to the histological type, serous ovarian cancer are recognized in 50% by CA 125 and CASA, in 36% by CA 72-4 and in 33% by CYFRA 21-1. In mucinous ovarian cancer, CA 72-4 with 43% has the highest number of the positive results, followed by CYFRA 21-1 with 36% and CA 125 and CASA with 21% (see table I and figure 2).

For the calculations of the combined sensitivities both markers had to fullfill the postulation of 95% specificity and at least one of the two markers had to show a true positive test result.

Combinations of two markers had a higher sensitivity in primary diagnosis of ovarian cancer when CA 125 II and CA 72-4 (58%) or CA 72-4 and CASA (57%) are used in combination. In serous ovarian cancer the combination of CA 125 II and CASA lead to a sensitivity of 61% versus 50% of the single determination, in mucinous ovarian cancer a small increase of sensitivity up to 47% was seen by combining CA 72-4 and CASA

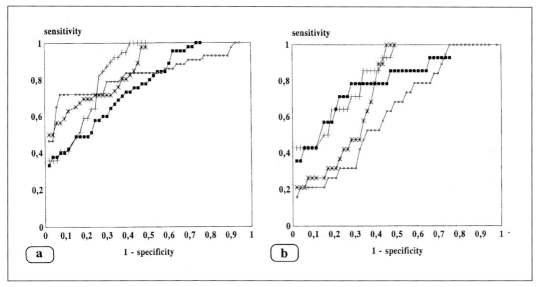

Figure 2. Receiver operating characteristic (ROC) curves; (a) serous (n = 53) and (b) mucinous (n = 27) ovarian cancer both versus benign gynecological diseases (n = 53); –□– CA 125 II, + CA 72-4, –*– CASA, –■– CYFRA 21-1.

(see table I). Sensitivities of the combinations are shown in table I.

In the follow-up of ovarian cancer, CA 125 II in serous ovarian cancer and CA 72-4 in mucinous ovarian cancer was confirmed as leading marker giving the best information about actual tumor activity. Only in cases where CA 125 II and CA 72-4 are negative in primary diagnosis, the additional determination of CASA seems to be suitable.

Conclusions

CA 125 II remains a marker of first choice for ovarian cancer, especially indicating serous ovarian cancer. CA 72-4 has the best sensitivity in mucinous ovarian cancer. CASA shows results comparable to CA 125 II in serous ovarian carcinomas and a slightly additive sensitivity to CA 72-4 in mucinous ovarian cancer. Therefore CASA can be regarded as a marker of second choice in ovarian cancer, especially if CA 125 II and CA 72-4 are negative.

CYFRA 21-1 shows no advantage in comparison with the other markers.

Following our results, the use of tumor markers in ovarian cancer can be summarized: Because of the lack of histological findings before the first therapy, at time of primary diagnosis the simultanous determination of CA 125 II and CA 72-4 is suitable; only if both markers are negative, the additional determination of CASA should be done.

For control of efficacy of therapy and follow-up care, the single determination of the preoperative positive marker, respectively the leading marker is sufficient; in cases of small primary tumor of serous histology and no marker expression, the combination of CA 125 II and CASA is suitable for follow up care.

In other histologies marker determination depends especially from histology (germ cell tumor, e.g.) and preoperative positive marker.

References

1 Meier W, Stieber P, Fateh-Moghadam A, Eiermann W, Hepp H (1987) CA 125 in gyncological malignancies. Eur J Cancer Clin Oncol 23:713

2 Meier W, Stieber P, Fateh-Moghadam A, Eiermann W, Hepp H (1988) CA 125 Serumwerte und histologischer Befund zum Zeitpunkt der Second-look-Laparotomie beim Ovarialkarzinom. Geburtsh Frauenheilk 48:331

3 Quaranta M, Lorusso V, Coviello M, Micelli G, Casamassima A (1988) CA 125 in the monitoring of

response to chemotherapy of ovarian carcinoma. Int J Cancer Suppl 3:68–70
4. Bayerl B, Meier W, Stieber P, Albiez M, Eiermann W, Fateh-Moghadam A (1990) Significance of CA 72-4 in the diagnosis of ovarian cancer. In: Klapdor R (ed) Recent results in tumor diagnosis and therapy. Zuckschwerdt, München, pp 111–112
5. Devine PL, McGuckin MA, Ramm LE, Ward BG, Pee D, Long S (1993) Serum mucin antigens CASA and MSA in tumors of the breast, ovary, lung, pancreas, bladder, colon and prostate – A blind trial with 420 patients. Cancer 72, 6:2007–2015
6. McGuckin MA, Ramm LE, Joy GJ, Free KE, Ward BG (1992) Preoperative discrimination between ovarian carcinomas, non-ovarian gynecological malignancy and benign adnexal masses using serum levels of CA 125 and the polymorphic epithelial mucin antigens CASA, OSA and MSA. Int J Gynecol Cancer 2:119–128
7. Stieber P, Hasholzner U, Bodenmüller H, Nagel D, Sunder-Plassmann L Dienemann H, Meier W, Fateh-Moghadam A (1993) CYFRA 21-1 - A new marker in lung cancer. Cancer 72, 3:707–713
8. Klapdor R (1992) Arbeitsgruppe Qualitätskontrolle und Standardisierung von Tumormarkertests im Rahmen der Hamburger Symposien über Tumormarker. Tumordiagn Ther 13

Address for correspondence:
Dr. med. Petra Stieber
Institut für Klinische Chemie
Klinikum Großhadern
Ludwig-Maximilians-Universität
Marchioninistraße 15
D-81377 München, Germany

Comparison of the cancer-associated serum antigen (CASA) with CA 125 – Specificity and sensitivity in benign and malignant disorders

[a]A.M. Malm, S.D. Costa, [a]J. Huober, [b]H.J. Roth, [a]I.J. Diel, [a]G. Bastert

[a]Department of Gynecology and Obstetrics, University,
[b]Laboratory Dr. Limbach and Partners, Heidelberg, Germany

Introduction

Tumor markers may be used as an adjunct to clinical examination and to imagine techniques to identify ovarian disease, specifically for early detection of ovarian cancer although their specificity and sensitivity are limited to 60–80%. Today, CA 125 is the most important tumor marker for ovarian cancer. The cancer-associated serum antigen (CASA) is a new mucin-derived tumor marker with a reported sensitivity of 58% for ovarian epithelial cancers. In the present study the tumor markers CASA and CA 125 were measured in sera from 231 patients with various benign and malignant diseases to compare their specificity and sensitivity.

Methods

CASA was determined in serum by a dual-determinant enzyme-linked immunosorbent assay (ELISA) using the anti-MUC1 core protein-reactive monoclonal antibodies BC2 (to capture mucin) and BC3 (to detect bound mucin). This assay was provided by medac GmbH, Hamburg. Serum CA 125 was determined using a standard EIA from Centocor. Cut-off values were 4 U/ml for CASA and 35 U/ml for CA 125.

Results

1. CASA and CA 125 were elevated at a similar rate (approximately 35%) in patients with cancers of the endometrium, cervix, colon, breast, liver, lung or pancreas and also in patients with diabetes mellitus, rheumatic disorders, COPD, renal insufficiency, hepatitis, liver cirrhosis, pancreatitis or pregnancy.

2. Only two of 41 patients with endometriosis had elevated CASA levels (5%) while 12 patients were CA 125-positive (29%), which is statistically significant (x^2-test: $p = 0.033$). If benign ovarian tumors were considered (15 endometriomas and nine solid tumors of other type) only two of 24 tumors were associated with elevated CASA values (8% false positive) but 11 of 24 patients were CA 125-positive (46%). This difference also was statistically significant (x^2-test: $p = 0.0001$).

3. In ovarian cancer 26 of 42 patients (62%) were CASA-positive as compared to 81% (34 of 42 patients) positive for CA 125. This difference was statistically not significant (x^2-test: $p = 0.08$).

4. If we use CASA and CA 125 in combination, we find a specificity of 96% (CASA > 4 U/ml and CA 125 > 35 U/ml) and a sensitivity of 88% (CASA > 4 U/ml or CA 125 > 35 U/ml).

Conclusions

CASA appears to be as sensitive as CA 125 for ovarian cancer (no statistically significant difference) but displays a significantly higher specificity (92% versus 54%) when there is an ovarian tumor. So CASA might contribute to define the nature of adnexal masses preoperatively and help planning a specific surgical procedure.

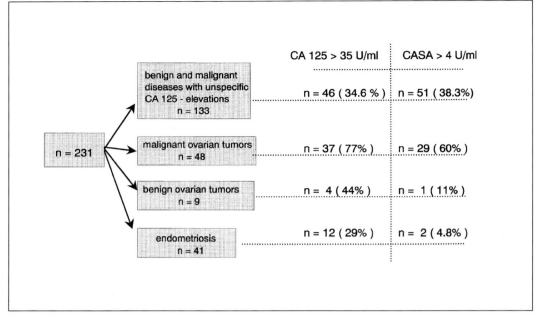

Figure 1. CASA and CA 125 values in benign and maligant disease.

References

1. Devine PL, McGuckin MA, Ramm LE, Ward BG, Pee D, Long S (1993) Serum mucin antigens CASA and MSA in tumors of the breast, ovary, lung, pancreas, bladder, colon, and prostate. Cancer 72:2007–2015
2. Layton GT, Xing PX, McKenzie IFC, Bishop JF, McGuckin MA (1991) Cancer associated serum antigen (CASA) and ovarian serum antigen (OSA): Two new tumor marker kits for detecting carcinoma-associated mucins. J Tumor Marker Oncol 6:9–17
3. McGuckin MA, Layton GT, Bailey MJ, Hurst T, Khoo SK, Ward BG (1990) Evaluation of two new assays for tumor-associated antigens, CASA and OSA, found in the serum of patients with epithelial ovarian carcinoma – comparison with CA 125. Gynecol Oncol 37:165–171
4. McGuckin MA, Ramm LE, Joy GJ, Free KE, Ward BG (1992) Pre-operative discrimination between ovarian carcinoma, non-ovarian gynecological malignancy and benign adnexal masses using serum levels of CA 125 and the polymorphic epithelial mucin antigens CASA, OSA and MSA. Int J Gynecol Cancer 2:119–128
5. Ward BG, McGuckin MA, Ramm LE, Forbes KL (1991) Expression of tumor markers CA 125, CASA and OSA in minimal/mild endometriosis. Aust NZ J Obstet Gynaecol 31:273–275
6. Ward BG, McGuckin MA, Ramm LE, Coglan M, Sanderson B, Tripcony L, Free KE (1993) The management of ovarian carcinoma is improved by the use of cancer associated serum antigen (CASA) and CA 125 assays. Cancer 71:430–438

Address for correspondence:
Dr. med. S. D. Costa
Universitätsfrauenklinik
Voßstraße 9
D-69115 Heidelberg, Germany

Tumor markers in gynecology

P. Kenemans[a], A.A. Verstraeten[a], G.J. van Kamp[b], J. Hilgers[a]

Departments of [a]Gynecology and Obstetrics and [b]Clinical Chemistry, Free University Hospital, Amsterdam, The Netherlands

Introduction

During the last decade, the hybridoma technology has provided several monoclonal antibodies, that are characterized by a highly specific binding to tumor associated molecules, such as hormones (e.g. hCG), mucins (e.g. the MUC-1 gene product) and mucin-like substances (e.g. the CA 125-glycoprotein).
Double determinant monoclonal antibody-based immunoassays have been developed for the quantification in serum of several of these clinically relevant tumor markers.

In the field of gynecological oncology the most important markers to date are:

- hCG in trophoblastic disease,
- CA 15-3 in breast cancer and
- CA 125 in ovarian carcinoma.

HCG and gestational trophoblastic disease (GTD)

GTD comprises a group of tumors derived from the trophoblast, after a conception. These tumors are characterized by the production of hCG, that can be specifically detected by serum immunoassays based on anti-βhCG subunit reactive antibodies. In many circumstances, this marker will allow initiation and termination of treatment based on the hCG marker alone, without histological proof.

Clinical applications are:

1. correct identification of patients with post-(hydatidiform) mole persistant disease by means of comparing with a normal hCG regression curve (1);
2. monitoring of (chemotherapeutic) treatment of patients with invasive moles and choriocarcinoma;
3. early detection of recurrence during follow-up.

A non-oncologic gynecological application is the monitoring of patients with an extra-uterine pregnancy, both during an expectant policy, hoping for spontaneous regression, as well as after conservative (e.g. laparoscopic or MTX-cytostatic) treatment.

CA 15-3 and breast cancer

The MUC-1 gene product (PEM, MCA, CA 15-3 antigen) which is overexpressed in many carcinomas, has been shown to provide the best breast cancer marker protein. It can be detected by various serum immunoassays, of which CA 15-3 is the best known (2).

Clinical applications are:

1. detection of residual (metastatic) or recurrent disease after primary treatment;
2. monitoring of second line treatment in patients with recurrent (metastatic) disease. The application is limited by a rather low positivity rate and the lack of predictive value.

However, recent investigations of our group (3, 4) have shown:

a. that in CA 15-3-test-negative patients the antigen is often present in the form of immune-complexes, bound by free anti-MUC-1 auto-antibody, and is therefore not detected;
b. that these circulating immune complexes and the serum level of free autoantibody might have important prognostic value as to treatment outcome.

CA 125 and ovarian carcinoma

Today, optimal management of patients with ovarian cancer is not possible without the CA 125 serum test (5). It should be realized, however, that marker values obtained with different commercial CA 125 kits can give discordant (6), and even discrepant results, as were found with the original Boehringer Mannheim (BM) Enzymun CA 125 assay (7).

Second generation CA 125 assays

We evaluated the newly introduced second generation CA 125 assays, the Centocor CA 125II IRMA and the BM Enzymun CA 125 II assay, that are one step heterologous double determinant solid phase assays utilizing the M11 mouse monoclonal antibody as capture antibody and as a tracer the radio-iodinated or enzyme-labeled OC 125 antibody, respectively.

In a technical evaluation, the Centocor CA 125 II IRMA revealed a fourfold increase in signal to noise ratio in the standard curve, intra- and inter-assay coefficients of variation (CVs) always smaller than 5% and 7%, respectively, and an improved linearity on dilution, with a minimal detectable dose of 0.34 U/ml (8).

For the BM Enzymun CA 125 II assay the standard line was found to be linear between the lowest, 0 U/ml, standard and the upper standard of 540 U/ml, with absorbances ranging from 0.148 to 2.539. Inter- and intra-assay CVs at the cut-off value of 35 U/ml were 5.5% and 4.3%, respectively. Linearity on dilution is excellent, with

Table I. Comparison of CA 125 assay results in healthy controls, and positivity rates in patients with benign and malignant conditions.

	Assay[a]	Min	Max	p95[b]	p99[c]	Percent	
						> 35 U/ml	> 65 U/ml
Healthy controls	CN CA 125	6.0	49	32.4	47.3	3.8	0
(n = 185)	CN CA 125 II	5.0	52	31.8	50.4	4.3	0
	BM CA 125 II	0.1	53	31.7	46.1	2.7	0
				Percent			
				> p95	> p99	> 35 U/ml	> 65 U/ml
Pregnancy (n = 51)	CN CA 125	2.0	78	19.6	9.8	17.6	2.0
	CN CA 125 II	5.0	86	23.5	7.8	19.6	2.0
	BM CA 125 II	4.0	73	19.6	7.8	11.8	3.9
Benign pelvic diseases	CN CA 125	1.0	507	27.1	18.8	26.4	14.6
(n = 144)	CN CA 125 II	5.0	476	36.8	18.1	30.6	17.4
	BM CA 125 II	0.1	460	26.4	18.1	23.6	15.3
Ovarian carcinoma	CN CA 125	1.0	18602	65.2	58.3	63.6	53.8
(n = 264)	CN CA 125 II	3.0	11985	66.7	56.8	64.8	52.3
	BM CA 125 II	0.1	14519	66.3	59.1	63.3	53.4
Other adeno-	CN CA 125	1.0	1530	16.1	14.5	16.1	8.1
carcinomas (n = 62)	CN CA 125 II	6.0	1058	19.4	14.5	17.7	11.3
	BM CA 125 II	0.1	966	16.1	14.5	16.1	9.7
Total study group	CN CA 125	1.0	18602	34.0	27.8	32.9	23.9
(n = 706)	CN CA 125 II	3.0	11985	37.1	26.9	34.6	24.2
	BM CA 125 II	0.1	14519	34.3	27.8	31.4	24.2

[a] CN CA 125: original CA 125 IRMA (Centocor); CN CA 125 II: Centocor CA 125 II IRMA; BM CA 125 II: Enzymun-Test® CA 125 II (Boehringer Mannheim)
[b] p95: 95th percentile
[c] p99: 99th percentile

Gynecology   127

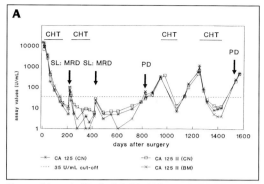 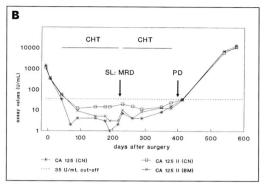

Figure 1A and 1B. Serial CA 125 measurements in two ovarian cancer monitored for course of disease during treatment and follow-up. CHT: chemotherapy (horizontal bars indicate the duration of the treatment); SL: second-look procedure; MRD: minimal residual disease; PD: progressive disease.

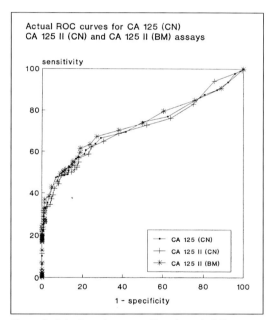 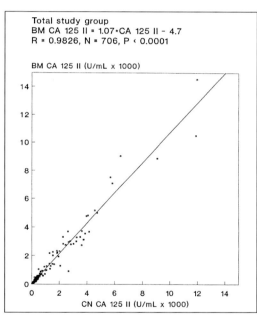

Figure 2. Actual receiver operating characteristic curves for the original CA 125 IRMA (CA 125 (CN)) (Centocor), the second generation CA 125 II IRMA (CA 125 II (CN)) (Centocor), and the Enzymun-Test® CA 125 II (Boehringer Mannheim) in patients with ovarian cancer (n = 264) versus patients with benign pelvic diseases (n = 144).

Figure 3. Scatter diagram of CA 125 assay results with the least-squares regression line (X-axis: the second generation CA 125 II IRMA (CN CA 125 II (centocor); Y-axis: the Enzymun-Test® CA 125II (Boehringer Mannheim).

a minimal detectable dose of less than 1.0 U/ml. In a clinical evaluation CA 125II assay values were determined in a total of 706 serum samples, including 185 samples of apparently healthy females and 264 samples of patients with cancer of the ovary.

In comparison to the original Centocor CA 125 IRMA, highly similar CA 125 distribution patterns were obtained with both CA 125 II assays, with equal reference ranges for healthy women and nearly identical positivity (> 35 U/ml) rates (table I), and comparable monitoring graphs of CA 125 assay values in the three assays and ROC-curves (figures 1 and 2, resp.). Least squares linear regression analysis in ovarian cancer patients (n = 216) showed for CA 125 assay values between 0–1000 U/ml slopes of 0.96 and 1.09, respectively: Centocor CA 125 II = 0.96*CA 125 IRMA + 13.6 (r = 0.8632, p = < 0.0001), Enzymun CA 125 II = 1.09*CA 125 IRMA + 6.1 (r = 0.8211, p = 0.0001).

For the total study group (n = 706), comparing both second generation assays directly, the regression equation was: Enzymun CA 125 II = 1.07*Centocor CA 125 II − 4.7 (r = 0.9826, p < 0.001) (figure 3). The problematic phenomenon of clearly discrepant results as found with the corresponding two homologous assays is not longer encountered with the heterologous type assays.

It can be concluded that this first technical and clinical evaluation of the two new CA 125 II assays shows their superior analytical performance, in addition to high qualitative and quantitative correlations with the original Centocor CA 125 test.

Clinical applications

Both the original OC 125-based homologous double determinant serum assays, as well as the above mentioned second generation heterologous double determinant CA 125 II assays, are currently widely applied in the following clinical situations:

1. Differential diagnosis of ovarian tumors: When used in combination with other diagnostic techniques, CA 125 determination has a value as a diagnostic adjunct in the differential diagnosis of patients presenting with a pelvic mass (9), especially in the discrimination of ovarian cancer patients from those with benign ovarian tumors (10) and from those with advanced colon cancer (11).
2. Monitoring of disease in ovarian cancer patients: Doubling or halving of CA 125 serum values correlates (in 87% of all cases) with tumor progression or regression, respectively.
3. Early prediction of outcome: Deviation of the ideal CA 125 regression curve predicts poor outcome within three months of cytostatic treatment after debulking surgery. The ideal CA 125 regression curve is characterized by a biological T 1/2 < 20 days and/or a CA 125 normalization within 90 days from initiation of treatment (12).
4. Tumor status after completion of first line treatment: Patients with CA 125 > 35 units/ml have (in 95% of all cases) still tumor present at second look surgery. However, patients with CA 125 ≤ 35 units/ml still have in 50% of all cases mostly minimal residual disease.
5. Early detection of recurrence: After a complete remission a rise of CA 125 precedes tumor recurrence in 75% of all patients with lead times up to more than one year, surpassing the CT-scan in cheapness and accuracy.

A non-oncologic gynecological application, currently under investigation, is monitoring for treatment in endometriosis.

References

1 Yedema CA, Verheijen RH, Kenemans P, Schijf ChP, Borm GF, Segers MF, Thomas ChM (1993) Identification of patients with persistent trophoblastic disease by means of a normal human chorionic gonadotropin regression curve. Am J Obstet Gynecol 68:787–92
2 Bon GG, Kenemans P, van Kamp GJ, Yedema CA, Hilgers J (1990) Review on the clinical value of polymorphic epithelial mucin tumor markers for the management of carcinoma patients. J Nucl Med Allied Sci 34 (suppl 3):151–62
3 Gourevitch MM, Mensdorff-Pouilly Sv, Litvinov SV, Verstraeten A, van Kamp GJ, Kenemans P, Hilgers J (1993) Circulating polymorphic epithelial mucin (PEM) might be included into immune complexes and not efficiently detected by the CA 15-3 assay. Abstract XXIst Meeting of the International Society for Oncodevelopmental Biology and Medicine, Jerusalem, Israel, November 7–11, p 50
4 Mensdorff-Pouilly Sv, Gourevitch M, Verstraeten A, van Kamp GJ, Kenemans P, Hilgers J (1993) Incidence of a humoral immune response against polymorphic epithelial mucin (PEM) in benign breast tumor and breast and ovarian cancer patients. Abstract XXIst Meeting of the International Society for Oncodevelopmental Biology and Medicine, Jerusalem, Israel, November 7–11, p 50
5 Kenemans P, Yedema CA, Bon GG, von Mensdorff-Pouilly S (1993) CA 125 in gynecological pathology – a review. Eur J Obstet Gynec Reprod Biol 49:115–124

6. van Kamp GJ, Verstraeten AA, Kenemans P (1993) Discordant serum CA 125 values in commercial immunoassays. Eur J Obstet Gynecol Reprod Biol 49:99–103
7. Kenemans P, Bon GG, Kessler AC, Verstraeten AA, van Kamp GJ (1992) Multicenter technical and clinical evaluation of a fully automated enzyme immunoassay for CA 125. Clin Chem 38:1466–1471
8. Kenemans P, van Kamp GJ, Oehr P, Verstraeten RA (1993) Heterologous double-determinant immunoradiometric assay CA 125 II: reliable second-generation immunoassay for determining CA 125 in serum. Clin Chem 39(12):2509–2513
9. Schutter EMJ, Kenemans P, Sohn C, Kristen P, Crombach G, Westermann R, Möbus V, Kaufmann M, Caffier H, Schmidt-Rhode P, Kreienberg R, Verstraeten AA, Cornillie F (1994) Diagnostic value of pelvic examination, ultrasound and serum CA 125 in postmenopausal women presenting with a pelvic mass, an international multicenter study. Cancer (in press)
10. Yedema CA, Massuger L, Hilgers J, Poels L, Thomas CMG, Kenemans P (1988) Pre-operative discrimination between benign and malignant ovarian tumors using a combination of CA 125 and CA 15-3 serum assays. Int J Cancer 3(suppl):61–67
11. Yedema CA, Kenemans P, Wobbes Th, Thomas CMG, Bon GG, Mulder C, Voorhorst FJ, Verstraeten AA, van Kamp GJ, Hilgers J (1992) Use of serum tumor markers in the differential diagnosis between ovarian and colorectal adenocarcinomas. Tumour Biol 13:18–26
12. Yedema CA, Kenemans P, Voorhorst F, Bon G, Schijf C, Beex L, Verstraeten A, Hilgers J, Vermorken J (1993) CA 125 half-life in ovarian cancer: a multivariate survival analysis. Br J Cancer 67:1361–1367

Address for correspondence:
Prof. Dr. P. Kenemans
Department of Gynecology and Obstetrics
Free University Hospital
P.O. Box 7057
NL-1007 11B Amsterdam, The Netherlands

Development of assays for determination of MUC-1 breast cancer antigen

O. Nilsson, B. Karlsson, L. Lindholm, A. Pettersson

CanAg Diagnostics AB, Gothenburg, Sweden

Introduction

The MUC-1 antigen is membrane anchored mucin type glycoprotein present in the cell membrane of normal and malignant epithelial cells of different organs, e.g. breast, lung, ovary and pancreas. The MUC-1 mucin has been identified by several independent groups and the antigen is known in the literature under many different names, e.g. PEM, PUM, episialin, Ca-1, PAS, ETA, EMA, HMFG etc (1, 2). The MUC-1 mucin is secreted from tumor cells, and serological determination of MUC-1 is used as a marker of breast cancer, and several commercial breast cancer assays measuring the MUC-1 breast cancer antigen are available under different "brand names", e.g. CA 15-3, CA 549, MCA. The MUC-1 mucin is a unique mucin as the protein core contains a transmembrane domain, a cytoplasmic domain, and an extra-cellular carbohydrate rich domain. The MUC-1 characteristic portion of the extra-cellular domain is a 20 amino acid sequence, which is repeated ≈ 20 – ≈ 80 times between different individuals. The polymorphism with respect to the number of the 20 amino acid tandem repeat (VNTR polymorphism), and the variation in glycosylation between individuals, different organs and between normal and malignant cells could explain the heterogeneity of the MUC-1 mucin. Monoclonal antibodies specific for the MUC-1 apoprotein have been shown to be directed against epitopes in the 20 aa tandem repeat sequence. Most of these antibodies detect an epitope containing whole or part of the following amino acid sequence [-PDTRP-].

The present paper describes the establishment of two new monoclonal antibodies reacting with the MUC-1 breast cancer antigen, and the use of the MAbs for the development of serological assays for determination of MUC-1 antigen.

Materials and methods

Establishment of MAb

Monoclonal antibodies were raised by i.p. immunization of Balb/c mice with the human adeno carcinoma cell line ZR 75-1. The mice were boostered 2–3 times with the same antigen, and fusions between spleenocytes and the P3x63-Ag8.653 myeloma cell line were performed 60–100 days after the priming as previously described (3). Hybridomas were initially screened by ELISA against the ZR75-1 cell line. Further screenings were performed by histochemistry on cryostate sections from normal and malignant tissues. MAb detecting secreted antigens were selected by an inhibition assay using spent medium from breast cancer cell lines and pools of normal human serum and serum from patients with advanced breast cancer as antigens.

Determination of epitope specificity

The chemical nature of the epitopes detected by the established MAb was characterized by chemical treatment (periodate, sialidase, PCA precipitation of extracts) of the ZR 75-1 cell line as described (4), and immunoblotting of ZR75-1 extract after SDS-PAGE. Glycolipids were isolated from ZR75-1 cell line, separated into gangliosides and neutral glycolipids, and tested for antigen reactivity by TLC-immunostaining and solid-phase binding assays as previously described (1).

Detailed epitope analysis of the Ma552 MAb was performed by determination of binding of the Ma552 MAb to solid-phase immobilized overlapping heptapeptides corresponding to the MUC-1 tandem repeat region (5, 6).

Development of serological assays

The antibodies were labeled with N1DTTA Eu chelate (Wallac Oy, Turku, Finland) according to *Hemmilä* et al. (7) and biotinylated using BNHS reagent according to standard procedures. The assays were developed as forward sandwich Delfia™ assays using biotinylated Ma552 MAb as catching antibody, and Eu labeled Ma552 or Ma695 MAb for detection. Streptavidin microtiter plates (Wallac Oy, Turku, Finland) were used for separation of the reactants. The assays were developed as two-step sandwich assays using the following assay procedure: 25 µl of sample (diluted 1/10 in assay buffer) + 100 µl of biotin MAb, 2.5 µg/ml, incubated in SA coated microtiterplates for 2 h with shaking; washing; addition of 100 µl Eu labeled Ma552 or Ma695 MAb, 2 µg/ml, and incubation for 1 h; after additional washing the Eu fluorescences were determined in an Arcus fluorometer after addition of 200 µl of enhancement solution. Correlation with commercial assays for determination of MUC-1 antigen was studied by analyses of 40 healthy females and 40 females with various stages of breast cancer using the CA 15-3 ELSA IRMA kit from CIS Bio-Industries, France, as reference.

Results and discussion

A number of hybridomas with relative specificity for breast cancer were established. Out of these

Table I. Histochemical staining of Ma552 and Ma695.

Tissue	Positive staining (positive/total)	
	Ma552	Ma695
Breast		
tumor	10/10	9/9
normal	4/4[a]	5/5[a]
Colon		
tumor	5/5	2/4
normal	3/4[a]	0/4
Normal tissues		
pancreas	l/l [c]	1/1[c]
spleen	0/1	0/1
liver	0/1	0/1
kidney	l/l [b]	l/l [b]

[a]Luminal staining, [b]staining of tubuli, [c]ducts positive

the Ma552 MAb and Ma695 MAb were selected owing to a relatively good histochemical specificity (table I), and that the MAbs detected epitopes co-expressed on a secreted antigen. Normal and tumor tissue from breast stained positive with the Ma552 and Ma695 MAbs, but in normal breast the staining showed a luminal staining commonly seen for mucin antigens. In colon the Ma552 MAb stained both normal and tumor tissue, while the Ma695 MAb only stained tumor tissue. Although the Ma552 MAb stained both normal and tumor tissue the staining was generally more intense in the tumor, and as in the normal breast tissue the staining of normal colon tissue was luminal.

The MA552 and Ma695 MAbs reacted with a PCA soluble high molecular antigen, > 200 kD, as shown by inhibition of binding of the Ma552 and Ma695 to ZR 75.1 cells using PCA soluble extracts as antigen, and by immunoblotting of extracts from ZR75-1 cell line separated by SDS-PAGE. The results indicated that the antigen in the ZR75-1 cell line showed characteristics typical of mucins. The epitope defined by the Ma695 MAb was sensitive towards mild periodate oxidation (1 mM periodate) and sialidase treatment of immobilized ZR75-1 cells. However, the antibody did not react with glycolipids isolated from ZR75-1 cells, which indicated that the Ma695 MAb recognized a sialylated carbohydrate epitope expressed in mucins.

The epitope defined by the Ma552 MAb was resistant towards periodate oxidation, indicating that the epitope was expressed in the polypeptide core of a mucin. The binding of the Ma552 MAb to heptapeptides corresponding to overlapping peptides of the MUC-1 tandem repeat 20 amino acid sequence showed that the Ma552 MAb recognized the [-TRPAPG-3] hexapeptide of the MUC-1 tandem repeat, (figure 1), (5). The binding of the Ma552 MAb was also inhibited by a peptide corresponding to the MUC-1 tandem repeat, but not by other peptides (5). These results strongly indicated that the Ma552 MAb recognized the MUC-1 apoprotein, and that the antigen recognized by the Ma552 and Ma695 MAb was the MUC-1 mucin antigen. The Ma552 MAb was less influenced by the glycosylation of the mucin as compared to other MUC-1 reactive antibodies e.g. SM3, and could be used for detection of the highly glycosylated MUC-1 antigen in colon cancer cell lines without prior deglycosylation of the antigen (5).

132 In Vitro Diagnosis

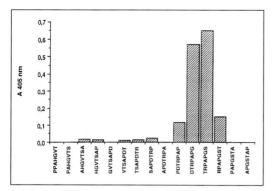

Figure 1. Epitope mapping of Ma552 MAb. The Ma552 MAb was reacted with immobilized synthetic sequence overlapping heptapeptides corresponding to the MUC-I tandem repeat in an ELISA (5, 6).

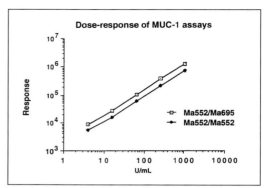

Figure 2. Dose-response of Ma552/Ma695 and Ma552/Ma552 immunofluorometric assays. Both assays were developed as two-step sandwich assays using biotinylated Ma552 MAb as catching MAb, and Eu labeled Ma552 resp. Ma695 MAb as tracer.

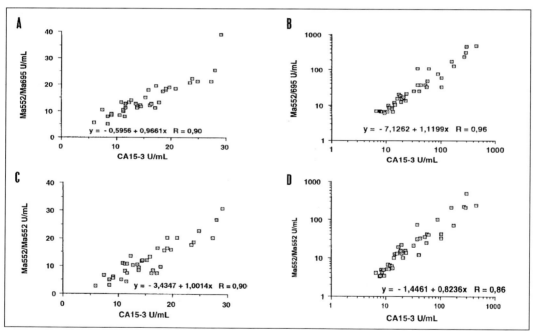

Figure 3. Correlation between CA 15-3, Ma552/Ma695 and Ma552/Ma552 assays. A) Ma552/Ma695 and CA 15-3 in healthy subjects; B) Ma552/Ma695 and CA15-3 in breast cancer; C) Ma552/Ma552 and CA 15-3 in healthy subjects; D) Ma552/Ma552 and CA 15-3 in breast cancer.

This difference in reactivity might be owing to that the Ma552 epitope did not contain a glycosylation site in the central part of the epitope.
The Ma552 MAb and Ma695 MAb were used for development of prototype immunofluorometric assays (IFMA), and used in a preliminary clinical evaluation. The Ma552 MAb was used as catching MAb both in a homologous assay with Eu labeled Ma552 as tracer, and in a heterologous assay using Eu labeled Ma695 MAb as tracer (figure 2). The Ma695 MAb could only be used in heterologous assays as a homologous Ma695 MAb assay resulted in a very low dose-response curve. The Ma695 MAb could be used either as catching

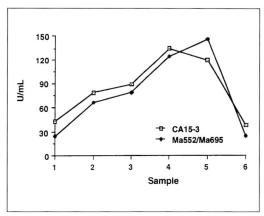

Figure 4. Serum levels of MUC-I antigen measured with CA 15-3 and Ma552/Ma695 assay during follow-up of a breast cancer patient.

MAb or tracer MAb together with Ma552 MAb, but the results presented in this paper are based on assays with the Ma695 MAb used as detecting MAb.

The Ma552/Ma552 and Ma552/Ma695 assays showed a good correlation with the commercial MUC-1 assay CA 15-3 both in healthy subjects and in patients with breast cancer (figure 3). In the primary evaluation the homologous Ma552 assay showed somewhat less sensitivity at 95 % specificity level compared to the CA 15-3 and Ma552/Ma695 assays; 43% sensitivity for CA 15-3 and Ma552/Ma695 and 34% sensitivity for the Ma552/Ma552 assay. Also during follow-up of patients with breast cancer the preliminary evaluation showed a close correlation of Ma552/Ma695 and CA15-3 assay (figure 4).

Based on the known specificity of the Ma552 and Ma695 MAb and the results of the preliminary clinical evaluation it is concluded that these MAb can be used for the development of assays for determination of breast cancer associated MUC-1 antigen.

References

1. Hilgers J, Zotter S, Kenemans P (1988) Polymorphic epithelial mucin and CA125-bearing glycoprotein in basic and applied carcinoma research. Cancer Rev 11–12:3–10
2. Taylor-Papadmitriou J, Gendler S (1988) Molecular aspects of mucins. Cancer Rev. 11–12:11–24
3. Lindolm L, Holmgren J, Svennerholm L, Fredman P, Nilsson O, Persson B, Myrvold H, Lagergard T (1983) Monoclonal antibodies against gastrointestinal tumor-associated antigens isolated as monosialogangliosides. Int Archs Allergy appl Immunol 71:178–181
4. Johansson C, Nilsson O, Baeckstöm D, Jansson E-L, Lindholm L (1991) Novel epitopes on the CA50-carrying Antigen: Chemical and Immunochemical studies. Tumor Biol 12:159–170
5. Baeckström D, Nilsson O, Price MR, Lindholm L, Hansson GC (1993) Discrimination of MUCl mucins from other Sialyl-Le a -carrying glyco-proteins produced by cblon carcinoma cells using a novel monoclonal antibody. Cancer Res 53:755–61
6. Price MR, Hudecz F, O'Sullivan C, Baldwin RW, Edwards PM, Tendler SJB (1990) Immunological and structural features of the protein core of human polymorphic epithelial mucin. Mol Immunol 27:795–802
7. Hemmilä I, Dakubu 5, Mukkala VM, Siitari H, Lövgren T (1983) Europium as a label in time-resolved immunofluorometric assays. Anal Biochem 237:335–340

Address for correspondence:
Dr. O. Nilsson
CanAg Diagnostics AB
P.O. Box 12136
S-402 42 Gothenburg, Sweden

Tissue polypeptide specific (TPS) antigen in benign and malignant gynecological diseases

G.C. Torre[a], V. Barbetti[e], M. Paganuzzi[e], C. Mazzei[c], M. Onetto[b], B. Bobbio[b],
M. Bruzzone[d], V. Lucchese[a], F. Boccardo[d], M. Gaffuri[e], R. Rembado[e]

[a]Department of Obstetrics and Gynecology, [c]Immunohemathological Service
[e]Nuclear Medicine Service, Ospedale Santa Corona, Pietra Ligure,
[b]Clinical Pathology, [d]Medical Oncology II,
Istituto Nazionale per la Ricerca sul Cancro, Genova, Italy

Introduction

In 1957 *Björklund* et al. (1) described an antigenic principle named tissue polypeptide antigen (TPA), a cell cycle product which is secreted into the body fluids by proliferating cells during the late S-phase and during the G2-phase of the cell division cycle. TPA was isolated from the residues of pooled tumors (2).

TPA is an index of cell proliferation or better a marker of proliferation which reflects the intensity of tumor cell proliferation, i.e. the number of new cells produced per time unit (2–4).

The monoclonal mapping of tissue polypeptide antigen revealed that it contained 35 different epitopes of which the M3 specific epitope constitutes the critical TPA specificity as related to cell proliferation (4).

The concentration of tissue polypeptide antigen can be determined by the recently introduced monoclonal TPS™ – IRMA assay. The release and extracellular concentration of TPS shows significant relationship with the synthesis of DNA as indicated by the incorporation of tritiated thymidine (4). Considering the interesting data reported, TPS is a marker of proliferative activity of different malignant diseases such as urological (5, 6), breast (7), gastrointestinal (8), cervical (9) and ovarian cancer (10). High concentrations of TPS are associated with progressive disease and low concentration with stable disease or remission (11).

The aim of this study was to investigate the TPS level and its distribution in gynecology and the possible role of TPS as tumor proliferation marker, in association with the specific gynecological tumor mass markers.

Material and methods

Patients

TPS was determined in a total of 718 sera of controls and patients with gynecological lesions. The control group consisted of 182 apparently healthy test subjects. Benign hepatic lesions may cause high levels of TPS as described by *Bremer* et al. (12). TPS was determined in 119 serum samples of women in pregnancy and in 417 patients with benign and malignant gynecological lesions. The benign pathology included 217 cases as follows: uterine myoma 48, cystic endometrial hyperplasia 19, polyps 20, cervicitis 6, C.I.N. 27, ovarian cyst 72, PID 11, vulvo-vaginal (craurosis, condylomata, Bartholin's gland abscess) 14.

The malignant pathology included 200 cases altogether divided as follows: vulvar 13, vaginal 3, ovarian 81, primary tumor 68 and relapse 13, endometrial 57, cervical 46. TPS levels were also analyzed in serum samples during postoperative follow-up in six benign and nine malignant gynecological lesions.

All the cases were HBsAg, HCV and HIV negative. Blood samples were drawn before any medical intervention, surgery or radiotherapy. One exception was post surgery sampling, where in the case of malignant gynecological lesions samples for TPS analysis were collected continuously. Furthermore we examined the behavior of the proliferation index in the immediate post surgery in order to have some indications about the serial controls and the reference values.

Blood samples were drawn from the cubital vein at 8.00 a.m. after overnight fasting, allowed to clot and centrifuged (3000 r.p.m., for 5 min).

After clotting the specimens were stored in aliquots in polyethylene test tubes, frozen and kept at −110 °C.

Assays

TPS concentrations in all serum samples were measured in duplicate – using a commercially, available TPS™ IRMA kit manufactured by BEKI Diagnostics AB, Bromma, Sweden.
This assay is based upon a polyclonal antibody for antigen capture and a monoclonal antibody M3 for antigen detection. The cut-off (M + 2SD) in this series of controls was 125 U/l.

Results

Pregnancy

Normal pregnancies, entire series, presented elevated levels of TPS in 59% of the patients and the specificity was 100% for ectopic pregnancies. The observed increase of the TPS signal was for the trimester I (0%), II (29%) and III (78%). In the gestosis of the third trimester the levels of TPS were positive in 63% of the patients prior to the elevation observed for the normals during the same period.

Benign gynecological pathology

In almost all the cases of benign pathologies investigated, the distribution of TPS serum levels remained within the normal range (cut-off 125 U/l) and only 7% (15/217) showed elevated TPS levels. The separated pathologies as demonstrated in table I, showed that the specificity was high, reaching 100% for the adnexal lesions, in the presence of both acute and chronic lesions. The uterine benign lesions of the cervix and of the corpus presented positivities of 6% (2/33) and 7% (6/87), respectively.
The ovarian pathology revealed a positivity of 7% (5/72) and a positivity of 14% (2/14) was observed for vulvovaginal lesions.

Malignant gynecological pathology

Patients with malignant gynecological pathologies showed elevated serum levels of TPS, preferably in the presence of ovarian neoplasia rather than in the other malignant gynecological pathologies (table II). The total sensitivity was 40% (79/200); the sensitivity varied between 39% (18/46) in cervicocarcinoma, 57% (46/81) in ovarian epithelial carcinoma, 57% (39/68) for primary lesions, 54% (7/13) for ovarian relapses, 15% (2/13) in vulvar carcinoma and 29% (13/57) in endometrial adenocarcinoma. TPS serum levels in patients with vaginal carcinoma were in the normal range.
No particular correlation was observed in the TPS levels of the cervicocarcinoma patients with the stages of the tumor. We observed elevated TPS levels in ovarian epithelial carcinoma patients in 62% (stage III) and 75% (stage IV), respectively. The incidence for the relapse was 54%.

Post surgery

Independent of the type of pathology, a significant decrease of presurgery elevated TPS levels was observed immediately after surgery. This decrease reached its minimum TPS value into the

Table I. Sensitivity of TPS in 217 patients with benign gynecological pathologies.

	No.	TPS > 125 U/l	Percentage
Cervix uteri	33	2	6.1
Corpus uteri	87	6	6.9
Vulvo-vaginal	14	2	14.3
Ovarian	72	5	6.9
Adnexa	11	0	0
Total	217	15	6.9

Table II. Sensitivity of TPS in 200 patients with malignant gynecological pathologies.

	No.	TPS > 125 U/l	Percentage
Cervicocarcinoma	46	18	39.1
Endometrial adeno ca.	57	13	28.8
Ovarian carcinoma	81	46	56.8
Vulvar carcinoma	13	2	15.4
Vaginal carcinoma	3	0	0
Total	200	79	39.5

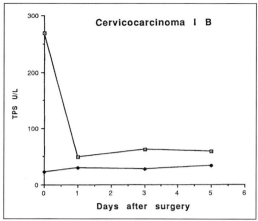

Figure 1. TPS serum levels monitored in two different patients with cervicocarcinoma IB after surgery.

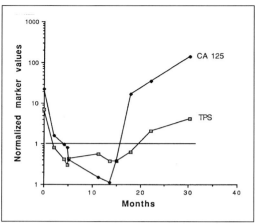

Figure 3. Normalized TPS and CA 125 marker levels (marker levels divided by respective cut-off) during follow-up of an ovarian cancer patient (C.A. 70 y), FIGO III.

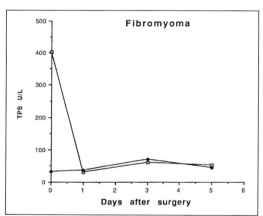

Figure 2. TPS serum profiles monitored in two different patients with fibromyoma after surgery.

normal range during the first 24 hours, without any correlation with the mass, the volume or the stage of the lesion (figures 1 and 2). This observation was characteristic for patients with both benign and malignant lesions. On the other hand some patients with benign and malignant pathologies showed presurgery TPS levels in the normal range without any statistical significant difference from the post surgery TPS levels (figures 1 and 2).

Monitoring

TPS revealed a good correlation with the evolution of the lesions during monitoring patients with ovarian cancer (figure 3). The TPS signal indicated a marked decrease (positive outcome for the patient) during the first months, followed by a stable period for about 15 months where the TPS values were within the reference limit. Subsequently a significant elevation of the TPS signal was observed (progression and death). CA 125 demonstrates a similar profile as with TPS in the ovarian cancer patient, but the rapid increase of the mucin mass marker is more pronounced (figure 3).

Discussion

TPS is related to the proliferative activity of the disease rather than to the tumor bulk (2). Elevated and increasing serum TPS levels were observed to be associated with the development of the lesion and particularly the metastatic lesion.
TPS displayed an excellent specificity in the presence of benign gynecological diseases and did not show alterations in case of acute or chronic female pelvic inflammatory diseases or other acute case of abdominal event as ovarian cyst in torsion.
The observed data in the gynecological pathology give further indications about the characteristics of TPS described as a proliferative marker, considering distribution with the stages reached from the neoplasia and the relapses.
The TPS level was not related to stage of the malignant lesion, and further more is independent of

the mass or volume of the involved organ. For the postoperative period, one interesting observation is the rapid decrease of the elevated presurgery levels independently of the benign or malignant type of the lesions. TPS showed a rapid decrease (within the reference level) during the first day after surgery, both in benign and in malignant gynecological lesions.

Klapdor et al. (13) showed that a normalization of TPS signal occurred after four hours following removal of the tumor in nude mice. The proliferative process of the postoperative period is sometimes affected by septic or other lesions such as inflammatory diseases in which case TPS may derive either from tissue or from cells surrounding the invasion as a defence mechanism. In ovarian carcinoma, TPS together with CA 125, offer prognostic information not available with CA 125 alone (14). It is now important to evaluate if the serum determination of TPS is useful in combination with CA 125 or SCC for ovarian, endometrial and cervical carcinom, as an additional test and if TPS can add a prognostic significance as indicated by *Dörffler* et al. (10) and *Caffier* et al. (14).

References

1. Björklund B, Björklund V (1957) Antigenicity of pooled human malignant and normal tissue by cytoimmunological techniques: Presence of an insoluble, heat-labile tumor antigen. Int Arch Allergy 10:153-184
2. Björklund B, Björklund V, Wiklund B et al (1973) A human tissue polypeptide related to cancer and placenta. I Preparation and properties. II Assay technique clinical studies of 1483 individuals with cancer and other conditions. In: Björklund B (ed) III Immunological techniques for detection of cancer. Bonniers, Stockholm, pp 134-187
3. Björklund B, Björklund V (1987) Biochemische und morphologische Grundlagen von TPA. In: Lütgens M, Schlegal G (eds) Tumormarkersystem CEA-TPA. Tumor Diagnostik, Leonberg, pp 14-30
4. Björklund B (1992) Tumor markers TPA, TPA-S and cytokeratins: A working hypothesis. Tumor Diagn Ther 13:78-80
5. Madersbacher S, Gregor N, Theyer G et al (1992) TPS is a useful epithelial proliferation and tumor marker. Am Urol Ass Ann Meeting J Urol 147: A 911
6. Oehr P, Liu O, Jin HY, El-Ahmady O, Nap M, Lackner B, Ota Y (1992) TPS: Biology and clinical value. In: Klapdor R (ed) Tumor associated antigens, oncogens, receptors, cytokines in tumor diagnosis and therapy at the beginning of the nineties. Zuckschwerdt, München, pp 213-218
7. Van Dalen, A (1992) TPS in breast cancer. A comparative study with carcinoembryonic antigen and CA 15-3. Tumor Biol 13:10-17
8. Kornek G, Pfeffel F, Schenck T et al (1992) TPS for monitoring chemotherapeutic response in gastrointestinal (GI) cancer. The 9th IATMO int conf on human tumor markers. J Tumor Marker Oncol 7:90
9. Gitsch G, Kainz Ch, Joura E et al (1992) Squamous cell carcinoma antigen, tumor associated trypsin inhibitor and tissue polypeptide specific antigen in follow-up of stage III cervical cancer. Anticancer Res 12:1247-1250
10. Dörffler P, Caffier H (1992) Comparison of the clinical value of tumor marker TPS and CA 125 regarding ovary carcinomas. In: Klapdor R (ed) Tumor associated antigens, oncogens, receptors, cytokines in tumor diagnosis and therapy at the beginning of the nineties. Zuckschwerdt, München, pp 103-106
11. Browning MCK, McFarlaney P (1992) Serum TPS concentrations in malignant disease. In: Klapdor R (ed) Tumor associated antigens, oncogens, receptors, cytokines in tumor diagnosis and therapy at the beginning of the nineties. Zuckschwerdt München, pp 208-212
12. Bremer K, Richter K, Bremer C, Kissing F (1992) Clinical value of TPS in breast cancer. In: Klapdor R (ed) Tumor associated antigens, oncogenes, receptors, cytokines in tumor diagnosis and therapy at the beginning of the nineties. Zuckschwerdt, München, pp 52-56
13. Klapdor R, Bahlo M, Pohlmann G (1992) Value of CA 19.9, CA 195, CEA and NSE in comparison to TPS for diagnosis of small tumors of the gastrointestinal tract and lung. Comparative studies in human and in nude mice rearing xenografts of human cancer. In: Klapdor R (ed) Tumor associated antigens, oncogens, receptors, cytokines in tumor diagnosis and therapy at the beginning of the nineties. Zuckschwerdt, München, pp 20-22
14. Caffier H, Kristen P (1993) Proliferative indexes (TPS alone or in relation to other tumor markers or/and other proliferation indexes). Proceedings of the International Symposium: CA 125 – Ten years later. 10-13th October 1993, San Remo, Italy. Anticancer Res 13 (5B):1644-1645

Address for correspondence:
Dr. G. C. Torre
Department of Obstetrics and Gynecology
Ospedale Santa Corona
I-17027 Pietra Ligure (SV), Italy

Urinary gonadotropin peptide (UGP) as a marker for gynecologic malignancies

R. P. Walker[a], V. Crebbin[a], J. Stern[b], J. Brown[b], S. Scudder[c], P. Schwartz[d]

[a]Ciba Corning Diagnostics, Alameda, CA, [b]Departments of Gynecologic Oncology and Obstetrics and Gynecology, University of California, San Francisco, CA, [c]Department of Oncology, University of California, Davis, CA, [d]Yale University Department of Gynecologic Oncology, New Haven, CT, USA

Introduction

UGP, also known as beta-core fragment or urinary gonadotropin fragment (UGF), is the core fragment of the beta subunit of human chorionic gonadotropin (hCG). It is a disulfide-linked heterodimeric protein of molecular weight 10.5 kD with a primary sequence identical to residues 6–40 and 55–92 of the beta subunit of hCG (1). The carbohydrate moieties of UGP are truncated relative to beta-hCG with only the core mannose, N-acetyl glucosamine and fucose residues remaining (2, 3). UGP has been demonstrated to be a highly stable protein in urine.

UGP is a major component of pregnancy urine (4), and it is also produced by a variety of trophoblastic and non-trophoblastic tumors. UGP is a pan-marker, and is present in the urine of patients with various malignancies, including colorectal, pancreatic, biliary, lung, and gynecologic cancers (5, 6, 7). UGP is expressed by ovarian, cervical, endometrial, and vaginal cancers in a stage-dependent manner (8, 9, 10).

Two mechanisms for the appearance of UGP in urine have been proposed. UGP can be secreted directly by tumor cells or tissues (11), or alternately is a product of renal degradation of circulating hCG species 12). UGP is not readily measurable in serum either due to its rapid clearance from the circulation, or because it is sequestered as a complex with another protein(s) rendering it undetectable by current immunological methods (13).

The objective of the present study was to evaluate the expression of UGP in normal patients, and patients with benign gynecologic disease and gynecologic cancer using the Triton UGP enzyme immunoassay (UGP EIA). The main focus was to determine the UGP levels in diagnosed ovarian cancer patients, and to compare the results to the established serum marker CA 125 to determine if the two markers were complimentary in detecting disease.

Patients and methods

Clinical specimens

A total of 866 spot urine samples were collected from 762 women at four clinics. Samples from 585 normal women and women with benign gynecologic and urologic disease were collected on a single occasion at the Department of Obstetrics, Gynecology and Reproductive Services at the University of California, San Francisco, and the Department of Oncology, University of California, Davis. Samples from 164 women with gynecologic malignancies were obtained from the Yale University Department of Gynecologic Oncology, the Department of Oncology, University of California, Davis, and the Department of Gynecologic Oncology, University of California, San Francisco. The majority of samples were obtained from women with active ovarian cancer, with 203 specimens obtained from 99 patients with active disease. Of the ovarian cancer patients, 84 patients were recruited with recurrent or persistent disease, 15 were recruited prior to primary laparotomy, and 24 of these patients donated serial urine and serum specimens over an average time period of 18 months.

Samples from patients recruited at the U.C. Davis and U.C. San Francisco clinics were obtained on a spot basis, and were collected without preservatives. The urine samples were frozen within four hours of collection. Samples from Yale University were collected and preserved as described previously (8). Paired plasma and urine samples were obtained in 153 instances from 79 cancer patients. CA 125 values from matched serum samples were obtained from the U.C. Davis and San Francisco clinics, or from Dianon Systems, Inc. in the case of the Yale samples.

UGP enzyme immunoassay

UGP was determined in freshly-thawed urine samples following centrifugation of the samples at 2000–3000 x g for ten minutes. Duplicate determinations were performed for each sample, and repeat assays were performed if the coefficient of variation of the replicates was greater than 15%. UGP was measured using an enzyme-linked immunoassay (Triton UGP EIA, Ciba Corning Diagnostics, Alameda, CA, USA). The Triton UGP EIA is a double-determinant enzyme immunoassay which utilizes a specific monoclonal capture antibody immobilized on a polystyrene tube and an affinity-purified polyclonal detection antibody labeled with horseradish peroxidase. The UGP EIA exhibited an analytical sensitivity of 0.2 fmol/ml, and the linear range of the assay was from 2 to 16 fmol/ml, intra- and inter-assay imprecision range from 4.28 to 5.65% and 5.60 to 7.53%, respectively, over the range of the assay. Excellent linearity of sample dilution was observed with pathological urine specimens, with linear regression analysis demonstrating a mean correlation coefficient of 0.997. The recovery of known amounts of UGP spiked at various levels into urine specimens ranged from 87 to 119%, with a mean of 102%. Cross-reactivity with known glycoprotein hormones and their subunits was less than 0.25%. Urine components including urea, creatinine, creatine, bilirubin, uric acid, vitamin C, urobilin, and blood did not interfere with the UGP EIA at levels exceeding the maximum expected values in pathological urines.

Normalization of sample UGP values

In order to account for variations in urine volumes, UGP values were normalized according to creatinine (Cr) concentration. The mean creatinine value for all urine was 1.04 mg/ml. After normalization for creatinine, the UGP values were reported in units of femtomole UGP per milligram creatinine (fmol/mg Cr).

Results

Distribution of UGP values in patient samples

UGP levels were determined in 788 spot urine samples from normal women, women with benign gynecologic and urologic disease and women with active gynecologic cancers. A range of UGP values from 0 to 567 fmol/mg Cr was observed in the urine of gynecological cancer patients of all stages, with a mean of 10.6 fmol/mg Cr (table I). The majority of samples in this group were from patients with ovarian cancer, and this group of

Table I. Expression of UGP in patients with active gynecological cancer. Number (%) of active gynecological cancer patients samples exceeding UGP level of 4 fmol/mg Cr: breakdown by type of malignancy.

	No. of patients	No. of samples	No. (%) of samples > 4 (fmol/mg Cr)	Mean UGP (fmol/mg Cr)	Range (fmol/mg Cr)
Ovarian	99	203	126 (62)	12.7	0 – 566.7
Cervical	31	41	14 (34)	5.4	0.5 – 40.6
Endometrial/ uterine/ fallopian tube	23	24	7 (29)	4.0	0.2 – 22.0
Vulva/vagina	11	13	7 (54)	6.0	0.4 – 21.9
Total	164	281	154 (55)	10.6	0 – 566.7

Table II. Expression of UGP in healthy women. Number (%) of samples from healthy women exceeding UGP level of 4 fmol/mg Cr.

	No. of patients	No. (%) exceeding 4 fmol/mg Cr	Mean UGP value (fmol/mg Cr)
Premenopausal	97	3 (3.1)	1.0
Postmenopausal	119	18 (15.1)	2.9
Total	216	21 (9.7)	2.2

Table III. Expression of UGP in women with benign gynecological disease. Number (%) of samples from women with benign disease exceeding UGP level of 4 fmol/mg Cr. Mean UGP level for all benign disease samples was 1.2 fmol/mg Cr.

Category	No. of patients	No. (%) exceeding 4 fmol/mg Cr
Abnormal bleeding/menorrhagia	22	1
Cysts	28	4
Condyloma	39	1
Dysplasia	25	2
Endometriosis	16	1
Fibroids	20	1
Myoma	23	1
Pelvic inflammatory disease/salpingitis	4	0
Urinary tract infection	12	1
Vaginitis/vulvitis/cervicitis	47	2
Amennorrhea/dysmennorhea	22	0
Other	30	4
Total[a]	288	18 (6.3%)

[a] 43 Postmenopausal, 245 premenopausal and perimenopausal

samples exhibited the greatest mean UGP level of 12.7 fmol/mg Cr. The mean UGP value for all normal women was 2.2 fmol/mg Cr (table II). When the normal female population was broken down according to menopausal status, a difference in the UGP distribution was observed, with the postmenopausal group showing a higher mean UGP value of 2.9 fmol/mg Cr relative to the UGP value of 1.0 fmol/mg Cr for the premenopausal group. The cohort of women with benign gynecologic and urologic disease consisted of 85% premenopausal and perimenopausal, and 15% postmenopausal subjects. The mean UGP value in these patients was 1.2 fmol/mg Cr (table III).

A cut-off of 4 fmol/mg Cr was chosen based on ROC curve analysis. A total of 9.7% of normal women exhibited elevated UGP values (table II). When analyzed according to menopausal status, normal premenopausal and postmenopausal women overexpressed UGP in 3.1% and 15.1% of cases, respectively. Of the gynecologic cancers, the highest level of UGP expression was observed in the ovarian cancer patients, with 62% of the samples exceeding the cut-off (table I). In patients with cervical, endometrial, and vaginal cancers, UGP values were elevated in 29–54% of the cases. In the benign gynecologic disease group, 6.4% of the samples exceeded the cut-off (table III). All categories of benign disease exhibited a low level of UGP overexpression.

The distribution of UGP values in samples from patients diagnosed with ovarian cancer as a function of clinical status is shown in table IV. The mean UGP value in each patient category increased from 6.4 fmol/mg Cr for patients in remission, to 7.6 fmol/mg Cr for patients with stable disease, to 10.1 fmol/mg Cr for patients with progressive disease, to 67.6 fmol/mg Cr for presurgical patients. The percent of samples exceeding the cut-off was similar for each category, except for the presurgical samples, in which 93% of the samples showed elevated UGP levels.

Table IV. UGP expression as a function of clinical status. Number (%) of active ovarian cancer patients samples exceeding UGP level of 4 fmol/mg Cr: breakdowm by clinical status.

Status	No. of patients	No. (%) of samples > 4 fmol/mg Cr	Mean UGP (fmol/mg Cr)	Range (fmol/mg Cr)
Regressive	13	8 (62)	6.4	0.3 – 12.6
Stable	52	33 (64)	7.6	0.5 – 35.1
Progressive	29	19 (66)	10.1	0.2 – 51.9
Presurgical	15	14 (93)	67.6	0.5 – 566.7
Total	109	74 (68)	16.4	0.2 – 566.7

Table V. Simultaneous determination of UGP and CA 125. Number (%) of samples exceeding UGP (fmol/mg Cr) and CA 125 (U/ml) levels in parallel urine and plasma samples from ovarian cancer patients: breakdown by histology.

Histology	No. of samples	UGP >4 fmol/mg Cr	CA 125 >35 U/ml	UGP > 4 fmol/mg Cr or CA 125 > 35 U/ml
Serous	98	57 (58)	64 (65)	80 (82)
Mucinous	4	4 (100)	3 (75)	4 (100)
Endometriod	20	14 (70)	9 (45)	15 (75)
Other[a]	11	7 (64)	4 (37)	8 (73)
Total	133	82 (62)	80 (60)	107 (81)

[a] Includes clear cell carcinoma, Brenner tumors, dysgerminoma, granulosa cell tumors, undifferentiated tumors, and tumors of mixed histology

Simultaneous determination of UGP and CA 125

UGP values and CA 125 values were obtained in 133 samples from 79 patients with active ovarian cancer. The distribution of these marker values as a function of histologic grade of disease is shown for a subset of these patients in table V. In all four categories encompassing both serous and non-serous disease, utilizing both markers simultaneously resulted in an increased sensitivity of detection of disease ranging from 19% to 37%, with an average of 28% over CA 125 alone. The greatest enhancement of sensitivity over using CA 125 was in the non-serous histologic disease categories.

Conclusion

UGP is overexpressed in a majority of patients with gynecologic malignancies. It compliments the CA 125 marker in that the sensitivity of detection of disease is increased when the two markers are used in tandem, and it has a low level of false-positive elevation in benign conditions. It is a highly stable marker that is measurable in urine. The UGP EIA is a highly sensitive and specific tool for further investigating the utility of UGP in the management of cancer.

References

1 Birken S, Armstrong EG, Kolks MAG, Cole LA et al (1988) The structure of the human chorionic gonadotropin beta core fragment from pregnancy urine. Endocrinol 123:572–583
2 Blithe DL, Wehmann RE, Nisula BC (1989) Carbohydrate composition of beta-core. Endocrinol 125: 2267–2272
3 Endo T, Nishimura R, Saito S, Kanazawa K et al (1992) Carbohydrate structures of beta-core fragment of human chorionic gonadotropin isolated from a pregnant individual. Endocrinol 130/4:2052–2058
4 Good A, Ramos-Uribe M, Ryan R, Kempers RD (1977) Molecular forms of human chorionic gonadotropin serum, urine and placental extracts. Fertil Steril 28:846–850
5 McGill J, Cole L, Nam JH, Thorson A (1990) Urinary gonadotropin fragment (UGF): A potential "marker" of colorectal cancer. J Tumor Marker Oncol 5:175–177
6 Alfthan H, Haglund C, Roberts P, Stenman UH (1992) Elevation of free β subunit of human chorio-

gonadotropin and core β fragment of human chorio-gonadotropin in the serum and urine of patients with malignant pancreatic and bilary disease. Cancer Res 52:4628–4633
7. Chen Y, Canfield RE, Flaster E, O'Connor J (1993) Abstract: Urinary HCG expression in lung cancer. The symposium on glycoprotein hormones: Structure, function and clinical implications. Santa Barbara, California
8. Nam JH, Cole LA, Chambers JT, Schwartz PE (1990) Urinary gonadotropin fragment, a new tumor marker: I. Assay development and cancer specificity. Gynecol Oncol 36:383–390
9. Cole LA, Nam JH (1989) Urinary gonadotropin fragment (UGF) measurements in the diagnosis and management of ovarian cancer. Yale J Biol Med 62:367–378
10. Norman RJ, Buck RH, Akar B, Mayet N (1990) Detection of a small molecular species of human chorionic gonadotropin in the urine of patients with carcinoma of the cervix and cervical intraepithelial neoplasia: Comparison with other assays for human chorionic gonadotropin and its fragments. Gynecol Oncol 37:254–259
11. Cole LA, Birken (1988) Origin and occurrence of human chorionic gonadotropin β-subunit core fragment. Mol Endocrinol 2: 825–830.
12. Wehmann RE, Blithe DL, Akar AH, Nisula BC (1990) Disparity between β-core levels in pregnancy urine and serum: Implications for the origin of urinary β-core. J Clin Endocrinol Metab 70:371–378
13. Kardana A, Cole LA (1990) Serum HCG β-core fragment is masked by associated macromolecules. J Clin Endocrinol Metab 71/5:1393–1395

Address for correspondence:
Dr. R. P. Walker
Ciba Corning Diagnostics
1401 Harbor Bay Parkway
Alameda, California, USA 94502

Prognostic value of serum fragments of cytokeratin 19 in patients with cervical cancer

K.N. Gaarenstroom[a], J.M.G. Bonfrer[b], C.M. Korse[b], M.E. Van Huizen[a], Th.J.M. Helmerhorst[c]

[a]Department of Gynecology of the Leiden University Medical Center, Leiden,
[b]Departments of Clinical Chemistry and [c]Gynecology of the Netherlands Cancer Institute, Amsterdam, The Netherlands

Introduction

Tumor markers can be a helpful tool in tumor diagnosis and follow-up of patients treated for malignant disease. Several serum markers have been investigated in cervical cancer. Squamous cell carcinoma antigen (SCC) seems to be the most valuable serum marker in case of squamous cell carcinoma of the uterine cervix (1, 2) However, a normal SCC level does not exclude the presence of tumor or recurrent disease (2). Therefore, it is important to search for new serum markers, which can reflect the amount of tumor burden or identify those patients at risk for early recurrence or poor survival.

Keratins represent a group of intermediate filament proteins (IFP) found in epithelial cells. The IFP are part of the intracytoplasmic matrix and provide internal stability to the cells. Cytokeratin 19 is an acidic subunit expressed in both normal and in malignant cervical epithelium (3) Fragments of keratins can be detected in human serum. It has been suggested that serum fragments of cytokeratins can be used as a marker of proliferation.

The objective of this study was to investigate the prognostic significance of serum fragments of cytokeratin 19, measured by CYFRA 21-1, in patients with cervical cancer. Pretreatment CYFRA 21-1 level was related to tumor stage and prognostic data.

Patients and methods

Patients

The study group comprised 78 patients with squamous cell cancer of the uterine cervix who were treated at the Netherlands Cancer Institute, Amsterdam, between 1984 and 1988. Patients were staged according to the FIGO criteria for gynecologic cancer. Two patients with FIGO stage Ia had been treated by cone biopsy of the uterine cervix. The other 76 patients had been treated by either radical hysterectomy and pelvic lymphadenectomy or primary radiotherapy. Clinical data were obtained from the medical files.

Histologic material was reviewed for tumor characteristics such as depth of infiltration, lymph-vascular space involvement, grade of malignancy and lymph node status. Tumor diameter was evaluated on histologic material if available or otherwise data of the clinical examinations were used.

The mean age of the patient group was 52 years (range 22–83) and the median follow-up was 65 months (range 6–97). Prognosis of patients was determined by disease-free interval and survival measured from the date of initial treatment.

CYFRA 21-1 enzyme-immunoassay

Pretreatment sera were tested for the presence of cytokeratin 19 fragments by the use of a double determinant enzyme-immunoassay (Boehringer Mannheim, Tutzing, Germany), referred to as CYFRA 21-1 (4). In this test two monoclonal antibodies (MoAb K 19.1 and BM 19.21) were used in an assay based on a 2-step sandwich principle. The test was considered positive if levels of CYFRA 21-1 were ≥ 1.2 µg/l. The 95 percentile for CYFRA 21-1 was found at this level in an apparently healthy population (5).

Statistical analysis

For statistical analysis the one-way analysis of variance was used. A p-value < 0.05 was regarded as indicating a significant difference. A stepwise procedure using Proportional Hazard regression analysis was used to identify prognostic factors with respect to disease-free interval and survival (death of disease). Three categories for CYFRA 21-1 levels were defined in order to create approximately equally sized groups. Lifetable calculations were performed using the product-limit method of Kaplan and Meier. Log transformed values of CYFRA 21-1 were used in the analysis.

Results

Table I shows the mean CYFRA 21-1 values in 78 patients with cervical cancer and the number of patients with an increased CYFRA 21-1 level in relation to FIGO stage. The correlation between CYFRA 21-1 level and FIGO stage was highly significant (p < 0.0001). CYFRA 21-1 concentration was elevated in all cases with stage III or IVa cancer.

Nine patients had residual tumor after treatment and in 21 of the 78 patients recurrent disease developed during follow-up. In the univariate Cox analysis FIGO stage (p = 0.0001), tumor size (p < 0.0001), grade of malignancy (p = 0.0045) as well as CYFRA 21-1 level (p < 0.0001) were significantly correlated with disease-free interval. An increased CYFRA 21-1 level was associated with the development of early recurrence (table II). However, after adjusting for tumor size, CYFRA 21-1 showed no additional prognostic value with respect to disease-free interval.

Twenty-nine patients died during follow-up. Prognostic factors in the univariate analysis for survival were: FIGO stage (p < 0.0001), tumor size (p = 0.0002), lymph node status (p = 0.001), and CYFRA 21-1 level (p < 0.0001). An increased CYFRA 21-1 level was correlated with a poor survival (table II). After controlling for FIGO stage, CYFRA 21-1 level lost its prognostic value with respect to survival.

Discussion

The aim of the present study was to investigate the prognostic value of the serum concentration of cytokeratin 19 fragments in cervical cancer patients and its applicability as a clinical marker. Pretreatment CYFRA 21-1 level was significantly correlated with FIGO stage. In the univariate analysis an increased CYFRA 21-1 level was associated with a poor prognosis. However, CYFRA 21-1 had no additional value over known prognosticators such as FIGO stage and tumor size in the multivariate analysis.

Thus far, the prognostic value of CYFRA 21-1 as a serum marker was only investigated in patients with lung carcinoma (6). A high CYFRA 21-1 level

Table I. Mean CYFRA 21-1 concentration, number and percentage of patients with an increased CYFRA 21-1 level in relation to FIGO stage.

FIGO stage	Ia	Ib	IIa	IIb	III	IVa
Total group no.	2	28	13	13	20	2
Mean CYFRA 21-1 value (µg/l)	1.02	1.20	2.94	4.09	11.50	13.42
No. (%) with CYFRA ≥1.20 µg/l	1 (50)	12 (43)	9 (69)	11 (85)	20 (100)	2 (100)

Table II. Two- and 5-year disease-free interval and survival rates according to pretreatment CYFRA 21-1 level in 78 patients with cervical cancer.

CYFRA 21-1 value	Disease-free interval (%)		Survival (%)	
	2-year	5-year	2-year	5-year
< 1.20 µg/l	87	82	95	81
1.20 - 2.24 µg/l	76	72	79	72
≥ 2.25 µg/l	37	32	46	36

was significantly correlated with advanced stage lung carcinoma and the presence of mediastinal lymph node metastases in this study. It is concluded that CYFRA 21-1 might be a useful serum marker in the management of patients with cervical cancer, but further investigation concerning its applicability in gynecologic practice is needed.

Acknowledgements

The authors thank *Dr. M.P.W. Gallee* for revision of the histology and *Dr. A.A.M. Hart* for the statistical analysis.

References

1. Farghaly SA (1992) Tumor markers in gynecologic cancer. Gynecol Obstet Invest 34:65–72
2. Montag ThW (1990) Tumor markers in gynecologic oncology. Obstet Gynecol Survey 45:94–105
3. Smedts F, Ramaekers F, Troyanovsky S, Pruszczynski M, Link M, Lane B, Leigh I, Schijf C, Vooijs GP (1992) Keratin expression in cervical cancer. Am J Pathol 141:497–511
4. Bodenmüller H, Stieber P, Banauch D, Hasholzner U, Dessauer H, Jaworek O (1992) Enzymun-test CYFRA 21-1: a new marker for NSCLC. Clin Chem 38:966
5. Rastel D, Ramaioli A, Clément M, Thirion B (1993) Evaluation of CYFRA 21-1 as tumor marker at the diagnosis step in the primary lung cancer. Eur J Cancer 6:243
6. Pujol JL, Grenier J, Daurès JP, Daver A, Pujol H, Michel FB (1993) Serum fragment of cytokeratin subunit 19 measured by CYFRA 21-1 immunoradiometric assay as a marker of lung cancer. Cancer Res 53:61–66

Address for correspondence:
Dr. K. N. Gaarenstroom
Department of Gynecology
Leiden University Medical Center
P.O. Box 9600
NL-2300 RC Leiden, The Netherlands

Clinical value of mammary serum antigen (MSA) as a tumor marker for breast carcinoma

G.M. Oremek[a], A. Vering[b], M. Stegmüller[b], U.B. Seiffert[a]

[a]Clinical-Chemical Central Laboratory, Center of Internal Medicine,
[b]Center of Gynecology, Klinikum of Johann-Wolfgang-Goethe-University, Frankfurt, Germany

Introduction

Breast cancer ranges at first place among malignant tumor diseases of women (1). The expectations of using tumor markers for screening purposes could not be fulfilled until today. Determination of tumor marker levels in serum samples preoperatively can assist to confirm the diagnosis. Furthermore, the effectivity of a therapeutical treatment (surgery, radiation and/or chemotherapy) can be monitored by tumor marker serum levels determined postoperatively. Further important information about the tumor behavior and clinical status can be obtained from this kind of analysis (2, 3, 4).

MSA serum levels were determined along with clinical parameters in order to detect a progressive disease of breast cancer patients as early as possible (8, 9).

Furthermore, tumor marker determinations can provide important information on the tumor behavior and tumor proliferation (5, 6, 7).

Material and methods

The reference region for MSA was determined by analysing 120 healthy individuals (100 women and 20 men) in the age of 18 to 65 years. In these persons twenty different parameters of clinical chemistry were measured and no pathological values were found, thus confirming the real state of health.

Principle of the procedure

Tests are performed on diluted sera which are pre-incubated with the monoclonal anti-MSA reagent (3E1.2). Any MSA present in the test specimen will combine with the monoclonal anti-MSA. The remaining free monoclonal antibody is then allowed to react with MSA coated onto microtiter strip wells.

The amount of 3E1.2 antibody bound to the coated microtiter strips is determined by the addition of a peroxidase-labeled anti-mouse IgM (Fc) conjugate followed by an enzyme substrate solution. The intensity of colour produced is inversely proportional to the amount of MSA in the test sample.

Results

The reference values for MSA in the control group of healthy women was between 10 U/ml and 40 U/ml with a mean value of 28 U/ml ± 9.3. In the reference group of healthy men the MSA concentrations in serum were between 2.5 and 17 U/ml and had a mean value of 7.5 ml ± 5.9.

Stability and precision

Serum samples of healthy individuals were stored at 2–8 °C for 24 hours. In comparison to MSA concentrations determined in fresh serum samples a decrease of 4.2% was observed. Serum samples that had been stored at –20 °C only showed a 2.7% decrease of the MSA concentrations.

The MSA concentration in one serum sample containing 25 U/ml MSA was determined ten times in the same run and a coefficient of variation (CV) of 3.4% was found (intra-assay variation).

One tumor marker control serum was analyzed ten times in duplicate in seperate runs and gave an interassay CV of 4.1%.

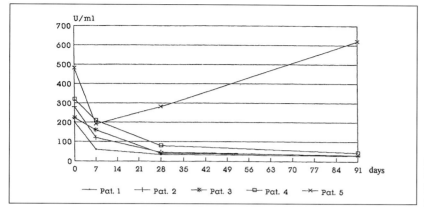

Figure 1. Postoperative MSA concentrations in patients with breast cancer.

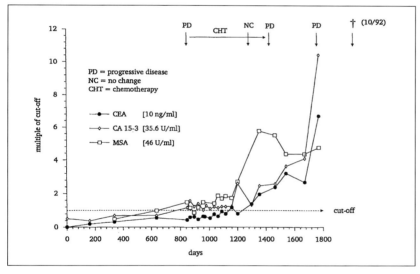

Figure 2. Monitoring of a breast cancer patient with MSA, CEA and CA 15-3 (pat. L.E.). Time interval: 25.06.87–16.05.92.

As in the case of other tumor markers, also for MSA an influence of chemotherapeutical drugs on the tumor marker level was observed, this means the tumor marker concentration decreases after addition of the chemotherapeutical drug e.g. Mitomycin C and Vindesin (10). A normalisation of the tumor marker concentration occurs 48 hours later. The MSA levels in breast cancer patients were between 17.5 U/ml and 485.5 U/ml with a mean value of 142.2 U/ml. Hence, the MSA concentrations were clearly elevated in comparison to the healthy control group.

Figure1 shows the postoperative MSA values of five patients with breast carcinoma. All patients show a significant reduction of MSA levels to the 7. day after surgery. Whereas the MSA levels in patients number 1–4 decrease further, there is a rapid increase in the MSA concentration in patient 5. This increase indicates a metastasis which could later be confirmed by sonography.

Figure 2 shows the disease course from the breast cancer patient L.E. in the time interval between June 1987 to May 1992. The primary tumor had been removed by surgery in 1994 and later occuring metastasis had been treated by radiation and Tamoxifen.

In this patient, the new tumor marker MSA was measured as well as the classical tumor markers CEA and CA 15-3 in order to monitor the disease course. This figure demonstrates the different expression dynamics of the three markers. Here, the real clinical status is especially clearly reflec-

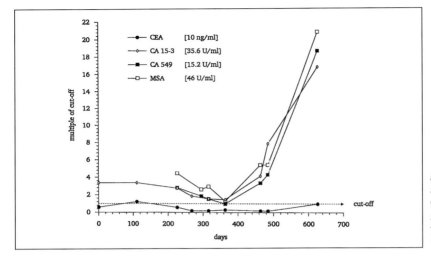

Figure 3. Monitoring of a breast cancer patient with MSA, CEA, CA 15-3 and CA 549 (pat. B.L.). Time interval: 10.06.1987–22.02.1989.

ted by the MSA serum values. The tumor progress is solely announced by a rapid increase of MSA before clinical manifestation.

The MSA expression dynamics can be different from the classical tumor markers or be similar as shown in figure 3.

Conclusions

The quality of the MSA ELISA is reflected by a very good intra- and inter-assay variation. A satisfactory stability of reagents is given. MSA provides important information by monitoring the disease course after surgery and under chemotherapy. Chemotherapeutical drugs lead to a decrease of the MSA concentrations, a normalization of MSA levels occurs 48 hours later.

References

1. Miller AB (1987) Breast cancer epidemiology, etiology and prevention In: Harris IR, Hellman S, Henderson IC, Kinne DW (eds) Breast diseases. Lippinscott, Philadelphia, pp 87–120
2. Kreienberg R, Möbus V (1992) Tumormarker in der Gynäkologie. Lab Med 16:21–26
3. Mai R, Kaesemann H, Caffier H (1991) Diagnostische Aussagekraft des MCA im Vergleich zum CA 15-3 beim Mammakarzinom. Tumordiagn u Ther 12:248–253
4. Stöckelhuber B, Stieber P, Lamerz R (1992) Influence of bone radiation on serum markers in breast cancer. In: Klapdor R (ed) Tumor associated antigens, oncogenes, receptors, cytokines in tumor diagnosis and therapy at the beginning of the nineties. Cancer of the breast–state and trends in diagnosis and therapy. Zuckschwerdt, München, pp 72–77
5. Cooper EH, Soletormös G (1992) A multicentre evaluation of CA 549 in breast cancer. Tumordiagn u Ther 13:91–94
6. Glaubitz M, Kupsch E (1993) Vergleich der Proliferationsmarker Ki-67 und Anti PCNA/Cyclin beim Mammakarzinom. Tumordiagn u Ther 14:187–193
7. Eichfeld U, Haerting J, Schwarz J (1993) Serumprolaktinspiegel primärer Mammakarzinome. Tumordiagn Ther 14:194–200
8. Stacker SA, Tjandra JJ, Walker CH, Thompson GH, McKenzie FC (1989) Purification and biochemical Characterization of a novel breast carcinoma-associated mucin-like glycoprotein (MSA). Br J Cancer 59:544–553
9. Tjandra JJ, Busmanis J, Russel JSR, Collins JP, Reed RG, Mc Kenzie JFC (1988) The association of mammary serum antigen (MSA) with the histopathological findings in localized breast cancer. Br J Cancer 58:815–817
10. Hoffmann W, Beisicht C, Weidmann B, Niederle N, Seeber S (1991) Kombinationstherapie des metastasierenden vorbehandelten Mammakarzinoms mit Mitomycin C und Vindesin. Tumordiagn u Ther 12:102–105

Address for correspondence:
Dr. med. G. M. Oremek
Zentrum der Inneren Medizin-Zentrallabor
Universitätskliniken
Theodor-Stern-Kai 7
D-60590 Frankfurt/Main, Germany

Time course of tumor markers MSA, CA 15-3 and CA 549 in patients with breast cancer

M. Meisel, W. Straube, C. Versümer

Department of Gynecology and Obstetrics, Ernst-Moritz-Arndt-University, Greifswald, Germany

Introduction

A suitable test for monitoring the course or to assist the diagnosis of all patients with breast cancer has not yet been described. While elevated tumor marker values are often associated with increased risk of disease progression or increased tumor volume, collectively their lack of specificity and sensitivity prevents their broad use.

We have used the recently developed MSA assay (mammary serum antigen) for the follow-up during management of cancer.

The competitive enzyme immunoassay detecting MSA utilizes the murine monoclonal antibody 3E1.2, which identifies a determinant present on a high molecular weight glycoprotein found in the serum of patients with breast cancer (1).

In addition we have studied the courses of CA 15-3 and CA 549, both classical tumor markers, which are suggested to have high sensitivity for mammary carcinoma.

The aim of this present study was to assess the individual and combined value of the MSA, CA 15-3 and CA 549 tests in the management of patients with breast cancer.

Material and methods

Serum samples of 12 patients with breast cancer were collected preoperatively and postoperatively throughout several months.

Serum was stored at −20° C until assay. MSA was determined by an enzyme immunoassay (medac, Hamburg, FRG), the cut-off level being 30 U/ml. CA 15-3 was determined by an enzyme immuno-assay (CIS-Isotopendiagnostik GmbH, Dreieich, FRG), the cut-off level being 25 U/ml. CA 549 was determined by an enzyme immunoassay (Hybritech, Köln, FRG) with a cut-off of 12.6 U/ml. All samples were tested in duplicate.

The clinical status of the patients was determined by means of clinical examination. The women have had full documentation of surgery.

Results

With the selected cut-off level of MSA positive values were ascertained preoperatively in five of 12 cases. Only in rare instances it was possible to get nearly the same time courses of MSA, CA 15-3 and CA 549. A well defined tendency and good correlation of MSA serum values regarding progression, metastatic formation and stability are found in 10 of 12 cases. For the interpretation four representative cases are described.

Case 1. Patient C.L.: Invasive ductable mammary carcinoma, G 3, p(T4b N1 M1). Ablatio mammae, axillary dissection, chemotherapy, exitus letalis a few months after surgery. Figure 1 shows the changes in tumor marker levels at the progressive disease, representative for three typical cases which came to a fatal end.

Case 2. Patient C.T.: Invasive ductable mammary carcinoma, G2, p(T1c No Mo). Tumor extirpation, axillary dissection, radiatio, chemotherapy, stability. Here the expected courses for MSA are shown (figure 2) beginning with pathological figures followed by a considerable decrease postoperative after surgery. It is interesting to note that six patients with advanced breast cancer had a raised MSA level but normal CA 15-3 and CA 549 levels, that are in 50% of the cases.

150   In Vitro Diagnosis

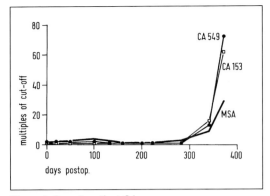

Figure 1. Case 1, patient C.L.

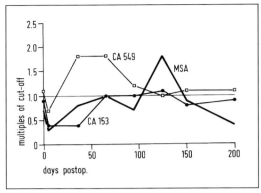

Figure 3. Case 3, patient H.M.

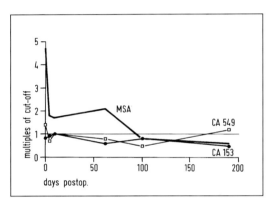

Figure 2. Case 2, patient C.T.

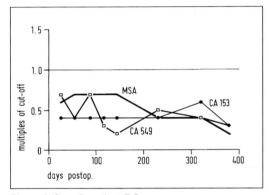

Figure 4. Case 4, patient E.S.

Case 3. Patient H.M.: Invasive ductable mammary carcinoma, G3, p(T2 No Mo). Tumor extirpation, chemotherapy, stability. Different tumor marker courses are found and remain unexplained. Only CA 549 shows an explicable time course, whereas MSA and CA 15-3 are mostly under the cut-off respectively with one exception to the rule. This could be estimated in two of twelve cases (figure 3).

Case 4. Patient E.S.: Medullary undifferentiated mammary carcinoma, G3, p(T3 No Mo). Ablatio mammae, axillary dissection, chemotherapy, stability. Similar time courses are demonstrated in all cases with levels below the cut-off in spite of the detected and confirmed tumor. Under such circumstances no marker is helpful for the screening process (figure 4).

Discussion

Several studies have shown that MSA is elevated in the sera of a high proportion of patients with breast cancer, compared to normal individuals, and that the levels are useful for monitoring patients with breast cancer (2).
Here, the MSA serum test has been compared to CA 15-3 and CA 549. It was found to improve in cases in which the well known tumor markers are not exprimed, see figure 2. In patients exhibiting elevated MSA as well as CA 15-3 and CA 549 levels mostly different time courses in these markers were found. This suggests that the antigenic determinants detected by the tests are different, and that they may be of additive value in the management of breast cancer patients. Studies are now in progress to define the clinical utility of the MSA test in monitoring breast cancer.

References

1 Stacker SA, Tjandra JJ, Pei-Xiang Xing, Walher ID, Thompson CH, McKenzie IEC (1989) Purification and biochemical characterisation of a novel breast carcinoma associated mucin-like glycoprotein defined by antibody 3E1.2. Brit J Cancer 59:544–553
2 Layton GT, Golder J, Johnston S et al (1991) Evaluation of an inhibition enzyme immunoassay kit for mammary serum antigen (MSA). J Tumor Marker Oncol 6:1–7

Address for correspondence:
Prof. Dr. W. Straube
Universitätsfrauenklinik
Wollweberstraße 1
D-17487 Greifswald, Germany

TPS compared to CA 15-3 and CEA in primary diagnosis of breast cancer

U. Heilenkötter[a], P. Jageila[a], M. Bahlo[b], R. Klapdor[b]
[a]Department of Gynecology, Johanniter-Hospital, Geesthacht,
[b]Internal Medicine, University Hospital, Hamburg, Germany

Introduction

TPS is discussed as a tumor marker of comparable sensitivity to CA 15-3 in advanced breast cancer (4). In the present study we now looked for the preoperative sensitivity of the tumor markers TPS, CA 15-3 and CEA in 61 patients suffering from malignant tumors of the breast at the time of primary diagnosis and compared the data with the rate of elevated levels in 76 patients with benign breast diseases. In addition, in some patients with advanced diseases we also measured these three markers in the follow-up of breast cancer.

Patients and methods

Benign breast diseases: n = 76, age 15–76 years, mean 44.6 years; n = 49 mastophathy, n = 20 fibroadenoma, n = 3 lipoma, one hemartoma and one cystadenoma phylloides benigna.
Malignant breast diseases: n = 61 years, age 35–85 years, mean 60.6 years; n = 33 nodal negative breast carcinoma (pTxpN-Mo), n = 10 nodal positive (pTxpN+Mo) without evidence for distant metastases and n = 18 patients with distant metastases (nine osseous, three hepatic, three pulmonal, two lymphatic and one osseous and hepatic metastasis).

TPS was determined radioimmunometrically (Beki, Biermann), CA 15-3 and CEA using an enzyme immunoassay (Enzymun, Boehringer Mannheim).
The following cut-offs were used: 55 and 95 U/l resp. for TPS, 26 U/ml for CA 15-3 and 3 ng/ml for CEA, and in addition, the cut-off values calculated on the basis of a 95% specificity for the 76 patients suffering from benign lesions of the breast: TPS: 156 U/l, CA 15-3: 22 U/ml and CEA: 4.3 ng/ml (table I).

Results and discussion

According to table II the sensitivity of the three tumor markers depends on the cut-off levels. On the basis of a cut-off level of 55 U/l for TPS this marker shows the highest sensitivity in primary diagnosis of breast cancer compared to CA 15-3 and CEA. On the basis of a cut-off level calculated on the basis of a comparable specificity (96%), however, CA 15-3 represents the most sensitive marker for breast cancer, followed by CEA and TPS.
In the follow-up TPS, however, may give additional information compared to CA 15-3 in some patients. Three typical follow-up studies are shown in figures 1-3.

Table I. TPS, CA 15-3 and CEA serum concentrations in 70 patients with benign tumors of the breast.

Marker	Cut-off (96% spec.)	Median	Minimum	Maximum	n
TPS (U/l)	156	48.4	10.5	212	70
CA 15-3 (U/ml)	22	10.7	3.9	25.5	70
CEA (ng/ml)	4.3	1.4	0.6	10.7	69

Table II. TPS, CA 15-3 and CEA: Preoperative sensitivity (%) for malignant breast tumors in 61 patients.

	TPS			CA 15-3		CEA	
Specifity (%)	55	78	96	96	100	93	96
Level	> 55	> 95	> 156 U/l	> 22	> 26 U/ml	> 3	> 4.3 ng/ml
Sensitivity (%)							
pTXpNoMo (n = 33)	23	11	4	22	3	16	13
pTxpN1Mo (n = 10)	60	30	10	30	20	20	10
pTxpNxM1 (n = 18)	83	72	44	72	67	61	50

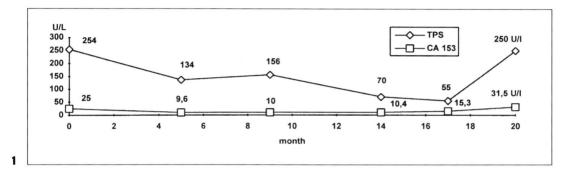

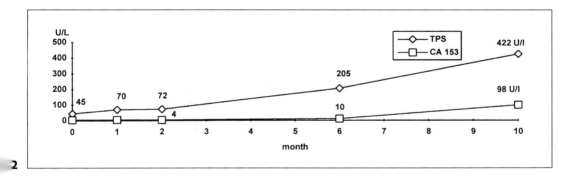

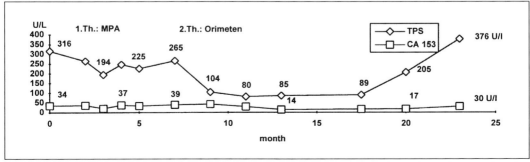

Figure 1–3. Examples for follow-up of patients suffering from breast cancer with TPS and CA 15-3. For explanation see text page 154.

Figure 1: TPS is reflecting response to therapy in a 67 years old patient suffering from breast cancer with osseous metastases treated with gestagens. The imaging methods show a stable disease, TPS a decrease into the normal range. The new progression in the imaging methods is also shown by TPS. In this case TPS represents a more valid parameter compared to CA 15-3 which shows a slight increase only in the case of the final rapid progressive disease.

Figure 2: Patient, 61 years of age, with hepatic metastases of breast cancer; six months after adjuvant chemotherapy a new increase of serum TPS indicated tumor relapse inspite of unsuspicious imaging methods. CA 15-3 showed a significant increase four months later together with liver failure due to progressive tumor disease.

Figure 3: This figure shows an initial decrease of TPS during a first line therapy of pulmonary metastasized breast cancer in a woman 59 years of age. After a new progress therapy with gestagens induced remission over a period of about ten months even in the imaging methods. Two months before the increase of CA 15-3 TPS already indicated the new tumor progress about 20 months after beginning of the follow-up study.

Summarizing, TPS seems to represent an unsuitable tumor marker for primary diagnosis of breast cancer because of the very low sensitivity on the basis of the 95% specificity for benign diseases of the breast.

In the case of advanced diseases TPS, however, seems to represent a valuable tumor marker for follow-up, in some cases indicating therapeutical efficacy and new tumor progress earlier and more valid than e.g. CA 15-3 and CEA.

References

1. Hoffmann L, Heinzerling LD, Bahlo M, Müller-Hagen S, Schäfer E (1986) CA 15-3 in der Kontrolle des klinischen Verlaufs beim metastasierten Mammakarzinom. In: Greten H, Klapdor R (eds) Klinische Relevanz neuer Monoklonaler Antikörper. 3. Hamburger Symposium über Tumormarker. Georg Thieme, Stuttgart New York, pp 239–245
2. Schröck R, Graeff H, Schmidt L (1986) CA 15-3 in der prä- und postoperativen Diagnostik des Mammakarzinoms. In: Greten H, Klapdor R (eds) Klinische Relevanz neuer Monoklonaler Antikörper. 3. Hamburger Symposium über Tumormarker. Georg Thieme, Stuttgart New York, pp 147–158
3. Stieber P (1992) TPS beim Mammakarzinom. Symposium: Zwei Jahre TPS-Assay. Bad Nauheim, Abstrakt p 25–26
4. van Dalen A (1991) Is TPS able to assist in decision making in breast cancer? In: Klapdor R (ed) Associated antigens, oncogenes, receptors, cytokines in tumor diagnosis and therapy at the beginning of the nineties. Zuckschwerdt, München, pp 86–88

Address for correspondence:
Dr. med. U. Heilenkötter
Gynäkologische Abteilung
Johanniter Krankenhaus
Am Runden Berge
D-21502 Geesthacht, Germany

The diagnostic efficiency of the tumor marker CA 549

J. Spitz, P. Benz, L. Ewald, Th. Rink, P. Berle

Division of Nuclear Medicine, Private Office RNS Wiesbaden and Clinic for Gynecology, Municipal Hospital HSK, Academic Hospital of J. Gutenberg University of Mainz, Wiesbaden, Germany

Introduction

Breast cancer is the most frequent malignant disease of women. Every 10th to 16th female is involved in this disease. 22% of all cancer patients have a breast cancer, the incidence ranging from 28 000 to 40 000 newly diagnosed cases per year. These facts make understandable why so much effort is put into the diagnosis and follow-up of breast cancer in women.

One of the measures is the estimation of so called tumor markers. Some of them are well known for years like CEA and CA 15-3. Tumor markers or better tumor associated antigens are used as indicators for tumor activity. Unfortunately, their sensitivity and specificity is limited except for some cases like β-HCG or PSA. This is due to the fact, that the tumor markers are derived from the cell membrane or cell structures which are present as well in benignant as in malignant tissues. Reason enough to look for improved tumor markers which – at their best – fulfill the characteristics of an ideal diagnostic tool:

1. high specificity combined with simple and quick handling to use it as a screening method, giving direct information about the tumor location,
2. high sensitivity to guarantee the necessary information about tumor existence and activity with a single diagnostic measure.

For many years CEA, CA 15-3 and other markers have been used as standard routine measures in breast cancer patients. Several others markers have been tested but did not improve diagnostic efficiency. Now again with CA 549 a tumor marker is available who claims to be of higher diagnostic quality than the established ones.

We therefore decided to use our large collection of specimens out of the routine diagnostic procedure from the last nine years, to compare the values of the CA 549 assay with the results of CEA and CA 15-3 on the basis of the documented clinical follow-up.

Material and methods

Specimen

Out of 1705 sera from 450 patients with established diagnoses by histology we used 1440 specimens from 423 patients. All had CEA, CA 15-3 and CA 549 estimated from the same specimen. After routine diagnostic procedure with CEA and CA 15-3 the specimens had been stored frozen at $-20°C$ until the time of the CA 549 estimation.

The following groups have been selected for statistical analysis.
Before surgery: 108 patients with benign gynecological diseases, 247 patients with breast cancer in various stages.
Follow-up control (< 7 years after surgery): 254 patients with 734 specimens (no evidence of disease), 301 patients with 419 specimens (progressive disease), 97 patients with 105 specimens (partial remission), 70 patients with 84 specimens (at the time of clinical relapse).

Assays

CEA (carcino-embryonal-antigen): Monoclonal radioimmunoassay (Riagnost Behring); (first and mostly established tumor marker especially for cancer of the GI-tract).

CA 15-3: Diagnostic assay which combines two monoclonal antibodies (DF3 and 11.5.D8) in a sandwich radioimmunoassay (CIS bio international).

CA 549: Sandwich radioimmunoassay with two antibodies. One is directed against milk fat globulin membrane, the other one against mucin like antigen (BC 4E 49). The assay Hybri-Brescan is produced by Hybritech Sa.

Results

Specificity

Based on 108 sera of patients with benign gynecological diseases we calculated a 90%, 95% and 98% specificity: CEA = 3.2, 5.2 and 5.9 ng/ml; CA 15-3 = 21.7, 23.0 and 24.3 ng/ml; CA 549 = 14.1, 15.0 and 17.3 U/l.

Further statistical evaluation was based on the product information of the kits using the following levels as cut-off: CEA = 5.0 ng/ml; CA 15-3 = 20.0 ng/ml; CA 549 = 12.0 U/l. These figures correspond to several publications (3, 6, 8) basing on a 95% specificity.

Sensitivity

Using these cut-offs we calculated the sensitivity of the three assays for the two most interesting patient subgroups.

1. Before surgery, all patients:
CEA = 0.13; CA 15-3 = 0.43; CA 549 = 0.33;
CEA + CA15-3 = 0.46; CEA + CA 549 = 0.37;
CA 15-3 + CA 549 = 0.49
Stage I/II: CEA = 0.08, CA 15-3 = 0.32, CA 549 = 0.20
Stage III: CEA = 0.16, CA 15-3 = 0.53, CA 549 = 0.47
Stage IV: CEA = 0.18, CA 15-3 = 0.45, CA 549 = 0.34

2. Time of relapse, all patients:
CEA = 0.29, CA 15-3 = 0.58, CA 549 = 0.54;
CEA + CA 15-3 = 0.60, CEA + CA 549 = 0.55,
CA 15-3 + CA 549 = 0.61
Stage I/II: CEA = 0.28, CA 15-3 = 0.56, CA 549 = 0.50
Stage III: CEA = 0.38, CA 15-3 = 0.71, CA 549 = 0.66
Stage IV: CEA = 0.28, CA 15-3 = 0.56, CA 549 = 0,52

In the subgroup with no evidence of disease (NED) all assays showed a limited number of false positive values: CEA = 3.8%; CA 15-3 = 27.3%; CA 549 = 19.2%, CA 15-3 + CEA = 28.9% CA 15-3 + CA 549 = 28.2% false positive.

Regression analysis for these three groups resulted in the following coefficients of correlation; before tumor surgery: CA 15-3 / CEA (r = 0.21), CA 15-3/CA 549 (r = 0.31); time of relapse: CA 15-3/CEA (r = 0.17), CA 15-3/CA 549 (r = 0.62); no evidence of disease: CA 15-3/CEA (r = 0.49), CA 15-3/CA 549 (r = 0.61).

Discussion

The re-evaluation of the specimen for CA 549 was done without knowledge of the values for CEA and CA 15-3. The 1440 sera were selected out of 1705 specimen of the years 1984–92 according to the following criteria: established diagnoses and availability of the values of both markers (CEA + CA 15-3).

Regarding the changes in postoperative care from strict in-house regiment to an extensive control in private praxis in the last years tumor markers got an important position in the follow-up of patients by the practitioner. But this may also lead to an unknown prevalence in our in-house patient groups and to difficulties in comparing our data with the results of other investigators. On the other hand the sera number is large enough to be representative and to give reliable results.

Summarising our data the following conclusions can be drawn:

1. CA 549 behaves similar to CA 15-3.
2. CA 549 is suitable for the detection and follow up of breast cancer.
3. CA 549 demonstrates better sensitivity compared to CEA.
4. CA 549 is not superior to CA 15-3.
5. CA 549 could replace CEA in breast cancer detection and follow-up control.
6. CA 549 in combination with CA 15-3 is – at least before surgery – superior to the combination of CA 15-3 with CEA.

Due to different cut-off values it is often difficult to compare results of calculations of sensitivity and specificity with those of other authors. *Bagni* et al. (1) also found a high correlation between CA 15-3 and CA 549 (r = 0.91). Our statement 3 was also found by *Cazin* et al. (4). Like other markers (CA 50 and MCA) CA 549 is suitable for the diagnosis and follow-up of breast cancer patients (1, 6). But obviously the assay gives not much additional information about the tumor activity compared to the established marker CA 15-3. This too was reported by *Cazin* et al. (4). As there is one recent report about a superior lead time of CA 549 (2) we shall re-evaluate our data with regard to that. Looking at the results of sensitivity at the time of relapse, it seems doubtful that we shall be able to support their findings.

In some publications the reported calculated sensitivity of CEA and CA 15-3 had been equal to ours, but often CA 549 has had higher ones (0.93–0.77) (3, 7, 8). As has already been pointed out, this may be related to different study populations. In this context it is important to keep in mind, that even though the estimation of CA 549 was done retrospectively, the specimen represent all the population from routine work up of our clinic for gynecology. So the study gets somewhat the character of a prospective one and cannot be compared with the results of selected cases in advanced stages of breast cancer.

Nevertheless with CA 15-3 and CA 549 two markers are now available, which can at least help to diagnose cancer relapse earlier then with the use of CEA alone. This was also shown by other studies (4, 5).

On the other hand as the prognosis of breast cancer, once the tumor has been diagnosed, still is very poor, much effort has to be made to improve earlier diagnosis. A new generation of tumor markers has to be developed which allows early detection and by that a real screening effort.

References

1 Bagni B, Cavallini AR, Indelli M, Malacarna P (1990) Evaluation of CA 549 in malignant neoplasms of the human breast. J Nu Med allied Sci 34:13–15
2 Beveridge RA, Kales AN, Koczyk K et al (1993) Prospective evaluation of CA 549 and CEA in predicting progression or recurrence of disease in breast cancer patients. J Tumour Marker Oncol 8:52
3 Blasco R, Rodriguez Cortasa MJ, Barbero EMA (1992) CA 549: The theorem of Bayes for obtaining cut-off values. Int J Biolog Markers 7:270
4 Cazin JL, Gosselin P, Boniface B (1992) An Evaluation of CA 549, a circulation marker of breast cancer, using a procedure for comparison with CA 15-3. Anti Cancer Res 12:719–724
5 Clocchiatti L, De Biasi F, Cartei G (1991) Evaluation of the circulating glycoprotein CA 549 in mammary cancer and other malignancies. Tumour 77:395–398.
6 Cooper EH, Laurence V, Hancock AK (1992) CA 549 (HybriBREScan) in breast cancer. J Nucl Med Allied Sci 34:91–94
7 Dnistrian AM, Schwartz MK, Greenberg EJ (1991) CA 549 as a marker in breast cancer. Int J Biol Markers 6:139–143
8 Zamagni C, Martoni A, Cacciari N (1992) CA 549 Serum level in breast cancer monitoring. Int J Biol Markers 7:217–221

Address for correspondence:
Priv.-Doz. Dr. med. J. Spitz
Abteilung für Nuklearmedizin
Privatpraxis RNS
Ludwig-Erhard-Straße 100
D-65199 Wiesbaden, Germany

CA 15-3 in the postoperative follow-up of breast cancer patients

D. Essmann-Seboth, I. Fuchs, R. Jakesz, G. Reiner, F. Zekert, M. Zekert

Department of Surgery I, University of Vienna Medical School, Vienna, Austria

Introduction

Just more than four years ago we reported on a clinical evaluation of the CA 15-3 enzyme immunoassay conducted at the laboratory of the First Surgery Department at the University Medical Center in Vienna. Since that time this marker (3) has been used in the follow-up of patients operated for breast cancer in an effort to find out whether it can offer information on recurrent or metastatic disease earlier than clinical findings or imaging techniques.

Patients and methods

70 patients with recurrent or metastatic lesions were available for evaluation of the value of CA 15-3 and CEA in the postoperative follow-up of breast cancer patients. Of these, 25 presented with bone metastases, 23 had lymph node involvement, 20 had developed local tumor regrowth or metastases at the original operative site, 13 showed lung and 9 liver metastases.

Results and discussions

In 29 of the 70 patients with recurrent and/or metastatic lesions, i.e. in almost 40% of cases, CA 15-3 was clearly elevated before clinical signs and symptoms or imaging modalities showed any abnormalities. The interval between the first elevated CA 15-3 level postoperatively and the detection and localization of recurrent or metastatic disease by clinical or imaging evidence varied considerably from 36 days in the best case to up to 737 days, i.e. almost two years. This goes to show that in some patients CA 15-3 was suggestive of recurrent disease long before other modalities raised any suspicion.

The correlation between CA 15-3 and other tumor markers was also of interest. Of 25 patients with confirmed bone metastases, 19 were found to show elevated CA 15-3 levels, while elevated CEA and alkaline phosphatase levels were only present in 15 and 9 cases, respectively. In two women alkaline phosphatase concentrations were borderline. In this subgroup of 25 patients, CA 15-3 was normal in six cases, while CEA and alkaline phosphatase were within normal ranges in 10 and in 14 patients, respectively.

Of our 13 patients with lung metastases, nine showed elevated CA 15-3 levels and six had elevated CEA levels. Normal CA 15-3 and CEA levels were noted in four and in seven patients, respectively.

The distribution of elevated and normal levels was less conclusive in the 23 patients with regional or distant lymph node involvement. In this subgroup CA 15-3 was elevated in eleven cases versus 7 for CEA. Twelve patients were normal for CA 15-3 and 15 had normal CEA levels.

This contrasts sharply with the distribution in the subgroup with liver metastases, which were found to be present in nine patients, all of whom showed elevated CA 15-3 levels.

As local recurrences in the skin or at the original operative site are easily accessible for clinical evaluation, CA 15-3 and CEA obviously play a less important role in their detection. In this subgroup the lesions were, in fact, diagnosed clinically in 19 of 20 cases. The number of patients with elevated CA 15-3 and CEA levels was the same as that of patients with normal levels.

The sensitivity and the specificity of CA 15-3 in breast cancer have been the subject of quite a number of studies and the acceptability of this tumor marker in the diagnosis of breast cancer has been given considerable thought. But few trials have so far been done to establish the potential advantages of CA 15-3 in the postoperative follow-up of breast cancer patients. Apparently the problem shared by all investigators has been that for these follow-up studies to be meaningful a fairly long follow-up time is needed in which patients are easily lost.

Hammer and coworkers (2) showed with statistical significance that the true benefit of tumors markers during scheduled postoperative follow-up examinations lies in the early detection of recurrent or metastatic lesions. *Bombardieri* and coworkers (1) also found CA 15-3 to be elevated four to 48 months before clinical or other investigations were suggestive of any abnormalities. We can not but endorse what *Prof. Knedel* (4) said shortly before his death: As attempts at an early detection of breast cancer have been vastly disappointing, the emphasis should be on follow-up monitoring after surgery.

More than that of other cancers, the diagnosis of breast cancer largely depends on the clinical examination, particularly on palpation, and on various imaging techniques. Once the primary tumor has been removed, these modalities are becoming less important so that alternative laboratory tests are needed to replace them. The earlier recurrent or metastatic lesions are suspected and the earlier further diagnostic studies can be initiated, the greater the chances of a successful outcome. This has prompted us to examine CA 15-3 in an effort of showing whether it was predictive of recurrent or metastatic disease earlier than other procedures.

References

1   Bombardieri E (1992) Eur J Cancer (England) 29A (1) 144-146
2   Hammer J et al (1992) Strahlentherapie Onkol 168 (2) 102–106
3   Jaworek D (1992) In: R Klapdor (ed) Tumor associated antigens, oncogenes, receptors, cytokines in tumor diagnosis and therapie at the beginning of the nineties. Cancer of breast – State and trends in diagnosis and therapy. Zuckschwerdt, München Bern Wien New York, pp 259–262
4   Knedel M (1992) (personal communication)

Address for correspondence:
Prof. Dr. F. Zekert
Universitätsklinik für Chirurgie
Klinische Abteilung für Allgemeinchirurgie
Währinger Gürtel 18–20
A-1090 Wien, Austria

The diagnostic value of the serum tumor markers CEA and CA 549 in patients with scintigraphically verified skeletal metastases of mammary carcinomas

Gertrud Alter, T. Mende
Clinic of Nuclear Medicine of the Martin-Luther-University, Halle-Wittenberg, Germany

Introduction

The most common localization of metastases of mammary carcinomas is the skeletal system. Bone scintigraphy has proven to be the best method for the detection of a skeletal metastasis due to its high sensitivity as well as the easily performed overall body scanning technique.

An early diagnosis of the presence of metastases is of great importance in establishing an adequate course of treatment or the change of an existing course of treatment, whereby the necessity of an improvement of the non-invasive diagnostic means are beyond question. Because of their low sensitivity tumor markers have not been successful in the early diagnosis of malignancies, but their existence can be used for the early diagnosis of recurrent cancer metastases.

For many years CEA has been an important part of follow-up tumor control and the monitoring of treatment. CA 549 is part of a series of new tumor markers which have been developed in search for a more perfect tumor marker.

In this study the question is examined, whether in patients with a verified mamma carcinoma showing an increase of the CEA and/or of the CA 549, one can expect the presence of skeletal metastases.

Patients and methods

119 female patients with carcinoma of the breast, who were regularly transferred to the Nuclear Medical Department of the University in Halle within the framework of an postoperative monitoring program, were included in the study.

The skeletal scintigraphy was performed three hours after i.v.-application of 99m-Tc-MDP in the normal planar technique with a big field camera of the Gamma Muvek company, and partly also with a small field camera Pho-Gamma IV from the Searle company.

Only clear negative scintigrams (n = 64) and clear positive scintigrams (n = 55) were included in the study, while patients with a questionable result were excluded.

The serum probes for the tumor marker assessment were taken on the day of the examination. CEA was assessed with the help of an luminescenc assays of the Behring AG, whereby the standard level is given as ≤ 5 ng/ml. The CA 549 assessment was performed with an immunradiometrical assay of Hybritech GmbH, whereby the standard level is < 12 U/ml.

Results

Of the 64 patients without metastases, 59 patients (92.2%) had normal CEA serum levels and 47 patients (73.4%) normal CA 549 levels (table I). In five patients (7.8%) the CEA level was above the normal level of 5 ng/ml, four patients of which

Table I. Sensitivity of the tumor markers CEA and CA 549 regarding skeletal metastases.

	Negative scintigrams		Positive scintigrams	
	n	%	n	%
CEA 0–5 ng/ml	59	92.2	26	47.3
CEA > 5 ng/ml	5	7.8	29	52.7
CA 549 0–12 U/ml	47	73.4	17	30.9
CA 549 >12 U/ml	17	26.6	38	69.1

Table II. Reaction of the tumor markers CEA and CA 549 depending on the scintigraphical findings.

	All positive scintigrams	Up to 6 metastases	General skeletal metastases
CEA > 5 ng/ml	52.7% (29/55)	33.3% (9/27)	71.7% (20/28)
CA 549 > 12 U/ml	69.1% (38/55)	51.8% (14/27)	85.7% (24/28)
CEA + CA 549	74.5% (41/55)	59.3% (16/27)	89.3% (25/28)

Table III. Average values of the tumor markers CEA and CA 549 in patients with scintigraphically verified bone metastases.

	Positive scintigrams			Negative scintigrams
	< 6 metastases	general	altogether	
CEA (ng/ml)	5.02	34.15	19.6	2.02
CA 549 (U/ml)	36.3	58.9	47.6	14.08

showed an increase in the so-called grey area (5–10 ng/ml). The CA 549 level had increased above the normal level of 12 U/ml in 17 patients (26.6 %), 12 patients of which showed an increase into the grey area (12–20 U/ml). Consequently, in the group of negative scintigrams only one patient showed a clear increase of the CEA level and five patients an increase of the CA 549 level. The specificity for CEA amounted to 92.2% and for CA 549 73.4%.
In the group of patients with scintigrafically proven metastases normal CEA concentrations were found in 26 of the 55 patients (47.3%) and 17 patients (30.9%) had a normal CA 549 concentration (table II).
Where up to six metastases had been verified in the bone scintigramm, even up to 66.6% of the patients had normal CEA levels and 48.2% normal CA 549 levels. With the existence of a general skeletal metastases the rate of patients with normal CEA levels sunk to 28.3% and with normal CA 549 levels to 14.3% (table II).
Increased CEA levels were registered in 29 patients (52.7%), of whom eight patients showed an increase in the grey area and 21 patients showed levels above the grey area (table II).
The CA 549 serum was found elevated in 38 patients (69.1%), of whom eight patients showed levels within the grey area and 30 patients had increased levels above the grey zone.
In case of general skeletal metastases, increased CEA levels were found in 71.4% and increased CA 549 concentrations in 85.7%. In the case of up to six bone metastases proven, only 33.3% of the patients showed increased CEA levels and 51.9% showed increased CA 549 levels (table II).
In the group of the positive scintigrams both tumor markers were increased in 47.3% and at least one tumor marker in 74.5% in the case of simultaneous determination.
With the existence of up to six metastases simultaneous determination resulted in an increase of at least one tumor marker in 59.3% with the proof of general skeletal metastases in 89.3%. Both tumor markers were increased in patients with general skeletal metastases of 67.8% and with the proof of up to six metastases they increased in 25.9% (table II).

Discussion

The results of the study show, that neither CEA nor CA 549 can provide a reliable statement about the existence of a skeletal metastasis, regarding the stated normal values.
Whilst we could find a higher specificity for CEA, in 47.3% of the patients with skeletal metastases normal serum concentrations were registered. In this study the sensitivity for CEA was 52.7%. Other authors described values of 55–58% (1, 3, 5). CA 549 showed in respect to the existence of skeletal metastases a higher sensitivity (69.1%), but with a lower specificity. Comparable values in the international literature are barely found. Only Zwirner (2) reported a sensitivity of the CA 549 of 60% with a mammary carcinoma in phase 4. With a combined determination of the tumor markers the sensitivity could be increased discretly from

69.1% with sole determination of the CA 549 to 74,5% in this study.

In contrast to this report the investigations of *Zwirner* show a clear increase in sensitivity in all phases of the illness by combined tumor marker determination (2).

The sensitivity of 89.3% which we found in our study with combined tumor marker determination regarding general skeletal metastases seems to come closer to the demands of a screening method for metastases, whereby it has to be taken into account, that already general skeletal metastases existed. In comparison, a sensitivity of only 59.3% was found in the group with less than six metastases with combined tumor marker determination.

High concentration causes suspicion of general skeletal metastases.

The average of the CEA levels of the patients with evidence for of up to six metastases shows a significant difference to the average of patients with general skeletal metastases. Only in patients with general skeletal metastases CEA values of over 30 ng/ml were found. As in the case of CEA also the average of the CA 549 levels varied between the patients free of metastases and those with a scintigraphical proof of metastases. But in the first group three patients were registered, who showed a CA 549 level of over 78 U/ml. With the existence of general skeletal metastases 35.7% of the patients showed values of more than 78 U/ml.

Summarizing, it can be said, that neither CEA, CA 549 nor their combined determinations are suitable screening tests for metastases.

But high serum levels should always be regarded as a hint to think about the existence of general skeletal metastases, whereby the sensitivity of CA 549 regarding skeletal metastasis is higher and a combined determination of both markers does not deliver a substantial increase in sensitivity.

References

1. Lamerz R, Dati F, Feller AC, Schnorr G (1988) Tumordiagnostik – Tumormarker bei malignen Erkrankungen. Behringwerke AG Marburg, Frankfurt/Main, p 90
2. Zwirner M, Mittmann S, Geppert M (1991) Clinical evaluation of new CA 549-test for monitoring breast cancer patients. In: Klapdor R (ed) 6. Hamburger Symposium über Tumormarker. Zuckschwerdt, München, pp 24
3. Heise J, Diziol P (1990) Tumormarker – praktischer Einsatz und klinische Bedeutung. Boehringer Mannheim GmbH
4. Bray KR, Gauer PK (1988) Correlation of serum levels of CA 549 to disease status in posttreatment serial samples rom breast cancer patients. J Clin Labor Analysis 2:134–137
5. Hoffmann L, Heinzerling D, Klapdor R, Bohler M et al (1986) CA 15-3, CA 125 und CEA in der Kontrolle des klinischen Verlaufs bei metastasierenden Mammakarzinom. In: Greten H, Klapdor R (ed) Klinische Relevanz neuer monoklonaler Antikörper. 3. Hamburger Symposium über Tumormarker. Thieme, Stuttgart, pp 239–245
6. Chigira M, Shinozaki T (1990) Diagnostic value of serum tumor markers in skeletal metastasis of carcinomas. Arch Orth Trauma Surg 109:247–251

Address for correspondence:
Dipl. med. Gertrud Alter
Klinik für Nuklearmedizin
Universität Halle/Wittenberg
Voßstraße 1
D-06110 Halle/Saale, Germany

Follow-up of breast cancer using CA 15-3 immunoluminometric determination

M. Drahovsky, Edith Greiner-Mai, D. Lentfer

Byk-Sangtec Diagnostica GmbH & Co. KG, Dietzenbach, Germany

Introduction

The tumor-associated antigen CA 15-3 is the tumor marker most frequently used in the follow-up of breast cancer. This is mainly due to its high sensitivity for metastatic carcinomas of the breast. The tests first developed for the detection of the CA 15-3 antigen were immunoradiometric assays (IRMA); so most clinical data published are based on this technique. Therefore, the quality of all non-radioactive detection methods is evaluated against these immunoradiometric tests. Giving the laboratory the possibility to compare the results obtained with a new assay to those obtained with a reference method is a prerequisite for using emerging technologies in cancer patient monitoring. In this study investigating the immunoluminometric (ILMA) determination of CA 15-3 with the LIA-mat® CA 15-3 assay, special consideration is given to this aspect.

Materials and methods

Immunoluminometric CA 15-3 assay

The LIA-mat® CA 15-3 (Byk-Sangtec Diagnostica) is a two-site immunoluminometric assay (sandwich principle). The monoclonal antibody 115D8 (1) is used for the coating of the solid phase (polystyrene tubes), the monoclonal antibody DF3 (2) is used for the tracer. Both antibodies react simultaneously with the CA 15-3 antigen forming a "sandwich" complex bound to the tube wall, which is detected by light emission.

Comparative CA 15-3 assays

Immunoradiometric determinations were carried out with CA 15-3 ELSA (CIS, 2-step method) and IRMA-mat CA 15-3 (Byk-Sangtec Diagnostica, l-step method) and immunoenzymatic determinations with CA 15-3 ENZELSA (CIS, 2-step method) and Enzymun CA 15-3 (Boehringer, 3-step method) according to manufacturers' instructions.

Materials tested

The following samples were included in the study: serum samples from blood donors, from normal pregnant and non-pregnant women, from patients with benign breast diseases and from breast cancer patients at different stages.

Results and discussion

Precision and reproducibility

The present study indicates that the immunoluminometric determination of CA 15-3 is highly consistent with the results obtained with two established immunoradiometric assays (correlation coefficients: 0.96–0.97). Precision studies with the ILMA compare favorable (intra-assay precision: mean CV = 5%, useful working range > 4.3 U/ml; inter-assay precision: CV < 10%) with the performances of the reference methods. In addition, the stability of the ILMA tracer is considerably extended compared to the stability of ^{125}I-labelled antibody. Shelf-life related imprecision is hardly noticeable.

To investigate the reproducibility, controls with low, intermediate and high CA 15-3 concentrations were measured over a period of several months, using different batches of reagents. Inter-assay coefficient of variation were markedly below 10% (65.37 U/ml: CV = 7.68%; 30.95 U/ml: CV = 7.54%; 16.95 U/ml: CV = 7.26%).

Lower detection limit and linearity upon dilution

To estimate the analytical sensitivity of the ILMA, the zero standard was measured five times, leading to a minimum detection limit below 0.3 U/ml (mean + 3 standard deviations).
Three samples with high CA 15-3 concentrations were serially diluted with the kit diluent. No departure from linearity was observed (r = 0.9971–0.9999).

Comparison with other methods

An excellent correlation of the ILMA was obtained with both IRMAs (figures 1a and 1b). The ILMA values were, however, slightly higher in the pathological range. A good correlation was also obtained with the Enzymun CA 15-3 (figure 1c) but, in this case, the trend was towards slightly lower results with the ILMA. More scattering was observed in the comparison with the ENZELSA CA 15-3 assay (figure 1d).

Reference range

Samples from four groups of subjects were evaluated with the ILMA (table I). Clinical data obtained are in close agreement with the literature (3, 4). Normal serum samples are found below 30 U/ml (mean value + 2 standard deviations). Benign breast disorders do not significantly influence CA 15-3 levels. Furthermore, the slight elevation of CA 15-3 observed in late pregnancy is consistent with the results of other studies.

Follow-up

Finally, retrospective studies obtained from repeated sampling in breast cancer patients support the equivalence of the ILMA, compared to the two IRMA reference methods. Figure 2 was selected as a representative example among a number of similar profiles.

Summary

Comparisons with established immunoradiometric assays were carried out to evaluate the per-

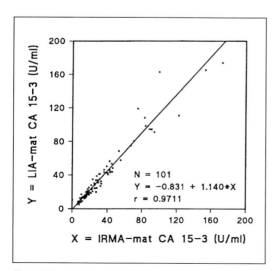

Figure 1a. Method comparison of patient samples. LIA-mat® CA 15-3 versus IRMA-mat CA 15-3.

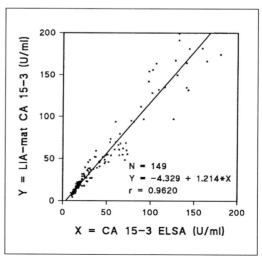

Figure 1b. Method comparison of patient samples. LIA-mat® CA 15-3 versus CA 15-3 ELSA.

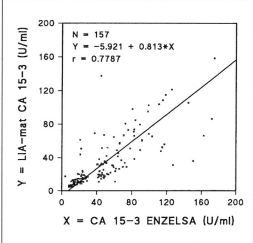
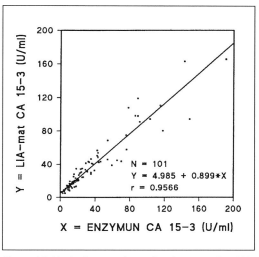

Figure 1c. Method comparison of patient samples. LIA-mat® CA 15-3 versus CA 15-3 ENZELSA.

Figure 1d. Method comparison of patient samples. LIA-mat® CA 15-3 versus ENZYMUN CA 15-3.

Table I. CA 15-3 serum levels in healthy subjects and in patients with benign breast diseases.

Subjects	Mean value	Limits of reference range	
	(50-percentile)	($\bar{x}$ + 2.5 D)	(95-percentile)
Healthy non pregnant women (n = 100)	13.4	31.7	31.9
Healthy pregnant women (n = 100)	18.6	42.1	36.6
Blood donors (male, female) (n = 200)	15.5	28.0	26.5
Benign breast diseases (n = 25)	14.7	32.5	27.8

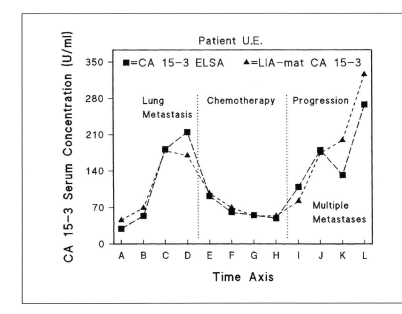

Figure 2. Follow-up of a breast cancer patient using parallel testing with LIA-mat® CA 15-3 and CA 15-3 ELSA.

formances of a new immunoluminometric assay (ILMA) for the determination of CA 15-3 in breast cancer patients.

The linear regression analysis demonstrates an excellent correlation between the ILMA and the two immunoradiometric assays.

Precision, dilution, linearity studies as well as clinical data obtained with normal and pathological subjects confirm the equivalence with the reference assays. This was confirmed by other authors (4, 5) for the fully automated performance of this assay on the LIA-mat® System 300.

References

1. Hilkens J, Bujis J, Hilgers J et al (1984) Monoclonal antibodies against human milk fat globule membranes detecting differentiation antigen of the mammay gland and its tumors. Int J Cancer 34:197–206
2. Kufe D, Inghirami G, Abe M et al (1984) Differential reactivity of novel monoclonal antibody (DF3) with human malignant versus benign breast cancer tumors. Hybridoma 33:223–232
3. Lelle R, Henkel E, Leinemann D et al (1989) Measurement of CEA, TPA, Neopterin, CA 125, CA 15-3, and CA 19-9 in sera of pregnant women, umbilical cord blood and amniotic fluid. Gynecol Obstet Invest 27:137–142
4. Villalta D, Borean M, Zannese L, Santini G (1990) Clinical evaluation of LIA-mat CA 15.3 in the breast pathology. J Nucl Med Allied Sci 34:237–241
5. Zucchelli G, Pilo A, Reum L et al (1990) A new chemiluninescence immunoassay for CA 15-3, CA 125, CA 19-9: evaluation using QC sera assayed in an interlaboratory survey. J Nucl Med allied Sci 34:222–228

Address for correspondence:
Dr. med. Edith Greiner-Mai
Byk-Sangtec Diagnostica
von-Hevesy-Straβe 3
D-63128 Dietzenbach, Germany

Survival time in breast cancer patients with osseous metastases after increase of CEA compared to CA 15-3

S. Krämer[a], A. Katalinic[b], W. Jäger[a]
[a]Department of Obstetrics and Gynecology,
[b]Institute for Medical Statistics and Documentation,
University of Erlangen-Nuremberg, Germany

Introduction

Previous studies have shown that in up to 80% of breast cancer patients the tumor associated antigens CEA and CA 15-3 increase when distant metastases develop (1, 2). It has also been noticed that not always both markers increase concommitantly but that in several patients either only CEA or CA 15-3 increases and that the other marker appears later during the course of the disease. That means that some tumor tissue is able to produce and secrete e.g. CEA and not CA 15-3. This could be interpreted as the expression of two distinct biological behaviors of metastatic breast cancer tissue. We speculated, whether this different biological behavior also finds its expression in different survival times. Therefore we analyzed the survival times of breast cancer patients who developed an increase of CEA and compared this with survival times of patients who developed an increase of CA 15-3. In order to obtain a reasonable homologous group we analyzed only patients with bone metastases, because that is the most common site of metastases in breast cancer patients (3).

Material and methods

129 breast cancer patients developed osseous metastases during follow-up examinations between August 1985 and May 1992. The diagnosis of metastases was established by bone scintigraphy and X-ray examination.
The records of each patient were reviewed for the following data: 1. time of detection of metastases, 2. time of tumor marker increase, 3. which tumor marker increased, 4. time interval between primary surgery and increase of tumor marker, 5. survival time from tumor marker increase until death.
In order to answer these questions the following criteria were used: 1. month when scintigraphy or x-ray revealed bone metastases (no other metastases should have appeared within the next three months), 2. month when tumor markers were elevated. The upper level of normal was defined as the 97th percentile of marker concentrations in previously operated metastases free breast cancer patients. The corresponding level for CEA was 6 µg/l (ELSA CEA, ID – CIS, Dreieich, Germany), and for CA 15-3 40 kU/l (ELSA CA 15-3, ID – CIS, Dreieich, Germany). 3. Isolated increase was only accepted when only one marker increased, without increase of the other marker within three months. Otherwise the increase was termed "combined". 4. and 5. Intervals were expressed in months, estimations of survival were calculated with the Kaplan-Meier method, and differences were calculated with the log-rank test. Furthermore the χ^2-test was used when appropiate. For all tests a niveau of 5% was accepted as significant.
Follow-up examinations were performed every three months within the first two years after primary surgery. Between two and five years after primary surgery follow-up examinations were performed in six month intervals. According to these different follow-up intervals two groups of patients were classified: Those patients with a tumor marker increase within the first two years after primary surgery were termed "group A", and those patients with a tumor marker increase after 2–5 years after primary surgery were termed "group B".

Results

Of the 129 patients with osseous metastases, three (2%) had no tumor marker increase. 24 patients were excluded from the analysis, because it was not possible to identify if an isolated or combined tumor marker increase had occured. Therefore 102 patients with bone metastases were eligible for analysis. According to the described definition 42 (41%) patients of the 102 patients with osseous metastases had an isolated CEA increase, 43 (42%) patients had an isolated CA 15-3 increase. In 17 (17%) patients both markers were elevated. In these 102 patients median survival time from tumor marker increase to death was 29 months. Patients with osseous metastases and an isolated CEA increase had a median survival of 31 months. Patients with an isolated CA 15-3 increase had a median survival of 29 months. This difference was not significant. The median survival time of patients with a combined increase of CEA and CA 15-3 was 27 months (figure 1). Differentiation according to group A and group B revealed a median survival time of 26 months for group A and a median survival time of 36 months for group B. This difference was significant (p < 0.01) (figure 2). Within the first two years after primary surgery (group A) 46 patients developed metastases. 19 of these patients had an increase of CEA, 27 patients an increase of CA 15-3. Between two and five years after primary surgery (group B) 28 patients developed metastases. 18 of these patients had an increase of CEA, ten patients an increase of CA 15-3. In group A significantly more patients presented with an increase of CA 15-3, while in group B significantly more patients presented with an increase of CEA (figure 3).

Discussion

Previous studies have shown that the median survival of patients with bone metastases is better than of patients with other sites of metastases (4,5). In our study we did not find any difference in median survival times of patients with bone metastases neither if CEA increased as first marker nor CA 15-3. We therefore conclude that the different biological behavior of bone metastases, i.e. either the production of CEA or CA 15-3 does not influence the prognosis of patients with osseous metastases. However, according to our statistical analysis the median survival of patients with osseous metastases within the first two years after primary surgery is worse than the survival time of patients who developed metastases after a postoperative period of two years. This difference, which was calculated as ten months was statistically significant, but we speculate that this was caused by the longer time intervals between tumor marker measurements in those patients, because they were only performed in six month intervals. However, we can not definitely exclude that there was a significant difference in survival time, which could be caused by the different localisation of bone metastases. This was not analyzed in our study. Nevertheless, it was interesting to note that most of the patients, who developed bone metastases during the first years after primary surgery, presented with an increase of CA 15-3. This should not be interpreted as if CA 15-3 producing metastases indicate an extremely aggressive tumor, because this conclusion was only derived from the ratio of 27 CA 15-3 producing tumors to 19 CEA producing tumors.

If these questions should be clarified further we would encourage a meta-analysis of the respective data of different research groups. However, in

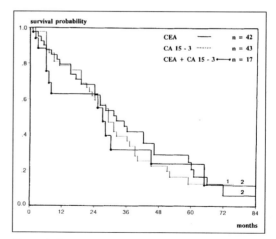

Figure 1. Estimation of survival probability according to Kaplan-Meier for patients with bone metastases. The solid line shows the curve for patients with an isolated increase of CEA, the dotted line shows the curve for patients with an isolated increase of CA 15-3. The survival curve of patients with an increase of both markers is shown as a solid line with dots.

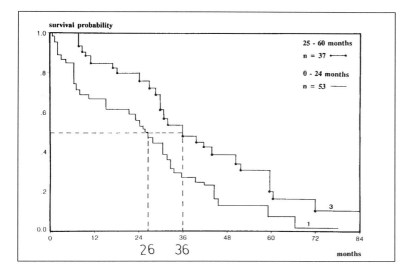

Figure 2. Estimation of survival probability according to *Kaplan-Meier* for patients with bone metastases. The solid line shows the curve for patients with bone metastases within the first two years after primary surgery, the solid line with dots shows the curve for patients who developed metastases between two and five years after primary surgery. The horizontal line delineates the median.

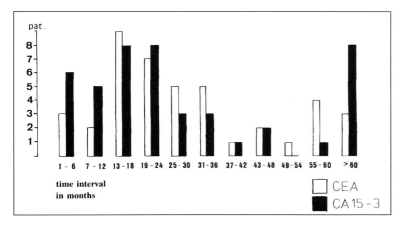

Figure 3. Distribution of patients with bone metastases according to the time interval of detection of metastases after primary surgery and according to the first marker increase.

our opinion the increase of CEA or CA 15-3 in metastatic breast cancer patients does not allow to draw any conclusion in regard to further prognosis.

References

1. Bon GG, Kenemans P, Yedema CA, van Kamp GJ, Nijman HW, Hilgers J (1990) Clinical relevance of the tumor marker CA 15.3 in the management of cancer patients. In: DJA Crommelin, H Schellekens (eds) From clone to clinic. Kluwer Academic Publishers, pp 111–122
2. Jäger W, Wildt L, Leyendecker G (1986) CA 15-3 and CEA serum concentrations in breast cancer patients. In: H Greten, R Klapdor (eds) Clinical relevance of new monoclonal antibodies. Thieme, Stuttgart, pp 167
3. Galarko CSB (1972) Skeletal metastases and mammary cancer. Ann R Coll Surg Engl 50:3–28
4. Hoogstraten B, Gad-El-Mawla N, Maloney TR (1984) Combined modality therapy for first recurrence of breast cancer: A SWOG study. Cancer 54:2248–2256
5. Scheid V, Buzdar AV, Smith TC, Hartobagyi GN (1986) Clinical course of breast cancer patients with osseous metastasis treated with combination chemotherapy. Cancer 58:2589–2593

Address for correspondence:
Dr. med. W. Jäger
Universitätsfrauenklinik
Universitätsstraße 21-23
D-91054 Erlangen, Germany

Is an increase of CA 125 in breast cancer patients an indicator of pleural metastases?

W. Jäger, A. Kissing, S. Cilaci, V. Palapelas, N. Lang

Department of Obstetrics and Gynecology, University of Erlangen-Nuremberg, Germany

Introduction

CA 125 is an established marker in ovarian cancer and has not gained any importance in the follow-up of breast cancer patients so far (1). However, we now report the cases of two patients which could indicate that CA 125 could be a very useful marker in metastatic breast cancer.

Case report 1

A 54 years old woman, who had been operated for breast cancer two years earlier presented with bone pain during follow-up. Bone scintigraphy described diffuse bone metastases which were also demonstrated by x-ray examination. No other metastases could be detected by chest x-ray or liver ultrasound at that time.

Since the primary tumor was hormone-receptor positive, tamoxifen treatment was started. Three months later the response to tamoxifen was classified as partial remission. After additional six months progression of the bone metastases was demonstrated after new metastases in the thoracic spine were found. A CAT-scan of the thoracic spine at that time further exhibited a small pleural effusion on both sides of the lung.

Consequently, treatment with tamoxifen was stopped and a combination chemotherapy of 5-FU, doxorubicin and cyclophosphamide (FAC) was initiated. Three months later partial remission of the bone metastases was noted. However, a small lung metastasis had appeared. The course of CEA and CA 15-3 of this patient is shown in figure 1. CA 15-3 levels always remained in the normal range during the entire observation period of twelve months. The CEA levels were in quite good accordance to the clinical impression: During the phase of stable disease CEA levels remained at 12 ng/ml, while the progression of the disease was indicated by the increase of CEA to 31 ng/ml. The effect of FAC was clinically classified as partial remission and was paralleled by a decrease of CEA to 17 ng/ml.

At the time of diagnosis of the bone metastases the CA 125 level was 110 U/ml (figure 2). The further course of the CA 125 levels, however, did not correspond to the clinical course. Ovarian metastases and ovarian cancer were considered extremely unlikely to cause the elevated CA 125 levels because of unsuspicious ultrasound and vaginal examination. Heart ultrasound did not exhibit pericardial effusion (2). During the next nine months of tamoxifen treatment, CA 125 levels dropped to 60 U/ml. At that time a pleural effusion was detected by the CAT-scan. After the therapy was changed from tamoxifen to FAC chemotherapy, the CA 125 levels increased to 150 U/ml within the next four weeks. Thereafter CA 125 levels dropped.

As no disease typically associated with an increase of CA 125 serum levels could be found in this patient, it must be suspected that the increase of CA 125 in this patient was caused by the metastatic breast cancer (3). Since the patient did not develop liver metastases and the bone metastases were soon progressive, these two sites of origin could be excluded. The pleural effusion at CAT-scan could indicate that a pleuritis carcinomatosa had developed but was not detectable at that time. It is tempting to speculate that the decrease of CA 125 during the following months was an effect of the tamoxifen treatment. This would then indicate that CA 125 could be a serum marker for assessment of response to tamoxifen treatment.

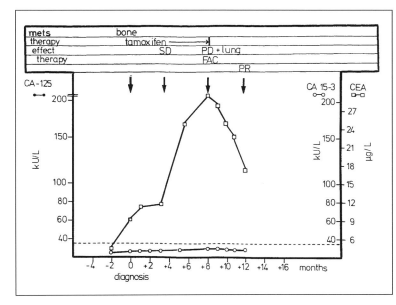

Figure 1. The course of CEA and CA 15-3 serum levels of case report 1. The following abbreviations were used: mets = location of metastases, SD = stable disease, PD = progressive disease, FAC = 5-fluorouracil, adriamycin, cyclophosphamide, PR = partial remission. The arrows show the time of clinical examination. Time scale is adopted to the time of detection of metastases.

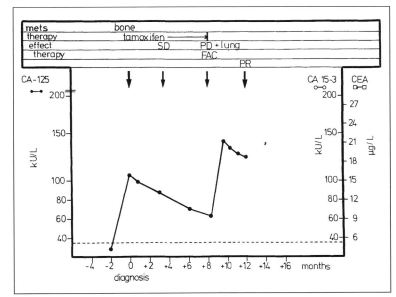

Figure 2. The course of CA 125 serum levels of the case report 1; for abbreviations see legend to figure 1.

Case report 2

A 62 year old woman, who had been operated for primary breast cancer three years earlier, presented with shortness of breath and cough during follow-up. Chest x-rays revealed a pleural effusion of the right side and two isolated lung metastases. She was punctured and 1l of serous fluid was removed. She was then placed on treatment; tamoxifen was chosen because the primary cancer has been estrogen-receptor positive. After three and after six months she was considered to be in complete remission. After nine months, however, bone metastases were detected, while the lung metastases were still in complete remission. At that point tamoxifen

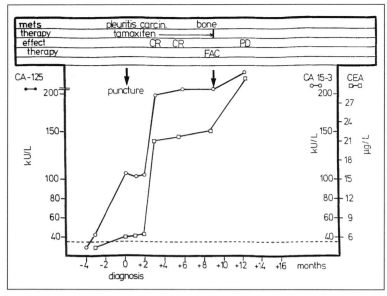

Figure 3. The course of CEA and CA 15-3 serum levels case report 2. The following abbreviations were used: mets = location of metastases, pleuritis carcin = pleuritis carcinoma, CR = complete remission, PD = progressive disease, FAC = 5-fluorouracil, adriamycin, cyclophosphamide. The arrows show the time of clinical examination. Time scale is adopted to the time of detection of metastases.

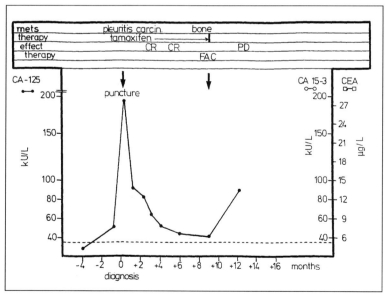

Figure 4. The course of CA 125 serum levels of the case report 2; for abbreviations see legend to figure 3.

treatment was stopped and the patient was given combination chemotherapy according to the FAC-regimen (see above).

At the time of diagnosis of the lung metastases, CEA and CA 15-3 were elevated (figure 3). The tumor markers increased substantially between the second and third months of tamoxifen treatment. One month before the detection of the lung metastases, CA 125 was elevated with a level of 50 kU/l (figure 4). When she presented with the symptoms of pleural effusion the CA 125 was 190 kU/l. An abdominal and heart ultrasound examination was performed before initiation of the FAC chemotherapy, which excluded ascites, ovarian tumors and pericardial effusion (2). In a specimen collected from the pleuropuncture the

CA 125 concentration was 350 kU/l. After puncture CA 125 levels gradually dropped during the following nine months to 40 kU/l. After change to FAC chemotherapy CA 125 levels increased again. The large increase of CA 125 coincided with the appearance of pleural effusion. It was shown that the pleural effusion contained high amounts of CA 125 and that within days after the puncture the CA 125 levels dropped (data not shown). This leads one to speculate that the CA 125 in the pleural fluid contributes at least in part to the CA 125 serum levels. Falling CA 125 levels did not correspond to the course of the bone metastases which were progressing during this time. On the other hand, the decrease of CA 125 during tamoxifen therapy did correlate with the complete response noted in the lung metastases.

Discussion

CEA and CA 15-3 are established tumor markers in breast cancer (4,5). However, the clinical information in measurements of these two markers are limited. They only can predict – with a high degree of reliability – wether the disease is in remission or in progression. They are not able to provide further differentiation of treatment response, e.g. according to an individual site metastases. These case reports, however, offer the possibility that CA 125 could be a marker in metastatic breast cancer which would indicate the response of one single site to treatment. The preliminary observations seem to indicate that the course of CA 125 in metastatic breast cancer is not associated to bone or liver metastases, but to lung and/or pleural metastases. That would offer the chance to assess selectively the response of the lung or pleura to treatment. One could argue that this could easily be obtained by chest x-ray or CAT-scans. However, the course of a serum tumor marker is easier to assess, because in diffuse metastatic disease it is sometimes difficult to decide whether progression, stable disease or remission prevails. Further studies should evaluate if the increase of CA 125 is caused by lung metastases alone or by involvement of the pleura. Preliminary observations seem to indicate that in isolated lung metastases without pleural effusion CA 125 does not increase in serum. These observations clearly need further investigation. If these data could be strengthened, CA 125 would be one of the most promising tumor markers – not only in ovarian cancer – but also in metastatic breast cancer!

Acknowledgement

The authors wish to thank *R. Melsheimer* from Centocor-Europe. His ideas were incorporated in the final manuscript.

References

1 Jäger W, Cilaci S, Merkle E, Palapelas V, Lang N (1991) Analysis of the first signs of metastases in breast cancer patients. Tumordiagn u Ther 12:60–64
2 Hopman EH, Helmerhorst TJM, Bonfrer JMG, Ten Bokkel Huinink WW (1993) Highly elevated serum CA 125 levels in a patient with cardiac failure. Eur J Obstet Gynecol Reprod Biol 48:71–73
3 Seckl MJ, Rustin GJS, Coombes RC (1992) CA-125 is not a useful marker in metastatic breast cancer. Br J Cancer 66:875–876
4 Kandylis K, Vassilomanolakis M, Baziotis N et al (1990) Diagnostic significance of the tumour markers! CEA, CA 15-3 and CA 125 in malignant effusions in breast cancer. Ann Oncol 6:435–438
5 Tsavaris N, Vonorta K, Sarafidou M et al (1992) Comparison of tumor markers CEA, CA 125, CA 15-3 and prolactin levels in patients with advanced breast cancer. Diagn Oncol 2:211–219

Address for correspondence:
Dr. med. W. Jäger
Universitätsfrauenklinik
Universitätsstraße 21-23
D-91054 Erlangen, Germany

A new chemiluminescence immunoassay for the detection of PEM in breast cancer sera

C. Schelp, S. Wege, P. Pfleiderer, K. Boßlet, N. Madry
Research Laboratories of Behringwerke, Marburg, Germany

Introduction

A new monoclonal antibody BW 835 (IgG1) has been generated after immunization of mice with breast cancer cell line MCF-7 and SW-613. This antibody has been studied for its immunoreactivity to mammary carcinomas. Recently we have developed a chemiluminescence immunoassay with this antibody for the quantification of polymorphic epithelial mucin (PEM) in breast cancer sera. The antigen is a mucin-like transmembrane glycoprotein, which contains a central region consisting of a sequential arrangement of genetically defined 20 amino acid peptides. The genetic polymorphism (hence the name PEM), causes the heterogenity of the antigen on a protein basis from individual to individual. Additionally, the complexity increases due to apparently different glycosylation patterns in tumor cells. So PEM has been proven to be an excellent marker for breast tumor monitoring (1–3).

Materials and methods

Polymorphic epithelial mucin: PEM was isolated from human milk.
Monoclonal antibodies: MAb BW 835 was generated by immunization of mice with breast carcinoma cell lines MCF-7 and SW 613; MAb B27.29 (Biomira Inc., Edmonton).

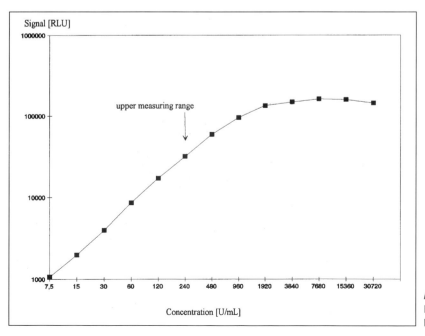

Figure 1.
BeriLux® BR high-dose hook behavior.

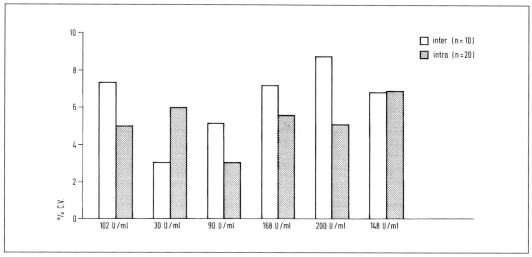

Figure 2. BeriLux® BR precision data.

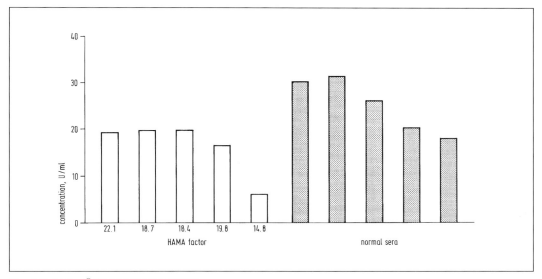

Figure 3. BeriLux® BR interference studies.

PEM-assay: The coated tube assay utilizes as catcher antibody the BW 835 and another monoclonal antibody, B27.29 (Biomira Inc.), labeled with an acridinium sulfonamide compound. The MAb BW 835 is adsorbed to the tubes. Into each of the tubes 200 µl incubation medium are pipetted. Then the tubes are incubated with 20 µl standards, controls, or serum samples for 1 h with shaking. After washing, the labeled mucin antibody B27.29 is added and incubated for 1 h with shaking. After the final wash step the sandwich complex formed is quantified by measuring the luminescent signal for 1 sec in a luminometer. The relative light units (RLU) correlate directly to the concentration of PEM or CA 15-3 antigen in the samples.

Specimen: Serum samples from healthy blood donors and patients with different malignant breast diseases were used in this study.

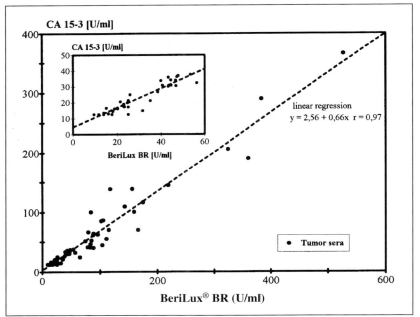

Figure 4.
BeriLux® BR correlation to a commercially available CA 15-3 assay.

Results

Assay evaluation – Precision, linearity, hook-effekt, HAMA-effect

The standard curve shows a good dose reponse in the measuring range from 0–200 U/ml. No high-dose hook effect occured in the 2-step assay up to 30.000 U/ml (figure 1).
Dilution of sera with diluent was used to test the linearity of the test system. Four serum samples (two above the measuring range) and the highest standard dilute linearly with recoveries between 91% and 111% over the whole measuring range.
The between-assay-variance (n = 10) for six samples (three tumor marker controls, two tumor sera and one normal sera spiked with PEM) in a range of 30–200 U/ml was found from 3–8%. The within-assay-variance (n = 20) ranged from 3–9% (figure 2).
Human anti-mouse antibody (HAMA) binding as seen in several tumor sera showed no interferences in this assay. Sera with high HAMA factors (Enzygnost®, HAMA micro, Behringwerke Marburg) exhibited results in the range of normal sera (figure 3). Analysis of a healthy blood donor group (n = 41) yielded a 5% percentile of about 30 U/ml.

Comparison of methods

65 human sera were measured with the BeriLux® BR and also with a commercially available CA 15-3 assay. At the beginning of each series, calibration curves were generated from duplicate determinations of the standards. Evaluations were performed using mean values. In the method comparison of BeriLux® BR against a commercially available CA 15-3 assay the values show a high degree of correlation. Correlation coefficients around 0.97 demonstrate that the correlation is very good, as is demonstrated in figure 4.

Conclusion

To perform an immunoluminometric assay we selected an appropriate second mucin antibody, the MAb B27.29, which was conjugated with a novel acridinium sulfonamide compound. The new BeriLux® Label has been synthesized to obtain:
- a fast light emission leading to a short measuring time,
- a high quantum yield to ensure a high sensitivity,
- an easy-to-handle-reagent with good stability and a long shelf life.

The good results ot the technical performance can be explained by the homogeneity of reagent and tubes, as well as the high accuracy and precision offered by the semi-automated test system. In comparison of methods, a good correlation was obtained with established tests. So we conclude, that this new non-isotopic BeriLux® assay would prove valuable for monitoring of breast cancer patients.

References

1. P Pfleiderer et al (1992) Characterization of a new anti-PEM monoclonal antibody detecting breast carcinoma associated mucin. In: R. Klapdor (ed) Tumor associated antigens, oncogens, receptors, cytokines in tumor diagnosis and therapy at the beginning of the nineties. Zuckschwerdt, München, pp 89–93
2. SJ Gendler et al (1991) Characterization and evolution of an expressed hypervariable gene for tumor-associated mucin, MUC-1. In: Ceriani RL (ed) Breast epithelial antigens. Plenum Press, New York, pp 15–24
3. J Hilkens et al (1992) Cell membrane-associated mucins and their adhesion-modulating property. TIBS 17:359–363.

Address for correspondence:
Dr. C. Schelp
Behringwerke AG
Diagnostische Abteilung
P.O. 1140
D-35001 Marburg, Germany

Are tumor marker changes in breast cancer reliable?

A. van Dalen[a], A. Blusse van OudAlblas[b], K.J. Heering[b], D.L. vd Linde[b]
Departments of [a]Nuclear Medicine and [b]Oncology, Groene Hart Ziekenhuis,
Bleuland Location, Gouda, The Netherlands

Introduction

Breast cancer has a high frequency of developing to the metastatic state. The International Union Against Cancer (UICC) has stimulated clear definitions of the disease state and of the response to therapy (1). It is obvious from these criteria that tumor marker values and other clinical chemistry data play a minor role. Only in the definition of complete response serological tests are mentioned. The definitions of partial response and no change are using the size of the metastatic site(s). This is very useful in measuring the response in i.e. patients with small cell lung cancer after the application of combined chemotherapy. However, in breast cancer patients with multiple bone metastases these criteria of PR or NC are hardly applicable. Moreover, in breast cancer patients many times different organs are involved and this makes the assessment of response even more complex. It is especially this situation which makes partial response and no change in breast cancer patients very difficult.

In the past tumor marker changes during treatment have been used to determine the effect of the applied treatment (2–4). However, not always the strict UICC criteria were applied, but also minimal remission (any improvement at the metastatic sites) and improvement of the performance (diminished complaints) were used as criteria. Besides, changes in the tumor marker values were not judged uniformally. Within the International Society of Oncodevelopmental Biology and Medicine (ISOBM) the discussion has started to develop strict tumor marker criteria which could then be related to UICC criteria (5). In a pilot study we correlated these strict criteria of tumor marker changes (progressive disease should be associated with an increase of more than 25% of the marker and a positive effect of treatment should cause a decrease of more than 50% of the marker) with UICC criteria (6). In this study we have increased the number of patients and we have also extended the time interval applying UICC criteria at month 3 and at month 6 after the start or the change of treatment in breast cancer patients with progressive metastatic disease.

Material and methods

In 88 patients 140 situations were analyzed when progressive disease was established according to UICC criteria (1). The treatment applied could be either hormonal or chemotherapy. Patients were included when distant metastases were discovered for the first time or when progressive disease was established during treatment. Patients with only locoregional recurrence i.e. skin metastases or locoregional lymph node metastases were excluded from the study.

The time interval between the sampling was variable and ranged from 0.5–3.0 months. The WHO criteria for progressive disease (PD), stable disease or no change (SD = NC), partial remission (PR) and complete remission (CR) were applied at month 3 and month 6 after the start of treatment. CA 15-3 was determined using an IRMA (CIS International), CEA by the ENZELSA method (CIS International) or the FEI method on the AIA 1200 (TOSOH) and TPS by the IRMA method (BEKI Diagnostics). Significant changes of tumor marker levels were defined as an increase of 25% or a decrease of 50% where at least one sample should have a level outside the reference range. The upper reference level used for CA 15-3 was 30 kU/l, for CEA 5 µg/l and for TPS 75 U/l.

Results

In table I the sensitivity of the markers is given at the start of the study (0-samples). In progressive disease the sensitivity for CA 15-3 was 77%, for CEA 69% and for TPS 81%, respectively. The number of significant changes of the tumor markers (+ 25% or – 50%) within the first episode after the start of the therapy (difference between sample 0 and sample 1) are given in table II. These numbers were calculated based on the initial number of elevated levels of the respective markers as represented in table I. After three months of treatment the clinical situation was described as 35 times PD, 98 times SD and 7 times PR. In the clinical situation of SD the number of patients in which the tumor markers had decreased (a decrease of more than 50% in the level) was in this period for CA 15-3 75%, CEA 65% and TPS 80%. When combining CA 15-3 and TPS in patients with initially elevated levels of one of the markers a decrease was registered for 90% of the patients with the clinical situation of stable disease (SD) at month 3. At months 6 the clinical diagnosis in 98 patients with stable disease had changed to nine patients with partial remission and 18 patients with progressive disease, leaving 71 patients with stable disease.

The tumor marker patterns in this type of patients are illustrated in figures 1 and 2. Figure 1 demonstrates a patient with progressive bone metastases detected at the start of the study (month 0). The patient was treated with Adriamycine and initially all markers with elevated levels decreased. During the observation period the clinical diagnosis was stable disease (SD). Nevertheless, at the end of the study a slight increase of CEA is registered (between 10 and 25%) and a clear increase of TPS (more than 25%). CA 15-3 is constantly decreasing from start to month 5. In figure 2 bone metastases and malignant pleural effusion were detected and the patient was treated with Tamoxifen. Initially only TPS was elevated, but after the start of treatment CEA and CA 15-3 started to increase during the first month. TPS decreased immediately after the start of therapy, followed by CA 15-3 and CEA. After three months the clinical observation revealed stable disease (SD). After seven months progressive disease was established (increase of pleural effusion). In the meanwhile TPS and CEA had increased, but CA 15-3 was still within the reference limit.

Discussion

The results of this study are not different from our pilot study (6). In this selective group of patients the initial sensitivity for metastatic disease is the same for the markers CA 15-3 and TPS with somewhat lower sensitivity of CEA (table I). The fast reaction of TPS after the start of therapy is confirmed in this study (table II). A multicenter study is being analyzed now to confirm these data. It is impossible within the context of this study to describe all kind of tumor marker patterns seen during hormonal or chemotherapy in metastasized breast cancer patients. However, an utmost important observation is the large number of patients with clinically stable disease according to UICC criteria after three months and still after six months. This problem is related to the criterion of a 50% reduction in size before partial remission is considered to be present. The combined use of CA 15-3 and TPS has a high sensitivity to detect metatatic disease and therefore could be a better parameter to indicate the effect of therapy. Figures 1 and 2 demonstrate the early decrease of tumor marker levels after the start of therapy in

Table I. Sensitivity of the tumor markers[a] CA 15-3, CEA and TPS in 88 patients with 140 episodes of progressive disease (PD) at the start of the study.

Marker	No. of elevated levels	Percentage
CA 15-3	108	77
CEA	97	69
TPS	113	81

[a]Cut-off CA 15-3: 30 kU/l; CEA: 5 µg/l and TPS: 75 U/l.

Table II. Sensitivity of increase ($\geq$ 25%) and decrease ($\geq$ 50%) after the first measuring interval correlated with UICC criteria at month 3.

Marker	No. of correlated changes	Percentage
CA 15-3	43	40
CEA	41	42
TPS	85	75

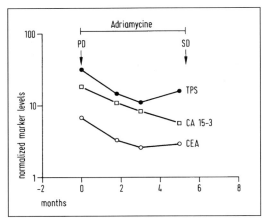
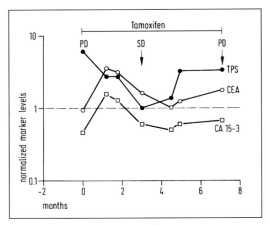

Figure 1. Normalized marker levels (marker levels divided by respective cut-off) in patient 1 during treatment of bone metastases who was in stable disease six months after the start of chemotherapy. PD = progressive disease and SD = stable disease.

Figure 2. Normalized marker levels (marker levels divided by respective cut-off) in patient 2 during treatment of bone metastases and malignant pleural effusion, who was in stable disease for three months, but demonstrated progressive disease at months 7 after the initiation of hormonal therapy. PD = progressive disease and SD = stable disease.

patients which are clinically considered to have stable disease. Figure 1 shows also an increase of TPS (and also of CEA to some extent) at the end of the study where clinically still stable disease is present. In our experience increasing marker values indicate progressive disease sooner than clinical findings (figure 2).

We conclude that SD is an insensitive 'golden standard' in breast cancer patients with bone metastases. Unless another clinical 'golden standard' will be developed, the reliability of tumor marker changes might be difficult to prove and consequently these changes will be attacked by invalid arguments.

References

1 Eckhardt S (1990) Diagnosis, staging and principles of management. In: Hossfeld DK, Sherman CD, Love RR, Bosch FX (eds) Springer, Berlin, pp 90–107

2 Safi F, Kohler I, Rottinger E and Berg HG (1991) The value of tumor marker CA 15-3 in diagnosing and monitoring breast cancer. A comparative study with carcinoembryonic antigen. Cancer 68:574–582

3 Dalen A van (1989) Tumour markers in breast cancer. Ann Chir Gynaecol 78: 54–64

4 Gion M (1992) Serum markers in breast cancer management. Breast 1:173–178

5 Bonfrer JMG (1990) Working group on tumor marker criteria (WGMTC). Tumor Biol 11:287–288

6 Dalen A van, Linde DL van der, Heering KJ, Blusse van OudAlblas A (1993) How can treatment response be measured in breast cancer patients? Anticancer Res 13:1901–1904

Address for corespondence:
Dr. A. van Dalen
Department of Nuclear Medicine
Bleuland Hospital
P.O. Box 1098
NL-2800 Gouda, The Netherlands

Is there still a relevance for measuring CEA during follow-up in breast cancer patients?

S. Krämer, G. Reinhardt, W. Jäger

Department of Obstetrics and Gynecology, University of Erlangen-Nuremberg, Germany

Introduction

Chest x-ray, liver ultrasound and bone scintigraphy are the established methods for detection of distant metastases in breast cancer patients. When the carcinoembryonic antigen (CEA) was first described and assays for serum measurements became available it was soon detected that about 60% of patients with metastatic breast cancer had elevated levels of this tumor associated antigen (1). However, it was noted, that elevated CEA levels could also be observed in some other circumstances which were not related to metastatic breast cancer. In this connection elevated CEA serum levels in patients with rheumatic diseases and heavy smokers are the most cited examples. The reasons for this elevation are still not fully explained today. When during the early 80ies the mucins were described as a group of proteins for following the course of breast cancer patients, it was found that one of these – CA 15-3 – was quiet a specific marker for the detection and follow-up of metastases in breast cancer patients. This specificity of CA 15-3 led to the discussion if there is still a relevance for measuring CEA for detection of metastases in breast cancer patients (2, 3).

Material and method

After primary surgery patients were submitted to our follow-up program. During the first two years after primary surgery the clinical examinations are usually repeated in three month intervals, thereafter in six month intervals. During those examinations, always a serum sample for tumor marker measurements was taken. The indications for screening examinations (chest x-ray, liver ultrasound and bone scintigraphy) were handled differently during these years. Between 1985 and 1990 screening examinations were performed in routinely defined time intervals, whereas after 1990 screening examinations were not routinely performed anymore, but only when CEA and/or CA 15-3 increased or the patient complained about symptoms (4). The critical concentrations of CEA and CA 15-3 were defined as the 97th percentile of marker concentrations in breast cancer patients who were without metastases during a period of at least two years after primary surgery. The corresponding levels for CEA were 6 µg/l and for CA 15-3 40 kU/l. When these levels were exceeded a screening examination was initiated. All tumor marker measurements were performed in duplicates. The intra- and interassay coefficients of variation were < 10%. The analysis which was based on the data of those patients was called »retrospective study«. These data were clearly separated from another study which we called the »prospective study«. In this study which we started in May 1986, tumor marker measurements were performed every month in a selective group of patients (5). If during follow-up CEA and/or CA 15-3 levels increased above the defined concentrations, patients were screened for metastases. Metastases were classified according to the first detected site of metastases. If within a time interval of three months other metastases at another site were detected the localisation was termed "multiple sites".

Results

During the time interval from August 1985 to May 1992 315 breast cancer patients developed distant metastases of their disease. The distribution

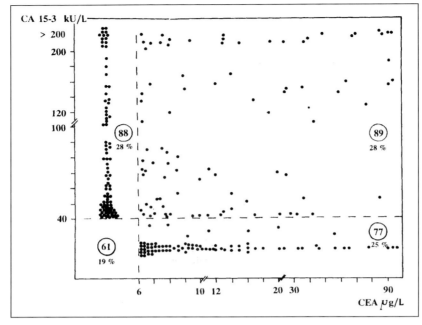

Figure 1. Distribution of CEA and CA 15-3 serum concentrations in 315 breast cancer patients at the time of diagnosis of metastases. The horizontal line shows the upper level of normal for CA 15-3 (40 kU/l), the vertical line shows the upper level of normal for CEA (6 µg/l).

of metastases according to the first site diagnosed in the "retrospective study" was as follows: bone 129 (41%), lung 76 (24%), liver 26 (8%), multiple sites 34 (11%), skin 45 (14%), brain 5 (2%). The concentrations of CEA and CA 15-3 at the time of detection of these metastases are shown in figure 1. In 61 (19%) patients metastases were detected without a tumor marker increase ("false negative"). In 166 (53%) patients CEA was elevated, and in 177 (56%) patients CA 15-3 was elevated. Only CEA was elevated in 77 (25%) patients, whereas only CA 15-3 was elevated in 88 (28%) patients. Both markers were elevated in 89 (28%) patients. In the "prospective study", where monthly measurements of CEA and CA 15-3 were performed, 61 patients developed metastases. The distribution of the sites of metastases in those 61 patients was as follows: bone 29 (48%), lung 15 (24%), liver 6 (10%), multiple sites 6 (10%), skin 3 (5%), brain 2 (3%). In 13 (21%) patients metastases were diagnosed without a tumor marker increase (»false negative«), while in 48 (79%) patients increasing tumor markers were observed before diagnosis of metastases. In 24 (40%) patients CEA was elevated at the time of diagnosis of metastases, while in 22 (36%) patients CA 15-3 was the elevated marker. The combined increase of both markers, however, was only observed in two (3%) patients.

Discussion

Previous studies gave evidence that an increase of CEA and/or CA 15-3 serum levels in breast cancer patients during follow-up could be an indicator for the development of distant metastases. Furthermore several investigations have shown that tumor markers can increase several months before the detectability of metastases (6). Since CA 15-3 exhibited a high sensitivity for detetion of metastatic breast cancer, it was discussed during recent years if the additional measurement of CEA would make sense (3).

According to the results of our study we still support the measurement of both markers. If only CA 15-3 measurements would have been performed during the follow-up of breast cancer patients according to our "retrospective study", metastases would have been suspected and detected in only 56% of patients, if only CEA would have been measured in only 53% of patients. It must be assumed that the percentage of patients with an elevated single marker would increase during longer observation time since most of the patients who developed an increase of e. g. CEA sooner or later also developed an increase of CA 15-3 and vice versa. However, our study showed that the combined measurement of both markers would led to the detection of metastases in up to 81% of all patients with distant metastases. Therefore the additional benefit of measuring the other marker for early detection of distant metastases is about 25%.

These results are on one side strengthened, on the other side diminished by the results of our "prospective study". In agreement with our "retrospective study", 79% of the breast cancer patients with distant metastases in the "prospective study" had already elevated tumor markers at the time of diagnosis of metastases. In other words also in the »prospective study« only 21% of all patients with distant metastases were detected without a tumor marker increase. In disagreement to the »retrospective study« the combined increase of both markers was a seldom event in the »prospective study«. In the »prospective study«, using monthly intervals of tumor marker measurements, more than 75% of the patients had an increase of one single marker. Again it was found that neither CEA nor CA 15-3 were absolutely dominant in the early detection of metastases, but 40% of patients developed an increase of CEA and 36% an increase of CA 15-3. In our opinion this difference between the studies was caused by the different time intervals in serum sampling, and it was shown that reliable clinical data can only be obtained from our »prospective study«.

These studies clearly show that CEA measurements have exactly the same relevance as CA 15-3 measurements during follow-up of breast cancer patients.

References

1. Lamerz R, Leonhardt A, Ehrhart H, v Lieven H (1980) Serial carcinoembryonic antigen (CEA) determinations in the management of metastatic breast cancer. Oncodevelop Biol Med 1:123–135
2. Krebs BP, Pons-Anicet D, Namer M (1987) CA 15-3 in breast cancer: A more specific and sensitive marker than carcinoembryonic antigen (CEA). In: Klapdor R (ed) New tumor markers and their monoclonal antibodies. Thieme, Stuttgart, pp 60–64
3. van Dalen A, Dupree HW, Heering KJ, v d Linde DL (1987) The determination of CA 15-3 during therapy monitoring of breast cancer patients. In: Klapdor R (ed) New tumor markers and their monoclonal antibodies. Thieme, Stuttgart, pp 105–112
4. Jäger W, Merkle E, Tulusan AH, Lang N (1991) Modifizierte Mammakarzinom-Nachsorge. Gynäkol Rundsch 31 (Suppl 2):296–299
5. Jäger W (1993) The early detection of disseminated (metastasized) breast cancer by serial tumor marker measurements. Europ J Cancer Prevent 2 (Suppl 3):133–139
6. Colomer R, Ruibal A, Salvador L (1989) Circulating tumor marker levels in advanced breast carcinoma correlate with the extent of metastatic disease. Cancer 64:1674–1681

Address for correspondence:
Dr. med. W. Jäger
Universitätsfrauenklinik
Universitätsstraße 21-23
D-91054 Erlangen, Germany

Cerebrospinal fluid TPA and CK-BB in comparison with cytology in diagnosing central nervous system metastases secondary to breast cancer

F. Bach[a], G. Söletormos[a,b], B. Bjerregaard[c], F. W. Bach[d], Th. Horn[c]

[a]Department of Oncology, [b]Clinical Chemistry and [c]Pathology, Herlev Hospital,
[d]Department of Clinical Chemistry, Gentofte Hospital, University of Copenhagen, Denmark

Introduction

In recent years, metastatic spread to the central nervous system (CNS) from breast cancer has been reported with increasing frequency, and autopsy studies have recorded metastatic spread to the CNS in approximately 35% of the patients. Only half of patients with meningeal carcinomatosis (MC) are diagnosed in vivo, and in 10% of the patients CNS symptoms may be the first manifestation of the disease or recurrence.

The diagnosis of MC is usually based on cerebrospinal fluid (CSF) cytology, however, no tumor cells are shown in nearly 30% of the patients by the initial lumbar puncture. Although the prognosis for patients with MC in general is poor, some carefully selected groups of patients seem to benefit from intra-cerebroventricular (ICV) cytostatic treatment. Using CSF from ICV reservoirs as assessment of response to treatment of MC, a large number of the CSF samples are categorized as "suspicious for malignancy", with a considerable degree of interobserver variability making monitoring of treatment difficult.

Three questions seemed apparent: 1. cytologic interobserver variability in the CSF from lumbar and ICV samples, 2. the presence of meningeal involvement despite a negative CSF cytology, 3. the significance of malignant cells in the CSF during treatment of MC from ICV reservoirs.

Patients and methods

Between June 1985 and January 1992, consecutive breast cancer patients suspected for CNS metastases were subjected to lumbar puncture. Cerebrospinal fluid was immediately analyzed for cell counts, and evaluated cytologically after cytocentrifugation. Simultaneously, samples for tumor marker investigation were collected, frozen and kept at –70° C until analysis. Based on the clinical course, neurological signs, CT-scans, cytology and autopsy findings, the patients were divided into two groups, with or without metastatic spread to the CNS.

Seventy-one patients included in the study had CSF tapped by lumbar puncture. Forty-three patients had no metastatic spread to the CNS. Twelve patients had brain metastases, five had both brain metastases and MC, and eleven patients had MC only. Seven of the patients with MC alone had an ICV reservoir inserted and received subsequent intrathecal treatment. From these seven patients additional 70 samples were obtained (table I).

Two senior pathologists reviewed the CSF samples retrospectively. The evaluation was performed blindly. Due to the clinical situation, in which especially ICV samples frequently are categorized as "suspicious for malignancy", the samples were classified as 1. with malignant cells, 2. suspicious cells or, 3. without malignant cells. In the clinical situation, however, a CSF sample classified as "suspicious for malignancy" is of limited value since it is important to determine simply whether a specimen is malignant or not. Subsequently, the observers were required to re-evaluate the

Table I. Distribution of CSF samples from 71 breast-cancer patients.

Absence of CNS metastases	43 patients
Parenchymal brain metastases	12 patients
Leptomeningeal carcinomatosis	16 patients
Total no. of lumbar punctures: 71	71 patients
Total no. of ICV punctures: 70	7 patients

samples categorized as "suspicious for malignancy" as either malignant or non-malignant.

Results and discussion

Interobserver variability of the 71 CSF samples from lumbar puncture showed a Kappa test value at 0.81. Eight specimens demonstrated suspicious cells by the primary cytologic evaluation. Subsequent reclassification of these "suspicious" eight samples into the groups containing malignant (three samples) or non-malignant cells (five samples) resulted in complete agreement between the two observers with no interobserver variability at all (Kappa test value, 1.0).
The evaluation of the CSF samples from ICV reservoirs demonstrated a large disagreement between the two observers. Among the 70 ICV samples, 36 (51%) were categorized as "suspicious for malignancy," 28 by observer no. 1 and 25 by observer no. 2. Subsequent reclassification of the 36 "suspicious" samples into malignant or non-malignant revealed a Kappa test value at 0.60. Focusing on the 36 "suspicious" ICV samples alone, both of the observers reclassified 13 samples as malignant and ten as non-malignant. In the remaining 13 samples, the observers contradicted each other (six versus seven samples were classified as malignant/non-malignant and vice versa) resulting in a Kappa test value as limited as 0.28. In 101 CSF specimens, both TPA and CK-BB values were determined. The samples originated from 35 patients without CNS metastases, 15 patients with parenchymal brain metastases and 11 patients with MC (seven patients with MC only and four patients with MC and parenchymal brain metastases).
Sixty-one samples were obtained with lumbar puncture and 40 samples by ICV reservoirs. TPA was elevated in 19 out of 26 patients with CNS metastases (73%) (median TPA value in patients with CNS metastases 500 U/l; without CNS metastases 2 U/l), and CK-BB was elevated in 17 out of 26 (65%) (median CK-BB value in patients with CNS metastases 0.42 U/l; without CNS metastases 0.12 U/l). These differences between patients with and without CNS metastases are significantly different, both according to TPA ($p < 0.00001$) and CK-BB ($p < 0.00003$) (Mann-Whitney test).
The correlated values of TPA and CK-BB from lumbar punctures are demonstrated in figure 1. Patients with parenchymal brain metastases and especially MC had raised activities of TPA and CK-BB, however, one patient with MC and three patients with brain metastases had both TPA and CK-BB activities below the cut-off values. The findings are significant ($p < 0.0001$) with a coefficient of correlation at 0.49 (Spearmans-Rho). Cut-off values employed; TPA 95 U/l, CK-BB 0.2 U/l.
Evaluating CSF activities of TPA and CK-BB when categorizing raised values of either TPA or CK-BB or both TPA and CK-BB as indicating malignancy, the sensitivity was 85% (95% confidence limits, 65% – 96%) and the predictive value of a negative test 90% (95% confidence limits, 76% – 97%) for having any CNS metastases. The specificity and the predictive value of a positive test was 100%. These combined findings (raised value of either TPA or CK-BB or both) are superior to the diagnostic abilities of either of the markers alone (TPA: sensitivity 73% (19/26), negative predictive value 83% (35/42) (CK-BB: sensitivity 65% (17/26), the negative predictive value 80% (35/44) (table II).

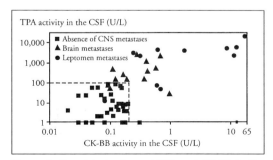

Figure 1. Correlated values of TPA and CK-BB in the CSF from lumbar puncture in 61 breast-cancer patients. Spearmans-Rho 0.49, p < 0.0001. Cut-off values employed: TPA 95 U/l, CK-BB 0.2 U/l.

Table II. Sensivity, specificity and predictive values of TPA and CK-BB in the CSF from lumbar punctures in 61 breast-cancer patients.

Test res./ diagn.	CNS metastases	No CNS true metastases
Positve test	22	0
Negative test	4	35

Sensitivity 22/26: 85%; specificity: 35/35 100; positive predictive value 22/22: 100%; negative predictive value 35/39: 90%

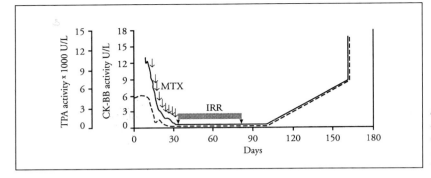

Figure 2. TPA and CK-BB activities in the CSF during treatment of meningeal carcinomastosis in breast cancer.

For what use is it?

I would like to demonstrate one case. Figure 2 shows the activities of TPA and CK-BB in the CSF during treatment of MC in female, age 37, who developed neurologic symptoms and underwent CT-scans of the brain and lumbar puncture. The scans gave no evidence of parenchymal brain metastases, whereas CSF contained tumor cells in the third lumbar puncture (TPA 5140 U/l, CK-BB 12.3 U/l (solid graph)). At day 15 following the first lumbar puncture the patient had a ICV reservoir inserted and began intrathecal treatment. Because of progressive neurologic symptoms and persistence of tumor cells in the CSF, the patient received whole-brain irradiation between day 32 and 83 including the entire neuraxis, with good response, nearly full relief of neurologic symptoms and disappearance of tumor cells (TPA 6 U/l, CK-BB 0.4 U/l). Subsequently the tumor cells recurred, the patient's general physical condition deteriorated and she died on day 178 (TPA 13730 U/l, CK-BB 16.9 U/l). Autopsy including the central nervous system demonstrated extented MC, but no parenchymal brain metastases was found just as the autopsy confirmed the absence of extracerebral malignant disease.

The diagnosis of MC may be difficult, and no single technique can exclude the diagnosis. In the search for better diagnostic methods, various biomarkers, among those TPA and CK-BB, have been determined. The finding of tumor cells in the CSF is generally considered diagnostic for MC, a routine the present study seems to support according to lumbar puncture. However, a breast cancer patient with non-malignant CSF cytology but raised activities of TPA and CK-BB needs further diagnostic considerations and repeated CSF examination.

Conclusion

Cytological evaluation of CSF obtained by lumbar puncture is a reliable procedure. In contrast, assessment of possible tumor cells in the CSF obtained by ICV reservoirs is of limited use. A large number of the cells are classified as "suspicious for malignancy" and the interobserver variability is significant. Tumor marker measurements (TPA and CK-BB) may be a very important supplement to cerebro-spinal fluid cytology.

Address for correspondence:
F. Bach, M.D.
Department of Oncology
Herlev Hospital
University of Copenhagen
Ringvej 75
DK-2730 Herlev, Denmark

In vitro analysis of CA 125 production and release by ovarian cancer cells

E. Beck[a], A. Moldenhauer[a], F. Kiesewetter[b], W. Jäger[a], L. Wildt[a], N. Lang[a]
[a]Department of Obstetrics and Gynecology, [b]Department of Dermatology,
University of Erlangen-Nuremberg, Germany

Introduction

The glycoprotein CA 125 is an antigenic determinant that is recognized by a monoclonal antibody (OC 125) which was raised against an established human ovarian cancer cell line (1). This antigen is expressed in more than 80% of all epithelial ovarian carcinomas (1, 2) and has been shown in a number of clinical trials to be a reliable marker during the follow-up of ovarian cancer patients (3, 4, 5).
According to clinical experience, rising CA 125 serum levels are always associated with a recurrence or a progression of the disease. In a recent in vitro study we found evidence, that the release of CA 125 into the culture supernatant by an ovarian cancer cell line could be associated with cell proliferation (6). We therefore assumed that CA 125 could be a marker for cell proliferation of ovarian cancer cells.
We now report on the release of CA 125 into the culture supernatant and the intracellular CA 125 concentrations of NIH:OVCAR 3 cells during exponential growth and during inhibition of cell proliferation by colchicine and cycloheximide.

Material and methods

Colchicine and Cycloheximide were obtained from Sigma Chemie (Deisenhofen, Germany), RPMI 1640 Medium, Trypsin/EDTA and bovine Insulin from Gibco BRL (Eggenstein, Germany), basal medium supplement (BMS) was purchased from Biochrom GmbH (Berlin, Germany). NIH:OVCAR cells were obtained from American Type Culture Collection (Rockville, USA).
Determination of CA 125 was performed with the ELSA CA 125 assay (ID CIS, Dreieich, Germany).

The intra-assay coefficient of variation was always less than 10%; the interassay coefficient of variation was in the range of 7.6 and 9.7%.
Cells were cultured in RPMI 1640 Medium, supplemented with 10% BMS, 2 mM glutamine, and 10 µg/ml bovine insulin and were passaged at weekly intervals according to standard laboratory procedures after detaching the cells with trypsin/EDTA.
For the experiments cells were plated in 24 well mikrotiterplates (Becton Dickinson, Heidelberg, Germany) at a density of 50,000 cells per well in 1 ml of complete medium and cultured for 48 h in a humidified atmosphere of 5% CO_2 at 37° C. Thereafter the culture medium was changed.
At each time point, the cells and culture supernatants of three wells were harvested. After removal of the supernatant, the cells were rinsed twice with plain RPMI 1640 medium and then they were detached completely with 200 µl of 0.05% trypsin, 0.02% EDTA (10 minutes, 37° C). Then 100 µl of complete culture medium were added in order to inactivate the trypsin, and a single cell suspension was generated by syringing the cells gently through a 26 gauge needle for at least 10 times. Finally the cells were counted in a hemocytometer applying the dye exclusion method with trypan blue. The cells of each well were counted three times in three different hemocytometers.
After the first 48 hours, the culture medium was changed every 24 hours in order to establish an exponential cell growth. Cells and culture supernatants were collected every 24 hours as described above. The culture supernatants of respective triplicates of wells were pooled and stored at −20° C until determination of the CA 125 was performed. Beginning 72 hours after the initiation of the exponential growth phase, the cells were treated

with either colchicine or cycloheximide (20 µg/ml in complete culture medium, respectively) or were continously cultured as described above. This treatment period lasted for a total of five days, during which the media were also changed every 24 hours.

For the determination of the intracellular CA 125 content cells were seeded at a density of $5 \cdot 10^5$ cells/ml in 250 ml cell culture flasks (Becton Dickinson, Heidelberg), and were incubated at 37° C in a humidified atmosphere of 5% CO_2 until the cell layers were almost 50% confluent. Then the medium was changed and the cells were cultured according to the methods described above, changing the medium every 24 hours, and adding cycloheximide and colchicine at the appropriate time points.

Cells and culture supernatants were harvested every 24 hours as already described. After detaching the cells completely (600 µl of 0.05% trypsin, 0.02% EDTA, 10 min, 37° C, 300 µl of complete medium to inactivate the trypsin) and counting an aliquot of the cell suspension in a hemocytometer, the cells were osmotically lysed by adding 1ml of destilled water and freezing this suspension immediately at −20° C in order to release the intracellular CA 125. Cell lysates and culture supernatants were stored at −20° C until the determination of the CA 125 was carried out.

For the estimation of the intracellular CA 125 concentrations, the cell lysates were thawed and the completeness of the cell destruction was checked by dye exclusion with trypan blue. Cell debris was removed by centrifugation (1000 x g, 10 min, 20 °C), and the resulting supernatant was measured with the ELSA CA 125 assay.

Results

Cell proliferation

Cell kinetics are shown in figure 1. Cell counts of untreated cells increased during the experimental period between days 5 and 10 steadily from 66.9 ± 1.8 · 10^3 cells/ml to 239.0 ± 30.9 · 10^3 cells/ml. Colchicine treated cells showed an increase in cell counts from 66.9 ± 4.4 · 10^3 cells/ml on day 5 to 84.9 ± 6.5 · 10^3 cells/ml on day 6, followed by a steep decrease in cell counts to 36.3 ± 2.7 · 10^3 cells/ml on day 7. Subsequentlcell counts increased again (68.1 ± 8.5 · 10^3 cells/ml on day 8) but finally decreased, reaching cell counts as low as 32.7 ± 5.6 · 10^3 cells/ml on day 10.

Cycloheximide treatment of the cells also lead to an increase in cell numbers between days 5 (60.0 ± 4.9 · 10^3 cells/ml) and 6 (84.3 ± 7.9 · 10^3 cells/ml), which was followed by a constant decrease in cell counts with a minimum of 41.9 ± 4.5 · 10^3 cells/ml on day 10.

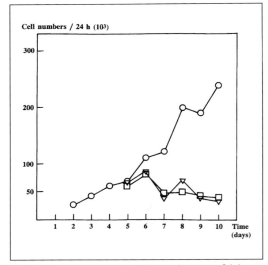

Figure 1. Cell kinetics: The cell-numbers per 24 hours are plotted versus time (○ untreated cells, ▽ colchicine treated cells, □ cycloheximide treated cells).

CA 125 release into the culture supernatant

The concentrations of CA 125 released during 24 hours by exponentially growing, colchicine and cycloheximide treated cells are shown in figure 2. The amount of CA 125 released into the culture supernatant by untreated NIH:OVCAR 3 cells increased from 34 U/ml on day 5 to 142m U/ml on day 10.

The CA 125 concentrations released by colchicine treated cells increased from 22.5 U/ml on day 5 to 68 U/ml on day 7, but thereafter a constant decrease in CA 125 release was noted, with only 17 U/ml beeing released on day 10.

Treatment with cycloheximide resulted in a constant decline of CA 125 release from 40 U/ml on day 5 to as low as 0.5 U/ml on day 10.

However, when we normalized the CA 125 concentrations realeased into the culture supernatant per single cell we found that untreated cells released almost constant amounts of CA 125 (range 4.7 ± 2.5 to $7.2 \pm 6.3 \cdot 10^{-4}$ U/cell) throughout the experiment (figure 3).

In contrast to these results obtained with exponentially growing cells, colchicine treatment lead to CA 125 concentrations released by a single cell in the range of 3.9 ± 0.6 and $25.0 \pm 3.7 \cdot 10^{-4}$ U per cell. However, the latter exceedingly high CA 125 concentration was measured during the phase of rapid cell destruction on day 7.

Those cells treated with cycloheximide showed a constant decrease in CA 125 release, which declined from $9.6 \pm 2.0 \cdot 10^{-4}$ U/cell on day 5 to $0.06 \pm 0.03 \cdot 10^{-4}$ U/cell on day 10.

Intracellular CA 125 concentrations

Concerning the intracellular concentrations of CA 125 that could be released from intact cells by osmotic cell lysis, we found that untreated cells contained between 3.1 ± 0.4 and $5.0 \pm 0.3 \cdot 10^{-4}$ U/cell. These values were alomost stable throughout the experimental period (figure 4). Colchicine treated cells contained between 2.8 ± 0.2 and $4.9 \pm 0.3 \cdot 10^{-4}$ U CA 125 per cell. Statistical analysis (Mann and Whitney test) showed that there was no difference in intracellular CA 125 content of untreated and colchicine treated cells.

Cycloheximide treatment of the cells resulted in a constant decline in intracellular CA 125 concentrations from $4.3 \pm 3.1 \cdot 10^{-4}$ U/cell on day 4 to $1.9 \pm 0.6 \cdot 10^{-4}$ U/cell on day 6, however, with a slight increase of values towards the end of the experiment ($3.4 \pm 2.3 \cdot 10^{-4}$ U/cell on day 7).

Discussion

The clinical value of serial CA 125 measurements for monitoring the treatment of ovarian cancer patients has been well established (1, 7). According to several authors, in more than 80% of ovarian cancer patients the preoperative CA 125 levels are elevated (8, 9). *Kenemans* et a.l (9) reviewing the literature found, that pretreatment levels of CA 125 were correlated to the tumor stage. According to these authors, only 41% of patients with stage I disease had CA 125 serum levels above the cut-off level of 35 U/ml whereas 93% and 97% of patients with stage III and IV disease respectively showed elevated CA 125 levels. Moreover it has been demonstrated that CA 125 serum levels correlate well with regression or progression of the disease (10, 11, 12). As reviewed in (9) almost all patients with CA 125 levels above 35 U/ml prior to second look laparotomy where found to have residual tumor. However, only 50% of patients with CA 125 levels within the normal range where free of tumor at the time of second look procedures.

With the data presented here we could clearly demonstrate, that the CA 125 levels released into the culture supernatant by exponentially growing NIH:OVCAR 3 cells increased almost in parallel to the increasing cell numbers. However, when the extra- and the intracellular CA 125 concentrations were standardized per single cell, almost constant levels of CA 125 were found throughout the experimental period.

Blockade of mitotic activity by colchicine lead to largely elevated levels of CA 125 released into the culture medium. This finding was also reflected by the CA 125 concentrations released per single cell. However, this rather temporary effect was correlated with a phase of rapid cell destruction which may have lead to large amounts of CA 125 released by dying cells, and consequently may have biased our calculations performed on the basis of intact cells. This assumption was supported by the fact, that no significant differences in intracellular CA 125 concentrations between exponentially growing cells and colchicine treated cells were found.

Although cell counts were constantly decreasing after the onset of the cycloheximide treatment, still a considerable number of viable cells were found after a treatment period of five days. During this treatment period cells released constantly decreasing amounts of CA 125 into the culture supernatant. This finding was also paralleled by decreasing intracellular CA 125 concentrations.

Conclusions

We would suggest, that according to our results, rising or elevated CA 125 (serum) levels rather reflect the total cell mass and are less likely related to cell proliferation. This seems to be well in accordance with the results of many clinical trials.

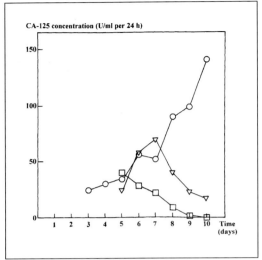

Figure 2. CA 125 concentrations released into the culture supernatant by untreated (○), colchicine (▽) and cycloheximide (□) treated cells per 24 hours.

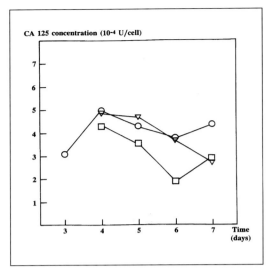

Figure 4. Intracellular CA 125 content per single cell (○ untreated cells, ▽ colchicine treated cells, □ cycloheximide treated cells).

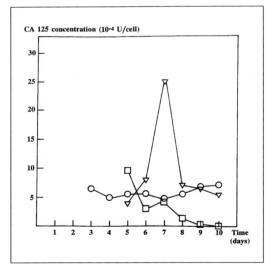

Figure 3. CA 125 concentrations released per single cell in 24 hours into the culture supernatant (○ untreated cells, ▽ colchicine treated cells, □ cycloheximide treated cells).

However, this hypothesis in our view needs to be investigated further including cell cycle analysis.
As most of the clinical trials comparing CA 125 levels prior to second look laparotomies and the clinical outcome in terms of residual tumor were performed immediately after cytotoxic chemotherapy, one could speculate on the basis of our results obtained with cycloheximide, that the false negative results obtained in about 50% of patients are due to an impaired protein synthesis by the tumor cells following chemotherapy.

References

1. Bast RC, Feeney M, Lazarus H, Nadler LM, Colvin NB, Knapp RC (1981) Reactivity of a monoclonal antibody with human ovarian carcinoma. J Clin Invest 68:1331–1337
2. Kabawat SE, Bast RC Jr, Welch WR, Covin NB (1983) Immunopathologic characterization of a monoclonal antibody that recognizes common surface antigens on human ovarian tumors of serous, endometrial and clear cell type. Am J Clin Pathol 79:98–104
3. Bast RC Jr, Knapp RC (1985) Monitoring epithelial ovarian cancer. Lab Med 16:315–318
4. Petru E, Sevin BU, Averette HE, Koechli OR, Perras JP, Hilsenbeck S (1990) Comparison ot three tumor markers: CA 125, lipid-asscociated sialic acid (LSA), and NB/70 K in monitoring ovarian cancer. Gynecol Oncol 38:181–186
5. Zurawski VR Jr, Orjaseter H, Andersen A, Jellum E (1988) Elevated serum CA 125 levels prior to diagnosis of ovarian neoplasia: Relevance for early detection of ovarian cancer. Int J Cancer 42:677–680

6. Beck E, Hofmann M, Kiesewetter F, Jäger W, Wildt L, Lang N (1992) Analysis of CA 125 release by ovarian cancer cells in vitro. In: Klapdor R (ed) Tumor associated antigens, oncogenes, receptors, cytokines in tumor diagnosis and therapy at the beginning of the nineties. Zuckschwerdt, München Bern Wien San Franzisco, pp117–121
7. Klug TL, Bast RC, Niloff JM, Knapp RC, Zurawski VK (1984) A monoclonal antibody immunoradiometric assay for an antigenic determinant (CA 125) associated with human epithelial ovarian cancer. Cancer Res 44:1048–1053
8. Crombach G, Zipell H, Würz H (1985) Erfahrungen mit CA 125, einem Tumormarker für maligne epitheliale Ovarialtumoren. Geburtsh Frauenheilk 45: 205–212
9. Kenemans P, Yedema CA, Bon GG, van Mensdorff-Pouilly S (1993) CA 125 in gynecological pathology – a review. Eur J Obstet Gynecol Reprod Biol 49: 115–124
10. Sevelda P, Salzer H, Dittrich Ch, Spona J (1985) Die klinische Bedeutung des Tumormarkers CA 125 für die präoperative Diagnostik und die postoperative Nachbetreuung von Patientinnen mit malignen Ovarialtumoren. Geburtsh Frauenheilk 45:769–773
11. Krebs HB, Goplerud DR, Kilpatrick SJ, Myers MB, Hunt A (1986) Role of CA 125 as tumor marker in ovarian carcinoma. Obstet Gynecol 67:473–477
12. Alvarez RD, To A, Boots LR, Shingleton HM, Hatch KD, Hubbard J, Soong SJ, Potter ME (1987) CA 125 as a serum marker for poor diagnosis in ovarian malignancies. Gynecol Oncol 26:284–289

Address for correspondence:
Dr. med. E. P. Beck
Universitätsfrauenklinik
Universitätsstraße 21-23
D-91054 Erlangen, Germany

Detection of the tumor-associated antigens CA 125, TPS, CA 72-4 and CASA in the supernatant of 25 human ovarian cancer cell lines

V. J. Möbus, D. G. Kieback, H.-J. Grill, R. Kreienberg
Department of Obstetrics and Gynecology, University of Ulm, Germany

Introduction

CA 125 is the most important marker for diagnosis and especially follow-up of ovarian cancer patients (1, 2). The marker is most sensitive in serous and undifferentiated carcinoma, but fails in endometrioid and mucinous carcinoma. A close correlation exists between the clinical course of the disease and the course of CA 125 levels. Nevertheless, the search for new tumor markers which supplement CA 125 in monitoring ovarian cancer is of clinical interest. New marker systems like TPS, CA 72-4 and CASA (3) have been introduced into clinical practice. The usefullness of these markers, especially in CA 125 negative patients, remains to be determined. It has been suggested that TPS correlates with tumor activity and not with tumor mass. The use of permanent ovarian cancer cell lines is a suitable method to clarify these questions.

Material and methods

Tumor marker levels were determined in 25 permanent human ovarian cancer cell lines, that were established in our own laboratory. 19 cell lines were derived from serous cystadenocarcinoma, two from undifferentiated carcinoma, one from clear cell carcinoma and one from a carcinosarcoma. Two cell lines were established from the ascites of patients with clinical suspicion of ovarian cancer that did not undergo exploratory surgery. Secreting pattern of the tumor markers, histology of xenotransplantation in nude mice and analysis of intermediate filament proteins by immunocytochemistry clearly demonstrate their origin from ovarian cancer.

The secretion of the tumor associated antigens in the supernatant was determined in proliferating and resting cells. The supernatant of exponentially growing cell cultures was collected on days 4, 6 and 8 and the cells were counted. Resting cells were defined as cell cultures which had reached confluence for at least one week. After a cell count the medium of resting cells was renewed and the supernatant collected after three days. The supernatant was spun at 1000 g for 10 min and stored at $-20\,°C$ until tested. The CA 125 levels in the supernatant were determined by a solid-phase RIA (CIS, Dreieich, Germany), the TPS levels by an immunoradiometric solid phase assay (Biermann Diagnostica, Bad Nauheim, Germany), the CASA (medac Diagnostica, Hamburg, Germany) and the CA72-4 (Boehringer Mannheim, Germany) levels were determined by an ELISA assay.

Results

The results of CA 125 analysis in the culture supernatant are shown in table I: 18 of 25 ovarian cancer cell lines were positive for the secretion of CA 125, seven lines were negative. Intra-individually the relative secretion of this tumor associated antigen is very stable with a maximum variability of a factor of 3.13. Marked variability was observed in CA 125 positive cell lines: CA 125 secretion of proliferating cells varied from 0.65 to 986 U/ml/$1 \cdot 10^6$ cells. In resting cells the secretion varied between 8.1 to 3281 U/ml/$1 \cdot 10^6$ cells. The secreted amounts differ up to a factor of 1509 between cell lines. The ratio of the increase in cell number to the increase of CA 125 concentration on the other hand was very stable: The highest

Table I. Secretion rate of CA 125 in U/ml/day/1·10⁶ cells for proliferating and quiescent cells and ratio of increase in cell number and increase in CA 125 concentration in the supernatant.

Cell line	CA 125 secretion rate (U/ml/day/1·10⁶ cells)				Increase of cell number/ increase of CA 125
	proliferating cells			quiescent cell	
	day 4	6	8	day 3	day 4–8
OV-MZ-la	24.20	50.60	23.30	n. e.	0.57
OV-MZ-lb	5.40	3.00	5.40	25.30	0.55
OV-MZ-lc	24.40	15.10	13.60	245.30	1.00
OV-MZ-2	4.20	0.90	0.23a	0.16	n. a.
OV-MZ-3	13.00	13.60	7.00	352.00	1.81
OV-MZ-4	2.20	0.50	0.20a	0.90	n.a.
OV-MZ-5	4.10	1.90	0.70a	10.4	n. a.
OV-MZ-6	1.70	0.65	1.10	8.45	2.1
OV-MZ-7b	3.18	3.90	5.00	13.00	0.71
OV-MZ-8	161.00	75.00	134.00	3281.00	1.23
OV-MZ-10	3.71	1.36	4.26	38.6	0.63
OV-MZ-11	92.80	122.40	51.00	n. e.	1.01
OV-MZ-12	5.00	1.20	0.95a	0.27	n. a.
OV-MZ-13	13.70	18.40	24.00	58.70	0.53
OV-MZ-15	3.90	2.50	3.60	23.30	2.86
OV-MZ-16	90.00	54.20	88.00	26.10	1.24
OV-MZ-17a	9.65	5.8	11.4	23.8	1.39
OV-MZ-18	5.30	4.40	4.40	8.10	0.68
OV-MZ-19	1.90	0.48	0.44a	0.66	n. a.
OV-MZ-21	520.00	261.00	606.00	904.80	0.47
OV-MZ-22	5.50	1.80	0.40a	0.20	n. a.
OV-MZ-25	1.82	0.85	0.51a	2.85	n. a.
OV-MZ-27	828.00	986.00	443.00	n. e.	0.77
OV-MZ-28	720.00	811.00	785.00	n. e.	1.15
OV-MZ-30	419.00	258.00	203.40	n. e.	0.58

[a] CA 125 negative cell lines; n. a. = not applicable, because the cell line is CA 125 negative; n. e. = not examined.

value of 2.86 is only sixfold higher than the lowest value of 0.47. This suggests a very close correlation between the cell number and the marker concentration in the supernatant.

The results of TPS analysis are shown in table II: The secretion of TPS in the proliferative and the stationary phase of the cell cycle, the ratio of the secretion of TPS to CA 125 and the relationship between increase in cell number and increase in TPS concentration in the supernatant are shown. All cell lines were positive for the secretion of TPS, especially the seven CA 125 negative cell lines.

The intra-individual variance of TPS secretion was greater than of CA 125 production (table IIa). Concurrent with CA 125 the secretion pattern also varies greatly between the lines. In the proliferative phase of the cell cycle values varied up to a factor of 696, in the quiescent phase of the cell cycle up to a factor of 3995. The ratio of the secretion of TPS to CA 125 was relatively stable. Again, in contrast to CA 125 the relationship between the increase in cell number and the increase in TPS concentration in the supernatant varied greatly from 0.2 to 6.7. Different from CA 125 we found no close correlation between tumor mass and marker secretion. In addition TPS was not preferentially secreted by rapidly proliferating cell lines. The medium TPS secretion of the five most actively growing cell lines (medium cell doubling time = 126.6 h) was 480 U/ml and thereby lower than the medium TPS secretion of the five most slowly growing cell lines (medium doubling time = 165 h) at 2617 U/ml.

Only two of the 25 cell lines were positive for CA 72-4. CASA was detectable in 6/25 cell lines with values ranging from 2.14 U/ml to 22.03 U/ml.

Table IIa. Secretion of TPS in the proliferative and the stationary phase of the cell cycle; proportion of the secretion of TPS/CA 125; ratio of increase in cell number and increase in TPS concentration in the supernatant.

Cell line	TPS secretion rate (U/l/day/1·10^6 cells)			
	proliferating cells			quiescent cells
	day 4	6	8	day 3
OV-MZ-1a	507.00	823.00	148.00	n. a
OV-MZ-1b	314.30	177.50	222.70	525.90
OV-MZ-1c	265.30	408.70	191.00	187.50
OV-MZ-2	2295.00	1485.00	1144.00	2571.60
OV-MZ-3	341.00	220.00	246.00	n. a
OV-MZ-4	7.80	7.50	14.80	92.20
OV-MZ-5	433.00	275.00	295.00	674.00
OV-MZ-6	222.00	278.00	478.00	4139.50
OV-MZ-7b	1205.00	1471.00	2405.00	6032.00
OV-MZ-8	1387.00	542.00	600.00	(23 475)
OV-MZ-10	368.00	180.00	274.00	332.70
OV-MZ-11	1012.00	872.00	117.00	n. a.
OV-MZ-12	413.00	781l00	1607.00	2707.00
OV-MZ-13	1805.00	809.00	n. a.	1858.00
OV-MZ-15	85.80	46.50	62.50	213.00
OV-MZ-16	533.00	554.00	1205.00	1662.00
OV-MZ-17a	176.00	239.00	277.00	331.00
OV-MZ-18	2071.00	3095.00	4282.00	2538.00
OV-MZ-19	51.30	36.00	116.90	178.60
OV-MZ-20	324.00	158.00	n. a.	301.0
OV-MZ-21	9689.00	4851.00	7122.00	624.80
OV-MZ-22	20.00	74.00	12.00	6.10
OV-MZ-23	219.00	454.00	2512.00	2616.00
OV-MZ-24	88.60	153.00	198.00	97.50
OV-MZ-25	1405.00	1298.00	1477.00	2444.00
OV-MZ-27	2800.00	4226.00	1456.00	n. a.
OV-MZ-28	2554.00	1168.0	1668.00	–
OV-MZ-30	11580.00	7297.00	8357.00	n. a.
OV-MZ-31	560.00	298.00	292.00	448.60

n.a. = not applicable

Whereas all of the seven CA 125 negative cell lines were positive for TPS, only one of the seven cell lines was positive for the secretion of CA 72-4 and none was positive for the secretion of CASA.

Discussion

Our in vitro data demonstrate that CA 125 continues to be the most important tumor marker in serous cystadenocarcinoma of the ovary. The marker correlated very closely with tumor mass independent of differences between the lines regarding their secreting behavior. This explains the well known clinical observation, that sometimes patients with early tumor stage exhibit highly elevated CA 125 levels and patients with advanced disease only low marker concentrations. In contrast to some clinical speculations (4) we can not confirm any positive relationship between tumor cell proliferation and secreting behavior of TPS. On the contrary: TPS secretion of slowly proliferating cell lines was greater than the secretion of fast proliferating cell lines. TPS may be useful in the follow-up of CA 125 negative patients because all CA 125 negative cell lines were TPS positive. The results of CA 72-4 and CASA analysis are disappointing. The clinical value of these tumor markers in monitoring ovarian cancer patients with serous or undifferentiated

Table IIb. Secretion of TPS in the proliferative and the stationary phase of the cell cycle; proportion of the secretion of TPS/CA 125; ratio of increase in cell number and increase in TPS concentration in the supernatant.

	Proportion of the secretion of TPS/CA 125				Increase of cell number/ increase of TPS
	proliferating cells			quiescent cells	
	day 4	6	8	day 3	
OV-MZ-1a	20.90	16.20	21.80	–	1.90
OV-MZ-1b	58.20	59.00	41.20	20.80	0.78
OV-MZ-1c	6.60	27.10	30.80	0.76	0.77
OV-MZ-2	n. a.	CA 125 neg.			0.37
OV-MZ-3	26.20	16.10	14.5	–	2.50
OV-MZ-4	n. a.	CA 125 neg.			0.58
OV-MZ-5	n. a.	CA 125 neg.			3.49
OV-MZ-6	130.00	427.00	434.00	490.00	0.20
OV-MZ-7b	379.00	377.00	481.00	464.00	0.28
OV-MZ-8	8.60	7.20	4.50	7.43	5.95
OV-MZ-10	99.20	132.00	64.30	8.60	0.77
OV-MZ-11	10.80	7.10	2.30	–	4.87
OV-MZ-12	n. a.	CA 125 neg.			1.68
OV-MZ-13	132.00	439.00	–	31.60	1.60
OV-MZ-15	22.00	18.20	17.40	9.10	6.7
OV-MZ-16	5.90	10.20	13.70	63.60	2.50
OV-MZ-17a	16.20	41.20	24.30	13.90	3.01
OV-MZ-18	390.00	703.00	973.00	313.00	0.27
OV-MZ-19	n. a.	CA 125 neg.			1.87
OV-MZ-20	6.57	6.17	–	4.70	1.46
OV-MZ-21	18.60	18.60	11.80	0.69	0.75
OV-MZ-22	n. a.	CA 125 neg.			3.48
OV-MZ-23	n. a.	CA 125 n. e.			0.10
OV-MZ-24	n. a.	CA 125 n. e.			0.25
OV-MZ-25	n. a.	CA 125 neg.			2.32
OV-MZ-27	3.38	4.27	3.29	–	0.99
OV-MZ-28	3.55	1.44	2.12	–	1.00
OV-MZ-30	27.60	28.20	41.00	–	0.45
OV-MZ-31	n.a.	CA 125 n. e.			1.07

n.a. = not applicable; n.e. not examined

carcinoma will probably be very limited, especially because they appear to be elevated only in a minority of CA 125 negative cell lines.

References

1 Bast RC, Hunter V, Knapp R (1987) Pros and cons of gynecologic tumor markers. Cancer 60:1984–1992
2 Möbus V, Kreienberg R, Crombach G, Würz H, Caffier H, Kaeseman H, Hoffmann FJ, Schmidt-Rhode P, Sturm G, Kaufmann M (1988) Evaluation of CA 125 as a prognostic and predictive factor in ovarian cancer. J Tumor Marker Onc 3:251–258
3 Mc Guckin MA, Layton GT, Bailey MJ, Hurst T, Khoo SK, Ward BG (1990) Evaluation of two new assays for tumorassociated antigens, CASA and OSA, found in the serum of patients with epithelial ovarian carcinoma-comparison with CA 125. Gynecol Oncol 37:165–171
4 Pravettoni G, Luporini AC, Marino P, Preatoni A, Buccheri G, Ferrigno D (1990) Evaluation of TPA serum levels in pulmonary tumor diseases. Correlation between TPSTM-IRMA value and clinical objectivity criteria. 7th International Conference on Human Tumor Markers, Kiew, USSR

Address for correspondence:
Priv.-Doz. Dr. V. J. Möbus
Universitätsfrauenklinik
Universität Ulm
Prittwitzstraβe 43
D-89075 Ulm, Germany

In Vitro Diagnosis

Lung

Enzymun-test CYFRA 21-1: Results of the clinical phase 1 multicenter study in bronchogenic carcinoma

W. Ebert[a], H. Dienemann[b], A. Fateh-Moghadam †[b], Ch. Müller[b], M.E. Scheulen[c],
N. Konietzko[d], Th. Schleich[e], E. Bombardieri[f], D. Banauch[g], W. Mühlhofer[g]

[a]Thorax-Clinic, Heidelberg, [b]University of Munich, [c]University of Essen, [d]Ruhrland-Clinic Essen,
[e]Klinikum of the City of Nuremberg, [f]Istituto Nazionale Tumori, Milano, Italy,
[g]Boehringer Mannheim GmbH, Mannheim, Germany

Introduction

In the last year, the new tumor marker assay CYFRA 21-1, later refered to as CYFRA, utilizing two monoclonal antibodies against well characterized epitopes of a water-soluble fragment of cytokeratin 19 was introduced by Boehringer, Mannheim (1). Subsequently, several papers have been published advocating CYFRA to be a useful adjunct for diagnosis purposes in patients with non-small cell lung cancer (NSCLC), in particular in those suffering from squamous cell carcinoma (3, 4, 5, 8, 9, 10).
In an international multicenter study, the CYFRA assay was evaluated against the well-established markers CEA, SCC, and NSE in 526 patients with benign chest diseases for specificity and in 244 untreated patients with lung cancer for sensitivity (2). The present paper describes the specificity of CYFRA regarding various forms of benign pulmonary diseases and its sensitivity for the primary diagnosis of patients with NSCLC in comparison with SCC and CEA. In addition, the utility of CYFRA as a test for monitoring response to treatment and for detecting relapse was investigated.

Material and methods

Serum samples were taken from 177 patients with NSCLC admitted to the following European Centers: Klinikum Großhadern University Munich, Thoraxklinik Heidelberg-Rohrbach, Tumorzentrum University Essen, Ruhrlandklinik Essen, Klinikum Nuremberg, Istitutio Nazionale Fumori Milano.
Of these 177 cases, 81 suffered from squamous cell carcinoma (mean age: 61.1, range: 32–78 years), 63 from adenocarcinoma (mean age: 60.0, range: 31–77 years) and 33 from other NSCLC (mostly large cell) (mean age: 57.1, range: 24–80 years). The reference group consisted of 526 patients with benign chest diseases (mean age: 52.1, range: 14–92 years) including acute inflammatory diseases (n = 37), tuberculosis (n = 132), chronic obstructive pulmonary diseases (COPD) (n = 171), bronchial asthma (n = 62), interstitial lung diseases (n = 68), and other benign pulmonary diseases (n = 50). The stage of the malignant disease was determined according to clinical staging after patients' passage of the diagnostic schedule (cTNM) and histological examination of surgical specimens (pTNM) following the UICC classification (6). Histological diagnosis was performed according to the guidelines of the WHO (11) and was based on the predominant cell type.
CYFRA assessment was done with the Enzymun-test CYFRA 21-1 of Boehringer, Mannheim (1). CEA was determined employing the CEA assays of Abbott (IMx), Roche (EIA), and Sorin (RIA). SCC antigen was measured using the test from Abbott (IMx and RIA). The cut-off values, defined as the 95th percentile of the group suffering from benign chest diseases, were set at 3.3 ng/ml for CYFRA, at 7.8 ng/ml for CEA, and at 1.9 ng/ml for SCC.
For the statistical evaluation, differences between two or more independent samples were tested using Kruskal-Wallis H-test (7).

Results

Figure 1 shows the distribution of CYFRA concentrations in respect of various forms of benign pulmonary diseases. The median values were higher in patients suffering from interstitial lung diseases, tuberculosis, and COPD compared to the other entities, but these differences did not reach a statistically significant level. The cut-off value, defined as the 95th percentile of CYFRA concentrations in the total benign population, was calculated to be 3.3 ng/ml. Taking this value into account, the specificity rates in the different forms of benign diseases were found as follows; acute inflammatory diseases: 86.5%, tuberculosis: 94.7%, bronchial asthma: 96.8%, COPD: 95.9%, interstitial lung diseases: 94.1%, other benign chest diseases: 98%.

Figure 2a shows the sensitivity values of CYFRA in comparison with CEA and SCC in respect to the histologies of NSCLC. The highest sensitivity values of CYFRA were observed in the total group of NSCLC, in squamous cell carcinoma, and in the group with other NSCLC. In adenocarcinoma, the positivity rate of CEA was slightly higher than that of CYFRA.

The sensitivity values of the marker assays in relation to the tumor stages are also presented in Figure 2b. The frequency of marker elevations in early stage (TNM I) was rather low.

Serial measurement of CYFRA was carried out in 72 patients under treatment. The correlation of rising CYFRA levels to the clinical status is presented in figure 3. Relapse was indicated by increasing CYFRA level prior to clinical signs of deterioration only in 25% of cases. A false-positive elevation of CYFRA concentrations have to be noted in 21% of patients.

Figure 4 shows an example of serial marker assays in the follow-up of a patients with unresectable adenocarcinoma.

Discussion

The sensitivity values of the marker assays described in the present study depend on cut-off values basing on the 95% specificity of a population suffering from benign pulmonary diseases. The rate of false-positive elevations of CYFRA varied across the different forms of benign diseases. The highest false-positive rate was observed in patients with acute inflammatory diseases (13.5%). False-positive elevations are not restricted to benign pulmonary diseases. Stieber et al. (9) have shown that false-positive results may also occur in benign disorders of the gastrointestinal tract, in benign gynecological disorders, in benign urological diseases or in patients with acute or chronic failure. As a consequence, those false-positive elevations have to be considered in the monitoring of lung cancer patients who suffer in addition from concomitant diseases.

In the 177 patients with untreated NSCLC, it was found that CYFRA was elevated more frequently than the well-established markers SCC and CEA. In particular, 58% of squamous cell carcinoma was indicated by CYFRA compared to 23% by CEA and 32% by SCC, thus confirming the results of previous studies (3, 4, 5, 8, 9, 10). CYFRA, therefore, can be considered as the marker of first choice for this cell type. In adenocarcinoma, however, CEA (44%) was found to be slightly superior to CYFRA (42%). Thus, a combination of both markers can be recommended for the diagnosis of this cell type.

The frequency of elevated CYFRA concentrations was rather low at an early stage of the disease (TNM I: 23%), thus limiting the practical use of CYFRA assays for early diagnosis. In patients with limited disease and not in individuals who have advanced, bulky tumors, marker determinations have the highest potential for clinical use.

It is generally agreed that the most fruitful application of tumor markers is in monitoring of therapy. The temporary effect of change to chemo- or radiotherapy was more or less directly indicated by CYFRA and the other markers. Despite this advantage, additional diagnostic procedures are still required for the confirmation of the clinical state, e.g. the markers were not able to differentiate between complete and partial remission.

Progressively increasing CYFRA concentrations predicted (25%) or accompanied (19%) clinical relapses in the follow-up studies of 72 patients. But there was also false-positive elevation of CYFRA levels in 21% of the patients, i.e. without any clinical signs of deterioration at least at time of the last observation. Thus, CYFRA seems to be not very helpful for a confident and early indication of relapse. Nevertheless, it should be stressed, that from a practical clinical point of view, rising marker levels often are the only sign of a primary malignant disease or tumor recurrence.

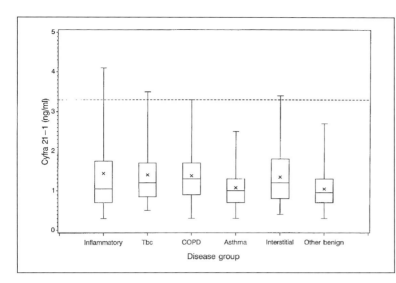

Figure 1. CYFRA concentrations in the various forms of benign pulmonary diseases. Data are presented as multiple box and whisker plots showing median value (horizontal line), mean value (x), upper and lower quartile and range (5th – 95th percentile).

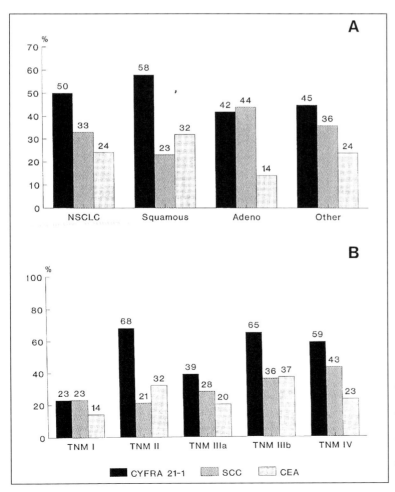

Figure 2. Elevated CYFRA (> 3.3 ng/ml), CEA (> 7.8 ng/ml), and SCC (> 1.9 ng/ml) levels in patients with NSCLC of different histological types (A). Elevated marker concentrations in patients with NSCLC according to TNM stages (B).

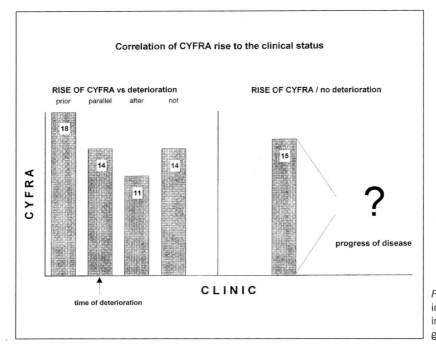

Figure 3. CYFRA levels in follow-up studies as indicators of tumor progression.

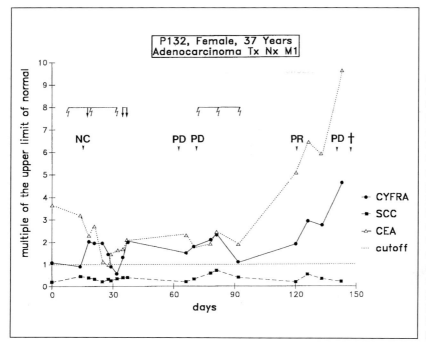

Figure 4. Monitoring of a patient with inoperable adenocarcinoma. In the initial phase of combined chemo- and radio-therapy, CYFRA and CEA levels declined for a very short period probably indicating response to therapy. In the final phase of the disease, CYFRA and CEA increased prior to clinical signs of progression despite partial remission as indicated by roentgenogram.
NC = no change,
PR = partial remission,
PD = progressive disease.

References

1. Bodenmüller H, Banauch D, Ofenloch B, Jaworek D Dessauer A (1992) Technical evaluation of a new automated tumor marker assay: The enzymun-test CYFRA 21-1. In: Klapdor R (ed) Tumor associated antigens, oncogenes, receptors, cytokines in tumor diagnosis and therapy at the beginning of the nineties. Cancer of the breast – State and trends in diagnosis and therapy. Zuckschwerdt, München, Bern, Wien, pp 137–138
2. Ebert W, Dienemann H, Fateh-Moghadam A, Müller Ch, Scheulen ME, Konietzko N, Schleich Th, Bombardieri E, Banauch D, Mühlhofer W (1994) CYFRA 21-1 in comparison with CEA, SCC and NSE in lung cancer. Results of an international multicenter study. Eur J Clin Chem Clin Biochem 32:189–199
3. Ebert W, Leichtweis B, Schapöhler B, Muley Th (1993) The new tumor marker CYFRA is superior to SCC antigen and CEA in the primary diagnosis of lung cancer. Tumor Diagn Ther 14:91–99
4. Ebert E, Muley Th, Leichtweis B, Bülzebruck H. CYFRA is the marker of the first choice in patients with squamous cell carcinoma. J Thorac Surg, in press
5. Hasholzner U, Stieber P, Fiebig M, Sunder-Plassmann L, Fateh-Moghadam A (1992) CYFRA – A new tumor marker for non-small cell lung cancer (NSCLC). In: Klapdor R (ed) Tumor associated antigens, oncogenes, receptors, cytokines in tumor diagnosis and therapy at the beginning of the nineties. Cancer of the breast – State and trends in diagnosis and therapy. Zuckschwerdt, München, Bern, Wien, pp 134–136
6. Hermanek P, Sobin L (1987) TNM Classification of malignant tumors. International Union against Cancer (UICC), ed 4, Springer, Berlin
7. Kruskal WH (1952) A nonparametric test for the several sampling problems. Ann Math Stat 23: 525–540
8. Pujol LJ, Grenier J, Daurés JP, Daver A, Pujol H, Michel FB (1993). Serum fragment of cytokeratin subunit 19 measured by CYFRA 21-1 immunoradiometric assay as a marker of lung cancer. Cancer Res 53:61–66
9. Stieber P, Dienemann H, Hasholzner U, Müller Ch, Poley S, Hofmann K, Fateh-Moghadam A (1993) Comparison of CYFRA 21-1, TPA and TPS in lung cancer. J Clin Chem Clin Biochem 31:689–694
10. Stieber P, Hasholzner U, Bodenmüller H, Nagel D, Sunder-Plassmann L, Dienemann H, Meier W, Fateh-Moghadam A (1993) CYFRA 21-1. A new marker in lung cancer. Cancer 72:707–713
11. World Health Organization (1981) Histological classification of lung tumors. Geneva, WHO

Address for correspondence:
Prof. Dr. med. W. Ebert
Thoraxklinik
Abteilung für Klinische Chemie und Bakteriologie
Amalienstraße 5
D-69126 Heidelberg, Germany

Radioimmunoassay of CYFRA 21-1 in 240 patients with untreated lung cancer

M. E. Scheulen[a], H. Klanig[a], J. K. Wiefelspütz[a], P. Kämper[a], B. Wagner[b], N. Konietzko[b], S. Seeber[a]

[a]Department of Internal Medicine (Cancer Research), West Germany Cancer Center,
[b]Ruhrlandklinik Essen, Germany

Introduction

In contrast to a number of solid tumors, where serum tumor marker evaluation is feasible with satisfactory sensitivity, up to now, there does not exist a tumor marker for the investigation of patients with non-small cell carcinoma (NSCLC).
We have analysed the water-soluble cytokeratin 19 fragment CYFRA 21-1 (CYFRA) in 162 patients with untreated NSCLC in comparison to 140 healthy blood donors (control 1) and 219 patients with benign lung diseases (control 2) for sensitivity and specificity, respectively.

Patients and methods

Patients

All 240 patients had histologically confirmed bronchogenic carcinomas und were not pretreated. They included 78 patients with small cell lung cancer (SCLC) and 162 patients with NSCLC: 75 squamous cell carcinomas (SCC), 61 adenocarcinomas (AC), 17 large cell carcinomas (LCC) and nine of other histology (OTH), respectively. Out of the 75 patients with squamous cell carcinomas 15 patients had stage I, 16 stage II, 26 stage IIIA, 11 stage IIIB and seven stage IV disease according to clinical staging (1).
A group of patients with benign lung diseases and a group of healthy blood donors separately served as controls. The 219 patients with benign lung diseases had emphysema, asthma, sarcoidosis, asbestosis, tuberculosis and bronchopneumonias. According to clinical and laboratory investigation, all 140 blood donors were not ill.

CYFRA RIA

All sera were stored at −80° C in tightly closed polypropylene tubes in the deep freezer in aliquots and only one time thawed for analysis.
The determination of CYFRA was performed with the Centocor CYFRA IRMA (Isotopen Diagnostic CIS, Dreieich), a monoclonal sandwich-assay composed of the two antibodies MAB 19-1 and MAB 19-21, which determines the soluble fragments of cytokeratin 19.

Statistical analysis

For the comparison of two independent groups the Mann-Whitney U-test was used (8). Differences between more than two groups were analysed with the variation analysis according to *Kruskal Wallis* (7).

Results

For CYFRA a cut-off (95%-confidence limit) of 1.1 ng/ml was determined for the 140 healthy blood donors (control 1) and of 2.2 ng/ml for the 219 patients with benign lung diseases (control 2), respectively.
Based on these two cut-off values the sensitivities of CYFRA were calculated for the different histological subtypes of lung cancer. According to table I sensitivities are highest for squamous cell carcinoma with 89% based on a cut-off of 1.1 ng/ml (control 1) and 68% based on a cut-off of 2.2 ng/ml (control 2), respectively.
When the data were further broken down according to the clinical stage of disease, in contrast to

Table I. Sensitivity of CYFRA in lung cancer according to histological subtype.

Histology	Number of patients	Control 1 (> 1.1 ng/ml)	Control 2 (> 2.2 ng/ml)
Total	240	172 (72%)	102 (43%)
SCLC	78	44 (56%)	20 (26%)
NSCLC	162	128 (79%)	82 (51%)
SCC	75	67 (89%)	51 (68%)
AC	61	41 (67%)	22 (35%)
LCC	17	13 (76%)	5 (29%)
OTH	9	7 (78%)	4 (44%)

Table II. Sensitivity of CYFRA in squamous cell carcinoma of the lung according to stage of disease.

Stage	Number of patients	Control 1 (> 1.1 ng/ml)	Control 2 (> 2.2 ng/ml)
Total	75	67 (89%)	51 (68%)
Stage I	15	10 (67%)	6 (40%)
Stage II	16	14 (88%)	11 (69%)
Stage IIIA	26	25 (96%)	19 (73%)
Stage IIIB	11	11 (100%)	8 (73%)
Stage IV	7	7 (100%)	7 (100%)

the other histological subtypes there was a significant correlation for the 75 patients with squamous cell carcinoma (table II).

Conclusions

In agreement with other investigations (2–6, 9–12) our study demonstrated that CYFRA is a tumor-associated antigen with a high overall sensitivity of 68% in squamous cell carcinoma of the lung when evaluated on the basis of a specificity of 95% in patients with benign lung diesease. Thus, it is the tumor marker of first choice in this histological subtype. Furthermore, CYFRA significantly correlates with the stage of disease. Therefore, it can be expected to be a pretreatment parameter of high prognostic value. This expectation has already been fulfilled in a study of Pujol and coworkers (9) and needs further confirmation by multivariate analysis of response or survival as an endpoint in correlation to the CYFRA serum levels, as compared to other potentially prognostic parameters before treatment.

References

1. Beahrs OH, Henson DE, Hutter RVP, Myers MH (eds)(1988) American Joint Committee on Cancer. Manual for Staging of Cancer. Philadelphia JB Lippincott, 3rd ed
2. Body JJ, Sculier JP, Raymakers N, Paesmans M, Ravez P, Libert P, Richez M, Dabouis G, Lacroix H, Bureau G, Rhiriaux J, Lecomte J, Brohée D, Mommen P, Frühling J, Klastersky J (1990) Evaluation of squamous cell carcinoma antigen as a new marker for lung cancer. Cancer 65:1552–1556
3. Buccheri GF, Ferrigno D, Sartoris AM, Violante B, Vola F, Curcio A (1987) Tumor markers in bronchogenic carcinoma. Superiority of tissue polypeptide antigen to carcinoembryonic antigen and carbohydrate antigenic determinant 19-9. Cancer 60:42-50
4. Dent PB, McCulloch PB, Wesley-James O, MacLaren R, Muirhead W, Dunnett CW (1978) Measurement of carcinoembryonic antigen in patients with bronchogenic carcinoma. Cancer 42:1484–1491
5. Ebert W, Leichtweis B, Schapöhler B, Muley T (1993) The new tumor marker CYFRA is superior to SCC antigen and CEA in the primary diagnosis of lung cancer. Tumordiagn Ther 14:91–99
6. Fischbach W, Rink C (1988) SCC-Antigen: ein sensitiver und spezifischer Tumormarker für Plattenepithelkarzinome? Dtsch med Wschr 113:289–293
7. Kruskal WH (1952) A nonparametric test for the several sampling problem. Ann Math Stat 23:525–540
8. Mann HB, Whitney PR (1974) On a test of whether one of two random variables is stochastically larger than the other. Ann Math Stat 18:50–60
9. Pujol J-L, Grenier J, Daurès J-P, Daver A, Pujol H, Michel F-B (1993) Serum fragment of cytokeratin subunit 19 measured by CYFRA 21-1 immunoradiometric assay as a marker of lung cancer. Cancer Res 53:61–66
10. Stieber P, Dienemann H, Hasholzner U, Müller C, Poley S, Hofmann K, Fateh-Moghadan A (1993) Comparison of cytokeratin fragment 19 (CYFRA 21-1), tissue polypeptide antigen (TPA) and tissue

polypeptide specific antigen (TPS) as tumor markers in lung cancer. Eur J Clin Chem Clin Biochem 31:689–694
11 Stieber P, Hasholzner U, Bodenmüller H, Nagel D, Sunder-Plassmann L, Dienemann H, Meier W, Fateh-Moghadan A (1993) CYFRA 21-1. A new marker in lung cancer. Cancer 72:707–713
12 van der Gaast A, Schoenmakers CHH, Kok TC, Blijenberg BG, Cornillie F, Splinter TAW (1994) Evaluation of a new tumour marker in patients with non-small-cell lung cancer: CYFRA 21-1. Br J Cancer 69:525–528

Address for correspondence:
Priv.-Doz. Dr. med. M. E. Scheulen
Innere Klinik und Poliklinik
(Tumorforschung)
Universitätsklinikum
Hufelandstraße 55
D-45122 Essen, Germany

Clinical applications of CYFRA 21-1 in patients with non-small cell lung cancer

A. van der Gaast, C. Schoenmaker, T.C. Kok, B.G. Blijenberg, T.A.W. Splinter

Departments of Medical Oncology and Clinical Chemistry,
University Hospital Rotterdam-Dijkzigt, The Netherlands

Introduction

In many countries lung cancer is the most common malignancy in men and the incidence in women is still rising. The prognosis of patients with non-small lung cancer heavily depends on the stage of disease. Only 25–30% of patients with tumors within the lung while the others have either locally advanced disease or distant metastases (1). Most disappointingly even the majority of patients who present with stage I or stage II non-small cell lung cancer relapse after initial surgery.

Chemotherapy in patients with non-small cell lung cancer can be employed in several settings such as adjuvant chemotherapy after surgery, neoadjuvant chemotherapy for patients with locally advanced disease and as palliative treatment for patients with metastatic disease. Unfortunately the impact of chemotherapy in patients with metastatic disease is small and seems to be restricted to those patients who respond to treatment. This latter fact underscores the importance of disease monitoring in these patients during chemotherapy.

The CYFRA 21-1 assay measures in serum a fragment of cytokeratin 19. We have evaluated the sensitivity, the prognostic value and the use of this marker for disease monitoring in patients with non-small cell lung cancer.

Material and methods

From 212 patients with a histologically proven non-small cell lung cancer serum samples were collected at diagnosis and during treatment for those patients receiving chemotherapy. The samples were stored at minus 70 °C until analysis. All patients were staged according to guidelines of the American Joint Committee on Cancer (2). Response to chemotherapy was assessed using standard WHO criteria (3). The following response criteria for the tumor markers were used: complete response = normalization of an elevated marker for at least one month; partial response = decrease of 65% or more of an elevated marker for at least one month; stable disease = less than 65% decrease or less than 40% increase of an elevated marker; progressive disease = more than 40% increase of an elevated marker level or a rise from below to above the cut-off level.

Serum CYFRA 21-1 assay values were determined using a solid-phase double determinant immunoradiometric assay as previously described (4). The cut-off value for CYFRA 21-1 used in this study was 3.3 ng/ml. This cut-off values correspond with a 96% specificity for the marker determined in 546 patients with non-malignant lung diseases. Differences between the medians of two groups were tested using Mann-Whitney's test. $P = 0.05$ was considered the limit of significance. Survival was recorded from the date of the first CYFRA 21-1 measurement to the date of death or last follow-up and survival curves were calculated according to the method of *Kaplan-Meier* (5). Single variable survival analysis was done with the log-rank test (6).

Results

Patient characteristics are listed in table I. Median values for all patients were 2.1 ng/ml (range 0.1–1057), for stage 3A 1.4 ng/ml (range 0.2–1057), for stage 3B 1.9 ng/ml (range 0.3–86), and for stage 4 2.1 ng/ml (range 0.1–92). Median values were significantly higher in stage 4 compared to stage 3A and 3B. The

Table I. CYFRA 21-1 in non-small cell lung cancer. Patient characteristics.

No. patients	212
Gender	
female	40 (19%)
male	172 (81%)
Median age (years)	59
range	29 – 81
Median performance (ECOG)	1
range	0 – 4
Stage	
1	5 (2%)
2	2 (1%)
3A	59 (28%)
3B	37 (17%)
4	109 (52%)
Histology	
adenocarcinoma	65 (31%)
squamous cell carcinoma	80 (38%)
large cell undifferentiated carcinoma	67 (32%)

sensitivity for all patients was 41%, for patients with adenocarcinomas 36%, for patients with squamous cell carcinoma 53%, and for patients with large cell undifferentiated carcinomas 32%.
The prognostic significance of CYFRA 21-1 for survival was determined in 199 patients with stage 3A, 3B and 4 disease. Patients with elevated levels of CYFRA 21-1 had a worse survival compared to patients with not elevated levels of CYFRA 21-1. The survival curves are shown in figure 1.
The value of CYFRA 21-1 in the use of disease monitoring during chemotherapy could be evaluated in 46 patients. These patients fulfilled the following criteria: 1. treated with chemotherapy, 2. a sufficient number of marker determinations during chemotherapy i.e. at least three serum samples, 3. evaluable lesions, and, 4. an elevated level of CYFRA 21-1 at the start of treatment. A total of 115 clinical evaluations were performed. A positive lead time of the marker, i.e. the change in the tumor marker preceded the results obtained by the clinical evaluation by one or two months, was observed ten times. On nine of these ten occasions the marker indicated already disease progression while the clinical response was stable disease. A negative lead time was observed once in a patient with progressive disease while the tumor marker met the criteria for progressive disease only four weeks later. Five evaluations yielded stable disease clinically and a partial or complete response of the marker. One patient had an increase of the marker level when clinical progression was documented but not sufficient enough to meet the criteria set for marker progression. The last discordant evaluation was in a patient who had progressive disease according to the marker but stable disease according to the WHO criteria.
A summary of the response evaluation according to the WHO criteria and according to the marker is listed in table II.
An example of the course of CYFRA 21-1 during chemotherapy is shown in figure 2.

Discussion

In this study we evaluated some clinical applications of the tumor marker CYFRA 21-1 in patients with non-small cell lung cancer. We found

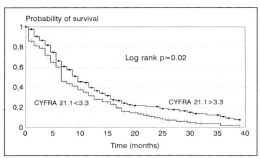

Figure 1. Survival curves of patients with NSCLC based on their CYFRA 21-1 levels.

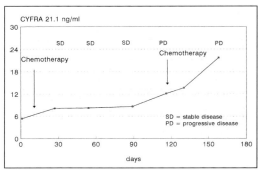

Figure 2. Course of CYFRA 21-1 during chemotherapy in patient with stage 3B squamous cell carcinoma of the lung.

Table II. Correlation between clinical response evaluation by standard WHO-criteria compared to reponse evaluation according to change in CYFRA 21-1 levels. Total number of evaluations: 107.

Marker response evaluation	Clinical response evaluation		
	progressive disease	stable disease	objective response
Progressive disease	25	1	
Stable disease	10	40	6
Objective response			25

that frequently elevated levels of this marker can be detected in the sera of patients with advanced non-small cell lung cancer, particularly in patients with squamous cell carcinomas. Higher median values of CYFRA 21-1 were observed in stage 4 disease compared to stage 3 disease which suggests that this marker gives an indirect reflection of the total tumor load. The fact that patients with an elevated CYFRA 21-1 serum level have a worse prognosis compared with patients with not elevated levels of CYFRA 21-1 is probably due to the association with the total tumor load. Most importantly we found that this tumor marker was very useful for disease monitoring during chemotherapy and that the changes in the tumor marker level correlated well with response evaluation according to the WHO criteria. Especially increasing levels of CYFRA 21-1 nearly always indicated disease progression and such knowledge is of great value in the management of patients with non-small cell lung cancer treated with chemotherapy.

Acknowledgement

We thank Centocor Diagnostic Europe for financial support for this study.

References

1. Ihde DC, Minna JD (1991) Non-small cell lung cancer. I. Biology, diagnosis, and staging. Curr Probl Cancer 15:61–104
2. American Joint Committee on Cancer (1988) In: Beahrs OH, Henson DE, Hutter RV, Myers MH (eds) Manual for staging of cancer. PA: Philadelphia, Lippincott, pp 115–122
3. WHO (1979) Handbook of reporting results of cancer treatment. Geneva. World Health Organization. Offset publication no 48
4. van der Gaast A, Schoenmakers CCH, Kok TC, Blijenberg BG, Cornillie F, Splinter TAW (1994) Evaluation of a new tumor marker in patients with non-small cell lung cancer: CYFRA 21-1. Br J Cancer, in press.
5. Kaplan EL, Meier P (1958) Nonparametric estimation from incomplete observations. J Am Stat Assoc 53:457–481
6. Mantel N (1966) Evaluation of survival data and two new rank order statistics arising in its consideration. Cancer Chemother Rep 50:163–170

Address for correspondence:
Dr. A. van der Gaast
Department of Medical Oncology
University Hospital Rotterdam-Dijkzigt
Dr. Molewaterplein 40
NL-3015 GD Rotterdam, The Netherlands

CYFRA 21-1, a non-small cell lung cancer tumor marker – Report of the first multicenter evaluation

D. Rastel

CIS bio International, Gif-sur-Yvette, France

Introduction

Cytokeratins are proteins of the intermediate filament family. Twenty known cytokeratins are part of the cytoskeleton of epithelial cells. They are not randomly distributed. CK 8, 18, 19 are preferentially found in epithelial cells of simple epithelium and overexpressed in cancer tissues (1). Their use as epithelial tumor markers in immunohistochemistry has been demonstrated for many years (2).

CYFRA 21-1 is an immunoradiometric assay developed with two monoclonal antibodies BM 19-21 and KS 19-1 for measuring only cytokeratin 19 fragments in serum (3).

The mechanism by which they are released in body fluids from tumors is still largely unknown. At the present time, the increase in the number of new substances roughly tested as tumor markers makes the clinician unable to choose which one to use in clinical practice. This is why the number of studies and the increase of informations after publication have to be included in the definition of a new tumor marker. It is the reason why a multicenter evaluation to establish the clinical characteristics of CYFRA 21-1 at diagnosis is the second step after a preliminary evaluation (4) to know more about this new tumor marker.

Material and methods

Serum from 711 blood donors, 546 benign lung diseases, and 621 lung cancers has been collected before any therapy in a multicenter retrospective trial including 11 centers (table I). Lung cancers were classified according to the WHO histological classification in 547 non-small cell lung cancers (277 squamous cell carcinomas, 172 adenocarcinomas, 98 large cell-undifferentiated carcinomas) and in 74 small cell lung cancers (5). Extension of the disease was evaluated according to the UICC criteria (6) and classification from American Thoracic society (7). 169 serum from other cancers (27 head and neck cancers, 56 digestive tract cancers, 63 gynecological cancers and 23 bladder cancers) were also tested for CYFRA 21-1. Overall sensitivity and specificity was shown by the means of curves adapted from CDA curves (8).

Results

CYFRA 21-1 shows a 99.9% specificity at 3.0 ng/ml in the 711 blood donors population. The highest value is 3.5 ng/ml. In benign diseases CYFRA 21-1 is shown to be elevated in chronic obstructive bronchopneumopathy and in chronic renal failure (figure 1). There is a slight elevation in case of liver disease only when cirrhosis was diagnosed but not in hepatitis (data not shown). These data prompt us to state that cytokeratin 19 is probably cleared by the kidney.

The overall sensitivity of CYFRA 21-1 in different types of lung cancer (figure 2) shows the best sensitivity for squamous type and the lowest one for small cell lung cancers. The 96% specificity which is at 3.3 ng/ml is chosen as the cut-off. This arbitrary cut-off represents in fact the first decrease of the slope of specificity with a loss of less than 10% sensitivity in the squamous cell lung carcinomas.

It is also shown that CYFRA 21-1 is much more elevated when the disease is extended (stages IIIb, IV) than when it is limited (stages I, II, IIIa) (figure 3). In other cancers, when 3.3 ng/ml is used as the cut-off, no more than 26% of cancers have elevated values (figure 4). The best sensitivities are for bladder cancers (26%), head and neck cancers (26%) and cervix cancers (21%).

Table I. The multicenter study group.

Splinter TWA, van der Gaast A, Blijenberg B	University hospital Rotterdam – Department of medical oncology Dr. Molewaterplein, 403015, GD Rotterdam, The Netherlands
Fombellida Cortazar JC, Genolla Subirats J	Servicio de Medicina Nuclear, Hospital de Cruces, Bilbao, Spain
Pecchio F, Rapellino M	Ospedale Maggiore S. Giovanni Battista - C. so Bramante, 88/90, 10100 Turin, Italy
Biersack HJ, Bieker RJ, Schultes BC, Loos U	Universitätsklinik für Nuklearmedizin, Sigmund-Freud-Straße 25, D-53127 Bonn, Germany
De Angelis G[a], Gianetti A[b]	[a]3e Department of C. Forlanini Chest Hospital, Via Portunese 332, 00149, [b]Central Laboratory of S. Camillo Hospital, Circonv. Gianicolense 87, 00152 Rome, Italy
Scheulen ME	Innere Klinik und Poliklinik (Tumorforschung), Westdeutsches Tumorzentrum, Universitätsklinik Essen, Hufelandstraße 55, D-45147 Essen, Germany
Tuchais C[a], Daver A[a], Tuchais E[b]	[a]CRLCC Paul Papin, [b]Service de Pneumologie CHRU d'Angers, 2 rue Moll, 49036 Angers, France
Gaillard G, Gachon F	CRLCC Jean Perrin, 58 rue Montalembert, BP 392, 63011 Clermont-Ferrand Cedex 1, France
Bonfrer JMG	Department of Clinical Chemistry, The Netherland Cancer Institute (Antoni van Leeuwenhoek Huis), Plesmanlaan 121, 1066 CX Amsterdam, The Netherlands
Larbre H	Institut Jean Godinot, 1 rue du Général Koenig, BP 171, 51056 Reims Cedex, France
Allende MaT, Fernandez Liana B, Ruibal A	Gabinete de Actos Cientificos, Hospital Central de Asturias, 33006 Oviedo, Spain

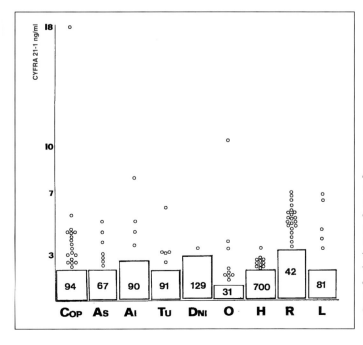

Figure 1. CYFRA 21-1 assay values (ng/ml) in benign lung diseases, healthy people, renal and liver diseases. (COP) chronic obstructive bronchopneumopathy; (AS) asthma; (AI) acute infectious bronchpneumopathy; (TU) tuberculosis; (DNI) diffuse non infectious interstitial pneumopathy; (O) other; (H) healthy people; (R) chronic renal failure; (L) cirrhosis and hepatitis (adapted from *Rastel D* et al (1994) Eur J Cancer 30A:601–606).

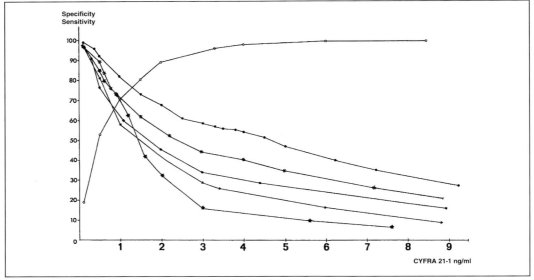

Figure 2. Overall sensitivity and specificity of CYFRA 21-1 in lung cancers by means of CDA curves. Specificity is based on 546 benign lung diseases: o—o. *—* non small cell lung cancers; ●—● squamous cell lung carcinomas; ▶—▶ adenocarcinomas; ■—■ large cell carcinomas; ★—★ small cell lung cancers (adapted from *Rastel D* et al (1994) Eur J Cancer 30A:601–606).

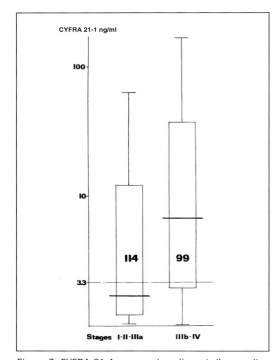

Figure 3. CYFRA 21-1 assay values (in ng/ml) according to stages in squamous cell lung carcinomas (n = 223). Bars represent 25th and 95th centiles; black line is the median and "T lines" are extremes.

Discussion

By testing CYFRA 21-1 in a well defined and large healthy and benign lung disease population we have got a good idea of the possible false positive increases of CYFRA 21-1 when it will be used in the follow-up of patients after therapy. We know that only progressive increase of tumor markers from the basic line (and not over the cut-off value) has to be taken into account in the follow-up of patients in order to detect relapses early. Nevertheless, we must keep in mind this cut-off (3.3 ng/ml) and the range of elevation of CYFRA 21-1 in benign lung diseases (up to 18 ng/ml) to be aware that false positive elevation could occur.

With this multicenter trial we established that the major fields in which CYFRA 21-1 will be used is non-small cell lung cancers and especially the squamous type. We know that CYFRA 21-1 is linked to the extension of the disease, reflecting the tumor burden. The difference between medians in limited diseases (stages I, II, IIIa) versus extended diseases (stages IIIb, IV) may be of help in staging cancer. On the other hand, the overlap of the two populations does not allow us to define any cut-off on which surgical decision could be made.

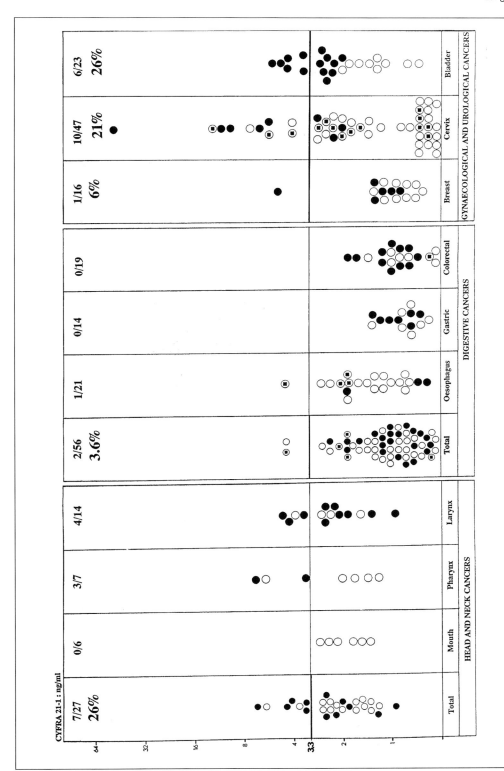

Figure 4. CYFRA 21-1 assay values (ng/ml) and CYFRA 21-1 sensitivities (%) in other cancers than lung: ○ stage I and II; ◉ stage III; ● stage IV.

In other cancers the sensitivity of CYFRA 21-1 remains very poor (less than 30%). CYFRA 21-1 will probably be of no important use in such cancers (bladder, cervix, head and neck) unless it will be possible to find a subgroup of patients in which it will add useful information. For this purpose we need further pilot studies.

Even if the control group (3.3 ng/ml cut-off) is probably not appropriate for other cancers, we can see that there is still a discrepancy between immunohistochemical results and serial measurements of a protein which is known to be basically expressed in all squamous carcinomas.

In conclusion, this evaluation shows that CYFRA 21-1 could be a useful tool in helping the clinician to manage lung cancer and especially non-small cell lung carcinomas before any therapy, knowing that CYFRA 21-1 has also an independent prognosis value (9).

References

1. Moll R, Franke WW, Schiller DL, Geiger B, Krepzer R (1982) The catalog of human cytokeratins: patterns of expression in normal epithelia, tumors and cultured cells. Cell 31:11–24
2. Broers JLV, Ramaekers FCS, Rot MK, Oostendorp T, Huysmans A, van Muijen GNP et al (1988) Cytokeratins in different types of human lung cancer as monitored by chain-specific monoclonal antibodies. Cancer Res 48:3221–3229
3. Roux F, Roux N, Ferrand V, Thomas P, Kleisbauer JP and G.F.P.C. (1993) A new tumor marker for lung cancer: CYFRA 21–1. J Tumor Marker Oncol 8(3):96
4. Tuchais C, Daver A, Tuchais E, Grenier J, Pujol JL, Rastel D, Clement M, Thirion B. (1993) Preliminary clinical evaluation of cytokeratin 9 fragment seric measurement by CYFRA 21-1 assay. In: Galteau MM, Siest G, Henny J (eds) Biologie prospective. Comptes Rendus du 8ème Colloque de Pont à Mousson. John Libbey Eurotext, Paris, pp 655–658
5. World Health Organization (1982) The World Health Organization histological typing of the lung tumors. 2nd ed. Am J Clin Pathol 77:123–136
6. Sobin LH, Hermanck-Hutter R (1988) Lung tumors. In: Hermanek P, Sobin LH (eds) International Union Against Cancer – TNM classification of malignant tumors. Springer, Paris, pp 71–76
7. Tisi GM, Friedman PJ, Peters RM et al (1982) American Thoracic Society clinical staging of primary lung cancer. Am Rev Respir Dis 125:659–664
8. Krouwer JS (1987) Cumulative distribution analysis graphs – An alternative to ROC curves. Clin Chem 33:2305–2306
9. Pujol JL, Grenier J, Daver A, Daurés JP, Pujol H, Michel FB (1993) Serum fragment of cytokeratin 19 measured by CYFRA 21-1 immuno-radiometric assay as a marker of lung cancer. Cancer Res 53:61–66

Address for correspondence:
Dr. D. Rastel
CIS bio International
B.P.32
F-91192 Gif-sur-Yvette, France

CYFRA 21-1, a new marker tested during follow-up of patients treated for adenocarcinoma of the lung

J.M.G. Bonfrer, C.M. Korse, P. Baas
The Netherlands Cancer Institute (Antoni van Leeuwenhoek Huis), Amsterdam, The Netherlands

Introduction

Lung carcinoma is the leading course of death due to cancer. At least four major histological types can be distinguished with a different prognosis (1). Adenocarcinoma is a significant but relatively small part of all non-small cell lung cancer. About 10–15% of all patients suffer from adenocarcinomas.

The growth rate of this histological type is relatively low, with a doubling time of ± 180 days. Tumor markers are not commonly used in the follow-up of patients with lung cancer. In non-small cell lung cancer neuron specific enolase (NSE) has been found to be a useful marker as it correlates well with tumor burden and prognosis (2).

In general, studies correlating clinical findings and CEA marker levels have been disappointing in NSCLC, but when applied to cases concerning adenocarcinomas the use of CEA in monitoring treatment of patients was reported to be satisfactory (3).

Tissue polypeptide antigen (TPA) has been proposed as a non-specific marker of proliferation. The assay measures cytokeratin fragments, mainly of CK 8, 18 and 19. Recently the CYFRA 21-1 assay was introduced. It detects fragments of CK 19 in serum (4). Results of the use of CYFRA 21-1 in non-small cell lung cancer were reported as encouraging (5). In this retrospective study we compared the results of two assays measuring fragments of cytokeratins, TPA and CYFRA 21-1, with the established marker for adenocarcinomas CEA, in the particular case of histologically proven adenocarcinomas of the lung.

Materials and methods

Twentythree patients (15 male/8 female, mean age 57) admitted in the Netherland's Cancer Institute to receive chemotherapy for adenocarcinoma of the lung were involved in this study. At least three serum samples of them were available for marker measurement. All patients were followed, after discontinuation of therapy, at intervals judged suitable by their physicians. A total of 130 samples were included. Per patient the number of samples varied from 3 to 19 with a median of 5. All patients had histologically proven adenocarcinoma of the lung.

Cytokeratin 19 fragments were measured with a solid phase sandwich radioimmunoassay utilizing 2 MoAbs, BM 29-21 and KS 19-1, (Cis-bio International, Gif-sur-Yvette Cedex, France). The between run variation was typically 9%. Of apparently healthy individuals 95% were given to have serum levels below 1.2 µg/l. TPA was measured with an IRMA (Byk-Sangtec Medical, Bromma, Sweden). We calculated an intra-variation coefficient of 8.5%. The reference value was given as 95 U/l and was based upon 200 apparently healthy individuals. In a log-normal distribution, 95% were found to have values below this concentration. CEA concentrations were determined with the ELSA-IRMA assay using monoclonal antibodies (Cis-bio International, Gif-sur-Yvette Cedex, France). The inter-variation coefficient was established in our laboratory as 12%. It was reported that 99% of presumably healthy subjects had values below 5 µlg/l. In a group of 43 smokers 95% had values below 7 µg/l (6). Statistical methods used were orthogonal regression analysis for the correlation study and receiver operating characteristic (ROC) curves for clinical comparisons.

Table I. Initial value of tumor markers.

	Value	Frequency	Percent
CYFRA 21-1 (µg/l)	< 3.3	15	65.2
	≥ 3.3	8	34.8
CYFRA 21-1 (µg/l)	< 1.2	6	26.1
	≥ 1.2	17	73.9
CEA (µg/l)	< 4.0	2	8.7
	≥ 4.0	21	91.3
TPA (U/l)	< 95	11	47.8
	≥ 95	12	52.2

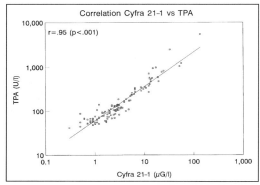

Figure 1. Correlation of CYFRA 21-1 versus TPA.

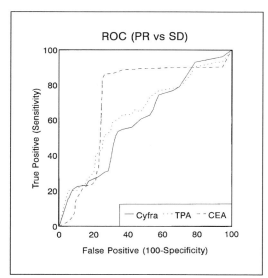

Figure 2. ROC curves discriminating between partial remission (PR) and stable disease (SD) of CYFRA, TPA and CEA.

Results

The initial value of CYFRA 21-1 was increased over the reference value for a normal population of 1.2 µg/l in 17 patients (74%). If a cut-off value of 3.3 µg/l was used, as recommended by the manufacturer, only 35% (8/23) of the results could be considered as positive. The corresponding CEA concentration was elevated (> 4 µg/l) in 21 cases (91%), while the TPA level was found higher than the upper reference level of 95 U/l in 52% (12/23) (table I).

Log values were used because of an asymmetric distribution. Although all correlations are significant, the r-value of CEA with both cytokeratin assays TPA and CYFRA 21-1 is 0.28. This is in contrast to the highly correlated results of TPA and CYFRA 21-1 ($r = 0.95$) as depicted in figure 1. The discriminative power of the markers between a partial remission (PR) and a stable disease (SD) is depicted by a ROC curve (figure 2). No difference could be demonstrated for both, CYFRA 21-1 and TPA. The serum level of CEA gave a better distinction between the two clinical stages as is seen by the fact that the CEA curve approaches the left upper curve.

Discussion

The availability of promising chemotherapy regimens has increased the demand for reliable parameters, which can be used in the follow-up of patients treated for NSCLC. A recently introduced assay, CYFRA 21-1, has been promoted as a parameter for non-small cell lung cancer (7). The assay is based on the specific determination of cytokeratin 19 fragments. The comparison of this assay with the long standing used TPA assay did not reveal a striking difference in performance as was shown by the correlation study and in the ROC curve. This is in contrast with earlier publications from *Stieber* et al. (8). This study however was directed to measure sensitivity and specificity in a single sample from patients with benign and malign lung disease.

We evaluated the clinical use of CYFRA 21-1 in the follow-up of patients treated for lung cancer using serial samples. *Van der Gaast* et al. also reported a highly significant inter-marker correlation for CYFRA 21-1 and TPA (9). In this group of patients with proven adenocarcinoma CEA performed better than both keratin markers in the differentiation between partial remission versus stable disease. This is in concordance with earlier publications showing a better correlation of CEA with disease status than TPA (3).

More recent data of marker studies during the follow-up of patients with adenocarcinoma of the lung are not available.

This limited and small study shows that the role of CYFRA 21-1 in follow-up of adenocarcinomas of the lung has to be evaluated in a more extensive way and may differ from its value in squamous cell carcinoma.

References

1. The World Health Organization of histological typing of lung tumors. 2nd ed (1982) Am J Clin Path 77:123–6.
2. Cooper EH, Splinter TAW, Brown DA et al (1985) Evaluation of a radioimmunoassay for neuron specific enolase in small cell lung cancer. Br J CA 52:333–8
3. Shinkai T, Saijo N, Tominaga K et al (1986) Serial plasma CEA measurements for monitoring patients with advanced lung cancer during chemotherapy. Cancer 57:1318–23
4. Bodenmüller H, Banauch D, Ofenloch Hänle B et al (1992) Technical and clinical evaluation of a new assay for NSCLC, the enzymun test CYFRA 21-1. Proc Am Ass Cancer Res 33:203
5. Pujol J, Grenier J, Daures J, Daver A. Puiol H, Michel F. (1993) Serum fragments of Cytokeratin subunit 19 measured by CYFRA 21-1 immunoradiometric assay as a marker of lung cancer. Cancer Res 53: 61–6
6. Sertour J, Ballesta A, Cianetti A, Molina R, Salard JL. (1988) Evaluation of one step monoclonal immunoradiometric assay for carcinoembryonic antigen (CEA). ISOBM XVIth International Congress Barcelona, September 25–9
7. Ebert W, Leichtweis B, Schapöhler B, Mule Y T (1993) The new tumormarker CYFRA is superior to SCC antigen and CEA in the primary diagnosis of lung cancer. Tumor Diagn u Ther 14:91–9
8. Stieber P, Dienemann H, Hasholzner U et al (1993) Comparison of CYFRA 21-1, TPA and TPS as tumor markers in lung cancer. Eur J Clin Chem Clin Biochem 31:689–94
9. Van der Gaast A, Schoenmakers CHH, Kok TC, Blijenberg BG, Cornillie F, Splinter TAW (1994) Evaluation of a new tumor marker in patients with nonsmall-cell lung cancer: Cyfra 21-1. Br J Cancer, 69:525–8

Address for correspondence:
Dr. J. M. G. Bonfrer
Antoni van Leeuwenhoek Huis
Plesmanlaan 121
NL-1066X Amsterdam, The Netherlands

Prognostic significance of TPS in patients with non-small cell lung cancer

A. van der Gaast, C. Schoenmaker, T.C. Kok, B.G. Blijenberg, T.A.W. Splinter

Departments of Medical Oncology and Clinical Chemistry,
University Hospital Rotterdam-Dijkzigt, The Netherlands

Introduction

The determination of prognostic factors in patients with malignant tumors may serve different purposes such as individual prognostication, choice of treatment, comparison of different trials or trialarms and gathering knowledge about the heterogeneity and biological behavior of the disease. Many of these factors are related to the total tumorload and/or site of metastases, the growth rate of the tumor and specific host factors. Also different treatments or better treatment modalities may influence the importance of established prognostic factors. In some instances the response to treatment may outweigh all other known prognostic factors.

The TPS assay measures in serum the M3 specific epitope of tissue polypeptide antigen. It has been claimed that serum TPS levels are related to the proliferation rate of a tumor. In this study we evaluated the prognostic significance of TPS serum levels for survival in patients with advanced non-small cell lung cancer and related it to other known prognostic factors.

Materials and methods

From 203 patients with histologically proven advanced non-small cell lung cancer serum samples were collected at diagnosis and stored at minus 70 °C until analysis. All patients were staged according to the guidelines of the American Joint Committee on Cancer (1). Nodal status was confirmed histologically or cytologically by mediastinoscopy, mediastinotomy or thoracotomy for those patients with stage 3A disease. Treatment in the patients was diverse and consisted of radiotherapy, chemotherapy or only supportive care.

TPS concentrations were measured with the TPS-ELISA kit (Beki Diagnostics AB, Bromma, Sweden).

Survival was recorded from the date of the TPS measurement to the date of death or last follow-up and survival curves were calculated according to the method of Kaplan-Meier (2). Single survival analysis was done with the log-rank test (3) and Cox's regression was used for the multivariate analysis (4).

Results

Patient characteristics are listed in table I.

The median value of TPS for all patients was 144 U/l (range 6–19208). Median values of TPS in stage 4 were significantly higher compared to stage 3 disease. The percentages of patients with a marker value above 100 U/l for all patients and according to stage are shown in figure 1.

In the univariate analysis performance status, stage of disease, lactate dehydrogenase, alkaline phosphatase and TPS all had a statistically significant association with survival. Patients with a histology of undifferentiated large cell carcinoma had also a significantly worse survival compared to patients with adenocarcinomas or squamous cell carcinomas. Age, weight loss, gamma-glutamyltranspeptidase and gender showed no statistically significant association with survival. Multivariate analyses revealed that stage of disease, performance status, histology and TPS were the most important prognostic factors. Addition of any of the other factors considered did not significantly improve the fit of the model. A tenfold increase of TPS was associated with a relative death rate of 1.9. The survival curves of patients based on their TPS levels are shown in figure 2.

Table I. Patient characteristics.

No. of patients	203	
Sex		
female	40	(20%)
male	163	(80%)
Median age (years)	59	
range	29–81	
Performance (ECOG)[a]		
0	34	(17%)
1	115	(58%)
2	43	(21%)
3	6	(3%)
4	2	(1%)
Stage		
3A	58	(29%)
3B	37	(18%)
4	108	(53%)
Histology		
adenocarcinoma	64	(32%)
squamous cell carcinoma	76	(37%)
large cell undifferentiated carcinoma	63	(31%)

[a]Missing data ECOG: n = 3

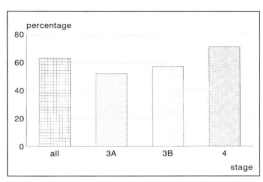

Figure 1. Percentage of patients with a TPS level > 100 U/l for all patients and according to stage.

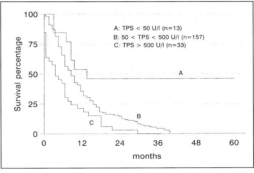

Figure 2. Survival curces of patients with NSCLC based on their TPS levels.

Discussion

Well known prognostic factors in patients with non-small cell lung cancer are: extent of disease, the performance status of the patient, weight loss, and gender in a number of studies. Several biochemical parameters such as alkaline phosphatase and lactate dehydrogenase have been related to the prognosis of a patient.

In this study we observed that frequently high TPS levels can be found in the sera of patients with non-small cell lung cancer. Multivariate analyses revealed that TPS was an independent prognostic factor for survival. Although higher TPS levels were found in stage 4 compared to stage 3 disease both stage of the disease and TPS were independent prognostic factors in the multivariate analysis. Further studies are warranted to elucidated the exact relation between TPS and the total tumorload, the growth rate of the tumor and treatment related factors.

Acknowledgement

We thank Beki Diagnostics AB, Bromma, Sweden, for providing the TPS-kits used in this study.

References

1 American Joint Committee on Cancer (1988) In: Beahrs OH, Henson DE, Hutter RV, Myers MH (eds) Manual for staging of cancer. PA: Philadelphia, Lippincott Co, pp 115–122
2 Kaplan EL, Meier P (1958) Nonparametric estimation from incomplete observations. J Am Stat Assoc 53:457–481
3 Mantel N (1966) Evaluation of survival data and two new rank order statistics arising in its consideration. Cancer Chemother Rep 50:163–70
4 Cox DR (1972) Regression models and life tables (with discussion). J Roy Stat Soc (B) 34:187–220

Address for correspondence:
Dr. A. van der Gaast
Department of Medical Oncology
University Hospital Rotterdam-Dijkzigt
Dr. Molewaterplein 40
NL-3015 GD Rotterdam, The Netherlands

CYFRA 21-1, TPA, TPAcyk and TPS versus CEA, CA 19-9, SCC and NSE in lung cancer

G. Gittermann[a], R. Klapdor[d], M. Bahlo[d], E. Kaukel[b], I. Beuerlein[c], N. Dahlmann[d], D. Jaworrek[e]

[a]Department of Nuclear Medicine, [b]Department of Pulmonology, [c]Department of Laboratory Medicine, [d]General Hospital, Harburg; Department of Internal Medicine, [e]University Hospital, Hamburg; BM Research Center, Tutzing, Germany

Introduction

Recently cytokeratin markers are attracting more and more clinical interest. Cytokeratins or cytokeratin fragments are released by epithelial cells and recent studies suggest a high sensitivity of assays measuring cytokeratin 19 especially in non-small cell lung cancer (NSCLC).

In order to evaluate the clinical relevance of these markers and in containing previous comparative studies we measured prospectively the serum concentrations of the tumor associated antigens CEA, CA 19-9, SCC and NSE and compared the results with those of the cytokeratin markers CYFRA 21-1, TPA, TPS and TPAcyk (1, 2, 3) in benign and malignant lung and gastrointestinal diseases.

Patients and methods

The studies were performed in 178 lung cancer patients (109 before primary treatment), in 30 healthy controls, in 28 patients with benign lung diseases and in 65 patients suffering from benign and malignant gastrointestinal disorders (n = 25 liver cirrhosis, n = 20 colon polyps, n = 20 pancreatic cancer). All lung cancer patients were splitted by histology and TNM-stage. The diagnoses were proven by histology.

The studies were done using CEA and CYFRA 21-1 (Enzymun EIA BM), SCC (EIA Abbott), CA 19-9 (Cobas Core Roche), NSE (RIA Pharmacia), TPA (LIA-mat Byk Sangtec), TPS (IRMA Beki), TPAcyk (IRMA medac).

Results and discussion

In contrast to healthy controls patients suffering from benign diseases of the lung and the gastrointestinal tract partly showed significantly elevated values for the cytokeratin markers (table I).

With respect to the 95% specificity in benign lung diseases the following tumor markers showed the highest sensitivity in lung cancer:

CEA with 38% for adenocarcinomas, CYFRA 21-1 with 49 and 62% for squameous and large cell carcinomas, NSE for small cell lung cancer.

Examples for stage relation are shown in figure 1a and 1b (table II).

CYFRA 21-1 shows a relation to stage in that way, that mainly stage IV patients are showing significantly elevated levels compared to the stage I–III patients (figure 1a). The difference is less pro-

Table I. Mean values ± SD for the cytokeratin markers measured in the study in healthy controls as well as in patients suffering from benign diseases of the lung and the gastrointestinal tract.

Marker	Controls	Benign	
		lung diseases	gastroint. diseases
CYFRA 21-1 (ng/ml)	1.2 ± 0.36	2.6 ± 0.56	3.6 ± 3.5
TPA (U/L)	59.2 ± 38.1	43.9 ± 17.9	447 ± 826
TPS (U/L)	60.0 ± 102	101 ± 80	1571 ± 4196
TPAcyk (ng/ml)	0.58 ± 0.35	1.26 ± 0.99	11.9 ± 29

Table II. Sensitivity of cytokeratin markers in comparison to CEA, CA 19-9, SCC and NSE in lung cancer disease in relation to the 95% specificity in healthy controls and benign lung diseases, respectively.

95% Specificity (benign diseases)		CEA > 4.5	TPA > 80	TPS > 216	CYF > 3.3	SCC > 3.4	NSE > 12.5	CA 19-9 > 53
Adeno-ca.	(n = 34)	38%	32%	18%	29%	3%	9%	18%
SCC	(n = 53)	19	40	19	49	25	30	8
LCC	(n = 23)	35	48	39	61	22	30	26
SCLC	(n = 55)	29	22	20	27	0	53	25
95% Specificity (healthy controls)		> 2.6	> 55	> 93	> 2.0	> 1.6	> 11.7	> 14.3
Adeno-ca.	(n = 34)	65%	44%	59%	59%	12%	9%	62%
SCC	(n = 53)	60	57	53	75	58	36	60
LCC	(n = 23)	65	83	74	83	43	30	65
SCLC	(n = 55)	56	36	49	60	7	53	64

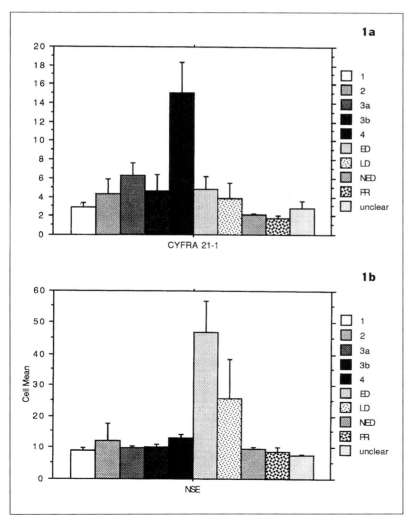

Figure 1. Mean values ± SD for CYFRA 21-1 (a) and NSE (b) in relation to tumor stage in 178 lung cancer patients (ED = extended disease, LD = limited disease, NED = no evidence of disease, PR = partial remission).

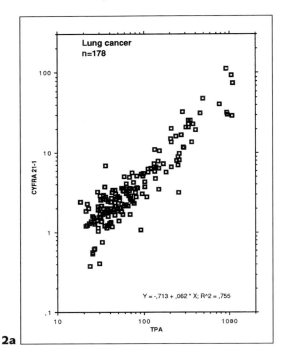
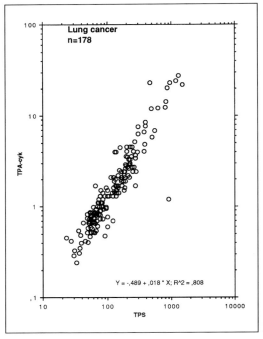
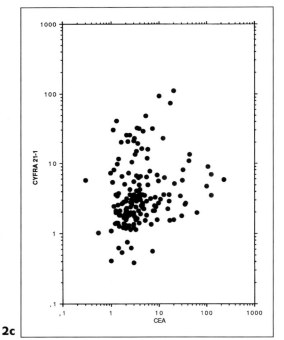
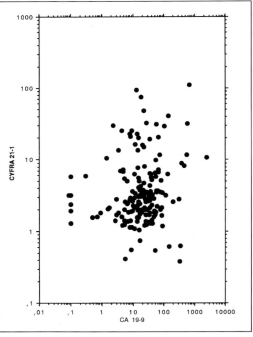

Figure 2. Evidence for a significant correlation between the serum concentrations of CYFRA 21-1 and TPA (a), TPS and TPA cyk (b), in contrast to the comparison between CYFRA 21-1 and the tumor associated antigens CEA, SCC and CA 19-9 (c, d, e) or between CYFRA 21-1 and NSE (f).

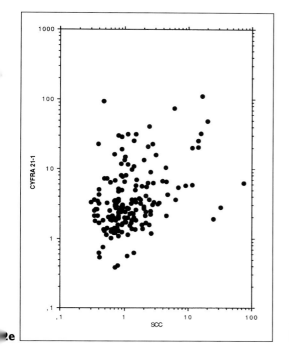
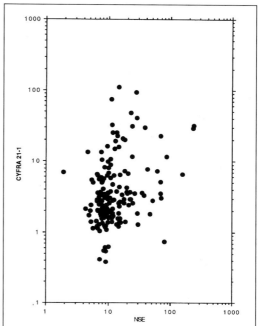

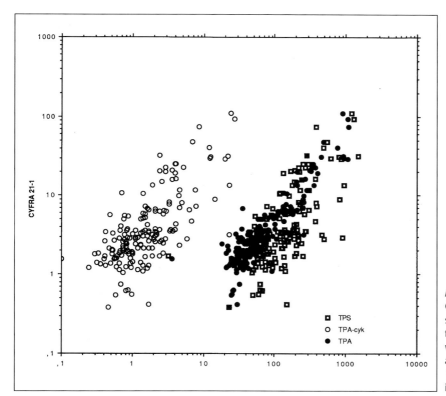

Figure 3. Comparison of the serum concentrations of CYFRA 21-1 with those of TPS and TPAcyk/TPA in 178 patients suffering from lung cancer.

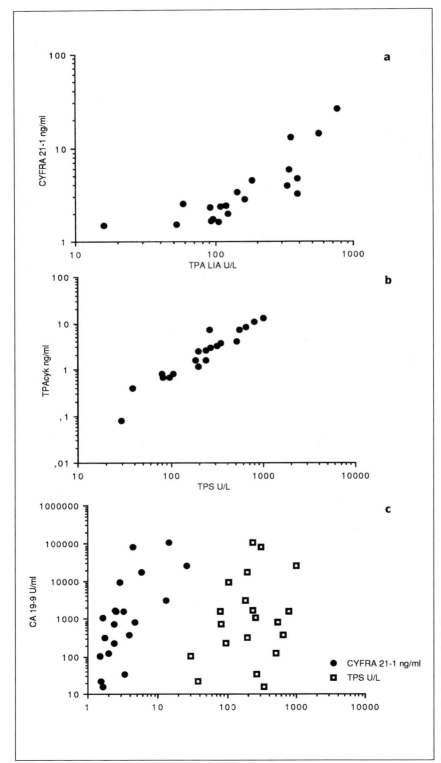

Figure 4. Comparison of the serum concentrations of CYFRA 21-1 with TPA (a), TPAcyk with TPS (b) and of CYFRA 21-1 and TPS with CA 19-9 (c) in 20 patients suffering from exocrine pancreatic cancer.

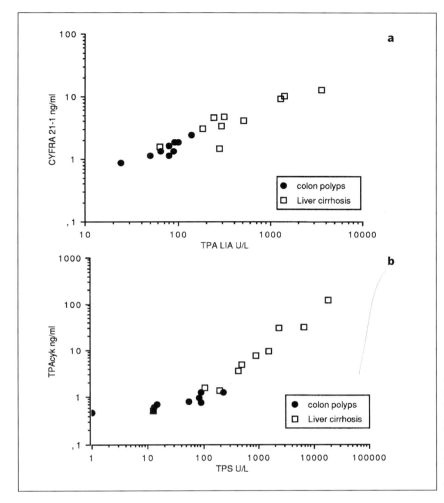

Figure 5. Comparison of the serum concentrations for CYFRA 21-1 with TPA (a) and TPAcyk with TPS (b) in 20 patients suffering from benign diseases of the gastrointestinal tract.

nounced for patients with limited and extended disease. Patients with NED or PR under treatment showed only slightly elevated levels.

In contrast, e.g. NSE showed no significant correlation to stage I–IV of the disease in our patients (figure 1b), whereas CEA, TPS and the others showed a correlation similar to CYFRA 21-1. Looking for a correlation between the various markers measured we find a significant correlation between CYFRA 21-1 and TPA as well as between TPS and TPAcyk in aggreement with immunological studies of other groups demonstrating that CYFRA 21-1 and TPA are measuring cytokeratin 19 alone and in addition to CK 8 and 18, respectively, in contrast to the monoclonal antibodies used in the TPS and TPA cyk assay mainly measuring cytokeratin 18.

However, we did not find a correlation between the cytokeratin markers and the tumor associated antigens CEA, CA 19-9 and SCC (figures 2a–f).

The correlation betweeen the assays measuring cytokeratin 19 fragments and cytokeratin 18 fragments are not so pronounced as the correlation between CYFRA 21-1 and TPA on the one hand or TPs and TPAcyk on the other hand (figures 3a, b)

A similar situation we also find for patients suffering from gastrointestinal cancer disease, like pancreatic cancer (figures 4a–c), as well as for patients suffering from benign diseases (figures 5a, b).

The results in patients suffering from benign gastrointestinal diseases also underline the necessity to calculate the sensitivity on the basis of the 95% specificity of benign diseases of the various organs of the gastrointestinal tract. Patients with colon polyps (median TPS 34 U/l, TPA 120 U/l, TPA cyk 0.77 ng/ml, CYFRA 21-1 1.3 ng/ml) e.g. show a significantly lower 95% specificity level than patients with liver cirrhosis (median TPS 679, TPA 304 U/l, TPA cyk 6.5 ng/ml, CYFRA 21-1 4.4 ng/ml) (figure 6a).

Summarizing, our data confirm CYFRA 21-1 as the most sensitive marker in NSCLC followed by CEA, and NSE as the most sensitive marker for SCLC. CYFRA 21-1 shows a narrow correlation to the TPA values, a less pronounced correlation to TPS and TPA cyk. In the case of simultaneous benign diseases of the gastrointestinal tract, however, one should take into consideraton that some benign diseases like liver cirrhosis may result in significantly elevated cytokeratin serum concentrations compared to benign lung diseases.

References

[1] Bahlo M, Strüven D, Klapdor R (1993) TPAcyk ELISA zur quantitativen Bestimmung des Tissue Polypeptide Antigen im Serum. Labor Med 16:24–26

[2] Boers JL, Ramaekers FC, Rot MK, Oostendorp T, Huysmans A, van Muijen GN, Wagenaar SS, Voojs GP (1988) Cytokeratins in different types of human lung cancer as monitored by chain-specific monoclonal antibodies.

[3] Hasholzner U, Stieber P, Fiebig M, Sunder-Plassmann L, Fatheh-Moghadam (1992) CYFRA – a new tumor marker for non-small cell lung cancer (NSCLC). In: Klapdor R (ed) Tumor associated antigens, oncogenes, receptors, cytokines in tumor diagnoses and therapy at the beginning of the nineties. 6th Symposium on Tumor Markers, Hamburg. Zuckschwerdt, München pp 130–133

Address for correspondence:
Prof. Dr. R. Klapdor
Medizinische Abteilung
Universität Hamburg
Martinistraße 52
D-20246 Hamburg, Germany

Can CYFRA 21-1 replace tissue polypeptide antigen (TPA)?
Studies on different patient groups including those with renal insufficiency

B. Lüdtke, G. Bahlmann, W. G. Wood

Institute for Clinical Laboratory Diagnoses,
Clinic of Hansestadt Stralsund, Stralsund, Germany

Introduction

Tissue polypeptide antigen (TPA) is a useful, though structurally ill-defined proliferation marker. It has been shown that TPA reacts with antibodies directed against cytokeratins 8, 18 and 19. This has led to the development of a new TPA immunometric assay in which monoclonal antibodies to cytokeratins 8, 18 and 19 have been used (TPA-M Kit, Byk-Sangtec, Dietzenbach, Germany). This kit has not been used in the present study.

Tissue polypeptide antigen is elevated during cell regeneration and proliferation (1) processes involving cytokeratins. For this reason, it was decided to compare CYFRA 21-1, a fragment of cytokeratin 19 defined by two monoclonal antibodies, with TPA levels in serum from healthy volunteers and different patient groups.

As TPA is known to be elevated in many patients with renal insufficiency (2), the question was posed as to whether CYFRA 21-1 serum levels were elevated in this group of patients. If not, CYFRA 21-1 would provide a marker for cell proliferation, which is independent of renal function.

Materials, methods and reference ranges

Tissue polypeptide antigen

Tissue polypeptide antigen was measured with the polyclonal immunoluminometric assay from Byk-Sangtec (LIA-MAT TPA Kit). Samples were measured in a semi-automatic 250-sample luminometer (LB 952 16T, E.G.&G.-Berthold, Bad Wildbad, Germany).

The median concentration found in healthy volunteers of both sexes between 16 and 65 years was 36 U/l (range 10–75 U/l), so that the reference range for this group was given as less than 75 U/l. No correlation was made with age and no cut-off levels were calculated. In view of the median age of hospitalised patients being around 60 years, this reference range must be treated with care.

CYFRA 21-1

CYFRA 21-1 was measured using the Enzymun Test System® ES 300 (Boehringer-Mannheim, Mannheim, Germany) and a fully automated immunoenzymometric assay.

The median value found in healthy blood donors was 1.22 µg/l (range 0.44–3.08 µg/l) so that a reference range of less than 3.1 µg/l was established. The same restrictions were applied on the use of this reference range as for TPA.

Groups of patients investigated

Patients attending the renal dialysis unit were measured before and after hemodialysis to examine the acute effects of this process. A correlation between TPA and CYFRA 21-1 was made on 66 samples, 50 taken before and after, and 16 either before or after dialysis.

A further group of patients attending the hematological-oncological out-patient clinic were also studied. They were divided into two different groups, those having a CYFRA 21-1 serum level lying within the reference range defined above, and those with elevated CYFRA 21-1. Other tumor markers were also determined as part of the routine diagnosis and follow-up in these patients.

Results and discussion

Table I and figure 1 show the results from the renal dialysis patients. In table I, which shows values from 15 patients, the serum creatinine values have been included as a measure of efficiency of the dialysis process. Tables II and III show the data from 20 patients with low CYFRA 21-1 levels and 15 with elevated levels. Figure 2 shows the correlation between CYFRA 21-1 and TPA in the patients shown in table III. Only patients with confirmed diagnosis or visual data (x-ray, CT, MRT) were included in this presentation. The data in the diagnosis columns was that at the time of the laboratory request.

It can be seen from table I that the behavior of CYFRA 21-1 and TPA is similar, values on average being 16% higher for TPA and 10% higher for

Table I. Serum TPA, CYFRA 21-1 and creatinine before (1) and after (2) dialysis together with percent changes. Concentration units: TPA = U/l; CYFRA 21-1 = µg/l; creatinine = µmol/l.

Pat. no.	TPA -1	TPA - 2	C 21-1 (1)	C 21-1 (2)	Creatinine -1	Creatinine -2	TPA diff %	C-21 diff%	Crea diff%
1	49	56	1.60	2.30	778	285	14.29	43.75	-63.37
2	82	121	3.13	4.28	1171	560	47.56	36.74	-52.18
3	105	63	3.41	2.64	701	218	-40.00	-22.58	-68.90
4	39	41	2.72	2.52	443	270	5.13	-7.35	-39.05
5	61	74	2.54	3.37	787	407	21.31	32.68	-48.28
6	66	100	2.34	2.85	615	312	51.52	21.79	-49.27
7	71	98	2.22	3.01	503	287	38.03	35.59	-42.94
8	81	100	3.13	3.73	1215	752	23.46	19.17	-38.11
9	146	187	4.86	5.37	838	454	28.08	10.49	-45.82
10	55	48	3.13	3.11	757	511	-12.73	-0.64	-32.50
11	80	90	4.30	5.51	590	143	12.50	28.14	-75.76
12	113	83	5.15	4.32	746	346	-26.55	-16.12	-53.62
13	89	76	3.57	3.19	1090	655	-14.61	-10.64	-39.91
14	111	129	4.72	4.84	935	384	16.22	2.54	-58.93
15	139	174	4.52	4.44	1011	393	25.18	-1.77	-61.13
Median	81	90	3.13	3.37	778	384	16.22	10.49	-49.27

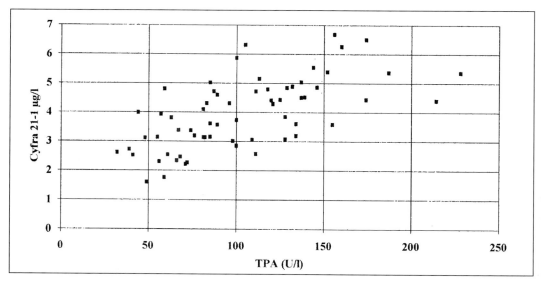

Figure 1. The relationship between TPA (x) and CYFRA 21-1 (y) in 66 serum samples from dialysis patients, taken before and after dialysis. The correlation is statistically significant at the level $p < 0.01$.

CYFRA 21-1 immediately after dialysis. This means that it is important in such patients to measure these analytes either before or after dialysis to standardise the comparability of results of within-patient control or follow-up. The creatinine values show those expected with an average drop of around 50% during dialysis.

Figure 1 shows a statistically significant correlation between TPA and CYFRA 21-1 in dialysis patients, both analytes behaving similarly in most cases. The concentrations of TPA in this collective are lower than those reported in the literature (3), although the relationship between the median concentration and the upper limit of the reference ranges was the same for both analytes.

Table II shows that in 18/20 patients CYFRA 21-1 and TPA gave results lying within the reference range, 2/20 patients having borderline TPA. This may represent the marginal additional reaction of cytokeratins 8 and 18 in these patients. Neuron

Table II. Tumor patients with normal CYFRA 21-1 levels. TPA and NSE levels and clinical diagnosis are given.

Pat. no.	CYFRA 21-1 (µg/l)	TPA (U/l)	NSE (ug/l)	Diagnosis
1	1.09	29	33.9	small cell lung carcinoma (SCLC)
2	1.26	27	10.1	adrenal tumor
3	2.82	34	36.4	SCLC
4	1.46	45	34.1	liver metastases - primary tumor unknown
5	0.92	23	22.2	SCLC
6	2.96	57	18.3	? SCLC
7	3.07	16	20.7	SCLC
8	2.83	36	13.5	lung tumor
9	3.09	18	13.9	? SCLC
10	2.05	15	18.1	vulva ca.
11	2.76	44	46.7	SCLC
12	2.34	51	8.5	? SCLC
13	2.62	36	18.9	? tumor
14	1.83	22	9.2	SCLC - post treatment
15	1.49	84	6.5	lung tumor
16	1.63	82	6.6	? lung tumor
17	2.19	32	8.6	? lung tumor
18	2.31	18	10.7	Tbc., pneumonia, ? lung tumor
19	2.22	64	10.5	lung tumor with metastases
20	2.53	72	10.5	bone metastases – primary bladder tumor

Table III. Tumor patients with elevated CYFRA 21-1 levels. TPA and NSE levels and clinical diagnosis are given.

Pat. no.	C 21-1 (µg/l)	TPA (U/l)	NSE (µg/l)	SCC (µg/l)	CEA (µg/l)	CA 19-9 (kU/l)	Diagnosis
1	34.5	1300	20.7		108	133	coecum ca.
2	17.1	367	13.6				bronchial ca. with metastases
3	22.9	409	12.3	19.9	21		squamous cell ca.
4	20.1	319	4.7				bronchial ca.
5	514	14400	48.8	0.6	14.2		CUP syndrome
6	10.7	118	16.5	0.6	<1	< 2	bronchial ca.
7	76.8	1470	16.8	0.2	9.9		bronchial ca.
8	8.2	112	11.7	1.7			bronchial ca.
9	8.8	138	5.1				neoplasm
10	7.3	52	4.9		66.7		colon ca. (pre-therapy)
11	6.4	46	5.2	1.9	680	< 2	bronchial ca.
12	11.9	124	8.3	1.7	6.7	< 2	bronchial ca.
13	34.4	274	12.7	0.8	39.9		? bronchial ca.
14a	18.5	167	9.3		1.28	58.8	bronchial ca. (20.1.93)
14b	32.9	729	8.3	2.5			bronchial ca. (27.1.93)

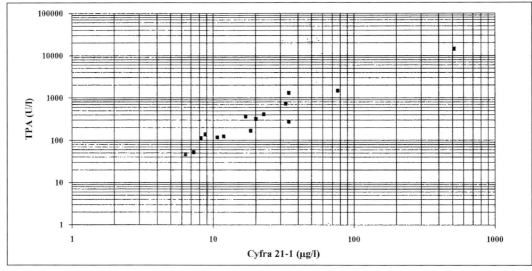

Figure 2. The relationship between CYFRA 21-1 (x) and TPA (y) in the 15 patients shown in table III. There is a clear linear relationship between both analyses. The double logarithmic scale has been chosen to demonstrate the distribution of values more clearly.

specific enolase (NSE) values are shown in table II as many patients were suspected of having a small cell lung carcinoma (SCLC).

Table III shows full concordance of TPA and CYFRA 21-1 in those cases with elevated CYFRA 21-1. This group consisted mainly of non-small cell bronchial carcinomata (NSCLC), or mixed tumors. Figure 2 confirms the close correlation between CYFRA 21-1 and TPA.

Conclusions

In the groups of patients studied here, it is possible to replace TPA by CYFRA 21-1, thus saving time and money in the laboratory. The choice of CYFRA 21-1 as analyte is that it has been defined by two monoclonal antibodies, thus standardising what is measured. The full automation of this analyte, together with the excellent precision (data not shown), allow singlicate determinations.

For those laboratories not possessing an Enzymun System ES 300, ES 600 or ES 700, but able to perform luminescence and radioisotopic measurements, TPA offers an alternative with comparable diagnostic sensitivity, which can only be improved by the introduction of the new TPA-M assay.

Finally, CYFRA 21-1 levels are also dependent upon renal function in the same way as TPA, a point which must be taken into consideration for renal dialysis patients and other patients with impared renal function.

References

1. Schultek T, Wood WG (1985) Tissue polypeptide antigen (TPA) as prognostic parameter in small-cell and non-small-cell bronchial carcinoma. Ärztl Lab 31:273–279
2. Wood WG, Werner A (1984) CEA, TPA and CA 125 levels in different patient groups with benign and malignant disease. Ärztl Lab 30:309–315
3. Stieber P, Dienemann H, Hasholzner U, Müller C, Poley S, Hoffmann K, Fateh-Moghadam A (1993) Comparison of cytokeratin fragment 19 (CYFRA 21-1), tissue polypeptide antigen (TPA) and tissue polypeptide specific antigen (TPS) as tumor markers in lung cancer. Eur J Clin Chem Clin Biochem 31:689–694

Address for correspondence:
Prof. Dr. med. W.G. Wood
Institut für Klinische Laboratoriumsdiagnostik
Klinikum der Hansestadt Stralsund
Postfach 103
D-18402 Stralsund, Germany

In: R. Klapdor (ed)
Current Tumor Diagnosis: Applications, Clinical Relevance, Research, Trends
Cancer of the Lung – State and Trends in Diagnosis and Therapy
© 1994 W. Zuckschwerdt Verlag München · Bern · Wien · New York

Biochemical characterization of CYFRA 21-1, a serum marker for monitoring of lung cancer

H. Bodenmüller[a], B. Ofenloch[a], B. Lane[b], D. Banauch[a], A. Dessauer[a]
[a]Boehringer Mannheim GmbH, Research Center Tutzing, Germany,
[b]The University of Dundee, Department of Anatomy and Physiology, Dundee, UK

Introduction

Enzymun-Test® CYFRA 21-1 is a new serum test for diagnosis and monitoring of non small cell lung cancer (NSCLC), especially squamous cell carcinoma. The development of this test was guided by clear biochemical principles.

Cytokeratins (CK) were chosen as a target group for the selection of the analyte because of its wide use in immunohistochemical tumor diagnosis (1). Since cytokeratins form the inner skeleton of the cell, they are poorly soluble in aequous solutions. The basic idea of the test development was to screen for the presence of soluble cytokeratin fragments in human sera with a possible relationship between cytokeratin concentration and malignant diseases.

Presently 20 members of the cytokeratin family are known, all of them have the same basic molecular structure (1): An α-helical, hydrophylic rod domain is flanked by two hydrophobic sections, the so-called head region (N-terminal) and tail region (C-terminal) of the molecule; the hydrophobic head and tail region do not form helical structures. According to their isolectric point, cytokeratins are divided in type I acidic (CK 9-20) and type II basic (CK 1-8) molecules. In vivo, type I and type II molecules form a 1:1 molecular complex, the so-called coiled-coil structure (figure1).

Methods and results

In order to select the best antibody combination for the test, a wide variety of monoclonal antibodies against different cytokeratins were tested (table I). The search concentrated on antibodies against cytokeratin 8, 18 and 19, however, also monoclonal antibodies reacting with a broad CK-specificity were tested. The selection was done exclusively according to clinical criteria by testing different sandwich combinations against carefully assembled serum panels. These panels contained samples from patients with malignant diseases with the emphasis on lung cancer and sera from patients with possibly interfering conditions, for instance benign lung diseases, autoimmune diseases, and inflammatory diseases of the GI tract.

By this way the combination of the two antibodies Ks 19.1 (3) and BM 19.21 was selected out of more than 200 different sandwich combinations. The best sensitivity for lung cancer together with the best specificity against the possibly interfering patient groups was achieved with Ks 19.1 as capture antibody and BM 19.21 as tracer antibody. The reactivity was tested with purified, single stranded preparations of CK 8, CK 18 and

Table I. Monoclonal antibodies against cytokeratins investigated during the development of Enzymun-Test® CYFRA 21-1.

Antibody	Specificity
a 4.1	CK 8
8.42	CK 8
17.2	CK 8
CK 2	CK 18
27 IV B 1	CK 18
27 I C 5	CK 18
Ks 19.1 // A 53-B / A 2	CK 19
Ks 19.2 // BM 19.21	CK 19
b 170	CK 19
pan 1-8	CK 1 – CK 8
LU 5	broad spec.
CAM 5.2	CK 8, CK 18, CK 19
K$_G$ 8.13	broad spec.
AE 1	CK 10, CK 14, CK 15, CK 16, CK 19

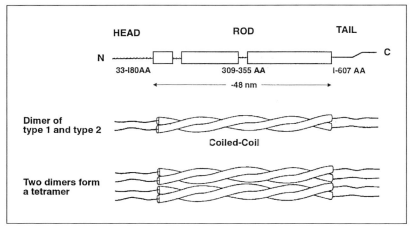

Figure 1. Principal structure of cytokeratins (according to Kartenbeck (2)).

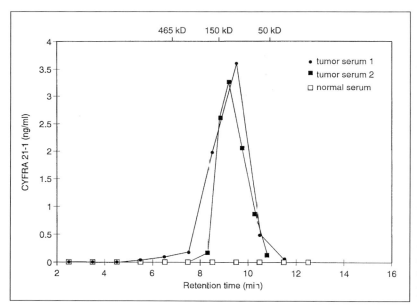

Figure 2. Size determination of the CYFRA 21-1 serum analyte after HPLC separation on a TSK 3000 column. The collected fractions were assayed in the Enzymun-Test® CYFRA 21-1.

Table II. Binding sites of the two monoclonal antibodies selected for Enzymun-Test® CYFRA 21-1.

	BM 19.21	Ks 19.1
CK 19	**qladvradserqnq** 348–361	**kaaledtlaetearf** 317–331
CK 18	elaqtraeggrqaq 348–361	kaslenslreveary 317–331
CK 8		rasleaaiadaeqrg 124–138

CK 19. Even against high concentrations of these analytes the antibodies reacted exclusively with CK 19, no cross reactivity against CK 8 or CK 18 could be observed.

Since the complete aminoacid sequence of CK 19 is known (4) the exact binding sites of both antibodies could be determined by epitope mapping. As shown in table II, both binding sites are close together on coil 2 of the cytokeratin 19 molecule. Sequence homologies exist for both epitopes; e.g. a homology on CK18 can be observed for the epitope of Ks 19.1. However, as stated before, no cross reactivity exists against CK 18 and CK 8.

As source of the standard material the human breast carcinoma cell line MCF-7 was used which is known to be especially rich in CK 8, 18 and 19. After isolation and purification of the CK fraction, the hydrophobic head and tail part were removed by a controlled digestion with chymotrypsin. After reconstitution the fragments of CK 8 and 18 or 19 rearranged in the coiled-coil structure. This preparation was used as standard material.

In order to get information about the size of the in vivo occurring serum analyte, three human sera, two from lung cancer patients and one from a normal healthy person, were analyzed under physiological conditions with HPLC technique. The elution pattern (figure 2) showed no signal for the normal serum sample. However, the two patient samples had an almost identical signal at 100 ± 10 kD. Since this is much higher than the molecular weight of the single stranded CK 19-fragment (40 kD), the serum analyte occurs obviously in an aggregated form, probably complexed with other cytokeratins from the type II fraction.

The work described above gave the solid biochemical basis for the test development of Enzymun-Test® CYFRA 21-1 (5). The selection procedure of two cytokeratin 19 specific antibodies with no cross reactivities and known epitope binding sites demonstrates clearly the necessity of a careful antibody selection according to clinical criteria.

References

1 Broers JLV et al (1988) Cytokeratins in different types of human lung cancer as monitored by chain-specific monoclonal antibodies. Cancer Res 48: 3221–3229
2 Kartenbeck J (1989) Intermediate filament proteins – diagnostic markers in tumor pathology. Interdisc Sci Rev 14:278–283
3 Conrad K et al (1988) Immunoblotting of monoclonal anti-cytoskeletal antibodies with cytoskeletal extracts of Hela and MCF-7 cells. Biomed Biochem Auto 47:697–703
4 Stasiak PC, Lane EB (1987) Sequence of cDNA coding for human keratin 19. Nucl Acids Res 15:10058
5 Bodenmüller H et al (1994) Lung cancer associated keratin 19-fragments: development and biochemical characterization of the new serum assay Enzymun Test® CYFRA 21-1. Int J Biol Markers, in press

Address for correspondence:
Dr. rer. nat. H. Bodenmüller
Forschungszentrum Tutzing
Boehringer Mannheim
Bahnhofstraße 9-15
D-82327 Tutzing/Obb., Germany

Secretion of CYFRA 21-1, TPS and TPA as well as CEA in relation to growth kinetics – Studies in nude mice bearing xenografts of human lung and pancreatic carcinomas

M. Rameken[a], M. Bahlo[a], A. Hassanein[a], R. Klapdor[a], A. von Osten[b], A. Niendorf[b]

[a]Department of Internal Medicine, [b]Department of Pathology, University Hospital, Hamburg, Germany

Introduction

In order to find an answer to the question recently discussed whether cytokeratin markers may be used as proliferation markers in clinical oncology we continued previous studies. In nude mice bearing xenografts of human carcinomas we studied the secretion behavior of the cytokeratin markers CYFRA 21-1 (2, 3), TPS and TPA in comparison to the tumor associated antigen CEA which is not discussed as a proliferation marker.

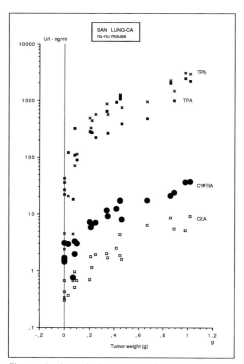

Figure 1. A typical example for the secretion behavior of the tumor markers CYFRA 21-1, TPA, TPS and CEA in relation to the tumor weight.

Methods

The studies were done in nude mice, females or castrated males, age 5–8 weeks, body weigt 20–30 g, bearing established xenografts of human pancreatic (n = 3) and lung carcinomas (n = 3).
In addition to tumor volume and tumor weigth the serum concentrations of CEA (Enzymun EIA BM), TPS (IRMA Beki), TPA (IRMA-mat Byk-Sangtec) and CYFRA 21-1 (Enzymun EIA BM) were measured. Immunohistochemically proliferation was studied using the MIB 1 assay. Necrosis rate was estimated in percent of tumor volume by microscopy.
In addition, we studied the effects of chemotherapeutic treatment for three weeks with mitomycin C, 2.4 mg/kg i.p. per week, and 5-fluorouracil, 80 mg/kg i.p. per week, on serum concentrations of the markers measured and on tumor volume/weigth in experiments with three different tumors.

Results and discussion

1. The measured tumor markers CYFRA 21-1, TPS and TPA as well as CEA show a significant correlation between the serum concentrations and the tumor volume up to volumes between 0.8 and 1.0 g. The results show no differences in the secretion behavior between CEA and the cytokeratin markers (figure 1).
2. The serum concentrations of the cytokeratin markers show a narrow correlation (figures 2a,b) and a less pronounced correlation to the serum concentrations of CEA (figure 2c).
3. As known from other studies the various human xenografts show significantly different secretion

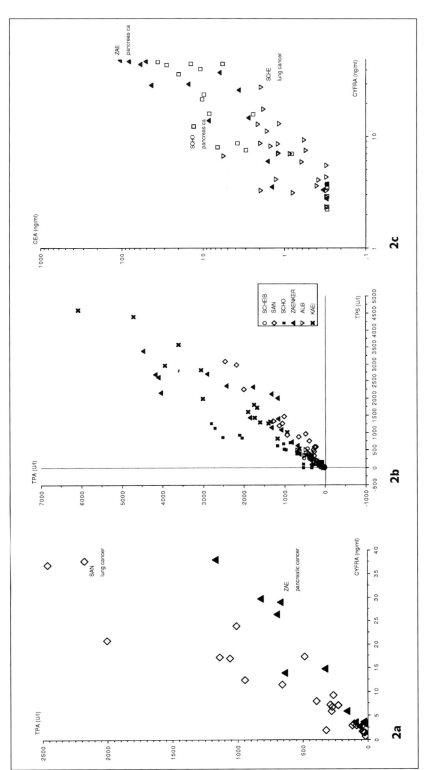

Figure 2. Evidence for a significant correlation between CYFRA 21-1 and TPA (a), TPA and TPS (b) and a less pronounced correlation between the cytokeratin marker CYFRA 21-1 and the tumor associated antigen CEA (c) in studies in nude mice bearing xenografts of lung (◇) and pancreatic (▲) carcinomas, respectively.

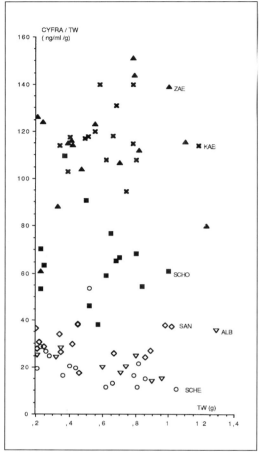

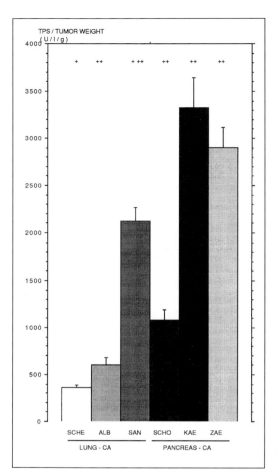

Figure 3. Demonstration of different individual secretion rates of CYFRA 21-1 in relation to the tumor weight for various human xenografts (lung carcinomas = open circles, pancreatic carcinomas = closed circles) – as it is also known for other tumor markers.

Figure 4. Secretion rates for TPS for the various human xenografts studied lacking a correlation to immunohistologically defined proliferation rate of the tumors (+/++/+++).

Table I. Necrosis and proliferation rates measured for the established xenografts used in this study.

Tumor	Necrosis	(%)	Proliferation
Sche	lung cancer	54	+
Alb	lung cancer	25	++
San	lung cancer	50	+++
Scho	pancreatic cancer	47	++
Kae	pancreatic cancer	42	++
Zae	pancreatic cancer	56	++

rates for the individual tumor markers as shown in figure 3 and 4.
4. The various tumors also show a different behavior with respect to necrosis rate and immuno-histochemical proliferation (table I and figure 4). Alltogether the studies do not confirm a correlation between the secretion of TPS into the serum and the immunohistochemically detected proliferation rate measured using the MIB 1 antibody.

In the studies looking for the secretion behavior of the measured tumor markers under chemotherapy with 5-fluorouracil and mitomycin C in comparison to untreated controls we did not find differences in the secretion behavior for the cytokeratin markers and the tumor associated antigen CEA in relation to tumor growth (figure 5).

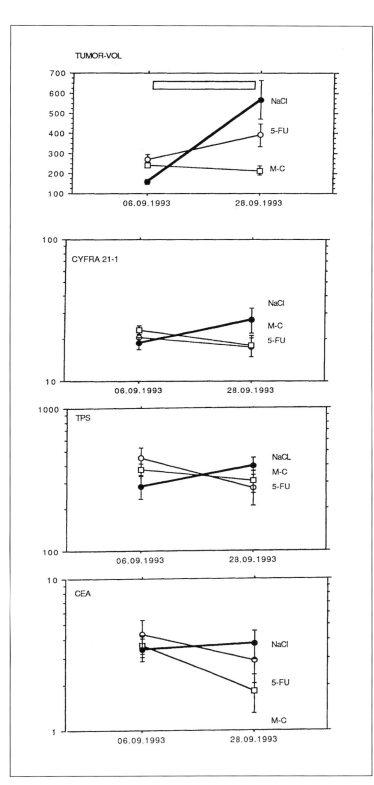

Figure 5. Evidence for a comparable secretion behavior of the studied cytokeratin markers and CEA even under treatment of the xenografts with mitomycin-C, 5-fluorouracil and NaCl (untreated controls).

Summarizing, we did not find relevant differences in the secretion behavior of cytokeratin markers and tumor associated antigens as could be expected from some previous discussions about TPS as a proliferation marker.

References

1. Bahlo M, Strüven D, Klapdor R (1993) TPAcyk ELISA zur quantitativen Bestimmung des Tissue Polypeptide Antigen im Serum. Labor Med 16:24–26
2. Boers JL, Ramaekers FC, Rot MK, Oostendorp T, Huysmans A, van Muijen GN, Wagenaar SS, Voojs GP (1988) Cytokeratins in different types of human lung cancer as monitored by chain-specific monoclonal antibodies.
3. Hasholzner U, Stieber P, Fiebig M, Sunder-Plassmann L, Fatheh-Moghadam (1992) CYFRA – a new tumor marker for non-small cell lung cancer (NSCLC). In: Klapdor R (ed) Tumor associated antigens, oncogenes, receptors, cytokines in tumor diagnosis and therapy at the beginning of the nineties. 6th Symposium on Tumor Markers, Hamburg. Zuckschwerdt, München, pp 130–133

Address for correspondence:
Prof. Dr. R. Klapdor
Medizinische Abteilung
Universitätskrankenhaus
Martinistraβe 52
D-20246 Hamburg, Germany

Embryonic NCAM isoform as a serum tumor marker in small cell lung cancer

Biochemical characterization and methods for detection

B. Auerbach[a], K. Takamatsu[a,e], A. Lang[b], R. Gerardy-Schahn[c], G. Jaques[d], N. Madry[a]

[a]Research Laboratories of Behringwerke AG, Marburg,
[b]Radiochemical Laboratory of Hoechst AG, Frankfurt, [c]Department of Medical Microbiology, Medical Highschool Hannover, [d]Department of Internal Medicine, University of Marburg, Marburg, Germany, [e]Current address: Department of Gynecology and Obstetrics, Saiseikai Kanagawaken Hospital, Yokohama, Japan

Introduction

According to histological criteria and from a clinical point of view, lung carcinoma are classified into two major subgroups, small cell lung cancer (SCLC) and non-SCLC (NSCLC). Patients suffering from SCLC have an especially poor prognosis due to early and widespread metastatic processes. On the other hand, SCLC is sensitive to initial chemotherapy and radiation, whereas the principal therapy of NSCLC is resection of the tumors. A marker which can help to distinguish between SCLC and NSCLC is therefore of utmost clinical importance.

The intercellular adhesion molecule "Neural Cell Adhesion Molecule" (NCAM), which is normally involved in neuron-neuron as well as nerve-muscle cell recognition, was shown to be an excellent immunohistochemical marker in small cell lung cancer (SCLC) (1). Various NCAM forms have been described, which differ in their molecular weights and glycosylation patterns (2). The so-called embryonic form of NCAM (eNCAM) is characterized by its long chains of alpha-2,8-linked N-acetyl-neuraminic acid monomers. This carbohydrate structure is reported to be unique for human proteins and represents the specific epitope for MAb 735 (3). The use of this MAb as capture antibody in an enzyme immunoassay enabled us to identify eNCAM as a valuable serum tumor marker in SCLC (4, 5). Here, we describe the molecular structure of the tumor-associated NCAM form in human serum. Also, we report on even more sensitive radioimmunoassay and luminescence immunoassay developed for improved detection of eNCAM.

Material and methods

eNCAM immunoassays

To improve the performance characteristics over the ELISA for detection of eNCAM described previously (4) we developed two more sensitive immunoassays, RIA-gnost eNCAM and eNCAM CIA, for routine use. For this, MAb 735 specifically binding embryonic NCAM form was adsorbed to polystyrene tubes and anti-NCAM MAb BW SCLC-1 (Behringwerke AG) labeled with ^{125}I or a chemiluminescent acridinium derivative, respectively, were used as tracer. The assay protocol of RIA-gnost eNCAM is briefly summarized in figure 1.

NSE RIA

The concentration of NSE (neuron-specific enolase) was measured using the radioimmunoassay kit from Pharmacia AB (Uppsala, Sweden).

Serum samples

The serum specimens from 221 patients with histologically confirmed SCLC were obtained before therapy. These sera as well as specimens from the control groups were rapidly frozen and stored at $< -20°$ C. From control experiments it is known that repetitive freezing and thawing cycles do not influence the NCAM concentration. NCAM in serum specimens is also stable for some days even at room temperature.

Table I. Number of serum specimens with increased eNCAM or NSE concentrations, respectively.

	n	NSE > 12.5 µg/l	NSE > 25 µg/l	eNCAM > 20 kU/l	NSE/eNCAM > 25 µg/l or > 20 kU/l
Controls	159	13 (8%)	2 (1%)	1 (1%)	2 (1%)
healthy blood donors	78	1 (1%)	0 (0%)	0 (0%)	0 (0%)
benign lung diseases	53	5 (9%)	0 (0%)	0 (0%)	0 (0%)
NSCLC	28	7 (25%)	2 (7%)	1 (4%)	2 (7%)
SCLC	221	134 (61%)	75 (34%)	113 (51%)	131 (59%)
limited disease	75	34 (45%)	11 (15%)	27 (36%)	32 (43%)
extensive disease	146	100 (68%)	64 (44%)	86 (59%)	99 (68%)

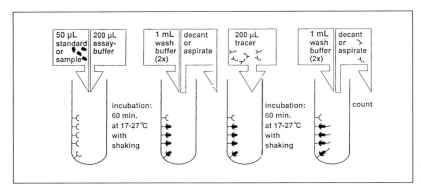

Figure 1. Assay protocol of RIA-gnost eNCAM.

Results and discussion

At least two different species of NCAM can be identified in human serum, a molecule with a molecular weight of 110–130 kD and a second tumor-associated form (150–180 kD) Both are characterized by the absence of epitopes for MAbs binding specifically to the intracellular domains of human NCAM indicating that they are truncated or secreted NCAM species. The only difference between these two forms – causing also the difference in the molecular weights – appears to be the presence of long chains of alpha-2,8-linked N-acetylneuraminic acid on the SCLC-associated NCAM form (= eNCAM) (5).

The polysialic acid-rich eNCAM has been recently found to be a potent serum tumor marker in SCLC: The high diagnostic specificity should enable a non-invasive diagnostic discrimination between SCLC and NSCLC and an elevated serum concentration of eNCAM indicates a poor prognosis. Further, it may be used as a valuable monitoring marker for therapy control and follow-up, respectively (4). On the basis of an identical diagnostic specificity of 99% for benign lung diseases and NSCLC (cut-off for eNCAM: 20 kU/l), eNCAM was shown to be a more sensitive SCLC marker compared to NSE (4) (table I). As eNCAM and NSE assays detect completely different molecules, measuring both markers (cut-off for NSE: 25 µg/l) might increase the diagnostic sensitivity for SCLC without significant loss of specificity (table I). An additional technical advantage over NSE, which is contained in large amounts by erythrocytes and thrombocytes, is the fact that hemolysis does not cause false positive eNCAM test results.

Both new immunoassays for detection of eNCAM, RIA-gnost eNCAM and eNCAM CIA, are characterized by their excellent intra- (1.6% – 4.1%, n = 10) and inter- (2.0% – 8.2%, n = 10) assay precision over the whole measuring range of 0 – 200 kU/l and the high analytical sensitivity (< 0.2 kU/l). Linearity and recovery studies produced results ±10% of the expected concentrations. No interferences were found with hemolytic, lipemic or heterophilic antibodies containing samples (figure 2a). Plasma specimens can also be measured instead of serum samples (figure 2b).

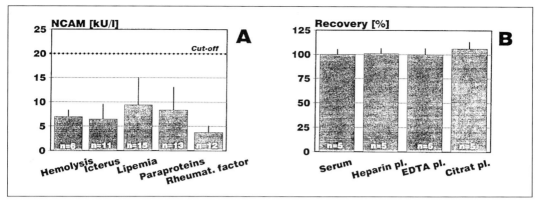

Figure 2. A. eNCAM concentration of various samples containing potentially interferring substances (m ± SD).
B. Recovery rate of eNCAM added to serum or plasma samples.

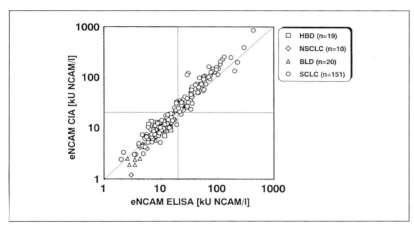

Figure 3. Correlation of eNCAM concentrations of different serum specimens determined with eNCAM CIA and eNCAM ELISA (4). The preliminary cut-off value of eNCAM (20 kU/l) is indicated as dotted line; HBD: healthy blood donors, NSCLC: non-small cell lung cancer patients, BLD: patients with benign lung diseases, SCLC: small cell lung cancer patients.

There is a good correlation between the different NCAM immunoassays and a slightly improved diagnostic sensitivity of the new eNCAM CIA/RIAgnost eNCAM in comparison to eNCAM ELISA originally used for the first preclinical trial (4) (figure 3).

Conclusions

A special form of NCAM carrying alpha-2,8-linked N-acetylneuraminic acid monomers, the so-called embryonic NCAM form or eNCAM, has been found to be a tumor-associated molecule in the serum of patients suffering from small cell lung cancer. New reliable immunossays detecting specifically this NCAM species have been developed and are now available for further investigations.

References

1. Kibbelaar RE et al (1989) J Pathol 159:23–28
2. Goridis C, Brunet JF (1992) Seminars in Cell Biology 3:189–197
3. Finne J et al (1987) J Immunol 138:4402–4407
4. Jaques G et al (1993) Cancer 72:418–425
5. Takamatsu K et al (1994) Cancer Res 54:2598–2603

Address for correspondence:
Dr. med. B. Auerbach
Forschungslabor der Behringwerke AG
Postfach 1140
D-35001 Marburg, Germany

Elevated serum levels of ICTP do not prove bone metastases in small cell lung cancer

W. Ebert, H. Brömmer, B. Schapöhler, Th. Muley

Thoraxklinik, Heidelberg-Rohrbach, Germany

Introduction

The ICTP antigen is a cross-linked carboxy-terminal telopeptide from mature type I collagen fibres. Its concentration was shown to correlate with bone resorption in metabolic bone disease involving high turnover (1) and destruction in rheumatoid arthritis (2). In multiple myeloma, ICTP was reported to function as a tumor-associated antigen reflecting very precisely the clinical data of the malignant disease of bone (3). In a group of 99 patients with bone pain due to metastases of prostate cancer, the serum ICTP concentration was above the reference interval in more than 70% of the patients (4).

In lung cancer, metastatic spread to bone occurs in 10% (5) to 35% (6) of cases at some time during the course of the disease. Radionuclide bone scan was found to be abnormal in as many as 40% of patients at this time. However, even with this form of examination, false-negative results can occur, metastases being detected on microscopic examination of the vertebrae in 10 of 80 autopsied patients who had normal technetium – 99m scans and skeletal roentgenograms shortly before death (7).

We, therefore, have investigated prospectively the clinical use of serum ICTP as an indicator of bone metastases in a group of patients suffering from small cell lung cancer (SCLC). The ICTP levels in SCLC patients with bone metastases, proved by skeletal roentgenogram, were compared to SCLC patients without evidence of bone metastases and control groups consisting of patients with benign chest diseases and healthy persons.

Material and methods

Serum samples investigated in this series were taken from 139 patients admitted to the Thoraxklinik Heidelberg.

Of these 139 patients, 52 (mean age: 60, range: 37–73 years) suffered from SCLC without evidence of bone metastases, 24 (mean age: 61, range: 45–72 years) from SCLC with bone metastases, 11 (mean age: 52, range: 33–69 years) from tuberculosis, 16 (mean age: 50, range: 19–83 years) from empyema thoracis, and 36 (mean age: 55, range: 27–75 years) from other benign chest diseases including idiopathic pulmonary fibrosis, chronic bronchitis, bronchial asthma, sarcoidosis, and pneumonia.

The control group consisted of 52 healthy persons (mean age: 43, range: 24–64 years). All individuals under study were of male sex to exclude rise of ICTP due to osteoporosis in postmenopausal women.

Bone metastases (BM+) in patients with SCLC were proved exclusively by skeletal roentgenogram or CT-scan. ICTP was assessed using the Orion Diagnostica Collagen ICTP RIA which is based on an antigen isolated from human femoral bone (8). For the statistical evaluation, differences betweeen two or more independent samples were tested using Kruskal-Wallis test (9).

Results

Figure 1 shows the distribution of serum ICTP levels in healthy persons, in patients with benign chest diseases, and in SCLC patients with and

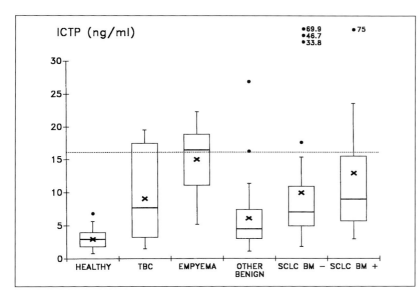

Figure 1. ICTP concentrations in the various study groups. Data are presented as multiple box and whisker plots showing median value (horizontal line), mean value (x), upper and lower quartile and range. Extreme values are plotted separately.

Table I. Results of multiple comparison of ICTP concentrations in the investigation of various study groups (Kruskal-Wallis) (9).

	TBC	Empyema	Other benign	SCLC BM-	SCLC BM+
Healthy	*	*	*	*	*
TBC		+	ns	ns	ns
Empyema			*	*	+
Other benign				*	*
SCLC BM-					ns

+p < 0.05, * p < 0.01, ns = not significant, BM + (-) = bone metastasis positive (negative)

those without bone metastases. The patients suffering from benign chest diseases are classified into the groups tuberculosis, empyema thoracis, and other benign disorders. The median values (5%, 95% percentiles) of ICTP levels for the groups: healthy persons, tuberculosis, empyema thoracis, other benign diseases, SCLC without bone metastases, SCLC with bone metastases were found to be 3.0 (0.9, 4.9), 7.7 (1.5, 19.6), 16.5 (5.2, 22.3), 4.5 (1.5, 16.1), 3.3 (7.1, 33.8), and 9.0 (3.1, 23.6) ng/ml, respectively. The ICTP levels of healthy persons were significantly lower than those of all the other groups (table I). There was also a significant difference between the group with other benign diseases and SCLC patients irrespective of the bone metastasis status. Except for empyema thoracis, there was no difference between tuberculosis and all the other groups. In contrast, the ICTP levels in patients with empyema thoracis were significantly higher compared to those in the other groups including SCLC patients with bone metastases. The ICTP levels in SCLC patients with bone metastases were higher than in those without metastases to the bone, but the difference did not reach a statistically significant level (p = 0.1).

Figure 2 shows sensitivity data obtained with the ICTP assay for the various study populations. These rates are based on a cut-off value which corresponds to the 95% percentile of ICTP concentrations in the group with other benign chest diseases. The highest sensitivity value was observed in empyema thoracis. In SCLC with bone metastases, only 21% of the cases could be identified by elevated ICTP concentrations. The rate of false-positive values in SCLC patients without metastases was about 8%.

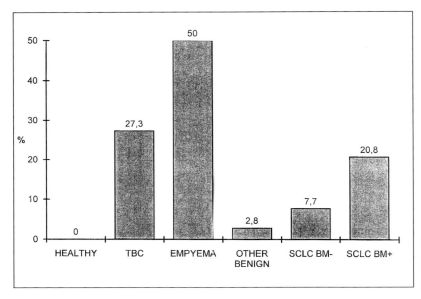

Figure 2. Elevated ICTP concentration (> 16.1 ng/ml) in the populations under study.

Discussion

Our results have shown that the ICTP assay is useless for the detection of bone metastases in patient suffering from SCLC. ICTP has been considered a biochemical marker of type I collagen degradation which occurs in osteolytic metastases (4). A roentgenographic analysis of the osseous system in patients with lung cancer (6) reported bone involvement in 35% of the cases. In roughly three quarters of these, the lesions were osteolytic, predominantly from squamous cell and large cell carcinoma. In the remaining quarter of patients, the metastases were predominantly osteoblastic, in all of these, the cell type was either SCLC or adenocarcinoma. Therefore, ICTP measurement might not be very suitable for the detection of osteoblastic bone metastases in SCLC. As a consequence, markers such as propeptide of type I procollagen (PICP) which reflect osteoblastic activity may be more useful indicators for this purpose.

The elevated ICTP levels in patients with tuberculosis may be derived from degradation of connective tissue due to foci of inflammation and necrosis in occupied portions of lung parenchyma. Studies of the enzyme content of tissue that compose tuberculous cavities have shown high protease activity which may cause degradation of connective tissue collagen type I (10). The most striking observation, however, was the finding of rather high ICTP concentrations in patients with empyema thoracis. The pleural fluid in empyema thoracis is characterized by a large number of neutrophiles. These inflammatory cells are supplied with a large array of proteolytic enzymes including collagenase and procollagenase (11). The active metallo-proteinase might be responsible for connective tissue remodelling within the pleural cavity resulting in increased concentrations of serum ICTP. It should be mentioned that patients with tuberculosis or empyema thoracis did not receive corticosteroids, nor was there any clinical sign of concomitant hyperthyroidism or hyperparathyroidism.

Acknowledgements

Donation of telopeptide ICTP RIA kits by Pharmacia-Biotech, Freiburg, is gratefully acknowledged.

References

1. Abramson SL, Malech HL, Gallin JL (1991) Neutrophils. In: Crystal RG, West JB et al (eds) The lung: Scientific foundations. Raven Press Ltd, New York, pp 553
2. Claim A (1965) Secondary malignant disease of bone. Br J Cancer 19:15

3 Covelli HD, Zaloznik AJ, Shekitka KM (1980) Evaluation of bone pain in carcinoma of the lung: Role of localized false-negative scan. JAMA 244:2625
4 Dannenberg AM jr, Sugimoto M (1976) Liquefication of caseous foci in tuberculosis. Am Rev Resp Dis 113:257
5 Elomaa I, Virkkunen P, Risteli L, Risteli J (1992) Serum concentration of the cross-linked carboxyterminal telopeptide of type I collagen (ICTP) is a useful prognostic indicator in multiple myeloma. Br J Cancer 66:337
6 Eriksen EF, Charles P, Melsen F, Mosekilde L, Risteli L, Risteli J (1993) Serum markers of type I collagen formation and degradation in metabolic bone disease. Correlation to bone histomorphometry. J Bone Miner Res 8:127
7 Hakala M, Risteli L, Manelius J, Nieminen P, Risteli J. Increased type I collagen degradation correlates with disease severity in rheumatoid arthritis, submitted
8 Kylmälä T, Tammela T, Risteli L, Risteli J, Taube T, Elomaa I (1993) Evaluation of the effect of oral clodronate on skeletal metastases with type I collagen metabolites. A controlled trial of the Finnish prostate cancer group. Eur J Cancer 29 A:821
9 Kruskal WH (1952) A nonparametric test for the several sampling problems. Ann Math Stat 23:525
10 Napoli LD, Hansen HH (1973) The incidence of osseous involvement in lung cancer, with special reference to the development of osteoblastic changes. Radiology 108:17
11 Risteli J, Elomaa I, Niemi S, Novamo A, Risteli L (1993) Radioimmunoassay for the pyridinoline cross-linked carboxyterminaltelopeptide of type I collagen: A new serum marker of bone collagen degradation. Clin Chem 39:635

Address for correspondence:
Prof. Dr. W. Ebert
Thoraxklinik
Abteilung Klinische Chemie und Bakteriologie
Amalienstraße 5
D-69126 Heidelberg, Germany

Clinical value of the tumor marker TPS versus TPA in different malignancies

W. Brenner[a], J. Zimmermann[b], K.H. Bohuslavizki[a], J.-U. Eberhardt[a], M. Clausen[a], E. Henze[a]

[a]Clinic of Nuclear Medicine, [b]Clinic of Radiotherapy, Christian-Albrechts-University of Kiel, Germany

Introduction

Today tumor markers are an important tool in the follow-up of cancer patients to determine response to therapy as well as to indicate tumor progression or relapse.

TPA, the tissue polypeptide antigen, originally described in 1957 by Björklund (1), is a serum component closely related to cytokeratins, especially cytokeratin 8, 18, and 19. It is proposed to be released from cells after mitosis as well as from dying tumor cells (2). Cell death occurs mainly in necrotic areas due to rapid tumor growth resulting in a decreased blood flow to the tumor mass. In both cases TPA indicates tumor growth. Therefore, TPA has been successfully utilized as a tumor marker for more than ten years.

Further investigations and monoclonal mapping of TPA revealed 35 different epitopes (3), of which the M3-epitope of cytokeratin 18 has been shown to be related to tumor progression activity correlating well with synthesis of DNA (4). Thus, a new assay for the so-called tumor proliferation marker tissue polypeptide specific antigen (TPS) was developed based upon a monoclonal antibody against the M3-antigen. However, it is not yet clear whether TPA or TPS is more appropriate to indicate tumor progression or relapse in the clinical follow-up of cancer patients.

Therefore, the aim of this study was to correlate TPA and TPS with concomitant clinical examinations in those tumor patients with discordant results of TPA and TPS in order to evaluate the clinical benefit of these two tumor markers.

Materials and methods

Following initial cancer treatment both TPA and TPS were measured in 65 tumor patients during routine clinical follow-up examinations. Patients were suffering from breast cancer (n = 22), lung cancer (n = 6), gastric (n = 2) and colorectal cancer (n = 8), head and neck malignancies (n = 6), ovarian (n = 4) and uterine (n = 7) carcinomas, cancer of the kidneys (n = 3), bladder cancer (n = 4) and prostatic carcinomas (n = 3).

Serum concentrations of TPA and TPS were measured with the polyclonal TPA immunoradiometric assay (IRMA) from Byk-Sangtec and with the monoclonal TPS IRMA from BEKI, respectively. Serum concentrations higher than cut-off levels of 95 U/l for TPA and 80 U/l for TPS were considered positive, while all values below the cut-off were defined negative.

In patients with discordant findings of TPA and TPS, the results were correlated with concomitant clinical investigations, i.e. physical examination, tumor markers like CEA, CA 19-9, CA 72-4, CA 125 and CA 15-3, sonography, bone scanning, conventional X-ray, and CT.

Results

Positive results of TPA were yielded in 14 out of 65 patients while TPS was positive in 28 out of 65 patients. In 51 patients concordant results of TPA and TPS were found: in 14 patients there were concordant positive results and in 37 cases both tumor markers revealed concordant negative values.

Table I. TPA and TPS in all 65 patients investigated.

TPS	TPA		
	positive	negative	Σ
Positive	14	14	28
Negative	0	37	37
Σ	14	51	65

Table II. Evaluation of 14 TPS-positive/TPA-negative patients (compare table I).

Results of further investigations	TPS-positive/ TPA-negative patients
Tumor progression	2
New metastasis	1
Secondary neoplasm	1
TU-marker elevation only	3
No progression	7
Total number	14

However, in 14 out of 65 patients discordant findings of TPA and TPS were obtained: in all cases TPS was positive indicating tumor progression or relapse while TPA serum concentrations were below the cut-off level mentioned above. In contrast, no patient showed positive TPA values when TPS was negativ. A summary of these results is given in table I.

In fact, patients with discordant TPA and TPS were of major interest for this study. Therefore TPA and TPS results of these patients were correlated with further diagnostic procedures. Clinical findings are summarized in table II. In seven out of 14 TPS-positive/TPA-negative patients there was clinical evidence of progression: In three cases metastasis could be proved. In one patient suffering from cancer of the kidneys bone metastasis in the sternum and os sacrum were seen by bone scanning and X-ray, in one case a lung metastasis of a known squamous cell carcinoma of the hypopharynx was found, and a suspected lymph node metastasis in a woman with breast cancer could be verified due to cytopathological investigations.

In one patient known to have ovarian cancer a secondary malignoma, i.e. a breast carcinoma, was proved by histopathological means.

In another three patients at least one more tumor marker such as CA 15-3, CA 72-4 or CEA was elevated, while ultrasonic or radiological investigations were negative.

In seven TPS-positive/TPA-negative patients there was no clinical evidence of tumor progression, relapse or metastasis so far.

Discussion

By measurement of both TPA and TPS serum concentrations in 65 tumor patients during clinical follow-up examinations concordant test results were obtained in 51 patients. To further evaluate differences of sensitivity and specifity of TPA and TPS concordant results mentioned above are of limited use.

However, in 14 out of 65 patients there were discordant TPA and TPS results. In all 14 cases TPS values were elevated, while TPA was below the cut-off level of 95 U/l.

In four out of these 14 TPS-positive/TPA-negative patients tumor progression or a secondary malignoma could be proved confirming four true positive results of TPS. Moreover, in another three TPS-positive/TPA-negative patients further tumor markers were elevated confirming the positive results of TPS. Due to the leadtime of tumor markers of several months these patients are expected to show a progression of their disease during the next time period. Therefore, a close clinical check-up of those patients is recommended urgently.

Surprisingly, of both tumor proliferation markers the monoclonal TPS assay seems to have a higher sensitivity than the polyclonal TPA assay.

Nevertheless, the clinical value of a tumor marker does not depend only on its high sensitivity. In addition, an equivalent specifity is necessary to prove a tumor marker to be a reliable tool for monitoring cancer patients.

In half of the TPS-positive/TPA-negative patients there was no clinical evidence of progressive disease due to all accompanying diagnostic procedures including other tumor markers. Because of the leadtime of tumor markers and because of the small number of patients in this study, it is not yet possible to assess the specifity of TPS and TPA.

In conclusion, additional investigations are necessary in order to further evaluate both sensitivity and specifity of TPS as well as of TPA and to prove the possibly higher sensitivity of TPS.

References

1 Björklund B, Björklund V (1957) Antigenicity of pooled human malignant and normal tissue by cytoimmunological techniques: Presence of an insoluble, heat-labile tumor antigen. Int Archs Allergy 10:153–184
2 Oehr P, Lüthgens M, Liu Q (1992) Tissue polypeptide antigen and specific TPA. In: Sell S (ed) Serological cancer markers. The Humana Press, Totowa, NJ, pp 193–206
3 Björklund B, Björklund V, Brunkener M, Grönlund H, Back M (1987) The enigma of a human tumor marker: TPA revisited. In: Cimino F (ed) Human tumor markers. de Gruyter, Berlin, pp 169–180
4 Björklund B (1992) Letters to the editor: Tumor markers TPA, TPA-S and Cytokeratins. Tumordiagn u Ther 13:78–80

Address for correspondence:
Dr. med. W. Brenner
Abteilung für Nuklearmedizin
Christian-Albrechts-Universität zu Kiel
Arnold Heller Straße 9
D-24105 Kiel, Germany

Determination of the tissue polypeptide antigen (TPA/TPS) with different commercially available assays

A methodological comparison

G.M. Oremek[a], U.B. Seiffert[a], D. Jonas[b]

[a]Clinical-Chemical Central Laboratory, Center of Internal Medicine, [b]Department of Urology, Center of Surgery, Klinikum of Johann-Wolfgang-Goethe-University, Frankfurt, Germany

Introduction

Looking for new specific tumor markers, a number of tumor associated cytokeratins were isolated within the last years. The diagnostic value of these cytokeratins was examined (1, 2, 3).

Cytokeratins are proteins with a molecular weight of 40 to 70 kD. They belong to the group of intermediate filaments and are components of normal epithelial cells and of tumors originating from epithelial tissues (4).

The intermediate filaments can be subdivided into five groups which are: cytokeratin, desmin, vimentin, GFAP and neurofilaments (1). Cytokeratins occur in different combinations in epithelial tissues; in a certain tissue type one or more cytokeratin pairs are expressed (5). Cytokeratin 8 and 18 have a molecular weight of 52 and 45 kD. A soluble fragment from cytokeratin 19, an acidic cytokeratin with a molecular weight of 40 kD, can be detected in the cytoplasm of malignomas with epithelial origin (6). Cytokeratins are expressed in all stages of epithelial tumors. The cytokeratin pair 8/18 is expressed in large quantities in different epithelia and carcinomas with epithelial origin (5, 7).

A relation between tissue polypeptide antigen (TPA) and cytokeratin 8, 18 and 19 could be demonstrated (8). It could be shown that monoclonal antibodies directed against the corresponding epitopes of cytokeratin 8, 18 and 19 could replace a polyclonal TPA antibody when applied singly or in pairs (7, 8).

TPA was first described by *Björklund* and *Björklund* in 1957 as a tumor associated antigen which is expressed in elevated concentrations in different malignant tumors (9). Elevated TPA concentrations are often found in patients with tumor progression and distant metastasis. The importance of TPAcyk for monitoring patients with endocrine and exocrine pancreas carcinomas was recently described (1, 10). The aim of this study was the comparison of different methods for the detection of TPA or TPS and the evaluation of the clinical value of TPA and TPS for monitoring the disease course of patients with urogenital carcinomas.

Materials and methods

Materials

One hundred serum samples from healthy individuals in the age of 18 to 65 years were analysed. In these persons twenty different parameters of clinical chemistry were measured and no pathological values were found, thus confirming the real state of health.

Furthermore 100 serum samples from patients with malignant and benign urological diseases were analyzed.

Methods

Six commercially available test kits for the determination of TPA were used (6) which are described more in detail in table I and table II.

Method 1 and method 2 are relatively new assays on the market and therefore the test principles are described below.

Method 3 to method 6 were performed according to the protocol of the producers.

Method 1: TPAcyk ELISA, medac GmbH Hamburg

The TPA ELISA is a solid phase sandwich assay. Specimens, standards and controls are incubated with a monoclonal anti-cytokeratin antibody mixture coated to wells, simultaneously with a

Table I. Test kit supplier and name of the assay.

Method	Name	Supplier/company
1	TPAcyk EIA	medac, Hamburg
2	TPAcyk IRMA	Serono, Freiburg
3	Prolifigen TPA IRMA	Byk-Sangtec, Dietzenbach
4	LIA-mat TPA Prolifigen	Byk-Sangtec, Dietzenbach
5	TPS IRMA	Hermann Biermann, Bad Nauheim
6	TPS EIA	Hermann Biermann, Bad Nauheim

Table II. Test principle and type of reaction.

Method	Test principle	Immunoreaction
1	enzyme-immunological solid phase sandwich assay	one-step
2	immunoradiometric solid phase sandwich assay	one-step
3	immunoradiometric solid phase sandwich assay	two-step
4	immunoluminometric solid phase sandwich assay	two-step
5	immunoradiometric solid phase sandwich assay	one-step
6	enzyme-immunological solid phasen assay	one-step

HRP-labeled antibody. During the incubation, both the immobilized antibody and the HRP-labeled antibody bind to the cytokeratin fragments forming a sandwich. The wells are washed and a substrate is added. The developed color is proportional to the concentration of the analyte. The time needed to perform the assay is 2.5 hours.

Method 2: TPAcyk IRMA, Serono Freiburg

The monoclonal TPAcyk IRMA is a solid phase immunoradiometric "sandwich"-ELISA.
Two different mouse monoclonal antibodies and a polyclonal horse antibody which is labeled with ^{125}I are used in the assay. The samples are incubated with the antibodies for four hours at room temperature. Antibody-antigen complexes are formed. Non-bound antibodies are removed by washing. The remaining radioactivity is counted with the "Riastar Hewlett Packard" - scintillation counter. The TPA concentrations are calculated via the standard curve.

Results

The reference values for healthy individuals (n = 100) were in the following ranges:
TPAcyk ELISA und TPAcyk IRMA: 0.3 ng/ml – 1 ng/ml
TPA LIAmat: 32 U/l – 90 U/l
TPA IRMA: 18 U/l – 95 U/l
TPS EIA und TPS-IRMA: 42 U/l – 155 U/l

There was a good correlation between the different methods as depicted in the following list:
TPAcyk ELISA / TPAcyk IRMA: r = 0.964
TPAcyk ELISA / TPA LIAmat: r = 0.950
TPAcyk ELISA / TPA IRMA: r = 0.940
TPAcyk ELISA / TPS IRMA: r = 0.913
TPAcyk ELISA / TPS EIA: r = 0.938

The results obtained with the TPAcyk assays were expressed in ng/ml and have to be multiplied with the factor 100 to receive the U/l value. The time needed to perform the TPAcyk ELISA is only 2.5 hours whereas at least four hours are needed for the performance of the other TPA/TPS assays.

Figure 1 shows the correlation between the TPA values determined by method 1 and method 2 for 41 patients with bladder carcinoma. In this case, the formula for linear regression is y = 0.87x + 2.38 and the correlation coefficient is r = 0.96.

Figure 2 shows the correlation between TPA and TPS-values from 39 bladder carcinoma patients determined with method 1 and method 5. The correlation coefficient is r = 0.95, the formula for linear regression is y = 1.07x - 8.87.

The correlation between method 1 and method 6 was determined for 40 patients with bladder diseases (figure 3). The correlation coefficient is r = 0.92, the formula for linear regression is y = 1.13x + 1.05.

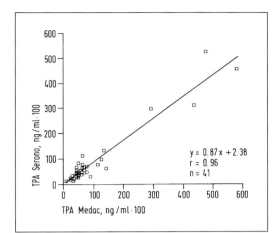

Figure 1. Correlation of TPA concentrations determined in patients with bladder carcinoma.

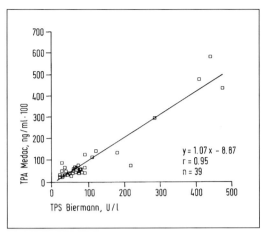

Figure 2. Correlation of TPA and TPS concentrations in patients with bladder carcinoma.

Conclusions

The performance of the TPAcyk ELISA is very fast and therefore the assay is very well suited for routine diagnostics. As the TPS assays, the TPAcyk ELISA shows a good precision for a manuell assay.

All assays show a good correlation with each other, especially those assays that use monoclonal antibodies.

References

1. Moll R, Schiller DL, Franke WW (1990) Identification of protein IT of the intestinal cytoskeleton as a novel type I cytokeratin with unusual properties and expression patterns. J Cell Biol 111:567–580
2. Lazarides E (1980) Intermediate filaments as mechanical integrators of cellular space. Nature 282:249–256
3. Bahr J, Carlsson K, Lüning B (1988) An epitope in coil 2B of cytokeratin 8. Acta Chem Scand B42: 442–447
4. Moll R, Franke WW, Schiller DL (1982) The catalog of human cytokeratins: Patterns of expression in normal epithelia, tumors and cultured cells. Cell 31:11–24
5. Quinlan RA, Schiller DL, Hatzfeld M, Achtstätter T, Moll R, Jorcano JL, Magin TM, Franke WW (1985) Patterns of expression and organisation of cytokeratin intermediate filaments. In: Wang E, Fishman D, Liem RRH, Sun TT (eds) Intermediate filaments. Ann N Y Acad Sci 455:282–306
6. Oremek GM, Seiffert UB (1994) Die Bedeutung von CYFRA 21-1 in der pneumologischen Differentialdiagnostik – Vergleichende Untersuchung mittels Enzymimmunoassay und Radioimmunoassay. Lab Med 18:100–104
7. Lüning B, Nilsson U (1983) Sequence homology between TPA and intermediate filament proteins. Acta Chem Scand B37:731–753
8. Hellerwick DM, Osborn M, Weber K (1990) On the nature of serological TPA; monoclonal ceratin 8, 18 and 19 antibodies react differently with TPA prepared from human cultured cells and TPA in human serum. Oncogene 5:1007–1017
9. Björklund B, Björklund V (1957) Antigenicity of pooled human malignant and normal tissues by cytoimmunological technique. Presence of an insoluble neat-labile tumor antigen. Int Arch Allergy 10:153–184
10. Bahlo M, Strüven D, Klapdor R (1993) TPAcyk-ELISA zur quantitativen Bestimmung des Tissue Polypeptide Antigen im Serum. GIT Lab-Med 16:24–26
11. Gitsch G, Kainz Ch, Joura E, Fröhlich B, Bieglmayr Ch, Tatra G (1992) Squamous cell carcinoma antigen, tumor associated trypsin inhibitor and tissue polypeptide specific antigen in follow up of stage II cervical cancer. Anticancer Res 12:1247–1250

Address for correspondence:
Dr. med. G. M. Oremek
Zentrum der Inneren Medizin
Zentrallabor
Universitätskliniken
Theodor-Stern-Kai 7
D-60590 Frankfurt/Main, Germany

Tumor markers profile in broncho-alveolar lavage in lung cancer

A. Khalifa[a], E.A. Mady[a,c], M.A. Tag El-Din[b], H.M. El-Dessouki[c]

[a]Oncology Diagnostic Unit, Faculty of Medicine, [b]Department of Chest, Faculty of Medicine, [c]Department of Biochemistry, Faculty of Science, Ain Shams University, Cairo, Egypt

Introduction

Lung cancer represents the most frequent tumor besides breast cancer and colorectal cancer (1). Early detection of bronchogenic carcinoma is important in the case of patients over the age of 45 years who smoke more than one half a package of cigarettes per day (2). Morbidity and mortality resulting from the failure to diagnose and treat this disease effectively are major problems (3). A problem in the diagnosis of lung cancer is the difficulty in detection of the disease. The sensitivity of diagnosis never exceeds 70% with a single marker (4). Broncho-alveolar lavage (BAL) is a widely used clinical procedure. Numerous studies have shown the advantage of using broncho-alveolar lavage in cytologic diagnosis of primary and secondary malignant neoplasms of the respiratory system (5). Recent studies on the determination of tumor markers in broncho-alveolar lavage fluid (BALF) have given reason to careful optimism (6).

This study has been carried out in order to evaluate the diagnostic usefulness of simultaneous determination of tumor markers CEA, CA 19-9, SCC-Ag and NSE in BALF of lung cancer.

Materials and methods

This study was carried out on 24 patients (22 males and two females). Their ages ranged from 38 to 65 years. Histological diagnosis revealed that there were 14 squamous cell carcinoma, four adenocarcinoma, three small cell carcinoma, one alveolar carcinoma and two breast cancer metastasis (table I). Broncho-alveolar lavage was carried out and BALF was stored at 20° C after centrifugation. The BALF was subjected to the assays of CEA, CA 19-9 and SCC-Ag were assayed using IMX-Micro particle immunoassay system (MEIA, Abbott), while NSE was assayed by the RIA method (ByK-Sangtec).

Results and discussion

The primary goal of this study was to investigate the possibility of differentiation between different histologic types of lung cancer by combined measurement of tumor markers CEA, CA 19-9, SCC-Ag and NSE in BALF (table II). SCC-Ag was significantly elevated in squamous cell carcinomas (mean 386 U/ml, 188 U/mg protein) compared to other histologic types except small cell carcinoma whith a mean value of 393 U/ml (218 U/mg protein) but this elevation was not significant due to the small number of cases (three only).

The elevation in SCC-Ag was more significant in more advanced stages of squamous cell carcinomas since it was increased three- and sevenfold in stages II and III than in stage I, respectively. This profound dominance of SCC-Ag in squamous cell carcinoma was confirmed also when relating its level with the protein content of the BALF (table II).

Table I. Histopathological classification of patients.

Histopathologic type	Number	Percentage
Squamous cell carcinoma	14	58
stage I	2	8
stage II	7	29
stage III	5	21
Adenocarcinoma	4	17
Small cell carcinoma	3	13
Alveolar carcinoma	1	4
Breast cancer metastasis	2	8

Table II. Mean values of tumor markers SCC-Ag, CA 19-9, CEA and NSE in broncho-alveolar lavage of different histopathlogical types of lung cancer.

Histopathologic type	SCC-Ag		CA 19-9		CEA		NSE	
	U/ml	U/mg prot.	U/ml	U/mg prot.	ng/ml	ng/mg prot.	U/ml	U/mg prot.
Squamous cell carcinoma	386	188	998	487	173	84	62	30
stage I	120	26	400	87	63	14	17	4
stage II	400	250	721	451	170	106	67	42
stage III	472	240	1624	824	220	112	76	39
Adenocarcinoma	32	43	1835	2531	597	824	10	14
Small cell carcinoma	393	218	314	174	45	25	171	95
Alveolar carcinoma	1.5	2.3	12	18	5	8	11	16
Breast cancer metastasis	58.5	98	36.5	61	18	30	8	13

These results are in accordance with those of *Hatakeyama* et al. (7) who obtained a highly significant level of SCC-Ag in squamous cell carcinoma. Also they are in agreement with those of *Niklinski* et al. (8) who observed a positive level of SCC-Ag in 50% of stage II and in 78.9% of stage III patients with squamous cell carcinoma of the lung.

CA 19-9 was highly significant in adenocarcinomas when compared to other histological types (mean 1835 U/ml, 2531 U/mg protein). It was detected also in squamous cell carcinoma with a significant correlation with increasing stage. *Asada* et al. (9) found that normal subjects have levels of CA 19-9 in BALF less than 1000 U/ml and levels between 1000 and 8000 U/ml in lung cancer patients. Also *Mizushima* et al. (10) found that CA 19-9 positive rate is best correlated with adenocarcinoma.

The level of CEA was also, as CA 19-9, highly significant in BALF of adenocarcinoma patients than the other histologic types, followed by squamous cell carcinomas which showed also a significant increase in CEA level with the advance of the disease. *Supervia* et al. (11) reported a positive level of CEA in BALF above 10 ng/ml. They obtained 91.48% specificity of CEA in determining adenocarcinoma in neoplastic effusions, whereas *de Diego* et al. (12) used 1000 ng/ml protein as a cutting point in BALF to obtain a specificity of 94%.

Also *Wesselius* et al. (13) obtained a mean value of CEA in BALF of 252 ± 47 ng/mg protein in 20 central lung cancer patients out of 48 patients.

NSE is said to be the most specific tumor marker in small cell lung cancer (SCLC) up to now (14). This was also evident in our study as we obtained the highest elevations of NSE level in the SCLC group (171 ng/ml, 95 ng/mg protein) compared to other histological types. These results are in accordance with those of *Lombardi* et al. (15) who found that NSE is of good help in diagnosing SCLC and with those of *Mizushima* et al. (10) who obtained a good correlation between NSE and SCLC.

Conclusion

Multiple tumor marker assays in BALF are of clinical significance in assisting the diagnosis of lung cancer. In this study the SCC-Ag levels were best correlated with squamous cell carcinoma, CA 19-9 levels with adenocarcinoma, CEA levels with adenocarcinoma, and NSE levels with small cell lung carcinoma. The multiple marker panels seemed to be more correlated than a single marker and may have a differential diagnostic value. Therefore, it appears that the simultaneous determination of SCC-Ag and CA 19-9 in BALF of squamous cell lung cancer patients would be more indicative than any single one of them. This is also true for CA 19-9 and CEA in adenocarcinoma and NSE in small cell lung cancer.

Acknowledgement

This work was supported by Abbott Diagnostic.

References

1. Hasholzner U, Stieber P, Fiebig M, Surder Plassmann L, Fateh-Moghadam A (1992) CYFRA–A new tumor marker for non-small cell lung cancer (NSCLC). In: Klapdor R (ed) Tumor associated antigens, oncogenes, receptors, cytokines in tumor diagnosis and therapy at the beginning of the nineties. Zuckschwerdt, München, pp 134–136
2. Weiss W, Baucot KR, Seidman H (1982) The Philadelphia pulmonary neoplasms research project. Clin Ches Med 3:243
3. Sieverberg E (1984) Cancer Statistics CA-34:7
4. Bernal SD, Speak JA (1984) Membrane antigen in small cell carcinoma of the lung defined by monoclonal antibody SMI. Cancer Res 44:265–270
5. Pirozynski M (1992) Broncho-alveolar lavage in the diagnosis of peripheral, primary lung cancer. Chest 102 (2):372–374
6. Ebert W, Stabrey A, Sibinger M, Schrenk M (1990) Value of pleural fluid hyaluronic acid and carcinoembryonic antigen determinations in the differentia dignosis between malignant mesothelioma and pleuritis carcinomatosa. Tumordiagn u Ther 12:1–6
7. Hatakeyama S, Nagai A, Kioi S, Arakawa M (1990) Clinical evaluation of combination assay of tumor markers in primary lung cancer patients. Nippon Kyobu 28(8):1053–1058
8. Niklinski J, Furman M, Landanski J, Kozlowski M (1992) Evaluation of squamous cell carcinoma antigen (SCC-Ag) in the diagnosis and follow up of patients with non-small cell lung carcinoma. Neoplasma 39(5):279–282
9. Asada K, Ogushi F, Tani K, Kawa Jik, Nakahira S, Yasouka S, Ogura T (1992) Measurement of CA 19-9 in bronchial lavage of fluid from patients with lung cancer. Nippon-Kyobu 30(9):1682–1686
10. Mizushima Y, Hirata H, Izumi S, Hoshinok, Konishi K, Morikage T, Maruyama M, Yamashita N, Yano S (1990) Clinical significance of the number of positive tumor markers in assisting the diagnosis of lung cancer with multiple tumor marker assay. Oncology 47(1):43–48
11. Supervia A, Guitart AC, Rubio J, Cornudell R (1992) Carcinoembryonic antigen in pleural effusion. Adenocarcinoma versus mesothelioma. Rev Clin ESP 190(2):69–71
12. de Diego A, Comore L, Sanchis J, Enguidanos MJ, Marco V (1990) Usefulness of carcinoembryonic antigen determintion in broncho-alveolar lavage fluid. A comparative study among patients with peripheral lung cancer, pneumonia, and healthy individuals. Chest 100(4):1060–1063
13. Wesselius LJ, Dark DS, Papasian CJ (1990) Airway carcinoembryomic antigen concentrations in patients with central lung cancer or chronic bronchitis. Chest 98(2):393–397
14. Cooper EH, Splinter TAW, Brown DA, Muers MF, Peake MD, Pearson SL (1985) Evaluation of a radioimmuno assay for neuronspecific enolase in small cell lung cancer. Br J Cancer 52:333–338
15. Lombardi C, Tassi GF, Pizzocolo G, Donato F (1990) Clinical significance of a multiple biomarker assay in patients with lung cancer. A study with logistic regression analysis. Chest 97(3):639–644

Address for correspondence:
Prof. Dr. A. Khalifa
Oncology Diagnostic Unit
Ain Shams Faculty of Medicine
ET-Abbassia, Cairo, Egypt

In Vitro Diagnosis

Urogenital Tract

Significance of the tumor markers TATI, NSE, CYFRA 21-1 and TPAcyk in carcinomas of the kidney

C. Schambeck[a], Petra Stieber[a], H. Hell[b], Ute Hasholzner[a], Karin Hofmann[a],
N. Schmeller[b], A. Fateh-Moghadam†[a]
[a]Institute for Clinical Chemistry, [b]Urological Hospital,
Ludwig-Maximilians-University, Munich, Germany

Introduction

Up to now there is not any reliable tumor marker available for follow-up care of patients with carcinomas of the kidney. However, *Labre* et al. described a sensitivity of 62% (versus healthy persons) for TATI (tumor-associated trypsin inhibitor) in 31 patients with cancer of the kidney (1). Sensitivities of 51% resp. 65% (versus healthy persons) were found for NSE (neuron specific enolase) in patients with cancer of the kidney by *Takashi* et al. (2) and *Kusama* et al. (3). We detected a sensitivity of 38% (versus benign urological diseases) for CYFRA 21-1 (cytokeratin 19 fragment) in urinary bladder cancer, resp. a 56% sensitivity for muscle invasive forms (4). Cytokeratin 8 and 18 detected by TPAcyk were shown to be frequent intermediate filaments in the proximal tubules of the kidney, the likely origin of renal cell cancer (5).
The aim of this study was to investigate the clinical significance of TATI, NSE and the cytokeratin markers CYFRA 21-1 (which proved to be a useful marker in urinary bladder cancer) and TPAcyk in carcinoma of the kidney.

Patients

We examined the sera of 39 patients with benign urological diseases and 71 patients with cancer of the kidney. All sera were collected pretherapeutically at an active stage of disease and were stored frozen at −80° C. Considering the reference group of patients with benign diseases urethral stones were diagnosed in 25 patients, renal stones in 11 patients and local inflammatory disease in three patients. According to the UICC staging system of 1987 the tumor patients were distributed as follows: six patients with stage I, 25 patients with stage II, 29 patients with stage III and 10 patients with stage IV. The stage of one patient could not be determined. Renal cell carcinomas were found in 69 patients and urothelium carcinomas in two patients.

Methods

The CYFRA 21-1 values were determined using the enzyme immunoassay on the automated test system ES 700 (Boehringer Mannheim). TPAcyk was analyzed by the EIA of medac (Hamburg), TATI by the RIA of Isotopen Diagnostik CIS and NSE by the RIA of Pharmacia.

Results

We defined the cut-off values based on 95% specificity versus the benign urological diseases (6): So we found for CYFRA 21-1 a cut-off value of 2.5 ng/ml, for TATI of 103 ng/ml, for NSE of 18.6 ng/ml and for TPAcyk of 4.7 ng/ml. Then a 11% sensitivity for TATI could be detected, a 10% sensitivity for CYFRA 21-1, a 7% sensitivity for NSE and a 4% sensitivity for TPAcyk. Considering stage III and IV cancers TATI, NSE and CYFRA 21-1 are more sensitive compared with stage I and II cancers (table I). The combination of TATI and CYFRA 21-1 resp. TATI and NSE led to the highest sensitivities compared with the other possible combinations: a 18% resp. a 17% sensitivity could be shown for these tumor marker combinations (table I). The distribution of the values divided by the cut-off value can be seen for each marker in

Table I. Marker sensitivity (%) at 95% specificity for carcinomas of the kidney.

Marker	Cut-off (ng/ml)	All (n = 71)	Stage I + II (n = 31)	Stage III + IV (n = 39)
TATI	103	11	3	18
CYFRA 21-1	2.5	10	7	13
NSE	18.6	7	3	10
TPAcyk	4.7	4	7	3
TATI or CYFRA 21-1	108/2.5	18	7	28
TATI or NSE	117/18.6	17	7	26
TATI or TPAcyk	117/4.7	14	7	20
CYFRA 21-1 or NSE	2.6/22.5	14	10	18
CYFRA 21-1 or TPAcyk	2.6/6.6	11	10	13
TPAcyk or NSE	8.3/22.5	9	7	10

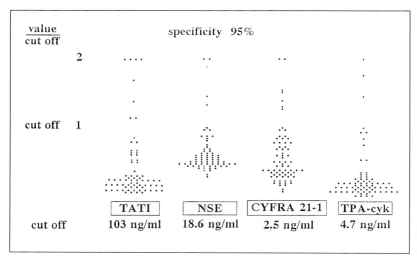

Figure 1. Distribution of the values in carcinomas of the kidney (n = 71).

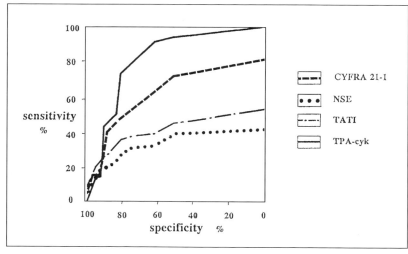

Figure 2. ROC curves for TATI, CYFRA 21-1, NSE and TPAcyk in carcinomas of the kidney (n = 71). The reference group consisted of patients with exclusively benign urological diseases (n = 39).

figure 1. As far as the sensitivity/specificity profile is concerned TPAcyk demonstrated the best discriminative power of all tumor markers investigated (figure 2).

Conclusions

Our investigations could not confirm the sensitivities described by *Labre* et al. (1), *Takashi* et al. (2) and *Kusama* et al. (3) for TATI and NSE.
The reference groups choosen by these authors exclusively consisted of healthy persons. Following the recommendations of the "Arbeitsgruppe für Qualitätskontrolle und Standardisierung von Tumormarkertests im Rahmen der Hamburger Symposien über Tumormarker" concerning evaluations of tumor marker tests (6) a reference group should include benign diseases causing problems in differential diagnosis (which means in this case benign urological diseases). Furthermore specificity versus this special reference group should be fixed at 95% in order to be able to compare different markers under the same conditions.
At this specificity of 95% the number of true positive test results for TATI and NSE was lower than 20% and therefore can not be recommended as tumor markers in cancer of the kidney. If requesting sensitivities of more than 50% for a clinically valuable marker the cytokeratin markers CYFRA 21-1 and TPAcyk were also disappointing.

This has also to be concluded for TPAcyk despite of the apparently good discriminative power of this marker reflected by the ROC curve.

References

1. Labre H et al (1990) Comparison of a new tumor marker, TATI, to other tumor marker in various cancers. J Tumor Oncol 5:305–311
2. Takashi M et al (1989) Evaluation of gammo-enolase as a tumor marker for renal cell carcinoma. J Urol 141:830–834
3. Kusama L et al (1991) Tumor markers in human renal cell carcinoma. Tumor Biol.12:189–197
4. Hasholzner U et al (1993) Die klinische Relevanz des neuen Tumormarkers CYFRA 21-1 bei Blasenkarzinomen im Vergleich zu TPA und TPS. Laboratoriumsmedizin 17:324–327
5. Moll R (1989) Intermediärfilamentmuster des Nephrons und des Urothels. Verh Dtsch Ges Path 73:314–320
6. Klapdor R (1992) Arbeitsgruppe Qualitätskontrolle und Standardisierung von Tumormarkertests im Rahmen der Hamburger Symposien über Tumormarker. Tumor Therapie 13:XIX–XXII

Address for correspondence:
Dr. med. Petra Stieber
Institut für Klinische Chemie
Klinikum Großhadern
Marchioninistraße 15
D-81377 München, Germany

Comparison between TPA and CA 50 expression in Egyptian bladder cancer patients

O. El-Ahmady[a], A. Gamal El-Din[a], Sanaa Eissa[b], Thanaa Helal[c], I. Khalaf[d]

[a]Tumor Marker Oncology Research Center and [d]Urology Department, Faculty of Medicine, Al-Azhar University, Oncology Diagnostic Unit, [b]Biochemistry and [c]Pathology Departments, Faculty of Medicine, Ain Shams University, Cairo, Egypt

Introduction

Tissue tumor markers are among the least studied biological parameters, where as much work has been done worldwide on serum tumor markers. In spite of this limited interest, the determination of tumor marker in tissue presents several areas of study: biological features of the tumor in order to register the individuality of the tumor and hence an individual therapy, choice of best tumor marker to use in follow-up and identification of occult metastasis (1). There is etiological association between bladder carcinoma (one of the most common types of cancer in Egypt) and urinary schistosomiasis and this causal association was postulated 80 years ago by *Ferguson*. Serum TPA is characteristic of carcinoma proliferation and increased levels of TPA are closely related to the progression of this type of tumor, on the other hand CA 50 is a tumor associated antigen which is defined by a monoclonal antibody raised against a colorectal carcinoma cell line (3, 4). By the immunohistochemical method the differentiated tumor cells were strongly stained for TPA, heavier than normal urothelial cells while undifferentiated neoplastic cells were less stained for TPA (5).
There is no relationship between TPA staining and the tumor staging or prognosis of the patients (6). Although serum TPA is very sensitive, it is not specific for screening purposes in diagnosis of urologic cancer (7). On the other hand, the urinary TPA is more sensitive than urine cytology for detection of bladder cancer and the combination of them will increase the accuracy of the diagnosis of bladder cancer (8). There is a good correlation between both serum and urinary TPA and stage, grade of the tumor in addion to the survival in bladder cancer patients (9, 10, 11, 12, 13).

Regarding CA 50 marker, serum levels can be considered as a useful marker in urologic malignancies with a sensitivity (47%) at 100% specificity in relation to control group, also, there is a correlation of high serum CA 50 levels with tumor invasion (13, 14). In the literatures, no findings concerning quantitative estimation of both TPA, CA 50 in bladder cancer are available. The aim of our work is to compare between the expression of TPA and CA 50 in bladder cancer tissue and their importance in the differential diagnosis of the high risk group.

Material and methods

This study was carried out on 246 individuals, 156 bladder cancer patients, 45 bilharzial patients and 45 normal healthy controls. Concerning the bladder cancer patients (n = 156), 136 of them were operable cases while the remaining 20 were inoperable cases. Five cases were T2, 116 cases were T3 and 15 cases were T4.
Blood samples and 24 h urine were taken 1–4 days preoperatively, sera were obtained by centrifugation of clotted blood samples, 10 ml of 24 h urine were centrifuged, adjusted to pH 7.3 ± 0.2 by 0.2 M NaOH or HCl and both stored at −20 °C until assayed.
In the bladder cancer group (operable cases n = 136), tissue samples from tumor and from normal tissue of the same bladder at least 5 cm distant from the tumor were obtained directly at the operating theatre, chilled on ice, dissected away from fat and necrotic tissue, washed with cold saline, quickly frozen and stored in deep freezer at −80 °C. A part of each sample was saved in 10% formaline solution for histopathological examination.

Tissue homogenization

The tumor tissue was weighed and finely chopped with a scalpel and scissors. The minced tissues were homogenized in 10 volumes of ice cold phosphate buffer. The tissue was homogenized by means of a whole glass homogenizer for 10–15 seconds at medium speed with 45–60 seconds elapsing between pulses. A small ice bath was kept around the cup of the homogenizer at all times. The subcellular fractions (cytosol and membrane) were separated according to figure 1.

Determination of cytosol and membrane protein

Protein concentration in cytosol membrane fractions was estimated by Bradford`s method. This method depends on the binding between protein and commassiee brilliant blue dye.

Determination of TPA and CA 50

Serum, 24 h urine cytosol, and membrane levels of TPA were determined using LIA-mat "TPA Prolifigen" kit supplied by AB Sangtec Medical, Bromma, Sweden. Also CA 50 levels were determined in the same fractions using RIA-gnost CA 50 kit supplied by Behring Werke, Marburg, Germany.

Results and discussion

Serum TPA correlates significantly with the proliferative activity (15). The mean cytosol and membrane TPA values of the malignant tissues of bladder cancer patients (6.33 ± 0.26, 26.12 ± 2.5 U/mg protein) were signifantly higher than those of normal tissue (2.56 ± 0.16, 3.91 ± 0.39 U/mg protein) (table I). Membrane TPA of the malignant tissue shows a very high mean value when

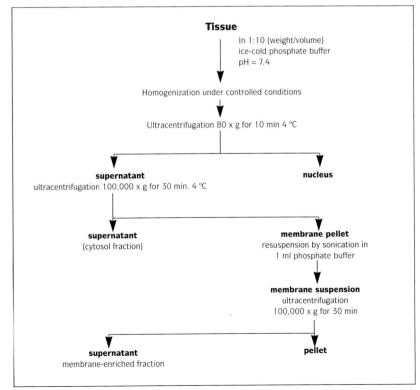

Figure 1. Schematic representation of subcellular fractions (cytosol and membrane fractions) preparation.

Table I. TPA U/mg protein (M ± S.E.) in normal and malignant tissues of bladder cancer patients.

	Cytosol		Membrane	
	M ± SE	range	M ± S.E.	range
Normal bladder tissue	2.6 ± 0.16	0.08 – 5.89	3.9 ± 0.39	0.12 – 19.3
Malignant bladder tissue	6.33[a] ± 0.26	1.15 – 12.91	26.1[a] ± 2.51	0.3 – 141.1

[a]Significant from normal tissue at $p < 0.01$

compared with that of cytosol. The c/m ratio for malignant tissue is lower than that of normal tissue which may be due to phenotypic characteristic of the tumor.

Our results are in accordance with those of *Senatore* et al. (5) and *Kaneko* et al. (6). Using immunohistochemical techniques they found that the concentration of TPA is higher in tumor tissue as compared to normal tissue specially in the differentiated tumors. The sensitivity of cytosol TPA for malignant tissue of bladder cancer patients was 56.5% at 100% specificity. For membrane TPA, the sensitivity was 39% at 100% specificity.

In relation to the histological type of the tumor, cytosol TPA showed the highest sensitivity (100%) in adenocarcinoma, followed by T.C.C. (82.5%), then S.C.C. (41.7%). These finding, agree with *Vogal* et al. (17) who reported that 100% of T.C.C. cases were TPA positive by immunohistochemical staining. There is no significant correlation between either cytosol or membrane TPA with the advancement of the disease which is in concordance with that of *Kaneko* et al. (6).

Cytosol and membrane TPA sensitivities were higher in lymph node positive tumors compared to lymph node negative group, this is due to aggressiveness lymph node positive tumors with more expression of TPA. Both serum and 24 h urine TPA mean values of bladder cancer patients were significantly higher than those of the normal and bilharzial group (tables II, III). Our study showed 100% sensitivity of 24 h urine TPA of bladder cancer patients at 100% specificity which is in accordance with that of *Costello* and *Kumar* (12). On the other hand, the sensitivity of serum TPA was 72% at 100% specificity. Regarding CA 50 marker, which is a tumor-associated antigen, it is proved that it is a useful marker in bladder cancer patients (13). Both cytosol and membrane CA 50 sensitivities of bladder cancer were much lower than those of TPA (12.1% and 15.3%, respectively) at 100% specificity (table IV). There is no correlation with stage or histologic grade of the disease. Both cytosol and membrane CA 50 sensitivities were higher in lymph node positive group than those in lymph node negative group. Both serum and 24 h urine CA 50 mean

Table II. 24 h urine TPA (M ± S.E.) in control, bilharzial and bladder cancer patients.

Urine TPA	Control group	Bilharzial group	Bladder cancer group
M ± S.E. (U/l)	60.6 ± 7.9	76.4 ± 9.5	3652.7[a] ± 163.9
Range	14–278	12–253	273–7810

[a]Significant from both normal and bilharzial groups at $p < 0.01$

Table III. Serum TPA (M ± S.E.) in control, bilharzial and bladder cancer patients.

Serum TPA	Control group	Bilharzial group	Bladder cancer group
M ± S.E. (U/l)	59 ± 3.7	80.9 ± 6.7	199[a] ± 14.6
Range	3.1 – 103.1	21.5 – 235.2	37 – 1210

[a]Significant from both normal and bilharzial groups at $p < 0.01$

values were significantly higher than those of the normal and bilharzial groups (tables V, VI). The sensitivity of 24 h urine CA 50 was 72.8% which was much lower for serum CA 50 (49.3%) at 100% specificity relative to the normal group. Evaluation of these two markers revealed potential application in 1. diagnosis of bladder cancer, specially 24 h urine TPA, 2. predicting prognosis. Tissue TPA was dependent on tumor size and nodal involvement which may indicate their usefulness as additional independent prognostic factors.

Table IV. CA 50 U/mg protein (M ± S.E.) in normal and malignant tissues of bladder cancer patients.

	Cytosol		Membrane	
	M ± SE	range	M ± S.E.	range
Normal bladder tissue	18.5 ± 2.4	0.7 – 92.6	51.8 ± 5.4	4.5 – 190
Malignant bladder tissue	40.9[a] ± 5.6	0.3 – 292	208.2a ± 48	0.63 – 4194

[a]Significant from normal tissue at $p < 0.01$

Table V. 24 h urine CA 50 (M ± S.E.) in control, bilharzial and bladder cancer patients.

Urine CA 50	Control group	Bilharzial group	Bladder cancer group
M ± S.E. (U/ml)	15.9 ± 1.8	16.9 ± 1.8	178.2[a] ± 13.1
Range	0.86 – 51.1	1.5 – 45.3	0.22 – 466

[a]Significant from both normal and bilharzial groups at $p < 0.01$

Table VI. Serum CA 50 (M ± S.E.) in control, bilharzial and bladder cancer patients.

Serum CA 50	Control group	Bilharzial group	Bladder cancer group
M ± S.E. (U/ml)	2.3 ± 0.23	2.95 ± 0.37	23.9[a] ± 4.2
Range	0.5 – 6.7	0.4 – 9.1	0.04 – 360

[a]Significant from both normal and bilharzial groups at $p < 0.01$

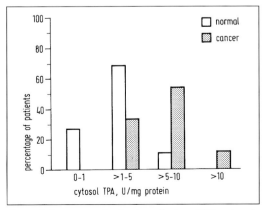

Figure 2. Frequency distribution of cytosol TPA values in normal and malignant bladder tissues.

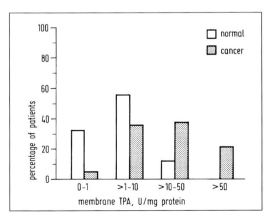

Figure 3. Frequency distribution of membrane TPA in normal and malignant bladder tissues.

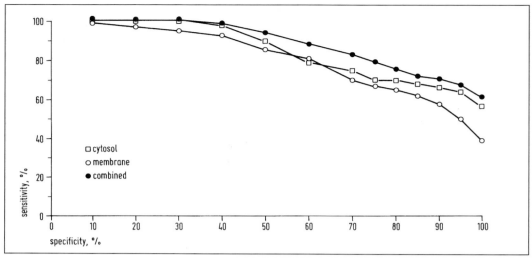

Figure 4. ROC curve for tissue TPA of bladder cancer patients.

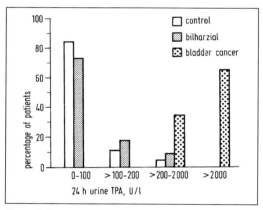

Figure 5. Frequency distribution of 24 h urine TPA values in normal, bilharzial and bladder cancer groups.

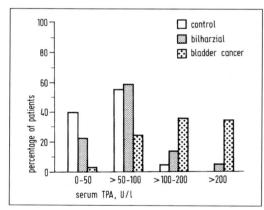

Figure 6. Frequency distribution of serum TPA values in normal and bladder cancer groups.

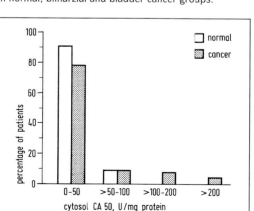

Figure 7. Frequency distribution of cytosol CA 50 values in normal and malignant bladder tissues.

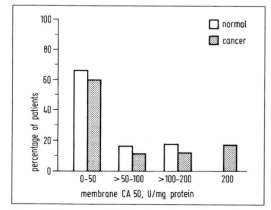

Figure 8. Frequency distribution of membrane CA 50 values in normal and malignant bladder tissues.

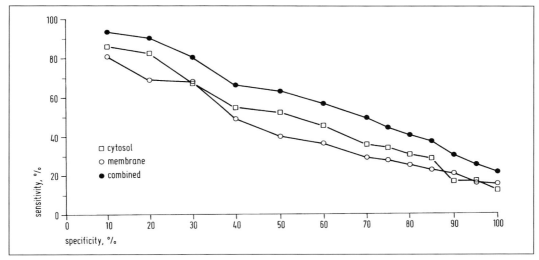

Figure 9. ROC curve for tissue CA 50 of bladder cancer patients.

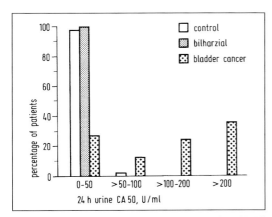

Figure 10. Frequency distribution of 24 h urine CA 50 values in normal, bilharzial and bladder cancer groups.

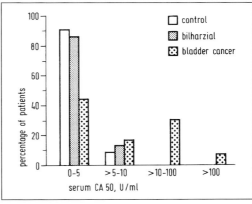

Figure 11. Frequency distribution of serum CA 50 values in normal, bilharzial and bladder cancer groups.

References

1 Massimo OG, Riccards M, Ruggero D, Luciano G, Gabriele M, Marco V, Orleo DM, Guiliano B (1986) Carcinoembryonic antigen, ferritin, tissue polypeptide antigen and CA 15-3 in breast cancer. Relationship between carcinoma and normal breast tissue. Intern J Biol Markers 1:33

2 Ferguson AR (1911) Associated bilharziasis and primary malignant diseases of the urinary bladder, with observations on a series of forty cases. J Pathol Bacteriol 16:76

3 Luning B and Nilsson U (1983) Sequence homology between tissue polypeptide antigen (TPA) and intermediate filament (IF) proteins. Acta Chem Scand B 37:731

4 Lindholm L, Holmgren J, Svennerholm L (1983) Monoclonal antibodies against gastrointestinal tumor-associated antigens isolated as monosialogangliosides. Int Arch Allerg Appl Immun 71:171

5 Senatore S, Zizzi L, Blasi C, Allieri G, Saccani-Jolli G, Gabrielli M, Uaccarelli S (1990) TPA in urinary bladder cancer cytology: a follow up study. Oncol 47(1):37

6 Kaneko K, Suzuki T, Takasaki C (1989) Immunohistochemical study of TPA in human urinary bladder tumors. Nippon-Hinyokika. Gukkai-Zasshi 80(10):1430

7 Isaka S, Musukagami T, Maruoka M, Shimazaki J, Murakami S, Oka M (1983) Serum tissue polypeptide antigen (TPA) in patients with urologic cancer. Nishinihon J Urol 45:1027

8. Isacson S, Andren-Sandberg A (1976) Tissue polypeptide antigen and cytology in cancer of the urinary bladder. 3rd International Symposium on Detection and Prevention of Cancer.
9. Oehr P, Adolphs HD (1989) Urogenital cancer. In: Lüthgens M, Schlegel G (eds) Clinical use of the tumor marker system CEA-TPA. Tumor Diagnostik, Leonberg, pp 99–119
10. Akiyama T, Tsujihashi H, Boku E, Nagai N, Malsuura T, Iguchi M, Yachiku S, Kurita T (1983) Tissue polypeptide antigen in urological malignancies. I. S. TPA in bladder cancer patients. Hinyokika Kiyo 29:1635
11. Tozuka K, Yonese Y, Nakagami Y, Minowa T, Hiraoka Y, Yamada N, Hikima N, Ishii Y, Tannowa K, Fujioka Y (1984) Evaluation of serum tissue polypeptide antigen (TPA) in patients with urological cancer. Gan To Kagaku Ryoho 11:1078 (abstract)
12. Costello CB, Kumar S (1986) Tissue polypeptide antigen (TPA): Usefulness in urological neoplasia Anticancer Res 6:713
13. Tizzani A, Cassella G, Cicigoi A, Piana P, Cerchier A, Pecchio F, Piantino P (1987) Tumor markers (CEA, TPA and CA 19-9) in urine of bladder cancer patients. Int J Biol Markers 2:121
14. Hershman MJ, Habib NA, Ferro MA, Williamson RCN, Wood CB (1987) The use of CA 50 radioimmunoassay test in diagnosis of urologic malignancy. Ann Meeting Am Surg Congress 53(12):691
15. Bradford MM (1976) A rapid and sensitive method for the quantitation of microgram quantities of protein utilizing the principle of protein dye binding. Anal Biochem 72:248
16. Björklund B (1978) Tissue polypeptide antigen (TPA): Biology, biochemistry, improved assay methodology, clinical significance in cancer and other conditions and future outlook. Antibiot Chemother 22:16
17. Vogal J, Oehr P, Maisey R, Adolphs HD (1988) Comparison between tissue antigen analysis and plasma determinations for TPA and CEA in transitional cell carcinomas and in tumor free urothelium of the urinary bladder. Cancer Detect Prev 2:389

Address for correspondence:
Prof. Dr. O. El-Ahmady
Tumor Marker Oncology Research Center
Al-Azhar University
2 Roshdy Street, Safeer Spuare
ET-Heliopolis, Cairo, Egypt

Plasma SCC (squamous cell carcinoma related antigen) levels in patients with bladder cancer

A. Katzenwadel, W. Schultze-Seemann, I. Struve, H. Sommerkamp

Department of Urology, University of Freiburg, Germany

Introduction

The squamous cell carcinoma related antigen (SCC antigen) is a subfraction of TA-4, a tumor-associated antigen which *Kato* and *Torigoe* (1) in 1977 first isolated from a squamous cell carcinoma of the cervix. SCC is one of 14 subfractions of TA-4, a glycoprotein with a molecular weight of 48 kD.

The biochemical properties of the originally described 14 subfractions of TA-4 were presented by *Kato* in 1984 (2). Two fractions proved to have different isoelectric points: a neutral TA-4 antigen, which was often found in non-malignantly altered squamous cells of the cervix, and an acidic TA-4, which was detected in tissue and serum of patients with squamous cell cancer of the cervix.

Since 1986, a radioimmunoassay (RIA) has been available, which measures only one of the subfractions. In addition, we use a microparticle enzyme immunoassay (MEIA), as well as an immunohistochemical method of identifying the antigen in tumor tissue.

Immunohistochemical investigations of various squamous cells of the upper aerodigestive tract have shown clear expression of TA-4 in the upper cell layers of normal squamous cells and in highly differentiated squamous cell carcinomas (3). In contrast, there is no TA-4 expression in dysplastic epithelium of the oral cavity and in undifferentiated carcinomas. *Kearsly* considers the expression of TA-4 indicating the degree of cellular differentiation of the squamous cells and not the cellular proliferation or malignant transformation. He goes so far as to claim that TA-4 expression can be used to judge the degree of heterogeneity of a tumor in morphologically identical tissues. Under the electron microscope TA-4 was detected in the tonofribrils in normal mucosa of the mouth and in squamous cell carcinomas.

As with most tumor markers, SCC has no specificity for discriminating between benign and malignant tissue (4). A number of benign gynecological diseases show raised SCC levels in a significant percentage of cases (5), as do patients with inflammatory lung disease and renal insufficiency. Nevertheless, the value of SCC for estimating the prognosis and monitoring the course of carcinoma of the cervix uteri is undisputed (6, 7, 8). Slightly to moderately raised SCC serum levels have been measured as well in the presence of a number of other squamous cell carcinomas (pharynx, larynx, palate, tongue, neck, lung) (9). However, in these cases SCC is of less relevance, because it does not have the same sensitivity and specificity as for cancer of the cervix.

Squamous cells and transitional cells have morphological similarities and it is suggested that they may have a common stem cell. Therefore, it was decided to evaluate SCC serum levels in transitional cell carcinomas of the bladder and urinary tract. In a first series *Takahashi* (10) measured SCC levels > 2 µg/l in 27% of his patients with urothelial carcinoma. Though no correlation between SCC serum levels and tumor stage and grade was found, changes in levels corresponding to the clinical course were determined. To date, there have been no reports that confirm these results or that assess the potential significance of SCC for transitional cell carcinoma. Since other tumor markers (TPA, CEA, p412) have also been shown to lack sensitivity, we investigated the value of SCC serum levels for diagnosing and monitoring the course of transitional cell carcinoma.

Material and methods

SCC was measured in the serum of 54 patients before the operation. 34 patients had a transitional cell carcinoma of the bladder or upper urinary tract of all stages (Ta-7, T1-5, T2-20, Cis-2). Only patients with transitional cell carcinoma were selected for evaluation, other histologies (urocystitis, dysplasia, squamous cell carcinoma) were excluded. The control group consisted of 20 patients without bladder tumor with the following urological diseases: condition after TCC control 4, urocystitis 2, BPH 5, prostate cancer 5, healthy subjects (erectile dysfunction) 3, 1 unknown primary tumor 1.

Serum samples were additionally taken after tumor resection (cystectomy, TUR) in 14 patients. In all patients blood was taken in the morning and centrifuged at 4.000 U/min, the serum was deep-frozen at −80 °C. SCC measurements were performed in a joint test procedure using a microparticle enzyme immunoassay (MEIA).

The analysis was performed in a fully automatic enzyme immunoanalyzer (IMX Abbott). The SCC test is a microparticle-immunoassay (MEIA) for the quantitative measurement of SCC antigen in serum or plasma. For the assay 200 µl serum were placed in a reaction cell. To construct an antigen antibody complex microparticles coated with antibodies and automatized with the patient sample were instilled into the reactor cell and incubated at 34 °C. After addition of a secondary antibody, an aliquot of the reaction mixture was transferred to a fiberglass matrix, which has a high affinity for the microparticles. By washing with buffer all of the unbound components were removed from the detection range. After application of a fluorescence dye (4-methylumbelliferryl phosphate) the secondary antibody was split off and the photometric measurement was performed.

Statistical evaluation

The data were presented using descriptive statistical methods (mean value, median, standard deviation). Significance was determined using the Wilcoxon-Mann-Whitney-U test.

Results

There were no significant differences in SCC serum levels between patients with transitional carcinomas and those in the urological control group (figure 1). In seven cases (five TCC, two control subjects) SCC plasma levels higher than 2.5 µg/l were measured. Renal insufficiency could be the explanation in four of these cases. In 14 patients with TCC and four control subjects serum levels were measured before surgery and after tumor removal (figure 2). The results were reproducible, independent of tumor stage and type of procedure performed (TUR, cystectomy). Therefore, it must be assumed that the SCC levels measured had no connection with the transitional carcinoma.

Discussion

Although it stems from the squamous epithelium, which is located throughout the body, the squamous cell-specific antigen (SCC) serves as a valid tumor marker only for squamous cell carcinoma of the cervix. SCC lacks the necessary sensitivity, especially for tumors of the aerodigestive tract. There are marked morphological similarities between squamous cells and transitional cells. It has even been suggested that they may have a common stem cell. Furthermore, they appear to react similarly to exogenous carcinogens in the nasopharynx, esophagus, and bladder, which is evident in multiple carcinomas or precancerous alterations and dysplasia.

Encouraged by these similarities, as well as initial results obtained by *Takahashi*, we compared SCC serum levels in patients with transitional cell carcinomas with those of a control group. No differences in SCC levels were found, the few SCC levels raised were related to renal insufficiency. Tumor removal did not bring about changes in SCC levels, which means that this marker is not adequate for follow-up of transitional cell carcinoma. This contradicts *Takahashi*'s findings.

In summary, a comparison of patients with urothelial carcinoma and urological control persons showed no significant differences in SCC serum levels. SCC levels were generally < 2.5 µg/l. SCC in the serum has proved to be an insensitive marker for transitional cell carcinoma, both for diagnostic as well as follow-up purposes.

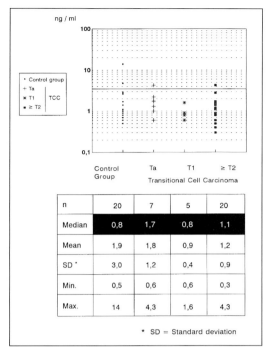

Figure 1. Plasma SCC-antigen in control group and in patients with transitional cell carcinoma of the bladder.

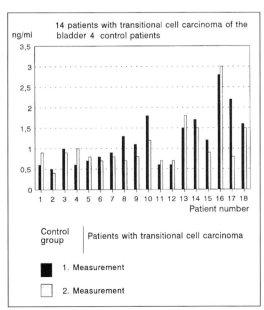

Figure 2. Pre- and post-surgical evaluation of plasma SCC-antigen levels in various patient groups.

References

1. Kato H, Torigoe T (1977) Radioimmunoassay for tumor antigen of human cervical squamous cell carcinoma. Cancer 40:1621–1628
2. Kato H, Nagaya T, Torigoe T (1984) Heterogeneity of a tumor antigen TA-4 of squamous cell carcinoma in relation to its appearance in the circulation. Gann 75:433–435
3. Kearsley JH, Stenzel DJ, Sculley TB, Cooke RA (1990) Cellular localisation of tumour antigen (TA-4) in normal, dysplastic and neoplastic squamous epithelia of the upper aerodigestive tract. Br J Cancer 61:631–635
4. Molina R, Filella X, Torres MD, Ballesta AM, Mengual P, Cases A, Balaque A (1990) SCC antigen measured in malignant and nonmalignant diseases. Clin Chem: 36/2, 251–254
5. Crombach G, Scharl A, Vierbuchen M, Würz M, Bolte A (1989) Detection of squamous cell carcinoma antigen in normal squamous epithelia and in squamous cell carcinomas of the uterine cervix. Cancer 63:1337–1342
6. Kato H, Tamai K, Morioka H, Nagai M, Nagaya T, Torigoe T (1984) Tumor-antigen TA-4 in the detection of recurrence in cervical squamous cell carcinoma. Cancer 54:1544–1546
7. Crombach G, Würz H, Horrmann F et al (1989) Bedeutung des SCC-Antigens in der Diagnostik und Verlaufskontrolle des Zervixkarzinoms. Eine kooperative Studie der Gynäkologischen Tumor-Marker-Gruppe (GTMG). Dtsch med Wschr 114:700–705
8. Meier W, Eiermann W, Stieber P, Fateh-Mogadam A, Hepp H (1989) SCC- und CEA-Verlauf als Prognosekriterium für das Ansprechen einer Chemotherapie beim Cervixkarzinom. Geburtsh Frauenheilkd 49:1050–1055
9. Fischbach W, Rink C (1988) SCC-Antigen: ein sensitiver und spezifischer Tumormarker für Plattenepithelkarzinome? Dtsch med Wschr 113:289–293
10. Takahashi Y, Shinoda I, Takeuchi T, Kuriyama M, Ban Y, Kawada Y (1988) Clinical assay of serum SCC-Ag in urothelial cancers. Intern J Biol Markers 3:15–18

Address for correspondence:
Dr. med. A. Katzenwadel
Urologische Universitätsklinik
Hugstetterstraße 55
D-79106 Freiburg, Germany

SCC (squamous cell carcinoma related antigen) in urine – A possible tumor marker in patients with transitional cell carcinoma

W. Schultze-Seemann, A. Katzenwadel, I. Struve, H. Sommerkamp

Department of Urology, University of Freiburg, Germany

Introduction

The clinical sign of transitional cell carcinoma of the bladder and upper urinary tract is usually hematuria. Tumor staging by means of imaging methods (sonography, computed tomography, magnetic resonance imaging) as well as diagnostic transurethral surgery carries a high rate of error. Attempts to minimize these staging errors by determining tumor markers were unsuccessful, since transitional cell carcinomas are very heterogeneous and monoclonal antibodies lack the necessary specificity (1).

None of the established tumor markers to date have shown sufficient sensitivity and specificity for transitional cell carcinoma. Only carcinoembryonic antigen (CEA), tissue polypeptide antigen (TPA), and P486 have achieved relative significance for the follow-up of bladder cancer. CEA and TPA are non-specific tumor-associated antigens, TPA is regarded as the »proliferation antigen«, whose synthesis takes place in epithelial cells in the S-phase (2). TPA lacks specificity, since the serum TPA level can also be raised in patients with benign diseases (virus infection, bacterial infection, hepatitis, cirrhosis of the liver) (2), which also show increased proliferation. There are a number of reasons for false-positive CEA serum levels (metabolism, lung, liver, colitis) (3, 4). Both tumor markers can be detected in urine, for reproducible measurements a number of conditions must be fulfilled (standardized collection periods, exclusion of benign diseases) (5). CEA measurements in the urine of women are worthless. TPA on the other hand can be determined in both genders. A number of benign diseases can affect the diagnostic sensitivity of TPA. The TPA levels in urine represent the proliferative activity of the transitional cell and thus are raised in patients with inflammatory disease. Nevertheless, sensitivity of TPA determination in urine and serum has been reported to be as high as 86% (6) when benign disease has been ruled out.

A number of monoclonal antibodies (14 III, 486 P3/12, T 138, etc.) are available for immunohistochemical and immunocytological examinations, however, due to the heterogeneity of transitional cell carcinoma a threshold of positive cells must be defined, which frequently increases sensitivity at the expense of specificity. SCC is the established tumor marker in the primary diagnosis and follow-up of neoplasms of the cervix uteri (7, 8). Because of the morphological similarities between transitional cells and squamous cells we conducted the first study on SCC serum levels in patients with transitional cell carcinoma. SCC proved to lack sensitivity. Since CEA and TPA are known to be expressed in urine (9), we addressed the detection of SCC in the urine of patients with transitional cell carcinoma in comparison with a normal population.

Materials and methods

Out of 65 patients with endoscopically confirmed bladder tumors, urine was collected between 7 and 11 a.m. prior to the scheduled operation (transurethral resection/cystectomy). A total of 10 ml was deep-frozen at −80 °C, specific weight was additionally measured.

The control group consisted of patients with a variety of other urological conditions (erectile dysfunction, no affection of the urinary tract n = 23, urolithiasis n = 32, urocystitis n = 7, condition after transitional cell carcinoma and BCG therapy n = 8). The determination of SCC in urine was performed by using a microparticle enzyme-

immunoassay (IMX, Abbott) in a joint test procedure.
Seventeen transitional cell tumors of all stages and different gradings with positive and negative SCC detection in urine were preserved in nitrogen and examined immunochemically (ABC technique) for SCC expression (McAB Lot 870, IgG/Abbott).

Statistical analysis

The data were presented using descriptive statistics (mean value, median, standard deviation). Significance was determined using the Wilcoxon-Mann-Whitney-U test.

Results

The control group with no disease of the urinary tract had SCC levels of < 2 µg/l, only in one case (long history of juvenile diabetes mellitus with renal insufficiency) 3.5 µg/l was measured. Patients with transitional cell carcinoma on the other hand showed increasing SCC levels (figure 1), with highly significant differences with regard to stages in comparison with the normal group (p = 0.0000001). The SCC levels were significantly higher in the presence of transitional cell carcinoma, independent of tumor stage, while the various T-stages differed only slightly (figure 3). The three benign conditions with considerably increased proliferative activity of the transitional cell (condition after transitional cell carcinoma and adjuvant BCG therapy, urolithiasis, urocystitis) were marked by raised urinary SCC levels (figure 2), which were significantly higher than those in the control group (p = 0.00005 to 0.0001). In terms of the urinary SCC levels the three benign conditions can not be distinguished from a transitional cell carcinoma. There were no significances (table I).
No quantitative evaluation of SCC expression was performed in the immunohistochemical preparations of bladder tumors, in half of the 17 stained tumors antibody binding was detected, which was confined to the cytoplasma (figures 4, 5), while undifferentiated tumors showed only minimal or no SCC expression.

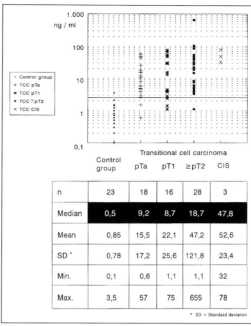

	Control group	Transitional cell carcinoma			
		pTa	pT1	≥pT2	CIS
n	23	18	16	28	3
Median	0,5	9,2	8,7	18,7	47,8
Mean	0,85	15,5	22,1	47,2	52,6
SD*	0,78	17,2	25,6	121,8	23,4
Min.	0,1	0,6	1,1	1,1	32
Max.	3,5	57	75	655	78

* SD = Standard deviation

Figure 1. Urine SCC-antigen levels of control patients and patients with transitional cell carcinoma of the bladder.

Table I. Statistical significance (p) of the differences between the urine SCC-Ag levels of patients with transitional cell carcinoma and benign urological diseases (Wilcoxon-Mann-Whitney-Test).

Patient groups			Significance (p)[a]
Control group	↔	TCC (total)	0.000001
Control group	↔	BPH	0.00005
Control group	↔	urocystitis	0.0001
Control group	↔	BCG instillation	0.0001
Control group	↔	urolithiasis	0.00005
Urocystitis	↔	TCC (total)	0.28 n.s.[b]
Urocystitis	↔	BCG instillation	0.46 n.s.[b]
Urocystitis	↔	urolithiasis	0.023
Urocystitis	↔	BPH	0.023
BCG instillation	↔	TCC (total)	0.16 n.s.
BCG instillation	↔	urolithiasis	0.015
BCG instillation	↔	BPH	0.015
Urolithiasis	↔	TCC (total)	0.16 n.s.[b]
Urolithiasis	↔	BPH	0.19 n.s.[b]
BPH	↔	TCC (total)	0.015

[a] p-Level for 95 per cent probability: 0.05;
[b] not significant: p > 0.05

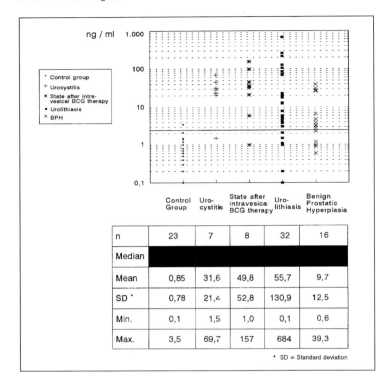

Figure 2. Urine SCC-antigen levels in a control group compared to patients with benign urological diseases.

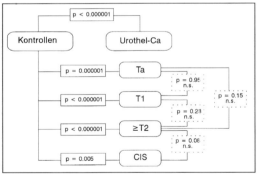

Figure 3. Significance of the differences between the urine SCC-Ag levels of a control group and various T-stages of TCC; Wilcoxon-Mann-Whitney-Test (p-level for 95 per cent probability: 0.05).

Discussion

The problem of tumor markers, which have been used to date in diagnosing transitional cell carcinoma, has often been the fact that threshold values had to be determined which increased sensitivity but at the expense of specificity. The same appears to apply for SCC detection in urine when one considers the highly positive values for the benign conditions named above, which, like malignant tumors, are associated with a considerably increased proliferation of transitional cells. Since these conditions all have typical clinical symptoms, however, the question arises how to distinguish between asymptomatic tumor patients and healthy subjects. Highly significant differences between all tumor stages and the normal population suggest that SCC could play an important role in tumor screening and monitoring. A number of other questions remain to be clarified, including the intra-individual reproducibility of urinary SCC levels. Initial controls indicate that there is only minimal SCC fluctuation, however, the number of subjects is too small to allow reliable conclusions. Furthermore, it must be determined whether resection of a superficial tumor can lead to a drop in SCC to levels found in healthy subjects. Preoperative and postoperative examinations of only 10 patients show that SCC levels decrease considerably after the resection of papillary tumors, while they drop only slightly or remain unchanged after palliative resection. Increases have not been measured. Another unanswered question is to

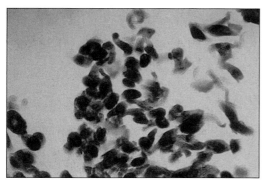

Figure 4. Positive staining for SCC in a Tcc Grade II (ABC-technique).

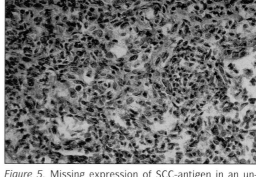

Figure 5. Missing expression of SCC-antigen in an undifferentiated bladder cancer.

what degree repeated measurements in the same subjects produce diverging results. Measurements repeated three and four times, in some cases months apart, confirm the reproducibility of the data. A final question concerns the temperature stability and the preparation of the urine, particularly whether fixatives have to be used to guarantee stability of the urinary SCC. Serial measurements done over several hours demonstrate a slow albeit continuous decrease of SCC levels.

It will be necessary in the near future to increase the number of subjects in the control group and to describe them exactly, and to analyze the sensitivity and specificity of urinary SCC in larger populations of patients with transitional cell carcinoma.

References

1. Arndt R, Dürkopf H, Huland H, Donn F, Loening T, Kalthoff H (1987) Monoclonal antibodies for characterization of the heterogenity of normal and malignant transitional cells. J Urol 137:758
2. Björklund B (1980) On the nature of clinical use of tissue polypeptide antigen (TPA). Tumor Diagnostik 1:9-10
3. Costanza ME, Das S, Nathanson R, Rule A, Schwartz RS (1974) Carcinoembryonic antigen. Report of a screening study. Cancer 33:583-590
4. Fraser RA, Ravry MJ, Segura JW, Go VLW (1975) Clinical evaluation of urinary and serum carcinoembryonic antigen in bladder cancer. J Urol 114:226-229
5. Adolphs HD, Oehr P (1982) Significance of urine and serum CEA determination for the diagnosis of urinary bladder cancer. Tumor Diagnostik 3:34-39
6. Oehr P, Adolphs HD, Odenthal U, Klein-Hitpass A, Kirsch J, Winkler C (1983) Verteilung, Sensitivität und Spezifität von TPA, TAG und TPAxTAG Marker-Produktwerten bei Patienten mit Blasenkarzinom. Tumor Diagnostik 4:179-181
7. Kato H, Tamai K, Morioka H, Nagai M, Nagaya T, Torigoe T (1985) Tumor antigen TA-4 in the detection of recurrence in cervical squamous cell carcinoma. Cancer 56:302-308
8. Crombach G, Würz H, Horrmann F et al (1985) Bedeutung des SCC Antigens in der Diagnostik und Verlaufskontrolle des Zervixkarzinoms. Eine kooperative Studie der Gynäkologischen Tumor-Marker-Gruppe (GTMG). Dtsch med Wschr 114:700-705
9. Adolphs HD, Oehr P (1984) Bedeutung der Serum- und Urin CEA und TPA Bestimmung für die Diagnose des Harnblasenkarzinoms.In: Bichler KH, Harzmann R (Hrsg) Das Harnblasenkarzinom. Springer, Berlin Heidelberg, pp 145-155

Address for correspondence:
Dr. med. W. Schultze-Seemann
Urologische Universitätsklinik
Hugstetterstraße 55
D-79106 Freiburg, Germany

sICAM-1 level in urine of bladder cancer patients

D. Rohde, D. Küsters, R. Sikora, G. Jakse
Oncological Research Laboratory, Department of Urology,
Technical University of Aachen, Germany

Introduction

The intercellular adhesion molecule 1 (ICAM-1, CD 54) represents a membran protein that is expressed on the surface of (8, 10, 41), stromal cells (9, 11), neural- (35), endothelial- (16) and epithelial cells (51). In addition it has been identified at neuroectodermal tumors (15, 19), skin cancer (42, 46), lymphoma and leukemia cells (28, 54), seminoma (47), epithelial carcinoma and adenocarcinoma (14, 24, 25, 49).
ICAM-1 is involved in several immunological cell-cell interactions by binding to the leucocyte-function-associated antigen-1 (LFA-1; CD11a/CD18) (5), Mac-1 (CD11b/CD18) (44) or CD43 (40). The molecule participates in the homotypic und heterotypic aggregation of T- und B-lymphocytes (32) and the activation of T- (memory-)cells by interaction with antigen presenting cells (APC) (30). Moreover the adhesion of ICAM-1 can influence antibody production (6) and support the CD3/TCR dependent lysability of tumor target cells by cytotoxic T-lymphocytes (CTL) (7, 29). In addition ICAM-1/LFA-1 can mediate morphological changes and the transendothelial migration of effector cells (12, 52).
Recently a soluble form of ICAM-1 has been characterized (43). The molecule designated sICAM-1 (cICAM-1) contains most but not all of the five extracellular domaines of the surface bound ICAM-1 (45). It binds to LFA-1 similary as ICAM-1 (41a). The mechanism for shedding of the antigen is still unknown. But it has been shown in vitro, that the concentration of sICAM-1 in cell culture supernatant correlates with the cellular expression of ICAM-1 (23, 42, 50).
Besides measurements in supernatant and serum sICAM-1 used to be detected in cerebrospinal fluid (17) and in bile (1). Significantly increased levels have been found in serum of patients with infections (25b, 33) or with an active auto-aggressive disease (18). Enhanced sICAM-1 values were described in serum of patients with malignant tumors as well (pancreas, stomach, colon, esophagus, gall bladder, melanoma, ovary, breast, renal cell carcinoma), preferentially in case of metastasis (3a, 17a, 50).
With regard to recent experimental data, that demonstrated a variable ICAM-1 expression on the surface of human transitional cell carcinoma in vitro (22) and on tissue specimen of bladder carcinoma (TCCB) (48), the aim of the present study was to evaluate, if sICAM-1 could be found in cell culture supernatant of established urothelial carcinoma cell lines and in serum of patients with a bladder cancer. In addition, it was of special interest to investigate, if sICAM-1 is expressed in human urine and if the observed urinary level would reflect phenotyp, tumor stage or the grade of malignancy of the corresponding tumors.

Materials and methods

Cell culture

Cell lines derived from human transitional cell carcinoma RT 112 (31), RT 112 CP (53), 647 V (13), HT 1376 (36), HT 1376-Eto (39) and J 82 (34) were routinely grown under cell culture conditions (7% CO_2; + 37 °C). Media (RPMI 1640, DMEM) were supplemented with 10–15% (v/v) fetal calf-serum, penicillin (100 IU/ml) and streptomycin (100 µg/ml) (GIBCO, Paisly, Scotland); the medium for RT 112 CP contained 3 µg/ml cis-platinum (medac, Hamburg, Germany).

$3 \cdot 10^5$ tumor cells were seeded per well of a 24 well-plate (Falcon) and incubated with 300 IU/ml rhu-interferon-α2a (Hoffmann-La Roche, Grenzach-Wylen, Germany) or rhu-interferon-γ (Rentschler, Laupheim, Germany) for 72 hours. Controls recieved supplemented cell culture medium without cytokines. Afterwards cell culture supernatants have been collected, centrifugated and stored at –80 °C. The number of corresponding cells per well was counted after trypsinization (Neubauer chamber).

Preparation and analysis of urine and serum

The first morning urine (40 ml) and serum (10 ml) of patients with a bladder carcinoma (n = 34) was collected before operation and processed within three hours (4 °C). Patients with signs of a systemic infection have been excluded.
Urine were screened with a dip stick test system (Combur 9, Boehringer, Mannheim, Germany) for erythrocytes/hemoglobin, leucocytes, nitrite, pH-value and the presence of protein, glucose, bilirubine and ketones; another probe was tested bacteriological (Department of Microbiology, Aachen). After pelletration of cellular components (1400 x g, 10 minutes) urinary supernatant was stored in aliquotes at –80 °C. Probes being screened for sICAM-1 expression have been quantified concerning their creatinine concentration as well (Department of Clinical Chemistry, Aachen).
Serum was cleared by centrifugation (3500 x g, 10 minutes) and stored at –80 °C. Hemolyzed or lipemic sera were rejected.
Material from healthy control persons (n = 10) was processed in a similar fashion.

Enzyme immunoassay

Humane sICAM-1 was measured with a specific sandwich enzyme immunoassay (Cellfree® ICAM-1 Test Kit; T Cell Diagnostics, Cambridge, MA, USA). The sensitivity of the assay is given with a detection limit of 0.3 ng/ml. The assay has been run in accordance to the test prescription. Serum was diluted 1 : 100; urine has been chosen undiluted or as a 1 : 100 diluted solution, whilst cell culture supernatant was used undiluted. Optical densities were read at a single wavelength of 492 nm. Resulting sICAM-1 concentrations (ng/ml) were calculated in respect of standard curves (0.56 ng/ml, 2.86 ng/ml, 5.89 ng/ml, 8.94 ng/ml ICAM-1). Each test solution has been run in duplicate.

Statistics

Concentration were condensed to mean values ($\bar{x}$), standard deviations (SD) and ranges. For significance calculations the student's t-test for unpaired variables was used with a significance level of $p < 0.05$. Correlations were calculated by Pearson's correlation analysis.

Results

A basal sICAM-1 expression was detected in the supernatants of 3/6 established cell lines of human transitional cell carcinoma (figure 1). There was no obvious difference between cell lines derived from grade 2 carcinoma (RT 112, RT 112 CP, 647 V) and grade 3 carcinoma (HT 1376, HT 1376-Eto, J 82).
Exposition to IFN-γ increased the concentration of sICAM-1 in initial sICAM-1-negative cell lines (RT 112, HT 1376-Eto) as well as in a sICAM-1-positive cell line (RT 112 CP). IFN-α was less effective in general but enhanced shedding of sICAM-1 from J 82 cells more sufficient than IFN-τ (figure 1).
The drug-resistant cell lines RT 112 CP and HT 1376-Eto expressed a higher basal or cytokine-induced sICAM-1 level compared to their parental cell lines. In addition they were most sensible to a stimulation with IFN-γ (figure 1).
Resected tumor specimen (n = 34) were classified in accordance to the WHO (Department of Pathology, Aachen) as transitional cell carcinoma (n = 32), squamous cell carcinoma (n = 1) and an oat cell bladder carcinoma (n = 1).
Urine analysis gave no evidence for bilirubine, ketones, glucose, nitrite or bacteria in any probe. Using the standardized test kit sICAM-1 could be reproducibly detected in urine as well as in 1:100 diluted serum. Dilution of the urinary probes (1:100) effected concentrations below the detection limit of the assay. The urinary sICAM-1 levels of volunteers (n = 2) reached a maximum in

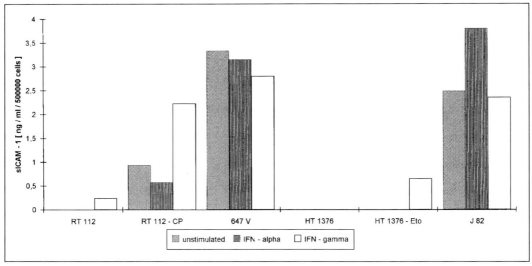

Figure 1. Expression of sICAM-1 in supernatants of cell lines from transitional cell carcinoma.

Table I. Results and statistics of sICAM-1 level in serum and urine of patients with bladder carcinoma.

Group	n	x̄	sICAM -1 urine (ng/ml) range	SD	x̄	sICAM-1 serum (ng /ml) range	SD
Control	10	2.54	0.0 – 6.0	1.82	259.00	160 – 370	66.53
Tu sum.	34	4.54	0.0 – 14.1	3.50	327.24	140 – 530	94.78
Ta	17	3.29	0.8 – 6.1	1.38	299.18	156 – 500	79.79
T1 – T4	17	5.85	0.0 – 14.4	4.44	355.00	140 – 530	102.42
T 1	10	6.59	0.6 – 14.1	4.66	342.50	140 – 515	101.08
T 2	5	5.40	0.0 – 12.7	4.89	414.00	345 – 530	74.62
T 3	1	1.80			170.00		
T 4	1	4.70			375.00		
G 1	12	3.95	0.8 – 14.1	3.40	316.25	180 – 500	87.39
G 2	15	4.34	0.6 – 10.8	2.63	301.33	140 – 425	67.97
G 3	7	5.99	0.0 – 12.7	5.18	405.00	170 – 530	119.93
M +	4	7.25	2.6 – 14.1	5.01	343.75	285 – 375	41.31
M –	30	4.18	0.0 – 12.7	3.20	325.97	140 – 530	98.45

Statistics
(significance level p < 0.05)

Group	n	Group	n	sICAM-1 urine	sICAM-1 serum
Tu sum.	34	control	10	p < 0.024	p < 0.016
Ta	17	T 1	10	p < 0.047	p < 0.278
Ta	17	T1 – T4	17	p < 0.048	p < 0.165
M +	4	control	10	p < 0.125	p < 0.025
M+	4	M –	30	p < 0.256	p < 0.534

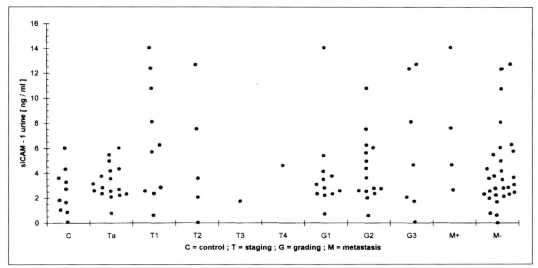

Figure 2. Urinary sICAM-1 level in accordance to tumor stage and grade of malignancy.

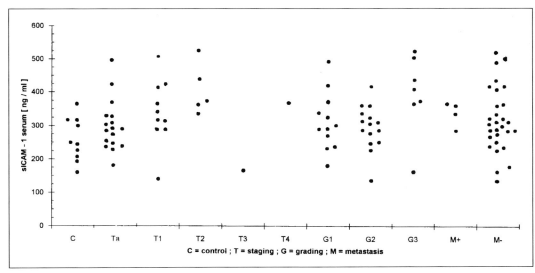

Figure 3. sICAM-1 serum level in accordance to tumor stage and grade of malignancy.

the morning (7 a.m.) compared to the evening values (9 p.m.) (data not shown).

The average concentration of sICAM-1 in the urine (u) of controls (n =10) was 2.54 ng/ml and in serum (s): 259 ng/ml, in contrast to bladder cancer patients (n = 34) with 4.54 ng/ml (u) and 327 ng/ml (s) respectively (figure 2). Urinary and serum sICAM-1 level of patients with a carcinoma (Tu sum.) were statistically enhanced in comparison to healthy volunteers and increased with tumor stage and grade of malignancy. Especially the concentrations of sICAM-1 in urine were significantly enhanced between cases of superficial carcinoma (pTa) and invasive bladder cancer (pT1, pT1-pT4) whereas corresponding serum level did not differ significantly (figure 2, 3). The presence of metastasis did not effect significantly higher sICAM-1 level in urine or serum than those being observed in patients with organ confined carcinoma (table I).

No correlation was found either between sICAM-1 concentrations in serum and urine (coefficient (k): 0.279) nor between urinary level and the presence of erythrocytes or leucocytes (k: 0.263–0.299), the pH or the urinary concentrations of creatinine and protein (k: 0.223–0.233).

Discussion

Recent studies have shown that ICAM-1 is expressed on the surface of cell lines and tissue specimen from human transitional cell carcinoma (21, 22, 46b, 48). The present study demonstrates that the soluble molecule (sICAM-1) is shed in supernatants from urothelial carcinoma cells in vitro, and could in addition be detected in urine and serum of patients with a bladder carcinoma. The observed serum concentrations of sICAM-1 were in the same range as Banks and co-workers recently published for a small group of six patients with a TCCB (3a). Increasing urine and serum sICAM-1 level both tend to indicate dedifferentiated and invasive tumors, as it has been suggested for the ICAM-1 expression on tissue specimen of invasive TCCB before (48). It was of particular interest, that preferentially the analysis of sICAM-1 level in urine tended to discriminate between superficial (pTa) and invasive (> pTa) bladder carcinoma, whereas no statistically significant difference was found between pTa tumors and controls ($p < 0.298$), or in regard to serum level. We suggest, that these findings may be due to an upregulation of ICAM-1 by the tumor cells themselves, by migration through the basement membrane (2b) and/or by an intensified immune or stromal response of the peritumoral microenvironment after invasion (48, 50).

The observed variable basal concentrations of shed sICAM-1 in supernatants of bladder carcinoma cells coincide with the reported quantity of ICAM-1-positive tumor cells in vitro (RT 112: 5%, J82: 63% (22), HT 1376: < 5% (48)). In addition, the stimulation of sICAM-1 shedding in supernatants of TCCB by cytokines similarly reflects the enhanced expression of ICAM-1 at the surface of bladder cancer cells after administration of interferons reported by other investigators (22, 46b, 48).

The interesting phenomenon that drug resistant cell lines shed a higher level of sICAM-1 as the corresponding parental tumor cells has been described for membrane bound ICAM-1-positive glioblastoma and colon cancer cells as well (37, 38). The definite role of sICAM-1 in tumorbiology of TCCB is at least still a part of speculations. Tomita and co-workers e.g. proposed that invading immunopotent mononuclear cells enhance the expression of membran-bound ICAM-1 on the surface of urothelial cancer cells by release of cytokines, and supported the view that this up-regulation should be associated with an increased tumor defense (48). In addition Jackson and co-workers demonstrated that the stimulation of ICAM-1 on TCCB by IFN-γ in vitro partially enhances the susceptibility and lysability of the tumor cells by lymphokin-activated killer cells (LAK-cells) (22). In contrast, it has been reported that the molecule sICAM-1 can inhibit the heterotypical adhesion and cytotoxicity of natural killer cells (NK-cells) and LAK-cells against target cells (3, 4, 50). It has been shown for example, that sICAM-1 derived from serum of patients with a melanoma inhibits the lysis of melanoma cells by NK-cells in vitro (2). Moreover, it has recently been reported that binding of sICAM-1 with LFA-1 can cause a de-adhesion of already adherend immunopotent effector cells (41a).

In conclusion, sICAM-1 can easily be detected by a simple and standardized assay. Urinary sICAM-1 level are suggested to be more sensitive to indicate early invasion of bladder carcinoma than serum level. Therefore the analysis especially of sICAM-1 in urine recommends itself as a tumor-marker for invasion of bladder carcinoma suitable for diagnosis and follow-up, but not as a marker for screening of superficial bladder cancer. Moreover, increased sICAM-1 level in case of invasion may indicate the potency of tumor cells to escape immunosurveillance and hereby to spread into an organism (3a). In addition, the fact that the sICAM-1 expression could be stimulated by biological response modifiers may offer the opportunity to estimate the efficay of an intravesical immunotherapy (IFN, BCG) by monitoring the urinary sICAM-1 level before, during or after a topic therapy.

References

1 Adams D, Mainolfi E, Elias E, Neuberger JM, Rothlein R (1993) Transplantation 55:83
2 Altomonte M, Gloghini A, Bertola G, Gasparollo A, Carbone A, Ferrone S, Maio M (1993) Cancer Res 53:3343
2b Anichini A, Mortarini R, Supina R, Parmiani G (1990) Int J Cancer 46:508
3a Banks RE, Gearing AJH, Hemingway IK, Norfolk DR, Perren TJ, Selby PJ (1993) Br J Cancer 68:122
3 Becker JC, Dummer R, Schmidt RE, Burg G, Hartmann AA (1992) Immun Infekt 20:62
4 Becker JC, Dummer R, Hartmann M, Burg G, Schmidt RE (1991) J Immunol 147:4398
5 Bierer BE, Burakoff SJ (1988) FASEB 2:2584
6 Boyd AW, Wawryk SO, Burns G (1988) Proc Natl Acad Sci USA 85:3095
7 Braakman E, Goedegebuure PS, Vreugdenhil RJ, Segal DM, Shaw S, Bolhuis RL (1990) Int J Cancer 46:475
8 Buckle A, Hogg N (1992). Eur J Immunol 20:337
9 Couffinhal T, Duplaa C, Labat L, Lamaziere JM, Moreau C, Printseva O, Bonnet J (1993) Arterioscler Thromb 13:407
10 Dougherty GJ, Murdoch S, Hogg N (1988) Eur J Immunol 18:35
11 Dustin ML, Rothlein R, Bhan AK, Dinarello CA, Springer TA (1986) J Immunol 137:245
12 Ebisawa M, Bochner BS, Georas SN, Schleimer RP (1992) J Immunol 149:4021
13 Elliot AY, Bronson DL, Stein N, Fraley EE (1976) Cancer Res 36:365
14 Ernstoff MS, Jaffee EM, Oeler T (1992) Nat Immun 11:17
15 Favrot MC, Combaret V, Goillot E, Tabone E, Boffet E, Dolbeau D, Bouvier R, Coze C, Michon J, Philip T (1991) Int J Cancer 48:502
16 Gerritsen ME, Kelley KA, Ligon G, Perry CA, Shen CP, Szczepanski A, Carley WW (1993) Arthritis Rheum 36:593
17a Harning R, Mainolfi E, Bystryn JC, Henn M, Merluzzi VJ, Rothlein R (1991) Cancer Res 51:5003
17 Hartung HP (1993) Ann Neurol 33
18 Hauschild S, Schmitt WH, Kekow J, Szymkowiak C, Gross WL (1992) Immun Infekt 20:84
19 Hong L, Imeri L, Opp MR, Postlethwaite AE, Seyer JM, Krueger JM (1993) J Neuroimmunol 44:163
20 Itami M, Takenoucki T, Tamaru J, Harigaya K, Mikata A (1991) Acta Pathol Jpn 41:277
21 Jackson AM, Prescott S, Hawkyard S, James K, Chisholm G (1993) Cancer Immunol Immunother 36:25
22 Jackson AM, Alexandrov AB, Prescott S, James K, Chisholm GD (1992) Immunology 76:286
23 Kageshita T, Yoshii A, Kimura T, Ono T (1992) J Dermatol 19:836
24 Kelly CP, O'Keane JC, Orellana J, Schroy III PC, Yang S, Lamont JA, Brady HR (1992) Am J Physiol 263:864
25 Koyama S, Ebihara T, Fukao K (1992) J Cancer Res Clin Oncol 118:609
25b Küster H, Degitz K (1993) Lancet 341:506
26 Larson RS, Corbi AL, Berman L, Springer T (1989) J Cell Biol 108:703
27 Leo R, Boeker M, Peest D, Hein R, Bartl R, Gessner JE, Selbach J, Wacker G, Deicher H (1992) Ann Hematol 64:132
28 Maio M, Pinto A, tarbone A, Zagonel V, Gloghini A, Marotta G, Cirillo D, Colombatti A, Ferrara F, Veochio LD, Ferrone S (1990) Blood 76:783
29 Makgoba MW, Sanders ME, Luce GEG, 6ugell EA, Dustin ML, Springer TA, Shaw S (1988) Eur J Immunol 18:637
30 Maraskovsky E, Toutt AB, Kelso A (1992) Int Immunol 4:475
31 Marshall CJ, Franks LM, Carbonell AW (1977) JNCI 5:1743
32 Mazerolles F, Lumbroso C, Lecomte O, Le Deist F, Fischer A (1988) Eur J Immunol 18:1229
33 Most J, Zangerle R, Herold M, Fuchs D, Wachter H, Fritsch P, Dierich MP (1992) J Acquir Immune Defic Syndr 6,3:221
34 O'Toole D, Price ZH, Ohnuki Y, Unsgaard B (1978) Br J Cancer 38:64
35 Powers JM, Liu Y, Moser AB, Moser HW (1992) J Neuropathol Exp Neurol 51:630
36 Rashee S, Gardner MB, Rongey RW, Nelson-Rees WA, Arnstein P (1977) JNCI 58:881
37 Reddy PG, Graham GM, Datta S, Guarini L, Moulton TA, Jiang H, Gottesman MM, Ferrone S, Fisher PB (1991) JNCI 83:1307
38 Rivoltini L, Cattoretti G, Arienti F, Matroianni A, Melani C, Colombo MP, Parmiani G (1991) Int J Cancer 47:746
39 Rohde D, Kapp T, Sikora R, Jakse G (1994) Urologie A 33 (Suppl 1): 118
40 Rosenstein Y, Park JK, Hahn WC, Rosen FS, Bierer BE, Burakoof SJ (1991) Nature 354:233
41a Rothlein R, Mainolfi EA, Czyjkowski M, Marlin SD (1991) J Immunol 147:3778
41 Ruco LP, Pomponi D, Pigott R, Gearing AJ, Baiocchini A, Baroni CD (1992) Am J Pathol 140:1337
42 Scheibenbogen C, Keilholz U, Meuer S, Dengler T, Tilgen W, Hunstein W (1993) Int J Cancer 54:494
43 Seth R, Raymond FD, Makgoba MW (1991) Lancet 338:3
44 Teixido J, Hemler ME, Greenberger JS, Anklesaria P (1992) J Clin Invest 90:358
45 Staunton DE, Marlin SD, Stratowa C, Dustin ML, Springer TA (1988) Cell 52:925
46 Taylor RS, Griffiths CEM, Brown MD, Swanson NA, Nickoloff BJ (1990) J Am Acad Dermatol 22:721

46b Temponi M, Romano G, D'Urso CM, Wang Z, Kekish U, Ferrone S (1988) Sem Oncol 15:595
47 Tomita Y, Kimura M, Tanikawa T, Nishiyama T, Morishita, Takeda M, Fujiwara M, Sato S (1993) J Urol 149:659
48 Tomita Y, Watanabe H, Kobayashi H, Nishiyama T, Tsuji S, Imai K, Abo T, Fujiwara M, Sato S (1993) Am J Pathol 143:191
49 Tomita Y, Nishiyama T, Watanabe H, Fujiwara M, Sato S (1990) Int J Cancer 46:1001
50 Tsujisaki M, Imai K, Hirata H, Hanzawa Y, Masuya J, Nakano T, Sugiyama T, Matsui M, Hinoda Y, Yachi A (1991) Clin Exp Immunol 85:3
51 van de Stolpe A, Caldenhoven E, Raaijmakers JA, van der Saag PT, Koenderman L (1993) Am J Respir Cell Mol Biol 8:340
52 van Kooyk Y, van de Wiel van Kemenade E, Weder P, Huijbens RJ, Figdor CG (1993) J Exp Med 177:185
53 Walker MC, Povey S, Parrington JM, Riddle PN, Knüchel R, Masters RW (1990) Eur J Cancer 26:742
54 Wang F, Gregory C, Sample C, Rowe M, Liebowitz D, Murray R, Rickinson A, Kieff E (1990) J Virol 64:2309

Address for correspondence:
Dr. med. D. Rohde
Urologische Klinik
Medizinische Einrichtung der RWTH Aachen
Pauwelstraße 30
D-52057 Aachen, Germany

Tissue polypeptide antigen (TPA) immunoradiometric assay (IRMA) in regional and systemic staging of transitional cell carcinoma (TCC) of the urinary tract

M.S. Soloway[a], F.S. Freiha[b], R.W. DeVere White[c], S.D. Graham[d],
D.L. Lamm[e], M. Feygin[f], L.N. Fischer[g]

[a]University of Miami School of Medicine, Miami, Florida; [b]Stanford University School of Medicine, Stanford, California; [c]University of California, Davis, School of Medicine, Sacramento, California; [d]The Emory University School of Medicine, Atlanta, Georgia; [e]West Virginia University, Morgantown, West Virginia; [f]DIANON Systems, Inc., Stratford, Connecticut, USA; [g]Santec Medical, Bromma, Sweden

Introduction

A number of methods have been advanced for the clinical staging of bladder cancer. These range from cystoscopic evaluation and biopsy to computed tomography (CT) or contrast enhanced magnetic resonance imaging (MRI) (1–8). All have as their objective the identification of disease that has already metastasized at diagnosis. At this point transurethral resection (TUR) or cystectomy can no longer be more than palliative and the prognosis is generally quite poor.

None of the staging methods is entirely satisfactory, however (2, 9–14).

Even with such techniques as laparoscopic lymphadenectomy, clinical understaging is a perennial problem in bladder cancer (2, 3, 9) leading to unwarranted surgical intervention and delays in possibly more appropriate systemic therapy. In addition to their inaccuracies, CT and MRI are expensive. Laparoscopy is both expensive and invasive.

A circulating tumor marker whose level correlated well with the extent of disease might provide an aid to staging that would be both non-invasive and relatively inexpensive. Tissue polypeptide antigen (TPA), the only marker so far to demonstrate significant clinical value in advanced bladder cancer, may be such an adjunct.

Circulating TPA appears to comprise proteolytic degradation products of cytokeratins (CKs) 8, 18, and 19 (15, 16). These CKs are characteristic of simple and stratified internal epithelium. While CKs themselves are insoluble, the fragments that make up the TPA complex are soluble. They may be released to the circulation in relatively large quantities during times of increased turn over of the internal epithelium, such as occurs in inflammatory conditions or in carcinomas (17). Plasma TPA levels have been shown to correlate with the growth of malignant tumors (18).

In a prospective study of patients with bladder cancer we examined the relationship between TPA levels and the presence of regional or distant metastases. We wished to determine whether the median TPA level in patients with disseminated disease was sufficiently different from the median level in local disease to discriminate between the two groups.

Patients and methods

This was a double-blind, prospective study carried out in the departments of urology of six university associated medical centres in different regions of the United States.

From October 1988 to August 1993, 373 consecutive patients with histologically confirmed transitional cell carcinoma and no history of malignancy other than TCC were enroled in the study. Informed consent was obtained from all patients. Of these subjects, 258 remained disease free (inactive) during the study and 115 had active disease, either at enrollment or during follow-up. Among the patients with active disease, 89 were male and 26 female, while 8 were less than 50 years old and 107 were 50 or more years of age. We excluded 15 of this group from analysis due to a history of malignancy other than TCC.

Serial blood samples were obtained from all patients, beginning with baseline samples at enrolment. All samples were assayed for TPA by Dianon Systems Inc. of Stratford, Connecticut, using an immunoradiometric assay supplied by AB Sangtec Medical of Bromma, Sweden (TPA IRMA). Clinical investigators were blind to the patients' TPA plasma values. Laboratory technicians performing the assays were blind to the patients' clinical status.

Patients were staged clinically and/or pathologically at enrolment according to the TNM system (1). Stages T2 and T3 were distinguished clinically according to whether a palpable mass or induration was detectable upon bimanual examination following the transurethral resection of the tumor. Stage N1 was determined pathologically as a solitary positive pelvic node less than 2 cm in diameter, stage N2 as one or more positive nodes 2–5 cm in diameter, and stage N3 as a fixed mass or a node more than 5 cm in diameter.

Patients scheduled for cystectomy at the time of their enrolment were staged pathologically from the surgical specimen. Patients enrolling with distant recurrences after earlier surgery were staged with CT, chest X-ray, and/or bone scan. Distant metastases (stage M1) were defined as any positive nodes or other metastases above the aortic bifurcation.

After definitive staging, patients were stratified by the extent of disease: superficial (confined to the mucosa or lamina propria), muscle-invasive (superficial or deep), with metastasis confined to the pelvis, or with distant metastases. They were then further grouped according to the presence or absence of dissemination.

Disease extent at staging was taken as the end point. The outcome variable was categorical dichotomous: metastatic disease present (1) or absent (0). The outcome variable was based on the results of pathological evaluation of surgical specimens or the results of CT, chest X-ray, and bone scan. The combined variable was used with the awareness that these staging techniques have different levels of diagnostic accuracy. The pathological stage was used in all cases for which both clinical and pathological stages were available for the same disease event.

We tested the null hypothesis (no differences between groups in median plasma TPA levels, with significance at $a = 0.05$) and the alternative hypothesis (median higher in patients with metastatic disease). A clinically important difference in median levels was defined as 60 U/l.

The following statistical procedures were used where appropriate: organisation of outcome variable as dichotomised variables, non-parametric unpaired Wilcoxon test for two-group comparison, and receiver operating characteristic (ROC) curve analysis.

Table I. Plasma TPA values in patients with active TCC of the urinary tract ($p < 0.000001$; Wilcoxon signed rank test was used for comparison of medians).

Extent of disease	Number of patients	Mean (SD)	Median	95% CI for median
Local disease	67	79.5 (57.2)	62.0	54.0–72.0
N+ or M+	33	419.8 (702.6)	179.0	126.0–252.0
Total	100			

Table II. Plasma TPA values in patients (active disease).

Extent of disease	Number of patients	Mean (SD)	Median
Superficial	48	73.7 (52.3)	57.0
Muscle-invasive	19	94.0 (67.3)	63.0
N+	22	399.0 (722.4)	171.0
M+	11	461.3 (693.5)	185.0
Total	100		

Results

Plasma TPA levels were strongly correlated with the presence or absence of metastatic TCC ($p < 0.000001$). The median level for the 67 patients with superficial disease or tumor confined to the muscle was 62 U/l, versus 179 U/l for the 33 patients with metastases. The means and 95% confidence intervals are shown in table I. Table II shows the two groups broken down by the four staging strata used. The within-group differences in medians were not significant.

Figure 1 shows the distribution of TPA values in the two groups above and below the medians. The five data points at the top of the scale in the metastasis group were actually considerably off scale and were not analysed at the 600 U/l level. The ability of TPA values to discriminate between disseminated and local TCC was further examined by ROC-curve analysis (figure 2). The optimal combination of 85% sensitivity and 79% specificity was achieved with a cut-off of 94 U/l (area under the curve = 0.85, $p < 0.000001$ with a one-tailed test).

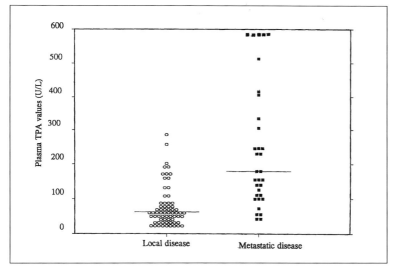

Figure 1. Plasma TPA in TCC patients (active disease).

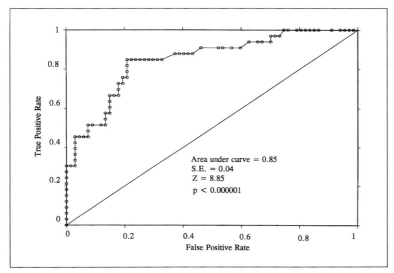

Figure 2. ROC curve for TPA as a diagnostic test for metastasis in TCC patients.

Discussion

The results of this study show that plasma TPA levels can serve as a sensitive and specific measure of the extent of disease in patients with carcinoma of the bladder. TPA may thus be suited for a role in the staging of advanced TCC.

Because of the complex, highly variable biology of bladder cancer, and the dismal prognosis once disease escapes beyond the bladder, staging of TCC remains worrisome. A welter of diagnostic modalities is now available. Each has significant strengths and limitations in bladder cancer staging (2).

Thus it is likely that most clinicians will continue to use a combination or algorithm of several staging methods (2, 8). In this setting TPA's discriminatory power could play a useful role. For example, in a patient with clinical T3A disease, a high level of TPA might suggest the need for carefu laparoscopic evaluation of regional nodes prior to scheduling cystectomy. A low value, on the other hand, would support going directly to laparotomy. This study was a preliminary test of TPA's ability to discriminate between metastatic and non metastatic TCC. Further studies will be required to properly delineate the analyte's clinical utility in the staging of advanced bladder cancer.

References

1. Droller MJ (1986) Transitional cell cancer: Upper tracts and bladder. In: Walsh PC, Gittes RF, Perlmutter AD, Stamey TA (eds) Campbell's Urology. 5th edition. WB Saunders, Philadelphia, pp 1343
2. See WA, Fuller JR (1992) Staging of advanced bladder cancer. Current concepts and pitfalls. Urol Clin North Am 19:663–683
3. Herr HW (1992) Staging invasive bladder tumors. J Surg Oncol 51:217–220
4. Malmstrom PU, Lonnemark M, Busch C, Magnusson A (1993) Staging of bladder carcinoma by computer tomography-guided transmural core biopsy. Scand J Urol Nephrol 27:193–198
5. Gerber GS, Rukstalis DB, Chodak GW (1993) The role of laparoscopic lymphadenectomy in staging and treatment of urological tumors. Ann Med 25:127–129
6. Barentsz JO, Ruijs SH, Strijk SP (1993) The role of MR imaging in carcinoma of the urinary bladder. Am J Roentgenol 160:937–947
7. Herr HW (1990) The role of surgery in initial staging and follow up. Prog Clin Biol Res 353:35–43
8. Gospodarowicz, MK (1994) Staging of bladder cancer. Semin Surg Oncol 10:51–59
9. Ovesen H, Iversen P, Beier Holgersen R, Hald T, Rasmussen, F, Steven K (1993) Extraperitoneal pelvioscopy in staging of bladder carcinoma and detection of pelvic lymph node metastasis. Scand J Urol Nephrol 27:211–214
10. Persad R, Kabala J, Gillatt D, Penry B, Gingell JC, Smith PJ (1993) Magnetic resonance imaging in the staging of bladder cancer. Br J Urol 71:566–573
11. Hawnaur JM, Johnson RJ, Read G, Isherwood I (1993) Magnetic resonance imaging with Gadolinium–DTPA for assessment of bladder carcinoma and its response to treatment. Clin Radiol 47:302–310
12. Olsen LH, Overgaard S, Frederiksen P, Ladefoged C, Ludwigsen E, Petri J, Poulsen JT (1993) The reliability of staging and grading of bladder tumors. Impact of misinformation on the pathologist's diagnosis. Scand J Urol Nephrol 27:349–353
13. Pathologists of the French Association of Urology Cancer Committee (1993) Lamina propria microinvasion of bladder tumors, incidence on stage allocation (pTa vs pT1): recommended approach. World J Urol 11:161–164
14. Hall RR, Prout GR (1990) Staging of bladder cancer: Is the tumor, node, metastasis system adequate? Semin Oncol 17:517–523
15. Mellerick DM, Osborn M, Weber K (1990) On the nature of serological tissue polypeptide antigen (TPA) monoclonal keratin 8, 18, and 19 antibodies react differently with TPA prepared from human cultured carcinoma cells and TPA in human serum. Oncogene 5:1007–1017
16. Pfaff M, O'Connor R, Vollmers HP, Müller-Hermelink HK (1990) Human monoclonal antibody against a tissue polypeptide antigen-related protein from a patient with a signet-ring-cell carcinoma of the stomach. Cancer Res 50:5192–5198
17. Carbin BE, Collins VP, Ekman P (1987) Tissue polypeptide antigen (TPA), some cytokeratins and epithelial membrane antigen (EMA) in normal, inflamed and malignant urothelium. Urol Res 15:191–194
18. Björklund B (1980) On the nature and clinical use of tissue polypeptide antigen (TPA). Tumordiagnostik 1:9–20

Address for correspondence:
Marina Feygin, M.D.
Dianon Systems, Inc.
200 Watson Boulevard
Stratford, CT 06497, USA

Use of TPS as a proliferation marker in studies of mammalian spermatogenesis

S. Blottner[a], A. Blottner[b], O. Hingst[a], D. Schadow[a]
[a]Institute for Zoo Biology and Wildlife Research, Berlin,
[b]Hospital Buch, Clinic for Nuclearmedicine and Endocrinology, Berlin, Germany

Introduction

Recently it has been shown that the tissue polypeptide specific antigen (TPS) is a cell cycle product released after mitosis in proportion to the number of new cells and time of growth (1, 2). The TPS secretion of living tumor cells correlated with proliferation activity measured by 3H-thymidine incorporation and protein synthesis activity (4–6). The release seems restricted to cell lines of epithelial origin.

The process of spermatogenesis in the seminiferous epithelium of testis is also characterized by high proliferation rates. The production of male germ cells is an important indicator for influences of ecological and anthropogenic factors on animal reproduction.

Characterization of this process by morphometric methods is difficult and time-consuming. Measurement of proliferation by 3H-thymidine incorporation (3, 8) or by immunohistochemical detection of the proliferation-associated Ki-67 antigen (9) promises informations about duration and localization of mitotic divisions during seminiferous epithelial cycle. However, our ability to quantify this process is rather limited.

The aim of the present study was to examine the use of TPS as a marker for quantitative characterization of testicular proliferation in several mammalian species.

Material and methods

Testes of different animal species were obtained by castration or after killing by euthanazation. Testis weights were measured and serum was collected. Aliquots of testicular parenchym (1–2 g) were minced and homogenized by tree times freezing/thawing in buffered solution and subsequent sonification at 4 °C for 1 min. Soluble proteins in supernatant were obtained after twice centrifugation (25 min at 2500 g and 25 min at 25 500 g, 4–6 °C). Different dilutions were used for the TPS-IRMA (Beki, Stockholm). The measured values were expressed in units/g testis (U/gT) and in units/g soluble protein (U/gP).

Additional, homogeneous suspensions of spermatogenic cells were prepared by pressing the parenchym through nylon mesh for counting of testicular spermatozoa and for subsequent fractionation of the different cell types in a Percoll density gradient in some cases. The discontinuos gradient consisted of six 1 ml-layers of 6 to 54% Percoll. Centrifugation of 1 ml suspension for 10 min at 500 g resulted in 5–6 fractions with different proportions of the cell types.

An other sample (0.5–1.0 g) of each testis was fixed in 2% paraformaldehyde in PBS and embedded in Technovit 8100. Serial sections (1.5–2 µm thick) were stained with hematoxyline-eosine. Ten round tubule sections per animal were evaluated microscopically: diameter and number of the different spermatogenic cells per cross section. The germ cells were identified on the basis of their nuclear morphology.

Epididymal spermatozoa were collected from minced caudae epididymis.

Results

Our preliminary results showed high species differences of detectable TPS-equivalent levels, suggesting different cross reactivity of the monoclonal antibody used in the test kit. The range varied between 6.4 ± 4.8 U/gP (Degu, n = 5) and 1416 ± 704 U/gP (roe deer, n = 10) in the analyzed adults of 16 species (table I).

Table I. TPS – Levels in testicular homogenates of adult mammals; examples without consideration of age, season or other factors.

Species	n	Units/g testis	Units/g sol. protein
Guinea pig (Cavia porcellus)	17	0.98 ± 1.74	12.17 ± 22.18
Degu (Octodon degus)	5	0.41 ± 0.28	6.41 ± 4.77
Domestic cat (Felis catus)	5	1.68 ± 0.82	36.12 ± 21.88
Puma (Felis concolor)	1	2.89	34.60
Leopard (Panthera pardus)	1	1.11	27.19
Racoon (Procyon lotor)	3	2.53 ± 0.41	58.97 ± 26.88
Goat (Capra hircus)	3	0.34 ± 0.15	6.81 ± 1.78
Sheep (Ovis ammon)	1	0.74	33.30
Blue sheep (Pseudois nayaur)	1	2.90	36.43
Roe deer (Capreolus capreolus)	10	96.78 ± 48.83	1416 ± 704
Sika deer (Cervus nippon)	5	4.52 ± 1.33	71.35 ± 20.12
Fallow deer (Dama d. mesopotamicus)	1	3.97	47.99
Kob (Kobus kob)	1	1.27	20.83
Oryx antelope (Oryx gazella)	2	0.46 ± 0.29	6.57 ± 3.90
Llama (Lama lama)	1	6.19	95.21
Monkey (Sanguinus fuscicollis)	1	16.98	30.33

TPS was related to the variable reproductive state of individuals and populations, as could be demonstrated with the examples of guinea pig and roe deer: Prepubertal and adult guinea pigs differed significantly in testis weight (0.44 ± 0.19 g and 1.69 ± 0.30 g), epididymal sperm concentration (no spermatozoa in juvenile animals) and numbers of spermatogenic cells per tubules sections (figure 1A). Consequently, they revealed significantly different TPS levels (figure 1B). The content of TPS in serum was lower than the detection limit of the assay (< 28 U/l) in most cases. The amount of testicular TPS estimated in adult guinea pigs seems to be influenced by the degree of inbreeding (variation between 24.10 U/gP of outbred animals and 4.14 U/gP of inbred animals). Testicular parameters in roe deer changed significantly from the pre-rutting (15th of may, n = 5) to the rutting period (15th of August, n = 5). Such alterations included the mean values of testis weights (15.39 and 19.68 g), of epididymal sperm reserve (0.108 · 10^9 and 1.535 · 10^9) as well as the number of spermatozoa per tubule sections (figure 2). The total TPS per testis, but also the amounts related to gram protein (1047 and 1748 U/gP) or to gram testis corresponded to the number of testicular spermatozoa. The levels in serum were lower by orders of magnitude (0.07–1.28 U/ml).

Remarkable testicular TPS has been found under conditions without production of testicular or epididymal spermatozoa, especially in cervids (Sika deer, see table I).

Furthermore, in growing fetal testis, available from the brown hare, the TPS level was much higher than the highest value of sexually active adults studied (64.7 U/gP and 39.7 U/gP, respectively).

The density gradient centrifugation of testicular cells from a goat provided a gradual enrichment of different spermatogenic cell types in the collected five fractions. Low levels of TPS were detected in cell-free supernatant, fractions I, II and fraction V containing spermatozoa (4.32–43.1 U/gP). The highest value was measured in fraction IV with the predominantly proportion of spermatocytes (138.2 U/gP).

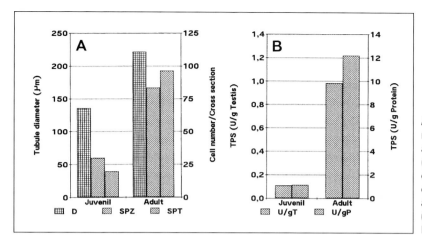

Figure 1. Testicular parameters of juvenile (n = 6) and adult guinea pigs (n = 17). A: Diameter of tubules (D), numbers of spermatozytes (SPZ) and round spermatides (SPT) per cross section. B: Testicular TPS.

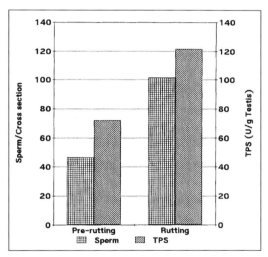

Figure 2. Number of spermatozoa per tubule cross section (10 per animal) and testicular TPS in the pre-rutting and rutting period of roe deer.

collection. The test does not require an injection of material in living animals or cell culture like in proliferation assays by incorporation of labelled thymidine or uridine. High TPS levels of growing testes (fetus, adults in pre-rutting period) and of isolated diploid spermatogenic cells qualify this polypeptide epitope as a marker for mitotic cell divisions.

The cross reactivity of the monoclonal mouse anti-human TPS antibody is obviously different in several animal species and seems to be better with decreasing relations to mouse, the antibody donor. (In mice TPS was undetectable.) Nevertheless, the distribution of TPS in a broad variety of mammals could be regarded as an indicator of the conservative mechanism of cell proliferation and gens encoding the regulating factors. Occurence of TPS in a variety of human tissues (7) might support such a hypothesis. Further investigations will be necessary to define the nature of this testicular antigen and to localize it exactly in the seminiferous tubules.

Discussion

The present results demonstrate that TPS can be detected in the seminiferous epithelium of several mammals. Advantages of the method used consist firstly in the simplicity of the assay and secondly in the possibility to get quantitative values from a representative sample size of homogenized testicular parenchym. The TPS measured reflects strictly the situation at the time of sample

Conclusion

The measurement of TPS in testicular parenchym could be a new, valuable parameter to quantify the spermatogenic proliferation. The characterization of this sensitive physiological process is relevant for studies of the reproductive status and its dependence on different conditions in selected mammals including zoo and wild animals.

References

1. Björklund B, Björklund V (1987) Biochemische und morphologische Grundlagen von TPA: Fortschritte in Richtung auf einen allgemeinen Marker für aktive Tumoren durch monoklonale Kartierung. In: Lüthgens M, Schlegel G (Hrsg) Tumormarkersystem CEA – TPA. Tumor Diagnostik Verlag, Leonberg, pp 14–30
2. Björklund B (1993) A conceptual approach to tumor antigen in the past and in the future with special reference to TPS. In: Ballesta AM, Torre GC, Bombardieri E, Gion M, Molina R (eds) Updating on tumor markers in tissues and biological fluids. Edizioni Minerva Medica, Torino, pp 651–669
3. Clermont Y, Trott M (1969) Duration of the cycle of the seminiferous epithelium in the mouse and hamster determined by means of 3H-thymidine and autoradiography. Fertil Steril 20:805–817
4. Madersbacher S, Schöllhammer A, Kramer G, Steiner G, Marberger M (1993) TPS in prostate cancer. Akt Urol 24:36–39
5. Madersbacher S, Gregor N, Theyer G, Steiner G, Marberger M (1992) TPS is a useful epithelial proliferation and tumor marker. J Urol 147:A911
6. Steiner G, Schöllhammer A, Madersbacher S, Marberger M (1993) Functional analysis of TPS. Symposium: Three years with the proliferation marker: TPS. Barcelona, February 4–6, p 49–54
7. Vogel J, Oehr P (1987) Immunhistochemischer Nachweis von TPA und CEA in menschlichen Geweben und Tumoren. In: Lüthgens M, Schlegel G (Hrsg) Tumormarkersystem CEA – TPA. Tumor Diagnostik Verlag, Leonberg, pp 47–60
8. Van Haaster LH, De Rooij DG (1993) Cycle of the seminiferous epithelium in the Djungarian hamster (Phodopus sungorus sungorus). Biol Reprod 48:515–521
9. Wrobel K-H, Kujat R, Lutz R (1993) Expression of the proliferation-associated Ki-67 antigen in bovine testicular tubular cells during the seminiferous epithelial cycle, demonstrated with the MIB-1 antibody. Andrologia 25:301–305

Address for correspondence:
Dr. rer. nat. A. Blottner
Institut für Zoo- und Wildtierforschung
Postfach 1103
D-10252 Berlin, Germany

Development of immunoassays specific for the different serological forms of PSA

O. Nilsson, U. Dahlen, B. Grundström, B. Karlsson, K. Nilsson

CanAg Diagnostics AB, Gothenburg, Sweden

Introduction

PSA is a 32 kD single chain glycoprotein serine protease with a chymotrypsin like specificity exclusively produced by the secretory epithelium of the prostate gland (1, 2). PSA is normally secreted into the seminal fluid, and plays a functional role in the cleavage of the seminal vesicle proteins and the liquefaction of the seminal coagulum (3). During normal conditions only a very low level of PSA is present in the blood stream, and increasing serum concentrations are indicative of prostatic pathology or trauma. Elevated levels of PSA are found in the majority of patients with prostatic cancer, and determination of PSA is today routinely used for detection and management of patients with prostatic cancer (4).

PSA has been shown to form stable complexes with different anti-proteases, and the dominating portion (~90%) of PSA in patient serum detectable with conventional immunoassays occurs in complex with α_1-antichymotrypsin (PSA-ACT) (5, 6, 7). However, large variations in the relation between free PSA and PSA-ACT complex between different individuals, and between benign and malignant prostatic disease have been noticed. Studies have also shown that the proportion of free PSA was higher in benign prostatic hypertrophy as compared to prostatic cancer (6, 8, 9), and that determination of the ratio between free PSA and total PSA significantly would increase the specificity for detection of prostatic cancer compared to the determination of total PSA alone (8). Specific determination PSA-ACT complex has also been suggested to give better discrimination between BPH and prostatic cancer (7, 15). Thus there is a need of assays specific for the different serological forms of PSA for the further clinical evaluation of the utility of specific determinations of the different serum forms of PSA.

In this paper different immunoassays for determination of total PSA (i.e. the sum of PSA-ACT and free PSA), free PSA and PSA-ACT are described. The characterization of an EIA for specific determination of both total PSA and free PSA is also described.

Materials and methods

Establishment of anti-PSA MAb

PSA-ACT complex was prepared by incubation of PSA with ACT (Biodesign International, ME, US) as described (5), and purified by size exclusion chromatography on Sephacryl S-100 (Pharmacia LKB Biotechnology, Uppsala, Sweden). Anti-PSA MAb were established by i.p. immunization of Balb/c mice with 3–5 doses of 5–20 µg of purified PSA or PSA-ACT complex in Ribi Adjuvant System (Ribi ImmunChem Research Inc, MT, US). Three to five days after the final booster dose hybridomas were obtained by fusion of spleen cells with the Ag8 myeloma cell line as described (10). The hybridomas were screened by incubation of the hybridoma medium in microtiter plates coated with affinity purified goat anti-mouse Ig (Jackson ImmunoResearch Lab, US), followed by incubation with purified PSA or PSA-ACT, and detection with rabbit anti-human PSA antisera (Dako AS, Copenhagen, Denmark). The established hybridomas were cloned by limiting dilution and monoclonal antibodies were produced by in vitro cultivation and purified by protein A affinity chromatography according to the manufacturers instruction. The isotype of the monoclonal antibodies were determined in solid-phase ELISA with goat anti-mouse Ig (G+A+M) as catching antibody and peroxidase labelled isotype specific rabbit anti-mouse IgG1, IgG2a, IgG2b, IgG3, IgA, and IgM as detecting reagents (Zymed Lab. Inc. CA, US). The specificity of the established hybridomas were determined in ELISA with the MAbs adsorbed to anti-mouse Ig solid-phase, which was incubated with serial dilutions of purified PSA, PSA-ACT and ACT, and detection with polyclonal anti-human PSA or anti-human ACT antisera (Dako AS, Copenhagen, Denmark), respectively.

Determination of dose-response and specificity of different anti-PSA MAb combinations

Each purified MAb was labeled with N1-DTTA Eu-chelate (Wallac Oy, Turku, Finland) to a specific activity of 4–7 Eu/IgG as previously described (11), and used as tracer in different IFMAs. The MAbs were also coated in microtiter plates, Nunc Maxisorp C12 Immuno-module plate (Nunc AS, Copenhagen, Denmark), as described (12), and used as solid-phase in the IFMAs. Dose-/response curves were determined in Delfia™ assays for all possible combinations of the anti-PSA MAb as follows: incubation of 25 µl of antigen (500, 100, 10, 5.1 and 0 ng/ml of free PSA, PSA-ACT complex or ACT) + 100 µl of assay buffer in anti-PSA MAb coated microtiter plates for 1 h; after washing 100 µl of Eu anti-PSA MAb, 1 µg/ml, was added and the incubation continued for additional 1 h; after additional washings and incubation with Enhancement Solution (Wallac Oy, Turku, Finland) the europium fluorescence was determined in an Arcus™ fluorometer. The specificity of the different assays was confirmed by determination of dose/response with purifed free PSA, PSA-ACT and ACT, and by determination of the PSA immunoactivity in the eluted fractions after separation of a mixture of purified PSA-ACT and free PSA on Sephacryl S 100.

Development of PSA EIA for specific determination of both free PSA and total PSA

PSA 10 MAb and PSA30 MAb were biotinylated using biotin caproate-N hydrosuccinimice ester from Sigma Chemical Co. The PSA 66 MAb was conjugated with horse radish peroxidase type VI (Sigma Chemical Co, MO, US) according to a modification of the original Nakone method (13). The standards were made by dilution of purified PSA in buffer matrix (50 mM Tris, 0.15 M NaCl, 60 g/l BSA, 0.5 g/l NaN_3, pH 7.5)), and calibrated against the Hybritech Tandem PSA RIA kit (Hybritech Inc., CA, US). For determination of total PSA 25 µl of standard/sample and 100 µl biotin PSA10 MAb was incubated for 1 h during shaking in streptavidin microtiter plates (Labsystems Oy, Helsinki, Finland), and for specific determination of free PSA 25 µl (or optional 50 µl) of standards/sample and 100 µl of biotin PSA 30 MAb was incubated for 1 h in streptavidin microtiter plates; after washing 100 µl of HRP PSA 66 MAb was added to all wells and the incubation continued for 1 h during shaking. The HRP activity was determined after washing and incubation with 100 µl TMB (tetramethyl benzidine) and measurement of absorbance at 620 nm. The cross reactivity between free PSA and total PSA of the assays was determined after separation of PSA-ACT and free PSA by size exclusion chromatography on Sephacryl S-100. Precision profile was determined from standards pipetted randomly in 12 replicates. The precision of analyses of patient samples during normal assay conditions were determined by calculation of CV% of duplicates from 92 clinical samples covering total PSA range from < 0.1– ~3000 µg/l, and free PSA from < 0.1– ~500 µg/l. The recovery of PSA was determined by addition of aliquots of highly elevated patient sample to normal male serum samples. The dilution linearity was studied by dilution of patient samples with the 0-standard. Correlation with Hybritech Tandem PSA RIA was determined in 92 subjects with benign and malignant prostatic disease.

Results and discussion

In this paper the term total PSA is used for the sum of free PSA and PSA ACT complex, and free PSA for the portion of PSA which do not occur in complex with anti-proteases. The term total PSA for free PSA + PSA-ACT is, however, somewhat inconsistent as it is known that in the serum PSA also occurs in complex with α_2-macroglubuline (α_2-M) (5). During complex formation with α_2-M the PSA molecule is totally covered by α_2-M, and

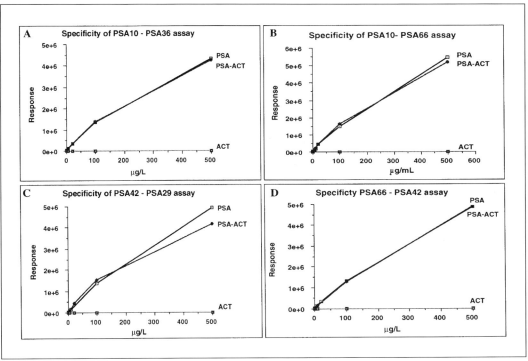

Figure 1. Dose/response and specificity of different IFMA for determination of total PSA. The assays were developed as two-step sandwich assays and the following assay protocol was used in all assays µl std./sample + 100 µl assay buffer, incubation 30 min; 100 µl Eu tracer MAb, 1µg/ml, incubation 30 min; 200 µl enhancement solution and measuement of Eu fluorescence in an Arcus Fluorometer. The specificity was determined by analyses of dose/response curves with purified PSA, PSA-ACT and ACT (0, 1, 5, 10, 100 and 500 µg/l respectively). A) PSA10 MAb solid-phase and Eu PSA36 MAb tracer. B) PSA10 MAb solid-phase and Eu PSA66 MAb tracer. C) PSA42 MAb solid-phase and EU PSA29 MAb tracer. D) PSA66 MAb solid-phase and Eu PSA42 MAb tracer.

the PSA-α_2-M complex is not detected in conventional two site immunoassays (for review on the reaction of PSA with anti-proteases, see (14)). The PSA-α_2-M complex may though be detected by immunoblotting using anti-PSA antibodies after separation by SDS-PAGE (9), but there are no quantitative data available on the proportion of PSA occurring as PSA-α_2-M complex in patient serum. Incubation of enzymatic active PSA and fresh human serum for 12–24 h results in 40% recovery of PSA immunactivity (6), suggesting that PSA-α_2-M may represent up to 60% of the "total" PSA in serum. The fraction of free PSA in serum would not likely represent the active serine protease, and may represent different forms of inactive PSA; possibly the zymogen form of the enzyme or the internally cleaved inactive form present in seminal plasma.

Totally 17 MAb recognizing epitopes exposed both in PSA-ACT complex and in free PSA, six MAb only reacting with free PSA, and 10 MAb reacting with PSA-ACT without reactivity with free PSA were established. The ten MAb react only with PSA-ACT detected epitopes of the ACT portion of the PSA-ACT complex, and thus were not specific for the PSA-ACT complex. Epitope mapping of PSA using the established MAbs showed a complex pattern of different epitopes, and at least seven major epitopes were detected (Nilsson et al., in preparation).

A large number of MAb combinations, selected among the 17 MAb recognizing both PSA-ACT and free PSA, could be used for the development of equimolar response assays for determination of total PSA (i.e. free PSA + PSA-ACT complex). Four combinations were further studied owing to the

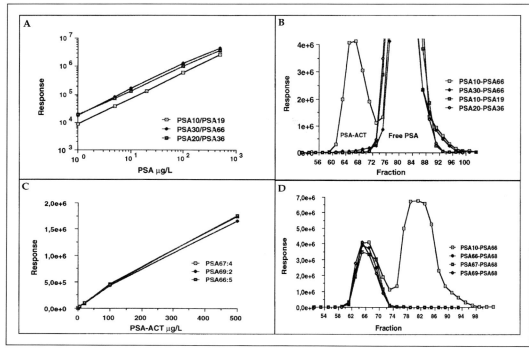

Figure 2. Dose-/response and specificity of free PSA and PSA-ACT specific assays. The specificity and cross reaction between free PSA and PSA-ACT of the different assays was tested by analyses of PSA immunoactivity in eluted fractions after separation of a mixture of ≈ 4 µg PSA-ACT and ≈ 40 µg free PSA on a Sephacryl S-100 column (1.0 x 60 cm) eluted with PBS, 10 mM benzamidine. The PSA10 – PSA66 assay was used as reference for PSA-ACT and free PSA. A) Dose-/response of free PSA assays: PSA10 + EuPSA19 PSA30 + Eu PSA66, PSA20 + Eu PSA36. The PSA19 MAb, PSA30 MAb and PSA20 MAb detected epitopes exposed only in free PSA. B) Specificity of the free PSA specific assays. C) Dose-/response of PSA-ACT assays using PSA 67 MAb, PSA69 MAb and PSA66 MAb as solid-phase and Eu PSA 68 MAb recognizing an epitope in ACT as tracer. D) Specificity of the PSA-ACT specific assays.

high sensitivity and fast kinetics obtained; PSA10 MAb + Eu PSA36 MAb, PSA10 MAb + EuPSA66 MAb, PSA66 MAb + Eu PSA42 MAb and PSA 42 MAb + EuPSA 29 MAb (figure 1A–D). The analytical sensitivity of the assays were < 0.01 µg/l using 25 µ/l of sample and 30 + 30 min incubation, when the analytical sensitivity was defined as the concentration corresponding to the response of the 0-std. + 2 times SD of the 0-standard. The assays showed also a high correlation with commercial PSA assay in preliminary clinical evaluations, r > 0.97 compared to PSA Delfia in 70 subjects with BPH and prostatic cancer.

The antibodies specific for free PSA could not be combined with each other in two-site sandwich assays. Thus for the development of assays specific for free PSA combinations of free PSA specific MAbs and MAb recognizing epitopes exposed both in free PSA and PSA-ACT complex were used. In figure 2 A and B the dose-/response and specificity of three assays specific for free PSA is shown. The sensitivities of the assays were < 0.05 µg/l using 25 µ/l samples using the same definition of analytical sensitivity as above. The cross reaction between free PSA and PSA-ACT were < 0.5% determined from the signal of the peak fraction of PSA-ACT in the equimolar response PSA10-PSA66 MAb total PSA assay and the signal of the same fraction in the free PSA specific assays after separation of PSA-ACT and free PSA on S-100 gel chromatography, figure 2 B. Preparations of PSA-ACT may contain small amounts of free PSA (up to 3–4% depending on storage conditions) thus determination of the response in fractions corresponding to PSA-ACT and free PSA directly after separation of free PSA

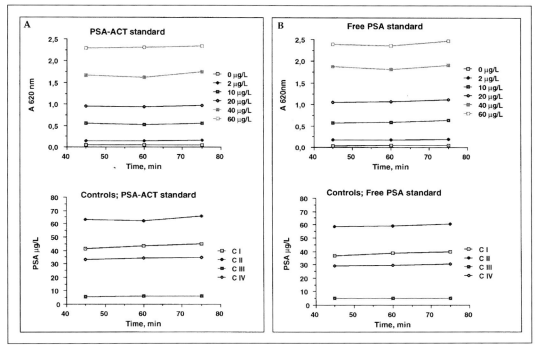

Figure 3. Kinetics of total PSA EIA using PSA-ACT and free PSA standards. The assay was performed according to the normal procedure except for the incubation time as indicated in the graphs. A) Kinetics of standards and control using PSA-ACT standard. B) Kinetics of standards and controls using free PSA standard.

and PSA-ACT by gelchromatography would give a more accurate estimation of the cross reaction between PSA-ACT and free PSA.
PSA-ACT specific assays were developed using MAb against total PSA as catching antibody and detection of the PSA-ACT complex with MAb against the ACT portion (figure 2 C and D). In these assays the cross reaction between PSA-ACT and free PSA was < 0.1% using antigen in buffer matrix, figure 2 D. Assays for PSA-ACT using anti-ACT Ab as tracer have shown to give an overestimation of the PSA-ACT concentration in a large proportion of patient samples, which may be explained by unspecific binding of ACT to the solid-phase leading to a falsely elevated signal with an anti-ACT tracer (15, 17). Thus this assay design may not be suitable for accurate determination of the concentration of PSA-ACT, particularly in the low region.
The EIA for specific determination of total and free PSA used two different biotinylated catching MAb, biotin PSA10 MAb specific for total PSA and biotin PSA30 MAb specific for free PSA, and the same tracer (HRP PSA66 MAb) was used for determination of both total PSA and free PSA. The standards were made by dilution of free PSA in buffer, which allowed the same standards to be used for determination of both free PSA and total PSA. The assay for total PSA showed an equimolar response and kinetics for free PSA and PSA-ACT (figure 3), which justifies that free PSA was used as standard also for determination of total PSA. The cross reaction between free PSA and PSA-ACT was < 0.5% in the free PSA EIA using the same method for determination of cross-reaction as shown in figure 2. The analytical sensitivity with 25 μl sample determined from 12 replicates of the 0-standard and 2 μg/l standard randomly pipetted was < 0.1 μg/l for both the total PSA and free PSA assays using the following formula for calculation of the analytical sensitivity: [(2 · SD of 0-std.)/(signal std. B-signal 0-std.) · conc. of std. B]. The precision-profile determined from random-pipetting of standards in 12 plicates gave a CV between 2–3.5% in the whole standard curve range for both the total PSA and the free

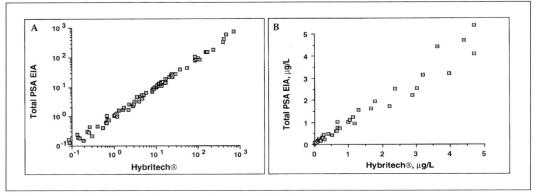

Figure 4. Correlation between total PSA EIA and Hybritech Tandem PSA RIA. The correlation was determined in 92 clinical samples from routin determination of PSA independent of clinical diagnosis of the patients. A) Hybritech Tandem PSA RIA < 1000 µg/l. Total PSA EIA = -1.4351 + 1.0222 Hybritech; R = 0.99, n = 87. B) Hybritech Tandem PSA RIA < 5 µg/ml. Total PSA EIA = 0.0409 + 0.9737 Hybritech; R = 0.98, n = 35.

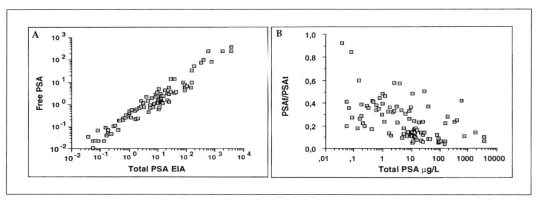

Figure 5. Relation between total PSA and free PSA in clinical samples. A) Correlation between free PSA EIA and total PSA EIA. Free PSA = 4.6077 + 0.0926 total PSA; R = 0.90. B) Ratio between free PSA and total PSA in relation to total PSA.

PSA EIA. Determination of CV% of duplicates of routine samples showed that > 85% of all duplicates had CV% < 7.5, and 95% showed CV% < 10% in the total PSA EIA, and in the free PSA EIA > 95% of duplicates with free PSA > 0.1 µg/l had CV% < 5%. The recovery of antigen was between 95–107% in the total PSA EIA, and 95–105% in the free PSA EIA. The dilution of patients gave also within the expected range for both total PSA and free PSA. The total PSA EIA showed an excellent correlation with the Hybritech Tandem PSA RIA both in the high and the low region, figure 4 A and B. The correlation between the total PSA EIA and free PSA EIA was: free PSA = 4.6077 + 0.0926 total PSA, R = 0.90, indicating that on average the free PSA fraction was 10% of total PSA (figure 5 A). However, when the ratio free PSA/total PSA was plotted against total PSA a large individual variation in the proportion of free PSA was found (figure 5 B), which is in agreement with previous reports in the literature (6). Even in the range total PSA > 200 µg/l, the proportion of free PSA varied considerably between different individuals; free PSA ~ 5–50% of total PSA. Although this study was not intended for comparison of free and total PSA in BPH and prostatic cancer a higher proportion of free PSA was found in the low total PSA region, which might support the previous reports of higher proportions of free PSA in BPH as compared to prostatic cancer (7–9). Studies have suggested that skewed response assays with a higher molar response for free PSA compared to PSA-ACT would give a better indication of disease regression and/or progression as compared to equimolar response assays (9, 16). The results from the samples analysed with our free and total PSA EIA showed large individual variations in the proportion of free PSA, which may suggest that determination of free PSA might give better information of changes in disease status compared to an equimolar response assay in some patients, but the opposite would be expected also in other patients.

Conclusions

Controlled studies with well documented clinical samples and highly specific assays for the different serological forms of PSA would be necessary for the evaluation of the clinical value of specific determination of the different serological forms of PSA in the diagnosis of prostatic cancer, and for follow-up of patients with prostatic cancer. The total and free PSA EIA described in this paper would be suitable assays for such studies, and further clinical studies are ongoing. The high affinity monoclonal antibodies specific for the different forms of PSA described in this paper would also be suitable for development of specific assays suitable for different assay formats.

Acknowledgement

The routine clinical samples used for comparison of Hybritech Tandem PSA RIA, total PSA EIA and free PSA EIA was kindly supplied by *Prof. G. Lindstedt,* Department of Clinical Chemistry, Sahlgren's Hospital, Gothenburg, Sweden.

References

1. Wang MC, Valenzuela LA, Murphy GP, Chu TM (1979) Purification of a human prostate specific antigen. Invest Urol 17: 159–163
2. Lilja H (1985) A kallikrein-like serine protease in prostatic fluid cleaves the predominant seminal vesicle protein. J Clin Invest 76:1899-1903
3. Lilja H, Oldbring J, Rannevik G, Laurell CB (1987) Seminal vesicle secreted proteins and their reactions during gelation and liquefaction of human semen. J Clin Invest 80:281–285
4. Oesterling JE (1991) Prostate specific antigen: A critical assessment of the most useful tumor marker for adenocarcinoma of the prostate. J Urol 145:907–923
5. Christensson A, Laurell CB, Lilja H (1990) Enzymatic activity of prostate specific antigen and its reactions with extracellular serine proteinase inhibitors. Eur J Biochem 194:755-763
6. Lilja H, Christensson A, Dahlen U, Matikainen MT, Nilsson O, Pettersson K, Lövgren T (1991) Prostate-specific antigen in serum occurs predominantly in complex with α_1-antichymotrypsin. Clin Chem 37:1618–1625
7. Christensson A, Björk T, Nilsson O, Dahlen U, Matikainen MT, Cockett ATK, Abrahamsson PA, Lilja H (1993) Serum prostate specific antigen complexed to α_1-antichymotrypsin as an indicator of prostate cancer. J Urol 150:100–105
8. Zhou A, Tewari PC, Bluestein BI, Caldwell GW, Larsen FL (1993) Multiple forms of prostate-specifc antigen in serum: Differences in immunorecognition by monoclonal and polyclonal assays. Clin Chem 39:2483–2491
9. Stenman UH, Leinonen J, Alfthan H, Ranniko S, Tuhkanen K, Alfthan O (1991) A complex between prostate-specific antigen and α_1-antichymotrypsin is the major form of prostate-specifc antigen in serum of patients with prostatic cancer: assays of the complex improves clinical sensitivity for cancer. Cancer Res 51:222-226
10. Lindolm L, Holmgren J, Svennerholm L, Fredman P, Nilsson O, Persson B, Myrvold H, Lagergard T (1983) Monoclonal antibodies against gastro intestinal tumour-associated antigens isolated as monosialogangliosides. Int Archs Allergy Appl Immunol 71:178–181
11. Hemmilä I, Dakubu S, Mukkala VM, Siitari H, Lövgren T (1983) Europium as a label in time-resolved immunofluorometricc assays. Anal Biochem 137:335–340
12. Nilsson O, Johansson C, Glimelius B, Persson B, Norgaard-Pedersen B, Andren-Sandberg A, Lindholm L (1992) Sensitivity and specificity of CA 242 in gastro-intestinal cancer. A comparison with CEA, CA 50 and CA 19-9. Br J Cancer 65:215–221
13. Tijssen P, Kurstak E (1984) Highly efficient methods for the preparation of peroidase and active peroxidase-antibody conjugates for enzyme immunoassays. Anal Biochem 136:451-457
14. Christensson A (1993) Prostate-specific antigen. Enzyme activity and reactions with extracellular protease inhibitors. Thesis, University of Lund

15. Leinonen J, Lövgren T, Voranen T, Stenman UH (1993) Double-label time resolved immunofluorometric assay of prostatic specific antigen and of its complex with α_1-antichymotrypsin. Clin Chem 39:2098–2103
16. Bluestein B, Zhou A, Tewari P, Comerci C, Schubert W, Larsen F (1992) Multi-site clinical evaluation of an automated chemiluminescent immunoassay for prostate-specific antigen (ACSTM PSA). J Tumor Marker Oncol 7:41–60
17. Wood WG, van der Sloot E, Böhle A (1991) The establishment and evaluation of luminescent-labeled immunometric assays for prostate specific antigen α_1-antichymotrypsin complexes in serum. Eur J Clin Chem Clin Biochem 39:787–794

Address for correspondence:
Dr. O. Nilsson
CanAg Diagnostics AB
P.O. Box 121 36
S-402 42 Gothenburg, Sweden

Clinical significance of free and complexed forms of PSA in prostate cancer

B. Bluestein, P. Tewari, A. Zhou, G. Caldwell, F. Larsen

Oncology Product Development, Ciba Corning Diagnostics Corp., East Walpole, Massachusetts, USA

Introduction

Although prostate specific antigen (PSA) has gained wide acceptance as a tumor marker to monitor successful therapy and disease recurrence in prostate cancer (PCa), only recently has it been determined that PSA exists in multiple forms in serum (1, 2). The predominant form of PSA detected by current immunoassays is as a complex to the proteinase – inhibitor, α_1-antichymotrypsin (ACT). This form, on average, contains about 80–90% of the total detectable PSA (Mr 100 kD) with the remaining PSA present as a free form (Mr 33 kD). While complexes to the higher molecular mass (Mr) inhibitor α_2-macroglobulin (A2M) have been prepared in vitro (3), immunoassays have not been able to measure these complexes in the serum of PCa patients, presumably due to blockage of reactive epitopes by the encapsulating protease inhibitor. Recently we have been able to identify A2M complexes in all PCa patients tested after solubilization with the anionic detergent, sodium dodecyl sulfate (SDS) followed by Western blot analysis using antibody to PSA (4). Christensson et al. (5) have provided preliminary evidence that measurement of the ratios of ACT complex/total PSA may improve specificity in differentiating benign prostatic hyperplasia (BPH) from PCa. Currently, at a cutoff level of 4 ng/ml using a monoclonal/ monoclonal assay (Tandem®, Hybritech®, Inc.), the false positive rate in differentiating BPH from PCa is ~78% (6).

Previously, in comparative serial monitoring studies comparing the Tandem assay with the Ciba-Corning ACS™ PSA assay, a polyclonal/ monoclonal assay performed on the ACS:180® automated chemiluminescent immunoassay system, we determined that ~ 30% of the patients exhibited an enhanced response in the ACS PSA assay compared to the dual monoclonal antibody based assay. Further, this enhanced response correlated well with clinical pathology including proportionality to tumor volume and tumor progression or regression (7). In order to explore the possibility that these responses were due to changes in the proportion of complexed and free PSA, we performed molecular sieve fractionation studies of serum from PCa patients at various time points during their disease progression. Purified PSA-ACT complexes and isolated free PSA were also analyzed by both assays in order to better understand differences in comparative responses of the various forms of PSA.

Patient samples and methods

Over 100 individual patients were monitored by both methods. Participating institutions and coordinators were: Memorial Sloan Kettering Cancer Center (New York, NY), Morton K. Schwartz; Tulane University Medical Center (New Orleans, LA), Sanda Clejan; Norwood Hospital (Norwood, MA), Vincent Andaloro; Stanford University Medical Center (Stanford, CA), Thomas A. Stamey and M.D. Anderson Medical Center Houston TX), Herbert Fritsche. Patient serum samples were fractionated by either Sephacryl S-200 or Superdex 200 gel chromatography (Pharmacia). Appropriate molecular mass markers were run in separate experiments to determine the mass of the forms of PSA as measured by the ACS PSA or Tandem PSA assays. Dose integration of eluted peaks allowed comparison of both the proportion of complex and free PSA as determined by each individual assay and also the relative relationship between assays in measuring each form.

Results

Determination of enhanced response in serial monitoring studies

As shown in figures 1–3, the enhanced response of the ACS PSA assay relative to the Tandem assay is based on a sharper slope rise with disease progression. That these differences go beyond issues of a uniform assay standardization bias is evidenced by the changing ACS Tandem ratio with disease progression and regression.

Analysis of in vitro prepared PSA-ACT complexes and free PSA

PSA purified from seminal fluid was complexed by addition to a sixfold molar excess of ACT followed by fractionation. As shown in figure 4, only 40% of the added PSA was complexed to ACT, as 60% eluted as the free form (33 kD). Additionally, while the complexed form reacted similarly in both assays (ACS/Tandem ratio 1.16), the free form reacted to a much greater extent in the ACS assay (ratio = 3.3.)

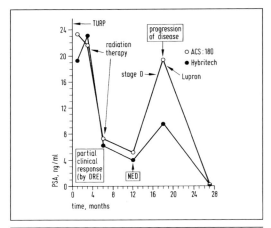

Month	ACS (ng/ml)	Tandem (ng/ml)	Ratio
1	23.3	19.3	1.2
4	21.7	23.1	0.94
7	7.3	6.1	1.2
13	5.2	4.0	1.3
18	19.3	9.4	2.05
27	0.29	0.33	0.9

Figure 2. Serial monitoring of patient 2936, stage C, transurethral prostatectomy and radiation therapy.

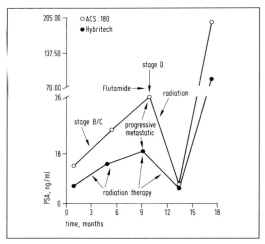

Month	ACS (ng/ml)	Tandem (ng/ml)	Ratio
1	13.2	7.0	1.9
5	23.8	14.0	1.7
9	35.2	17.8	2.0
13	5.4	4.3	1.3
17	201	88.9	2.3

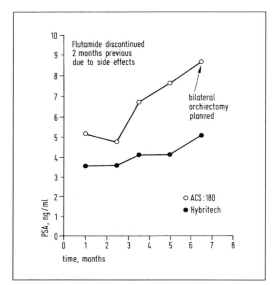

Figure 1. Serial monitoring of patient 1087768, stage BI organ confined PCa post hormonal therapy.

Figure 3. Serial monitoring of patient 3399, stage D, hormonal and radiation therapy.

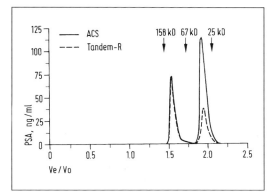

Figure 4. Fractionation of PSA-ACT prepared in vitro. Purified PSA from seminal fluid was reacted with pure ACT followed by fractionation. Only 40% of seminal fluid PSA is capable of forming complexes, hence the presence of free PSA.

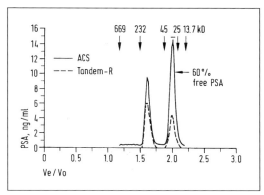

Figure 6. Elution profile of free and complexed forms of PSA from patient 3399 (figure 3) at month 17. Free PSA represents 60% of the toal PSA as determined by the ACS assay and is quantitated as 3.8 times the Tandem value.

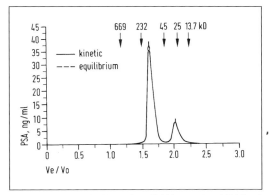

Figure 5. "Typical" PCa patient (84% complex 16% free) fractionation on Superdex followed by measurement in the ACS PSA assay as performed on the ACS:180 (7.5 min – kinetic) versus a four hour incubation (equilibrium) demonstrating identical recovery of both forms of PSA.

Effect of kinetics in the ACS PSA assay on reactivity to different forms of PSA

Since the ACS PSA assay is a short incubation assay (7.5 minutes), studies were undertaken to determine if the variability in the reactivity of the complex and free forms was due to differences in the kinetics of reaction. For example, could potential steric hindrance by ACT slow down the rate of reaction of antibodies to PSA? The ACS assay was manually reacted for 4 hours at 37 °C to assure equilibrium conditions. When calibrated under indentical conditions, dose integration of a "typical" PCa patient wherein 84% PSA was complexed and 16% was free resulted in superimposable profiles for both peaks demonstrating that differences in reactivity by the ACS assay for complex and free forms was not due to the short incubation time which appears to be a condition approaching equilibrium (figure 5).

Increasing amounts of free form during PCa disease progression

In order to better understand the ACS/Tandem PSA ratios in patient serum, sera from months 9 and 17 from the patient depicted in figure 3, were fractionated. Compared to the "typical" PCa sample (85% complex, 15% free from PSA) both samples demonstrated an increase proportion of free PSA. At month 9, this proportion was 48% of the total, while at month 17, the proportion rose to 60% of the total PSA (figure 6). During this interval, the intact serum ACS/Tandem ratio rose from 2.0 to 2.3, a change proportional to the increase intree PSA. At month 13, PSA levels fell to low levels in both assays in response to radiation therapy. The intact serum ratio fell to 1.3, presumably due to a reduction in the free form. Unfortunately, using current fractionation techniques, this level of PSA (4–5 ng/ml) was too low to chromatograph with analytical recovery.

Discussion

Results of studies presented here suggest the following. First, differences in the way the ACS PSA assay measures complex and free forms of PSA compared to the Tandem assay are not due to differential kinetic reactivity. It appears that even at 7.5 minutes, the ACS assay is at equilibrium. This is not unexpected in that the assay uses a high concentration of microscopic paramagnetic particles as the solid phase. Unlike fixed surface antibody coated tube, coated bead or glass fiber filter reactions, the use of a suspension of high surface area particles reduces the diffusional path length sufficiently to allow a situation approaching solution kinetics. This phenomenon coupled with a 37 °C reaction temperature and a high concentration excess of reactive antibodies maximally pushes these reactions, via mass action, toward rapid equilibration.

How then to account for the increased reactivity toward the free form of PSA compared to the dual monoclonal assay? There are two possible alternatives or combinations, both of which relate to multiple epitopes on the PSA molecule and the epitope restriction that can result when a dual monoclonal assay is used. The first possibility is that there are epitopes on PSA that are masked when complexed with ACT. In this instance, the polyclonal tracer antibody would amplify the signal from the free form of PSA when epitopes were exposed. Recent studies by *Nilsson* et al. suggest that there are at least nine epitopes on PSA, two of which may be blocked by interaction with ACT (8). The second aspect relates to whether or not these epitopes are spatially arranged in an identical fashion on all PSA molecules or whether there is microheterogeneity amongst different PSA molecules. If all molecules had the same spatial arrangement of epitopes, then one would expect that the ratio of ACS/Tandem for the free form of PSA would be a constant, regardless of the patient. In fractionation studies performed on PCa patients thus far, this does not appear to be the case as the ratio of ACS/Tandem for the integrated free PSA peak varies from 2 to 4fold.

For this reason, there is a strong possibility that a dual monoclonal assay is underestimating the free form of PSA that is present. The observation that alternative forms of PSA may be missed by a monoclonal assay, was first put forth by *Stephenson* et al. (9). Using the Yang Proscheck™ PSA assay, they found that the polyclonal/monoclonal ratio of PSA values from stage C PCa patients varied from 1.2 to 2.3 (Proscheck/Tandem-R). Variations in this ratio from patient to patient confirmed that a consistent bias, which would be expected if only a difference in standardization was at issue, was not the cause; rather, there were genuine discrepancies in how the two assays recognized PSA. These investigators were able to demonstrate a statistically significant relationship between nodal status and the polyclonal/monoclonal PSA ratio, with higher ratios correlating with positive nodes. They suggested that polyclonal PSA assays may be reacting with forms of PSA undetectable in strictly monoclonal assays. Finally, since the Yang assay is an equilibrium competitive binding assay with either a 4 hour or overnight incubation, kinetic issues of variable reactivity of complex – and free forms are an unlikely consideration as the source of variation in comparison between the two assays.

Regardless of the actual biochemistry, the empirical clinical findings are clear. In over 100 patients followed by both assays, responses to disease recurrence or failed therapy tracked each other similarly. However, in approximately 30% of these cases, the ACS PSA assay demonstrated an enhanced response showing increased rates of change in PSA values compared to the Tandem assay. Therefore, the ability to maximally detect all forms of PSA may help in the evaluation of early recurrence, and differentiation of latent versus aggressive PCa.

References

1. Lilja H, Christensson A, Dahlen U et al (1991) Prostate-specific antigen in serum occurs predominantly in complex with α_1-antichymotrypsin. Clin Chem 37:1618–1625
2. Stenman U-H, Leinonen J, Alfthan H et al (1991) A complex between prostate-specific antigen and α_1-antichymotrypsin is the major form of prostate-specific antigen in the serum of patients with prostatic cancer: assay of the complex improves clinical sensitivity for cancer. Cancer Res 51:222–226

3. Christensson A, Laurell CB, Lilja H (1990) Enzymatic activity of prostate-specific antigen and its reactions with extracellular serine proteinase inhibitors. Eur J Biochem 194:755–763
4. Zhou AM, Tewari PC, Bluestein BI et al (1993) Multiple forms of prostate-specific antigen in serum: differences in immunorecognition by monoclonal and polyclonal assays. Clin Chem 39(12):2483–2491
5. Christensson A, Bjork T, Nilsson O et al (1993) Serum prostate-specific antigen complexed to α_1-antichymotrypsin as an indicator of prostate cancer. J Urol 150:100–105
6. Southwick PC, Catalona WJ, Richie JP et al (1993) Evaluation of prostate-specific antigen (PSA) and digital rectal examination (DRE) for early detection of prostate cancer: results of a multicenter study of 6,630 men. Clin Chem 39:1195
7. Bluestein B, Zhou A, Tewari P et al (1992) Multi-site clinical evaluation of an automated chemiluminescent immunoassay for prostate specific antigen (ACS™ PSA). J Tumor Marker Oncol 7:41–60
8. Nilsson O, Nilsson K, Dahlen B et al (1993) Epitope mapping of PSA and development of assays for the determination of different isoforms of PSA. J Tumor Marker Oncol 8(3):110
9. Stephenson RA, Greskovich FJ, Fritsche HA et al (1991) Ratio of polyclonal-monoclonal prostate specific antigen levels: discrimination of nodal status in prostate tumors that produce low marker levels. Urol Clin North Am 18:467–471

Address for correspondence:
Dr. B. Bluestein
Oncology Product Development
Ciba-Corning Diagnostics Corp.
333 Coney Street
East Walpole, MA 02032, USA

Free PSA analyzed by chromatofocusing, molecular sieving and immunological methods

P. R. Huber[a], B Strittmatter[a], A. Maurer[b], H. P. Schmid[c]

[a]Kantonsspital Basel, Hormone Laboratory DZL, [b]Roche Diagnostic Systems, a Division of Hoffmann-La Roche, Ltd, [c]Kantonsspital Basel, Department of Urology, Basel, Switzerland

Introduction

The quantification of serum PSA has proven to be very useful in the screening and early detection of prostate carcinoma. However, the collectives of patients with benign hyperplasia of the prostate (BPH) and early stages of prostate carcinoma (P-CA, stages T1 and T2; TNM-classification) are often intermixed and presently no commercially available PSA test kit can distinguish between them.

Therefore, it would be very useful to find a system capable of distinguishing between benign hyperplasia of the prostate (BPH) and prostate carcinoma (P-CA).

Analysis of sera by molecular sieving by our group (1) and figure 1 and others (2, 3) revealed two main immunological active species with molecular weights of 100 and 36 kD. The Swedish group of Lilja and Stenman (2, 3) identified the 100 kD molecule to be a complex between alpha-1-antichymo-trypsin and PSA. By introducing a novel immunoassay system based on their findings they claimed to be able to clearly distinguish between patients with P-CA and those with BPH by introducing a ratio of complexed versus free (uncomplexed) PSA. The ratio is said to be higher in P-CA than in BPH (2, 3).

Using a test system of our own, we were unable to repeat these experiments which led us to further study the question at hand (1).

We concluded that a study going into more details on the characteristics of free PSA in serum might be helpful to find out why PSA remains free in the presence of such large excess of serum alpha-1-chymotrypsin.

Efficacy of different PSA test systems to detect free and complexed PSA

To this end we analyzed a pool of sera from patients with high PSA content in order to establish the efficiency of different test systems to detect free and complexed PSA (figure 1).

As expected, the competitive assay of Yang® using a polyclonal antiserum detected a nearly 50/50 proportion of complexed and free PSA at a rather high concentration level. The same distribution with only half the peak PSA concentrations was obtained with the test systems of Roche Cobas® Core and Ciba-Corning ACS-180®. Both tests use saturation assays involving either two different monoclonal, F5 and 1AF 5–6 in Cobas Core® PSA and MAb F5 and a polyclonal antiserum in the ACS:180. From this we conclude that the antisera used in these two systems bind to more or less the same epitopes on the PSA molecule in both the free and the complexed form as does the competitive polyclonal test system by Yang® albeit with less high affinity. In addition we found that Wallac's Delfia® test recognizes more (approx. 80 %) of the complexed form and less (approx. 20 %) of the free form of PSA. Contrary to Stenman and coworkers who used the same technology as Wallac's Delfia but not necessarily the same antisera we assume from the outcome of our experiment (figure 1) that the ratio of the complexed to the non-complexed form is not so much dependent on the clinical finding of P-CA or BPH but much more on the type of antisera employed in the test system and on the nature of the PSA in the sample. Individual characteristics of the peak distribution have been omitted by our approach of using a pool of sera with high PSA content. Therefore only the binding characteristics to the two peaks of the different test systems are detected.

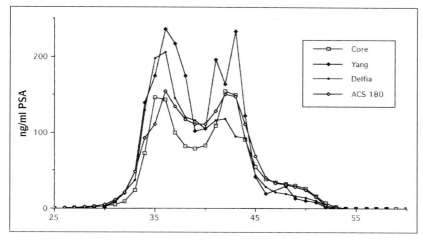

Figure 1. Discriminative antibody binding to free and complexed PSA by different commercially available test systems. (S–300 (1.54 x 45 cm); serum pool, P-CA patients).

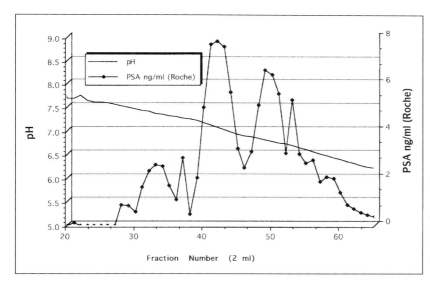

Figure 2. Free (uncomplexed) PSA from prostate carcinoma serum pool analysed by chromatofocusing. Detection of isoenzymes by PSA - EIA (Cobas® Core).

Chromatofocusing and epitope mapping

In a further experiment we analyzed PSA from a P-CA serum pool by chromatofocusing and epitope mapping (figures 2 and 3).
To detect the free PSA fractionated by the chromatofocusing process, which separates proteins according to their isoelectric point, we used the Cobas Core® system. We found free PSA having a strong microheterogeneity as described for seminal PSA by Wang (4) and by our group (5). Free PSA can be fractionated into at least five isoenzymes in the pH range between 6.0 and 8.0 revealing a main peak at pH 7.0 corresponding to the isoelectric point of PSA at pH 6.9 described in the literature. In the process of chromatofocusing the complexed form of PSA is strongly bound to the ionic exchange support. It only can be eluted from the column at pH below 6 in the presence of high salt (1 M NaCl) yielding highly purified PSA-alpha-1-chymotrypsin complex. Epitope mapping of the fractions of free PSA analyzed by chromatofusing reveals that different monoclonal and polyclonal antibodies react with varying affinity to the five most prominent isoenzymes found in free PSA. All antisera detect the

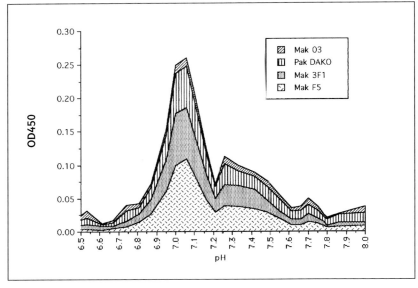

Figure 3. Differential binding of monoclonal and polyclonal antisera to isoenzymes of free (uncomplexed) PSA resolved on chromatofocusing column (cf. figure 2) Mak: monoclonal antibody; Pak: polyclonal antibody; DAKO: Anti-PSA (Nr. A 562) DAKO-Patts, Denmark); signal antibody: 1A5-6 POD conjugate.

isoenzymes between pH 6.9 to pH 8 with various strength disclosing that not all isoenzymes carry the same number of epitopes as the main peak at pH 7 (figure 3).

Conclusions

It is very important to take into account that different monoclonal antisera react with differing affinity to their respective binding sites or epitopes. Therefore varying signals depending on the antibody-antigen reaction will be obtained. This can be seen from the preliminary chromatofocusing experiments carried out on individual patients sera where we find various binding to the different isoenzymes. This may account for the different results for the total amount of PSA so often observed when one sample is examined by several methods.

The results shown demonstrate that caution should be taken when claiming that with the simple comparison of free to complexed PSA, sera from patients with either BPH or P-CA can be distinguished. This is especially so as there is no proof at hand that BPH tissue and P-CA tissue should secrete PSA molecules with different affinities for the protease inhibitor ACT present in such large excess.

References

1. Maurer A, Huber PR (1992) Interaction of prostate specific antigen with alpha-1-antichymotrypsin. In: Klapdor R (ed) Tumor associated antigens, oncogenes, receptors, cytokines in tumor diagnosis and therapy at the beginning of the nineties. Zuckschwerdt, München, pp 321–327
2. Lilja H et al (1991) Prostate-specific antigen in serum occurs predominantly in complex with alpha-1-chymotrypsin. Clin Chem 37:1618–1625
3. Stenman UH et al (1991) A complex between prostate-specific antigen and alpha-1-chymotrypsin is the major form of prostate-specific antigen in serum of patients with prostatic cancer: Assay of the complex improves clinical sensitivity for cancer. Cancer Res 51:222–226
4. Wang MC (1982) Prostate antigen of human cancer patients. In: Busch H, Yeoman LC (eds) Methods in Cancer Research. Acad Press, London, XIX, pp 179–197
5. Huber PR (1987) Prostate specific antigen. Experimental and clinical observations. Scand J Urol Nephrol 104:33–39

Address for correspondence:
Priv.-Doz. Dr. P. R. Huber
Kantonsspital Basel
Hormonlabor DZL
CH-4031 Basel, Switzerland

Combined estimation of free and complexed PSA – First clinical results

J. Spitz[a], P. Benz[a], M. Köllermann[b]

[a]Division of Nuclear Medicine, Private Office RNS, Wiesbaden,
[b]Clinic of Urology, Municipal Hospital HSK, Wiesbaden, Germany

Introduction

The estimation of the prostate-specific antigen (PSA) in the specimens of patients suffering from prostate cancer has proved to be of high efficiency in the diagnostic follow-up procedure. PSA complexed to α_1-antichymotrypsin represents the dominant form of PSA in the sera of patients and normals (7). Different portions of uncomplexed (free) form of PSA also exist in the sera of patients with prostate cancer and benign prostate hyperplasia. Depending upon the degree of PSA complexion, various assays, using monoclonal or polyclonal antibodies, differ in immunorecognition of total PSA in serum (4, 6, 7, 10).

Recently data have been presented suggesting that the use of at least one polyclonal antibody in the measurement of PSA may be either advantageous or complementary to an assay composed of only MAbs, as the epitope recognition of monoclonal antibodies may be too restrictive in the measurement of heterogeneous forms of PSA (11).

This study reports the results of measurements with an established dual monoclonal reference assay in comparison with a new developed non-isotopic, chemoluminescent assay for PSA, based on both monoclonal and affinity purified polyclonal Abs in a single test system.

Material and methods

Assays

Tandem® PSA: Manual, dual monoclonal immunoradiometric assay, Hybritech Inc. San Diego, CA.
ACS PSA: Automated polyclonal / monoclonal immunochemiluminometric assay formated for use with the Ciba Corning ACS 180 system; Ciba-Corning Diagnostics Corp., East Walepole, MA.

Specimens

64 patients with 430 specimen collected between January 1989 and November 1993. All specimens derived from routine diagnostic procedure, using Hybritech Tandem® PSA, and were frozen at –20 °C until further evaluation.

The selection criteria of specimen for this study out of a large number of 6000 frozen sera were the following: length of follow-up time and apparent changes of PSA values from normal to pathologic values or vice versa. All patients had a histologically proven diagnosis either by biopsy or by resection.

Results

The re-evaluation for PSA was done in duplicates of the 430 specimen within one day due to the high performance of the fully automated ACS 180 system. The values were calculated without knowledge of the Tandem® PSA values and then submitted to statistical analysis.

Both assays showed an excellent overall correlation (r = 1.00) for the range from 0.1 – 3500 ng PSA/ml.

This was also found for the range from 0.1 – 4.0 ng/ml (n = 224), the slope being almost 1.0 with a minimal offset (figure 1).

The following linear regression was calculated: ACS = 0.94 x Hybritech + 0.11 (r = 0.94).

Looking for the range from 4.0 – 20.0 ng/ml (n = 81) the r-value decreased to r = 0.88 and the slope went up (figure 2). The linear regression

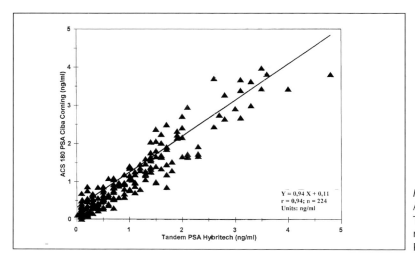

Figure 1. Comparison of ACS PSA values (y) with Tandem® values (x) for the range from 0.1 – 4.0 ng PSA/ml (ACS).

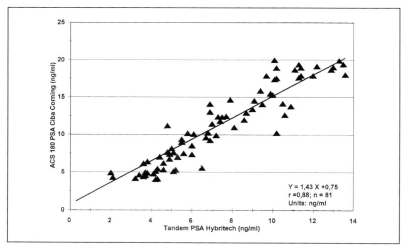

Figure 2. Comparison of ACS PSA values (y) with Tandem® PSA values (x) in the range from 4.0 – 20.0 ng PSA/ml (ACS).

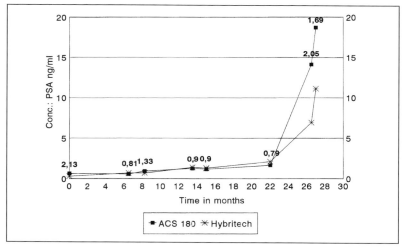

Figure 3. Follow-up controll of a 73 year old patient for 39 months after radical prostatectomy. The numbers within the drawing do not represent the absolute PSA values at the different investigation times but the ratios ACS PSA/Tandem® PSA.

was calculated as: ACS = 1.43 x Hybritech + 0.75. Selecting the values between 20 and 3500 ng/ml (n = 123) the slope was lower and the offset greater, the linear regression being: ACS = 1.27 x Hybritech + 7.2 (r = 0.99).

The direct comparison of individual values gave the following results: After radical prostatectomy patients showed comparably low PSA values (< 0.4 ng/ml) in both assays, the ACS values being more differentiated in this very low range. In case of tumor progression ACS values rose more pronounced in all cases. This increased rate of change becomes evident by calculating a ratio PSA ACS/PSA Hybritech. Within the normal range (< 4.0 ng) these ratios usually were near 1.0. In cases of tumor progress the ratios were as high as 2.0 (figure 3).

Discussion

As could be clearly demonstrated by recent publications (3, 7, 9, 11) PSA is predominantly present in sera of patients as high molecular weight complexes with endogeneous protease inhibitors (in about 85% of the patients) but also as uncomplexed free PSA molecules in about 15% of the patients. Although serum PSA is complexed, different stages of disease and different patients produce different ratios of complexed and free PSA (9).

The results of the analyses presented here strongly suggest a greater reactivity (i.e. greater clinical sensitivity) of the ACS PSA assay compared to the Tandem® assay, possibly due to the described about 3-fold reactivity of the former test to uncomplexed forms of PSA.

The reason for the observed differential reactivity is not completely understood today but could at least partially be explained by the use of a polyclonal antibody in the ACS assay recognizing multiple epitopes on the PSA molecule (4). The finding that alternative forms of PSA in patient sera may be missed by a test design employing only monoclonal antibodies has already been discussed by different authors (10, 11).

Regardless the underlying still controversially discussed biochemistry of different PSA forms in patient sera and their recognition by different commercial assays the clinical findings of this study are clear. In more than 60 patients longitudinally followed by the Tandem® and the ACS PSA assays responses to disease recurrence or to failed or successful therapy tracked each other quite similarly. However, in a substantial portion of the analysed patients enhanced response of the ACS PSA showing increased ranges of changes in PSA values (ACS PSA/ Tandem® PSA ratio) compared to the Tandem PSA® assay could be demonstrated. This enhanced reactivity correlated well with the observed clinical pathology. Similar findings were reported including proportionality to volume and progression or regression of the respective tumour (11).

Conclusion

The optimal recognition of all forms of PSA could be of great importance to successfully identify early progression or recurrence of prostate cancer and/or better predict its metastatic potential in the future. Our results indicate that the PSA values of the ACS system seem to provide such additional informations. Further clinical studies on a larger patients scale have to be carried out to evaluate the full range of diagnostic efficiency of free PSA in serum.

On the other hand after a long period of high inter-assay comparability for PSA values the new technique of ACS to estimate also uncomplexed PSA makes it necessary to label the results of each PSA estimation with the name of the applied kit, to enable correct interpretation during follow-up control.

References

1 Bluestein BI, Zhou AM, Tewari PC et al (1992) Multi-site clinical evaluation of an automated chemiluminescent immunoassay for prostate specific antigen (ACS PSA). J Tumor Marker Oncol 7:41–60
2 Chan DW, Bruzek DJ, Oesterling JE et al (1987) Prostate specific antigen as a marker for prostate cancer: a monoclonal and a pollyclonal immunoassay compared. Clin Chem 33 1916–1920
3 Christenson A, Laurell CB, Lilja H (1990) Enzymatic activity of prostate-specific antigen and its reactions with extracellular serine protease inhibitors. Eur J Biochem 194:755–763
4 Chu TM, Kawinski E, Hibi N et al (1989) Prostate specific antigen identified with monoclonal antibodies. J Urol 141:152–156

5. Graves HCB, Wehner N, Stamey TA (1990) Comparison of a polyclonal and a monoclonal immunoassay for PSA: need for an international antigen standard. J Urol 144:1516–1522
6. Hortin GL, Bahnson RR, Draft M et al (1988) Differences in values abtained with 2 assays of prostate specific antigen. J Urol 139:762–765
7. Lilja H, Christensson A, Dahlen U et al (1991) Prostate specific antigen in serum occurs predominantly in complex with α_1-antichymotrypsin. Clin Chem 73:1618–1625
8. Lilja H, Cockett AT, and Abrahamson PA (1992) Prostate specific antigen predominantly forms a complex with α_1-antichymotrypsinogen in blood: Implications for procedures to measure prostate specific antigen in serum. Cancer 70:230–234
9. Stenman UH, Leionen J, Alfthan H et al (1991) A complex between prostate specific antigen and alpha1-antichymotrypsin is the major form of prostate specific antigen in serum of patients with prostate cancer: Assay of the complex improves clinical sensitivity for cancer. Cancer Res 51:222–226
10. Stephenson RA, Geskovich FJ, Fritsche HA et al (1991) Ratio of polyclonal-monoclonal prostate – specific antigen levels: Discrimination of nodal status in prostate tumors that produce low marker levels. Urol Clin North Amer 18:467–471
11. Zhou AM., Tewari PC, Bluestein Bl et al (1993) Multiple forms of prostate specific antigen in serum: Differences.in immunorecognition by monoclonal and polyclonal assays. Clin Chem 39:2483–2491

Address for correspondence:
Priv.-Doz. Dr. med. J. Spitz
RNS
Ludwig-Erhard-Straβe 100
D-65199 Wiesbaden, Germany

Early diagnosis of recurrent prostate cancer after radical prostatectomy by a new and simple ultrasensitive PSA-detection

Edith Huland, D. Hübner, A. Haese, H. Huland

Department of Urology, University Hospital, Hamburg, Germany

Introduction

PSA is a sensitive serum marker for prostate cancer (1). Serum values of PSA in patients after radical prostatectomy decrease within several days after the operation to zero values because of the unique organ specificity. The most sensitive detection of residual prostate cancer is the measurement of PSA (2). Unfortunately common PSA assays have flat calibration curves so that the detection of patients with recurrent cancer is late (4).

The basic idea of our new ultrasensitive PSA-assay is to increase the analytical sensitivity of standard assays through a modification of patients sera. This is achieved by reduction of water content and measurement of defined concentration steps. The present study shows first results of this new ultrasensitive detection of PSA in patients who underwent radical prostatectomy. The reliability of this method is proven by positive (sera of patients with BPH and prostate cancer) and negative (female sera) controls.

Patients and methods

Aliquots of patients sera are distributed in four different test tubes. One tube was used for immediate – native – measurement of the probe, the three others were weighted to determine the exact weight of the probe. Then a lyophilization was performed overnight (Lyovac GT 2). After freeze drying serum was weighted again and partially rehydrated with aqua dest. to achieve the desired concentration of 2fold, 3fold, and 4fold, e.g. if 10 g of serum were in the test tube before freeze drying the desired total weight of the probe would be 2.5 g and the water to be added is calculated by subtracting the dry weight of the probe from the desired total weight. Calculation was performed by a computer directed procedure which adjusted the real weights and calculated correspondingly. After redilution weight was determined again and real redilution factor calculated. Subsequent measurement was performed in triplicate by an Abbott IMX Assay, a fully automated procedure. For evaluation the mean value of three measurements was used.

178 sera from patients after radical prostatectomy (35–1416 days) were collected, PSA values in native sera were determined immediately. Concentration of sera to 2fold, 3fold and 4fold was performed and the PSA values were determined in each serum probe. Further 20 female sera served as negative controls. Measurements for PSA values in native serum and after complete lyophilisation and partial redilution in 2fold, 3fold and 4fold concentrations were performed and compared to native values.

PSA of male patients (PSA values ranged between 0.10–55.40 ng/ml) with different diseases (BPH, prostatitis and prostate cancer) were measured in native serum without any pretreatment. Subsequently probes of these patients were completely lyophilized over night and rediluted to 1fold (complete redilution), 2fold, 3fold, 3,5fold and 4fold concentrations. Afterwards PSA values were determined. Alltogether 318 sera of this patient group served as positive controls. The redetection rate for each serum was calculated and compared with native measurements and give the information about the reliability of PSA values in concentrated serum.

Results

Interpretation of PSA measurements after concentration based on results of concentration studies in sera with detectable PSA levels

Positive: 1. Sera which show after any concentration PSA values positive according to standard definition in sera without concentration. For the Abbott IMX Assay we have used a borderline of = > 0.10 ng/ml as standard definition of beeing positive.

2. Sera which are measured below standard cut-off line (< 0.1 ng/ml) in concentrated probes are defined to be positive if they show a continuous increase in three measurements: the native, the 2fold, and 4fold concentrated samples.

Suspicious: Values below the standard cut-off line for positivity e.g. ≤ 0.1 ng/ml which show a 2.5 times or more increase of PSA value after 4fold concentration of patients serum compared to native serum PSA values.

Table I. A total of 48 sera from 178 sera were evaluated to be positive according to definition 1 and 2. Standard measurement detects 16 from 178. All sera positiv in standard evaluation have increasing PSA values in subsequent concentration steps. Positive results showed in 10 sera as typical examples. Ultrasensitive PSA detection in native and lyoconcentrated sera of patients after radical prostatectomy (RP)

Serum no.	Days after RP	PSA value of native sera	PSA value of lyoconcentrated sera		
			2fold	3fold	4fold
	(d)	(ng/ml)	(ng/ml)	(ng/ml)	(ng/ml)
74	70	0.00	0.01	0.06	0.08
124	551	0.00	0.02	0.04	0.06
95	357	0.00	0.00	0.02	0.04
160	265	0.01	0.03	0.03	0.06
168	81	0.01	0.02	0.02	0.03
156	199	0.02	0.14	0.23	0.32
211	203	0.04	0.15	0.27	0.29
115	129	0.07	0.15	0.27	0.29
278	82	0.19	0.37	0.53	0.64
248	290	1.49	3.01	4.37	5.60
Total n = 48	average $\bar{x} = 234$	average $\bar{x} = 0.29$	average $\bar{x} = 0.60$	average $\bar{x} = 0.89$	average $\bar{x} = 1.05$
	range (d) 60–572	range 0.00–4.27	range 0.00–8.18	range 0.01–12.10	range 0.02–15.07

Table II. Measurement of PSA containing sera (0.10–55.40 ng/ml) of patients with prostatic carcinoma, benign prostatic hyperplasia (BPH) and prostatitis before and after complete lyophilization and complete or partial rehydration. The percentage of recovery of the total PSA (= 100%) in the different concentration steps and the range is given.

	Samples n	PSA values in native serum range (ng/ml)	Average redetection (%)	SD	range (%)
PSA 1-fold (compl. redilut.)	25	0.31–55.40	99.23	6.82	80.35–107.44
PSA 2-fold (partl. redilut.)	101	0.10–33.17	97.21	6.77	82.52–122.99
PSA 3-fold (partl. redilut.)	79	0.10–33.17	91.68	9.11	67.56–115.70
PSA 3.5-fold (partl. redilut.)	30	0.10–33.17	84.94	9.60	64.81–101.49
PSA 4-fold (partl. redilut.)	79	0.10–33.17	81.15	9.06	64.79–103.19

Negative: All others.

PSA values of 178 concentrated sera (2fold, 3fold and 4fold) of 95 patients after radical prostatectomy were measured. Blood of patients was taken about every 3–6 months after the operation. Using a cut-off line of 0.10 ng/ml and more for the definition of a serum probe being positive for PSA, 16 of 178 sera judged positive in standard measurements. By including the concentrated serum probes into this evaluation 48 sera have to be judged to be positive according to the above definition. All sera positive in standard evaluation are also positive in the concentrated evaluation. That means, additional 32 of 178 sera reached detectable levels. Examples for measurements are given in table I. According to the definition above 29 sera which were negative in standard measurements had to be considered for suspicious PSA serum values. The remaining 101 serum samples showed negative results according to the definition, 65 of these sera had 0.00 ng/ml in all concentration steps, 36 samples presented measurable values but without any increasing tendency in subsequent concentrations. Sera of 20 female control persons were measured native and after subsequent concentration steps for their PSA values. All determinations were negative before and after concentration steps of sera.

Measurement of sera of patients with different diseases such as BPH, prostatitis and proven prostate cancer with PSA values between 0.31–55.4 ng/ml served as positive controls and showed high recognition of PSA after lyophilization and complete or incomplete redilution and measurement of serum samples. 25 sera with native PSA values of 0.31–55.40 ng/ml were measured before and after complete lyophilization and complete redilution. Compared to native measurement an average of 99.23% of PSA (range 80.32–107.44%) was redetected. Further 289 sera were evaluated after partial redilution to 2fold, 3fold, 3,5fold and 4fold concentrations. In such concentrated probes redetection rates decreased to values between 97.21 and 81.15%. The more the sera were concentrated the less PSA was redetected. Compared to native sera a clear increase in sensitivity, however, was still achieved.

Discussion

Our data clearly show that complete lyophilization and complete redilution (average redetection rate > 99%, range 80.35%–107.44%) does not influence the PSA values measured with the Abott IMX. The range given in table II shows that up to 103.19% can be redetected in the 4fold concentrated sera, allowing a 4fold increase in sensitivity, while the lowest range with redetection of 64.79% in the 4fold concentration still gives about a 2.5 times increase. These data show that the use of defined increasing concentration steps of patient serum allows a quite reliable detection of PSA in serum concentrations where standard assays fail. The definition 1 of being positive by simply using the standard cut-off lines for the concentrated values are simple and self evident. The second definition which is the detection of a continuous increase in such concentrated probes which are below the standard cut-off line should give additional information in the lower PSA values. Thus recurrent prostate cancer in patients after radical prostatectomy could be detected much earlier (3).

The described method to manipulate the patients' probe and not the method of determination will allow routine laboratories to continue to use their standard assay. It does not require the acquisition of additional technology or the additional training of personel and is therefore very easy to establish. Furthermore it can be combined with other supersensitive detection assays.

Our data show that the sensitivity can be increased specifically to a factor 4 and in addition "grey zone samples" can be defined by performing continuously increasing concentration steps and measuring each single step. This new detection method is extremely simple, reliable and could give highly valuable information at an early stage of recurrent prostate cancer.

References

1 Lange PH, Ercole CJ, Lightner DJ, Fraley EE, Vessella R (1989) The value of serum prostate specific antigen determinations befor and after radical prostatectomy. J Urol 141:8732
2 Morgan WR, Zincke H, Rainwater LM, Myers RP Klee GG (1991) Prostate specific antigen values

after radical retropubic prostatectomy for adenocarcinoma of the prostate: Impact of adjuvant treatment (hormonal and radiation). J Urol 145:319
3. Graves HC, Wehner N, Stamey TA (1992) An ultrasensitive radioimmunoassay for prostate specific antigen. Clin Chem 38:1
4. Stamey TA, Graves HCB, Wehner N, Ferrari M, Freiha FS (1993) Early detection of residual prostate cancer after radical prostatectomy by an ultrasensitive assay for prostate specific antigen. J Urol 141:787

Address for correspondence:
Dr. med. Edith Huland
Urologische Universitätsklinik
Hamburg-Eppendorf
Martinistraße 52
D-20246 Hamburg, Germany

Prostate specific antigen as a screening test for prostate cancer

F. Donn[a], P. Kondziella[a], H. Becker[a], K. Hannemann-Pohl[b]
[a]Department of Urology, [b]Department of Clinical Chemistry,
Marienkrankenhaus, Hamburg, Germany

Introduction

The early detection of prostate cancer has long been the goal of urologists. Many believe that moving the point of diagnosis backward in time, so that the prostate cancer is diagnosed earlier than usual, means that the treatment will be more effective than treatment occuring at the usual time. It is believed that those screening programs will result in a decline in prostate cancer mortality rates. Traditionally, the early detection of prostate cancer in asymptomatic men depends on digital rectal examination, but recently PSA measurement and transrectal ultrasonography become available. The prospect of using these techniques in widespread screening or early dedection programs has generated considerable controversy by published reports. Unfortunately, the presumption of effectiveness may not be correct, and the value of prostate cancer screening program must be established. In an attempt to detect prostate cancer when the disease was still localised, this screening procedure was done for men over the age of 55 years.

Patients and methods

500 asymptomatic patients who did not have a prior urologic history of disease were screened for the presence of early prostate cancer by PSA measurements. Prostate specific antigen (PSA) and rectal examination were the front-line tests. All PSA determinations were made on routine serum samples using the PSA-IRMA-Count of DPC (Diagnostic Products Corporation). According to the manufacture's recommendations, the expected range for PSA in unaffected men using this assay is zero to 1.95 ng/ml and 4.15ng/ml. Ultrasonography and ultrasound guided biopsies were performed for men with suspicious findings on either tests. Ultrasonography was performed in real-time using Bruel & Kjaer Model 1846 equipment.

Results

The average age of the men was 61.3 years. 10% were 55–59 years of age, 30% were 60–64, and 60% were 65–70. The data in table I report the PSA values for all groupes. 4% of men (55-59 years of age) had elevated PSA levels being submitted to ultrasound guided biopsy. But no cancer was found. 13.3% of men (60–64 years of age) had elevated PSA levels. In those patients a non-palpable cancer was found by TRUS in a small area. The lesion was staged as A1. 22% men (65–70 years of age) had elevated PSA levels (4.0–10 ng/ml and >10 ng/ml). All of them were submitted to biopsy. 14 men had positive biopsies staged as localised prostate cancer (table II). PSA levels were elevated in 18%. PSA levels were measured false-positive in 15%. The detection rate for prostate cancer was 3% (figure 1). In the 55 to 59, 60 to 64 and 65 to 70-year age groups cancer was detected in 1.5%, 4.4% and 4.5%, respectively. In our screened groups, none of 15 patients with prostate cancer had bone metastases or clinical evidence of lymph node metastases.

Discussion

PSA is a simple easily performed test. Patients may more readily accept a blood test compared to the more invasive digital rectal examination or

Table I. Test results according to age and PSA level.

Age	Total		0-4 ng/ml		4-10 ng/ml		> 10 ng/ml	
	no.	%	no.	%	no.	%	no.	%
55-59	50	100	48	96	2	4	0	0
60-64	150	100	127	84.7	20	13.3	3	2
65-70	300	100	235	78.3	45	15	20	6.7
Total	500	100	410	82	67	13.4	23	4.6

Table II. Test results according to age, PSA (> 4 ng/ml), digital rectal excamination (DRE), transrectal ultrasonography (TRUS) and TRUS-guided biopsy.

Age	PSA > 4 ng/ml		DRE		TRUS		Biopsy	
	no.	%	no.	%	no.	%	no.	%
55-59	2	100	0	0	0	0	0	0
60-64	23	100	0	0	1	4.3	1	4.3
65-70	65	100	0	0	12	18.5	14	21.5
Total	90	100	0	0	13	14.4	15	16.7

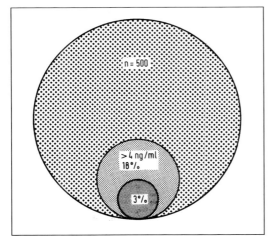

Figure 1. Early dectection rate of prostate cancer in asymptomatic men by PSA screening.

transrectal ultrasound. The detection rate in our screened group was 3% and reflected the age-related increase. Other investigatiors using PSA as the initial test in early detection of prostate cancer were reported in the literature (1, 2, 3, 4, 5, 6, 7, 8, 9). In spite of these results, the value of prostate cancer screening is still unproven. The number of undetected prostate cancer because of normal PSA levels are still unknown. Digital rectal examination has a limited ability to detect tumors of small volume that are most likely to be confined to the prostate. Thus, it may not confer enough advantage at the present time detecting those tumors with the greatest potential for cure.

It is not merely sufficient to show that screening detects cancers more early; early detection may not lead to improve survival, if treatments are ineffective or cancers detected are either latent or already incurable. First, the mortality for prostate cancer has not declined in the past thirty years. Second, the disease is asymptomatic during its most curable stages, making early detection difficult. Third, upper age limits have not been set, but it is generally agreed that routine screening is not desirable in men with a life expectancy of less than 10 years; therefore, the upper age limit should be 70 years.

The idea of screening is simple, the clinical practice of screening is complex. The initial screening examination appears to detect cancers at somewhat earlier clinical stage than they are detected in unscreened patients. For screening to be effective, a high sensitivity and specificity is needed. This criterion is especially important due to the relatively low incidence of prostate cancer. The incidence of all early lesions is strongly dependent on age. The specifity of a screening test is even more important than its sensitivity.

The present protocol design does not allow determination of the sensitivity or specifity of

PSA. Sensitivity implies knowledge not only of the true positive cases but also the false negatives, and this latter statistic can only be ascertained by performing serial section of the prostates of individuals in whom cancer was not detected by PSA. The available data suggest that the most practical PSA threshold is 4 ng/ml. Lower cut-offs lead to more biopsies with a low yield of cancer; higher cut-offs detect more cancers too late.

PSA, using a normal range of 4.0 ng/ml, fails to detect localised prostate cancer in 30 to 40% of cases reflecting the 78.7% sensitivity and 59.2% specifity. This diagnostic sensitivity is similiar to that found in the literature (10, 11, 12, 13, 14, 15, 16, 17, 18, 19, 20, 21).

In the general population, approximately 80% of all prostate cancers are less than 0.5 ml in volume, and the most of these go undetected. In most patients, the current study indicates that it would require approximately 12 years for a 0.5 ml cancer to reach 4 ml in volume if its doubling time was four years.

Lowering the threshold for "normal" PSA will improve sensitivity but specifity also will be lowered. PSA already has a poor specifity because several benign conditions produce an abnormal value (22, 23, 24, 25, 26). The most common reasons for false-positive (for cancer) elevations are BPH and prostatitis. Men with BPH have PSA elevations in 21% to 86% of cases. Therefore, PSA elevations are not specific for prostate cancer, and a normal PSA level do not exclude the presence of cancer. Since BPH is more prevalent than prostate cancer, differentiation between men with prostate cancer and BPH would avoid subjecting a large number of men with lower PSA levels to unnecessary work-up and the psycholological trauma associated with cancer suspicion.

An important question that remains to be answered is whether screening for prostate cancer can prolong survival. The incidence of prostate cancer is known to rise with increasing age. Thus close to 50% of men in the eighth decade of live have microscopic evidence of prostate cancer at autopsy. Detecting prostate cancer in asymptomatic men by mass screening it is argued that patients may be diagnosed and treated who would never normally require any therapy for this disease because their tumors are slow growing and they would die of another cause (27, 28, 29, 30).

Conclusions

We have found that PSA as the initial test in men older than 50 years is limited as a solitary screening test for prostate cancer because of the limitations of both sensitivity and specifity. A normal PSA value in combination with normal sonographic findings indicates an almost negligible risk of prostate cancer. The combination of normal digital rectal examination and normal ultrasound findings but high PSA value may indicate the presence of a transition zone cancer and diagnostic transurethal resection might be considered. But there is also a high risk of a high psychological morbidity due to a relative high frequency of false positive test results.

At present time, widespread implementation of screening programmes for prostate cancer cannot be recommended. The implementation of a pilot study of prostate cancer screening using comprehensive data monitoring would provide invaluable information to clarify the probabilities used in this study.

References

1 Brawer MK, Chetner MP, Beatie J, Buchner DM, Vesella RL, Lange P (1992) Screening for prostatic carcinoma with prostate specific antigen. J Urol 147: 841–845

2 Labrie F, Dupont A, Suburu R, Cusan L, Tremblay M, Gomez J-L, Emond J (1992) Serum prostate specific antigen as pre-screening test for prostate cancer. J Urol 147:846–852

3 Mettlin C, Lee F, Drago J, Murphy G (1991) The American Cancer Society National Prostate Detection Project: Findings on the detection of early prostate cancer. Cancer 67:2949–2958

4 Babaian RJ, Mettlin C, Cane, Murphy G, Lee F, Drago J (1992) Findings of the American Cancer Society National Prostate Cancer Detection Project: The relationship of prostate-specific antigen to digital rectal examination and transrectal ultrasonography. Cancer 69:1195–1200

5 Babaian RJ, Camps JL, Frangos DN, Ramirez EI, Tenny DM, Hassel JS, Fritsch HA (1991) Monoclonal prostate-specific antigen in untreated prostate cancer: Relationship to clinical stage and grade. Cancer 8:2200–2206

6 Babaian RJ, Miyashita H, Evans Rb, Ramirez E (1992) The distribution of prostate specific antigen in men without clinical or pathological evidence of

prostate cancer: Relationship to gland volume and age. J Urol 147:837-840
7. Ballentine HC, Pearson JD, Metter EJ, Brant LJ, Chan DW, Andres R, Fozard Walsh PC (1992) Longitudinal evaluation of prostate-specific antigen levels in men with and without prostate disease. JAMA 267:2215-2220
8. Carter HB, Person JD, Metter EJ, Brand LJ, Chan DW, Andres R, Fozard JL, Walsh PC (1992) Longitudinal evaluation of prostatic specific antigen levels in men with and without prostate disease. JAMA 267:2215-2220
9. Brawer MK, Beatie J, Wener MH, Vesella RL, Preston SD, Lange P (1993) Screening for prostatic carcinoma with prostate specific antigen: Results of the second year. J Urol 150:106-109
10. Kuriyama M, Wang MC, Papsidero LD, Killian CS, Shimaro T, Valenzuela L, Nishiura T, Murphy GP (1980) Quantitation of prostate-specific antigen in serum by a sensitive enzyme immunoassay. Cancer Res 40: 4568-4662
11. Yang N (1984) Diagnostic and prognostic application of prostate-specific tissue markers: Prostate antigen (PA) and prostatic acid phosphatase (PAP). Clin Chem 30:1057
12. Liedtke R, Batjer JD (1984) Measurement of prostate-specific antigen by radioimmunoassay. Clin Chem 30:649-652
13. Hudson MA, Bahnson RR, Catalona WJ (1989) Clinical use of prostate specific antigen in patients with prostate cancer. J Urol 142:1011-1017
14. Stamey TA, Yang N, Hay AR (1987) Prostate specific antigen as a serum marker for adenocarcinoma of the prostate. N Engl J Med 317:909-916
15. Pons-Anicet O, Ramaioli A, Namer M (1988) Evaluation of prostate-specific antigen in prostate cancer. Amer J Clin Oncol (CCT) 11 (suppl 2):871
16. Caty A, Gosselin P, Cazin, JL (1988) Significance of PSA and PAP in patients with or without prostatic cancer. Amer J Clin Oncol (CCT) 11 (suppl 2):863
17. Guillet J, Role C, Duc AT (1988) Prostate specific antigen (PSA) in the management of 500 prostatic patients. Amer J Clin Oncol (CCT) 11 (suppl 2):861
18. Cooner WH, Mosley BR, Rutherford CL (1988) Clinical application of transrectal ultrasonography and prostate specific antigen in the search for prostate cancer. J Urol 139:758-761
19. Cooner WH, Mosley BR, Rutherford CL Jr, Beard JH, Pond HS, Terry WJ, Igel TC, Kidd DD (1990) Prostate cancer detection in a clinical urological practice by ultrasonography, digital rectal examination and prostate specific antigen. J Urol 143:1146-1154
20. Brawer HK, Lange PH (1989) Prostate-specific antigen: Its role in early detection, staging, and monitoring of prostatic carcinoma. J Endourol 3:227
21. Gustafsson O, Norming U, Almgard L-E, Fredriksson A, Gustavsson G, Harvig B, Nyman CR (1992) Diagnostic methods in the detection of prostate cancer: A study of a randomly selected population of 2,400 men. J Urol 148:1827-1831
22. Ercole CJ, Lange PH, Mathisen M, Chiou RK, Reddy PK, Vesella RL (1987) Prostatic specific antigen and prostatic acid phosphatase in the monitoring and staging of patients with prostate cancer. J Urol 138:1181-1184
23. Oesterling JE, Chan DW, Epstein JI, Komball AW, Bruzek DJ, Rock RC, Brendler CB, Walsh PC (1988) Prostate specific antigen in hte preoperative and postoperative evaluation of localised prostatic cancertreated with radical prostatectomy. J Urol 139:766-772
24. Cooner WH, Mosley BR, Rutherford CL, Jeff JR, Beard JH, Pond HS, Bass RB, Terry WJ (1988) Clinical application of transrectal ultrasonography and prostate specific antigen in the search for prostate cancer. J Urol 139:758-761
25. Hudson MA, Bahnson RR, Catalona WJ (1989) Clinical use of prostate specific antigen in patients with prostate cancer. J Urol 142:1011-1017
26. Catalona WJ, Smith DS, Ratliff TL, Dodds KM, Coplen DE, Yuan JJJ, Petros JA, Andriole GL (1991) Measurement of prostate-specific antigen in serum as a screening test for prostate cancer. New Engl J Med 324:1156-1161
27. Johanson JE, Adami HO, Anderson SO, Bergström R, Holmberg L, Krusemo UB (1992) High 10-year survival rate in patients with early, untreated prostatic cancer. JAMA 267:2191-2196
28. Whitmore WF JR (1984) Natural history and staging of prostate cancer. Urol Clin North Am 11:205-220
29. Epstein JI, Paull G, Eggleston JC, Walsh PC (1986) Prognosis of untreated stage A1 prostatic carcinoma: A study of 94 cases with extended follow-up. J Urol 136:837-839
30. Blute ML, Zincke H, Farrow GM (1986) Long-term follow-up of young patients with stage A adeno-carcinoma of the prostate. J Urol 136:840-843

Address of correspondence:
Dr. med. F. Donn
Abteilung für Urologie
Marienkrankenhaus
Alfredstraße 9
D-22087 Hamburg, Germany

Clinical use of serum prostate specific antigen (PSA)

F. Donn, P. Kondziella, H. Becker, K. Hannemann-Pohl
Department of Urology, Department of Clinical Chemistry,
Marienkrankenhaus, Hamburg, Germany

Introduction

PSA was first described by *Wang* et al. (1). The molecular weight was estimated to be 33–34 kD by SDS-polyacrylamide gel electrophoresis.
By sequence homology, PSA is homologous with serine protease of the kallikrein family (2). Its in vivo substrate is identified as a structural protein with a molecular weight of 52 kD involved in the gelatinous entrapment of ejaculated spermatozoa (3). *Kuriyama* et al. (4) were the first to show the potential prognostic and monitoring capability of serum PSA. Using a sensitive enzyme immunoassay, elevated levels of circulating PSA were found in prostate cancer patients. The clinical utility of PSA is most profoundly revealed in prognosis evaluation, in disease monitoring, and in differential diagnosis of metastatic lesions secondary to prostate performed by commercial methods of Yang Laboratories (5) and Hybritech Incorporated (6). The purpose of this study was to correlate serum PSA levels in patients with BPH and with prostate cancer at different stages by the IRMA-Count PSA assay from Diagnostic Product Corporation (DPC).

Materials and methods

Serum samples from 600 men without evidence of prostate cancer, 100 women, 300 men with pathologiocally confirmed BPH by transurethral resection and prostatectomy and 137 patients with prostate cancer were measured with the sensitive immunometric IRMA-Count PSA assay. The staging categories used are pathological categories according WHO. PSA levels in patients with regionally confined prostate cancer were obtained before pelvic lymphadenectomy and radical retropubic prostatectomy in 42 patients with clinical, apparently localised prostate cancer. The IRMA-Count PSA assay used biotin-coated tubes so that sandwich formation can occur in the liquid phase and the 125y-labeled antibody-PSA complex becomes immobilized on the cell wall after complex formation.

Results

The values in all healthy subjects under 40 years of age, and of all women were less than or equal to 4.0 ng/ml. Consequently, 4.0 ng/ml was selected and established as the appropriate cut-off concentration to differentiate normal from elevated PSA-levels. A serum level of > 4.1 ng/ml or greater was selected as a substantiated elevation. Results obtained in BPH patients are summarized in table I. Of these patients 24% had PSA levels greater than 4 ng/ml. All patients with PSA levels greater than 4 ng/ml preoperatively had normal levels postoperatively. Results obtained in patients with prostate cancer are summarized in table II. 60% organ-defined prostate cancers showed significantly elevated serum levels of PSA although no quantitative difference in PSA levels was demonstrated between BPH and stages A and B prostate cancer. Patients with stages C and D prostate cancer, however, showed significantly elevated levels indicating the relation of prostate tumor size either intracapsular or extracapsular and serum PSA level. These results show that PSA is useful for staging prostate cancer but not for screening the disease. Therefore, determinations of serum PSA is very useful in detecting residual and recurrent disease in patients undergoing therapy. The concentration of serum PSA is also proportional to the volume of BPH without

Table I. PSA serum levels in patients with BPH.

	No.	0 – 4.0	4.01 – 10.0	> 10.01
BHP	100% (300)	76% (226)	22% (66)	2% (6)

Table II. PSA serum levels in patients with prostate cancer in relation to tumor stage.

	No.	0 – 4.0	4.01 – 10.0	> 10.01 – 20.0	> 20.01
Stage T1, 2 N0 M0	42 (100%)	40%	24%	34%	2%
Stage T3 N0 M0	95 (100%)	19%	21%	15%	45%
Stage T4 N1,2 M1	90 (100%)	10%	12%	21%	57%
Total	227				

prostate cancer and decreases after resection of BPH tissue.

Discussion

As with other tumor-associated markers, the primary objective of PSA is for the diagnosis of prostate cancer. The ideal tumor marker should possess high specifity, high senitivity, organ specifity and correlation with the tumor stage or tumor mass. The criteria of 100% specifity and sensitivity have not been fulfilled by PSA. As already known a low cut-off value indicates a high sensitivity and a low specifity, a high value a low sensitivity and a high specifity. Even if the cut-off value may be increased in order to differentiate more exactly between malignant and benign disease these criteria have not yet been fullfilled.
As to staging for prostate cancer both false positives and false negatives will be detected. The frequency of false results will depend on the cut-off level selected for PSA. Although there are no set conditions how the cut-off value should be calculated, we believe as others the cut-off value of 4 ng/ml is considerd to be the best reference in PSA-tests. PSA is a specific product of prostatic tissue. Men without prostate glands should not have detectable PSA in their serum. But some women have been found to have endogenous antibody to PSA, who will interfere with all PSA immunoassys including enzyme immunoassays, immunoradiometric assays and radioimmuno-assays. But this is yet no problem because there is no clinical indication for PSA testing in women. Lacking PSA synthesis is often described to undifferentiated tumors as a rule. In metastasizing prostate cancer, normalizing PSA levels reflect the often curative effect of secondary treatment.

Both RIAs and IRMAs have been developed for PSA and most of the clinical data reported in the literature are derived from an RIA and an IRMA (7, 8, 9, 10, 11, 12). No clear superiority of one over the other is apparent. Widely used are the Pros-Check assay (Yang Laboratories, Bellevue, U.S.A.) and the Tandem-R-test (Hybritech, San Diego, U.S.A) and the Diagnostic Products IRMA-Count assay. The manufacturers list the normal reference ranges in males as 0– 4.0 ng/ml. On the upper limit of normal or 4.0 ng/ml 70% sensitivity and 77% specifity are obtained. Lower cut-offs lead to more biopsies with a low yield of cancer, higher cut-offs detect more cancers too late. If the PSA level is elevated, sytematic biopsies should be performed. If one waits for the PSA level to rise above 10 ng/ml before recommending a biopsy, more than half of the cancers detected already will have spread, and the prognosis will be less favorable. Researchers have reported the reference ranges for these assays to start at zero with an upper limit anywhere from 2 to 12.
Recognizing the clinical impact of PSA detection several manufacturers released new available tests with altered analytical principles. Hybritech's monoclonal antibody to PSA has been adapted to the Stratus analyzer in a fluorescence immuno-assay or PSA has been adapted to the IMx analyzer (Abbott). In general, the methodological differences between PSA assays are significant, so that misinterpretation of a change in PSA values due to samples being assayed in different laboratories are possible. Thus, it cannot be taken

for granted that the clinical utility of immunoassay kits are similiar.

The former RIAs now have almost completely been replaced by the IRMAs, which have a much better theoretical sensitivity, and where the appropriate assay specifity can be achieved by the use of two monoclonal antibodies in a sandwich assay.

Like many laboratory PSA methods the IRMA-Count PSA assay is a specific in vitro laboratory test for determining circulating serum PSA. The assay protocol is simple and straightforward. Within-assay precision, between-assay precision and assay sensitivity are routine quality control parameters. The test offers good precision and recovery of PSA. Equipment and calibration and data interpretation are factors affecting the performance characteristics of every in vitro laboratory test. An international standard for PSA is still lacking. But it is important for the future that PSA immunoassays should be standardized in the range of 0–10 ng/ml PSA because this range is critical concerning sreening programs on early prostate cancer. It is apparent that the optimal assay configuration would be an assay that detects free and complexed PSA to alpha-1-antichymotrypsin and alpha-2-macroglobulin.

Evaluation of our data indicates that over 60% of stage A and B had elevated levels of serum PSA, and it is important to notice that nearly 40% of cancers were detected in men who had PSA levels within normal limits. Our data and those from ohters (10, 11, 12, 13) have shown that if an upper limit of normal of 4.0 ng PSA/ml is chosen 40 per cent of all known prostate-confined malignancies remain undetected. If an upper limit of normal or 10.0 ng PSA/ml is chosen, only 34 per cent of patients with known A1, B1, and B2 cancer are indentified. Improving the sensitivity to detect all tumors in a population leads to a significant reduction in specifity. Thus, patients (symptomatic or asymptomatic) with abnormal serum PSA may have a very high probability of having clinically undiagnosed early stage prostate cancer. This objective has been very encouraging. But the elevation of serum PSA only indicates that there is an increased level of antigen in the circulation. As already known this may be the result of a primary or secondary cancer, or it may due to BPH or prostatitis. Because PSA may be elevated in some patients with BPH, its use as a screening modality for localised prostate cancer is somewhat limited. But in the case of benign conditions, the levels of PSA range in our study from within the normal test limit to levels of PSA as high as 10 ng/ml, in general, however, somewhat lower than in patients with prostate cancer. In our experience, as PSA increases, the probability of prostate cancer also increases. Our data as well as those from other investigators have shown that levels of PSA in BPH overlap with PSA levels present in patients with prostate cancer.

PSA, using a normal range of 4.0 ng/ml, fails to detect localised prostate cancer in 40% of cases reflecting 78.7% sensitivity and 59.2% specifity of the PSA assay. This diagnostic sensitivity is similiar to that found in the literature (10, 11, 13). Most of them are micro-focal cancers that may not need treatment. Approximately 80% of all prostate cancers are less than 0.5 ml in volume, and the most of these go undetected.

PSA already has a poor specifity because several benign conditions produce an abnormal value (14, 15, 16, 17, 18, 19, 20). The most common reasons for false-positive (for cancer) elevations are BPH and prostatitis. Men with BPH have PSA elevations in 24%. Therefore, PSA elevations are not specific for prostate cancer, and a normal PSA level do not exclude the presence of cancer. Since BPH is more prevalent than prostate cancer, differentiation between men with prostate cancer and BPH would avoid subjecting a large number of men with lower PSA levels to unnecessary work-up and the pschyolological trauma associated with cancer suspicion.

References

1 Wang MC, Valenzia LA, Murphy GP, Chu TM (1979) Purification of a human prostate specific antigen. Invest Urol 17:159–163
2 Watt KW, Lee PJ, Tinkulu TM, Chan WP, Loor R (1986) Human prostatic specific antigen: Structural and functional similarity with serine proteases. Proc Natl Acad Sci (U.S.A.) 83:3166–3170
3 Lilja H (1985) A kallikrein-like serine protease in prostatic fluid cleaves the predominant seminal vesicle protein. J Clin Invest 76:1899–1903
4 Kuriyama M, Wang MC, Papsidero LD, Kilian CS, Shimano T, Valenzuela L, Nishiura T, Murphy GP, Chu TM (1980) Quantitation of prostate-specific

antigen in serum by a sensitive enzyme immunoassay. Cancer Res 40:4568–4662
5. Yang N (1984) Diagnostic and prognostic application of prostate-specific tissue markers: Prostate antigen (PA) and prostatic acid phosphatase (PAP). Clin Chem 30:1057
6. Liedtke R, Batjer JD (1984) Measurement of prostate-specific antigen by radioimmunoassay. Clin Chem 30:649–652
7. Hudson MA, Bahnson RR, Catalona WJ (1989) Clinical use of prostate specific antigen in patients with prostate cancer. J Urol 142:1011–1017
8. Stamey TA, Yang N, Hay AR (1987) Prostate specific antigen as a serum marker for adenocarcinoma of the prostate. N Engl J Med 317:909–916
9. Pons-Anicet O, Ramaioli A, Namer M. (1988) Evaluation of prostate-specific antigen in prostate cancer. Amer J Clin Oncol (CCT) 11 (suppl 2):871
10. Caty A, Gosselin P, Cazin JL (1988) Significance of PSA and PAP in patients with or without prostatic cancer. Amer J Clin Oncol (CCT) 11 (suppl 2):863
11. Guillet J, Role C, Duc AT (1988) Prostate specific antigen (PSA) in the management of 500 prostatic patients. Amer J Clin Oncol (CCT) 11 (suppl 2):861
12. Cooner WH, Mosley BR, Rutherford CL (1988) Clinical application of transrectal ultrasonography and prostate specific antigen in the search for prostate cancer. J Urol 139:758–761
13. Brawer HK, Lange PH (1989) Prostate-specific antigen: Its role in early detection, staging, and monitoring of prostatic carcinoma. J Endourol 3:227
14. Armitage TG, Cooper EH, Newling DW, Robinson MR, Appleyard I (1988) The value of measurement of serum prostate specific antigen in patients with benign prostatic hyperplasia and untreated prostate cancer. Br J Urol 62:584–589
15. Ercole CJ, Lange PH, Mathisen M, Chiou RK, Reddy PK, Vesella RL (1987) Prostatic specific antigen and prostatic acid phosphatase in the monitoring and staging of patients with prostate cancer. J Urol 138:1181–1184
16. Myrtle KR, Klimley PG, Ivor LP, Bruni JF (1986) Clinical utility of prostate specific antigen (PSA) in the managment of prostate cancer. Advances in Cancer Diagnostics, Hybritech Inc, pp 1–9
17. Oesterling JE, Chan DW, Epstein JI, Komball AW, Bruzek DJ, Rock RC, Brendler CB, Walsh PC (1988) Prostate specific antigen in the preoperative and postoperative evaluation of localized prostatic cancer treated with radical prostatectomy. J Urol 139:766–772
18. Cooner WH, Mosley BR, Rutherford CL, Jeff JR, Beard JH, Pond HS, Bass RB, Terry WJ (1988) Clinical application of transrectal ultrasonography and prostate specific antigen in the search for prostate cancer. J Urol 139:758–761
19. Hudson MA, Bahnson RB, Catalona WJ (1989) Clinical use of prostate specific antigen in patients with prostate cancer. J Urol 142:1011–1017
20. Catalona WJ, Smith DS, Ratliff TL, Dodds KM, Coplen DE, Petros JA, Andriole GL (1991) Measurement of prostate-specific antigen in serum as a screening test for prostate cancer. N Engl J Med 324:1156–1161

Address for correspondence:
Dr. med. F. Donn
Abteilung für Urologie
Marienkrankenhaus
Alfredstraße 9
D-22087 Hamburg, Germany

Evaluation of prostate specific antigen (PSA) and digital rectal examination (DRE) for early detection of prostate cancer

Results of a multicenter study of 6630 men

C. Darte[a], P.C. Southwick[b], W.J. Catalona[c], J.P. Richie[d], F.R. Ahmann[e], M.A. Hudson[f],
P.T. Scardino[f], R.C. Flanigan[g], J.B. deKernion[h], T.L. Ratliff[c], L.R. Kavoussi[d],
B.L. Dalkin[e], W.B. Waters[g], M.T. MacFarlane[h]

[a]Hybritech Europe, Liège, Belgium; [b]Hybritech Inc., San Diego, CA;
[c]Washington University School of Medicine, St. Louis, MO;
[d]Harvard Medicine School, Boston, MA; [e]University of Arizona College of Medicine, Tucson, AZ;
[f]Bayfor College of Medicine, Houston, TX; [g]Loyola University Medicine Centre, Chicago, IL;
[h]UCLA School of Medicine, Los Angeles, CA, USA

Introduction

Prostate cancer is the second cause of cancer death (1). Unfortunately, the majority of prostate cancers have spread beyond the gland when first diagnosed using the conventional detection method, digital rectal examination (DRE) (2–4). Recent reports show that prostate specific antigen (PSA) detects a significant number of cancers missed by DRE (4, 5, 6).

A multicenter evaluation was conducted to compare the efficacy of DRE and PSA in the detection of prostate cancer and to determine if PSA would significantly increase the detection of potentially curable organ-confined cancers when added to DRE.

Subjects and methods

6630 male volunteers aged 50 or over were enrolled into this prospective study at six medical centers. Exclusion criteria were a prior history of prostate cancers, accute prostatitis or urinary tract infection.

All men underwent determination of serum PSA concentration (Hybritech Tandem®-E PSA Immunoenzymetric Assay (Photon ERA®) or Tandem®-R PSA Immunoradiometric Assay) and digital rectal examination (DRE).

Men with normal PSA levels (0–4 ng/ml) and normal DRE findings, or DRE findings that were abnormal but benign (including enlargement with a normal consistency), were not further evaluated. If either the PSA concentration was elevated (> 4 ng/ml) or the DRE was suspicious for cancer (including induration), or both, subjects underwent four (quadrant) transrectal ultrasound (TRUS)-guided needle biopsies (2-apex, 2-base). Suspicious TRUS findings (including hypoechoic areas in the posterior peripheral zone) were recorded, but TRUS results were not used to determine whether a biopsy was performed. All four quadrants were biopsied even if no suspicious areas on DRE or TRUS were present.

If cancer was detected, clinical tumor stage was recorded. For subjects treated with radical prostatectomy or lymphadenectomy, the pathologic tumor stage was recorded.

Results

As shown in figure I, 15% (983) of the men had PSA > 4 ng/ml (Tandem-E or Tandem-R), 15% (982) had a suspicious DRE result, and 26% (1710) had either PSA > 4 ng/ml or a suspicious DRE.

1167 biopsies were performed and 264 cancers were detected. As illustrated in figure II, PSA detected significantly more cancers than DRE (82% versus 55%, p < 0.0001). If biopsy had required TRUS verification, nearly 40% of the cancers would have been missed.

The cancer detection rate was 3.2% for DRE, 4.6% for PSA, and 5.8% for the two methods

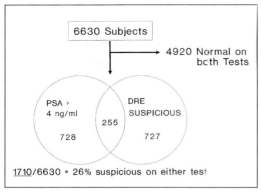

Figure 1. PSA determination and DRE in men aged 50 or over.

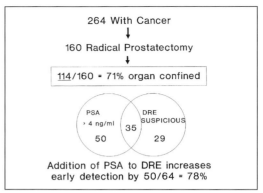

Figure 3. Comparison of PSA and DRE for organ-confined prostate cancer detection effectiveness.

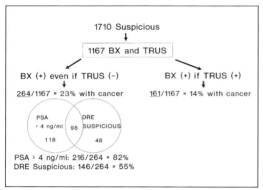

Figure 2. Comparison of PSA, DRE and TRUS for prostate cancer detection effectiveness (BX: TRUS-guided needle biopsy).

combined. Positive predictive value was 32% for PSA, and 21% for DRE.
Figure 3 shows that of the 160 patients who underwent radical prostatectomy and pathological staging, 114 had early, potentially curable organ-confined cancer. PSA detected significantly more organ-confined cancers than DRE (75% vs 56%, p < 0.05). The addition of PSA to DRE increased the detection of early cancers by 78%.

Discussion

In conclusion, this evaluation has demonstrated that PSA is a more powerful predictor of prostate cancer than DRE. A biopsy should be considered if either PSA is superior to 4 ng/ml (Hybritech Tandem PSA) or DRE is suspicious, even if TRUS is normal.
This study has also evidenced that the addition of PSA to DRE enhances early detection of organ-confined and potentially curable prostate cancer.

References

1. American Cancer Society. Cancer facts and figures (1992) Atlanta, GA: American Cancer Society
2. Boring CC, Squires TS, Tong T (1993) Cancer statistics. CA Cancer J Clin 43:7–26
3. Catalona WJ, Bigg SW (1990) Nerve-sparing radical prostatectomy: Evaluation of results after 250 patients. J Urol 143:538–544
4. Catalona WJ, Smith DS, Ratliff TL et al (1991) Measurement of prostate-specific antigen in serum as a screening test for prostate cancer. N Engl J Med 324:1156–1161
5. Brawer MK, Chetner MP, Beatie J, Buchner DM, Vessella RL, Lange PH (1992) Screening for prostatic carcinoma with prostate specific antigen. J Urol 147:841–845
6. Cooner WH, Mosley BR, Rutherford CL et al (1990) Prostate cancer detection in a clinical urological practice by ultrasonography, digital rectal examination, and prostate specific antigen. J Urol 143:1146–1154.

Address for correspondence:
Dr. C. Darte
Hybritech Europe
Parc Scientifique du Sart Tilman
Allee des Noisetiers 12
B-4031 Liège, Belgium

Clinical relevance of PSA values in urine

J. Spitz[a], P. Benz[a], Th. Bickert[a], M. Köllermann[b]
[a]Division of Nuclear Medicine, Private Office RNS Wiesbaden,
[b]Clinic for Urology, Municipal Hospital HSK, Wiesbaden, Germany

Introduction

The estimation of PSA-levels in blood is well established and of great importance and interest for the diagnosis and follow-up of prostate cancer in various stages. For many years little was known about PSA in urine. In 1985 *Graves* (4) was the first to report about 15 male controls, all of which showed high PSA values in the urine while 15 female controls had no PSA in their urine. After *Trembley* at al. (15) had supported these findings in 1987, *De Vere White* et al. (1) again draw attention to urine PSA in 1992. They investigated midstream urine of 43 patients after radical resection of the prostate and postulated that PSA in urine might be a potential tumor marker.

On the other hand there is a growing number of publications about PSA in extra prostate localisation, i.e. periurethral glands (2, 3, 7, 9, 10) even in females (10, 14).

To get a better understanding of this phenomenon, we decided to take a closer look at the technical aspects and clinical usefulness of PSA estimation in urine.

Material and method

All investigation were done with a commercial immunoradiometric assay (Tandem PSA, Hybritech) without modifications of the kit.
1. Estimation of PSA levels in urine specimens of normal men and women were done, looking for circadian rhythms, 24h values and various influences (stability, reproducibility, ejaculation, location of excretion).
2. Specimens of 64 patients (median age 70 years) with cancer of the prostate in stage A-C were analysed for PSA levels as well in blood as in urine before (n = 8) and after radical prostate resection (in 14 patients more than three years after). The resection rims were screened histologically for cancer cells. Endocrine therapy was started in 75% of patients.

Results

Technical aspects

The technical performance was as good in urine as in blood. The lowest detection limit was estimated to be 0.3 ng PSA/ml of urine. Reproducibility of values was excellent with low variations in all cases.

To evaluate the linearity of the assay in urine conditions defined amounts of PSA (standards of the Hybritech assay) were added to the urine specimen of two women without detectable PSA levels and then diluted (1:2, 1:5, 1:10, 1:20, 1:100, 1:200, and 1:500). The triplicate estimations showed a good linearity over the whole range of the test.

Five urine samples were stored for one week. The PSA levels of the samples had been chosen for various ranges. A basic PSA estimation was performed in all cases before freezing the specimen. Further checks followed after 16 hours at room temperature as well as after three and six days by thawing and freezing the corresponding sample. We found a good reproducibility in all cases without any dependence from the PSA content of the respective specimen.

Clinical studies

The urine PSA determination in 15 healthy men (aged between 27 and 68 years) led to PSA

Table I. Patient groups after radical resection of the prostate with regard to therapy and PSA levels in blood and urine. Column A: Patients with positiv margin and therapy. 13 have no PSA in urine nor in blood while 5 are positiv. B: From 8 patients without therapy 6 are PSA positiv in urine. C: From 12 patients with therapy, 11 have no detectable PSA level. D: Despite being margin negativ 14 of 17 patients are positiv for PSA in urine. Line 1+2: In 55 patients regardless margins and therapy, only 7 are positiv for serum PSA.

PSA levels	Margin + therapy +	Margin + therapy −	Margin − therapy +	Margin − therapy −
Serum > 0.3	2	0	0	0
Serum + urin > 0.3	3	0	0	2
Urin > 0.3	0	6	1	12
All levels < 0.3	13	2	11	3
	A	B	C	D

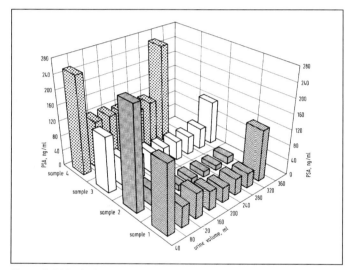

Figure 1. PAS distribution in four fractionated urine samples. Typically the first and the last fraction contained the highest amount of PSA.

No PSA was found in the urine of two men collected by nephrostoma. The patient group after radical resection of the prostate was divided into subgroups for better evaluation of influence of histological results and therapeutical effects (table I). Only five out of 27 patients without chemo- and hormone therapy demonstrated urine PSA values below 0.3 ng/ml, the positive ones having values up to 8.3 ng PSA/ml urine.

Out of the 36 patients with therapy 32 patients showed values below 0.3 ng PSA/ml in their urine. By statistical analysis (exact Fisher Test) we found a high significance between PSA in midstream urine and therapy (2.24 E-5 $< p <$ 7.39 E-10). Urine PSA levels in both groups were not dependent on histological criteria of the resected material (tumor free margins or not) ($p = 0.50–0.69$).

No correlation could be found between PSA values in serum and urine as well as between intraindividual values in the urine pre- and post- resection. Follow-up time after radical resection of the prostate is too short to give statistical results. We were able to follow-up six patients without therapy after radical resection of the prostate for four to 15 months (mean five months). Five patients demonstrated constantly elevated values in the urine (0.3–10.0 ng/ml) without regard to the histological finding at resection margin. PSA

values between 2.9 and 442 ng/ml (mean 97.5 ng/ml). In women all but one values were below 0.1 ng/ml.

Fractionated collection and estimation of PSA in urine specimens of two volunteers over 24 hours resulted in large variations of values without clear pattern. Fractionating a single sample at a given time resulted highest levels in the first and last portion of the sample (figure 1). Midstream values were as representative as a 24h collection.

With regard to the large physiologic variations the influence of ejaculation seems to be of minor importance.

values in serum of these patients stayed below 0.3 ng/ml corresponding to the clinical findings of no tumor recurrence. In one case of evident tumor relapse again no correlation was found with PSA values in urine ($0.263 < p < 1.0$). On the other hand PSA in the serum did show a correlation between elevated PSA values and tumor recurrence ($p = 6.96$ E-06).

Discussion

The estimation of PSA in urine is technically simple and reproducible on the basis of a commercial assay. It is not excreted by the kidneys (6, 11). It is independent from residual tumor tissue after radical resection of prostate cancer. Supported also by the clinical and histological findings of other groups we conclude, that PSA in urine is produced by extraprostatic sources which seem to be located in periurethral glands and highly dependent on endocrine therapy (5, 7, 9, 13).

In correspondence with a recently published paper (15) we were unable to extract from our patient data a diagnostic benefit of urine PSA values in patients with cancer of the prostate. Instead of that, serum PSA values proved again to be of high clinical reliability (8, 12).

Regarding these arguments the clinical benefit of PSA values in urine seems to be very questionable although a final answer can only be given by a long term prospective study. This should be based on initial values after resection of the prostate followed by regular controls in defined intervals. To simplify the collecting procedure, initial stream samples can be used (5, 13).

For the moment a practical indication for a PSA determination in urine might be the control of patient compliance during endocrine therapy.

References

1 DeVere White RW, Meyers FJ, Soares SE, Miller DG, Soriano TF (1992) Urinary prostate specific antigen levels: Roll in monitoring the reponse of prostate cancer to therapy. J Urol 147:947–951
2 Frazier HA, A Humphrey P, Buchette JL, Paulson DF (1992) Immunoractive prostatic specific antigen in male periurethral glands. J Urol 147:246–248
3 Golz R, Schubert GE (1989) Prostatic specific antigen: Immunoreactivity in urachal remnants. J Urol 141:1480–1482
4 Graves HCB, Sensabaugh GF, Crim D, Blake ET (1985) Postcoital detection of a male specific semen protein. N Engl J Med 312 6:338–343
5 Iwakiri J, Grandbois K, Wehner N, Graves HCB, Stamey T (1993) An analysis of urinary prostate specific antigen before and after radical prostatectomy: Evidence for secretion of prostate specific antigen by the periurethral glands. J Urol 149: 783–786
6 Kabalin JN, Hornberger JC (1991) Prostate specific antigen is not excreted by human kidney or eliminated by routine hemodialysis. Urol 37:308–310
7 Kamoshida S, Tsutsumi Y (1990) Exraprostatic localization of prostatic acid phosphatase and prostate specific antigen: distribution in cloacogenic glandular epithelium and sex–dependent expression in human anal gland. Hum Pathol 21:1108–1111
8 Lange PH, Ercole CJ, Lightner DJ, Fraley EE, Vessella R (1989) The value of serum prostate specific antigen determinations before and after radical prostatectomy. J Urol 141:873–879
9 Nowels K, Kent E, Risho K, Oyasu R (1988) Prostate specific antigen and acid phosphatase-reactive cells in cystitis cystica and glandularis. Arch Pathol Lab Med 112:734–737
10 Pollen JJ, Dreilinger A (1984) Immunohistochemical identification of prostatic acid phosphatase and prostate specific antigen in female periurethral glands. Urology 23:303–304
11 Semjonow A, Rathert P (1992) Evidence for extra-renal elimination of prostate specific antigen. Prostate cancer 349
12 Stamey TA, McNeal JE, Freiha FS, Redwine E (1988) Morphometric and clinical studies on 68 consecutive radical prostatectomies. J Urol 139: 1235–1241
13 Takayama TK, Vessella RL, BrawerR M K, True LD, Noteboom J, Lange PH (1994) Urinary prostate specific antigen levels after radical prostatectomy. J Urol 151:82–87
14 Tepper SL, Jagirdar J, Heath D, Geller SA (1984) Homology between the female paraurethral (Skene's) glands and the prostate. Arch Pathol Lab Med 108:423–425
15 Tremblay J, Frenette G, Tremblay RR, Dupont A, Thabet M, Dubé JY (1987) Excretion of three major prostatic secretory proteins in the urine of normal men and patients with benign prostatic hypertrophy or prostate cancer. The Prostate 10:235–243

Address for correspondence:
Priv.-Doz. Dr. med. J. Spitz
Abt. Nuklearmedizin
Privatpraxis RNS
Ludwig-Erhard-Straße 100
D-65199 Wiesbaden, Germany

Cytokeratin fragments – A release product from growing prostate cancer cells?

Å. Silén[a], S. Nilsson[b], B. Wiklund[a], L. Lennartsson[b]

[a]AB IDL ImmunoDevelopLab, Borlänge,
[b]University of Uppsala, University Hospital, Department of Oncology, Uppsala, Sweden

Introduction

In simple epithelia four major cytokeratin (CK) polypeptides have been identified so far (CKs 7, 8, 18 and 19). Cytokeratins form pairs (type I + type II) and in these cells the most frequent combinations are 8:18; 8:18, 19; 7, 8:18, 19 (2, 4, 6).
The smallest cytokeratin pair, 8 and 18, is found in large quantities in simple, ductal and glandular epithelium, pseudo-stratified epithelium, transitional epithelium and carcinomas arising therefrom. Cytokeratins 8 and 18 have pI values of 6.1 and 5.7 respectively and molecular weights of 52 kD and 45 kD respectively (4, 5, 7).
Cytokeratin 8 has at least three major epitopes where one of the epitopes is potentially repetitive. For cytokeratin 18, at least five antigenic sites have been found. One specific site, widely conserved among mammalian species, has been designated C-04 (9, 11).
In the culture medium of the human mammary epithelial cell line MCF7, known to contain CKs 8, 18 and 19, proteolytic fragments of cytokeratins have been found (1).
The in vitro and in vivo behavior of cytokeratins is extraordinarily complex and many unexpected results occur with the use of anti-cytokeratin antibodies. Cross reactivity may occur due to sequence homologies between the different cytokeratins. Masking of epitopes has been reported and in formalin treated paraffin embedded tissues, the cytokeratins are sometimes cross-linked and require enzymatic treatment to unmask the epitopes. Conformation dependent cytokeratin epitopes have been found where the monoclonal antibody (Ks 18.18) specific for cytokeratin 18 is non-reactive with many cytokeratin 18 preparations but reacts strongly with heterotypic coil-coil complexes between cytokeratins 8 and 18 (3).

Materials and methods

The anti-cytokeratin 8 antibody (6D7 IgG1 kappa) and the anti-cytokeratin 18 antibody (3F3 IgG1 kappa) have been tested for their specificity in Western blot. The antibody 6D7 reacts with intact cytokeratin 8, with a minor cross reactivity with intact cytokeratin 18. The 3F3 antibody reacts with intact cytokeratin 18. Both antibodies reacts extensively with fragments of the corresponding cytokeratin but show no cross reactivity with either of the fragments of cytokeratin 18 or cytokeratin 8, respectively.
Cells from the DU145 cell line were obtained from ATCC (American Tissue Culture Collection) and were cultured in 12-wells plates in RPMI 1640 with 10% fetal calf serum and 1% glutamine. To each well, 100 000 cells were added and as soon as the cells had fixed to the bottom of the plate, one set of plates were irradiated with 10 Gy. The other set was not irradiated. The cells were allowed to grow for seven days and samples were taken at days 1, 2, 3, 4, and 7. During days 2–4 three samples were taken each day. Each sample was analyzed for total number of cells, viability and the concentration of cytokeratin fragments (TPAcyk).
The cytospun DU145 cells were allowed to dry in air (60 min RT) and fixed with methanol for 10 min at RT. Before addition of the primary antibody (10 µg/ml in PBS incl. 0.5 % BSA), the cells were washed with PBS incl. 0.5 % BSA and incubated for 30 min at RT. A fluorescein labelled anti-

mouse IgG antibody (Dako, Denmark) diluted (1:20) in PBS was added and incubated for 30 min at RT. A few drops of glycerol were added before UV microscopic examination (5 sec).

For the estimation of cytokeratin fragments, the TPAcyk ELISA (AB IDL, Sweden) was used. The assay is a "sandwich" type with a 1:1 mixture of monoclonal antibodies directed against cytokeratins 8 and 18 covalently bound to the wells of a microtitration plate. The standard in the assay consists of purified and solubilized human cytokeratins 8 and 18. One hundred µl of the standard/control/specimen and 100 µl of the HRP-tracer (horseradish peroxidase) antibody are added to the wells and incubated for two hours at 37 °C. After rinsing, an OPD-substrate (orthophenylene-diamine) is added and, after 30 minutes at RT, the reaction is terminated by the addition of sulphuric acid and the absorbance at 490 nm is read. A TPAcyk tumor marker control serum was assayed in parallel with all the serum samples.

The antibody PCNA, PC10 (Dako, Denmark) was used to label proliferating cells. PCNA (proliferating cell nuclear antigen) was originally defined as an intranuclear polypeptide whose synthesis reaches its maximum during the S-phase of the cell cycle. The antibody reacts with proliferating cells in all human tissues. The antibody was diluted according to manufacturer's recommendation.

Mice of the NMRI type were obtained from Boomholts gård, Denmark. The mice had an average weight of 25 g. Approximatly 30 million DU145 cells were inoculated per amimal. The cells, inoculated at one place subcutaneously in the flank of the animal were allowed to grow for 14 days. The tumors were excised and frozen to −80° C.

Results

The two anti-cytokeratin MAbs were found to be highly reactive with the prostate cancer cell line DU145 in immunofluorescence with both methnol fixed and cytospun cells. The cells exhibited a typical cytoskeletal structure for intermediate filaments. With the cytokeratin 8 antibody (6D7), we found a number of (typically 2–8) clearly visible dots within the cells when the antibody was reacted with methanol fixed cytospun cells. These

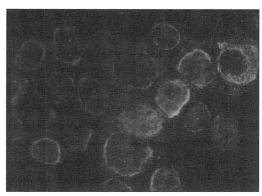

Figure 1. Anti-cytokeratin 8 reacted with methanol fixed DU145 cells.

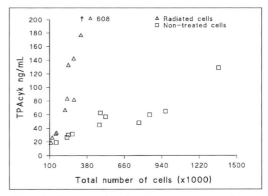

Figure 2. Concentration in the supernatant of cytokeratin fragments released from growing DU145 prostate cancer cells.

dots were not found when the cells were reacted with the anti-cytokeratin 18 antibody (3F3)(figure 1). The viability of the non-radiated cells has more than 97% during the first four days and dropped to 86% on the seventh day. The irradiated cells looked markedly different under the microscope and also exhibited high viability (> 95%) during the first four days and dropped to 82% on the seventh day. The data indicated a quite normal doubling-time of 27 hours for non-irradiated cells and approximately 46 hours for the radiated cells. We estimated the concentration of cytokeratin fragments using the TPAcyk assay in the supernatant of growing DU145 cells, both non-irradiated and irradiated with 10 Gy. The release of cytokeratin fragments to the supernatant increased with an increasing number of cells. The concentrations were found to range from 19 ng/ml

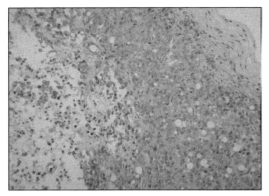

Figure 3. Immunohistology of in nude mice implanted DU145 tumor. A marked reactivity for the anti-cytokeratin 8 antibody with the outer viable parts of the tumor was found.

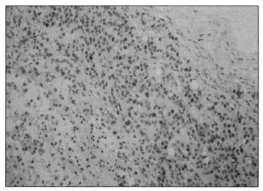

Figure 4. Immunohistology of in nude mice implanted DU145 tumor with the PCNA antibody. The PCNA antibody reacts with proliferating cells.

(day 1) to 129 ng/ml (day 7) for non-irradiated cells. We did not find any significant concentration of cytokeratin fragments in the growth medium (RPMI 1640). Irradiated cells known to have increased cell membrane permeability, exhibited concentrations ranging from 18 (day 1) to 608 ng/ml (day 7) (figure 2).

Non-irradiated cells released about 8 ng/ml to the supernatant when the number of cells doubles from 100 to 200 000 compared to approximately 83 ng/ml for irradiated cells.

Immunohistology of the implanted tumor illustrated a marked reactivity for the anti-cytokeratin 8 (6D7) antibody with the outer viable parts of the tumor which contain most of the proliferating cells as detected by the PCNA antibody (figures 3 and 4). The reactivity of the anti-cytokeratin 18 (3F3) antibody was essentially the same but the reactivity was not as pronounced with the viable parts as with the 6D7 antibody.

Discussion

Not much is known about the assembly and disassembly of the intermediate filaments in epithelial cells. Granular keratin aggregates similar to our findings have previously been observed during mitosis of epithelial cells. Partially successful attempts have been made to induce the disruption of the filaments by cold hypotonic buffer, pretreatment with phorbol esters etc. to be able to further investigate these intracellular granular keratin aggregates. Additional factors in the growth medium are probably essential for the formation of these granules (10).

One possible explanation for the difficulty of detecting these granules in all mitotic epithelial cells could be that the epitopes are mainly expressed by heterotypic complexes of intermediate filaments in the aggregates. One murine antibody (Ks18.18) has been shown to strongly react with heterotypic complexes between cytokeratin 18 and notably cytokeratin 8. The same antibody is also reactive with the spheroidal bodies of mitotic cells and has been used to demonstrate the existence of a soluble heterotypic cytokeratin 8 and 18 complex (3).

Our data illustrate a marked release of soluble cytokeratin fragments from growing prostate cancer cells expressing epitopes reactive with the monoclonal antibodies 6D7 and 3F3. Approximately ten times more of these soluble fragments are released from cells that are irradiated. Radiation is known to cause a change in the permeability of the cell membranes. A release from dead cells cannot explain the findings of increasing very high concentrations of cytokeratin fragments in the supernatant. Initially and during the first day, the viability of the cells is very high, nearly 100%. There is an initial very high correlation (about 0.9) between the concentrations found and the number of cells. We speculate that the soluble cytokeratin fragments express epitopes detected by the TPAcyk assay and that these epitopes originate from a pool of fragments of cytokeratins 8 and 18 in the form of heterotypic complexes in the cells.

The immunohistology data indicate that epitopes related to epitopes of native cytokeratins 8 and 18 are expressed by viable parts of the tumor. In particular the 6D7 antibody reacts with epitopes expressed by viable cells and a very low reactivity was found with the necrotic parts of the tumor. This is in contrast to the anti-cytokeratin 8 antibody TS1 which in a similar experiment exhibited a marked reactivity with the necrotic parts of the tumor (8).

We postulate that these monoclonal antibodies (3F3 and 6D7), and in particular the anti-cytokeratin 8 antibody (6D7), recognize epitopes on cytokeratin fragments released by dividing cells. Further studies to evaluate these monoclonal antibodies are in progress.

References

1. Chan R, Rossitto PV, Edwards BF, Cardiff RD (1986) Presence of proteolytically processed keratins in culture medium of MCF-7 cells. Cancer Res 46:6353–6359
2. Franke WW, Schiller DL, Moll R, Winter S, Schmidt E, Engelbrecht I, Denk H, Krepler R, Platser B (1981) Diversity of cytokeratins: differentiation-specific expression of cytokeratin polypeptides in epithelial cells and tissues. J Mol Biol 53: 933–959
3. Franke WW, Winter S, Schmid E, Söllner P, Hämmerling G, Achtstätter T (1987) Monoclonal cytokeratin antibody recognizing a heterotypic complex: Immunological probing of conformational states of cytoskeletal proteins in filaments and solutions. Exp Cell Res 173:17–37.
4. Moll R., Franke WW, Schiller DL, Geiger B, Krepler R (1982) The catalog of human cytokeratins: Patterns of expression in normal epithelia, tumors and cultured cells. Cell 31:11–24
5. Osborn M, Weber K (1983) Tumour diagnosis by intermediate filament typing: a novel tool for surgical patology. Lab Inv 48:372–394
6. Quinlan RA, Cohlberg JA, Schiller DL, Hatzfeld M Franke WW (1984) Heterotypic tetramer (A2D2) complexes of non-epidermal keratins isolated from cytoskeleton of rat hepatocytes and hepatoma cells. J Mol Biol 178:365–388
7. Quinlan RA, Schiller DL, Hatzfeld M, Achtstätter T, Moll R, Jorcano JL, Magin TM, Franke WW (1985) Patterns of expression and organization of cytokeratin intermediate filaments. In: Wang E, Fishman D, Liem RRH, Sun TT (eds) Intermediate filaments. Ann NY Acad Sci 455:282–306
8. Riklund KE, Makiya R, Sundström B, Bäck O, Henriksson R, Hietala S-O, Stigbrand T (1991) Inhibition of growth of HeLa cell tumours in nude mice by 125I-labeled anticytokeratin and antiPLAP monoclonal antibodies. Anticancer Res 11:555–560
9. Sundström B, Nathrath WB, Stigbrand T (1989) Diversity in immnunoreactivity of tumor-derived cytokeratin monoclonal antibodies. J Histochem Cytochem 37(12):1845–1854
10. Tölle HG, Weber K, Osborn M (1987) Keratin filament disruption in interphase and miotic cells – how is it induced? Eur J Cell Biol 43(1):35–47
11. Vojtesek B, Staskova Z, Nenutil R, Lauerova L, Kovarik J, Rejthar A, Bartkova J, Bartek J (1989) Monoclonal antibodies recognizing different epitopes of cytokeratin 18. Folia Biologica (Praha) 373–382

Address for correspondence:
Dr. Å. Silén
AB IDL ImmunoDevelopLab
Box 766
S-78127 Borlänge, Sweden

Tandem® Ostase™ – An IRMA for bone alkaline phosphatase evaluated in breast and prostate cancer

E.H. Cooper[a], D.A. Purves[a], M.-J. Yerna[b]

[a]Department of Chemical Pathology, University of Leeds, Leeds, UK,
[b]Hybritech, Europe, Liège, Belgium

Introduction

Breast and prostate cancer are the most common sources of bone metastases, which predominantly involve the axial skeleton. The development of bone metastases produces local changes in the normal balance between new bone formation by osteoblasts and its remodelling by the lytic action of osteoclasts that maintain the steady state of bone and mineral metabolism. Prostate cancer cells stimulate the local activity of osteoblasts so that the metastases tend to be sclerotic, breast cancer cells produce a mixed reaction by osteoblasts and osteoclasts resulting in sclerotic and lytic metastases. Bone metastases cause pain, restricted movement, fractures or may be asymptomatic. They are usually diagnosed by bone scintigraphy using technetium-99m labelled bisphosphonates and conventional radiology. Recently assays for several biochemical indicators of bone metabolism have become available, they include osteocalcin, bone alkaline phosphatase (BAP) and procollagen types I and III reflecting bone synthesis, and the urinary excretion of pyridinoline cross links as an indicator of lytic activity (1, 2).

We have investigated the relationships of BAP, tumor markers and clinical status in prostate and breast cancer. BAP was measured by Tandem double monoclonal immunoradiometric assay (Tandem® Ostase™, Hybritech, Liège) (3.) The normal range is 3–19 ng/ml with a tendency for the value to rise within this range in women following the menopause. BAP has a cross reactivity with liver alkaline phosphatase of < 15% (4.)

Prostate cancer

An investigation was made of 156 patients. In 19 patients following radical prostatectomy, with a PSA < 0.1 ng/ml and a negative bone scan the BAP was 11.2 + 3.3 ng/ml (mean, SD) and in 30 patients with negative bone scans who were under observation or treated by hormone manipulation the BAP was 8.9 + 4.5 ng/ml. Repeated measurements (3–4 times) of BAP in 16 patients who remained scan negative during a two year period showed limited intra-individual variation. Except in two cases, none of the levels were greater than 20 ng/ml. In 39 patients with positive bone scans at presentation 83% had a BAP > 20 ng/ml (range 8 ≥ 1000 ng/ml), and 2/36 (5.5%) of the scan negative patients had a BAP > 20 ng/ml. Figure 1 illustrates the way in which the combination of BAP and PSA at the time of bone scan helps to indicate whether an equivocal bone scan appearance is likely to be due to metastases. Paget's disease is a strong stimulus for osteoblastic activity and a high BAP.

In metastatic disease the tumor burden at presentation, as estimated from the bone scan and the nadir of the PSA level 3–6 months after commencing hormone therapy are powerful prognostic indices, a low tumor burden and a PSA nadir returning to the normal range are usually accompanied by a prolonged remission (5, 6, 7). Figure 2 shows the distribution of BAP stratified according to the PSA nadir at six months after commencing hormone therapy. Note the persistently raised BAP in half the patients with a PSA nadir of > 50 ng/ml. This data indicates that the switch-off of drive to the osteoblasts from the

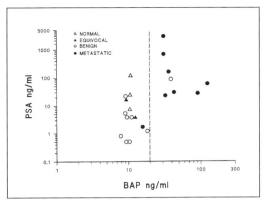

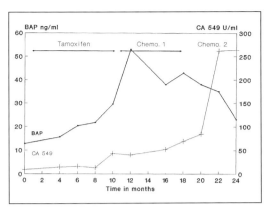

Figure 1. Combination of serum BAP and PSA estimated in patients with prostate cancer at the time of referral for bone scan (in collaboration with Dr. R. Bury).

Figure 3. Time course of CA 549 and BAP in a patient with breast cancer and extensive bone metastases.

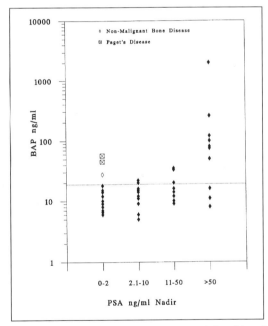

Figure 2. Metastatic prostate cancer relationship of serum BAP and PSA nadir six months after commencing hormone therapy.

tumor cells and the osteoblastic activity in remodelling the bone has largely stopped after six months in patients with moderate tumor burdens. Measurement of the BAP shortly after commencing hormone therapy may show an elevation of the level during the so called flare response of increased tumor activity.

Longitudinal studies of 39 patients with bone metastases for 12 to 60 months indicated a concordant rise and fall of PSA and BAP in 85%, although the direction of change was similar there was considerable variation in the relative rates of change of PSA and BAP. Discordant behavior of these markers was seen when there was local or lymph node progression in the absence of advancing bone disease or when progression occured in patients with tumors that were poor producers of PSA during the hormone resistant phase. Longitudinal studies indicated that in the absence of specific symptoms the combination of PSA and BAP could be used instead of repeated bone scans.

Total alkaline phosphatase (TAP), in the range of normal – 3 x normal, was correlated to BAP $r = 0.89$, for higher levels of TAP the correlation was $r = 0.94$

Breast cancer

The combination of the breast cancer marker CA 549 (HybriBREScan™ Hybritech, Liege) and BAP were examined in the sera of 125 patients with breast cancer, 49 with bone metastases, 25 with metastases in sites other than bone and 40 who were tumor free. CA 549 was measured by an double monoclonal IRMA with an upper limit of normal of 12 U/ml (8.)

In 40 patients who were tumor free after treatment of a primary breast cancer the median BAP

Table I. The distribution of serum BAP (Ostase) in breast cancer.

Status	Number	Median	BAP (ng/ml) Q1	Q3	range
Stage III N+ve	20	6.7	5.0	7.8	3–13
Tumor-free	20	7.6	4.4	9.6	4–14
Bone metastasis (limited)	16	10.6	6.8	12.1	5–40
Bone metastasis	33	18.7	11.2	22.0	4–87
Non-bone metastasis	25	8.4	5.9	13.4	3–63

was 7.1 ng/ml with a range of 3–16.5 ng/ml. Repeated annual measurements for 5–6 years in 11 patients showed a low intra-individual variation but a wide range of individual median levels across the normal range.

Table I shows the levels of BAP in various subgroups of patients with breast cancer. It will be seen that the high risk group Stage III with positive nodes (scan negative) had a normal BAP but when there was limited spread to the skeleton the levels of BAP rose but the interquartile range remained within the normal range. A further increase occured in patients with widespread metastatic involvement of the skeleton, but only 40% had levels > 20 ng/ml, which contrasts with the stronger response in prostate cancer.

In 20 patients with bone metastases longitudinal studies were carried out of BAP and CA 549 levels over a 4–60 months period. Several patterns of change of BAP and CA 549 levels were observed. In 13/20 patients (65%) the changes in BAP and CA 549 were concordant, in six patients (30%) who responded to treatment there was a 2 – 3 month delay in lowering BAP compared to the fall of CA 549 level. Seven patients showed changes in BAP and CA 549 that were independent; in two of them the rise in BAP was a sign of disease progression while the CA 549 remained in normal limits. Figure 3 is an illustrative patient, RK aged 61 years, presented with a stage III breast cancer treated by mastectomy and tamoxifen. 14 months later (time 0) she complained of upper thoracic pain but there was no evidence of bone metastases, 14 months later she had evidence of widespread bone metastases. Note the different time courses of the BAP and CA 549 during the development of the metastases and their response to treatment.

Discussion

Earlier studies of biochemical markers in bone metastases have given controversial results. Whilst there is general agreement that indicators of bone formation (osteocalcin and BAP) and bone remodelling (urinary hydroxyproline excretion) are abnormal in widespread disease, they do not add greatly from what can be infered from TAP. Furthermore confusion can occur when comparing the various assays for osteocalcin (9), and those for BAP were either laborious electrophoretic separations or lectin precipitation with intrinsic problem of standardisation.

Consequently they have not been adopted for the monitoring of breast or prostate cancer with bone metastases.

This study has shown that BAP as measured by the Tandem® Ostase™ assay provides an opportunity for the close monitoring of bone alkaline phosphatase that is independent of the effects of hepatic metastases, an important feature in breast cancer, although liver metastases are rare in prostate cancer. The sensitivity of the assay becomes evident in longitudinal studies when highly significant changes can occur within the normal range, which cannot be interpreted with certainty using TAP as many factors including treatment can affect liver function in breast and prostate cancer. Clearly the response of BAP in relation to the bone tumor burden estimated by the number of hot spots in the scintigram is greater in prostate than breast cancer. Both breast and prostate cancer are hormone dependent characterised by relatively long periods of survival despite the presence of bone metastases. During the management of the disease several treatment regimes may be tried, especially in breast cancer where chemotherapy is a realistic option. Other treatments may be directed to palliate the painful effect of the bone disease, they include bisphosphonates, radioactive strontium and hemibody irradiation. The preliminary study has shown that tumor markers and BAP can indicate the pattern of change of the tumor burden, whatever its site, and the local effects of the bone metastases which can show a variety of changes throughout the patients' illness. BAP provides an accurate picture of osteoblastic activity and can be substituted for repeated bone scans, especially when the patient is asymptomatic.

References

1. Deftos LF (1991) Bone protein and peptide assays in the diagnosis and management of skeletal disease. Clin Chem 37:1143–1148
2. Cooper EH, Jones RG (1993) Biochemical markers of bone metastases. Tumour Marker Update 5:1–4
3. Hill CS, Wolfert R (1990) The preparation of antibodies which react preferentially with human bone alkaline phosphatase and not liver alkaline phosphatase. Clin Chim Acta 186:315–321
4. Kress BC (1993) (personal communication) Hybritech, San Diego, California
5. Cooper EH, Armitage TG, Robinson MRG et al (1990) Prostatic specific antigen and the prediction of prognosis in metastatic prostatic cancer. Cancer 66:1025–1028
6. Soloway MS, Hardeman SW, Hickey D et al (1988) Stratification of patients with metastatic prostate cancer based on extent disease on initial bone scan. Cancer 61:195–202
7. Martzkin H, Eber P, Todd B et al (1992) Prognostic significance of changes in prostate-specific markers after endocrine treatment of stage D2 prostatic cancer. Cancer 70:2302–2309
8. Cooper EH, Forbes MA, Hancock MAK et al (1992) Serum alkaline phosphatase and CA 549 in breast cancer with bone metastases. Biomed Pharmacother 46:31–8
9. Masters PM, Cooper EH, Purves D, Jones RG Commercial assays for osteocalcin show clinically discordant results. Clin Chem 40:358–363

Address for correspondence:
Dr. E. H. Cooper
Department of Chemical Pathology
University of Leeds
Leeds LS2 9JT, UK

Skeletal alkaline phosphatase and total alkaline phosphatase as serum markers for bone metastases

A. Semjonow[a], H.J. Adomeit[b], P. Rathert[b]

[a]Clinic and Policlinic of Urology, Wilhelms-University of Westfalen, Münster,
[b]Clinic of Urology and Children's Clinic of Urology, Düren, Germany

Introduction

Identification and quantitation of alkaline phosphatase in serum of patients with prostatic cancer is commonly performed for diagnosis of bone metastases. However, it is difficult to distinguish between the liver and bone isoenzymes which are the most clinically relevant using procedures such as electrophoresis and/or urea and heat denaturation. We present our experience with an immunoradiometric assay for determination of skeletal alkaline phosphatase (1) as compared to total alkaline phosphatase in a population comprising of patients with liver diseases or prostatic carcinoma with or without bone metastases.

Patients and methods

The study was done with frozen sera from patients being followed because of prostatic carcinoma on an ambulatory basis and with sera from patients with liver disease collected in the same time period. Serum concentrations of skeletal alkaline phosphatase (double monoclonal immunoradiometric assay, Tandem-R Ostase, Hybritech) were compared to the concentrations of total alkaline phosphatase (EC 3.1.3.1 Boehringer Mannheim[1]; normal range ~258 IU/l) and prostate specific antigen (double monoclonal immunoradiometric assay, Tandem-R PSA, Hybritech; normal range < 4–10 ng/ml) in 75 patients with prostatic carcinoma and 18 patients with liver disease. Of the 75 patients with prostatic carcinoma 26 had positive and 49 had negative bone scans. In each case the interval between serum asservation and bone scan was less than two weeks.

Results

The median skeletal alkaline phosphatase level in 49 men with negative bone scans was 8.1 µg/l whereas it was 33.8 µg/l in the 26 men with positive bone scans. In 18 patients with liver disease the median skeletal alkaline phosphatase level was 9.3 µg/l. The median total alkaline phosphatase level in the group with negative bone scans was 167 IU/l whereas it was 447 IU/l in the group with positive bone scans. In the patients with liver disease the median total alkaline phosphatase level was 341 IU/l. Applying upper limits of normal of 12 µg/l for skeletal alkaline phosphatase and 258 IU/l for total alkaline phosphatase the following results were obtained.

Total alkaline phosphatase

Pathological concentrations were found in 19 of 26 patients with bone metastases and 5 of 49 patients without bone metastases. 16 of 18 patients with liver disease exceeded the normal range. Figure 1 shows the distribution of total alkaline phosphatase levels related to diagnosis.

Skeletal alkaline phosphatase

Pathological concentrations were found in 19 of 26 patients with bone metastases and 6 of 49

---

[1]p-nitrophenylphosphate + $H_2O \xrightarrow{AP}$ phosphate + p-nitrophenol

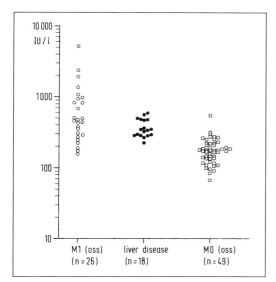

Figure 1. Distribution of total alkaline phosphatase levels in patients with prostate cancer with (M1 (oss)) and without (M0 (oss)) bone metastases and patients with liver disease.

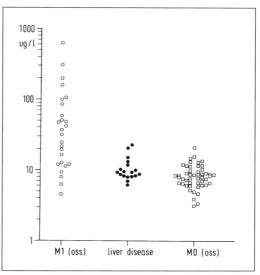

Figure 2. Distribution of skeletal alkaline phosphatase levels in patients with prostate cancer with (M1 (oss)) and without (M0 (oss)) bone metastases and patients with liver disease.

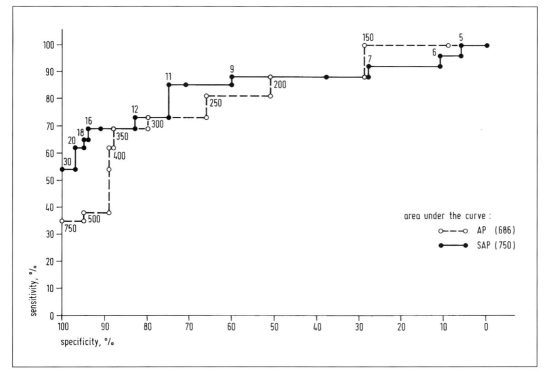

Figure 3. Receiver operating characteristic curves for skeletal alkaline phosphatase and total alkaline phosphatase comparing sensitivity for identification of bone metastases. The area under the curves denotes the diagnostic accuracy.

patients without bone metastases. Four of 18 patients with liver disease exceeded the normal range. Figure 2 shows the distribution of skeletal alkaline phosphatase levels related to diagnosis. Receiver operating characteristic (ROC) curves for skeletal alkaline phosphatase and total alkaline phosphatase comparing sensitivity and specificity for identifying bone metastases in 26 of the 93 patients under investigation are shown in figure 3. The area under the curves denotes the diagnostic accuracy.

Prostate specific antigen

Following hormonal treatment six of the 26 patients with prostatic carcinoma and bone metastases showed markedly elevated skeletal alkaline phosphatase levels although concentrations of the prostate specific antigen ranged below 4 ng/ml.

Conclusion

Applying upper limits of normal that are equal sensitive in detecting bone metastases, skeletal alkaline phosphatase reveals a higher specificity than total alkaline phosphatase (figure 3) in a patient population including elevations of alkaline phosphatase due to advanced liver disease. At the current status of our investigations we do not recommend routine performance of skeletal alkaline phosphatase, but it is shown to be helpful in the evaluation of high total alkaline phosphatase levels of doubtful origin.

Reference

1 Hill CS, Wolfert RL (1989) The preparation of monoclonal antibodies which react preferentially with human bone alkaline phosphatase and not liver phosphatase. Clin Chim Acta 186:315

Address for correspondence:
Dr. A. Semjonow
Klinik und Poliklinik für Urologie
Westfälische Wilhelms-Universität
Albert-Schweitzer-Straße 33
D-48149 Münster, Germany

HCG and free hCGβ as markers in trophoblastic and non-trophoblastic tumors

B. Saller[a], R. Hoermann[a], G. Reichel[b], G. Spoettl[b], M. Grossmann[b], K. Mann[a]

[a] Department of Clinical Endocrinology, University of Essen,
[b] Department of Internal Medicine II, Klinikum Großhadern, University of Munich, Germany

Introduction

Human chorionic gonadotropin (hCG) is a member of the glycoprotein hormone family which also includes LH, FSH, and TSH. The glycoprotein hormones are made up of two dissimilar non-covalently linked subunits termed alpha (α) and beta (β). Within a species, the α-subunit of all members of this hormone family has an identical amino acid sequence. The biological specificities are confered by the β-subunits, which are structurally unique, although showing some degree of sequence homology. The β-subunit of hCG (hCGβ) differs from those of the other glycoprotein hormones by the presence of a 24-amino acid carboxyterminal polypeptide extension (CTP). Moreover, hCG contains the largest amount of carbohydrates comprising approximately 30% of its mass. Physiologically, hCG is synthesized by the trophoblastic cells of the placenta during pregnancy, where it has an important role in maintaining corpus luteum function during the first weeks of gestation (1, 2). Under pathological conditions, hCG is produced in large quantities by various tumors of trophoblastic origin such as hydatidiform mole, choriocarcinoma or testicular cancer. In the diagnosis and follow-up of these tumors, hCG has become a well established and highly useful tumor marker (3, 4).

The following sections will give a short overview on hCG and its free β-subunit in trophoblastic and non-trophoblastic tumors.

Determination of hCG

During recent years, monoclonal antibodies have become available to develop highly sensitive and specific methods for determination of hCG. These procedures recognize either the heterodimer hCG without cross reacting with free hCGβ ("hCG assays") or they recognize both, hCG and free hCGβ ("hCG+hCGβ assays"). Moreover, methods have been developed that specifically measure the free β- or α-subunit of hCG with neglegible cross reactivities with intact hCG (5).

The use of these specific assays in samples from pregnant women and from patients with trophoblastic tumors has given further insight in the secretion of hCG under physiological and pathological conditions. It could be shown, that in most samples, not only the intact hCG molecule but also its free subunits can be detected (6). Additionally, further biochemical characterization of hCG-immunoreactivity has led to the detection of various modified forms of hCG and its subunits in biological fluids.

One of these altered hCG forms is the core fragment of hCGβ (hCGβcf) which represents a 10 kD two-chain polypeptide lacking the amino acid sequences 1–5, 41–54 and 93–145. HCGβcf accounts for the majority of hCG-immunoactivity in urine samples.

More recently, nicks or missing peptide linkages could be identified in a proportion of hCG molecules, particularly between the residues 45–46 and 47–48 of hCGβ (7). Nicked hCG (hCGn) differs from hCG in its physical and immunological properties. As a result of these differences, some monoclonal hCG antibodies can not detect nicked hCG molecules which may cause false negative results from monoclonal hCG assays (8). However, since hCGn is more abundant in urine than in serum samples this seems not to have a critical impact on the routine use of serum hCG as a tumor marker.

HCG and hCGβ in non-seminomatous and seminomatous testicular cancer

In patients with non-seminomatous testicular cancer the overall incidence of elevated serum hCG levels determined with "hCG+hCGβ-assays" is approximately 40 to 60%. Thereby, the frequency of elevated hCG levels is correlated with tumor stage ranging from approximately 15% in patients with stage I disease up to approximately 90% in patients with stage III disease (9). The serum concentrations of hCG in patients with non-seminomatous testicular cancer range up to 3,000,000 IU/l. In these patients, the intact hCG molecule is almost exclusively secreted together with free hCGβ leading to a high degree of correlation between these two parameters (10).

In patients with seminomatous testicular cancer, the incidence of elevated hCG levels is approximately 20-40% (so-called "hCG-positive seminoma") (11). In these patients, hCG levels determined with "hCG+hCGβ-assays" usually do not exceed 1000 IU/l and hCG levels of more than 5000 IU/l are rather incompatible with diagnosis of pure seminoma. In contrast to non-seminomatous testicular cancer, the levels of hCG and hCGβ are not well correlated in seminoma samples. In approximately 30% of patients with "hCG positive seminoma", the free β-subunit can be detected in the absence of intact hCG and in approximately 20% the intact hCG molecule is found in the absence of free hCGβ (12).

The occurrence of isolated hGCβ secretion in patients with seminomatous testicular cancer establishes the need for the determination of free hCGβ in these patients. HCGβ can be measured either with an assay procedure which is sensitive for hCG and hCGβ ("hCG+hCGβ-assays") or by a separate hCGβ-assay (10). Interestingly, in patients with seminomatous testicular cancer the incidence of elevated hCG or hCGβ levels can be increased up to 75% when samples are taken from testicular vene during orchiectomy instead of peripheral vene (13).

During the follow-up, the determination of hCG provides a sensitive and specific means of monitoring the response to surgery, radiation or chemotherapy (14). Regression lines for the disappearance of hCG from blood following successful therapy have been established. Apparent hCG half lives longer than three days indicate the presence of residual hCG producing tumor. A transient marker increase in hCG serum concentrations shortly after chemotherapy, however, indicates lysis of the tumor and should not be confused with tumor progression (15).

It is important to know that a tumor which originally produces hCG may well change its behavior and becomes marker-negative during follow-up. Vice versa, a hCG negative primary tumor may occasionally be able to generate hCG positive metastases.

In summary, hCG is a highly sensitive and specific tumor marker in patients with testicular cancer. HCG immunoreactivity should be determined by assay procedures which measure both, the intact hCG molecule and its free β-subunit. Due to the occurrence of isolated hCGβ elevations, this is particularly important in patients with pure seminoma.

Principally, the determination of hCG has to be done simultaneously with AFP as both markers are independent indicating the presence of different tumor types.

Prognostic implications of hCG-determinations

The prognosis of patients with testicular germ-cell tumors has greatly improved since the introduction of cis-platin based chemotherapy together with improved staging and follow-up procedures. Nevertheless, approximately 20-30% of patients fail to achieve complete response to chemotherapy or experience a relapse after being in complete remission (17).

Several studies have focused on the evaluation of prognostically relevant pretreatment parameters, that will allow the identification of patients with a low probability of achieving complete response to chemotherapy (18-22). The best established and most important prognostic factor is the extent of disease. Other variables identified so far are the patients' age, extragonadal primary site, histopathologic cell type, number and size of metastases and the levels of various tumor markers, particularly hCG, AFP and also LDH. From the various multivariate analyses on prognostic factors in non-seminomatous germ-cell tumors it became clear, that the level of serum hCG is one of the most important prognostic factors in metastatic testicular cancer. There is general agreement that higher hCG-levels at presentation confer a worse prognosis. Although the cut-off level below or above which the prognosis is significantly better or worse is not well defined, most studies found hCG-levels greater than 1000 IU/l associated with a poor prognosis.

In addition to the absolute pretreatment levels of hCG, some studies have measured hCG at two points of time between orchiectomy and the start of chemotherapy to calculate tumor marker production and the marker-production doubling-time (22). Thereby, a short marker-production doubling-time indicates rapid tumor growth and is associated with poor prognosis. Another approach is to study tumor marker regression rates during chemotherapy as a prognostic variable. Prolonged apparent half lives turned out to indicate poor treatment response (23).

In patients with seminomatous testicular cancer, it is still not well established whether "hCG-positive" seminoma are associated with poor prognosis. The preliminary results of a large German multicenter study argues against the assumption, that elevated hCG-levels in patients with seminomatous testicular cancer indicate poor treatment response.

HCG in gestational trophoblastic disease

HCG is secreted in nearly all cases of gestational trophoblastic disease such as hydatidiform mole, invasive mole and choriocarcinoma (24, 25, 26). In these patients, hCG levels ranging up to 1,000,000 IU/l can be found and a close correlation exists between hCG levels and tumor burden. Nevertheless, in most cases, a single hCG measurement cannot reliably distinguish between tumorous hCG production and normal pregnancy. In hydatidiform moles, the diagnosis is established by the typical ultrasound findings together with high hCG concentrations (27). After the complete evacuation of moles, hCG levels decrease and characteristically reach the normal range within three to twelve weeks. An increase, persistence or lower than expected fall of hCG values strongly indicate the presence of invasive mole or choriocarcinoma.

Additionally, weekly hCG determinations are highly useful for the monitoring of disease response if chemotherapy is needed. Similarly to patients with testicular cancer, high pretreatment serum levels of hCG seem to indicate a high likelihood of treatment failure in patients with choriocarcinoma.

The determination of free hCGβ in addition to hCG by highly specific assays may be of some additional value since the ratio of hCGβ to hCG has been shown to be higher in patients with moles and particularly in those with choriocarcinoma than in normal pregnancy.

HCG in non-trophoblastic tumors

In patients with various non-trophoblastic tumors such as cancers of the cervix, ovary, pancreas, stomach, colon, liver, lung, breast, kidney, bladder as well as lymphomas, serum concentrations of hCG immunoreactivity have been reported in up to 50% (28–31). In contrast to tumors of trophoblastic origin, these tumors frequently produce hCGβ in the absence of the intact hCG-molecule. Free hCGβ and hCGα have been found to be elevated in malignant endocrine gastroenteropancreatic tumors.

The levels of hCGβ concentrations in these patients are usually much lower than in trophoblastic tumors. Moreover, established tumor markers like CEA or CA 19-9 are usually superior with respect to their sensitivities.

In patients presenting with pleural effusion or ascites measurement of hCGβ may be a useful marker for the differentiation between benign and malignant disease (32).

References

1 Pierce JG, Parsons TF (1981) Glycoprotein hormones: structure and function. Annu Rev Biochem 50:465
2 Hussa RO (1981) Human chorionic gonadotropin, a clinical marker: review of its biosynthesis. Ligand Review 3:6
3 Mann K, Saller B, Hoermann R (1993) Clinical use of hCG and hCGβ determinations. Scand J Clin Lab Invest Suppl 216:97
4 Bates SE (1991) Clinical application of serum tumor markers. Ann Int Med 115:623
5 Stenman UH, Bidart JM, Birken S, Mann K, Nisula B, O'Connor J (1993) Standardization of protein immunoprocedures. Choriogonadotropin. J Clin Lab Invest (suppl) 216:42

6. Ozturk M, Bellet D, Manil L, Hennen G, Frydman R, Wands J (1987) Physiological studies of human chorionic gonadotropin (hCG), ahCG and βhCG as measured by specific monoclonal immunoradiometric assays. Endocrinol 120:549
7. Cole LA, Kardana A, Andrade GP, Gawinowicz MA, Morris JC, Bergert ER et al (1991) The heterogeneity of human chorionic gonadotropin (hCG). III The occurrence and biological and immunological activities of nicked hCG. Endocrinol 129:1559
8. Kardana A, Cole LA (1992) Polypeptide nicks cause erroneous results in assays of human chorionic gonadotropin free β-subunit. Clin Chem 38:26
9. Bosl GJ, Lange PH, Fraley EE et al (1981) Human chorionic gonadotropin and alphafetoprotein in the staging of non-seminomatous testicular cancer. Cancer 47:328
10. Saller B, Clara R, Spöttl G, Siddle K, Mann K (1990) Testicular cancer secretes intact human chorionic gonadotropin (hCG) and its free beta-subunit: evidence that hCG (+hCG-beta) assays are the most reliable in diagnosis and follow up. Clin Chem 36: 234
11. Lange PH, Nochomovitz LE, Rosai J, Fraley EE, Kennedy BJ, Bosl G (1980) Serum alpha-fetoprotein and human chorionic gonadotropin in patients with seminoma. J Urol 124:472
12. Mann K, Siddle K (1988) Evidence for free beta-subunit secretion in so-called human chorionic gonadotropin-positive seminoma. Cancer 62:2378
13. Saller B, Mumperow E, Dettmann R et al (HCG/HCG-beta immunoactivity in testicular vein samples from patients with pure seminoma. Exp Clin Endocrinol 101 (suppl):167.
14. Seckl MJ, Rustin GJ, Bagshawe KD (1990) Frequency of serum tumour marker monitoring in patients with non-seminomatous germ cell tumours. Br J Cancer 61:916
15. Horwich A, Peckham MJ (1986) Transient tumor marker elevation following chemotherapy for germ cell tumors of the testis. Cancer Treat Rep 70:1329
16. Mann K, Saller B (1992) Tumour markers as prognostic factors in testicular cancer. Aktuelle Onkologie 78:177–185
17. Murphy P, Johnson DH (1991) Staging and prognostic factors in non-seminomatous testicular cancer. Hematol Oncol Clin North Am 5:1233
18. Aass N, Klepp O, Cavallin Stahl E et al (1991) Prognostic factors in unselected patients with non-seminomatous metastatic testicular cancer: a multicenter experience. J Clin Oncol 9:818
19. Jensen JL, Venner PM (1992) Predictive factors for outcome in treatment of metastatic non-seminomatous germ cell tumors. Urology 39:237
20. Mead GM, Stenning SP, Parkinson MC et al (1992) The Second Medical Research Council study of prognostic factors in non-seminomatous germ cell tumors. Medical Research Council Testicular Tumour Working Party. J Clin Oncol 10:85
21. Sesterhenn IA, Weiss RB, Mostofi FK et al (1992) Prognosis and other clinical correlates of pathologic review in stage I and II testicular carcinoma: a report from the Testicular Cancer Intergroup Study. J Clin Oncol 10:69
22. Gerl A, Clemm C, Lamerz R, Mann K, Wilmanns W (1993) Prognostic implications of tumor marker analysis in advanced non-seminomatous germ cell tumors. Eur J Cancer 29:961
23. Toner GC, Geller NL, Tan C, Nisselbaum J, Bosl GJ (1990) Serum tumor marker half-life during chemotherapy allows early prediction of complete response and survival in non-seminomatous germ cell tumors. Cancer Res 50:5904
24. Soper JT (1990) Gestational trophoblastic neoplasia. Curr Opin Obstet Gynecol 2:92
25. Miller DS, Lurain JR (1988) Classification and staging of gestational trophoblastic tumors. Obstet Gynecol Clin North Am 15:477
26. Ozturk M (1991) Human chorionic gonadotropin, its free subunits and gestational trophoblastic disease. J Reprod Med 36:21
27. Berkowitz RS, Goldstein DP (1988) Diagnosis and management of the primary hydatidiform mole. Obstet Gynecol Clin North Am 15:491
28. Braunstein GD, Vaitukaitis JL, Carbone PP, Ross GT (1973) Ectopic production of human chorionic gonadotrophin by neoplasms. Ann Int Med 78:39
29. Kuida CA, Braunstein GD, Shintaku P, Said JW (1988) Human chorionic gonadotropin expression in lung, breast, and renal carcinomas. Arch Pathol Lab Med 112:282
30. Senba M, Watanabe M (1991) Ectopic production of beta-subunit of human chorionic gonadotropin in malignant lymphoma. Zentralbl Pathol 137:402
31. Marcillac I, Troalen F, Bidart JM et al (1992) Free human chorionic gonadotropin beta subunit in gonadal and nongonadal neoplasms. Cancer Res 52:3901
32. Hoermann R, Gerbes AL, Spoettl G, Jungst D, Mann K (1992) Immunoreactive human chorionic gonadotropin and its free beta subunit in serum and ascites of patients with malignant tumors. Cancer Res 52:1520

Address for correspondence:
Dr. med. B. Saller
Abteilung für klinische Endokrinologie
Universitätsklinikum Essen
Medizinische Einrichtungen der GHS
Hufelandstraße 55
D-45122 Essen, Germany

Tumor marker in the supernatant of primary germ cell culture – A new test system for detection of vital tumor cells

T. Otto[a], C. Fuhrmann[b], M. Goepel[a], S. Krege[a], H. Rübben[a]

[a]Department of Urology, [b]Department of Radiobiology,
University of Essen, Medical School, Essen, Germany

Introduction

The persistance of vital tumor is of great prognostic and therapeutic value in patients with germ cell tumors (4, 6, 10). The surgical removement of residual lesions after chemotherapy is mandatory. The complete histopathological examination of enlarged residual tumor mass in serial sections is not possible for a routine procedure. We proofed additional methods to detect vital germ tumor cells and used primary culture technique to measure the expression of tumor markers, i.e. human choreon gonadotropine (HCP) and alpha fetoprotein (AFP) in the supernatant of 30 primary tumors and 21 secondary lesions.

Materials and methods

51 caucasian patients, 19–37 (median age 27) years old, underwent surgery at the Department of Urology, University of Essen, and tissue samples (1 ccm) were immediately brought into medium (MEM + Earle's salt + FCS 20%). The specimens were mechanically and enzymatically disaggregated (collagenase/dispase PBS – 1 mg enzymes/ml PBS, 30–60 min). The centrifugated pellet (5 min, 1000 rpm) is brought into medium (MEM + Earle's salt + FCS 20% + transferrin + insulin + hydrocortison + EGF + refobacin). Cell suspension (20 ml/75 qcm) is incubated (37 °C, 5% CO_2).
Measurement of AFP and β-HCG is performed in the cell culture supernatant by fluorescence sandwich immunoassay (Firma Stratos) using monoclonal antibodies against AFP and β-HCG.

Results

We measured increased levels of AFP and/or β-HCG in the supernatant of ten primary tumors. The corresponding serum level of β-HCG/AFP was increased in only seven patients (table I).
All patients with metastatic disease have shown a seroconversion after inductive chemotherapy before surgical removement of residual retroperitoneal tumor mass. The pathologist revealed in 19/20 metastatic lesions necrosis or fibrosis only and in 1/20 specimens vital tumor cells. We found increased levels of HCG or AFP in the supernatant of 4/20 metastatic lesions (table II).

Table I. Tumor marker level in the supernatant of primary germ cell tumors in correlation to the corresponding serum level of HCG and AFP.

	n	Primary tumors HCG ↑/ AFP ↑ (increased)
Serum	18	7
Cell culture	18	10
Control[a]	10	0

[a]Supernatant of fibroblast cell culture, four different bladder cancer cell lines, normal germ cell culture

Table II. Tumor marker level in the supernatant of retroperitoneal metastatic lesions in correlation to the corresponding serum level of HCG and AFP.

	n	Metastasis HCG ↑/ AFP ↑ (increased)
Serum	20	0
Cell culture	20	4

Table III. Clinical outcome of patients with metastatic disease according to the marker expression of AFP and HCG in the supernatant of residual lesions.

	AFP / HCG	
	normal	increased
Progression	0	3
No evidence of disease	16	1
Median follow-up 12 months		

After a median follow-up of 12 months 3/4 patients with increased marker expression in the supernatant developed early tumor progression. 16/20 patients who have shown a normal marker expression in cell culture supernatant are without evidence of disease (table III).

Discussion

Determination of beta human chorionic gonadotropine (β-HCG) and alpha fetoprotein (AFP) is mandatory for the diagnosis and follow-up of patients with non-seminomatous germ cell tumors (NSGT). After inductive chemotherapy most of the patients even with advanced disease (LUGANO stage II c, III) will reveal seroconversion of tumor markers. But in case of initially enlarged retroperitoneal tumor mass residual tumor remains after primary chemotherapy. It is not possible to distinguish preoperatively between non-malignant residual tissue and vital tumor (1, 2, 3, 6, 8,). Subsequent retroperitoneal lymphadenectomy (RPLA) remains mandatory in all cases with residual retroperitoneal disease (2, 4, 5, 9). The histopathological examination of residual lesions after chemotherapy is of great prognostic and therapeutic importance. According to the histopathological finding of vital tumor adjuvant chemotherapy is mandatory (7). But the histopathological examination of enlarged residual lesions in serial sections is impossible for a routine procedure.

We proofed additional methods to detect vital germ tumor cells and used a primary culture system to detect tumor marker in the cell culture supernatant. We found in the majority of the primary germ cell tumors (10/18) an increased tumor marker level in the supernatant. Only a limited number of metastatic lesions (4/20) were marker positive in the cell culture system. Interestingely 3/4 patients with positive marker expression developed early tumor progression though these specimens were regarded as fibrosis only. According to these results we found that primary culture assay is a powerful additional technique in the examination of chemotherapeutically treated metastatic lesions and yield information in addition to standard histopathology in 20% of the patients.

Summary

From 1991–1993 we performed cell culture analysis of 51 different germ cell tumors. We investigated 8 seminomas and 43 non-seminomatous germ cell tumors; 30 tumors were primary cancers and 21 were metastatic retroperitoneal lesions after chemotherapy.

Primary culture was successful in 30/51 tumors (59%). We revealed increased human choriongonadotropine (HCG) levels in the supernatant of primary germ cell culture in 70%; alpha fetoprotein was increased in 37%.

Cell culture technique yielded information in addition to standard histopathology in 20% of the metastatic lesions. 3/4 patients with positive cell culture assay and the histopathological finding of necrosis in the retroperitoneal specimen developed early tumor progression. Primary culture assays are powerful additional techniques in the examination of germ cell tumors.

References

1. Donohue JP, Rowland RG, Kopecky K (1987) Correlation of computerized tomographic changes and histological findings in 80 patients having radical retroperitoneal lymph node dissection after chemotherapy for testis cancer. J Urol 137:1176–1179
2. Fossa SD, Aass N, Ous S (1989) Histology of tumor residuals following chemotherapy in patients with advanced nonseminomatous testicular cancer. J Urol 142:1239–1242
3. Hoekstra H, Hogeboom WR, Sleyfer DT, Mooyaart EL and Schraffordt Koops H (1989) Comparison of MRI and CT imaging in staging and treatment evaluation of retroperitoneal metastases of non-seminomatous testicular tumors. 5th European Conference on Clinical Oncology, abstr P-0808

4. Otto T, Goepel M, Seeber S, Rübben H (1993) Verzögerte RLA in der Behandlung fortgeschrittener nichtseminomatöser Germinalzelltumoren. Urol [A] 32:189–193
5. Pizzocaro G, Salvioni R, Pasi M, Zanoni F, Milani A, Pilotti S, Monfardini S (1985) Early resection of residual tumor during cisplatin, vinblastine, bleomycin combination chemotherapy in stage III and bulky stage II nonseminomatous testicular cancer. Cancer, 56:249–255
6. Qvist HL, Fossa SD, Ous S, Høie J, Stenwig AE, Giercksky KE (1991) Post-chemotherapy tumor residuals in patients with advanced nonseminomatous testicular cancer. Is it necessary to resect all residual masses? J Urol 145:300–303
7. Schmoll HJ, Seeber S (1993) Aktuelle Entwicklungen in der Chemotherapie fortgeschrittener Hodentumoren Urol [A] 32:207–216
8. Stomper PC, Jochelson MS, Garnick MB, Richie JP (1985) Residual abdominal masses after chemotherapy for nonseminomatous testicular cancer: correlation of CT and histology. AJR 145:743
9. Tonkin KS, Rustin GJS, Wignall B, Paradinas F, Benenett M (1989) Successful treatment of patients in whom germ cell tumour masses enlarged on chemotherapy while their serum tumour markers decreased. Eur J Cancer Clin Oncol 25:1739–1743
10. Wood DP JR, Herr HW, Heller G, Vlamis V, Sogani PC, Motzer RJ, Fair WR, Bosl GJ (1992) Distribution of retroperitoneal metastases after chemotherapy in patients with nonseminomatous germ cell tumors. J Urol 148:1812–1816

Address for correspondence:
Dr. med. R. T. Otto
Urologische Klinik
Universität Essen
Hufelandstraße 55
D-45122 Essen, Germany

In Vitro Diagnosis

Varia

Serum NCAM:
A potential new prognostic marker for multiple myeloma

U. Kaiser[a], G. Jaques[a], B. Auerbach[b], K. Havemann[b]

[a]Department of Hematology/Oncology, Philipps-University Marburg,
[b]Research Laboratories of Behringwerke AG, Marburg, Germany

Introduction

The neural cell adhesion molecule NCAM is a membrane bound glycoprotein characterized by five immunoglobulin domains and the occurence of sialinic acids (1). In humans NCAM was first isolated in the neural system. Heterogenity of different variants suggests biological function (2). NCAM was shown to be identical with CD 56 (3) which is expressed on the surface of natural killer cells, subsets of T-cell lymphomas (4) and myeloma cells but not on normal plasma cells (5, 6).

Soluble NCAM was first demonstrated in the supernatant of glioma cells (7). A clinical value of serum NCAM as a potential marker for small cell lung cancer could recently be demonstrated (8). The expression of NCAM on myeloma cells but not on normal plasma cells and the necessity for new prognostic parameters in plasma cell dyscrasias led us to investigate serum NCAM in patients with myeloma.

Methods and patients

Serum embryonic NCAM was determined with an enzyme immunoassay developed by the Research Laboratories of Behringwerke AG, Marburg, Germany. Two monoclonal antibodies, MoAb 735 which detects the long chains of alpha-2,8-linked acetylneuraminic acids (9), and BW SCLC-I were employed.

The studies were performed in 32 healthy blood donors, seven patients with monoclonal gammopathy. 70 patients with multiple myeloma were classified according to the staging system proposed by Salmon and Durie (10). 58 patients who were under treatment or under observation were classified according to their response to therapy.

Results and discussion

32 healthy blood donors had serum NCAM levels below 20 U/ml. Hyperlipemia, paraproteinemia and hyperbilirubinemia did not interfere. Seven patients with monoclonal gammopathy of undetermined significance (MGUS) had NCAM levels below 20 U/ml (mean 8.5, median 9.5).

14 patients with stage I had a mean serum NCAM level of 14.9 U/ml (median 10.9), 18 patients with stage II had a mean NCAM level of 28.8 U/ml (median 15.4) and 38 patients with stage III had a

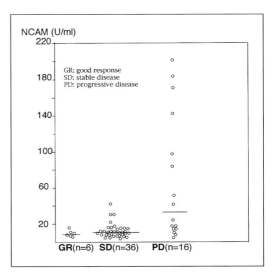

Figure 1. Serum NCAM levels in patients with multiple myeloma grouped according to response of therapy; — = median NCAM.

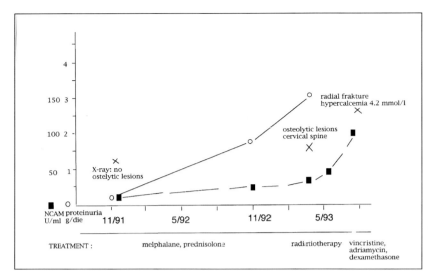

Figure 2. Serial serum NCAM in a patient with kappa light chain myeloma.

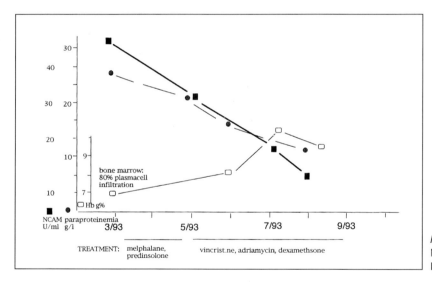

Figure 3. Serial serum NCAM in a patient with IgA lambda myeloma.

mean NCAM level of 32.2 U/ml (median 11.7). Six patients who were classified as good responder according to the classification propcsed by *Michielis* (11) (disappearance or reduction of paraprotein > 75%) had a mean NCAM level of 8.1 (median 6.9). None of them had NCAM > 20 ml/U. Among 36 patients who had stable disease (25–75% reduction of paraprotein) 11% (n = 4) had NCAM levels > 20 U/ml. Mean NCAM level was 12.5 (median 11).

16 patients were assigned to progressive disease (no reduction in paraprotein, new lytic lesions, anemia or hypercalcemia). 56% (n = 9) had NCAM levels > 20 U/ml. Mean NCAM level was 33 U/ml (median 68.3). Differences in serum NCAM levels were significant when patients were grouped according to their response to therapy (Wilcoxon Test, p = 0.0003) (figure 1). Serial NCAM measurements in patients demonstrated a good correlation between NCAM levels and response to therapy (figure 2, 3).

In conclusion, serum NCAM may be a potential valuable marker for monitoring therapy in multiple myeloma.

References

1. Cunningham BA, Hemperly JJ, Murray BA, Prediger EA, Brackenbury R, Eddelman GM (1987) Neural cell adhesion molecule: structure, immunoglublin-like domains, cell surface modulation, and alternative RNA splicing. Science 236:799
2. Goridis C, Brunet JF (1992) NCAM; structural diversity, function and regulation of expression. Semin Cell Biol 3:189
3. Lanier LL, Testi R, Bindl J, Phillips JH (1989) Identity of Leu-I9 (CD56) leucocyte differentiation antigen and neural cell adhesiion molecule. J Exp Med 169:2233
4. Kern WF, Spier CM, Hannemann EH, Miller TP, Matzner M, Grogan TM (1992) Neural cell adhesion molecule-positive peripheral T cell lymphoma: a rare variant with a propensity for unusual sites of involvement. Blood 79:2432
5. van Camp B, Durie BGM, Spier C, de Waele M, van Riet I, Vela E, Frutiger Y, Richter L, Grogan TM (1990) Plasma cells in multiple myeloma express a natural killer cell-associated antigen: CD 56 (NKHI; LeuI9). Blood 76:377
6. Barker HF, Hamilton MS, Ball J, Drew M, Franklin IM (1992) Expression of adhesion molecules LFA-3 and N-CAM on normal and malignant plasma cells. Br J Haematol 81:331
7. Gower HJ, Barton CH, Elsom VL, Thompson J, Moore S, Dickson G, Walsh FS (1988) Alternative splicing generates a secreted form od NCAM in muscle and brain. Cell 55:955
8. Jaques G, Auerbach B, Pritsch M, Wolf M, Madry N, Havemann K (1993) Evaluation of serum neural cell adhesion molecule as a new tumor marker in small cell lung cancer. Cancer 72:4181
9. Kibbelaar RE, Moolenaar CEC, Michalides RJAM, Bitter-Suermann D, Addis BJ, Mooi WJ (1989) Expression of the embryonal neural cell adhesion molecule N-CAM in lung carcinoma. Diagnostic usefulness of monoclonal antibody 735 for the distinction between small cell lung cancer and non-small cell lung cancer. J Pathol 159:23
10. Durie BGM, Salmon SF (1975) A clinical staging system for multiple myeloma. Cancer 36:842
11. Michielis JJ (1992) Multiple myeloma: prognostic factors and treatment modalities. Neth J Med 40:254

Address for correspondence:
Dr. med. U. Kaiser
Zentrum Innere Medizin
Hämatologie/Onkologie
Baldinger Straße
D-35033 Marburg, Germany

Clinical significance of the labeling index in multiple myeloma compared with beta-2-microglobulin, thymidine kinase and bone marrow histology

C. Schambeck[a], A. Fateh-Moghadam[a], R. Bartl[b], R. Lamerz[c], M. Wick[a]

[a]Institute of Clinical Chemistry, [b]Medical Clinic III, [c]Medical Clinic II,
Ludwig-Maximilians-University, Munich, Germany

Introduction

Currently there is no single parameter permitting always an early diagnosis of multiple myeloma. A decision to therapy can be difficult from case to case. Prognostic factors help to assess requirement of therapy. Survival of myeloma patients is often very different due to the growth rate of tumor cells and myeloma complications.

The study of the proliferation kinetics described by the so called labeling index (LI%) provides a key to determine tumor growth. The LI% corresponds to the percentage of plasma cells in the S-phase related to all counted plasma cells. S-phase plasma cells can be detected by antibodies against bromodeoxyuridine inserted in the replicating DNA instead of thymidine. Durie et al. (1), Hofmann et al. (2) and Latreille et al. (3) demonstrated a LI% > 1% to be associated with poor survival.

The aim of this study was to compare the diagnostic significance of LI% with other clinical parameters such as serum beta-2-microglobulin (β2M) and serum thymidine kinase (TK) also indicating proliferation as well as bone marrow histology.

Patients

Bone marrow specimen of 62 patients with a monoclonal gammopathy were analysed as well as peripheral blood of two patients with massive plasma cell leukemia for determination of LI%. Diagnosis of "benign monoclonal gammopathy" (BMG) or smouldering myeloma (SM) was established in 20 patients. Active untreated myeloma was found in 17 cases. The myeloma had been treated at least for more than six weeks ago in 27 cases. Criteria for BMG, SM, progressive (active) or therapy-resistant disease can be found in (4).

Blood was drawn parallel to bone marrow aspiration to measure β2M and TK. Sera were frozen at $-80°$ C when the parameters were not immediately determined. Other 25 patients with BMG or SM served as a reference group to define the cut-off value for TK.

Methods

For measuring LI% mononuclear cells of bone marrow aspirate obtained by Ficoll-Paque were incubated one hour at 37 °C in RPMI 1640 containing 10% fetal calf serum, 1% Glutamine, 1% penicillin-streptomycin, 10 µM bromodeoxyuridine and 1 µM fluorodeoxyuridine. The cells were fixed for 30 minutes in 70% ethanol for perforating the membrane. The cells were incubated with BU-1 (BU-1 was kindly provided by Dr. Gonchoroff and Dr. Kyle, Mayo Clinic Rochester (USA)) 1:4 for 30 minutes at room temperature (flow cytometry) or 1:1 one hour at 4 °C (microscopy). BU-1 is an antibody against Bromodeoxyuridine without requiring denaturating agents (5). The cells were then incubated with FITC labeled goat anti human kappa or lambda from SBA (1:720 for flow cytometry or 1:30 for microscopy) and PE labeled goat anti mouse IgG from SBA (1:180 for flow cytometry or 1:10 for microscopy) for 30 minutes at room temperature (flow cytometry) or at 4 °C (microscopy). The steps were interrupted by thoroughly washing with PBS. The cells on a Bio-rad adhesion slide were read in a Zeiss fluorescence microscope or the suspended cells were measured by a flow cytometer (FACScan from Becton Dickinson). LI% values obtained by the established microscopic method were used in the following analyses.

TK was measured by means of the "prolifigen"-radioenzymeassay from Sangtec medicals, Bromma (Schweden). β2M was determined by the "IMx β2-microglobulin"-enzyme immunoassay from Abbott, North Chicago (USA).

The bone marrow biopsies were classified according to the system of Bartl (6). The prognostically favourable cell types "Marschalko" and "Small Cell" were summarized as cells of "low grade malignancy". Cells of "intermediate grade malignancy" comprise the cell types "Cleaved", "Polymorphous" and "Asynchronous" representing a moderate survival rate.

Differences among patients' groups were analysed by means of the test of Wilcoxon, Mann, Whitney. Correlations were investigated according to the Spearman correlation procedure.

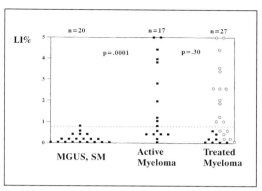

Figure 1. Labeling index versus disease status. Open circles indicate therapy-resistant or progressive cases.

Results

There was a significant difference of the proliferation kinetics considering smouldering and active untreated myelomas (p = 0.0001). Defining the cut-off value based on 100% specificity versus SM and BMG (according to a LI% = 0.8%) a 53% sensitivity resulted for active untreated myelomas. All treated patients with a LI% > 0.8% were proved to be therapy-resistant or progressive. Six of 19 such patients however did not show an elevated S-phase part (figure 1). Defining the cut-off value for β2M = 3.5 mg/l (Crea < 1.8 mg/dl) and for LI% = 0.8% β2M and LI% were both low in 20 patients with BMG or SM (r = 0.33, p > 0.05). Also no correlation of these parameters could be found in the 17 active untreated myelomas (r = 0.18, p > 0.05). In nine cases β2M or LI% and in four cases both β2M and LI% were increased. In four cases none of the parameters was elevated.

Our analysis demonstrated a significant correlation between TK and LI% (r = 0.64, p < 0.001, n = 34). Our reference group showed an average TK = 5.3 IU/ml, δ = 3.3. We fixed the cut-off value at 10 IU/ml according to 96% specificity. Then we found low or high values for both parameters in 25 patients. A high TK but low LI% was observed

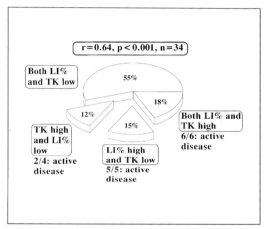

Figure 2. Labeling index and thymidine kinase; cut-off TK = 10 IU/ml, LI % = 0.8.

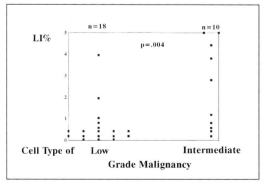

Figure 3. Labeling index and bone marrow histology according to the classification of Bartl in untreated (smouldering or active) myelomas.

in four patients (two of them had active disease). A high LI% but low TK could be found in five patients characterized by active disease (figure 2). Considering all patients with SM or active untreated disease there was a striking difference between the two histologic groups (p < 0.004): The low grade malignancy myelomas were generally characterized by a low LI% contrary to the intermediate grade malignancy myelomas. Two patients with "Marschalko" cell type demonstrated a LI% > 2%. There were also intermediate grade myelomas with low LI% (figure 3).

Discussion

The proliferation kinetics in multiple myeloma offer a prognostic indicator established by former studies. Our data confirm the good discrimination of smouldering and active myelomas shown by studies of *Greipp* and *Boccadoro* (7, 8). Considering patients with monoclonal gammopathy a LI% > 0.8% indicates an active myeloma with 100% specificity. Although all treated patients with an increased kinetics were judged resistant or progressive, also patients were found to be therapy-resistant or progressive despite a low LI%. A negative result despite of disease progression can be caused by puncture location, repeated aspiration or a great tumor bulk. Growth seems to be self-limiting in cases of an extensive tumor mass. Except in smouldering myelomas β2M and LI% do not reflect disease in a congruent manner. Both parameters uncover different aspects of the tumor: growth and tumor load. Both parameters were shown to be independent by means of a larger database by *Boccadoro* et al. (9).

First of all the significant but moderate correlation between TK and LI% is not astonishing. TK represents the key enzyme of the salvage pathway for DNA synthesis. Endogeneous thymidine is reutilized and therefore linked with proliferation. Also the false nucleotid and thymidine analogon bromodeoxyuridine is inserted by this enzyme. Both parameters bear prognostic relevance. Nevertheless TK and LI% cannot be used in the same manner. TK is much influenced by viral diseases, considerable circadian variations and other effects (10). LI% identifies exclusively the proliferation compartment of myeloma and is unlike TK independent of tumor burden.

There is a significant correlation between LI% and the grade of malignancy according to the classification of *Bartl*. In untreated patients with a high LI% plasma cells of intermediate grade of malignancy were mostly detected. But there are myelomas characterized by both mature plasma cells and a high LI% and vice versa.

Summary

The LI% is a helpful factor in completing other established parameters. A synopsis of markers describing tumor biology (LI%, load, grade) tumor products (β2M, immunoglobulin) and tumor complications (anemia, osteolyses, hypercalcaemia, azotaemia a.s.o.) enalbes a more reliable assessment of disease activity in multiple myeloma.

References

1. Durie BGM, Salmon SE, Moon TE (1980) Pretreatment tumor mass, cell kinetics and prognosis in multiple myeloma. Blood 55:364–372
2. Hofmann V, Salmon SE, Durie BGM (1981) Drug resistance in multiple myeloma associated with in vitro incorporation 3H-thymidine. Blood 58:471–476
3. Latreille J, Barlogie B, Johnston D, Drewinko B, Alexanian R (1982) Ploidy and proliferative characteristics in monoclonal gammopathies. Blood 59:43–51
4. Fateh-Moghadam A, Wilmanns W (1992) Multiples myelom. In: Krück et al (eds) Therapiehandbuch. Urban & Schwarzenberg, München
5. Greipp PR, Witzig TE, Gonchoroff NJ (1985) Immunofluorescent plasma cell labeling indices (LI) using a monoclonal antibody (BU-1). Am J Haematol 20:289–292
6. Bartl R, Frisch B, Fateh-Moghadam A, Kettner G, Jaeger K, Sommerfeld W (1987) Histologic classification and staging of multiple myeloma. Am J Clin Path 87:342–355
7. Boccadoro M, Gavarotti P, Fossati G et al (1984) Low plasma cell 3H-thymidine incorporation in monoclonal gammopathy of undetermined significance (MGUS), smouldering myeloma and remission phase myeloma: a reliable indicator of patients not requiring therapy. Br J Haematol 58:689–696
8. Greipp PR, Kyle RA (1983) Clinical, morphological and cell kinetic differences among multiple myeloma, monoclonal gammopathy of undetermined

significance and smoldering multiple myeloma. Blood 62:166–171

9 Boccadoro M, Durie BGM, Frutiger Y et al (1987) Lack of correlation between plasma cell thymidine labelling index and serum beta-2-microglobulin in monoclonal gammopathies. Acta Hematol 78:239–242

10 Hallek M, Wanders L, Strohmeyer S, Emmerich B (1992) Thymidine kinase a tumor marker with prognostic value for non-Hodgkin's lymphoma and a broad range of potential clinical applications. Ann Hematol 65:1–5

Address for correspondence:
Dr. med. M. Wick
Institut für Klinische Chemie
Klinikum Großhadern
Marchioninistraβe 15
D-81377 München, Germany

Soluble interleukin-2 receptors, serum thymidine kinase and beta-2-microglobulin as tumor markers in therapy monitoring and follow-up of patients with high-grade non-Hodgkin's lymphoma

O. Micke[a], U. Schäfer[a], Ch. Wilken[b], F.J. Prott[a], B. Wörmann[c], W. Hiddemann[b]

[a]Department of Radiotherapy and Radiation Oncology,
[b]Department of Internal Medicine A, Münster,
[c]Department of Hematology and Oncology, Göttingen, Germany

Introduction

The outcome of patients with high-grade non-Hodgkin's lymphoma (NHL) has improved over the past ten years through intensified chemotherapy and adjuvant radiation treatment (1). Therefore therapy monitoring and follow-up of patients with NHL became more important.

Diagnosis and staging is conventionally done by histology, laboratory parameters, clinical examination and imaging (CT, MRI, Ultrasound). In therapy monitoring and follow-up the addition of serum tumor markers may be useful, if an elevation of tumor marker levels predicts relapse earlier than conventional diagnostic methods can do. Furthermore the initial tumor marker level and the decrease of tumor levels under therapy may reflect in vivo sensitivity to chemotherapy and be related to the final outcome (9).

Soluble interleukin-2 receptor (sIL-2R), serum thymidine kinase (sTK) and beta-2-microglobulin (β2M) have been described as tumor markers in NHL (3, 4, 5, 6, 7). Their levels were related to tumor burden and disease activity. Soluble interleukin-2 receptors are released from activated lymphoid cells in vitro and in vivo (8).

sTK is an intracellular enzyme of the nucleic acid metabolism increased in diseases with high cell turnover, for example hematological disorders (3, 6).
β2M is a small subunit of the MHC-1 complex and is also increased in the serum of patients with malignant lymphomas (4, 6) and in diseases with decreased glomerular filtration.

As we could recently show a high sensitivity of sIL-2R and sTK in patients with high-grade NHL (7), we investigated in this study wether sIL-2R, sTK and β2M are suitable as tumor markers in therapy monitoring and follow-up of patients with high-grade NHL.

Material and methods

Two non-crossreactive anti-IL-2R antibodies B-G3 and B-F2 were used for measuring sIL-2R levels with an ELISA of the sandwich type as described by *Rubin* et al. (8). The antibodies had been generated by Dr. J. Wijdens (Besançon, France). sTK and beta2M were determined using commercial kits. sTK was measured with a REA (radio enzyme assay) of Byk-Sangtec and β2M with fluoroimmunoassay of Pharmacia.

The cut-off-level was defined as the average of 80 healthy normal volunteers plus the twofold standard deviation. It was 645 U/l for sIL-2R, 5 U/l for sTK and 3.0 mg/l for beta2M.

30 untreated patients with a newly diagnosed high-grade NHL from 5/87 to 12/92 were included in this study. 17 patients were male, 13 female. Median age was 58.5 years with a range from 20 to 77 years.

The distribution of the histological subgroups according to the Kiel classification were: 13 patients with centroblastic lymphoma, 11 with T-cell-lymphoma and six immunoblastic lymphoma Stages of disease according to the criteria of staging adopted at the Ann Arbor symposium on Hodgkin's disease were: one patient with stage I, five with stage II, four with stage III and 20 with stage IV. The patients were homogeneously treated with the COPBLAM/IMVP-16 scheme (2). They received three cycles of COPBLAM, in case of a good response five cycles. If the response to COPBLAM was inadequate, treatment was immediately switched to IMVP-16, otherwise after the fifth cycle COPBLAM, i.e. a total of 3–5 cycles.

Blood was drawn before starting chemotherapy and during chemotherapy before every new cycle, i.e. monthly. During follow-up tumor marker levels were measured all three month.

Under this regimen 24 patients achieved a complete remission, three patients a partial remission and three patients progressed under therapy. Ten patients relapsed during the observation period.

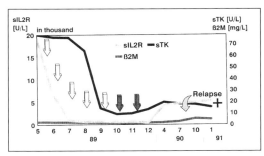

Figure 1. Patient 1, 29 years old male, T-cell-lymphoma IV B.

Results

Mean pretherapeutic serum levels of sIL-2R (5225 U/l) and sTK (37.9 U/l) were significantly elevated against normal controls. Pretherapeutic elevation of tumor marker levels was found in sIL-2R and sTK in 97% of all patients, in β2M in 37%. We like to present typical curves of tumor marker levels in relation with the clinical presentation and course of the patients.

The first patient (figure 1) is a 29 years old male suffering from a stage IV B T-cell-lymphoma. Initially he had a good response to chemotherapy and achieved a complete remission evaluated by imaging and clinical examination. The serum levels of sIL-2R and sTK decrease to values at lower range. Ten months later the patient presented with a thoracic recurence of disease shown by CT-scan (figure 2). Four months before presentation of relapse an elevation of serum levels of sIL-2R and sTK could be observed. The patient finally died from his disease.

The second patient (figure 3) is a 66 years old male with a centroblastic lymphoma stage IV B. The patient responded well to chemotherapy and achieved a stable complete remission. Until the end of the observation period no relapse could be observed. The serum levels of sIL-2R and sTK of this patient rapidly decreased to normal values.

Relating the curves of the serum levels of sIL-2R, sTK and β2M with the clinical course and the staging examinations sIL-2R showed in 90% of patients a good correlation, sTk in 80% a good correlation and β2M in 37%.

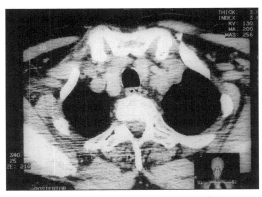

Figure 2. Patient 1, computertomography of the upper mediastinum showing bilateral paratracheal masses as a manifestation of a lymphonodular relapse.

10/30 patients relapsed during the observation period. In 8/10 patients sIL-2R and sTK showed an elevation of serum levels before manifestation of recurrence. In 2/10 patients β2M showed an elevation of values. The mean leading time was 4.1 months.

Discussion

In the present paper we could demonstrate, that sIL-2R and sTK show in a high percentage of patients a good correlation with the clinical course of patients. In case of good response to chemotherapy serum levels of sTK and sIL-2R often dramatically decrease to levels at the lower range. In a stable complete remission normal values of sTK and sIL-2R were observed. Recurrence of disease was predicted in 80% patients by significant elevation of serum levels of sIL-2R or sTK.

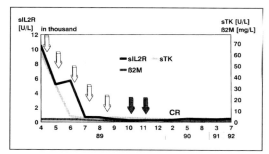

Figure 3. Patient 2, 66 years old male, centroblastic lymphoma IV B.

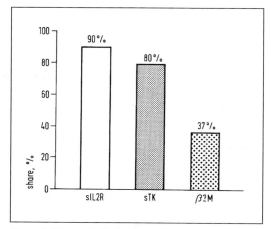

Figure 4. Share of initially elevated serum levels.

Gronowitz et al. (3) also showed in a longitudinal studies of sTK levels in 19 NHL patients that sTK levels increase with progression of disease, decreases during succesful therapy, and finally increases during relapse.
Similar results were found by *Harrington* et al. (5) for sIL-2R levels. They showed in group of 35 patients with both high-grade and low-grade lymphoma that serum sIL-2R levels correlate with disease activity and tumor size.
Our results indicate that sIL-2R and sTK support additional information in therapy monitoring and follow-up of patients with high-grade NHL.
In cases where there is an elevation of sTK or sIL-2R levels without a suspicion of recurrence of disease in clinical presentation the intervals of follow-up should be shortened or additional sometimes more invasive diagnostic means should be considered.

On the other hand in those cases, when image studies show findings of unclear dignity, sTK and sIL-2R may be helpful for the correct evaluation of these unclear findings.

Conclusion

In our study we could show that sIL-2R and sTK seem to be uselful markers in therapy monitoring and follow-up of patients with high-grade NHL.

References

1 Brittinger G, Bartels H, Common H, Dühmke E, Engelhard M, Fülle HH, Günzer U, Gyenes T, Heinz R, König E, Meuser P, Pralle H, Themel H, Musshoff K, Stacher A, Brücher H, Herrmann F, Ludwig WD, Pribilla W, Burger - Schüler A, Löher GW, Gremmel H, Oertel J, Gerhartz H, Köppen KM, Boll I, Huhn D, Binder T, Schoengen A, Nowicki L, Pees HW, Scheurlen Pg, Leopold H, Wannenmacher M, Schmidt M, Löffler H, Michelmeyer G, Thiel E, Zettel R, Rühl U, Wilke HJ, Schwarze EW, Stein H, Feller AC, Lennert K (Kieler Lymphomgruppe) (1986) Klinische und prognostische Relevanz der Kiel-Klassifikation der Non-Hodgkin-Lymphome. Onkologie 9:118–125

2 Engelhard M, Meusers P, Brittinger G, Brack N, Dornoff W, Enne W, Gassmann W, Gerhartz H, Hallek M, Heise J, Hettchen W, Huhn D, Kabelitz K, Kuse R, Lengfelder E, Ludwig F, Meuthen I, Radtke H, Schadeck C, Schöber C, Schumacher E, Siegert W, Staiger HJ, Terhardt E, Thiel E, Thomas M, Wagner T, Willems MG, Wilmanns W, Zwinger T, Stein H, Tiemann M, Lennert K (1991) Prospective multicenter trial for the response-adapted treatment of high-grade non-Hodgkin's lymphoma: Updated results of the COP-BLAM/IMVP-16 protocol with randomized adjuvant radiotherapy. Ann Onc 2 (suppl 2):177–180

3 Gronowitz JS, Hagberg H, Källander CFR, Simonsson B (1983) The use of deoxythymidine-kinase as a prognostic marker in the monitoring of non Hodgkin's lymphoma. Br J Cancer 47:487–495

4 Hagberg H, Kilander A, Simonsson W (1983) Serum beta 2-microglobulin in malignant lymhomas. Cancer 51:2220–2225

5 Harrington DS, Patil K, Lai PK, Yasadu NN, Ip ST, Weissenburger DD, Lindner J, Purtilo DT (1988) Interleukin 2 receptors in patients with malignant lymphoma. Arch Path Lab Med 132:3172–3175

6 Lehtinen T, Lehtinen M, Aaran RK, Laine S, Hakala T, Leinikki P (1988) Serum levels of thymidine

kinase, beta-2-microglobulin and herpesvirus antibodies in patients with newly diagnosed lymhoma. J Tumor Marker Oncol 3:259–268

7   Micke O, Wilken C, Hiddemann W, van de Loo J, Wörmann B (1992) Sensitivity of soluble interleukin-2 receptors, serum thymidine kinase and beta-2 microglobulin in patients with high-grade Non-Hodgkin-Lymphoma. In: Klapdor R (ed) Tumor associated antigens, oncogenes, receptors, cytokines in tumor diagnosis and therapy at the beginning of the nineties. Zuckschwerdt, München, Bern, Wien, New York, pp 405–408

8   Rubin LA, Kurman CC, Fritz ME, Biddison WE, Boutin B, Yarchoan R, Nelson DL (1985) Soluble interleukin-2 receptors are released from lymphoid cells in vitro. J Immunol 132:3172–3175

9   Wagner DK, Kiwanuka J, Edwards BK, Rubin LA, Nelson DL, Magrath IT (1987) Soluble interleukin-2 receptor levels in patients with undifferentiated and lymphoblastic lymphomas: Correlation with survival. J Clin Oncol 5:1262–1274

Address for correspondence:
Dr. med. O. Micke
Klinik und Poliklinik für Strahlentherapie
Radioonkologie
Universität Münster
Albert-Schweitzer-Straße 33
D-48129 Münster, Germany

Serum level of soluble interleukin-2 receptor is a marker for disease activity in cutaneous T-cell lymphoma (CTCL)

L. Kowalzick, I. Köhler, K. Meißner

Clinic of Dermatology of the University Hamburg-Eppendorf, Hamburg, Germany

Introduction

Interleukin-2 (IL-2) is produced by T-lymphocytes after stimulation with antigen or mitogen (1). It stimulates the proliferation and differentiation of activated T-cells, natural killer cells, other cytotoxic cells, B-cells and monocytes (2, 3). IL-2 binds to receptors on the surface of these cells the expression of which are stimulated by antigens or mitogens (4). Two types of IL-2 receptors were demonstrated: the low affinity receptor (also called Tac) of 55 kD that is also part (alpha-chain) of the high affinity receptor which additionally consists of a 75 kD protein (beta-chain) (5). Activated T- and B-lymphocytes and monocytes were shown to shed a soluble form of the 55 kD protein after stimulation in vitro (6). The serum levels of soluble interleukin-2 receptor (sIL-2R) is known to parallel T-cell activation (7). Elevated levels of sIL-2R have been demonstrated in patients suffering from diseases associated with T-cell affection or activitation as Hodgkin's disease, HTLV-1-associated T-cell leukemia, hairy cell leukemia, HIV-infection, rheumatic arthritis, lupus erythematosous, psoriasis and atopic dermatitis (8–15).

Elevated levels of cell sIL-2R were found in patients with cutaneous T-cell lymphoma (mycosis fungoides, Sézary syndrome). It was demonstrated, that serum levels do correlate with the clinical stage of this disease, although patient numbers in some stage groups were small or no controls were included in the published studies (figure 1a–c) (16–18). Photochemotherapy (oral methoxypsoralene plus UV-A irradiation) has been shown to be an efficient treatment modality both in early CTCL and psoriasis (19, 20). In this study we investigated sIL-2R serum levels in patients with CTCL of the small cerebriform type (mycosis fungoides, MF) before and during photochemotherapy in order to answer the question wether clinical improvement correlates with descreasing of sIL-2R levels as a marker of disease activity in cutaneous T-cell lymphoma. To exclude a general effect of photochemotherapy on sIL-2R serum levels, patients with psoriasis were included as controls.

Patients and methods

Patients: Seven patients with CTCL of the small cerebriform cell type (mycosis fungoides) in stage (21) Ia + b and IIa (stage Ia = 1, stage Ib = 5, stage IIa = 1) were included (m = 3, f = 4, age 55.3 ± 12.4 years). Nine patients with disseminated psoriasis were included (m = 5, f = 4, age 57.0 + 10.3 years).

Controls: Control serum samples were collected from 17 healthy volunteers (m = 9, f = 8, age 33.1 + 8.8 years).

Photochemotherapy: PUVA-treatment was done administering 8-methoxypsoralene (8-MOP, Meladinine, Basotherm, Biberach a.d.R., Germany) orally two hours before irradiation in a dose of approx. 0.5mg/kg bodyweight. UV-A irradiation was done with a Waldmann PUVA 4000 bed (Waldmann, Schwenningen, Germany, Emax = 355 nm) four times per week for at least 25 treatments. Later the number of irridiation per week was reduced according to the clinical improvement. Total UV-A doses were 167 ± 87 J/cm^2 in the patients with CTCL and 122 ± 59 J/cm^2 in the psoriasis group. No further specific systemical or topical treatment was given during the study.

Serum sIL-2R essay: Before onset of PUVA-treatment and after every tenth irradiation 20 ml EDTA blood were collected from the patients

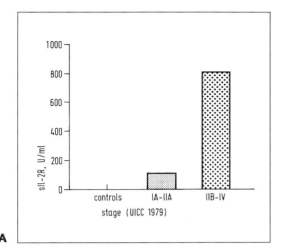
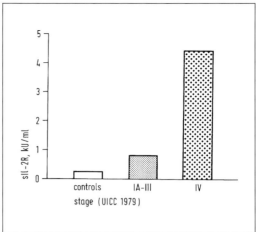
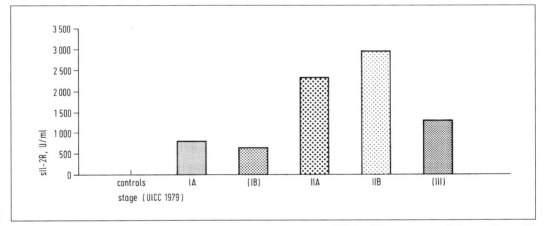

Figure 1A-C. Reported (16–18) means of sIL-2R levels in patients with CTCL in different stages of disease. Bars with designation in brackets refer to stage groups with only few cases included.

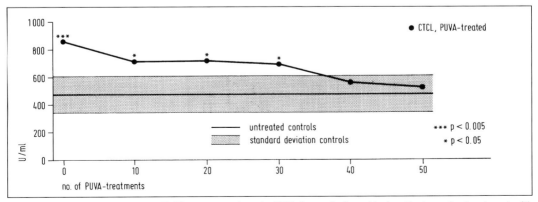

Figure 2. Time course of serum sIL-2R concentrations in CTCL (mycosis fungoides) patients under treatment with photochemotherapy (PUVA); (n = 7, normal range n = 19).

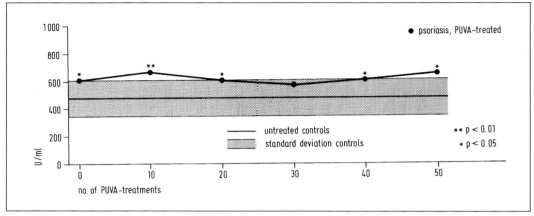

Figure 3. Time course of serum sIL-2R concentrations in psoriasis patients under treatment with photochemotherapy (PUVA); (n = 9, normal range n = 19) (compare to figure 2).

Configuration and aliquotation of serum samples was performed within 1 hour after collection. Aliquots were stored at −70 °C until measurment. All serum aliquots were examined at the same time. ELISA for sIL-2R was performed by using a test kit (Cellfree, T Cell Sciences, Cambridge, MA, USA) according to established methods (22). Extinction was measured at 450 nm.
Statistics: Normal range of sIL-2R was defined as single standard deviation of control samples. Student's T-test was used in order to detect significantly elevated sIL-2R levels at different time points of treatment in both diseases.

Results

Clinically, all our patients responded well during photochemotherapy: 5/7 patients with CTCL and 7/9 patients with psoriasis showed a complete remission under PUVA-treatment. The serum levels of sIL-2R before and during photochemotherapy are shown in figure 2 (CTCL) and figure 3 (psoriasis). Before onset of the therapy sIL-2R values were significantly elevated both in CTCL (858 ± 413 U/ml, $p < 0.005$) and in psoriasis (606 ± 243 U/ml, $p < 0.05$) compared to healthy controls (475 ± 143 U/ml). During photochemotherapy mean sIL-2R levels continously decreased in patients with CTCL, reaching normal values after 50 irradiations (529 ± 183 U/ml). Significantly elevated sIL-2R was not measured any longer after the 30th irradiation in CTCL patients corresponding clinical improvement. In contrast, clinical improvement under photochemotherapy did not correlate with a change (i.e. decrease) of serum sIL-2R levels in psoriasis patients. Significantly elevated values were detectable even after 50 irradiations (658 ± 134 U/ml, $p < 0.05$).

Discussion

In our present study we can confirm results of other authors (10, 16) in that we found significantly elevated levels of serum sIL-2R in both CTCL and psoriasis before treatment. Our data with psoriatic control patients show that photochemotherapy itself does not generally exert a decrease in serum sIL-2R levels. In contrast to our findings in psoriasis, clinical improvement parallels with decrease of sIL-2R levels in our CTCL patients treated with photochemotherapy. Normal range values were detected after achievement of complete or partial remission.
In CTCL, skin biopsies also show frequently up to 25% IL-2R (CD25+) positive T-cells in the dermis and epidermis (23, 24), which diminish the following clinically effective therapy, although it is unclear, whether malignant T-lymphoid cells or inflammatory cells were stained. Furthermore, the numbers of CD25+ T-cells in skin, lymph nodes and peripheral blood do not correlate (25).
However, beside from the known correlation of the stage of the active disease, we conclude from the correlation of clinical remission with normaliz-

ing of the serum sIL-2R levels, that this parameter is a good marker for disease activity and for assessement of therapeutic efficacy in patients with CTCL.

References

1. Grabstein KS, Dowes S, Gillis S, Urdal D, Larsen A (1986) Expression of interleukin-2, interferon gamma and the IL-2 receptor by human peripheral blood lymphocytes. J Immunol 136:4503–4508
2. Cantrell DA, Smith KA (1984) The interleukin-2/ T-cell system: A new cell growth model. Science 224:1312
3. Suzuki R, Handa K, Itoh K, Kuzmazi K (1983) Natural killer cells as a responder to interleukin-2. J Immunol 130:981–992
4. Kaplan Dr, Bracialo V, Braciale TJ (1984) Antigen-dependent regulation of interleukin-2 receptor on cloned human cytotoxic T-lymphocytes. J Immunol 133:1966–1969
5. Robb RJ, Greene WC (1987) Internalisation of interleukin-2 is mediated by the beta chain of the high affinity interleukin-2 receptor. J Exp Med 165:1205–1206
6. Rubin LA, Kurman CC, Fritz ME, Biddeson WE Boutin B, Yardochan R, Nelson DL (1985) Soluble interleukin-2 receptors are released from activated human lymphoid cells in vitro. J Immunol 135:3172–3177
7. Prince HE, Kleinman SH, Maino VC, Jackson AL (1988) In vitro activation of T-lymphocytes from HIV-seropositive blood donors. Soluble interleukin-2 receptor production parallels cellular IL-2R expression and DNA synthesis. J Clin Immunol 8:114–118
8. Gause A, Roschansky V, Tschiersch A, Schmits A, Diehl V, Pfreundschuh M (1990) The prognostic value of low pretreatment serum interleukin-2 receptor in patients with Hogkin's disease. J Cancer Res Clin Oncol 116:3208
9. Greene WC, Leonhard WJ, Depper JM, Nelson DL, Waldmann TA (1986) The human interleukin-2 receptor: normal and abnormal expression in T-cells and in leukemias induced by the human T-lymphotropic retroviruses. Ann Intern Med 105:560–575
10. Kapp A, Piskorski A, Schöpf E (1988) Elevated levels of interleukin-2 receptor in sera of patients with atopic dermatitis and psoriasis. Brit J Dermatol 119:707–710
11. Nelson DL (1986) Soluble interleukin-2 receptors. Analysis in normal individuals and in certain disease states. Fed Proc 45:377
12. Schulte C, Meurer M (1989) Soluble IL-2 receptor seruim levels – a marker for disease progression in patients with HIV-1 infection. Arch Dermatol Res 281:299–303
13. Symons JA, Wood NC, DiGiovine FS, Duff GW (1988) Soluble IL-2 receptor in rheumatoid arthritis: correlation with disease actiuvity, IL-1 and IL-2 inhibition. J Immunol 141:2612–2618
14. Wagner DK, Kiwanuka J, Edwards BK, Rubin LA, Nelson DL, Margrath IT (1987) Soluble interleukin-2 receptor levels in patients with undifferentiated lymphoblastic lymphomas: correlation with survival. J Clin Oncol 5:1262–1274
15. Wüthrich B, Joller-Jemelka H, Helfenstein U, Grob PJ (1990) Levels of soluble interleukin-2 receptors correlate with severity of atopic dermatitis. Dermatologica 181:92–97
16. Kaudewitz P, Josimovic-Alasevi O, Diamantstein T, Eckert F, Klepzig K, Burg G (1988) Soluble IL-2R receptor serum levels in cutaneous T-cell lymphoma – correlation with clinical status and IL-2 receptor in cutaneous infiltrates. J Invest Dermatol 91:386
17. Dummer R, Posseckert G, Nestle F, Witzgall R, Burger M, Becker JC, Schäfer E, Wiede J, Sebald W, Burg G (1992) Soluble interleukin-2 receptors inhibit interleukin-2 dependent proliferation and cytotoxicity: Explantation for diminished natural killer cell activity in cutaneous T-cell lymphomas in vivo? J Invest Dermatol 98:50–54
18. Bernengo MG, Fierro MT, Novelli M, Lisa F, Appino A (1993) Soluble interleukin-2 receptor in Sézary syndrome: its origin and clinical application. Brit J Dermatol 128:124–129
19. Gilchrest BA, Parrish JA, Tanenbaum L, Haynes HA, Fitzpatrick TB (1976) Oral methoxypsoralen photochemotherapy of mycosis fungoides. Cancer 38:683–689
20. Wolff K, Fitzpatrick TB, Parrish JA, Gschnalt F, Gilchrest B, Hönigsmann H, Pathak MS, Tanenbaum L (1976) Photochemotherapy for psoriasis with oral 8-methoxypsoralen. Arch Dermatol 112:943–959
21. Bunn PA, Lamberg SJ (1979) Report of the comittee on staging and classification of contaneous T-cell lymphomas. Cancer Treat Rep 63:725–728
22. Goldstein AM, Marcon L, Cullen BR, Nelson DL (1988) A competetive enzyme-linked immunoassay for the measurement of soluble human interleukin-2 receptors. J Immunol Methods 107:103–109
23. Klaerskog L, Scheynius A, Tjernlund U (1986) Distribution of interleukin-2 receptor bearing lymphocytes in the skin: A comparative study of allergic and irritant contact dermatitis, tuberculin reaction and contaneous T-cell lymphoma. Acta Derm Venerol (Stockh) 66:193–199
24. Meissner K, Löning T, Rehpennig W (1991) Mycosis fungoides und Sézary-Syndrom: Diagnostische und prognostische Relevanz der Expression zellulärer Antigene. Hausarzt 42:84–91
25. Küng E, Meissner K, Löning T (1988) Cutaneous T-cell lymphoma: immunohistochemical study on activation, proliferation and differentiation associated antigens in lymph nodes, skin and peripheral blood. Virchows Archiv A Pathol Anat 413:539–549

Address for correspondence:
Dr. med. L. Kowalzick
Universitätshautklinik
Martinistraße 52
D-20246 Hamburg, Germany

Neopterin is an indicator of metastatic disease in patients with choroidal melanoma

H. Gerding, G. Cremer-Bartels, K. Krause, H. Busse

Department of Ophthalmology, University of Münster, Münster, Germany

Introduction

In recent years the role of neopterin as an indicator of activated cell-mediated immunity has clearly been established in a variety of clinical disorders (7, 9, 13, 14). One of the major medical applications of neopterin analysis is the monitoring of tumor associated cellular reactions in patients with different kinds of malignant neoplastic diseases. Neopterin-positivity is regularly associated with hematological neoplasias. The magnitude of significantly increased serum or urinary neopterin levels seems to be rather variant in solid malignancies (8, 10, 12). There have been some representative examples of a well established correlation between the staging of solid tumors and neopterin levels (12). In cutaneous malignant melanoma elevated neopterin levels are indicating metastatic disease (10). Both, choroidal and cutaneous melanoma, share some immunological properties (4). The longterm prognosis of choroidal melanoma is much better so that it seems worthwhile to look for a correlation between the occurence of metastases and neopterin levels.

Material and methods

Urinary neopterin excretion was determined in the urine of 110 patients with a malignant melanoma of the choroid. The clinical situation of these patients was classified as: a) untreated, b) incomplete tumor regression after brachytherapy with [106]Ru/[106]Rh-applicators, c) presumed complete tumor regression after brachytherapy, d) metastatic disease, e) delayed diagnosis of metastases during follow up or orbital infiltration at the time of analysis. Only patients with a clinical follow-up of 14 months were enroled in the study. The results of tumor patients were compared with those from age and sex-matched healthy volunteers (n = 92). Samples of all tumor patients and healthy volunteers were collected between 9 and 12 o'clock a.m. in order to avoid any bias by circadian variations (15). The determination of urinary neopterin was performed under oxidative conditions by fluorometric HPLC-detection (350/450 nm). Samples were analysed according to Goldberg's (6) modification of the Fukushima and Nixon (5) procedure. Immediately after collection 1ml of each specimen was incubated with 300 µl of 1 mol/l HCl and 200 µl of 5g/l J_2/10g/l KJ in 0.1 mol/l HCl in darkness. One hour later 200 µl ascorbic acid was added to reduce excess iodine. Further purification was perfomed with Dowex H⁺ (50 WX 8, 100–200 mesh). Urinary creatinine concentrations were determined with the Boehringer kit No. 124192 (Boehringer/Mannheim). All pterins used as references were from Dr. Schircks (Jona/Switzerland). The quality parameters of neopterin determination (standard solution) were evaluated as: lower detection limit = 13 pmol/l, recovery = 97.7%, non-linearity ≤ 2%, variation coefficients of within-run imprecision = 0.9%, variation coefficient of between-day imprecision = 2.7%.

Results

Basic statistical information on the examined groups of patients and healthy controls are listed in table I. At the time of urine collection two of the

Table I. Age and sex ratio of the study groups.

	n	Age (years) mean ± SD	Age range (years)	Sex ♀ : ♂
Tumor patients	110	61.4 ± 11.8	48 – 88	59 : 51
Healthy controls	92	59.2 ± 12.5	47 – 84	48 : 44

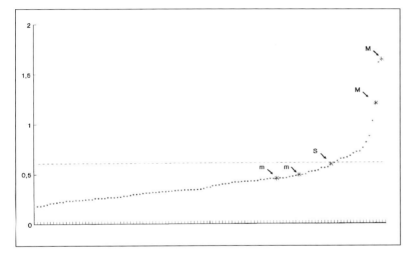

Figure 1. Neopterin excretion in urine of 110 patients with a choroidal melanoma (mmol/mol creatinine). (-----) = Upper limit (mean + 2 SD) of healthy controls. M→∗ = Patients with metastatic disease at the time of analysis. m→∗ = Patients with later diagnosis of metastases during clinical follow-up (7 and 10 months after neopterin analyses). S→∗ = Patient with transscleral infiltration of the orbit at the time of analysis.

Table II. Average excretion of neopterin in urine of patients with malignant melanoma of the choroid and in healthy controls. Two patients with metastatic disease are not included in this table.

	n	Neopterin (mean ± SD) µmol/mol creatinine
Untreated tumor patients	21	377 ± 165
Partial tumor regression	37	419 ± 223
Complete tumor regression	50	399 ± 174
Healthy controls	92	410 ± 101

melanoma patients presented metastatic disease (stage IVb) and one patient a transscleral infiltration of the orbit. In two further patients metastases were diagnosed during the clinical follow-up period. The analytical results of neopterin excretion in tumor patients compared to the normal range of healthy volunteers (mean + 2 standard deviations) are shown in figure 1. Results of the majority of patients were below the upper normal limit. Neopterin in urine of those two patients with verified metastatic disease (M→∗ in figure 1) were greatly elevated. Neopterin excretion of two other patients with a latency of diagnosed metastases (M→∗ in figure 1) and the one patient with orbital tumor infiltration at the time of analysis (S→∗ in figure 1) rank near the upper normal limit. The results of neopterin measurements grouped according to the tumor state are listed in table II. The results of patient groups without metastatic disease were not significantly different compared to healthy normals according to the F-test (ANOVA) at a $p < 0.1$.

Discussion

The determination of urinary neopterin excretion in patients with a malignant melanoma of the choroid showes a relative low percentage of elevated concentrations beyond the upper limit. This result resembles the situation of other malignant neoplastic diseases (2, 11, 16) and infers that neopterin is not a suitable tool as a marker for the diagnosis or differential diagnosis of this kind of tumor. The missing of an indicator effect of neopterin regarding the primary malignant melanoma of the choroid may perhaps be the result of the relative low tumor mass at the time of discovery compared to other malignant diseases. Second, the missing of a neopterin elevation in reaction to the primar tumor may be a consequence of subnormal immunreactivity at least in a subgroup of patients as previously reported (1, 3). Although the number of critical cases in this series was relatively low it seems that neopterin is informative with respect to metastatic spread of choroidal melanomas. The magnitude of neopterin concentrations in these patients is so far above and well discriminated from the upper normal limit that neopterin can be regarded as a helpful tool in the diagnosis of metastatic stage in patients with this kind of malignant disease.

References

1. Dieckhues B, Schmitz G (1986) T4- und T8-Lymphozytenbestimmungen beim malignen Melanom der Aderhaut und ihre Bedeutung für die Diagnostik. Fortschr Ophthalmol 83:480
2. Dhondt JL, Hayte JM, Bonneterre J, Adenis L, Demaille A, Ardouin P, Farriaux JP (1982) In: Wachter H, Curtius HC, Pfleiderer W (eds) Biochemical and clinical aspects of pteridines. W de Gruyter, Berlin, pp 133-140
3. Flynn K, Feldberg NT, Koegel A, Hager R, Shields JA, Augsburger JJ, Donoso LA (1986) Lymphocyte subpopulation before therapy in patients with uveal malignant melanoma. Am J Ophthalmol 101:160
4. Folberg R, Donoso LA, Atkinson B, Ernst C, Herlyn M, Arbizo VV (1985) An antimelanoma monoclonal antibody and the histopathology of uveal melanomas. Arch Ophthalmol 103:275
5. Fukushima T, Nixon JC (1980) Analysis of reduced forms of biopterin in biological tissues and fluids. Anal Biochem 102:176
6. Goldberg M, Gasser F, Merkenschläger M (1989) Studies and comparison of urinary pteridine patterns in dogs and cats and their alteration in various neoplasias and virus infections. Pteridines 1:29
7. Hausen A, Fuchs D, Reibnegger G, Werner ER, Wachter H (1989) Neopterin in clinical use. Pteridines 1:3
8. Iino T, Watanabe H, Gyure WL, Mazda T, Mieno H, Tsusue M (1993) In: JE Ayling, MG Nair, CM Baugh (eds) Chemistry and biology of pteridines and folates. Plenum, New York, pp 243-246
9. Müller MM, Curtius HC, Herold M, Huber C (1991) Neopterin in clinical praxis. Clin Chim Acta 210:1
10. Mura P, Barriere M, Papet Y, Reiss D, Camenen I, Vaillant L, Lorette G (1989) The clinical significance of urinary neopterin in the follow-up of patients after excision of malignant melanoma. Pteridines 1:19
11. Reibnegger G, Fuchs D, Hausen A, Wachter H, Bichler E, Böheim K (1982) In: Wachter H, Curtius HC, Pfleiderer W (eds) Biochemical and clinical aspects of pteridines. Vol 1, W de Gruyter, Berlin, pp 207-215
12. Reibnegger G, Bichler A, Fuchs D, Hausen A, Werner ER, Wachter H (1986) In: Wüst G (ed) Tumormarker. Aktuelle Aspekte und klinische Relevanz. Steinkopf, Darmstadt, pp 284-288
13. Wachter H, Fuchs A, Hausen A, Reibnegger G, Werner ER (1989) Neopterin as marker for the activation of cellular immunity: Immunological basis and clinical application. Adv Clin Chem 27:81
14. Wachter H, Fuchs D, Hausen A, Reibnegger G, Weiss G, Werner ER, Werner-Feldmayer G (1992) Neopterin, biochemistry, methods, clinical application. W de Gruyter, Berlin
15. Wever RA, Cremer-Bartels G, Krause K, Gerding H (1991) In: Blau N, Curtius HC, Levine RA (eds) Pterins and biogenic amines in neurology, pediatrics, and immunology. Lakeshore Publ, Grosse Pointe, pp 119-134
16. Wiegele J, Margreiter R, Huber C, Dworzak, E, Fuchs D, Hausen A, Reibnegger G, Wachter H (1984) In: Pfleiderer W, Wachter H, Curtius HC (eds) Biochemical and clinical aspects of pteridines. Vol 3, W de Gruyter, Berlin, pp 417-424

Address for correspondence:
Priv.-Doz. Dr. med. H. Gerding
Abteilung für Augenheilkunde
Universität Münster
Domagkstraße 15
D-48129 Münster, Germany

Quantitative determination (ELISA) of pyruvate kinase type tumor M2 – A new tumor marker

U. Scheefers-Borchel[a], H. Scheefers[a], A. Michel[a], H. Will[a], G. Fischer[b], D. Basenau[b], N. Dahlmann[c], R. Laumen[d], S. Mazurek[e], E. Eigenbrodt[e]

[a]ScheBo Tech GmbH Wettenberg, [b]Center for Pathology of the University of Göttingen, [c]Center Laboratory of General Hospital Hamburg-Harburg, [d]Clinic Seltersberg, [e]Institute of Biochemistry, Veterinary Medicine of the University of Gießen, Germany

Introduction

Tumor formation is generally linked to increased aerobic glycolysis. There are multiple steps involved in the generation of cells with aerobic glycolytic capacities. Some steps include the switch in the isoenzyme equipment and an increase in total enzymatic capacities. Studies on a variety of tumors either of animal or human origin demonstrate that all tumors so far investigated are equipped with a special isoenzyme called pyruvate kinase type tumor M2 (Tu M2-PK) (1, 2). We were able to produce specific monoclonal antibodies to Tu M2-PK which do not crossreact with other pyruvate kinases (type L, R, M1 and M2). In contrast to other pyruvate kinases which mainly exist in a tetrameric form Tu M2-PK occurs in a dimeric or monomeric form that is phosphorylated in serine and tyrosine by onc-gene coded kinases (3, 4).
We produced two monoclonal antibodies against different epitopes of Tu M2-PK. By means of these antibodies a sensitive immunoassay has been developed for the quantitative determination of Tu M2-PK in sera of tumor patients (5).

Methods

Quantitative Determination of Tu M2-PK: The test is a two step sandwich immunoassay using one monoclonal antibody coated to microtiter plates (6 x 16 determinations) and a second monoclonal antibody conjugated to HRP (ScheBo Tech GmbH, Wettenberg). After incubation of five standards and samples (serum) for 60 minutes and a washing step the HRP conjugated antibody was added for 60 minutes. The unbound conjugate was removed by a second washing step. After addition of ABTS (ready to use) the absorbance was measured photometrically after 45 minutes at 405 nm and Tu M2-PK concentrations were calculated from the standard curve.

Patients

Sera of 195 blood donors served as control group. 800 sera from patients with different diseases of the lung have been collected over a period of nine months and Tu M2-PK concentration has been determined in these sera in a blind study. After that a doctoral candidate looked up the diagnosis of these patients in the clinic files. In addition sera of patients with tumors other than lung were analyzed in a prospective study.

Results

In order to determine the intra-assay precision of the quantitative determination of Tu M2-PK sera from six patients with different concentrations of Tu M2-PK were measured 20-fold. The ranges of variation coefficients were between 2.4% and 7% with a mean value of 3.5%. When six sera with different concentrations of Tu M2-PK have been measured on ten different days the variation coefficients of the inter-assay precision ranged between 3.3% and 7.5% with a mean value of 5.8%.

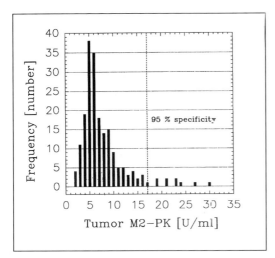

Figure 1. Tu M2-PK concentration in sera of 195 blood donors. The histogram shows the frequency (actual numbers) versus Tu M2-PK concentration (U/ml). A cut-off value of 17 U/ml corresponds to 95% specificity.

Table I. Summary of Tu M2-PK determination in patients with different diseases of the lung. Sensitivities have been calculated at a cut-off value of 22.5 U/ml.

	Total number	False negative
Tumor (untreated)	116	46
adenocarcinoma	30	12
squamous cell carcinoma	60	17
small cell carcinoma	26	17
	Total number	False positive
Non tumor	142	14
benign	37	2
TBC and inflammation	105	12

Prevalence = 45%, negative predictive value = 83%, positive predictive value = 73%, efficiency = 77%.

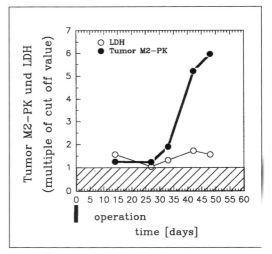

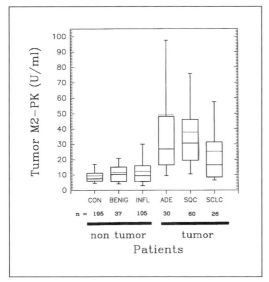

Figure 2. Concentration of Tu M2-PK in the various study groups (blood donors and patients with benign and malignant diseases of the lung). Data are presented as multiple box and whisker plots showing median value (horizontal line), mean value (dashed line) and upper and lower quartile. CON = blood donors, BENIG = patients with benign diseases of the lung, ADE = patients with adenocarcinoma, SQC = patients with squamous cell carcinoma, SCLC = patients with small cell lung carcinoma.

Figure 3. Follow-up study of a patient with progressive large cell carcinoma of the lung (stadium M1). The cut-off value was set to 22.5 U/ml. Tu M2-PK (●) has been determined by ELISA, LDH has been measured enzymatically (○).

The distribution of Tu M2-PK in sera of 195 blood donors is shown in figure 1. Statistical analysis (normality test according to Kolmogorov-Smirnov failed) showed that the distribution of Tu M2-PK in sera of blood donors is a non-gaussian. A cut-off value of 17 U/ml corresponds to 95% specificity of blood donors.

The clinical significance of Tu M2-PK was evaluated in sera from patients with benign and

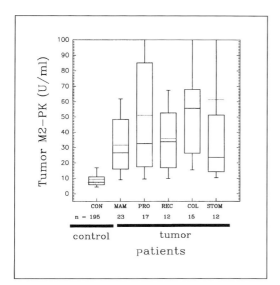

Figure 4. Concentration of Tu M2-PK in blood donors and patients with different malignant diseases (box and whisker plots). CON = blood donors, MAM = mamma carcinoma, PRO = prostata carcinoma, REC = rectum carcinoma, COL = colon carcinoma, STOM = stomach carcinoma.

malignant diseases of the lung. The sera were not from selected patients but reflected the patients from the Lung Clinic at the University of Gießen. More than 800 sera were analysed. For statistical analysis sera from tumor patients were only included if patients have not received a tumor therapy. Statistical multiple comparison of different patients groups has been done according to *Kruskal-Wallis* one way anova on ranks.
In figure 2 the distribution of Tu M2-PK concentration in sera of blood donors, patients with benign lung diseases, TBC and inflammation in comparison to patients with different histological cell typs of lung cancer is shown. Values for the 50% percentiles (median) were: blood donors = 7.5 U/ml; patients with benign diseases of the lung (sarcoidosis, fibrosis and asthma) = 10.2 U/ml; TBC and inflammation = 9.5 U/ml; adenocarcinoma = 27.1 U/ml; squamous cell carcinoma = 30.2 U/ml; small cell lung carcinoma = 16.9 U/ml. It could be shown by the Mann-Whitney rank sum test that there is a statistically significant difference ($p < 0.001$) between the group with benign diseases of the lung and the tumor group.
In table I the data of the clinical study are summarized. A cut-off value of Tu M2-PK of 22.5 U/ml corresponds to 95% specificity of patients with benign diseases (sarcoidosis, fibrosis, asthma, n = 37).
This cut-off value corresponds to 89% specificity in patients with inflammation or tuberculosis (n = 105). All patients with benign diseases of the lung were included in this study, also those with multiple diseases. The highest sensitivities (72%) could be measured in patients with squamous cell carcinoma (n = 60). In patients with adenocarcinoma (n = 30) the sensitivity was 60%. The sensitivity for small cell carcinoma was 35%. The sensitivity of this group increased to 80% when only patients with extensive disease have been taken into calculation (data not shown). Because patients included in this study were not selected but reflected the common distribution of patients in that clinic, the efficiency (75%), the negative predictive value (83%) and the positive predictive value (73%) at a prevalence of 45% could be determined (table I).
From several tumor patients several blood samples had been taken under tumor therapy over a period of several months. It could be demonstrated that the determination of Tu M2-PK might be well suited for follow-up studies after operation or under tumor therapy (figure 3).
A second clinical study demonstrates that Tu M2-PK significantly increases also in sera of tumor patients other than lung.
In this study sera from following tumor patients were analyzed: mamma carcinoma (n = 23), prostata carcinoma (n = 17), rectum carcinoma (n = 12), colon carcinoma (n = 15), stomach carcinoma (n = 12).
The distribution of Tu M2-PK concentrations in respect to different types of cancer in comparison to blood donors is illustrated in figure 4. Statistical analysis by the Mann-Whitney rank sum test showed that there is a statistically significant difference ($p < 0.001$) between each tumor group and the group of blood donors. The values for the 50% percentiles were 26.6 U/ml for mamma carcinoma, 32.7 U/ml for prostata carcinoma, 33.9 U/ml for rectum carcinoma, 55.7 U/ml for colon carcinoma, 23.8 U/ml for stomach carcinoma and 7.5 U/ml for blood donors.
Summarizing, we have produced monoclonal antibodies against a special isoenzyme of pyruvate kinase, called pyruvate kinase type tumor M2 (Tu M2-PK). By means of these antibodies a sensitive

immunoassay has been developed. In contrast to other pyruvate kinases which mainly exist in a tetrameric form Tu M2-PK exists in a dimeric or monomeric form. The onc-gene coded pp60-src tyrosinekinase phosphorylates the isoenzyme at the amino acid tyrosine (3).

In addition phosphorylation of serine is induced by growth factors. These phosphorylations induce the breakdown of tetrameric pyruvate kinase to the dimeric and monomeric form.

Monoclonal antibodies used in the immunoassay only detect Tu M2-PK and do not crossreact with other pyruvate kinases.

The quantitative determination of Tu M2-PK measures a changed metabolic state which is specific for tumor cells. Therefore the Tu M2-PK assay is not organ specific. The clinical study with 800 patients with different lung diseases showed that Tu M2-PK significantly increases in tumor patients in comparison to the benign control group with a p-value of < 0.001 (*Kruskal-Wallis* one way anova on ranks).

We could further demonstrate that even in tumor stadium I and II of NSCLC patients Tu M2-PK increased significantly (data not shown).

In patients with SCLC only patients with extensive disease showed an increase of Tu M2-PK.

It could be shown in this study that Tu M2-PK might be a valuable tool for therapy control and follow-up of lung cancer patients. A prospective study with patients other than lung cancer also demonstrated a significantly increase of Tu M2-PK (figure 4).

Studies are in progress to correlate the diagnostic sensitivity of Tu M2-PK with other established tumor markers. Especially for lung cancer patients with NSCLC Tu M2-PK will be correlated with the new tumor marker CYFRA 21-1 (6).

References

1. Eigenbrodt E, Reinacher M, Scheefers-Borchel U, Scheefers H, Friis R (1992) Double role for pyruvate kinase type M2 in the expansion of phosphometabolite pools found in tumor cells. Critical Reviews in Oncogenesis 3 (1, 2):91–115
2. Fischer G, Holzrichter S, Reinacher M, Heinrichs M, Dembowski J, Eigenbrodt E (1989) Immunhistochemische Darstellung der L- und M2-Pyruvatkinase in primären Nierenzellkarzinomen und deren Metastasen. Verh Dtsch Ges Path 73:422–427
3. Presek P, Reinacher M, Eigenbrodt E (1988) Pyruvate kinase type M2 is phosphorylated at tyrosine residues in cells transformed by Rous sarcoma virus. FEBS Letters 242:194–198
4. Oude Weernink PA, Rijksen G, van der Heijden MCM, Staal GEJ (1990) Phosphorylation of pyruvate kinase type K in human gliomas by a cyclic adenosine 5'-monophosphate-independent protein kinase. Cancer Res 50:4604–4610
5. Mazurek S, Scheefers-Borchel U, Scheefers H, Michel A, Fischer G, Basenau D, Dahlmann N, Laumen R, Eigenbrodt E (1993) Die Bedeutung der Pyruvatkinase in der Onkologie. notabene medici 3:97–104
6. Stieber P, Hasholzner U, Bodenmüller H, Nagel D, Sunder-Plassmann L, Dienemann H, Meier W, Fateh-Moghadam A (1993) CYFRA 21-1, a new marker in lung cancer. Cancer 72:707–713

Address for correspondence:
Dr. rer. nat. U. Scheefers-Borchel
ScheBo Tech GmbH
Bahnhofstraße 6
D-35435 Wettenberg, Germany

In Vitro Diagnosis

New Assays

Cobas® Core CA 72-4 EIA: Analytical performance of a fast and automated determination for TAG-72 antigen on the Cobas® Core immunochemistry analyzer

V. Henne, S. Jung, M. Schmutz
Roche Diagnostic Systems, a Division of F. Hoffmann-La Roche Ltd., Basel, Switzerland

Introduction

Tumor-associated glycoprotein TAG-72 is a protein of high molecular weight (220–400 kD) with mucin-like properties. The isolation of TAG-72 was first described by Colcher et al. due to its reactivity with the monoclonal antibody B72.3 (1, 2), which was prepared against a membrane-enriched fraction of human mammary carcinoma. The epitope recognized by the B72.3 antibody is a repetitive sialo-oligosaccharide structure (3). The second monoclonal antibody, termed CC-49, which is also reactive to an oligosaccharide epitope on TAG-72 was developed using pure antigen for the immunisation (4). It has been shown that the TAG-72 antigen is different from other tumor-associated glycoproteins such as carcinoembryonic antigen (CEA), CA 19-9, CA 125, or CA 15-3 (5). Assays employing the combination of these two monoclonal antibodies have been established for the detection of TAG-72 in human serum and are termed CA 72-4. Clinical studies demonstrated that highly elevated serum levels of TAG-72 are mainly observed in patients suffering from gastric cancer (6, 7) and that the clinical sensitivity of this marker is superior to CEA or CA 19-9 (6).

The Cobas® Core CA 72-4 EIA is a new, non-competitive enzyme-immunoassay which employs the two monoclonal antibodies B72.3 and CC-49 in the original test configuration developed by Centocor (Malvern, PA, USA). In comparison to other CA 72-4 assays, the test has a very short total incubation time and can be performed with the Cobas® Core EIA semi-automated system or on the Cobas Core® Core Random Access Analyzer. A high analytical sensitivity, the low sample volume and excellent precision for serum samples are further aspects of the automated determination of CA 72-4 with this assay.

CA 72-4 assay design

The main characteristics of the Cobas® Core CA 72-4 EIA are summarized in table I. The two-step enzyme immunoassay based on the sandwich principle has a total incubation time of 75 minutes. The four standards cover a measuring range from 1 to 100 U/ml for serum or plasma samples. The assay employs the monoclonal antibodies B 72.3 and CC-49 in the normal configuration which is also used by the Centocor-IRMA. The CC-49 antibody is used for capturing in conjunction with the horse-radish peroxidase labeled B72.3 antibody for tracing. Reliable results can also be obtained for very low CA 72-4 concentrations due to the high analytical sensitivity of the assay which is less than 0.3

Table I. Main characteristics of the Cobas® Core CA 72-4 EIA assay design.

Test principle:	two-step-assay, non-competitive, enzyme immunoassay
Total assay time:	75 min
Measuring range:	1–100 U/ml
Capturing antibody:	CC-49
Conjugate antibody:	B 72.3
Sample:	serum; plasma
Analytical sensitivity:	< 0.3 U/ml
High-dose hook effekt:	> 15,000 U/ml
Specificity:	no detectable interferences with: CEA, CA 19-9, CA 125, MCA only low interference with CA 15-3

Table II. Reproducibility of automated CA 72-4 determinations on the Cobas® Core Analyzer ntra-assay coefficient of variation was calculated from 12-fold measurement; the reproducibility of the test between test series was calculated from duplicate determination of the sample in 12 independent test runs.

Intra-assay precision

Sample	Mean	CV (%)
Serum 1	6.7 U/ml	4.7
Serum 2	14.1 U/ml	3.2
Serum 3	44.3 U/ml	2.2
Serum 4	73.3 U/ml	5.5

Inter-assay precision

Sample	Mean	CV (%)
Serum 1	4.6 U/ml	4.9
Serum 2	10.3 U/ml	4.5
Serum 3	29.1 U/ml	3.7
Serum 4	41.8 U/ml	3.0
Serum 5	59.3 U/ml	3.0
Serum 6	79.5 U/ml	3.1

Table III. CA 72-4 recovery rates from spiked blood donors. The recovery rates were calculated from the amount of CA 72-4 antigen added to blood donor samples and that value measured.

Antigen added (U/ml)	Measured value (U/ml)	Recovery (%)
12.0	11.5	96
15.0	14.4	96
50.0	47.0	94
85.0	78.8	93

of CA 72-4 antigen is not influenced by other known carbohydrate proteins used for oncological purposes, the specificity of the antibody combination has been tested. No interferences were detected with CEA, CA 19-9, MCA or CA 125 and only slight interference was found with CA 15-3.

Precision

It is well known that the precision for the quantitation of most oncological carbohydrate antigens from serum samples may be a problem. Therefore, the coefficients of variation (CV) for the intra-assay and the inter-assay precisions were determined for sets of serum samples on the

U/ml. CA 72-4 serum concentrations of patients suffering from gastric cancer normally do not exceed 10,000 U/ml, and no high-dose hook effect could be observed below a concentration of 15,000 U/ml. To guarantee that the quantitation

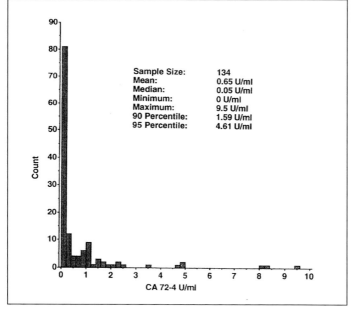

Figure 1. Frequency distribution of CA 72-4 levels in 134 blood donors.

Cobas® Core Analyzer (table II). In the intra-assay precision study the CVs for four sera were calculated from 12-fold replicates each. For CA 72-4 concentrations ranging from 6.7 to 73.3 U/ml, CVs from 4.7 to 5.5% were obtained, but were mostly below 5%.

For investigating the inter-assay precision, six sera were run on the Cobas® Core Analyzer for duplicate determinations in twelve independent runs. The CV-profile was similar to that obtained for the within-run precisions. The CVs in this investigation were clearly below 5%.

Recovery rates from spiked blood donors

The recovery rates of spiked CA 72-4 antigen to blood donor sera were determined as demonstrated in table III For this investigation a known amount of CA 72-4 pure antigen was added to blood donor sera with CA 72-4 concentrations less than 1.0 U/ml. Afterwards, the CA 72-4 contents of the prepared sera were measured. The values obtained were percentually related to the CA 72-4 amounts added.
The calculated recovery rates ranged between 93 and 96%.

Determination of sera from blood donors

Randomly selected sera (n = 134) from apparently healthy blood donors were determined in the Cobas® Core CA 72-4 EIA. The measured CA 72-4 levels were distributed as illustrated in figure 1. The CA 72-4 values ranged from 0 to 9.5 U/ml, with a mean value of 0.65 U/ml. The cut-off value which corresponds to the 95% percentile was calculated by statistical analysis. A value of 4.6 U/ml was obtained.

Determination of sera from cancer patients

The Cobas® Core CA 72-4 EIA can be performed on the Cobas Core random access analyzer as well as in a semi-automated version employing the same set of assay reagents. The equivalence between these two different methods is shown in figure 2. For this experiment 71 samples taken from patients with benign and malignant gastrointestinal carcinoma were assayed in duplicate on the Cobas® Core Analyzer and in parallel with the semi-automated test version. The patient values of these sera ranged between 0.1 and 82.2 U/ml. Corresponding data pairs were compared by

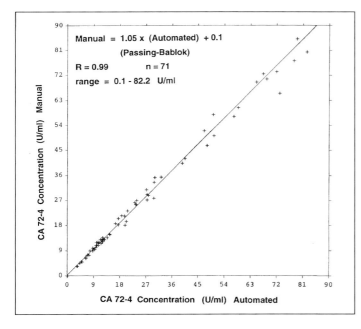

Figure 2. Comparison of the semi-automated (Cobas® Core EIA system) to the fully automated (Cobas® Core Analyzer) CA 72-4 determination for sera of patients with several benign and malignant gastrointestinal diseases.

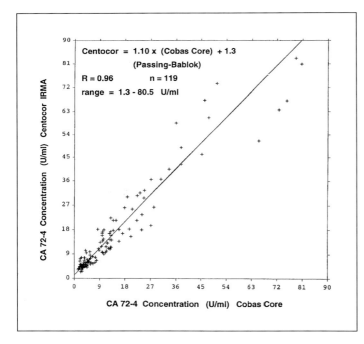

Figure 3. Comparison of the CA 72-4 determinations on the Cobas® Core Analyzer to the Centocor-IRMA method for sera of patients with several benign and malignant gastrointestinal diseases.

statistical analysis using the method of *Passing* and *Bablock*. The results showed an excellent correlation as indicated by the coefficient of correlation of 0.99. The slope of the regression line was close to 1.

A similar investigation was also carried out on 119 patient sera by comparing results generated with the Cobas® Core Analyzer to those obtained with the CA 72-4 radioimmunometric assay from Centocor, which is considered to be the reference assay for CA 72-4. As shown in figure 3, the patient values ranged from 1.3 to 80.5 U/ml. Also in this case the values generated with both assays correlated well (R = 0.96). The Cobas® Core values were only 10% lower than the corresponding data obtained with the Centocor assay as indicated by the slope of the regression line (1.10).

Conclusion

The Cobas® Core CA 72-4 is a two-step enzyme immunoassay with a very short total incubation time, which makes its performance very suitable for the automated determinations that can be carried out on the Cobas® Core Analyzer. The high accordance of this method to the semi-automated version allows the switching from one version to the other without any complication for patient monitoring. The low sample volume also may help to reduce possible matrix effects of the serum sample. The high analytical sensitivity and the excellent reproducibility offers the advantage to determine CA 72-4 concentrations over the whole measuring range with a high degree of reliability. In contrast to many other carbohydrate proteins (CA 19-9, CA 15-3, CA 125) the CA 72-4 determination exhibits a very good accordance between different methods, i.e. EIA versus IRMA.

References

1. Colcher D, Horan Hand P, Nuti M, Schlom JA (1981) A spectrum of monoclonal antibodies reactive with human mammary tumor cells. Proc Natl Acad Sci USA 78:3199–3203
2. Johnson VG, Schlom J, Paterson AJ, Bennett J, Magnani JL, Colcher D (1986) Analysis of a human tumor-associated glycoprotein (TAG-72) identified by monoclonal antibody B72.3. Cancer Res 46:850–857
3. Kjeldsen T, Clausen H, Hirohashi S, Ogawa T, Iijima H, Hakomori S (1988) Preparation and characterization of monoclonal antibodies directed to the tumor-associated o-linked sialosyl-2- 6a-n-acetyl-

galactosaminyl (sialosyl-tn) Epitope. Cancer Res 48:2214–2200
4. Gero EJ, Colcher D, Ferroni P, Melsheimer R, Giani S, Schlom J, Kaplan P (1989) CA 72-4 Radioimmunoassay for the detection of the TAG-72 carcinoma-associated antigen in serum of patients. J Clin Lab Anal 3:360–369
5. Paterson AJ, Schlom J, Sears HF, Bennett J, Colcher D (1986) A Radioimmunoassay for the detection of a human tumor-associated glycoprotein (TAG-72) using monoclonal antibody B72.3. Int J Cancer 37:659–666
6. Heptner G, Domschke S, Domschke W (189) Comparison of CA 72-4 with CA 19-9 and carcinoembryonic antigen in the serodiagnostics of gastrointestinal malignancies. Scand J Gastroenterol 24:745–750
7. Ohuchi N, Takahashi K, Matoba N, Sato T, Taira Y, Sakai N, Masuda M, Mori S (1989) Comparison of serum assays for TAG-72, CA 19-9 and CEA in gastrointestinal carcinoma patients. Jpn J Clin Oncol 19:242–248

Address for correspondence:
Dr. rer. nat. V. Henne
Roche Diagnostic Systems
a Division of F. Hoffmann-La Roche Ltd.
CH-4002 Basel, Switzerland

CA 72-4 in gastrointestinal malignancies – Experience with a new assay

D. Lentfer, Edith Greiner-Mai, M. Drahovsky

Byk-Sangtec Diagnostica GmbH, Dietzenbach, Germany

Introduction

TAG 72 (CA 72-4), a mucinous-type glycoprotein, was discovered by *Colcher* et al. in 1981 (1). This cancer-associated mucin shows high serum concentrations in patients suffering from gastric cancer, colorectal cancer and mucinous-type ovarian cancer (2–5). Moreover, CA 72-4 appears to possess the highest sensitivity of all known tumor markers in gastric cancer (6). Therefore, its determination is an important tool in the follow-up of such patients. IRMA-mat® CA 72-4, a recently developed coated-tube-format test, was evaluated in this study. The technical quality and the clinical value were compared to those of other commercial CA 72-4 assays.

Materials and methods

IRMA-mat® CA 72-4

The new immunoradiometric assay (Byk-Sangtec Diagnostica) is based on the coated-tube technique and uses a ^{125}iodine label for detection. Two monoclonal antibodies, cc49 (solid phase) and B72.3 (tracer) are used in this "sandwich"-type assay (7, 8). Trapping and detection of the CA 72-4 antigen are performed in a two-step-incubation protocol (figure 1). The fully automated performance of the assay is possible with the RIA-mat® 280.

Comparative CA 72-4 assay

For comparison, the immunoradiometric tests CA 72-4 IRMA (Centocor), CA 72-4 ELSA (CIS) and the immunoluminometric assay LIA-mat® CA 72-4 (Byk-Sangtec Diagnostica) were used. All assays were performed according to the instruction manuals.

Serum samples

The following samples were included in the study: 65 sera from apparently healthy males and females, from 51 patients with benign gastrointestinal diseases (colorectum, duodenum, liver, pancreas), 65 with gastric cancer, 33 with colonic and 39 with pancreatic carcinoma respectively.

Results and discussion

Precision, reproducibility and linearity upon dilution

The results of the present study indicate the good comparability of the IRMA-mat® CA 72-4 with other CA 72-4 assays. Very good precision and reproducibility were obtained with the IRMA-mat® CA 27-4. This is demonstrated by the precision profile of duplicate determinations (mean CV = 8.9%; working range > 2.6 U/ml) and the reproducibility profile of control and pool sera (18.4 U/ml: CV = 5.7%; 15.6 U/ml: CV = 4.6%; 5.7 U/ml: CV = 7.6%) (figures 2 and 3). For linearity studies, high-titred CA 72-4 samples were diluted with the kit diluent. A strictly linear response was observed over the whole standard range (r = 0.9965 – 0.9985) (figure 4).

Comparison with other methods

Comparisons between the IRMA-mat® CA 72-4 and other CA 72-4 assays were run with low and

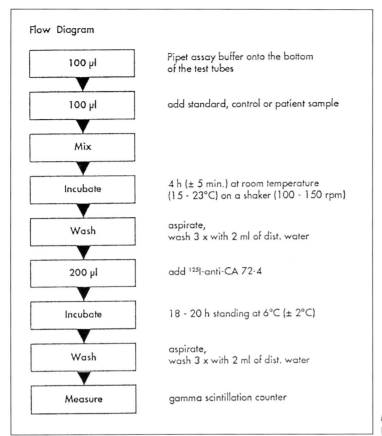

Figure 1. Flow diagram for IRMA-mat® CA 72-4.

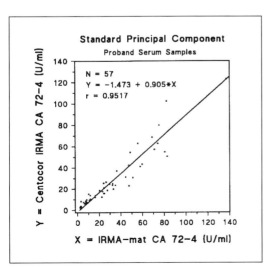

Figure 2a. Correlation IRMA-mat® CA 72-4 versus IRMA CA 72-4 (Centocor).

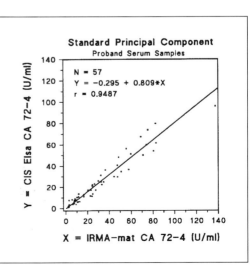

Figure 2b. Correlation IRMA-mat® CA 72-4 versus CA 72-4 ELSA (CIS).

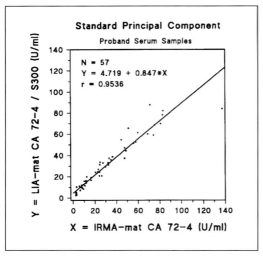

Figure 2c. Correlation IRMA-mat® CA 72-4 versus LIA-mat® CA 72-4.

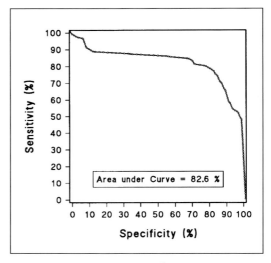

Figure 3a. ROC curve IRMA-mat® CA 72-4. Negatives: benign gastrointestinal diseases, n = 41; positives: malignant gastrointestinal diseases, n = 68.

high-titred samples from all three groups. Good correlations were found with both IRMAs and the ILMA (figure 2 a-c; correlation coefficient r = 0.95).

Reference range

To determine the reference range, samples from healthy male and female subjects and from patients with benign gastrointestinal diseases were used. In the healthy volunteers with a mean at 2.20 U/ml, the 95-percentile was found at 5 U/ml. It was striking that men showed lower CA 72-4 serum values than women (95-percentile: 4.1 U/ml versus 6.1 U/ml). The benign group – mean at 2.21 U/ml and 95-percentile at 8.4 U/ml showed elevations up to 10 U/ml in hepatitis and liver cirrhosis.

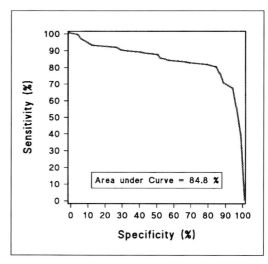

Figure 3b. ROC curve LIA-mat® CA 72-4. Negatives: benign gastrointestinal diseases, n = 41; positives: malignant gastrointestinal diseases, n = 68.

Follow-up

The ROC analysis revealed an excellent discrimination between the benign and malignant groups when measured with the IRMA-mat® CA 72-4. This was in accordance with other methods (figure 3 a,b). Finally, retrospective studies from repeated sampling in gastric cancer patients support the equivalence of the IRMA-mat® CA 72-4 with other commercial CA 72-4 assays (figure 4).

Summary

TAG 72, a mucinous-type glycoprotein, was discovered by *Colcher* et al. in 1983. It appears to possess the highest sensitivity of all known tumor markers for gastric cancer. The IRMA-mat® CA 72-4 assay (Byk-Sangtec Diagnostica) is based on the "sandwich principle". It uses both of

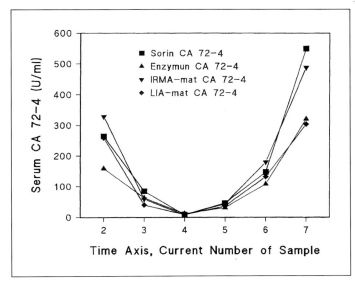

Figure 4. Follow-up of a patient with gastric cancer.

Colcher's antibodies, cc49 for the solid phase (coated tubes) and B72.3 for the tracer (^{125}I-labeled). The incubation is done according to the conventional 2-step method. This study describes the technical data of the new assay: << 10% for intra- and inter-assay precision, 95–105% recovery upon dilution. The IRMA-mat® CA 72-4 shows a good comparability with other radioactive and non-radioactive methods (correlation coefficient: 0.95). Sera from healthy subjects are found below 4 U/ml. Benign diseases of the gastrointestinal tract do not lead to remarkable elevations in CA 72-4 serum levels. Retrospective studies show the consistency of IRMA-mat® CA 72-4 results with the clinical status and with results from reference methods.

References

1. Colcher D, Horan Hand P, Nuti M, Schlom J (1981) A spectrum of monoclonal antibodies reactive with human mammary tumor cells. Proc Nat Acad Sci USA 78:3199–3203
2. Byrne DJ, Browning MCK, Cushieri A (1990) CA 72-4: A new marker for gastric cancer. Br J Surg 77:1010–1013
3. Guadagni F, Rosselli F, Cosinelli M et al (1993) TAG-72 (CA 72-4 Assay) as a complementary serum tumor antigen to carcinoembryonic antigen in monitoring patients with colorectal cancer. Cancer 72:2098–2106
4. Bayerl B, Stieber P, Albiez M et al (1990) Significance of CA 72-4 in the diagnosis of ovarian cancer. In: Klapdor R (ed) Recent results in tumor diagnosis and therapy. Zuckschwerdt, Munich, pp 111–112
5. Soper JT, Verda J, Hunter MD et al (1990) Preoperative serum tumor-associated antigen levels in women with pelvic masses. J Obstet Gyn 75:249–254
6. Brandt B, Liffers E, Sasse W, Assmann G (1992) CA 72-4: The tumor marker for gastric carcinoma. In: Klapdor R (ed) Tumor associated antigens, oncogenes, receptors, cytokines in tumor diagnosis and therapy at the beginning of the nineties. Zuckschwerdt, Munich, pp 10–12
7. Paterson AJ, Schlom J, Sears HF, Bennett J, Colcher D (1986) A radioimmunoassay for the detection of a human tumor-associated glycoprotein (TAG-72) using monoclonal antibody B 72.3. Int J Cancer 37(5):659–666
8. Klug TL, Sattler MA, Colcher D, Schlom J (1986) Monoclonal anitbody immunoradiometric assay for an antigenic determinant (CA 72) on a novel pancarcinoma antigen (TAG-72). Int J Cancer 38(5): 661–669

Address for correspondence:
Dr. Edith Greiner-Mai
Byk-Sangtec Diagnostika GmbH
Von Hevesy-Straße 3
D-63128 Dietzenbach, Germany

Immunoluminometric determination of CA 72-4 in the follow-up of gynecological tumors

T. Heinze[a], R. Theunissen[b], Edith Greiner-Mai[c], D. Lentfer[c]

[a]Department of Gynecology, FU Berlin, Klinikum Rudolf Virchow of the University,
[b]Hospital Neukölln, Berlin, [c]Byk-Sangtec Diagnostica GmbH, Dietzenbach, Germany

Introduction

The determination of the tumor-associated mucinous-like glycoprotein CA 72-4 is frequently used in the follow-up of patients with gastrointestinal (1, 2) and mucinous ovarian carcinomas (3, 4). The aim of our study was the evaluation of CA 72-4 in the follow-up of gynecological carcinoma. We measured CA 72-4 in sera of patients with carcinoma of the ovary, uterus, cervix and other parts of the female genital tract, in case of benign diseases, and in case of pregnancy. We compared the new immunoluminometric determination of CA 72-4 (LIA-mat®, Byk-Sangtec Diagnostica) with the established immunoradiometric method (ELSA, CIS Diagnostica). Furthermore, the follow-up in some patients with gynecological tumors was simultaneously tested with both methods.

Materials and methods

Immunoluminometric CA 72-4 assay

The new LIA-mat® CA 72-4 (Byk-Sangtec Diagnostica) is based on the "sandwich" principle. The monoclonal antibodies cc49 and B72.3 (5, 6) are used for the solid phase (coated tubes) and for the detection (luminescence-labelled tracer) respectively. Both antibodies react simultaneously with the CA 72-4 antigen to form the sandwich, which is detected by light emission. The assay can be performed either manually or fully automatically on the LIA-mat® System 300.

Comparative CA 72-4 assay

The immunoradiometric determination was carried out with the CA 72-4 ELSA (CIS Diagnostica). Serum samples were taken from 82 apparently healthy postmenopausal women, 60 women in all terms of pregnancy, 53 women with benign gynecological diseases (endometriosis, breast tumor, adnexitis, myoma, ovarian cysts, myomatosis of the uterus) and 168 patients with malignant gynecological tumors (ovarian, uterine, collum and cervical cancer).

Results

Precision, reproducibility and comparability

The immunoluminometric determination of CA 72-4 was shown to correlate well with the established immunoradiometric determination (correlation coefficient r = 0.946). The values for LIA-mat® CA 72-4 were slightly higher, especially in the pathological range (figure 1). The precision data obtained for the LIA-mat® CA 72-4 show the reliability of this assay (mean intra-assay CV = 5.8%, useful working range > 1.7 U/ml). The high long-term reproducibility was shown with controls measured over a period of several months (inter-assay and inter-lot precision 58.7 U/ml: CV = 9.3%; 18.6 U/ml: CV = 7.3%; 91 U/ml: CV = 8.8%; 5.8 U/ml: CV = 7%). Shelf-life-related imprecision was hardly noticeable.

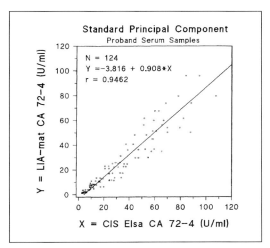

Figure 1. Correlation LIA-mat®CA 72-4 versus CA 72-4 ELSA.

Linearity upon dilution and high-dose hook behavior

Four samples with high CA 72-4 concentrations were diluted serially with the kit diluent. Strict linearity over the whole standard range was found in all cases (r = 0.997–0.999). One-step assays bear the risk of a high-dose hook effect. Therefore, high-titred serum samples were used for detection. The LIA-mat® CA 72-4 showed a high-dose hook risk at concentrations > 8,500 U/ml, which is believed to be uncritical in routine use.

The aim of this study was the investigation of CA 72-4 as a gynecological tumor marker. Therefore, only female subjects were included for reference (table I).

CA 72-4 in postmenopausal women

95% of the subjects were found to have concentrations < 6.15 U/ml. Rarely, concentrations can be found up to 12 U/ml.

CA 72-4 in pregnancy

Slight elevations in CA 72-4 levels were seen in the group of pregnant women and the 95-percentile was found at 8.3 U/ml. No rise in CA 72-4 levels occurred in relation to pregnancy terms. It remains to be clarified whether or not there is a relation between elevated CA 72-4 levels and high-risk pregnancies.

CA 72-4 and benign gynecological disorders

The majority of patients with benign disorders exhibited concentrations below 5 U/ml, however, elevations up to 20 U/ml were also observed. The 95-percentile for this group was found at 9.5 U/ml. Reference ranges for CA 72-4 have so far been determined for a mixed cohort of males and females which is reasonable for gastric cancer. Earlier results from the measurement of approximately 200 blood donors revealed a cut-off at 4 U/ml. In the present study, however, in which only female subjects were included as reference, higher values were obtained. Therefore, a slightly higher cut-off may be considered for gynecological tumors. This is also reported by other authors (7), however, further investigations are necessary.

CA 72-4 and gynecological malignancies

Moderate elevations up to 10 U/ml or 20 U/ml were seen to be caused by non-malignant disorders and during pregnancy. This should be taken into consideration when using CA 72-4 as a tumor marker in gynecology. The subjects included in this study are not necessarily representative of the patient spectrum seen in clinical practice. Therefore, the results obtained here

Table I. Serum CA 72-4 levels in healthy women and patients with benign gynecological diseases.

Subjects	Mean value (U/ml)	95-Percentile (U/ml)	Range (U/ml)
Healthy postmenopausal women (n = 82)	2.55	6.15	0–12
Healthy pregnant women (n = 60)	2.23	8.3	0–12
Benign gynecological diseases (n = 53)	3.01	9.5	0–20

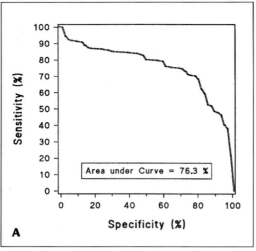
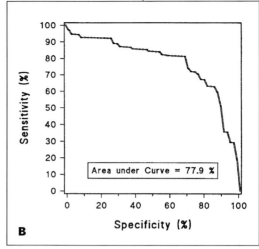

Figure 2. A) ROC curve LIA-mat® CA 72-4. B) ROC-curve CA 72-4 ELSA. (Negatives: benign gynecological diseases, n = 53; positives: malignant gynecological diseases, n = 146).

should only be used for the comparison of methods rather than for the determination of absolute ranges of diagnostic specificity and sensitivity. The ROC analyses clearly show the good comparability of both CA 72-4 methods. The differences between the LIA-mat® CA 72-4 and the IRMA assay were only marginal (figure 2 a, b). The equivalence of both methods was also demonstrated by retrospective studies obtained from repeated sampling in ovarian cancer patients (figure 3). A good consistency was found between CA 72-4 serum levels and response to therapy. Thus, the immunoluminometric determination of CA 72-4 can be used as a supplement to the established tumor markers in gynecological tumors.

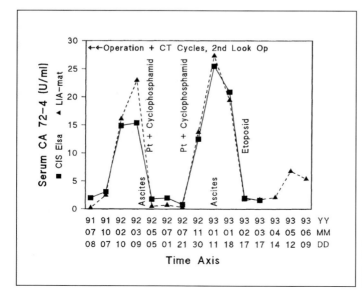

Figure 3. Follow-up of a patient with serous-papillary ovarian cancer, parallel testing with LIA-mat® CA 72-4 and CA 72-4 ELSA.

Conclusions

The immunoluminometric determination of CA 72-4 is highly consistent with the results obtained with the established IRMA method. Precision studies are also in good agreement with the results obtained with the IRMA. Elevated levels of CA 72-4 were not only expressed by ovarian cancer but also by other gynecological tumors. Rarely, CA 72-4 is also elevated in pregnancy and in some cases of benign diseases. Finally, our results show the equivalence of both methods in the follow-up of gynecological tumors. For both assays, a good conformity was found between CA 72-4 serum levels and therapy response. We conclude that the immunoluminometric determination of CA 72-4 is a valid method which can be used in addition to the established tumor markers in gynecological tumors.

References

1. Byrne DJ, Browning MCK, Cushieri A (1990) CA 72-4: A new tumor marker for gastric cancer. Br J Surg 77:1010–1013
2. Gero E, Colcher D, Ferroni P et al (1989) CA 72-4 radioimmunoassay for the detection of the TAG-72 carcinoma-associated antigen in serum of patients. J Clin Lab Anal 3:360–369
3. Bayerl B, Stieber P, Albiez M et al (1990) Significance of CA 72-4 in the diagnosis of ovarian cancer. In: Klapdor R (ed) Recent results in tumor diagnosis and therapy. Zuckschwerdt, Munich, pp 111–112
4. Soper JT, Verda J, Hunter MD et al (1990) Preoperative serum tumor-associated antigen levels in women with pelvic masses. J Obstet Gyn 75:249–254
5. Klug TL, Sattler MA, Colcher D, Schlom J (1986) Monoclonal anitbody immunoradiometric assay for an antigenic determinant (CA 72) on a novel pancarcinoma antigen (TAG-72). Int J Cancer 38(5):661–669
6. Paterson AJ, Schlom J, Sears HF, Bennett J, Colcher D (1986) A radioimmunoassay for the detection of a human tumor-associated glycoprotein (TAG-72) using monoclonal antibody B 72.3. Int J Cancer 37(5):659–666
7. Filella X, Molina R, Jo J et al (1992) Tumor associated glycoprotein-72 (TAG-72) levels in patients with non-malignant and malignant diseases. Bull Cancer 79:271–277

Address for correspondence:
Dr. Dr. med. T. Heinze
Abteilung für Gynäkologie
Universitätsklinikum Rudolf Virchow
Freie Universität Berlin
Pulsstraße 4
D-14059 Berlin, Germany

Improved CA 125 determinations using two different monoclonal antibodies

W. Uhl, B. Denk

Boehringer Mannheim GmbH, Werk Penzberg, Test-Development, Penzberg, Germany

Introduction

First generation CA 125 immunoassays, using OC 125 as the only antibody for the capturing system as well as for detection, were prone to false positive readings resulting from interfering factors in the serum matrix (1–3). Extended internal investigations, comprising various modifications to the test format and the addition of many different "blocking agents" demonstrated the complexity of the phenomenon. Using a combination of two antibodies (MAbs) with separate binding sites on the antigen proved to be the most effective way to eliminate or significantly reduce this problem.

Our new ENZYMUN-Test® CA 125 II is a 1-step sandwich assay, still using HRP-labeled OC 125 as the signal antibody. Different from the established method, however, biotinylated MAb M 11 is now applied to attach reaction complexes, as formed with the antigen in the sample, to the walls of streptavidin coated tubes. Addition of the chromogen ABTS® yields a colored product that can be measured in ENZYMUN-Analyzers®.

With the exception of the lyophilized enzyme conjugate, all reagents are liquid and ready to use. The assay can be run with either serum or plasma material; a sample volume of 70 µl is required. Each test takes 150 min to perform, including 60 min for color development. The measuring range extends from 0 to 500 U/ml. Samples exceeding this concentration may be diluted with the seperately provided diluent (table I).

Methods and patients

The comparison bases on comparative studies using the ENZYMUN-Test CA 125 and the ENZYMUN-Test CA 125 II. In addition to the "routine" samples for the technical characterization of the test, 25 "outlier" sera were used to specifically investigate the problem of false positive readings. For the most part, the specimens had been obtained from external labs reporting results not in accordance with the clinical situation of the patient or with RIA reference values. With only a few exceptions, the already assigned concentrations from RIA methods had to be accepted without the possibility of further verification.

Results

Standardization / method comparison studies

Reference standardization of ENZYMUN-Test® CA 125 II is against the established generation of the test to guarantee consistent recoveries with either version of the assay. The study comprised a total of 99 sera distributed over the whole concentration range. Measurements were done

Table I. Characterization of ENZYMUN-Test® CA 125 II (changes/improvements over 1. generation test in bold print).

Product name	ENZYMUN-Test® CA 125 II
Antibodies	
Solid phase	**M 11 (biotinylated)**
Detection	OC 125 (HRP)
Reference test	ENZYMUN-Test® CA 125
Measuring range	0–500 U/ml
Detection limit	< 3 U/ml (+ 2 SD)
Sample material	serum/plasma
Sample volume	70 µl
Incubation time	**90 min + 60 min**
Hook effect	not observed
Applications	ES 700, ES 600, ES 300, ES 33

on four different ES 600 instruments in four independent runs at each site. Regression analysis is based on the method described by Pasing and Bablok (4, 5). Figure 1 demonstrates the conformity of both test generations after the adjustment resulting from standardization. With a slope of "1" and an offset close to "0" (0.02 U/ml), no systematic deviation is to be apprehended from a switch to the new assay. The cut-off value remains at 35 U/ml.

There is also excellent comparability with the CA 125 II IRMA from Centocor. This second generation test now also uses M 11 as a sandwich partner for OC 125. In a method comparison study comprising 54 samples, the equation y = 0.39 + 0.96x was calculated for the regression line. The correlation coefficient r = 0.992 reflects the close conformity between both systems.

Precision/detection limit

Intra-assay precision data are based on n = 20 replicate measurements of sera and controls. With both lots of reagents employed, CVs ≤ 6% around and below the cut-off, and CVs ≤ 3.1% at higher concentrations were obtained.

The detection limit was determinated according to "Kaiser". Twenty replicates each of standard A were measured in three independent runs on different ENZYMUN-Anlayzers®. The means calculated from the individual series were 0.8 U/ml for the ES 600 and 2.2 U/ml for the ES 300 instruments. Inter-assay precision studies were as well performed on both ES 600 and ES 300 analyzers. Data were collected from 10 resp. 12 individual runs. CVs are < 10% below the cut-off, for higher concentrations CVs of < 4. 5% were found (table II).

Recalibration

The comparison of full calibration and 1 point recalibration data reflects a very consistent performance level with regard to recovery and precision. Data obtained with four sera and two controls are virtually identical. The lack of any shift in concentration values, neither in the lower nor in the upper part of the measuring range, clearly proves the stability of the calibration curve.

Interfering factors ("Outliers")

For a series of 25 samples, reported to yield falsely elevated readings with EIAs, determinations of antigen concentrations were repeated internally. Both generations of ENZYMUN-Tests® CA 125 were applied, results are compared to RIA data as reference values (table III).

Samples 1, 11 and 13 were not confirmed as outliers (EIA: > cut-off/RIA: < cut-off), five sera could not be rechecked with the "old" test because ofthe limited volume. In 14 samples the concentration clearly dropped below the decision level with ENZYMUN-Test® CA 125 II. For sera 17+18 the reading was not (completely) reduced to a "normal" value. The external RIA results, however, indicate a pathological concentration as well. Of the remaining elevated samples that did not or only partially respond, only no. 5, 6 and 20 had a confirmed normal reference value (no. 19 borderline).

Unfortunately, no clinical background information is avaiable for these three specimens and there is no experimental confirmation of the RIA data. Even if taken as real outliers without further proof, the gross result clearly demonstrates the almost completely eliminated susceptibility of the ENZYMUN-Test® CA 125 II to this type of interference.

Hook effect

The absorption pattern of two highly pathological sera with CA 125 antigen concentrations of 35,000 U/ml and 11,000 U/ml respectively, was monitored prior to and after dilution. No hook effect was observed in either case.

Linearity

Three human sera with elevated CA 125 antigen concentrations were gradually diluted with the CA 125 II diluent. Considering the limited range of pathological concentrations, there is no need to restrict the maximum possible dilution factor. Dilutions into the lower part of the measuring range should not result in concentrations below the cut-off (35 U/ml) to avoid recoveries deviating by more than ± 10% from the expected value.

Table II. Precision profile of ENZYMUN-Test® CA 125 II.

Intra-assay precision

Lot A

Sample	Pool 1	Pool 2	Pool 3	Pool 4	Control low	Control high
Mean (U/ml)	16.2	32.6	82.2	199	27.9	86.6
SD	0.97	0.78	1.51	3.94	0.69	0.03
CV (%)	6.0	2.4	1.8	2.0	2.5	2.3

Lot B

Sample	Pool 1	Pool 2	Pool 3	Pool 4	Control low	Control high
Mean (U/ml)	18.3	36.8	64.9	132	347	424
SD	1.01	1.6	1.9	4.1	9.74	11.8
CV (%)	5.5	4.4	3.0	3.1	2.8	2.8

Inter-assay precision

ES 600

Sample	Serum 1	Serum 2	Serum 3	Serum 4	Control low	Control high
Mean (U/ml)	15.2	24.1	88.5	208.1	28.6	86.6
SD	1.09	2.06	3.54	9.24	1.28	2.07
CV (%)	7.2	8.6	4.0	4.4	4.5	2.4

ES 300

Sample	Serum 1	Serum 2	Serum 3	Serum 4	Control low	Control high
Mean (U/ml)	10.1	18.0	24.1	76.6	146.7	213.5
SD	0.97	1.78	1.84	2.70	4.89	7.59
CV (%)	9.6	9.9	7.6	3.5	3.3	3.6

Detection limit

ES 600

Signal (E): mean	0.090		0.092	0.079
SD	0.003		0.005	0.003
CV (%)	3.4		5.0	4.0
Mean + 2 SD	0.096		0.101	0.085
Conc. (U/ml)	0.72		0.95	0.67
Mean			0.8 U/ml	

ES 300

Signal (E) mean	0.113		0.108	0.139
SD	0.06		0.012	0.011
CV (%)	5.1		11.2	8.1
Mean + 2 SD	0.124		0.133	0.162
Conc. (U/ml)	1.18		2.40	2.92
Mean			2.2 U/ml	

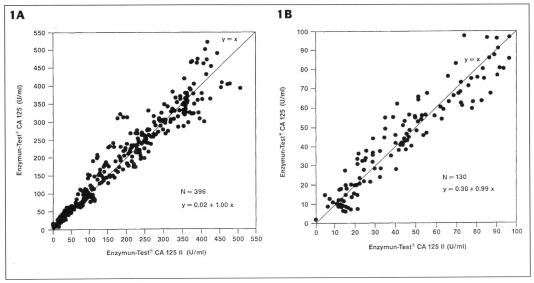

Figure 1. Method comparison data as obtained from ENZYMUN-Test® CA 125 II reference standardization: 0–500 U/ml (1A) and 0–100 U/ml (1B).

Table III. Recovery of sera with reported false positive readings; results from both generations ENZYMUN-Test® CA 125 and different RIAs.

Serum no.	CA 125 II (U/ml)	CA 125 "old" (U/ml)	RIA (U/ml)
1	20.9	31.2	–
2	17.9	220	9.7
3	16.8	273	8.8
4	13.2	> 800	(5.0/IMX)
5	64.9	106	29.1
6	80.8	110	23.5
7	15.9	366	–
8	8.9	–	–
9	17.7	58.5	–
10	> 800	> 800	817
11	5.2	9.7	–
12	26.3	44.9	–
13	7.8	22.3	–
14	3 13	201	205
15	4.7	87.4	–
16	11.4	–	56.0
17	40.8	–	65.0
18	123	–	48.0
19	302	494	37.6
20	11 0	535	"normal"
21	3.7	77.0	"normal"
22	4.9	90.0	"normal"
23	14.5	–	15.0
24	10.5	457	12.1
25	23.4	1500	< 25

Conclusion

After the availability of M 11 as a sandwich partner to the established OC 125 antibody, our first generation ENZYMUN-Test® CA 125 was redeveloped, with special emphasis on improvements to precision and interference problems.

EMZYMUN-Test® CA 125 II is again based on the well approved streptavidin-tube technology with biotinylated and HRP-conjugated reagents. The murine MAb M 11 is used as the capture antibody, replacing OC 125 on the solid phase. As a result, problems with false positive readings ("outliers") could be almost completely eliminated and a number of performance criteria improved. Thus, incubation times were shortened from 180/60 min to 90/60 min. Better precision at the low end combined with the introduction of a "true" zero standard allowed to lower the detection limit from 10 U/ml to 3 U/ml. The sample volume was cut by 30% to now 70 µl. Markedly reduced matrix effects, more stable calibration curves and an extended dilution linearity generally inproved the robustness of the test. Standardization against ENZYMUN-Test® CA 125 first generation ensures the required comparability to the earlier introduced version of the assay.

References

1. Weber Th, Käpyaho KI, Tanner P (1990) Endogenous interference in immunoassays in clinical chemistry. Scand J Clin Lab Invest 50, suppl 201:77–82
2. Boermann OC, Segers MFG, Poels LG, Kenemans P, Thomas CMG (1990) Heterophilic antibodies in human sera causing falsely increased results in the CA 125 immunofluorometric assay. Clin Chem 36/6:889–891
3. Hashimoto T, Ohba-N, Nishibu M, Matsubara F (1990) The immunoglobulin M (IGM) effect on CA 125 enzyme-immunoassay. Clin Chem 36/6:1120
4. Pasing H, Bablok W (1983) A new biometrical procedure for testing the equality of measurements from two different analytical methods; application of linear regression procedures for method comparison studies in clinical chemistry. Part I. J Clin Chem Clin Biochem 21:709–720
5. Pasing H, Bablok W (1983) Comparison of several regression procedures for method comparison studies and determination of sample sizes. Application of linera regression procedures for method comparison studies in clinical chemistry. Part II. J Clin Chem Clin Biochem 22:431–445

Address for correspondence:
Dr.-Ing. W. Uhl
Boehringer Mannheim GmbH
Nonnenwald 2
D-82372 Penzberg, Germany

CA 125 mechanized microparticle enzyme immunoassay (MEIA)

A clinical and methodical evaluation

Ute Hasholzner[a], Petra Stieber[a], L. Baumgartner[b], Heike Pahl[a], W. Meier[b], A. Fateh-Moghadam †[a]

[a]Institute for Clinical Chemistry, [b]Gynecological Clinic,
Ludwig-Maximilians-University, Munich, Germany

Introduction

Since almost ten years CA 125 is considered to be a sensitive and valuable marker in follow-up care and monitoring of therapy-efficacy of ovarian cancer. We wanted to answer the question, whether the CA 125 II RIA is comparable to three automated systems of CA 125 detection concerning methodical and clinical aspects.

Patients and methods

CA 125 II was measured as RIA (Centocor, USA) and automated as CA 125 MEIA (Abbott) on the IMx® system, Enzymun® CA 125 II EIA (Boehringer) on ES 700 and CA 125 II EIA (Roche) on Cobas® Core system according to manufacturers' instructions.

Investigation was done retrospectively in 338 patients' sera stored at –70° C: 79 patients had an ovarian carcinoma at the time of primary diagnosis, 18 a relapse of ovarian cancer and 46 determinations were done in the follow-up of ovarian cancer patients. 42 patients were suffering from another cancer (22 cervical cancer, 20 gastrointestinal tumors) and nine underwent an immunoscintigraphy, five of these had positive HAMA-factors at time of examination.

The reference group included 28 healthy women as judged by clinical investigation and clinical chemistry parameters, 28 pregnants women, 62 sera of patients suffering from benign gynecological and 26 from benign gastrointestinal diseases.

Results

Intra-assay imprecision varied between 6 and 8% for RIA II, 1.5–4.2% for MEIA, 2.1–6.5% for EIA (Boehringer) and about 3.4% for EIA (Roche). Inter-assay imprecision was 5.4–10.2% for the RIA II, 3.7–6.9% for MEIA, 6.0–8.7% for Boehringer and 4.7–8.4% for Roche. The lowest detectable dose (calculated as mean plus double standard deviation) was 0.15 U/ml for Centocor, 1.57 U/ml for Abbott, 0.98 U/ml for Boehringer and was not done for Roche.

The correlation of the assays in general was very good: benign gynecological diseases correlation was from 0.99 (Centocor/Boehringer and Boehringer/Roche) to 0.98 (Abbott/Boehringer and Abbott/Roche), in ovarian cancer it was 0.98 (Boehringer/Roche) respectively 0.99 (Centocor/Abbott). Only in healthy subjects correlation showed a greater range from 0.47 (Centocor/

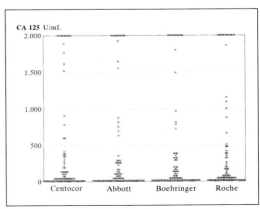

Figure 1. Dot plot: CA 125 in ovarian cancer at the time of primary diagnosis (n = 79).

Table I. Sensitivities (%) and specificities (%) of four CA 125 assays at different cut-off values (35 U/ml and 65 U/ml) and at a specificity of 95% versus the reference group of benign gynecological diseases; prim. diag. = primary diagnosis, benign g.d. = benign gynecological diseases.

CA 125 cut-off (U/ml)	Marker	Specificity		Ovarian cancer			
		healthy	benign g.d.	prim. diag.	relapse	serous	mucinous
35	Centocor	89	65	83	61	73	50
35	Abbott	93	77	72	61	78	36
35	Boehringer	93	62	72	61	78	32
35	Roche	89	63	80	67	81	40
65	Centocor	96	84	67	61	67	18
65	Abbott	100	89	64	61	69	23
65	Boehringer	100	84	68	61	69	18
65	Roche	96	81	68	56	72	23
156	Centocor	100	95	50	33	47	18
125	Abbott	100	95	60	39	53	14
168	Boehringer	100	95	60	39	53	9
179	Roche	100	95	60	44	56	14

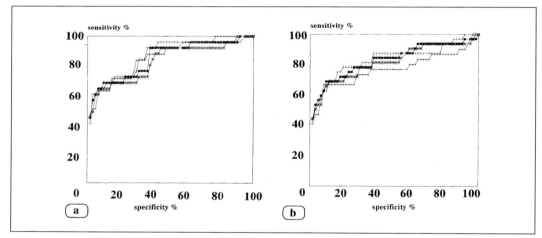

Figure 2. Receiver operating characteric (ROC) curves. a) Ovarian carcinoma at time of primary diagnosis, n = 79. b) serous ovarian carcinoma, n = 32, both versus benign gynecological diseases, n = 62; —□— = CA 125 II Centocor; —+— = CA 125 Abbott; —*— = CA 125 II Boehringer; —■— = CA 125 II Roche.

Abbott), 0.58 (Abbott/Roche), 0.74 (Abbott/Boehringer) to 0.886 (Centocor/Boehringer and Centocor/Roche) and 0.946 (Boehringer/Roche). Regarding dot plots (figure 1) of all and special diagnoses, Abbott shows most points low and Roche most points high.

Fixing specificity at 95% we found a cut-off value of CA 125 II for healthy persons of 51.8 U/ml for Centocor, 41.1 U/ml for Abbott, 35.9 U/ml for Boehringer and 45.7 U/ml for Roche; for pregnants we found a cut-off value at 95% specificity from 86.7 U/ml (Centocor), 38.3 U/ml (Abbott), 51.6 U/ml (Boehringer) and 67 U/ml (Roche); for benign gynecological diseases the cut-off was 156 U/ml for RIA II, 124.9 U/ml for MEIA, 168 U/ml for Boehringer and 179.2 U/ml for Roche, for benign gastrointestinal diseases 864 U/ml for Centocor, 594.5 U/ml for Abbottt, 589.6 U/ml for Boehringer and 890 U/ml for Roche. Basing our calculations for sensitivities on the specificity of 95% versus benign gynecological diseases as clinical relevant reference groupe, the sensitivity for primary diagnosis of ovarian cancer was 50% for RIA II and 60% for all three automatized systems – this can also be seen in ROC curves (figure 2) –, for relapses a sensitivity of 33% for RIA II, 39% for Abbott II and Boehringer and 44% for Roche was found. In literature and producer instructions often cut-off values of 35 U/ml and 65 U/ml are used. To make our results comparable with those, the resulting sensitivities and specificities in 35 and 65 U/ml are listed in table I (table1).

Human anti-mouse antibodies (HAMA) seem not to disturb all four assays. In the follow-up of cancer patients in general all CA 125 assays showed comparable values, CA 125 Roche in general the highest values compared to CA 125 Centocor, CA 125 Boehringer little higher and CA 125 Abbott lower. In singular cases values can be different. Consequently a control of the last value or simultaneous determination with both assays has to be demanded when changing the method to establish the new niveau of marker in the follow-up.

All three automatized systems are faster and easier to handle and show better reproducibility than the RIA II.

Conclusions

Following the results of clinical and methodical evaluation and ROC curves MEIA CA 125 is comparable to the two other automatized systems from Boehringer and Roche which are investigated and show slightly better discrimination between benign and malign gynecological diseases than the CA 125 II RIA.

References

1 Meier W, Stieber P, Fateh-Moghadam A, Eiermann W, Hepp H (1987) CA 125 in gynecological malignancies. Eur J Cancer Clin Oncol 23:713

2 Meier W, Stieber P, Fateh-Moghadam A, Eiermann W, Hepp H (1988) CA 125 Serumwerte und histologischer Befund zum Zeitpunkt der Second-look-Laparotomie beim Ovarialkarzinom. Geburtsh u Frauenheilk 48:331

3 Quaranta M, Lorusso V, Coviello M, Micelli G, Casamassima A (1988) CA 125 in the monitoring of response to chemotherapy of ovarian carcinoma. Int J Cancer: Suppl 3:68–70

4 Klapdor R (1992) Arbeitsgruppe Qualitätskontrolle und Standardisierung von Tumormarkertests im Rahmen der Hamburger Symposien über Tumormarker. Tumordiagn u Ther 13

Address for correspondence:
Dr. med. Petra Stieber
Institut für Klinische Chemie
Klinikum Großhadern
Marchioninistraße 15
D-81366 München, Germany

Evaluation of a new CA 125 assay: The LIA-mat CA 125 II

J.M.G. Bonfrer, E. Jansen, H.M de Feij-de Graaf, C.M. Korse

The Netherlands Cancer Institute (Antoni van Leeuwenhoek Huis), Amsterdam, The Netherlands

Introduction

After the introduction ten years ago of the CA 125 tumor marker, the use of this assay has become widespread in clinical practice (1). Although the initial publications focused mainly on monitoring patients with epithelial ovarian carcinoma (2), other applications were described in rapid succession.
The OC 125 MoAb was first described in 1981. It was obtained by immunizing BALB/C mice with the OVCA 433 cell line which was isolated from ascites of a patient with a serous papillary cystadenocarcinoma. Recently new CA 125 II assays were introduced in which the CA 125 capture antibody is now a new murine MoAb M-11 with a higher avidity for epitopes of the CA 125 molecule (3). We compared three new CA 125 II kits (4).

Materials and methods

Assay procedures

The LIA-mat CA 125 II (Byk-Sangtec, Dietzenbach, Germany) is a heterologous assay using M-11 as solid phase and OC 125 as tracer Ab, utilizing a covalently bound isoluminol derivative as signal. The signal is proportionate to the amount of CA 125 antigen in the sample. The LIA-mat assay was processed on a LIA-mat 300 System.
The CA 125 II IRMA-mat (Byk-Sangtec) is a radioimmunoassay based on the sandwich principle. In this one step assay the M-11 antibody is used as a solid phase (coated tube) and the OC 125 as tracer (^{125}I label).
The CentocorR CA 125 II (Centocor, Malvern, PA, USA) is a one step "sandwich" assay as described for the IRMA-mat but uses polystyrene beads coated with the M-11 clone as solid phase. The tracer is the ^{125}I labeled murine monoclonal OC 125.
Samples were centrifuged within one hour and stored at $-20\,°C$ the same day when not processed immediately.
All routine determinations were performed as duplicates, according to the manufacturer's instructions.

Sample collection

Test samples were collected from three different groups.
Group A (n = 28): Apparently healthy women age between 25 and 57 years (mean 39); no abnormal levels were found when their sera were tested for a set of biochemical parameters according to the criteria of the "Working Group on Quality Control and Standardisation of the Hamburg Symposium" (5).
Group B (n = 160): 1. Patients with primary tumors stage I to IV of the cervix (n = 30) endometrium (n = 25) ovarium (n = 37); 2. samples from patients treated for ovarian cancer (n = 96).
Group C (n = 80): Unselected serum samples from routine requests, mainly from ovarian and breast carcinoma patients, in order of receipt.

Results

Comparisons

One sample had to be rejected because of an inappropriate duplicate result. In the comparison of the different assays none of the remaining results had to be considered as an outlier

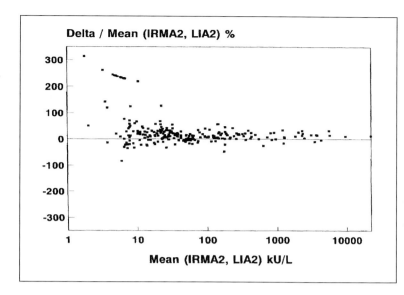

Figure 1. Correlation of IRMA-mat und LIA-mat. Depicted is the difference between the result of a sample measurement of both assays as a percentage of the mean of two results.

according to the difference in outcome between assays in relation to the mean. This graph is shown in figure 1 for the LIA-mat II and the IRMA-mat II assay.

Distribution of CA 125 values

We measured CA 125 concentrations in group A (normal population) with the LIA-mat and IRMA-mat CA 125 II assay. We used serum as well as EDTA and heparin plasma.
The distribution of CA 125 values is asymmetric. The median, 90 and 99 percentiles are given in table I. There was no significant correlation found between age and CA 125 levels in this small group of mainly pre-menopausal women. The way of blood collection had no demonstrable significant influence on the result. The CA 125 concentrations measured in serum from patients with different gynecological malignancies determined with the new assays show that very high levels of the antigen are mainly found in ovarian carcinomas. The mean value differed significantly from the other groups ($p < 0.001$) (table II).

Precision

The intra-assay variation for all assays was calculated from the duplicates of all test samples using an exponential regression of the log concentration. This gives a good indication of the assay precision under practical conditions. A variation below 10% is considered to peg out a useful working range. We found that the Centocor II assay can be used over the complete standard range (0-500) while the LIA-mat II and IRMA-mat II kits have a lower limit of about 10 kU/l.

Reproducibility

Reproducibility was estimated by introducing a panel of three control sera in each series. The

Table I. CA 125 concentration in a normal population. The normal population consisted of 28 apparently healthy females (group A). All samples were assayed in one run.

CA 125 assay	n	Median	Percentiles (kU/l)	
			90	99
IRMA2				
serum	28	14.5	30.8	52.7
heparin plasma	28	15.0	37.1	52.0
EDTA plasma	28	14.0	31.5	42.1
LIA2				
serum	28	12.2	28.7	48.3
heparin plasma	28	11.8	29.7	47.3
EDTA plasma	28	10.8	30.4	43.7

Table II. CA 125 concentration in sera from ovarian and non-ovarian malignancies determined by three CA 125 assays.

	Non-ovarian (n = 102)			Ovarian (n = 149)		
	mean	std. dev.	max.	mean	std. dev.	n > max.[a]
IRMA2	64	166	1405	1333	3592	31
LIA2	52	134	1000	1161	3159	33
CENT	47	105	870	884	2335	33

[a]Number of samples over maximum value of non-ovarian cancer

Table III. Correlations from log-linear regression analysis. The assay mentioned in the top heading is taken as the x-component.

n = 251	LN-CENT	LN-IRMA2	LN-LIA2
LN-CENT		0.9912 (y = 0.08 + 0.92 x)	0.9624 (y = 0.78 + 0.82 x)
LN-IRMA2	0.9913 (y = −0.01 + 1.06 x)		0.9652 (y = 0.78 + 0.88 x)
LN-LIA2	0.9624 (y = −0.59 + 1.13 x)	0.9652 (y = −0.55 + 1.06 x)	

inter-assay variation was calculated from means between runs. The coefficients of variation ranged between 14% for the IRMA-mat II in the kit control to 5.7% for the kit control of the Centocor II assay. Mean CVs were 9.5% for the LIA-mat, 9.3 for the Centocor assay and 13% for the IRMA-mat.

Linearity

We tested all assays for their linearity performance. For that purpose five patient samples were diluted with 0-standard and kit diluent. All dilutions showed an excellent linear relationship, ranging in the IRMA-mat II and LIA-mat II assay. The average r-value was 0.994 for the manual IRMA-mat and 0.997 for the automated LIA-mat test.

High-dose hook effect (H.D.H)

We studied the high-dose hook phenomenon with serum and an ascites sample. By diluting serum samples and plotting the signal values we could calculate the likely threshold above which the effect will occur. In this way a concentration of 20.000 kU/l was assessed as a general limit applicable for all five assays studied. The ascites fluid tested gave rise to a H.D.H effect at similar concentration.

Correlation studies

For this purpose we used the samples of group B and C totaling 251 after the rejection of the incorrect duplicate. A matrix of the results is given in Table III. Secondly, we selected a range from 0–100 kU/l, because changes in this area may have important clinical consequences. A specific example of how the comparability of results of linear regression analyses may change, depending on the range under examination, is given in figure 2. The regression lines in both of the above mentioned ranges were almost parallel, but there was a significant difference of about 50 kU/l in intercept.

Conclusions

The introduction of a second monoclonal antibody in the CA 125 assay has probably been dictated by the search for a better sensitivity and specificity. This may be important when the CA 125 assay is implemented in treatment of

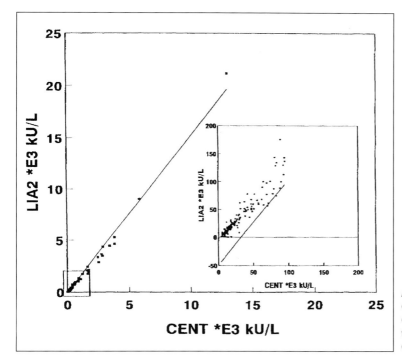

Figure 2. Regression analysis. Comparison of LIA-mat II and Centocor. The insertion shows the correlation in the range 0–200 kU/l.

endometriosis when smaller changes of CA 125 levels may have clinical impact (6). An improved sensitivity is expressed by a wider working range and we indeed found that the precision of the novel kits at lower levels is generally better. The small amount of rejected duplicate measurements justify in our opinion the singular measurement of CA 125 concentrations on the automated system. This will enhance the cost-effectiveness of the kit tremendously.

A major factor in the quality of follow-up studies is the reproducibility of assay results. The automated CA 125 assay scores much better than its manual counterpart but not better than the manual Centocor assay. The occurrence of the high dose hook effect in all assay systems is a well known cause of concern.

In our evaluation of the sampling mode it became evident that the bias of a serum – or plasma matrix on the results is minimal. The same holds for the freezing procedure, which is not an unexpected finding, because it is well known that large glycoproteins are relatively stable in a protein matrix.

The 95 percentile of about 50 kU/l of our small selection of apparently healthy females indicate that there may be a need to reconsider the reference value of 35 kU/l as has been used previously. The value of 35 kU/l was introduced by *Bast* et al. (2). It was the 99 percentile of a large group of 888 healthy persons including only 351 females. The reference value might have to be adjusted although the clinical benefit of such an adjustment is doubtful.

References

1. Bates SE (1991) Clinical applications of serum tumor markers. Ann Int Med 115(8):623–638
2. Bast RC Jr, Klug TL, St John E, Jenison E, Niloff JM, Lazarus H, Berkowitz RS, Leavitt T, Griffiths CT, Parker L, Zurawski VR Jr, Knapp RC (1983) A radioimmunoassay using a monoclonal antibody to monitor the course of epithelial ovarian cancer. N Eng J Med 309:883–887
3. Hardardottir H, Parmley TH, Quirk JG Sanders MM, Miller FC, O'Brien TJ (1990) Distribution of CA 125 in embryonic tissues and adult derivatives of the

fetal periderm. Am J Obstet Gynecol 163:1925–1931
4 Bonfrer JMG, Baan AW, Jansen E, Lentfer D, Kenemans P (1994) Technical evaluation of three second generation CA 125 assays. Eur J Clin Chem Clin Biochem 32:201–207
5 Klapdor R (1992) Arbeitsgruppe Qualitätskontrolle und Standardisierung von Tumormarkertests in Rahmen des Hamburger Symposium über Tumormarker. Tumordiagn u Ther 13
6 Pittaway DE (1990) The use of serial CA 125 concentrations to monitor endometriosis in infertile women. Obstet Gynecol 163:1032–1037

Address for correspondence:
Dr. J.M.G. Bonfrer
Algemeen Klinisch Laboratorium
Plesmanlaan 121
NL-1066 CX Amsterdam, The Netherlands

Immunoassays for the CA 125-related antigen using new monoclonal antibodies

K. Nustad[a], O. Nilsson[b], B. Kierulf[a], T. Varaas[a], K. Thrane-Steen[a], E. Paus[a], C. Okkenhaug[a], K. H. Olsen[a], O. P. Børmer[a]

[a]Central Laboratory, Norwegian Radium Hospital, Oslo,
[b]CanAg Diagnostics AB, Gothenburg, Sweden

Introduction

Assays for the ovarian cancer marker CA 125, first described by *Bast* et al. (for review, see *Jacobs* and *Bast* (3)), have proved to be of great practical value in the management of patients with various forms of epihelial ovarian cancer.

The antigen molecule itself has to this day only been partly characterized, apparently being a high molecular weight glycoprotein or mucin composed of subunits of approx. 200 kD. The large complex can certainly be expected to express more than one type of antigenic determinant or epitope, but this has not been studied systematically so far. The term CA 125 should therefore in principle be restricted to the epitope recognized by the monoclonal antibody (MAb) OC 125, while the complete molecule might be denominated the CA 125-related antigen.

The first generation of CA 125 assays all used the proprietary monoclonal MAb OC 125, usually in the format of homologous sandwich immunometric assays. In a concerted action, most commercial vendors of CA 125 assays have recently introduced another MAb, M11 (4), to be used as the catcher antibody in their various assays. OC 125 is still used as the tracer MAb to quantitate CA 125. These new heterogeneous CA 125 II assays are analytically more robust and sensitive than the former version, still yielding the same important clinical information.

Here we will report the development of several other monoclonal antibodies against the CA 125 related antigen, and also a preliminary evaluation of their use in new immunoassays.

Materials and methods

Reagents and procedures

Antibody OV 185, reacting with the CA 125-related antigen and used by us as an accessory reagent, was kindly supplied by CanAg AB (Gothenburg, Sweden).

Immunoglobulin class and subclass determinations were performed by double diffusion in agarose gel, using specific antisera (Miles Laboratories).

Antibodies were radiolabeled with ^{125}I by the Iodo-Gen method, as described (5), or with Europium for the Delfia assay format as described in the Wallac (Turku, Finland) Eu labeling kit insert.

Solid-phase antibodies were prepared by adsorption onto wells of microtiter plates, or onto monodisperse polymer particles (Dynabeads M280, Dynal, Norway), as likewise described (2). For the Delfia assays, biotinylated MAb was adsorbed onto streptavidin-coated microtiter plates (Wallac).

Preparation of the CA 125-related antigen

Ascites from ovarian cancer patients, drawn at therapeutic laparocentesis, was precipitated with increasing concentrations of ammonium sulfate. The fraction precipitating from 40 to 60% saturation was collected by centrifugation, and dissolved in a minimal volume of water. After dialysis against phosphate-buffered saline, pH 7.4 (PBS), the preparation was subjected to gel

Table I. Epitope group and Ig class characteristics of the antibodies.

Antibodies	Inhibits binding to CA 125 of antibody		IgG subclass
	OC 125	OV185	
K93, K95	+	−	1
K100	−	−	2a
K90, K91, K94, K101, K102	−	+	1
K92, K96, K97	−	+	2a

Table II. Testing of antibody combinations for use in immunometric assays. Numbers given are the percentage bound of tracer antibody (horizontal) when incubating with a semipurified CA125 from human ascites in microtiter wells coated with SAM (Sheep-Anti-Mouse Ig) and the various solid phase antibodies (vertical). Antibodies are grouped according to their epitope group specificities.

	K93	K95	K100	K90	K91	K92	K94	K96	K97	K101	K102
K93	8	3	0	30	28	6	18	10	16	35	14
K95	2	0	1	28	26	6	15	9	14	28	13
K100	2	5	0	19	13	4	10	6	9	17	8
K90	14	23	3	3	7	2	2	2	2	12	2
K91	11	18	2	6	0	1	3	3	3	1	2
K92	0	12	1	17	8	1	6	4	5	12	5
K94	12	19	2	7	6	2	1	1	1	11	1
K96	12	17	2	6	4	2	1	0	0	8	1
K97	11	17	2	4	3	1	0	0	1	7	1
K101	11	19	2	6	0	1	2	3	3	1	2
K102	12	18	2	7	5	2	1	1	1	10	1

chromatography on a Biogel A-15m column. Fractions were collected, and their CA 125 content monitored with a homologous immunoradiometric assay employing the OV 185 monoclonal antibody. Most CA 125 activity appeared in fractions corresponding to the void volume. These were pooled, demonstrating a specific activity of approx. 950 kU of CA 125 (measured by the Abbott IMX CA 125 assay) per mg of protein (measured by BCA Protein Assay Reagent, Pierce Chemical Co.) using bovine serum albumin (Sigma) as the standard.

Production of monoclonal antibodies

Female Balb/c mice were immunized intraperitoneally, and spleen cells were hybridized with NSO myeloma cells, as described (1), except that the antigen preparation used for immunization was adsorbed onto immunobeads (Dynospheres M280, Dynal, Norway, carrying antibody OV 185) before injection.

Hybridoma supernatants were screened by incubation in microtiter wells coated with polyclonal sheep anti mouse immunoglobulins (SAM). After washing with PBS, wells were incubated with a diluted CA 125 containing human ascites. Unbound material was again washed away, and bound monoclonal antibody presenting the antigen was detected with radiolabeled MAb OV 185. This step was performed in the presence of an excess of irrelevant mouse IgG1 (the same IgG subclass as for OV 185), in order to block unspecific binding of this tracer MAb directly to the solid-phase SAM.

Positive clones were subcloned twice, expanded, and used for ascites production in Pristan-primed

Balb/c mice. Monoclonal antibodies were then purified from mouse ascites by protein A chromatography.

Epitope mapping

Cross inhibition experiments were performed in microtiter wells, essentially as described (2). However, as the purified antigen preparation could not be adsorbed directly onto plastic, an indirect binding via an adsorbed MAb was employed. In order to circumvent the interpretation problems caused by the solid-phase antibody, the experiments were repeated with solid-phase MAbs of different epitope specificities.

Selection of antibody pairs for use in immunometric assays

Antibodies were added to wells of microtiter plates, previously coated with SAM. After 1 h incubation the plates were washed, and semi-purified CA 125 was added (0.1 ml of a 200 kU/l preparation, containg an excess of irrelevant mouse MAb of the same Ig sublass as the tracer MAb to be used in the next step). After another 1 h incubation the wells were washed, and ^{125}I-labeled MAb was added (10 ng, approx. 100,000 cpm, in 0.1 ml). After a final 1 h incubation, wells were washed, separated, their radioactivity counted, and results calculated as percent of total radioactivity bound. All possible combinations of solid-phase and tracer MAbs were tested in this way (table II).

Comparison of assays in patient and reference populations

Prototype assays and the CIS CA 125 II assay (CIS Bioindustries) were compared using serum samples from 47 ovarian cancer patients in various stages, 49 blood donors, 24 patients undergoing surgery for benign diseases, and from 25 apparently healthy women aged 60 to 70 years.

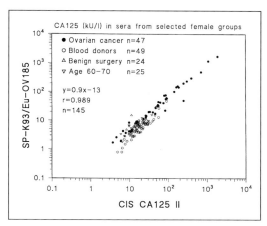

Figure 1. Comparison of CA 125 values measured with a prototype new immunofluorometric assay (solid-phase MAb K93, Eu-labeled OV 185) and with the CIS CA 125 II assay kit, in sera from reference and patient populations.

Results and discussion

After the initial screening procedure, eleven MAbs (denominated K90–K97 and K100–K102) were found to be of possible interest for analytical use. The cross-inhibition experiments revealed their epitope specificities to fall into two main groups (table I), one similar to OC 125, the other to the CanAg MAb OV 185. Antibody K100 may represent a third group, as it gave no significant inhibition in these experiments. Table I also shows results of the Ig class and subclass determinations, demonstrating that four of the MAbs were of the IgG2a subclass, presumably not suitable as solid-phase MAbs due to complement interference with serum samples (1).

The large experiment where all possible MAb combinations were screened for immunoassay use gave several interesting results (table II). First, it is seen that in homologous assays, i.e. when the same MAb was used both as catcher and tracer MAb, practically no signal was obtained. This may seem surprising, as homologous CA 125 assays using MAb OC 125 have been in routine use for many years. In supplementary experiments, both with microtiter wells and Dynabeads M280, we found that the observed binding in such assays was extremely dependent on the amounts of MAb coupled to the solid phase (data not shown). This may explain why various earlier commercial CA 125 assays, all using the OC 125 MAb, tended to give surprisingly different results with patient samples.

It is also seen that the strongest signals in general were achieved when the solid-phase (catcher) and the tracer MAb reacted with different epitope groups (upper right and lower left fields in table II). Antibody K100 works reasonably well as a solid-phase MAb, using OV 185-like MAbs as tracers, but it gives practically no binding when used under reverse conditions, i.e. as a tracer MAb itself. This may be due either to an epitope group specificity different from the OC 125-like MAbs, or to a low affinity not suitable for tracer applications. Such a low affinity could also explain why no inhibition was found with his MAb in the cross inhibition experiments (table I).

The most promising combinations, as read from table II, would be MAbs K90, K91, or K101 used as tracers, with K93 or K95 (having an OC 125-like specificity) as catcher MAb. In preliminary evaluations, these antibody combinations have been found to give rapid and robust assays both in the immunoradiometric assay format, using Dynabeads M280 and ^{125}I-labeled tracer, and in the Delfia format with microtiter wells and Eu-labelled tracer.

These assays have, however, not yet been evaluated with clinical samples. We therefore illustrate the use of our new antibodies by results obtained in a cooperation with CanAg AB. Here, our K93 was used as the solid-phase MAb, and their Eu-labelled OV 185 was employed as tracer in a Delfia assay format. Figure 1 demonstrates the excellent correlation (r = 0.989) between this prototype assay and the CIS CA 125 II assay.

Our results so far clearly indicate that this field, where the assays until now have been dominated by proprietary antibodies, are about to be »opened« for new immunoassays, measuring the same molecular antigen. We are now active in initiating an international workshop on monoclonal antibodies against the CA 125-related antigen. If successful, the workshop will contribute also to the understanding of this quite elusive tumor marker molecule, and possibly also give us a name for it that may be more meaningful than the current CA 125.

Acknowledgement

Parts of the work were supported by Norwegian Cancer Society.

References

1 Börmer OP (1989) Interference of complement with the binding of carcinoembryonic antigen to solid-phase monoclonal antibodies. J Immunol Methods 121:85–93
2 Börmer OP, Nustad K (1990) Selection of monoclonal antibodies for use in an immunometric assay for carcinoembryonic antigen. J Immunol Methods 127:171–178
3 Jacobs I, Bast RC (1989) The CA 125 tumour-associated antigen: a review of the literature. Hum Reprod 4:1–12
4 O'Brien TJ, Raymond LM, Bannon GA, Ford DH, Hardardottir H, Miller FC, Quirk JG (1991) New monoclonal antibodies identify the glycoprotein carrying the CA 125 epitope. Am J Obstet Gynecol 165:1857–1864
5 Paus E, Börmer O, Nustad K (1982) Radioiodination of proteins with the Iodogen method. In: Radioimmunoassay and related procedures in medicine. International Atomic Energy Agency, Vienna, pp 161–171

Address for correspondence:
Dr. K. Nustad
Central Laboratory
Norwegian Radium Hospital
N-0310 Oslo, Norway

New monoclonal antibodies for determination of the ovarian cancer associated antigen CA 125

O. Nilsson[a], E.-L. Jansson[a], U. Dahlen[a], K. Nilsson[a], K. Nustad[b], T. Högberg[c], L. Lindholm[a]

[a]CanAg Diagnostics AB, Gothenburg, Sweden,
[b]Central Laboratory, Norwegian Radium Hospital, Oslo, Norway,
[c]Department of Gynecological Oncology, University Hospital Lund, Lund, Sweden

Introduction

The CA 125 antigen, originally defined by the Oc 125 MAb (1), has been characterized as a high molecular weight mucin like glycoprotein or glycoprotein complex with an apparent molecular weight between $\approx 200 - > 10,000$ kD. The biochemical characterisation of the CA 125 antigen show a relative low carbohydrate content, abundant presence of both N- and O-linked carbohydrates, and relative low proportions of serine and threonine in the protein back bone, which suggest that the CA 125 antigen is not a typical mucin. The large variation in apparent molecular weight of the antigen has been suggested to be owing either to that the CA 125 antigen consists of multiple subunits of ≈ 200 kD in size, or may be due to break down of the naturally occurring CA 125 antigen (2, 3).

Serological determination of the CA 125 ovarian cancer associated antigen has proven to be a valuable tool in the management of patients with epithelial ovarian cancer, and determination of CA 125 is today accepted as the first choice tumor marker for epithelial ovarian cancer (2, 3). The first generation of CA 125 assays were developed as homologous sandwich immunometric assays based on the Oc 125 MAb. Recently double determinant assays have been introduced using the M-11 MAb (4) as catching antibody and labelled Oc 125 MAb as tracer antibody. These assays show clear technical advantages as compared to the original homologous Oc 125 MAb assays without changing the clinical information of the assays (5). Additional MAb reacting with the CA 125 antigen have been established and used for development of assays of CA 125 (2). In this paper the establishment of three new MAbs reacting with protein determinants of the CA 125 antigen and the development of homologous and heterologous immunoflurometric assays for the determination of CA 125 antigen is described.

Materials and methods

Establishment of anti CA 125 MAb

The mucin fraction from tumor of epithelial ovarian cancer was partially purified by extraction with PBS containing 0.1% Triton X-100 and 1 mM PMSF, precipitation of bulk proteins with 0.6 M PCA, and S-300 Sephacryl size exclusion chromatography of the PCA soluble fraction. The elution of the mucins from the S-300 column was monitored by determination of CA 50 activity, and the CA 50 containing fractions were pooled and concentrated by ultrafiltration. The CA 125 concentration in concentrated mucin fraction was determined with commercial CA 125 kit obtained from CIS BioIndustries, France.

The Ov 185 MAb was established by i.p. immunization of Balb/c mice with 10,000 CA 125 U in complete Freunds adjuvant, and fusion of spleen cells from the immunized mice with Ag 8 myeloma cells as described (6). Primary screening was performed in an ELISA with the immunization antigen adsorbed to the wells of the microtiter wells for positive selection of clones, and sialyl Lewis a pentaglycosylceramide, coated in the microtiter wells for negative selection. The Ov 197 and Ov 198 MAb were established in a similar way except that the screening was performed by incubation of the hybridoma supernatants in microtiter wells coated with affinity purified polyclonal antisera against mouse IgG + M (Jackson Immunoresearch Lab. Inc, US). The wells were then incubated with 100 µl CA 125 antigen (≈ 500 U/ml), and after washing the bound CA 125 antigen was detected by incubation with 100 µl of biotinylated Ov 185 MAb, 1 µg/ml, and detection with HRP streptavidin (Vector Laboratories, US). The selected clones were cloned twice, and monoclonal antibodies were produced by in vitro cultivation, and purified by Protein A affinity chromatography according to the manufacturers recommendation (BioProcessing, Durham, UK).

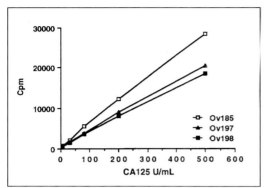

Figure 1. Co-expression of OV 185, Ov 197, Ov 198 and Oc 125 epitopes. Ov 185, Ov 197 and Ov 198 MAb were coated in Nunc Star tubes, and used as solid-phase in immunoassays using CA 125 standards and 125 labeled Oc 125 MAb as tracer obtained from CIS ELSA IRMA CA 125 kit. The coated tubes were incubated with 50 µl of standards and 100 µl assay buffer (50 mM TBS, 0.5 g/l BSA, 0.1 g/l Tween 40, pH7.8) for 2 h; after washing the CA 125 ELSA IRMA tracer was incubated in the tubes for additional 2 h.

Co-expression with Oc 125 epitope, epitope mapping and chemical characterization of epitopes

Co-expression of the Ov 185, Ov 197, Ov 198 and Oc 125 epitopes was tested using components from the CIS CA 125 ELSA IRMA kit. The dose-response using the standards of the CIS kit was tested with Ov 185 MAb, Ov 197 MAb or Ov 198 MAb coated in Nunc Star tubes (Nunc AS, Copenhagen, Denmark) as solid phase and the ^{125}I Oc 125 MAb included in the kit as tracer. Inhibition of binding of labeled Ov 185, Ov 197 and Ov 198 MAb to solid phase CA 125 antigen by unlabelled MAb were performed in microtiter wells as described (7, 8).

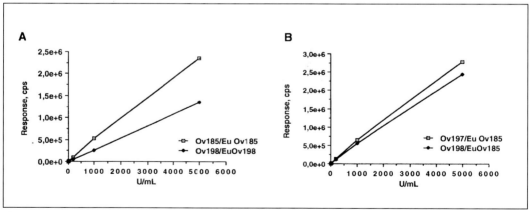

Figure 2. Dose-response of homologous and heterologous IFMAs for determination of CA 125 antigen. A) Homologous Ov 185 MAb and Ov 198 MAb assays. Assay procedure: 50 µl standard + 100 µl biotin Ov 185 or Ov 198 MAb, 0.75 µg/ml, incubated for 2 h in streptavidin coated microtiterplates. After washing 100 µ/l Europium labelled Ov 185 or Ov 198 MAb, 1 µg/ml, was added and the incubation continued for 1 h. The bound Eu was determined in an Arcus fluorometer after addition of 200 µ/l enhancement solution. B) Heterologous Ov 197/Ov 185 MAb and Ov 198/Ov 185 MAb assays. Assay procedure: 25 µl standard + 100 µl biotin Ov 197 or Ov 198 MAb, 1.5 µg/ml, incubated for 2 h in streptavidin coated microtiterplates. After washing 100 µl Eu labeled Ov 185 MAb, 1 µg/ml, was added and the incubation continued for 1 h. The bound Eu was determined in an Arcus fluorometer after addition of 200 µl enhancement solution.

The chemical nature of the epitopes was studied by periodate oxidation of CA 125 antigen immobilized in microtiter plates as described previously (9), and by proteolysis of partially purified CA 125 antigen with trypsin. The trypsin digested CA 125 antigen was used as antigen to inhibit the binding of the MAbs to solid-phase immobilized CA 125 antigen.

Development of immunoassays for determination of CA 125 antigen

The MAbs were labeled with N1DTTA Eu chelate (Wallac Oy, Turku, Finland) as previously described (10), and biotinylated according to standard procedures using the caproate derivative of BNHS. The Ov 185, Ov 197 and Ov 198 MAb

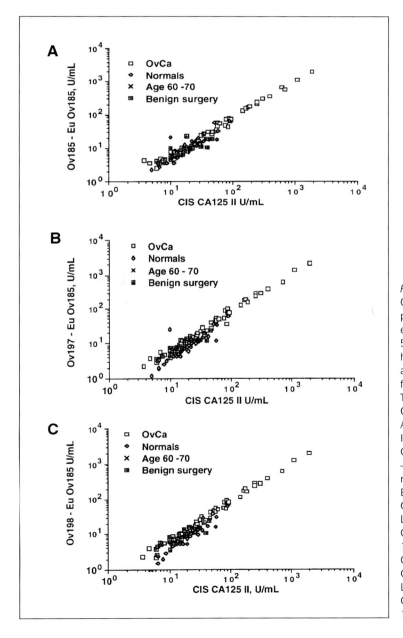

Figure 3. Correlation with CA 125 II. The correlation was performed in 47 subjects with epithelial ovarian cancer, 50 female blood donors, 25 healthy females aged 60–70 y, and 25 females surgical treated for non-malignant disease. The IFMAs were compared with CIS CA 125 II ELSA IRMA. A) Homologous OV 185 MAb IFMA. Linear correlation: Ov 185/Ov 185 IFMA = $-12{,}4004 + 1.06$ CA 125 II; $r = 99$; B) Heterologous Ov 197/Ov 185 MAb IFMA. Linear correlation: Ov 197/Ov 185 IFMA = $-14{,}1634 + 1.16$ CA 125 II; $r = 0.99$; C) Heterologous Ov 198/Ov 185 MAb IFMA. Linear correlation: Ov 198/Ov 185 IFMA = $-10.8459 + 1.08$ CA 125 II; $r = 0.99$.

were used in different combinations in two-step immunofluorometric assays (IFMA) using biotinylated MAB incubated in streptavidin coated microtiter plates (Wallac Oy, Turku, Finland) as solid phase. Preliminary clinical performance of the assays was compared with CA 125 ELSA IRMA and with CA 125 II ELSA IRMA kits (CIS Bio Industries, France).

Results and discussion

The Ov 185, Ov 197 and Ov 198 MAb used as solid-phase showed a linear dose-response using standard and tracer from commercial CA 125 kits (figure 1), which clearly demonstrated that the Ov 185, Ov 197, Ov 198 and Oc 125 epitopes were co-expressed on the CA 125 antigen in standards of commercial CA 125 kit. The dose-response with Ov 185 and Oc 125 was almost twice that obtained using Ov 197 or Ov 198 MAb as solid-phase, which may suggest that the epitope defined by the Ov 185 MAb and the Oc 125 epitope were located distantly from each other, while the Ov 197 and Ov 198 epitopes may be located close to the Oc 125 epitope causing steric hindrance between the antibodies.

The Ov 185, Ov 197 or Ov 198 MAbs did not significantly inhibit the binding of labelled Oc 125 MAb to solid-phase CA 125 antigen indicating that the epitopes defined by these MAb were not identical to the Oc 125 epitope. The inhibition studies showed also that the Ov 185, Ov 197 and Ov 198 MAb did not inhibit each other, and would thus recognize three different epitopes. In the study by Nustad et al. three epitope groups including Oc 125 and Ov 185 like epitopes were detected in the CA 125 antigen (8), and the Ov 197 and Ov 198 MAb may represent additional epitopes. The epitopes defined by the Ov 185, Ov 197 and Ov 198 MAb were of proteineous nature as the antibodies were not sensitive for periodate oxidation of the antigen.

IFMAs were developed with all possible homologous or heterologous combinations of the three MAbs. Homologous assays could be developed using all three antibodies, but the best response was obtained using the Ov 185 MAb (figure 2A). The homologous assays were sensitive for the concentration of the catching MAb, and the signal could be almost completely "inhibited" using high concentrations of the catching MAb, which may suggest that in contrast to e.g. the CA 19-9 antigen there were relatively low numbers of

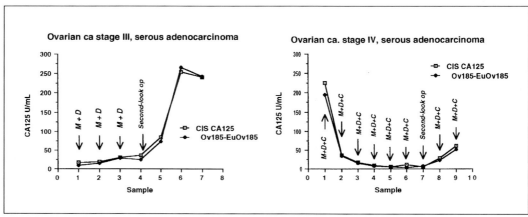

Figure 4. Follow-up patients with epithelial ovarian cancer with CA 125 and homologous Ov 185/Ov 185 IFMA. Left: Ovarian cancer stage III, seropapillary adenocarcinoma. First sample taken at the 4th treatment with Melphalan + Doxorubicin; 2nd and 3rd sample at treatment 5 and 6 with Melphalan + Doxorubicin. The second-look operation showed tumors >3 cm. The patient died in progressive disease 19 months after diagnosis. Right: Ovarian cancer stage IV, seropapillary adenocarcinoma. Samples 1–6 taken at the treatment 1–6 with Melphalan + Doxorubicin + Cisplatin. Second-look operation showed numerous positive nodules. The patient died 16 months after diagnosis in progressive disease.

repeating epitopes available in the CA 125 antigen. The best dose-response was obtained using double determinant assays using combinations of either Ov 197 or Ov 198 MAb together with Ov 185 MAb (figure 2B). In our studies the most robust assays were obtained when the Ov 197 or Ov 198 MAb were used as solid-phase antibodies and the Ov 185 MAb was used as tracer antibody in two-step sandwich assays. In the opposite configuration, i.e. the Ov 185 MAb used as the catching MAb, the assays were more sensitive to the concentration of catching MAb suggesting that binding of the CA 125 antigen to the Ov 185 MAb may lead to changes of the CA 125 antigen resulting in diminished exposure of the Ov 197 or Ov 198 epitopes. The prototype double determinant assays showed in preliminary clinical evaluations close correlation with CA 125 and CA 125 II assays, $r > 0.95$ (figure 3 and 4), which further support that these antibodies recognize epitopes exposed on the same antigen as the Oc 125 epitope.

The results of this study and the study by *Nustad* et al. demonstrate (8) that different new epitopes can be detected in the CA 125 antigen using monoclonal antibodies, and that combinations of these antibodies may be used for development of sensitive immunoassays for determination of the CA 125 antigen.

The new antibodies may also be of value for further biochemical characterization of the CA 125 antigen, and for studies whether CA 125 antigen from different tissues or serum from different clinical conditions would differ in the exposure of epitopes.

References

1 Bast R, Feeney M, Lazarus H, Nadler L, Colvin R, Knapp R (1981) Reactivity of a monoclonal antibody with human ovarian carcinoma. J Clin Invest 68: 1331–1337
2 Kenemans P, Yedema CA, Bon GG, van Mensdorff-Pouilly S (1993) CA 125 in gynecological pathology – a review. Eur J Obst Gynecol Reprod Biol 49:115–124.
3 Jacobs I and Bast Jr RC (1989) The CA 125 tumour-associated antigen: a review of the literature. Hum Reprod 4:1–12
4 O Brien T, Raymond L, Bannon G, Ford D, Hardardottir H, Miller F, Quirk J (1991) New monoclonal antibodies identify the glycoprotein carrying the CA 125 epitope. Am J Obstet Gynecol 165: 1857–1864
5 Kenemans P, van Kamp GJ, Oehr P, Verstraeten RA (1993) Heterologous double-determinant immunoradiometric assay CA 125 II: reliable second generation immunoassay for determining CA 125 in serum. Clin Chem 39:2509–2513
6 Lindolm L, Holmgren J, Svennerholm L, Fredman P, Nilsson O, Persson B, Myrvold H, Lagergard T (1983) Monoclonal antibodies against gastrointestinal tumour-associated antigens isolated as monosialogangliosides. Int Archs Allergy Appl Immunol 71:178–181
7 Børmer OP, Nustad K (1990) Selection of monoclonal antibodies for use in an immunometric assay for carcinoembryonic antigen. J Immunol Methods 127:171–178
8 Nustad K, Nilsson O, Kierulf B, Varaas T, Thrane-Steen K, Paus E, Okkenhaug C, Hauge Olsen K Børmer OP (1994) Immunoassays for the CA 125 related antigen using new monoclonal antibodies. In: Klapdor R (ed) Current tumor diagnosis: Applications, clinical relevance, research, trends. Zuckschwerdt, München, pp 397–400
9 Johansson C, Nilsson O, Baeckstöm D, Jansson EL, Lindholm L (1991) Novel epitopes on the CA, 50-carrying antigen: Chemical and immunochemical studies. Tumor Biol 12:159–170
10 Hemmilä I, Dakubu S, Mukkala VM Siitari H, Lövgren T (1983) Europium as a label in time-resolved immunofluorometricc assays. Anal Biochem 137:335–340

Address for correspondence:
Dr. O. Nilsson
CanAg Diagnostics AB
P.O. Box 12136
S-402 42 Gothenburg, Sweden

Consistency of Tandem® PSA dual-monoclonal assay and its clinical importance

M. Meyer, C. Darte, M. Wilmet, R.L. Sokoloff, H.G. Rittenhouse, R.L. Wolfert

Hybritech Europe S.A., Liège, Belgium, Hybritech Inc., San Diego, USA

Introduction

Prostate specific antigen (PSA) has become an established marker in the diagnosis and follow-up of prostate cancer patients. Some critical elements, recently described, can impact the accuracy of PSA results and, therefore, on the clinical value of the results. Three of these critical elements are:

1. The serum PSA circulating forms and the way these forms are recognized by different test methods. PSA is a protease and as such will be bound by any of several protease inhibitors when released into the blood (1, 2, 3, 4). The major form of PSA found in patient serum is equimolarly complexed with the protease inhibitor α_1-antichymotrypsin (PSA-ACT). The second major detectable form of PSA in serum is the free, uncomplexed form of PSA (f-PSA). Since it is not bound by inhibitors, it is felt that its "active" site is either not available or is inactive. The last major form of PSA is bound to α_2-macroglobulin (AM). A2M completely encloses PSA and therefore, it is considered as immunologically occult. The equal recognition of PSA forms is emerging as an essential criterion for PSA assays (5). Equimolar assays see both major PSA forms (f-PSA and PSA-ACT) the same, and report changes only when changes occur in overall PSA concentrations.

2. PSA is a member of a larger family of kallikrein proteins, some of which have remarkable amino acid homology to PSA, such as hGK-1 (human glandular kallikrein) or PRK (pancreatic renal kallikrein). hGK-1, like PSA, appears to be prostate-specific based on presence of m-RNA transcripts. PRK can be elevated in several pathological conditions. Therefore, the high level of homology of PRK and PSA can be problematic in an assay system incorporating polyclonal antibodies.

3. New tests combinations, such as the PSA measurement and the digital rectal examination, lead to an earlier prostate cancer detection and to longer patient follow-up. This is a true clinical and analytical challenge since PSA assays need to be consistent year after year.

Prostate cancer long-term monitoring

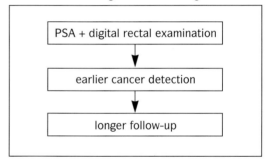

Methods

Equimolar recognition of PSA forms

PSA purified from seminal fluid was incubated 3 hours at 37° C with ACT, during which the enzymatically active portion of PSA (60%) complexed to ACT. The incubation products (f-PSA and PSA-ACT complex) were fractionated by HP-size exclusion chromatography and three samples containing 100% free PSA, 100% PSA-ACT and 50/50% free to bound PSA were prepared. The PSA molar concentration of the three solutions was adjusted to identical levels. After dilution with 1 ml of the sample diluent of the assay to be tested, a concentration of 4 ng/ml was obtained. The Tandem PSA (Hybritech) and IMx® PSA (Abbott Laboratories) assays were analyzed with these three samples.

Long-term consistency of results

A real time study made on Tandem PSA during six years and hundreds of manufacturing lots, using Lyphochek (Biorad) controls, Gilford Control (Ciba-Corning Diagnostic Division) and human sera, was done to assess the ability of this assay to accurately follow patients during long periods of time.

Results

Equimolar recognition of PSA forms

The Tandem PSA assays show consistent results for the three samples tested while IMx® PSA demonstrates a preferential recognition of the free PSA form compared to the complexed form, giving results between 3 and 6 ng/ml (figure 1).

An earlier detection of prostate cancer, made possible by the combined PSA and digital rectal examination testing, will lead to earlier treatment and longer patient follow-up. Therefore, the long-term consistency of PSA results with Tandem PSA was analyzed.

A real time study made on Tandem PSA during six years (1987–1993) and hundreds of manufacturing lots demonstrated an excellent consistency of results when using two commercial controls (Biorad Lyphochek and Gilford) and four human sera at different concentration levels. The coefficients of variation were ranging between 2.0 and 4.2% confirming the ability of this assay to follow accurately patients during long periods of time (figure 2).

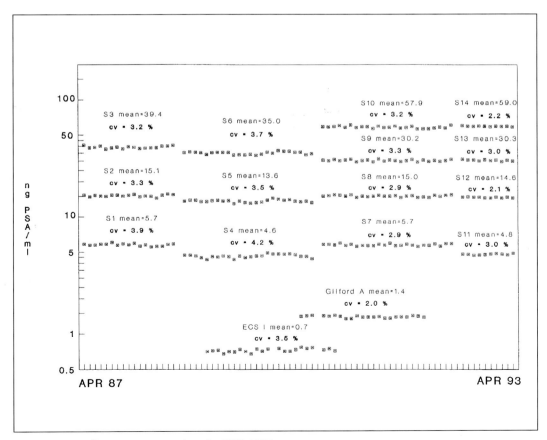

Figure 1. Tandem® PSA consistency of results 1987–1993.

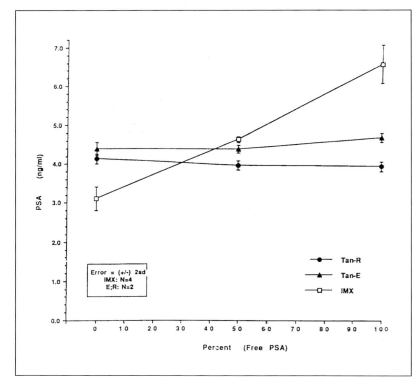

Figure 2. Recognition of PSA forms. Comparison of Tandem® PSA versus Tandem-E PSA versus IMx® PSA 100% PSA-ACT; 50/50% free PSA/PSA-ACT; 100% free PSA.

Discussion

At least three factors can influence the accuracy of PSA determinations: the way an immunoassay recognizes the PSA circulating forms, the antibodies' specificity for PSA, and the long-term performance and stability of the assay.

Several authors (2, 3, 4) have demonstrated the variability of the free to total PSA ratio from patient to patient.

It is crucial that the PSA assay used to monitor prostate cancer measures free PSA and PSA-ACT equivalently: an apparent change in PSA concentrations must correspond unequivocally to a total PSA change. With a non-equimolar assay, the PSA change observed can be either due to a true PSA change or to a modification of the free to bound PSA ratio.

According to *Graves* (6), the optimal assay configuration would be an assay that detects free and complexed PSA in equal molar ratios. This assay is not affected by complexation of PSA; the assay gives true molar value of PSA in the sample regardless of the ratio of free to complexed PSA that is present in the sample.

It has also been realized that PSA is only one member of a large family of kallikrein proteins, some of which have remarkable amino acid homology to PSA (80% for human glandular kallikrein and 60% for pancreatic renal kallikrein). A recent publication reported that, out of 22 women with renal cell carcinoma, six demonstrated elevated PSA levels with a polyclonal assay but not with Tandem PSA dual-monoclonal. The authors concluded that these falsely elevated results were probably due to cross-reaction with a highly homologous protein (7).

With the equimolar PSA measurement, the dual-monoclonal antibody specificity and the demonstrated long-term consistency of the results, Tandem PSA incorporates the necessary features for an accurate and precise prostate cancer patient management.

References

1. Christensson A, Laurell CB, Lilja H (1990) Enzymatic activity of prostate-specific antigen and its reaction with extracellular serine proteinase inhibitors. Eur J Biochem 194:755–63
2. Stenman UH, Leinonen J, Alfthan H, Rannikko S, Tuhkanen K, Alfthan O (1991) A complex between prostate-specific antigen and alpha1-antichymotrypsin is the major form of prostate-specific antigen in serum of patients with prostatic cancer: assay of the complex improves clinical sensitivity for cancer. Cancer Res 51:222–6
3. Lilja H, Christensson A, Dahlén U, Matikainen M-T, Nilsson O, Pettersson K et al (1991) Prostate-specific antigen in serum occurs predominantly in complex with alpha-1-antichymotrypsin. Clin Chem 37:1618–25
4. Christensson A, Björk T, Nilsson O, Dahlén U, Matikainen T, Cockett AT et al (1993) Serum prostate-specific antigen complexed to α_1-antichymotrypsin as an indicator of prostate cancer. J Urol 150:100–5
5. Graves HCB (1993) Issues on standardization of immunoassays for prostate-specific antigen: a review. Clin Invest Med 16:416–25
6. Graves HCB (1993) Standardization of immunoassays for prostate-specific antigen. Cancer 72:3141–44
7. Pummer K, Wirnsberger G, Pürstner P, Stettner H, Wandschneider G (1992) False positive prostate specific antigen values in the sera of women with renal cell carcinoma. J Urol 148:21–23

Address for correspondence:
M. Meyer
Hybritech Europe S.A.
Parc Scientifique du Sart Tilman
Allée des Noisetiers 12
B-4031 Liège, Belgium

Automated chemiluminescence immunoassay for prostate specific antigen (PSA)

Marketa Drahovsky, U. Fritsch, R. Schlett, M. Mack, M. Oed, L. Reum

Byk-Sangtec Diagnostica, Dietzenbach, Germany

Introduction

Prostate specific antigen (PSA) is a single chain 33 kD glycoprotein belonging to the kallikrein family produced by normal, benign and malignant prostatic epithelial cells (1).

The monitoring of PSA concentrations in serum has become indispensable in the clinical management of patients with primary or recurrent prostate cancer (2, 3). Early diagnosis of prostate cancer and radical treatment are essential to improve prostate cancer prognosis (4, 7).

Material and methods

The LIA-mat® PSA is a two-site immunoluminometric assay (sandwich principle). Highly specific monoclonal antibodies are used for coating the solid phase (coated tubes) and for the tracer. The antibodies were produced using conventional methods, purified by affinity chromatography and characterized by Western blot analysis. The combination of these antibodies used in the LIA-mat® PSA assay allows to recognize free PSA and the PSA α_1-antichymotrypsin complex (5, 6). The anti-PSA tracer conjugate consists of the antibody and a covalently bound isoluminol derivative. The tracer-PSA-complex bound to the tube wall in the immunological reaction is detected by a light reaction. Oxidation of isoluminol is started by the automatic injection of alkaline peroxide solution and catalyst solution into the test tubes. Due to the fast kinetic of the luminogenic reaction the luminescence is measured immediatelly by photocounting in the fully automated analyzer LIA-mat® S300. The light signal measured in RLUs (relative light units) is directly proportional to the amount of PSA present in standard and sample.

The use of the isoluminol derivative label does not interfere with the antigen antibody reaction.

The LIA-mat PSA assay protocol is as follows: pipet 50 ml standard, control or patient sample, add 150 ml anti-PSA tracer conjugate, mix, incubate while shaking (100 – 150 rpm) for 2 (± 5 min) at room temperature (18–25 °C), aspirate, wash three times with 2 ml of 0.9% NaCl solution, measure the luminescence for 5 sec in the luminometer.

The LIA-mat® PSA assay was developed to be performed manually and for the use in the fully automated luminescence immunoassay analyzer LIA-mat® S300.

Results and discussion

Reproducibility

LIA-mat® PSA intra- and inter-assay reproducibility was determined at multiple points on the calibration curve for the patient sera and controls (figures 1, 2).

Sensitivity

To estimate the analytical sensitivity of the LIA-mat® PSA, the zero standard was measured ten times, leading to a minimum detection below 0.05 ng/ml (3SD).

Linearity and recovery

For the linearity and recovery the correlation coefficient (r) from the linear regression analysis was between 0.98–0.99.

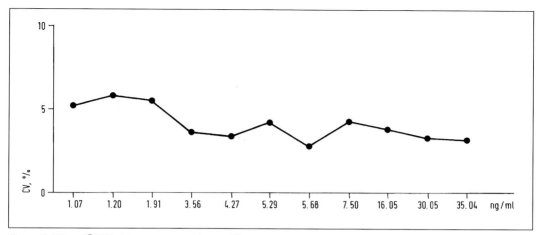

Figure 1. LIA-mat® PSA: intra-assay precision profile.

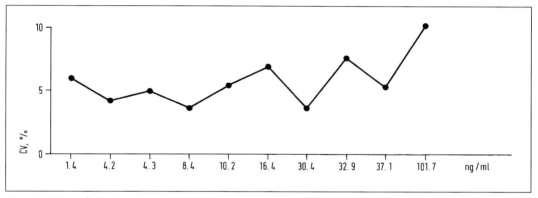

Figure 2. LIA-mat® PSA: inter-assay precision profile.

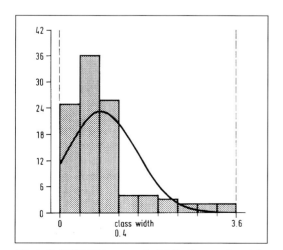

Figure 3. IRMA-PSA, normal distribution, male adults n = 104.

Table I. Analytical recovery. A patient's serum was spiked with different amounts of PSA.

Measured value n/ml	Expected value ng/ml	Recovery %
91.10	90.11	101
68.80	72.41	95
37.40	37.01	101
19.40	19.31	100
11.20	10.46	107
6.70	6.03	111
4.25	3.82	111

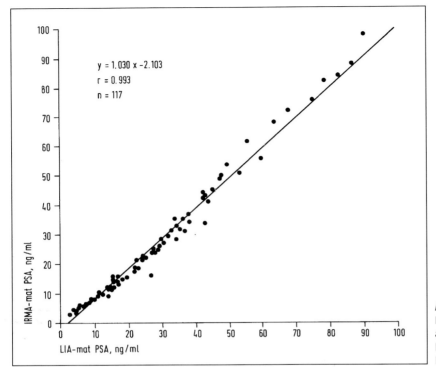

Figure 4. Linear regression analysis between LIA-mat® PSA and IRMA-mat® PSA.

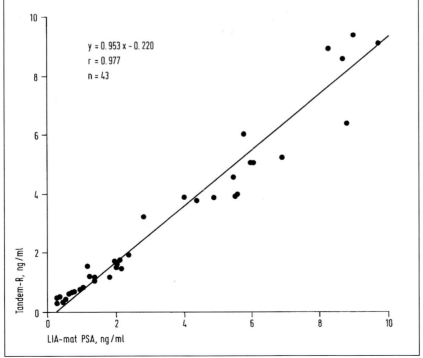

Figure 5. Linear regression analysis between LIA-mat® PSA and Tandem® PSA Hybritech. Concentration range between 0–10 ng/ml.

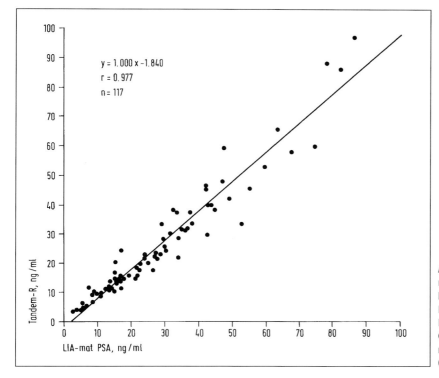

Figure 6. Linear regression analysis between LIA-mat® PSA and Tandem® PSA Hybritech. Concentration range between 0–100 ng/ml.

Distribution of normal values

In 95% of healthy male adults serum PSA concentrations below 3.0 ng/ml (cut-off) were found with the LIA-mat® PSA.

High-dose hook effect

LIA-mat® PSA demonstrates no high-dose "hook effect" up to 10,000 ng/ml.

Comparison with other methods

Results obtained by LIA-mat® PSA are in excellent correlation with our in-house IRMA-mat® PSA and the Tandem® PSA assay of Hybritech (figure 4, 5, 6).

Conclusion

Comparison with established immunoradiometric assays was carried out to evaluate the performances of the new immunoluminometric assay LIA-mat® PSA for the determination of PSA in prostate cancer patients. Excellent correlation between the LIA-mat® PSA and the two immunoradiometric assays was found.

In conclusion the new LIA-mat® PSA fully automated immunoassay will contribute well to the clinical management of patients with prostate cancer.

References

1. Wang MC, Valenzuela LA, Murphy GP, Chu TM (1979) Purification of a human prostate specific antigen. Invest Urol 17:159–63
2. Stamey TA, Yang N, Hay AR, McNeal JE, Freiha FS, Redwine E (1987) Prostate specific antigen as a serum marker for adenocarcinoma of the prostate. N Eng J Med 317:909–16
3. Oesterling JE (1991) Prostate specific antigen: A critical assessment of the most useful tumor marker for adenocarcinoma of the prostate. J Urol 145:907–23
4. Catalona WJ et al (1991) Measurement of prostate specific antigen in serum as a screening test for prostate cancer. N Eng J Med 324:1156–61

5 Stenman UH, Leinonen J, Alfthan H, Rannikko S, Tuhkanen K, Alfthan O (1991) A complex between prostate specific antigen and alpha1-antichymotrypsin is the major form of prostate specific antigen in serum of patients with prostatic cancer: assay of the complex improves clinical sensitivity for cancer. Cancer Res 51:222–226

6 Lilja H, Christensson A, Dahlen U, Matikainen MT, Nilsson O, Pettersson K et al (1991) Prostate specific antigen in human serum occurs predominantly in complex with a1-antichymotrypsin. Clin Chem 37:1618–25

7 Graves HCB (1992) Prostate specific antigen comes of age in diagnosis and management of prostate cancer. Clin Chem 38/10:1930–32

Address for correspondence:
Marketa Drahovsky
Byk-Sangtec Diagnostika GmbH
Von Hevesy-Straβe 3
D-63128 Dietzenbach, Germany

Evaluation of the LIA-mat® PSA assay

B. G. Blijenberg[a], Edith Greiner-Mai[b]
[a]Academic Hospital Rotterdam-Dijkzicht, The Netherlands,
[b]Byk-Sangtec Diagnostica GmbH, Dietzenbach, Germany

Introduction

Prostate-specific antigen (PSA) is a glycoprotein with a molecular weight of 30 kD (amino acids plus 6.9% carbohydrate) which is organ-specific (1). PSA is the most important and clinically useful marker for prostate cancer. It can lead to the diagnosis of clinically significant prostate cancers at an early stage and is an excellent predictor of the pathological stage (2, 3).

When PSA is measured in the serum of patients with prostate cancer, very little is free and most is complexed with α_1-antichymotrypsin (ACT) (4, 5, 6). In the new Byk-Sangtec PSA procedure both the solid-phase antibody and the detecting antibody showed an approximately 100% cross-reactivity with the PSA-ACT complex.

In the absence of an internationally accepted standard preparation, the LIA-mat® method was calibrated using the Hybritech Tandem-R as reference method.

Materials and methods

The LIA-mat® PSA is a two-site immunoluminometric assay (sandwich principle, 1-step incubation, 2 hours at room temperature). Highly specific monoclonal antibodies are used for the coating of the solid phase (coated tubes) and for the tracer. The combination of these antibodies used in the LIA-mat® PSA assay allows the detection of free PSA and the PSA-α_1-antichymotrypsin complex.

The anti-PSA tracer conjugate consists of an antibody and a covalently bound isoluminol derivative. The tracer-PSA complex bound to the tube wall in the immunological reaction is detected by a light reaction. Oxidation of isoluminol is started by the automatic injection of alkaline peroxide solution and catalyst solution into the test tubes. Since there is an immediate emission of photons, which vanishes within seconds (< 20 sec), the luminogenic reaction is started in the luminometer (automated analyzer LIA-mat® System 300). The light (425 nm) produced by the reaction is measured in the photomultiplier of the luminometer. The light signal measured in RLUs (relative light units) is directly proportional to the amount of PSA present in standard and sample.

For comparison, the immunoenzymatic assay IMx® PSA (Abbott Diagnostics) and the immunoradiometric assay IRMA-mat® PSA (Byk-Sangtec Diagnostica) were used. The assays were performed according to the manufacturer's procedure.

In the study, serum and plasma samples were used from apparently healthy male and female blood donors, patients with benign prostatic diseases and patients with prostate cancer (different stages and after prostatectomy).

Results

Precision and reproducibility

The LIA-mat® PSA intra-assay precision profile was obtained by measurement of serum samples in duplicate. The mean CV remained well below 10% (mean CV = 3.3%) and the lower limit of the useful working range < 0.1 ng/ml underlines the high technical quality of the assay.

The LIA-mat® PSA inter-assay precision was determined by 10 replicates at multiple points on the calibration curve for commercial control sera. Excellent CV values ranging between 2.5 and

6.9% were obtained (29.2 ng/ml: CV = 2.5%; 8.15 ng/ml: CV = 5%; 4 ng/ml: CV = 4.1%; 1.35 ng/ml: CV = 6.8%).

Linearity upon dilution

For dilution linearity, patient's sera and controls were diluted with the kit diluent. This test revealed strict linearity over the whole standard range (r = 0.997).

Comparison with other methods

The correlation study was performed by comparing serum values from patients with benign and malignant prostatic disease measured with the LIA-mat® PSA, IMx® PSA, and IRMA-mat® PSA. In all cases, a very good correlation was found at low and high PSA levels (r = 0.99 and r = 0.97 resp., figures 1 a, b).

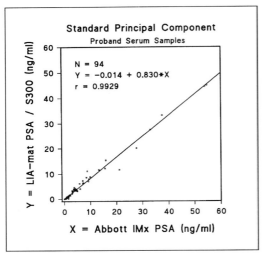

Figure 1a. Correlation LIA-mat® PSA versus IMx® PSA.

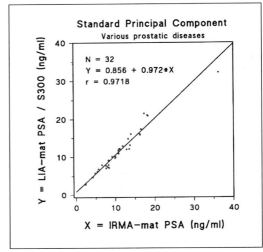

Figure 1b. Correlation LIA-mat® PSA versus IRMA-mat® PSA.

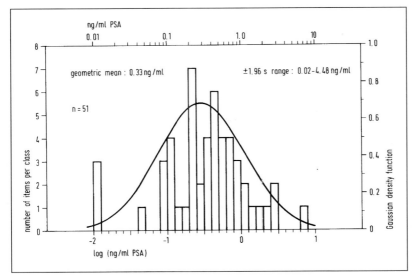

Figure 2. LIA-mat® PSA reference range in healthy men.

Table I. Serum PSA (ng/ml) in patients after radical prostatectomy.

LIA-mat® PSA	IMx® PSA
0.08	0.17
0.00	0.00
0.00	0.00
0.00	0.00
0.00	0.00
0.00	0.00
0.00	0.00
0.07	0.20
0.00	0.00
0.00	0.07
0.00	0.00
0.00	0.00
0.00	0.02
0.00	0.00
0.22	0.32
0.00	0.00
0.00	0.00
0.00	0.00
0.51	0.69
0.00	0.00
0.05	0.23
0.00	0.00
0.00	0.00
0.00	0.00

Reference range

A restricted check of reference values was performed with sera from 51 male and 30 female blood donors. It revealed values lower than 3 ng/ml for 50 samples (minus one of uncertain clinical status, figure 2). The female sera gave results as 0 ng/ml. For the male donor group, serum and plasma samples were cross-checked, revealing no influence on different matrices (r = 0.994). Sera from 24 prostatectomized patients did not show any values exceeding 0.5 ng/ml (table I).

Discussion

In this evaluation, the newly developed Byk Sangtec assay LIA-mat® PSA was tested. Preliminary results, analytical as well as clinical, showed a favourable performance. Concerning the coefficients of variation, we found excellent results. For the lower detection limit, important for the assessment of prostatectomized men, we found a value below 0.1 ng/ml which is the state-of-the-art. A proof with 24 samples from this category showed excellent results as compared with the Abbott IMx data. A restricted check of the reference values revealed that the generally accepted cut-off value of 4 ng/ml can be applied. A comparison study with other methods, especially with the Abbott IMx showed good correlations. This holds true for randomly chosen specimens as well as clinically described sera (benign prostatic hyperplasia and prostate carcinoma at various stages).

Summary

This study reports the results of evaluations performed on the newly designed LIA-mat® PSA. An analytical as well as clinical evaluation was performed at the University Hospital Rotterdam, The Netherlands. For the lower limit of the useful working range, we measured less than 0.1 ng/ml. Inter-assay precision was assessed by ten replicates of various commercial control samples. At level 1.3 ng/ml, we found CVs of 6.9% for the LIA-mat® PSA. At higher levels, 4.8 and 29 ng/ml respectively, we found results between 2.9 and 5.9%. A restricted check of the reference values with 51 randomly chosen male donor samples revealed values lower than 3 ng/ml for 50 samples. Thirty female donor samples, also randomly chosen, gave results as 0 ng/ml.

A correlation study was performed by comparison with Abbott IMx using samples taken from patients with benign prostate hyperplasia and prostate carcinoma at various stages. In all situations, a very good correlation was found. In conclusion: All data available show that the LIA-mat® PSA is a valid alternative for use in the routine determination of PSA.

References

1. Wang MC, Valenzuela LA, Murphy GP, Chu TM (1979) Purification of a human prostate specific antigen. Invest Urol 17:159–163
2. Stamey TA, Yang N, Hay AR, McNeal JE, Freiha FS, Redwine E (1987) Prostate specific antigen as a serum marker for adenocarcinoma of the prostate. N Eng J Med 317:909–916

3. Armbruster DA (1993) Prostate specific antigen: Biochemistry, analytical methods, and clinical application. Clin Chem 39:181–195
4. Christensson A, Björk T, Nilsson O et al (1993) Serum prostate specific antigen complexed of α_1-antichymotrypsin as an indicator of prostate cancer. J Urol 150:100–105
5. Stenman UH, Leinonen J, Alfthan H, Rannikko S, Tuhkanen K, Aofthan O (1991) A complex between prostate specific antigen and α_1-antichymotrypsin is the major form of prostate specific antigen in serum of patients with prostatic cancer: assay of the complex improves clinical sensitivity for cancer. Cancer Res 51:222–226
6. Lilja H, Christensson A, Dahlen U, Matikainen MT, Milsson O, Petterson K et al (1990) Prostate specific antigen in human serum occurs predominantly in complex with α_1-antichymotrypsin. Clin Chem 37:1618–1625

Address for correspondence:
Dr. Edith Greiner-Mai
Byk-Sangtec Diagnostika GmbH
Von Hevesy-Straße 3
D-63128 Dietzenbach, Germany

Tumor necrosis factor p55 and p75 measured in sera of prostatic cancer patients using Cobas® Core

P.R. Huber[a], H.P. Schmid[b], C. Stremmel[b], H. Gallati[c], A. Maurer[d], M. Thein[d]

[a]Kantonsspital Basel, Hormone Laboratory DZL, [b]Kantonsspital Basel, Department of Urology,
[c]Pharma Research, F. Hoffmann-La Roche & Cie,
[d]Roche Diagnostic Systems, a Division of F. Hoffmann-La Roche Ltd, Basel, Switzerland

Introduction

Tumor necrosis factor (TNF-a) also called Cachectin and Lymphotoxin (TNF-β) (1,2) are pluripotent cytokines. Activated macrophages are the main source of the TNF activity, however other cells are capable to produce TNF as well (3). Both cytokines TNF-α and TNF-β exert their biological activity by two types of receptor proteins situated in the cell membrane of a multiude of cells and cell types. From in vitro experiments it is known that cancer cells express these two types of receptor proteins for TNF on their surface (5, 6). Probably by proteolytic cleavage (11). The extracellular moieties of both receptors are probably sheared off proteolytic cleavage and are shed into circulation (soluble TNFR; sTNFR). The sTNFRs are still able to actively bind TNF-a and TNF-β and therefore lend themselves as possible diagnostic tools. The expression of TNFR on the surface of different cancer cells in vitro, their shedding into circulation, the stability of the proteins in solution and the availability of simple and straightforward assay systems to measure sTNFR p55 and p75 led us to study the distribution of these proteins in the serum of prostate cancer patients.

Patients and methods

Patients sera for routine estimation PSA were subjected to the subsequent quantification of sTNFR and Neopterin. The study population consisted of in- and out-patients visiting the urological clinic for prostatic disfunction, for radiation therapy or post surgery surveillance as well as of patients receiving LHRH treatment.

Sera from blood donors were used as controls. In addition sera from patients with various non-prostatic illnesses, were included to establish the effect of potential tissue inflammation. All these patients had a concommittant examination for prostatic growth and a determination of serum PSA (upper limit for normal controls 3.5 ng/ml and patients with benign hyperplasia of the prostate (BPH) 14 ng/ml).

Soluble Tumor necrosis factors (sTNFR) p 55 and p 75 were determined by the ELIBA technique (Cobas® Core; F. Hoffmann-La Roche Basel, Switzerland). In brief, monoclonal anti human TNFR antibody (TNFR p55:htr-20;TNFR p75:utr-4) bound to a polystyrene support (polystyrene beads) is reacted with either recombinant TNFR standard or natural TNFR from the sample. Simultaneously human r-TNF-α-horse radish peroxidase conjugate is added. Subsequently the immuno reaction is quantitated by color development from TMB (tetramethyl benzidin/H_2O_2) reacted with the bound enzyme. The sensitivity of both assays was 100 pg/ml. Prostate specific antigen (PSA) was estimated with the commercially available test system from DELFIA (Wallac Oy, Turku, Finnland)) which uses two monoclonal antibodies. Neopterin was measured by RIA (Henning, Germany).

Results and discussion

Figure 1 summarizes the results for TNFR p55 obtained in sera of blood donors, patients with non-prostatic illness (NPI), patients with BPH or P-Ca. The levels of sTNFR p55 in blood donor sera patients was significantly different from the levels found in sera of NPI ($p < 0.001$), BPH

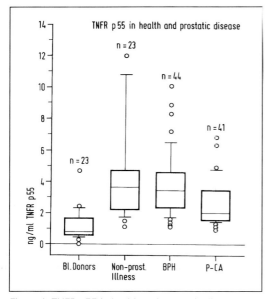

Figure 1. TNFR p55 in health and prostatic disease.

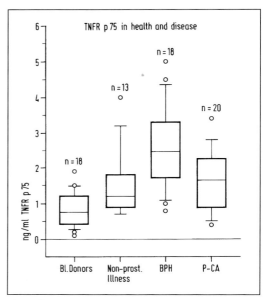

Figure 2. TNFR p75 in health and prostatic disease.

($p < 0.001$) and P-Ca ($p < 0.001$) patients. Significant differences were also observed when BPH and P-Ca sera were compared ($p < 0.01$). Interestingly the mean concentration of sTNFR p55 was lower than in NPI or BPH. We analyzed the data in some more detail and found a prominent decrease in sTNFR p55 concentrations in patients with P-CA staged T1 and/or T2 ($p < 0.01$) compared to BPH or P-Ca of stage T3 ($p < 0.01$) and T4 respectively. As shown in figure 2 the same increase of serum concentrations of sTNFR p75 from blood donors to BPH patients ($p < 0.001$) as for sTNFR p55 can be observed. Again P-Ca patients in comparison to BPH-patients have a tendency ($p = 0.02$) to decreased serum concentration of sTNFR p75. Once more we observed the trend to lower values in patients with untreated and treated prostate carcinomas staged T1 and T2 and albeit only two cases of untreated prostate carcinomas staged a) T3N1 M0 with sTNFR p75 1.0 ng/ml and sTNFR p55 2.0 ng/ml, PSA 43.2 ng/ml, and b) T3 NxM1 with sTNFR p75 0.4ng/ml and sTNFR p55 1.4 ng/ml, PSA 8.0 ng/ml were included.

Overall the simultaneously measured serum PSA follows the well described pattern of NPI < BPH < P-Ca. For BPH patients we observed a strong correlation of $r = 0.436$ ($p < 0.005$) for sTNFR p55 and serum PSA. In patients with P-Ca sTNFR p55 correlated well with PSA ($p < 0.001$). For sTNFR p75 in BPH there is no significant correlation whereas in the P-Ca group a significant correlation between these two parameters PSA and TNFR p75 was observed: ($r = 0.514$ ($p < 0.01$)).

In patients with NPI serum PSA was well within the limit of 14 ng/ml indicating that these patients did not suffer from a prostatic carcinoma. Only a few patients showed PSA levels well above the 3.5 ng/ml. The higher levels of serum p55 fragment are probably caused by illness of non-prostatic origin. The p75 fragment on the other hand never increased drastically above its normal limit. The group of prostate carcinoma patients include treated and untreated cases. This is reflected by the fact that several collectives of patients can be distinguished. First a group of patients with low PSA and low p55 and p75 fragment concentrations indicating an inactive disease. A second group with normal PSA and elevated mostly above normal sTNFR p55 concentrations. The third small group of patients shows both high PSA levels and higher than normal levels of sTNFR p55 but not sTNFR p75 indicating enhanced activity on the tissue level.

Figure 3 shows the distribution of PSA, TNFR p55 and p75 and the other macrophage product

New Assays 421

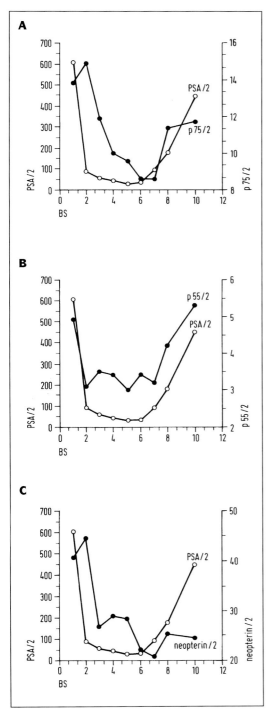

Figure 3. Data from TNFR prostate therapy. A. Patient no. 2 (see text), time course of PSA and p75. B. Time course of PSA and p55. C. Time course of PSA and neopterin. BS: number of blood sampling.

neopterin over time of an LH-RH analogue treated patient with advanced prostate carcinoma. In this patient a concurrent fall and rise of the single serum parameters is observed. This is not always seen. In three of the four patients treated with LH-RH analog PSA went from very high to low but detectable levels parallel with suppressed testosterone activity. At the same time two other patients showed erratic reactions of both TNFR fragments and neopterin for unknown reasons. The observed peaks were not superimposable. It is important to note that smooth distribution patterns over time were observed in two patients for sTNFR fragment and neopterin concentration whereas in two patients erratic patterns were seen in the other two patients.

The method to measure sTNFR in serum described in this study involves highly specific monoclonal antibodies to detect the soluble forms of TNF receptor p55 or p75. The detection of the immune reaction by binding enzyme labelled TNF to the naturally occurring binding site is new. Aderka et al. (7) described the serum concentrations of soluble TNF receptors in several types of carcinomas including breast, colon, pancreas, stomach and ovary, but not P-Ca. PSA has been widely accepted as the tumor marker for prostate carcinoma, but it cannot clearly distinguish between BPH and early stages of P-Ca. As it seems to be generally accepted serum PSA is strongly associated with tumor size in the prostate. As the TNFRs are associated with the autoimmune reaction to tumors, the sTNFR could reflect the autoimmune reaction of the body towards the tumor and the probable inflammation connected to it.

The distribution pattern of the two sTNFRs p55 and p75 in the different groups of prostate lesion examined was surprisingly parallel indicating the same mechanism of secretion reacting to similar stimuli but the source not necessarily being the same.

Activated macrophages seem to be the main source of TNF and also of neopterin (8, 9). As TNFR p75 is described in the literature to be attributed to the hematopoietic cell system (10) and TNFR p55 to the more epithelial tissues (3) we intended with the simultaneous estimation of neopterin to disclose the different sources of the receptor fragments.

Based on the findings presented here the source of soluble TNFR remains still unclear. From the data presented here we observed the reaction of the patient's immune system as it reacts to tumor growth.

At the present stage of research sTNFR quantification does not lend itself as diagnostic tool to differentiate BPH from P-Ca.

References

1. Beutler B, Cerami A (1986) Cachectin and tumor necrosis factor as two sides of the same biological coin. Nature 320:584–588
2. Beutler B, Cerami A (1988) Cachectin (Tumor Necrosis Factor): A macrophage hormone governing cellular metabolism and inflammatory response. Endocrin Rev 9:57–66
3. Loetscher H, Pan YCE, Lahm HW, Gentz R, Brockhaus M, Tabuchi H, Lesslauer W (1990) Molecular cloning and expression of the human 55 kd tumor necrosis factor receptor. Cell 61:351–359
4. Brockhaus M, Schoenfeld HJ, Schlaeger EJ, Hunziker W, Lesslauer W, Loetscher HR (1990) Identification of two types of tumor necrosis factor receptors on human cell lines by monoclonal antibodies. Proc Natl Acad Sci (USA) 87:3127–3131
5. Hohmann H, Remy R, Brockhaus M, van Loon APGM (1989) Two different cell types have 5/different major receptors for human tumor necrosis factor (TNF alpha). J Biol Chem 5/264:14927–14934
6. Porteu F, Brockhaus M, Wallach D, Engelmann H, Nathan CF (1991) Human neutrophil elastase releases a ligand binding fragment from the 75 kDa tumor necrosis factor (TNF) receptor. J Biol Chem 266:18846–18853
7. Aderka D, Engelmann H, Hornik V, Skornick Y, Yoram L, Wallach D, Kushtai G (1991) Increased serum levels of soluble receptors for tumor necrosis factor in cancer patients. Cancer Res 51:5602–5607
8. Beutler B, Greenwald D, Hulmes J, Chang M, Pan YCE, Mathieson J, Ulevitch R, Cerami A (1985) Identity of tumor necrosis factor and the macrophage-secreted factor 9/cachectin. Nature 316:552–554
9. Fuchs D, Hansen A, Rebnegger G, Werner ER, Dierich MP, Wachter H (1988) Neopterin as a marker for activated cell mediated immunity. Immunol Today 9:150–155
10. Heller RA, Song K, Onasch MA, Fischer WH, Chang D, Ringold GM (1990) Complementary DNA-cloning of a receptor for tumor necrosis factor and demonstration of a shed form of the receptor. Proc Natl Acad Sci (USA) 87:6151–6155

Address for correspondence:
Priv.-Doz. Dr. P. R. Huber
Kantonsspital Basel
Hormonlabor DZL
CH-4031 Basel, Switzerland

A new monoclonal antibody based immunoassay for tissue polypeptide antigen

Preliminary clinical results

M. Correale[a], H. Arnberg[b], P. Blockx[c], E. Bombardieri[d], M. Castelli[e], G. Encabo[f], M. Gion[g], R. Klapdor[h], S. Nilsson[b], H. Reutgen[i], G. Ruggeri[j], F. Safi[k], M. Stegmuller[l], A. Vering[l]

[a]Istituto Oncologico, Bari, Italy, [b]Akademiska Sjukhuset Uppsala, Sweden, [c]UIA Nuclear Medicine Department, Edegem, Belgium, [d]Dipartimento di Medicina Nucleare, Istituto Nazionale per la Cura e lo Studio dei Tumori, Milano, Italy, [e]Istituto Sperimentale Oncologia »Regina Elena«, Roma, Italy, [f]Valle Hebron Hospital, Barcelona, Spain, [g]Centro Regionale per lo Studio degli Indicatori Biochimici di Tumore, Ospedale Civile, Venezia, Italy, [h]Universitätskrankenhaus Eppendorf I., Medizinische Klinik Hamburg, Germany, [i]Fachkrankenhaus für Lungenheilkunde, Berlin, Germany, [j]III Laboratorio Analisi Chimico-Cliniche, Spedali Civili, Brescia, Italy, [k]Universitätsklinik Ulm-Safranberg, Chirurgische Abteilung, Ulm, [l]Universitätsfrauenklinik, Frankfurt, Germany

Introduction

Tissue polypeptide antigen (TPA) is a molecular complex of cytokeratin 8, 18 and 19 (1, 2). The more than decennial use of quantification of TPA in sera from cancer patients has shown to be of large value as a support for diagnosing a patient with a suspicious tumor as well as assisting in staging of the tumor and monitoring the treatment of the patient (3). A new assay for TPA (TPA-M IRMA) has been developed (4). It makes use of three monoclonal antibodies, recognizing epitopes on cytokeratin 8, 18 and 19. A comprehensive effort to document this new TPA assay in the clinic is presently under way. These studies are aimed at evaluating whether the new monoclonal TPA assay could represent a valid alternative to classical polyclonal TPA assay in the determination of cytokeratin 8, 18, and 19. This is a preliminary report on the findings of this international multicentre investigation.

Patients and methods

This clinical evaluation has been multicentric and multinational in several European countries (TPA-M European Study Group), in patients with newly diagnosed lung, breast, colorectal and urinary bladder cancers. The clinical importance of the TPA determination, by means of both the classical polyclonal (Prolifigen TPA IRMA-Sangtec Medical, Bromma, Sweden) and of the new assay based on monoclonal antibodies (Prolifigen TPA-M IRMA-Sangtec Medical, Bromma, Sweden), was assessed in four cross sectional studies. The procedure of the polyclonal and of the new monoclonal TPA assays are summarized in table I.

The monoclonal TPA-M IRMA assay has been carefully validated by the manufacturer and the correlation with polyclonal was determined. The test proved to be robust, with minimal influence from variation of assay parameters: incubation time and temperature. The high-dose hook effect can be seen only at titres exceeding 100,000 U/l. The correlation coefficient between the polyclonal and the monoclonal assay, as reported by the manufacturer, was very good with a correlation coefficient of 0.98.

Those markers generally considered as reference markers for the above mentioned malignancies, CEA and NSE for lung, CA 15-3 for breast and CEA and CA 19-9 for colorectal tumors (all IRMA assays, NSE by Sangtec Medical; CEA, CA 19-9 and CA 15-3 by Byk Sangtec Diagnostica), as well as other cytokeratin markers, namely TPS (TPS IRMA, Beki Diagn.), CYFRA (CYFRA 21-1, Boehringer Mannheim) TPAcyk (TPAcyk IRMA, IDL), have been also determined.

Table I. Procedure of the TPA IRMA assay and of the TPA-M IRMA assay.

TPA IRMA (polyclonal)	TPA-M IRMA (monoclonal)
100 µl sample + 100 µl diluent + antibody bead	100 µl sample + 200 µl tracer + antibody bead
incubate 4 h with shaking	incubate 2 h with shaking
wash twice with saline	wash 3 times with 2-3 ml deionized water
200 µl tracer	–
incubate for 17–20 h	–
wash twice with saline	–
count activity	count activity

Table II. Sensitivities at 95% specificity (from ROC curve analysis). Cut-off expressed in U/l for TPA-M, TPA and TPS, in U/ml for CA 15-3 and CA 19-9, and in ng/ml for CYFRA, CEA and NSE; sens. = sensitivity (%).

	Lung		Breast		Colonrectum		Bladder	
	cut-off	sens.	cut-off	sens.	cut-off	sens.	cut-off	sens.
TPA-M	63	70	89	17	72	45	61	55
TPA	82	70	130	11	100	62	77	64
TPS	130	52	150	10	134	27	116	30
CYFRA	2.6	69	2.2	11	2.1	28	1.8	57
TPAcyk	–	–	1.3	9	–	–	–	–
CEA	7.2	28	–	–	4.3	45	–	–
NSE	8.5	58	–	–	–	–	–	–
CA 15-3	–	–	33	11	–	–	–	–
CA 19-9	–	–	–	–	22	31	–	–

Results

This report covers the results from a preliminary analysis performed on a total of 561 patient data. A final statistical evaluation from the complete patient data base, which accounts over 700 subjects, will be the object of a final report. Serum samples were obtained from 160 healthy subjects, 198 patients with non malignant disease (94, 47, 28 and 29 with benign diseases of the lung, breast, colonrectum and urinary bladder, respectively) and 203 patients suffering from malignant tumors (57, 59, 35, 52 with malignancies of the lung, breast, colonrectum and urinary bladder, respectively).

The mean + SD TPA-M value in control subjects was 32.5 + 19.5 U/l. The median value was 29.75 U/l. 95% of the control subjects resulted to have values below 77 U/l.

The sensitivity and specificity data as well as data from ROC curve analysis (summarized in table II) indicated that TPA, polyclonal as well as monoclonal, resulted as a marker with high sensitivity (50 to 80%) in lung, colorectal and urinary bladder carcinoma, at 95% specificity. Although CYFRA 21-1 showed a good sensitivity for lung tumor cancer (70%), expecially for epidermoid carcinoma (80%), these values resulted to be identical to those of TPA. In breast cancer, the majority of patients had disease in very early stages and thus the sensitivity of the markers was relatively low. TPA-M as well as TPA polyclonal serum levels in stage III and IV patients resulted significantly higher than those measured in stage 0 to II patients. A similar discriminating power was also shown in urinary bladder cancer patients.

Conclusions

Among the cytokeratin markers, TPA resulted as the marker with the widest range of clinical applications, and in the localization studied, it was the most sensitive marker. Monoclonal TPA seems to offer an interesting alternative to TPA polyclonal, with improved technical characteristics and comparable performances when used in the clinic.

References

1. Sundstroem B, Stigbrand T (1994) Cytokeratins and Tissue Polypeptide Antigen. Int J Biol Markers 9:102–108
2. Mellerik DM, Osborn M, Weber K (1990) On the nature of serological tissue polypeptide antigen (TPA); monoclonal keratin 8, 18, 19 antibodies react differently with TPA prepared from human cultured carcinoma cells and TPA in human serum. Oncogene 5:107–1017
3. Montinari F, Luporini G (1993) The Tissue Polypeptide Antigen. In: Ballesta AM, Torre CC, Bombardieri E, Gion M, Molina R (eds) Updating on tumor markers in tissues and in biological fluids. Minerva Medica, Torino, Italy, pp 639–650
4. Brundell J, D'Amico Y, Sundstrom B (1993) TPA IRMA-M. A new assay for TPA based on monoclonal antibodies. J Tum Marker Oncol 8:71

Address for correspondence:
Dr. M. Correale
Istituto Oncologico
via Amendola, 209
I-70126 Bari, Italy

A standardized protocol for determination of TPA in urine by a monoclonal assay and its clinical significance

L. N. Fischer[a], B. E. Carbin[b], M. Bäcklander[a], A. C. Lanneskog[a], B. Sundström[b]

[a]Sangtec Medical, Bromma, [b]Karolinska Hospital, Stockholm, Sweden

Introduction

The world-wide financial crisis for medicine has made it necessary to reduce the costs in areas that are felt to be urgent. Thus, the number of cystoscopic follow-up investigations in bladder cancer patients to detect local recurrence has been greatly reduced in the last years. To compensate for this, a simple and inexpensive laboratory investigation to detect recurrent local bladder cancer is urgent. Earlier investigations (1–7) indicated that the determination of TPA, an established tumor marker, in urine would be suitable, but no standardized procedure for TPA determination in urine has been available. We report here on one part of a research program aiming to develop standard protocols for TPA in urine and evaluating them clinically.

On a previous occasion we reported about a standardized protocol for determination of TPA in urine with the polyclonal TPA IRMA assay (8, 9). The assay was based on a procedure suggested by *Yoshida* et al. (10) where Tween 40 is added to improve assay characteristics. The purpose of this investigation was to standardize the protocol for a monoclonal TPA IRMA.

Method

The standard TPA-M IRMA kit from Sangtec Medical, Bromma, Sweden was used. 10 ml 24 hour urine was centrifuged at 1,500–2,000 rpm for 10–15 min. 50 μl of Tween 20 was added per 10 ml of urine. For the assay, 50 μl of the pretreated urine and 150 μl of kit diluent were added to the test tube. 200 μl tracer and the antibody-coated bead were added and incubated under agitation for 2 h at RT, then washed with 3 x 2 ml 0.9% NaCl. As standards the standards of the kit are used, treated in accordance with the kit instruction and were read in a gamma counter. The test result must be multiplied by 2 to compensate for the dilution.

Results and discussion

In the validation of the test procedure, the kinetics was found to be stable: Variation of the first incubation step from 3 to 5 hours does not change the value measured in the samples, figure 1. The temperature changed the values marginally, but it is recommended that the temperature is maintained at 22 ± 2 °C (figure 2). The assay was not sensitive to variation in the pH of the sample, and therefore it was not considered to be necessary to adjust the pH of the urine samples (figure 3). The dilution and recovery tests indicate that the assay measures correctly. One example of a dilution curve is given in figure 4, and one example of a recovery experiment is reported in table I. The imprecision analysis shows that the measurement is stable and reproducible. One aspect of the measurement, that is particularly important for the clinical evaluation is the stability of samples against freezing and thawing. Figure 5 demonstrates that repeated freezing and thawing does not alter the value significantly. The method validation thus demonstrates that the method is robust and reliable.

The preliminary clinical validation gives values lower than those obtained in the polyclonal assay. The average value for normal subjects is 130 U/l, as compared to 250 U/l for the polyclonal TPA assay. For patients with benign disease, the averages are 260 U/l for the monoclonal assay and 370 U/l for the polyclonal assay. This is in

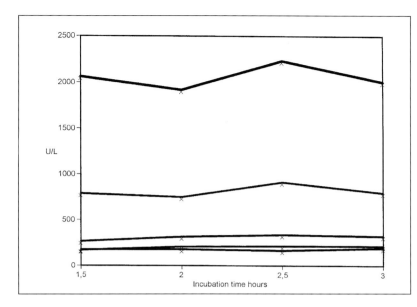

Figure 1. Assay dependence on incubation time, demonstrating stable conditions for 3 to 5 hours incubation.

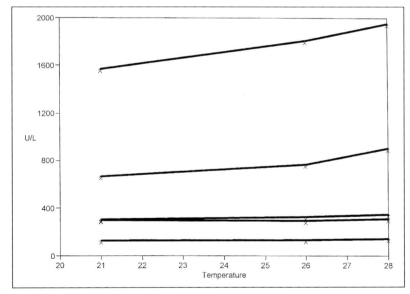

Figure 2. Assay dependence on incubation temperature, demonstrating stable conditions in the range 21–28 °C.

contrast to the assay in serum, where the polyclonal and the monoclonal assays give nearly the same values both in normal and in pathological samples. Also in patient samples, the monoclonal assay gives a lower value than the polyclonal assay, although the difference is not as marked as in normal subjects and patients with benign disease (see figure 6). The separation between samples from healthy subjects and patients with TCC of the urinary bladder is thus even better than that observed with the polyclonal assay. Patients with bladder cancer stage GI are different from those with benign disease, $p < 0.05$, those with stage GII disease different from those with benign disease with a significance of $p < 0.025$, those with stage GIII disease differ from those with benign disease with a significance of $p < 0.005$.

It should be added, that a few normal subjects have TPA values considerably higher than the remainder. We thus found one normal person with

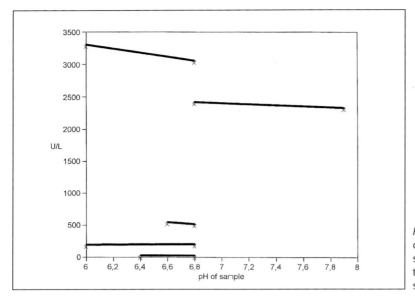

Figure 3. Assay dependence on the sample pH, demonstrating that no adjustment of sample pH is required.

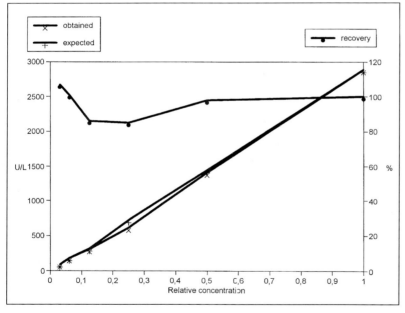

Figure 4. Example of dilution curve, demonstrating that the assay dilutes linearly.

Table I. Recovery of TPA added to urine with a low initial titre.

U/l added	U/l obtained	U/l expected	Recovery (%)
0	54		
141	248	196	127
204	272	258	105
294	346	348	99
401	416	454	92

TPA value 512. In those cases, chronic persistent bacteriuria was present.

The method described is robust and reliable for determination of TPA in urine. It is suitable as a supplement for the follow-up of patients treated for bladder cancer, to detect recurrent local disease. The number of patients in the clinical evaluation is still small, and the investigation will therefore continue.

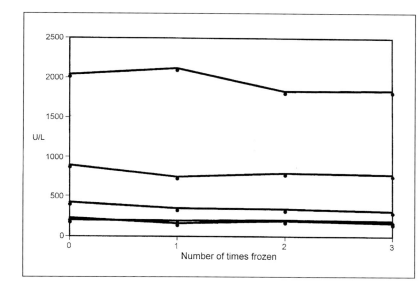

Figure 5. Assay dependence on freezing and thawing, demonstrating that the samples can be frozen and thawn repeatedly without influencing the assay.

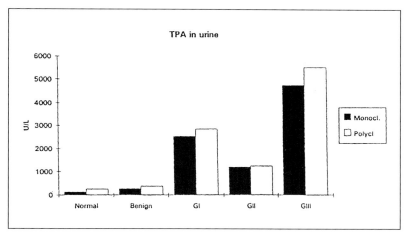

Figure 6. TPA in the urine of bladder cancer patients with different histological grade, related to normal subjects and patients with benign disease. The outcome of assays with monoclonal and a polyclonal assay are compared.

References

1. Andren-Sandberg A, Isacson S (1975) Tissue polypeptide antigen in the urine correlated to urinary cytology in cancer vesicae urinariae – a pilot study (meeting abstract) Scand J Immunol 4:7-747
2. Oehr P, Adolphs HD, Altmann R (1984) Clinical use of TPA in cancer of the urinary bladder using CEA for comparison: In: Peeters H (ed) Protiede biol fluids. Proc Colloq 31. Pergamon Press Oxford, pp 483–486
3. Kumar S, Costello CB, Glashan RW, Björklund B (1981) The clinical significance of tissue polypeptide antigen (TPA) in the urine of bladder cancer patients. Br J Urol 53:6 578–581
4. Costello CB, Kumar S (1986) Prognostic value of tissue polypeptide antigen in urological neoplasia. Anticancer Res 6:4 713–716
5. Carbin BE, Ekman P, Eneroth P, Nilsson B (1989) Urine TPA (tissue polypeptide antigen), flow cytometry and cytology as markers for tumor invasiveness in urinary bladder carcinoma. Urol Res 17:5 269–272
6. el-Ahmady O, Hamza S, Aboul-Ela M, Halim AB, Oehr P (1990) The value of tissue polypeptide antigen in Egyptian bladder cancer patients. In: Klapdor R (ed) Recent results in tumor diagnosis and therapy. Zuckschwerdt, München, pp 230–236
7. Tizzani A, Casetta G, Piana P, Cavallini A (1990) Tumor-associated antigens in diagnosis and follow-

up of superficial bladder carcinomas (meeting abstract) European Urol; 18 Suppl 1:69
8   Fischer LN, Carbin BE, Bäcklander M, Lanneskog AC, Sundström BE (1993) A standardised protocol for determination of TPA in urine. 10. IATMO International Conference, Bonn, Germany
9   Fischer LN, Carbin BE, Bäcklander M, Lanneskog AC, Sundström BE (1993) TPA in urine from patients with bladder cancer and controls. 10. IATMO International Conference, Bonn, Germany
10 Yoshida M, Morimoto S, Uekado Y, Yasukawa S, Aoshi H, Yoshida T, Ebisuno S, Ohkawa T (1989) Clinical studies on urinary tissue polypeptide antigen (TPA): problems and improvement in determination (jpn). Hinyokika Kiyo 35, 2:217–223

Address for correspondence:
Dr. med. L. N. Fischer
AB Sangtec Medical
Box 20045
S-16102 Bromma, Sweden

Serum cytokeratin antigen (CKA):
An enzyme immunoassay for quantitative measurement of serum cytokeratins in carcinoma

G. Ayanoglu, D. Chen, K. Sverlow

Triton Laboratories, Division of Ciba Corning Diagnostics Corp., Alameda, California, USA

Introduction

Cytokeratins released from simple epithelia can be detected in biological fluids. Extracellular, soluble cytokeratin polypeptides were first shown to be shed into the MCF-7 mammary tumor cell line culture media (1). Subsequently, their presence was demonstrated in the urine of cancer patients and in the sera of tumor bearing mice (2–5). The exact mechanism for the release of these antigens is not yet understood. These peptides were shown to contain epitopes related to cytokeratins 8, 18 and 19, which are normally expressed in simple epithelium. However, they were smaller and more acidic than their counterparts (2). We have developed an enzyme immunoassay by using monoclonal antibodies which specifically detect small molecular weight cytokeratins and their proteolytic fragments. We determined the serum cytokeratin levels in normals and various carcinomas of simple non-squamous epithelium origin.

Methods

Monoclonal antibodies were generated using MCF-7 cell intermediate filament extracts and screened for their reactivity with cytokeratin 8, 18, 19 and their proteolytic fragments by western blots. Cytokeratins were purified from MCF-7 serum free culture medium by affinity chromatography using a cytokeratin monoclonal antibody (Clone UCD/6.11). The assay utilized a monoclonal antibody (Clone B10) on a microtiter plate and a horseradish peroxidase conjugated monoclonal antibody (Clone DS) as the label. The assay procedure involved incubation of 50 µl sample with the solid phase antibody, a wash step and a second incubation with the label antibody. Following a second wash, tetramethylbenzidine/H_2O_2 was added. The reaction was stopped after 10 minutes and the intensity of the colored product was measured spectrophotometrically at 450 nm. Calibrators were prepared from affinity purified cytokeratins of MCF-7 cell culture medium. Patient samples and serum from healthy individuals were obtained from NCI Diagnostic Serum Bank. Additional samples were obtained from various sources.

Results

The final CKA assay had a range of 0-50 ng/ml of cytokeratin with a sensitivity of less than 2 ng/ml. Intra-assay coefficients of variation for two serum controls (n = 24) with mean values of 7.5 and 17.0 ng/ml were 4.1% and 5.7% respectively. Normal serum was found to have low levels of cytokeratin. Mean values of three different normal panels (n = 184) fell below 3 ng/ml. There was no association of age or sex with the marker levels in normal and disease groups except in advanced colorectal carcinoma where a negative correlation was observed between age and the CKA values. Cytokeratin levels were significantly elevated over normal levels in a high percentage of carcinomas including colorectal, bladder, ovarian, and breast carcinoma groups. The highest sensitivity in preoperative groups was observed in advanced ovarian and advanced bladder carcinomas, with positive rates of 77% and 62% respectively (table I, II). In these groups CKA elevations were significant with respect to their control groups, both normals and the benign conditions (p < 0.001). CEA elevation was not significant in these two cancers. CKA displayed significant elevations

Table I. Sensitivity and specificity of CKA and CEA for ovarian cancer, benign and neoplasms. Estimated sensitivity/specificity based on minimum classification error (median value versus healthy (n = 68), versus benign (n = 34)).

CKA	CEA
0.82	0.30
0.77/.95	0.14/0.95
0.69/.91	0.23/0.91

Advanced ovarian cancer

n = 35	CEA + (23%)	CEA – (77%)
CKA +	7	20
CKA –	1	7

Ovarian benign and neoplasms

n = 34	CEA + (9%)	CEA – (27%)
CKA +	0	9
CKA –	3	22

Table II. Sensitivity and specificity of CKA and CEA for bladder cancer, benign and neoplasms. Estimated sensitivity/specificity based on minimum classification error (median value versus healthy (n = 68), versus benign (n = 28)).

CKA	CEA
(0.62)	(0.32)
0.52/0.90	0.24/0.99
0.76/0.89	0.55/0.75

Advanced bladder cancer

n = 29	CEA + (21%)	CEA – (62%)
CKA +	5	13
CKA –	1	10

Bladder benign and neoplasms

n = 28	CEA + (18%)	CEA – (14%)
CKA +	1	3
CKA –	4	20

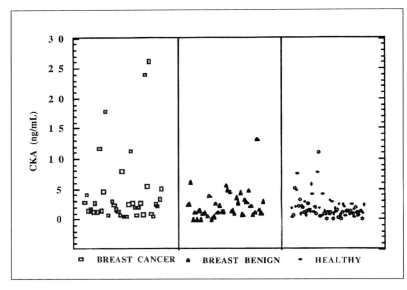

Figure 1. Frequency plot of breast carcinoma, breast benign diseases and healthy control.

in breast cancer group over only healthy women (figure 1), whereas CEA showed elevation in breast cancer with respect to both control groups (data not shown). Neither marker showed significant elevations in testicular cancer group (n = 20). In colorectal cancer the sensitivities of 51, 37, and 34% were obtained with Dukes' stages D, C, and B (figure 2) respectively. The specificity was greater than 90 % in all three cases. As expected CEA was the first predictor in all colorectal cancer comparisons, while CKA marginally increased the predictive power in advanced and stage C versus healthy controls (table III). Because CEA is such an effective marker for colorectal cancer, little improvement was achieved. Nevertheless, CKA detected 75% CEA negative Dukes' D, 58% Dukes' C and 30% Dukes' B (figure 3). This corresponds to an increased combined sensitivity to 94% in Stage D, 77% in stage C and 60% stage B.

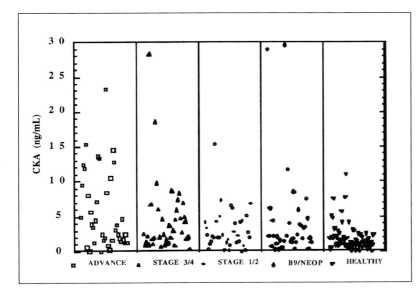

Figure 2. Frequency plot of colorectal carcinoma (Dukes' stages), benign and healty control.

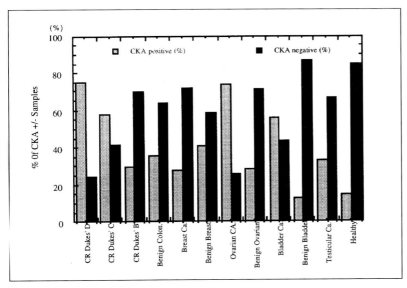

Figure 3. Complementarity of CKA to CEA negative samples.

Conclusions

CKA EIA is a sensitive immunoassay which quantitates extracellular cytokeratin polypeptides originated primarily from simple epithelium. CKA is elevated in various carcinomas, including colorectal, breast, ovarian and bladder carcinomas. CKA could prove valuable in monitoring carcinoma, and for the detection of recurrent disease. Further studies are needed to determine the clinical utility of CKA as a potential marker.

Acknowledgement

Serum sample panel was provided by the NCI Diagnostic Serum Data Bank, Bethesda, Maryland, USA. Partial data analysis was carried out by the Information Management Services, Serum Diagnostic Bank.

Table III. Sensitivity and specificity of CKA and CEA for colorectal cancer at various Dukes' stages. Estimated sensitivity/specificity based on minimum classification error (median value versus healthy (n = 68), versus benign (n = 34)).

Dukes' B	
CKA	CEA
0.48	0.38
0.34/.91	0.40/.99
0.97/.15	0.57/.85

Dukes' C	
CKA	CEA
0.54	0.45
0.37/0.94	0.37/0.99
0.97/0.21	0.63/0.85

Dukes' D	
CKA	CEA
0.62	1.06
0.51/0.90	0.74/0.97
0.60/0.65	0.83/0.88

References

1. Brabon AB, Williams JF, Cardiff RD (1984) A monoclonal antibody to a human breast cancer protein released in response to estrogen. Cancer Res 44:2704–2710
2. Chan R, Rossitto PV, Edwards BF, Cardiff RD (1986) Presence of proteolytically processed ceratins in the culture medium of MCF-7 cells. Cancer Res 46:6353–6359
3. Rossitto PV, Chan R, Edwards BF, Cardiff RD (1986) A quantitative immunoradiometric assay that detects a soluble form of cytokeratin No.18 in serum. 2nd International Workshop on Monoclonal Antibodies and Breast Cancer. Abstr no 57
4. Rossitto PV, Chan R, Strand M, Miller CH, Baker WMC, Deitch AD, deVere White R, Cardiff R (1988) Characterization of urinary ceratin number 18 using a new assay. J Urol 140:431–435
5. Nargessi RD, Sverlow K, Schneider D, Ralston S (1989) Two-site immunometric assay for determination of urinary cytokeratin-18. Clin Chem 35,6:1198

Address for correspondence:
G. Ayanoglu, Ph. D.
Triton Laboratories
Division of Ciba Corning Diagnostic Corp.
1401 Harbor Bay Parkway
Alameda, CA 94502, USA

Evaluation of a new AFP assay

J. M. G. Bonfrèr[a], R. Lodewijks[a], E. Jansen[a], D. Lentfer[b]

[a]The Netherlands Cancer Institute (Antoni von Leeuwenhoek Huis), Amsterdam, The Netherlands,
[b]Byk-Sangtec Diagnostica, Dietzenbach, Germany

Introduction

Alphafetoprotein (AFP) is a glycoprotein mainly produced in the liver and in the yolk sac of the fetus. It is an important parameter in prenatal diagnostics (1) as well as in the monitoring of patients suffering from testicular or liver cancer (2, 3). Being one of the oldest routinely used markers, new AFP assays need to meet high demands in terms of precision, reproducibility and correlation to established methods. A new luminescence-based AFP assay has recently been developed. We compared the new LIA-mat® AFP with the assay previously used in our laboratory and three commonly used automated tests.

Materials and methods

Assays used

Both assays, LIA-mat® AFP "new" and "old" (Byk-Sangtec Diagnostica, Dietzenbach, Germany) are based on the "sandwich principle". Two specific monoclonal antibodies are used for the solid phase (coated tubes) and for detection (isoluminol labelled tracer). The sandwich-complex is formed in a one-step reaction. For detection, oxidation of isoluminol is started by the automated injection of alkaline peroxide and catalyst solution into the test tube. The immediate light emission (425 nm) is measured by the photomultiplier of the luminometer. The signal is proportional to the amount of AFP antigen in samples and standards. The LIA-mat® AFP assays were processed in the fully automated system LIA-mat® S 300.
Two immunoenzymatic assays (MEIA AFP IMx, Abbott, USA and Enzymun AFP Boehringer Mannheim, Germany on ES300) and another immunoluminometric assay (Berilux AFP, Behring, Marburg, Germany on LIA-mat® S 300) were determined automatically on the respective systems. With the exception of MEIA AFP IMx, which is calibrated in ng/ml, all assays are calibrated in IU/ml (MRC 72/225). The accepted conversion for MEIA AFP is 1 IU = 1.21 ng.

Control sera

Kit controls, Lyphocheck control sera (BioRad) and pooled patients' sera were used.

Sample collection

Altogether, 250 sera, derived from 60 well-defined healthy adults, 28 pregnant females, and 162 patients with oncological or non-oncological diseases, were applied.

Results and discussion

Precision, reproducibility and comparability

The determination of intra-assay variation from duplicate determination by quadratic exponential regression revealed the data given in table one showing high precision of the LIA-mat® AFP "new" over the whole standard range.
The long-term (two months) inter-lot reproducibility of LIA-mat® AFP "new" for different control sera showed the reliability of the assay (conc. 171 IU/ml, CV% 7.0; 11.6 IU/ml, CV% 3.0; 19.2 IU/ml, CV% 2.6). Shelf-life related imprecision was hardly noticeable.

Table I. Precision data.

Assay	Mean CV (%)	Useful working range (CV < 10%)
LIA-mat® AFP "new"	4.43	0.31 –> 600
LIA-mat® AFP "old"	2.97	0 –> 600
MEIA AFP	5.22	2.17 – 315
Enzymun AFP	2.85	0.01 –> 150
Berilux AFP	5.22	0.57 –> 800

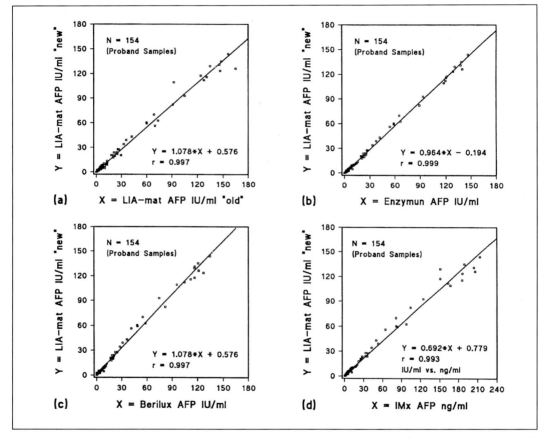

Figure 1. Method comparison by standard principal component. a) Correlation LIA-mat® AFP "new" versus LIA-mat® AFP "old". b) Correlation LIA-mat® AFP "new" versus Enzymun AFP. c) Correlation LIA-mat® AFP "new" versus Berilux AFP. d) Correlation LIA-mat® AFP "new" versus MEIA AFP IMx.

No differences in the measuring level were seen in a comparison of serum and plasma (heparin, EDTA) determinations.
The LIA-mat® AFP "new" showed an excellent correlation with all assays (figure 1, r ≥ 0.98). Differences in the measuring level were only obtained for MEIA AFP IMx.

Linearity upon dilution and high-dose hook effect

Five samples with high AFP concentrations were serially diluted with the kit diluent. All dilutions showed an excellent linear relationship in the LIA-mat® AFP "new" over the whole standard range (figure 2, r = 0.997–0.999).

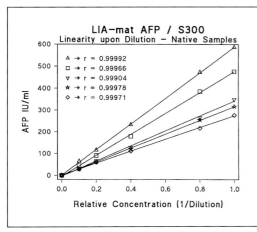

Figure 2. LIA-mat® AFP linearity studies.

Summary

A new AFP sandwich assay based on the LIA-mat® principle has been developed by Byk-Sangtec Diagnostica (Dietzenbach, Germany). The technical evaluation of this new AFP test revealed excellent data for intra- and inter-assay precision (mean CV% 4.4 versus CV% < 7%) and a high analytical sensitivity (< 0.3 IU/ml). A high-dose hook effect was only found beyond 36,000 IU/ml. The dilution linearity revealed high precision throughout the standard range (r = 0.999). Using sera from healthy and pregnant subjects as well as from patients with benign or malignant disorders, an excellent correlation (r ≥ 0.98) was obtained with the previous LIA-mat® AFP assay and three commonly used AFP assays.

The high-dose hook phenomenon was studied with high-titred serum samples, which were diluted with kit diluent. The risk of a high-dose hook effect appeared at concentrations above 36,000 IU/ml.

Distribution of AFP values in a normal population

To assess the possible impact of a change in method on the upper limit of reference values, the AFP serum levels in a small group of healthy male and female (pregnant and non-pregnant) controls were determined. The overall range of values was from < 0.3 IU/ml to 10.4 IU/ml with a median at 1.85 IU/ml and the 95-percentile at 8.05 IU/ml. The values obtained for plasma were slightly lower (median: 1.6 IU/ml; 95-percentile: 7.4 IU/ml).

References

1 Spencer K, Macri JN, Anderson RW, Aitken DA, Berry E, Crossley JA, Wood PJ, Coombes EJ, Stroud M, Worthington DJ, Doran J, Barbour H, Wilmot R (1993) Analyte immunoassay in neural tube defect and Down's syndrome screening – Results of a multicentre clinical trial. Ann Clin Biochem 30:394–401

2 Piantino P, Arrigoni A, Brunetto M, Bindro T (1989) Alpha-fetoprotein in hepatic pathology and hepatocarcinoma. J Nucl Med Allied Sci 33:34–38

3 See WA, Cohen MB, Hoxie LD (1993) Alpha-Fetoprotein half-life as a predictor of residual testicular tumor – Effect of the analytic strategy on test sensitivity and specificity. Cancer 71:2048–2054

Address for correspondence:
Dr. J. M. G. Bonfrèr
Antoni van Leeuwenhoek Ziekenhuis
Plesmanlaan 121
NL-1066 CX Amsterdam, The Netherlands

Development of an enzyme immunoassay for determination of the tumor-associated antigen CA 242

U. Dahlen, B. Karlsson, L. Lindholm, O. Nilsson

CanAg Diagnostics AB, Gothenburg, Sweden

Introduction

CA 242, defined by the CA 242 MAb, is a novel and unique tumor-associated sialylated carbohydrate epitope characterized by high tumor specificity and sensitivity when used as a tumor marker in pancreatic and colorectal cancer (1-6). Immunochemical studies show that CA 242 is different from other known tumor associated mucin antigens such as CA 19-9, CA 50, B72.3, STN, SLEX, CA 12-5 and CA 15-3 (7). Histochemical studies have shown high tumor specificity of the CA 242 epitope and staining of normal tissues were rarely seen (8–10). The CA 242 epitope is expressed on the same mucin apo protein(s) as Sialyl Lewis[a] (S-Le[a]), i.e. the CA 19-9 epitope (7, 11). The mucin antigen probably carries more CA 242 epitopes in malignant disease as compared with S-Le[a], and the relative expression of CA 242 in benign disease is lower than that of S-Le[a].

This paper describes the development of an EIA method for the determination of CA 242 antigen in serum and plasma.

Materials and methods

Establishment of MAbs

Monoclonal antibodies C242 (IgG1) and C241 (IgG1) MAbs were raised by immunization of Balb/c mice with the human adenocarcinoma cell line Colo-205 and fusion between spleenocytes and the Sp 2/0 myeloma cell line (7). The C241 MAb was specific for Sialylated Lewis[a] as demonstrated by TLC immunostaining and solid-phase binding assays as described (7). The C242 MAb detected an sialylated carbohydrate epitope expressed in mucin antigens as shown by periodate oxidation, sialidas treatment and alkaline borohydride reduction (7).

Test design

The C241 MAb was biotinylated using Biotin caproate-N-hydrosuccinimide ester (Sigma Chemical Co, MO, US), and the C242 MAb was conjugated with horse radish peroxidase Type VI (Sigma Chemical Co, MO, US) according to a modification of the original Nakane method (12). The standards were made by dilution of cell culture supernatant from SW1116 cell line in buffer matrix (50 mM Tris, 0.15 M NaCl, 60 g/l BSA, 0.5 g/l NaN_3, pH 7.5), and calibrated against an in-house reference preparation of CA 242 antigen with the arbitrarily defined concentration 500 U/ml. The assay was developed as a two-step sandwich assay with the following protocol: 25 µl of standard/ sample and 100 µl biotin C241 MAb, 1 µg/ml, was incubated for 2 h during shaking in streptavidin microtiter plates (Labsystems Oy, Helsinki, Finland); after washing 100 µl of HRP C242 MAb, 2 µg/ml, was added and the incubation continued for 1 h during shaking. The HRP activity was determined after washing and incubation with 100 µl TMB (3, 3', 5, 5' tetramethyl-benzidine) addition and measurement of absorbance at 620 nm. Precision profile was determined from standards pipetted randomly in 12 replicates. The recovery of CA 242 was determined by addition of aliquots of highly elevated patient sample to normal serum samples. The dilution linearity was studied by dilution of patient samples with the sample diluent. The CA 242 concentration was determined in 920 samples from healthy individuals and benign and malignant diseases. Method comparison between the CA 242 EIA kit with CA 242 Delfia kit was tested in 145 samples from healthy individuals and subjects with benign and malignant gastrointestinal disease.

Results and discussion

There are two assays for CA 242 available on the market, CA 242 Delfia (Wallac Oy, Turku, Finland) and the CA 242 EIA described in this paper, both assays have the same two-step sandwich configuration with a monodonal antibody specific for sialylated Lewis[a] (S-Le[a]), i.e. CA 19-9, as the catching MAb, and labeled C242 MAb for specific detection of the CA 242 epitope. Thus from the assay design it is obvious that the CA 242 assays determine S-Le[a] containing mucin antigen(s) i.e CA 19-9 antigen, expressing the CA 242 epitope. CA 242 has in a number of reports shown to have a higher tumor specificity compared to CA 19-9 and CA 50, while the sensitivity in pancreatic cancer of CA 242 and CA 19-9 is similar, and a higher sensitivity of CA 242 in colorectal cancer has been reported (1–6). In the CA 19-9 and CA 242 assays the same antigen is determined, i.e. S-Le[a] containing mucin(s), and the differences in sensitivity and specificity seen between CA 19-9, CA 50 and CA 242 would reflect differences in expression of the S-Le[a] and CA 242 epitope.

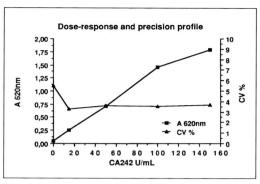

Figure 1. Standard curve and precision profile for CanAG CA 242 EIA.

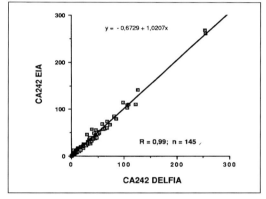

Figure 2. Correlation between CA 242 EIA and CA 242 Delfia™ for blood donors and various and malignant diseases.

Performance characteristics of the assay

The precision profile determined from analyses of standards and control samples pipetted randomly in replicates of 12 showed a CV of < 5% in the whole standard curve range, figure 1. The interassay reproducibility of three control samples analysed in four duplicates during three days showed a total CV < 3%. The detection limit of the assay was less than 1 U/ml, defined as the concentration corresponding to the mean of the absorbance values for the 0-standard plus two standard deviations of the 0-standard determination (mean + 2 SD). The assay was developed as a two-step sandwich, and therefore a high-dose hook effect should not be expected. This was also confirmed with samples up to 150,000 U/ml. Patient samples showing elevated CA 242 concentration were serially diluted with sample diluent and analyzed. The coefficient of correlation between CA 242 concentration and dilution was better than 0.95. The obtained values were in the range 93–109% of expected values. For determination of recovery human serum and plasma samples were analyzed before and after addition of known amounts of CA 242 antigen. Recovery of CA 242 antigen were in the range of 88–107%.

Method comparison

The coefficient of correlation between CanAg CA 242 EIA and CA 242 Delfia™ (Wallac Oy, Turku, Finland) was determined in 70 blood donors and 75 subjects with benign and

Table I. Distribution of CA 242 values (U/ml) in healthy subjects and in malignant and non-malignant diseases, determined with CanAg CA 242 EIA.

	n	0–20	21–30	31–150	>150
Healthy subjects	200	92.5	6.0	1.5	–
Benign disease					
ulcerative colitis	38	97.4	2.6	–	–
polyps	62	95.2	1.6	3.2	–
hepatopancreatobilary disease[a]	87	79.3	12.6	8.0	–
inflammatory disease[b]	74	89.2	5.4	5.4	–
Malign disease					
Colorectal ca.					
Dukes A	36	86.1	2.8	11.1	–
Dukes B	72	62.5	9.7	26.0	2.8
Dukes C	57	54.4	22.8	14.0	8.8
Dukes D	65	30.8	6.2	26.1	36.9
pancreatic ca.	61	39.5	9.9	11.6	39.0
other carcinomas[c]	69	81.2	11.6	5.7	1.4
non-carcinomas[d]	99	86.9	6.1	7.1	–

[a] Pancreatitis, liver chirrhosis, obstructive biliary diaease, sclerosing cholangitis; [b] reumatiod arthritis, pnemonia; [c] lung ca., prostatic ca., breast ca.; [d] lymphomas, melanomas

malignant diseases. The coefficient of correlation was better than 0.98 in both blood donors and in the subjects with benign and malignant diseases. The correlation for blood donors and patient samples are shown in figure 2.

Clinical data

CA 242 concentration was determined in sera from 200 healthy subjects and in 720 individuals with various malignant and non-malignant diseases, table I. The CA 242 level in healthy subjects was 8.0 + 6.7 U/ml with a mean value of 6.4 U/ml and the 95th percentile 21.7 U/ml.

Conclusion

The CA 242 assays are double determinant assays, and therefore the robustness of the assay should be expected to be better compared to a homologous assay. The technical evaluation of the CA 242 EIA showed good technical performances, and the method comparison between the CA 242 Delfia and CA 242 EIA showed also a good correlation and agreement in absolute values. This should be compared to the problems of discordant results with different assay configurations in homologous assays for determination of CA 19-9 antigen. Thus from a purely technical point of view the introduction of a double determinant assay for determinantion of the 19-9 mucin(s) should improve the technical quality of the assay. From a clinical point of view the specific determination of the CA 242 epitope would also lead to a clinical improvement of assays for 19-9 mucin(s) with less number of false positives particularly in benign pancreatohepatobiliary disease (1–6). The CanAg CA 242 EIA will be an additional tool for further clinical evaluation of this new tumor marker for the management of patients with gastrointestinal and pancreatic cancer.

References

1 Johansson C, Nilsson O, Lindholm L (1991) Comparison of serological expression of different epitopes on the CA50 carrying antigen CanAg. Int J Cancer. 48:757
2 Nilsson O, Johansson C, Glimelius B, Persson B, Norgaard B, Andren-Sandberg A, Lindholm L (1992) Sensitivity and specificity of CA 242 in gastrointestinal cancer. A comparison with CEA, CA 50 and CA 19-9. Br J Cancer 65:215

3. Röthlin MA, Joller H, Largiader F (1993) CA 242 is a new tumor marker for pancreatic cancer. Cancer 71:701
4. Kuusela P, Haglund C, Roberts PJ (1991) Comparison of a new tumor marker CA 242 with CA 19-9, CA 50 and carcinoembryonic antigen (CEA) in digestive tract disease. Br J Cancer 63:636
5. Pasanen, PA, Eskelinen M, Partanen K, Pikkarainen P, Penttilä I, Alhava E (1992) Clinical value of serum tumour markers CEA, CA 50 and CA 242 in the distinction between malignant versus benign disease causing jaundice and cholestasis; results from a prospective study. Br J Cancer 65:731
6. Haglund C, Lundin J, Kuusela P, Roberts PJ (1994) CA 242 – A new tumour marker for pancreatic cancer. A comparison with CA 19-9, CA 50 and CEA. Br J Cancer, in press
7. Johansson C, Nilsson O, Bäckström D, Jansson E-L, Lindholm L (1991) Novel epitopes on the CA 50 carrying antigen: Chemical and immunochemical studies. Tumor Biol 12:159.
8. Haglund C, Lindgren J, Roberts PJ, Kuusela P, Nordling S (1989) Tissue expression of the tumour associated antigen CA 242 in benign and malignant pancreatic lesions. A comparison with CA 50 and CA 19-9. Br J Cancer 60:845
9. Ouyang Q, Vilen M, Ravn Juhl B, Grupe Larsen L, Binder V (1987) CEA and carbohydrate antigens in normal and neoplastic mucosa. Acta Pathol Microbiol Immunol Scand Sect A 95:177
10. Johansson C (1991) CA 242 and other monoclonal antibodies defining novel human colorectal carcinoma associated epitopes. Thesis, University of Göteborg
11. Baeckström D, Hansson GC, Nilsson O, Johansson C, Gendler SJ, Lindholm L (1991) Purification and characterization of a membrane-bound and a secreted mucin-type glycoprotein carrying the carcinoma-associated sialyl-Le^a epitope on distinct core proteins. J Biol Chem 266:21537
12. Tijssen P, Kurstak E (1984) Highly efficient and simple methods for the preparation of peroxidase-antibody conjugates for enzyme immunoassays. Analyt Biochem 136:451

Address for correspondence:
Dr. B. Karlsson
CanAg Diagnostics AB
P.O. Box 121 36
S-402 42 Gothenburg, Sweden

Monitoring of oncological patients with an automated luminescence-labeled immunoassay for ferritin

Marketa Drahovsky, D. Lentfer, P. Völcker

Byk-Sangtec Diagnostica GmbH, Dietzenbach, Germany

Introduction

Ferritin has since long been discussed and used as a tumor marker for a spectrum of malignant situations, especially leukemias and lymphomas, but also for solid tumors such as hepatomas and carcinomas of the breast, pancreas or lung.

It has been postulated that transferrin is a growth factor in malignancy and that the uptake of transferrin into proliferating malignant cells causes a loss of circulating transferrin. In consequence, the resulting hypotransferrinemia will lead to a decrease in iron uptake into the erythropoietic precursors resulting in an increased flow of iron to the reticuloendothelial iron stores, which is accompanied by an increased serum ferritin concentration. By this mechanism, the degree of hyper-ferritinemia very closely parallels the severity of tumor related anemia (1, 2).

The administration of recombinant human erythropoietin offers a possibility for the treatment of myeloma associated anemia. The efficacy of treatment is well reflected by a decrease in the originally elevated ferritin levels (3, 4).

Another cause of anemia is to be found in the adverse effects of some chemotherapeutic anti-tumor regimens on the erythropoietic system, especially high-dosage cisplatin. Both these effects (5, 6, 7) as well as the beneficial ones of erythropoietin administration on therapy-induced anemia (8) can reliably be monitored by the determination of serum ferritin.

Assay procedure for LIA-mat® Ferritin on the LIA-mat® System 300

Recently, a newly developed non-isotopic immunoassay for the determination of human ferritin in blood has been introduced: LIA-mat®, Ferritin. It is a coated-tube immunometric assay (sandwich principle) with a one-step incubation employing a pair of monoclonal antibodies for the capturing and the tracer antibody. The tracer is labelled with an isoluminol derivative, which is triggered for the emission of light by the addition of alkaline hydrogen peroxide and a catalyst (table I). The assay can be performed manually or with the instrumentation specially designed for the fully auto-mated performance of LIA-mat® assays, viz. LIA-mat® System 300. LIA-mat® Ferritin is calibrated in ng/ml ferritin against the NBSB reference standard preparation 80/602 (liver ferritin), with a standard range from 0 to 1000 ng/ml. Its cross-reactivity with spleen ferritin approximates 60%, that with heart ferritin is below 10%.

Results

Normal ranges were established from the combined data of several investigations with LIA-mat® Ferritin; they are between 19 and 370 ng/ml for adult men and between 7 and 94 ng/ml for

Table I. LIA-mat® Ferritin flow diagram.

1. Pipet 25 µl standard or sample into antibody-coated test tube
2. Add 300 µl anti-ferritin tracer conjugate
3. Mix, incubate for 2 hours at room temperature while shaking
4. Aspirate, wash 3 times with 0.9 % saline
5. Luminometer: Measure light emission triggered by "in situ" injection of starter reagents; measuring time: 5 sec

premenopausal women. Performed on the LIA-mat® System 300, excellent precision and reproducibility are obtained with the LIA-mat® Ferritin, as is demonstrated by the precision profile of duplicate determinations (figure 1) and by the profile of inter-assay reproducibility of control and pool sera (figure 2). The mean intra-assay CV of duplicate determinations of around 3% over the whole concentration range is in accordance with an excellent lower limit of the working range of only 0.02 ng/ml, i.e. the concentration where the mean CV passes below the 10% line. Inter-assay CVs ranging between 4 and 9% underline the long-term stability of assay results.

The high technical quality of LIA-mat® Ferritin is further demonstrated by the results of dilution experiments revealing a strictly linear response over the whole standard range (figure 3). Comparisons of the LIA-mat® Ferritin results with those of other established ferritin assays were based on groups of both sexes and covering healthy subjects as well as patients with neoplastic and/or hematological diseases. A high degree of consistency was obtained with the two isotopic assays, IRMA-mat® Ferritin (figure 4) and Behring RIA-gnost Ferritin (figure 5), as was with the non-isotopic assay Abbott IMx Ferritin (figure 6). Slightly deviating results, esp. concerning the level of calibration, were found for two other non-isotopic assays, namely Boehringer Enzymun Ferritin (figure 7) and Kodak Amerlite Ferritin (figure 8).

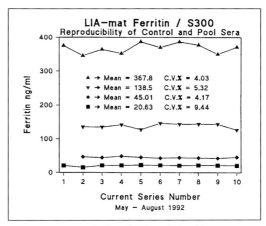

Figure 2. Reproducibility of LIA-mat® Ferritin.

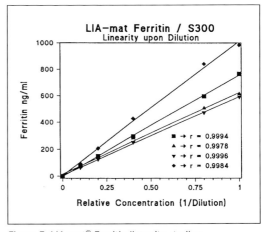

Figure 3. LIA-mat® Ferritin linearity studies.

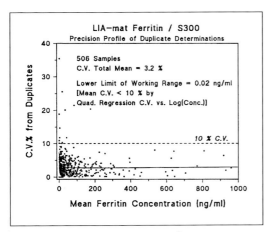

Figure 1. Precision profile of LIA-mat® Ferritin.

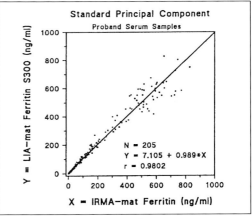

Figure 4. Correlation LIA-mat® Ferritin versus IRMA-mat® Ferritin.

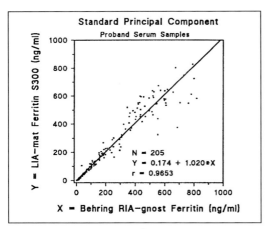

Figure 5. Correlation LIA-mat® Ferritin versus RIA-gnost Ferritin.

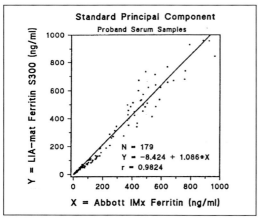

Figure 6. Correlation LIA-mat® Ferritin versus IMX Ferritin.

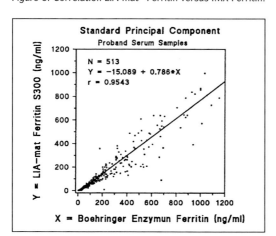

Figure 7. Correlation LIA-mat® Ferritin versus Enzymun Ferritin.

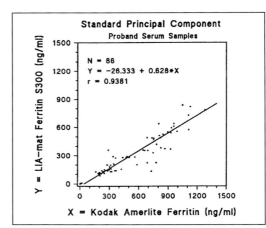

Figure 8. Correlation LIA-mat® Ferritin versus Amerlite Ferritin.

Conclusions

The determination of ferritin in cancer patients is a valuable means for monitoring the effects and side-effects of cancer therapy and should therefore be considered not only in those cases where the tumor activity itself affects serum ferritin concentration, but also for the monitoring of chemo-therapeutic regimens, which might cause impairment to the erythropoietic system. The LIA-mat, Ferritin assay, either performed manually or fully automatically on the LIA-mat, System 300, is an outstanding tool for this purpose.

References

1. Aulbert E, Jakob M, Kurschel E (1989) Die Anämie bei malignen Tumorerkrankungen. V. Die Beziehung zwischen der tumorbedingten Hypotransferrinämie und dem Grad der Anämie. Onkologie 12:81–89
2. Aulbert E, Kurschel E, Jakob M (1989) Die Anämie bei malignen Tumorerkrankungen. VI. Sekundäre Siderose durch die Umverteilung des für die Hämoglobinsynthese nicht verwertbaren Eisens in die Eisenspeicher. Medizinische Klinik 84:421–428
3. Ludwig H, Fritz E, Kotzmann H et al (1990) Erythropoietin treatment of anemia associated with multiple myeloma. New Engl J Med 322:1693–1699
4. Oster W, Herrmann F, Gamm H et al (1990) Erythropoietin for the treatment of anemia of malignancy associated with neoplastic bone marrow infiltration. J Clin Oncol 8 956–962

5. Pollera CF, Ameglio F, Nardi M et al (1990) Dose and schedule effects of cisplatin on the related acute iron changes. Oncol 47:133–138
6. Sartori S, Nielsen I et al (1991) Early and late hyperferremia during cisplatin therapy. J Chemother 3:45–50
7. Milman N, Sengelov H, Dombernowsky P (1991) Iron status markers in patients with small cell carcinoma of the lung. Relation to survival. British J Cancer 64:895–898
8. Oster W, Herrmann F, Cicco A et al (1990) Erythropoietin prevents chemotherapy-induced anemia: case report. Blut 60:88–92

Address for correspondence:
Marketa Drahovsky
Byk-Sangtec Diagnostica GmbH
Von Hevesy-Straβe 3
D-63128 Dietzenbach, Germany

Technical and clinical evaluation of seven tumor marker assays based on ELISA technology – Results of a multicenter study

Anne-Ch. Kessler
Evaluation Department for Immunology Systems, Boehringer Mannheim GmbH, Tutzing, Germany

Introduction

An international comparative study on tumor marker tests has been performed in 25 laboratories from seven European countries. The object of this study was to examine the analytical reliability and reproducibility of the Boehringer Mannheim assays under uniform instrumental and experimental conditions. Included in the study were the currently commercially available ENZYMUN-Test tumor markers CEA, AFP, CA 15-3, CA 19-9, CA 72-4, CA 125 II and CYFRA 21-1. Measurements were carried out on the fully automated ENZYMUN-Test Systems ES 300 and ES 600, in the majority of cases as single determinations using one-point recalibration.

Patients and methods

In this study all participating laboratories were provided with ENZYMUN-Test CEA, AFP, CA 15-3, CA 19-9, CA 72-4, CA 125 II and CYFRA 21-1. For these enzymimmunoassays streptavidin-coated tubes and biotinylated antibodies were used. All kits were taken from current production batches. For comparison studies assays of the following producers have been used: ABBOTT, Baxter, Centocor, CIS, Roche, Sorin and Tosoh. The assays were performed using the procedure and systems recommended by the kit manufactures.
The accuracy and lot to lot stability of the Boehringer Mannheim assays were checked by comparing results with already existing findings from inter-laboratory surveys in 1992. The inter-laboratory study controls TM 2/92, A and B were kindly made available for this study by the German Society for Clinical Chemistry.

The reproducibility of the measurements obtained was checked using the following materials: Boehringer Mannheim kit controls, level low and level high for CA 15-3, CA 19-9, CA 72-4, CA 125 II and CYFRA 21-1; tumor marker controls, level 1, level 2 Precinorm IM, Precipath IM (partly). BIORAD, Lyphocheck (partly). Serum samples were taken from the routine of each laboratory. Altogether about 15,000 sera have been determined.

Results

For the determination of intra-assay precision the target coefficient of variation (CV) less than 5% was confirmed in 93% of all series (all n = 258). Only at concentration ranges well below the cut-off region CVs >5% were obtained. For precision inter-assay the target CV less than 10% was confirmed in 87% of all series (all n = 185). An example is shown in figure 1.
The agreement of the results with those of the previous interlaboratory survey 1992 is remarkably good (table I). The medians are identical in some instances.
Results of CA 125 II are divergent. Values obtained in the survey 1992 were determined with the first generation of CA 125 II, now all laboratories used the second generation. The recovery is in expected ranges.
High human sera have been diluted with the diluents of the kits ENZYMUN-Test CA 15-3, CA 19-9, CA 72-4, CYFRA 21-1 and the separate diluents for CEA. The results confirm an excellent linearity.
In comparison studies patients samples were measured using Boehringer Mannheim assays in

Table I. Inter-laboratory survey. Results obtained from this study (study) in comparison to the recovery of the official trial (TM 2/92 A and B).

ENZYMUN-Test®

TM 2/92 A		16%	med.	84%	n
CEA	TM 2/92	13.3	14.4	15.0	66
	study	13.0	14.5	15.3	25
CA 15-3	TM 2/92	14.0	15.9	17.8	51
	study		17.3		7
CA 19-9	TM 2/92	10.7	14.2	16.1	47
	study	12.8	14.6	17.2	13
CA 125	TM 2/92[a]	18.9	22.9	30.5	31
	study[b]	12.6	15.0	17.9	12
AFP	TM 2/92	7.6	8.8	9.8	27
	study		9.5		9
TM 2/92 B					
CEA	TM 2/92	5.9	6.5	6.7	66
	study	6.0	6.5	7.1	25
CA 15-3	TM 2/92	11.8	13.4	15.4	51
	study		15.5		7
CA 19-9	TM 2/92	11.8	15.1	16.8	47
	study	13.7	15.2	18.4	13
CA 125	TM 2/92[a]	18.6	22.5	26.6	31
	study[b]	13.9	14.9	16.7	12
AFP	TM 2/92	13.5	15.2	16.3	27
	study		16.9		9

[a] 1st generation
[b] 2nd generation

Table II. Reference values. Results of the study in comparison to the values given in the package insert.

Parameter	Package insert		Results of the study		
	95%	99%	n	95%	99%
CEA (ng/ml)	4.6	5.7	351	3.38	4.36
CA 15-3 (U/ml)	22	30	44	20.7	21.4
CA 19-9 (U/ml)	22	37	166	21.5	34.4
CA 72-4 (U/ml)	6.7	9.8	135	4.5	9.34
CA 125 II (U/ml)	35	65	104	21.7	35.4
CYFRA 21-1[a] (U/ml)	3.3		298	8.8	
AFP (IU/ml)	5.5	9.6			

[a] Based on a benign lung disease

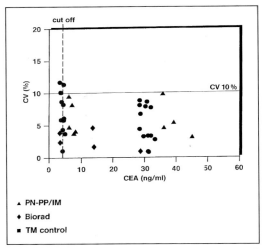

Figure 1. Precision inter-assay. The mean values of 42 results obtained from 16 laboratories (x-axis) were plotted against the corresponding coefficient of variation (y-axis).

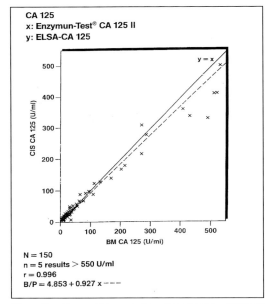

Figure 2. Comparison study. Correlation between ENZYMUN-Test CA 125 II and ELSA-CA 125, CIS 2nd generation.

parallel to the routine method of the laboratory. The results confirm the well known fact, that comparable data are not always obtained due to the differing test principles and the absence of standardisation. But it is remarkable, all 29 comparison studies show correlation coefficients (r) in the range 0.920–1.000. Figure 2 gives an example of the correlation of CA 125 II.

Part of the study was to control and to confirm the reference values of the seven tumor marker kits of Boehringer Mannheim. The reference values based on the 95th percentiles of healthy subjects were determined and calculated by repeating the previous procedures. The official reference values (package insert) were well confirmed by this study, see table I.

The reference range of ENZYMUN-Test CYFRA 21-1 is based on the 95th percentile of benign lung diseases. Results of this studies were higher than values collected during the evaluation of the assay. Possibly in benign lung diseases the ratio of acute to chronic infections is of higher importance for the cut-off calculation than realised before.

Conclusion

The usefulness of tumor markers for "follow-up studies" - the monitoring of surgery or treatment - was underlined by particular good quality of the Boehringer Mannheim assays in regard to analytical reliability and reproducibility, like data on intra-assay-precision with CVs < 5%, inter-assay precision < 10%, confirmation of the analytical lower detection limit, confirmation of the reference ranges, linear results by dilution experiments and for lot-to-lot reproducibility expressed by a repetition of an official inter-laboratory survey.

The few outlying results were explained by technical faults (e.g. extremely hot summer temperatures, installation - difficulties of few ES Systems).

In comparison studies to various producers the correlation is remarkably better than one year before, none coefficient of correlation (r) was below 0.920.

Address for correspondence:
Anne-Ch. Kessler
Boehringer Mannheim GmbH
Banhofstraβe 9-15
D-82327 Tutzing, Germany

Performance of tumor marker assays on the true Random Access Immunochemistry Analyzer Cobas® Core

P. Pfleiderer, Ph. Giradin, V. Henne, A. Maurer
Roche Diagnostic Systems, a Division of Hoffman-La Roche Ltd., Basel Switzerland

Introduction

The fully automated Cobas Core Immunochemistry Analyzer has been developed to meet the laboratories needs of today. The system offers the advantages of a true random access instrument performing immunoassays in various diagnostic fields. Among the immunochemical parameters, the tumor markers have become of great importance as adjunctive tools for routine cancer diagnosis. The key application of these assays remains the monitoring of cancer patients during therapy or the follow-up period. In recent years assay automation has increased strongly due to higher sample throughput in the laboratory. Besides economic reasons it is obvious that automation is also improving the performance of the assays. In the following we want to give a status report of tumor marker tests on the Cobas Core and to show the use of the system for routine cancer diagnostics.

The instrument

The Cobas® Core Immunochemistry Analyzer is a true random access instrument for immunoassays. It utilizes big bead technology as solid phase, horse-radish peroxidase as marker enzyme and 3,3',5,5'-tetramethyl-benzidine (TMB) as substrate. One-step and two-step sandwich assays as well as competitive assays can be run on the Cobas® Core.
The Cobas Core instrument can handle a wide variety of immunochemical assays including virological, thyroid, fertility and tumor marker tests. This is due to the remarkable degree of flexibility concerning incubation times, pipetting schemes and sample volume.

Samples and reagents are positively identified by a barcode reader. Samples are placed on the instrument in sample racks. Biocups (dead volume < 150 µl), Eppendorf tubes or Sarsted 3.5 ml secondary tubes (dead volume < 200 µl) may be used. Primary tubes may also be placed directly on the instrument.

The instrument design allows continuous loading of samples and reagents without affecting test-work flow. Having switched on the instrument it is possible to start testing samples after only a few minutes warm-up time. Depending on the parameter first results can be obtained in 30 minutes. They can be inspected or printed immediately after the end of the determination of the particular sample.

Standard curves of the individual tests can be stored on the instrument and used for up to two weeks. Up to three standard curves can be stored for each parameter. Automatic calibration curve correction is also be available.

Table I. Key features of the Immunochemistry Analyzer Corbas® Core.

True random access
Real-time STAT
Extensive range of high quality reagents
Primary or secondary tube sampling
Auto pre- and post-dilution[a]
Flexible rack system
Continuous reloading of samples and reagents
Up to 10 on-line reagents[a]
Ready-to-use reagents
Level detection
Integrated bidirectional interface
One- or two-point recalibration
Positive ID of samples and reagents
Excellent sensitivity and specificity
Profile and conditional profile[a]

[a] In development

Table II. Cobas Core tumor marker menu.

Test	Total assay time	Range	Analytical sensitivity
Cobas Core AFP	30 min	0–200 IU/ml	< 0.5 IU/ml
Cobas Core CEA	45 min	0–50 ng/ml	< 0.2 ng/ml
Cobas Core Ferritin	30 min	0–1200 ng/ml	< 0.8 ng/ml
Cobas Core β-hCG	45 min	0–200 mIU/ml	< 2.0 mIU/ml
Cobas Core β2-M	35 min	10–18000 ng/ml	< 3.0 ng/ml
Cobas Core MCA	55 min	0–50 U/ml	0.2 U/ml
Cobas Core NSE	45 min	0–200 ng/ml	1.0 ng/ml
Cobas Core CA 125 II	45 min	0–540 U/ml	< 1.0 U/ml
Cobas Core CA 19-9	75 min	0–400 U/ml	2.2 U/ml
Cobas Core PSA	30 min	0–120 ng/ml	< 0.2 ng/ml
[a]Cobas Core CA 15-3	75 min	0–200 U/ml	<1.0 U/ml
[a]Cobas Core Ca 72-4	75 min	1–100 U/ml	< 0.3 IU/ml

[a]Available late 1994

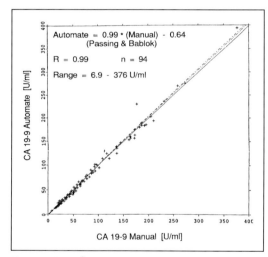

Figure 1. Cobas® Core CA 19-0 EIA. Equivalence between manual and automate measurements for patients sera.

For quality control a confidence range is given for a kit control. If the value falls outside these limits, the result is flagged.

The user-friendly, multi-dialog software allows easy communication with the instrument. The instrument can be connected to a computer via a RS 232 interface and bidirectional communication with the host computer is possible.

Tumor marker line

The Cobas Core offers a complete line of tumor marker tests for comprehensive diagnostics of cancer diseases (table II). Starting with the first classical marker CEA in 1974 the tumor marker line has been enlarged according to the progress of cancer research. Up to now ten of the most important tumor marker tests are available. In late 1994 CA 15-3 and CA 72-4 will be added to the tumor marker line.

The tests are characterized by short incubation times, broad measuring ranges and good analytical sensitivity for reliable testing. The generally short incubation times allow a high throughput and a better workflow in the laboratory. All these assays can also be performed semiautomatically (Cobas Core EIA system) resulting in excellent agreement with the automated version (figure 1).

A basic condition for reliable tumor marker assay development is the careful choice of antibodies. Quality, kinetics and specificity are important aspects which have to be taken into consideration when choosing the right antibody combination. A good example is the determination of prostate specific antigen, which is shown to circulate in the sera of patients with prostate malignancy. The antigen is predominantly found in tumor sera as a complexed form with alpha-1-antichymotrypsin. Despite some controversies about the ratios of these forms it has become normal practice to offer tests which are able to detect both forms (figure 2). As a consequence, the Cobas Core assays utilize (with the exception of NSE) monoclonal antibodies to gain the highest specificity and to avoid undesirable cross-reactions.

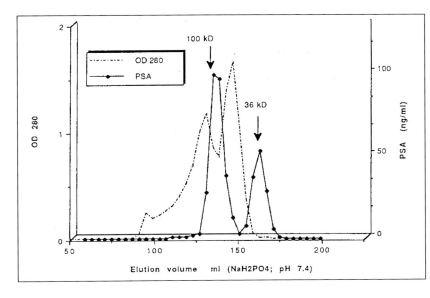

Figure 2. Cobas® Core PSA EIA. Elution profile of patient serum with prostate cancer and chromatographed on a Sephacryl S-300 column. PSA concentration was determined by Cobas Core PSA EIA (1).

Table III. Cobas Core Feritin EIA. Precision on Cobas Core: Intra-assay precision was calculated by measuring three sera as 11-fold determinations. Inter-assay precision was calculated by measuring the same sera as duplicates over 11 runs.

Serum	Intra-assay mean (ng/ml)	CV (%)	Inter-assay mean (ng/ml)	CV (%)
A (low)	80	1.9	76	1.7
B (medium)	230	2.2	209	2.3
C (high)	750	2.4	765	2.6

Automation of immunoassays results not only in more economic testing, but also in an improved reliability. The combination of state-of-the-art technology coupled with optimized assays in standardized conditions, results in excellent CVs and the very reproducibility needed for reliable monitoring (table III).

Conclusions

The Cobas Core Random Access Immunochemistry Analyzer is ideally suited for laboratories with high sample throughput. Several parameters can be run in parallel and continuous reloading of samples and reagents is possible. Due to the high flexibility and easy communication with the instrument it facilitates the organization of laboratory. The actual hands-on-time is short compared to other automated systems. The Cobas Core offers a complete line of highly specific assays for tumor marker diagnosis.

Reference

1 Maurer A, Huber P (1992) Interaktion von Prostata spezifischem Antigen mit alpha-1-Antichymotrypsin in vitro. Diagnostica Nachrichten 2:1112

Address for correspondence:
P. Pfleiderer
Roche Diagnostic Systems
a Division of Hoffmann-La Roche Ltd.
CH-4002 Basel, Switzerland

β2-Microglobulin enzyme immunoassay (Cobas® Core) – A methodical and clinical evaluation

Susanne Poley[a], A. Fateh-Moghadam †[a], V. Nüssler[b], Heike Pahl[a]

[a]Institut for Clinical Chemistry, [b]Medical Clinic III, Klinikum Großhadern,
Ludwig-Maximilians-University Munich, Germany

Introduction

β2-microglobulin (β2-m) is a low-molecular-weight protein of 11,800 daltons. β2-m is identical to the light chain of the histocompatibility antigen (HLA) system and can therefore be demonstrated on the membrane of all cells in the body. The serum β2-m rises in patients with renal malfunction, because it is freely filtered through the glomerular membrane and further reabsorbed in the proximal tubule. Increased β2-m levels are also found in various malignant and inflammatory diseases. In lymphoproliferative disorders such as multiple myeloma (MM) and low-grade non-Hodgkin's lymphomas (NHL) the serum concentration of β2-m correlates with tumor mass and is a useful prognostic indicator and parameter of response to treatment. When tested for efficiency in recognizing patients with poor (average survival time < 1 year) and good (average survival time > 5 years) prognosis, serum β2-m was the best parameter.

Following the methodical evaluation we investigated in a retrospective study the clinical significance of a new β2-m enzyme immunoassay (EIA) on Cobas® Core system (Hoffmann-La Roche) in comparison to the well established microparticle enzyme immunoassay (MEIA) on IMx system (Abbott).

Patients

As reference group we investigated the sera of 81 clinically and by terms of clinical chemistry healthy persons ranging in age from 20 to 76 years and sera of 42 patients with renal failure. As tumor patients we investigated the sera of 108 persons (aged between 23 and 84 years) with monoclonal gammopathies (3 monoclonal gammopathies of undetermined significance, 91 MM, 14 macroglobulinemia) and 11 patients with different NHL (8 chronic lymphatic leukemia, 1 centrocytoma, 1 centroblastoma, 1 lymphoblastoma). All sera were collected at an active stage of disease (primary diagnosis or recurrent disease). In addition serum β2-m-levels were measured in 29 follow-ups of patients with malignant lymphoma (24 MM, 4 macroglobulinemia, 1 B-CLL). The patients with MM were staged according to the classification of *Durie* and *Salmon*.

Methods

The Cobas® Core β2-microglobulin EIA (Hoffmann-La Roche) is a one step solid phase enzyme immunoassay with competitive inhibition. The microparticle enzyme immunoassay on IMx system (Abbott) is based on a "sandwich"-type immunoassay.

Any association of β2-m levels with stage of myeloma was assessed using Mann-Whitney one-way, non-parametric analysis of variants. Relationships between β2-m and other biochemical parameters were done by correlation analysis.

Results

Methodical results

The methodical evaluation showed a very high precision for both assays (table I) and a good linearity of β2-m EIA between 1–18 mg/l.
The EIA on Cobas® Core had a strong correlation to the MEIA on the IMx-system. The coefficient of

correlation of all groups without renal failure was 0.99 (figure 1). The assays showed in the group of renal failure a lower coefficient of correlation of 0.87. One reason could be the influence of matrix effects. Patients with renal malfunction had the highest β2-m concentrations (60 mg/l) and a correlation with serum creatinine could be demonstrated (r = 0.445).

Clinical results

In healthy persons the MEIA β2-m concentrations were normally distributed between 0.6 and 2.3 mg/l. Higher β2-m values were measured with the EIA-assay in healthy controls ranging between 1.0 and 3.3 mg/l. We fixed the cut-off at 97.5 percentage. In 97.5% of the normal healthy controls, β2-m MEIA-values were then below 1.8 mg/l and β2-m EIA-values were below 3.0 mg/l. Taking into account these mentioned cut-off values 52% of IgG-MM, 46% of IgA-MM, 50% of macroglobulinemia, 57% of Bence-Jones-MM, 86% of IgD-MM and 91% of different NHL had elevated β2-m serum concentrations with the Cobas® Core EIA. There was no significant difference in the distribution of β2-m between the immunoglobulin classes G, A and M. Higher β2-m levels in Bence-Jones- and IgD-MM could be related to the general worse prognosis of this myeloma types. Quantity of monoclonal immunoglobulins did not correlate with serum β2-m values. This indicates the independence of immunoglobulin and β2-m synthesis in spite of their homology.

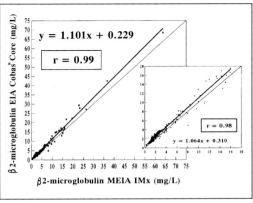

Figure 1. Correlation of β2-microglobulin EIA Cobas® Core and MEIA IMx of all groups without renal failure. The small picture shows a limited scale up to 18 mg/l.

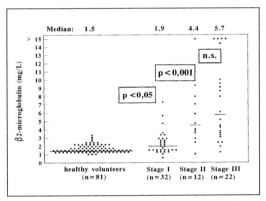

Figure 2. Dependence of β2-microglobulin levels on clinical stage according to the classification of Salmon and Durie.

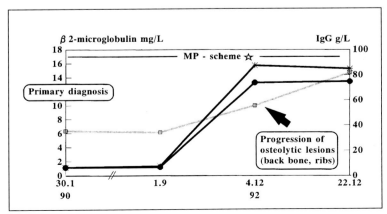

Figure 3. Follow-up of serum β2-microglobulin and monoclonal IgG in a patient with multiple myeloma.
S.B.1941 female, ● β2-MEIA, ✱ β2-EIA, □ IgG,
☆ MP-scheme = Melphalan + Prednison (according to Alexanian).

Table I. Coefficients of variancy for 20 determinations of low, medium and high β2-microglobulin concentrations within one assay and from day to day.

β2-m (mg/l)	Intra-assay CV%		Inter-assay CV%	
(n = 20)	EIA	MEIA	EIA	MEIA
Low (1.2)	2.2	2.7	3.4	4.2
Medium (3)	2.9	3.3	3.2	7.2
High (10)	5.9	4.2	7.7	4.6

Using the staging classification of *Durie* and *Salmon* (based on myeloma cell mass) we found a good correlation between stage and survival. Based on this stratification patients with high cell mass myeloma (stage II and III) had significantly higher β2-m levels than those with low cell mass in stage I (figure 2). Seven patients with smouldering myeloma showed β2-m concentrations within the normal range. Furthermore we have observed a significant difference between β2-m levels of healthy controls and those of patients in stage I. Due to these findings high β2-m concentrations could be indicative of malignancy, whereas low levels do not exclude a malignant gammopathy.

Serial measurements showed in 16 cases a decrease of β2-m with response to chemotherapy and low levels in stable remission. In ten cases relapse or progression of osteolyses was associated with increasing and elevated β2-m concentrations (figure 3). The clinical course of four patients with Bence-Jones-MM and one patient with B-CLL lacking monoclonal immunoglobulin was documented by serum β2-m (figure 3). Only three cases had a disagreement between β2-m and the final clinical outcome with monoclonal immunoglobulin giving more information.

Summary

In conclusion serum β2-m is an extremely useful marker in initial stratification and follow-up of patients with multiple myeloma, macroglobulinemia and other non-Hodgkin's lymphomas. β2-m is the best prognostic marker in multiple myeloma independent of the paraprotein concentration.

Determination of β2-m in serum with the enzyme immunoassay on Cobas® Core (Roche) system is a method with a very good precision and shows a strong correlation to the microparticle enzym-immunoassay on IMx (Abbott).

References

1. Bartl R, Frisch B, Diem H, Mündel M, Nagel D, Lamerz R, Fateh-Moghadam A (1991) Histologic, biochemical, and clinical parameters for monitoring multiple myeloma. Cancer 68:2241–2250
2. Bataille R, Grenier J, Sany J (1984) Beta-2-microglobulin in myeloma: Optimal use for staging, prognosis, and treatment – A prospective study of 160 patients. Blood 63:468–476
3. Diem H, Fateh-Moghadam A, Lamerz R (1993) Prognostic factors in multiple myeloma: role of β2-microglobulin and thymidine kinase. Clin Invest 71:918–923
4. Durie BGM, Salmon SE (1975) A clinical staging system for multiple myeloma. Cancer 36:842–854
5. Litam P, Swan F, Cabanillas F, Tucker SL, McLaughlin P, Hagemeister FB, Rodriguez MA, Velasquez WS (1991) Prognostic value of serum β-2 microglobulin in low-grade lymphoma. Int Med 114:855–860

Address for correspondence:
Dr. med. Susanne Poley
Institut für Klinische Chemie
Klinikum Großhadern
Ludwig-Maximilians-Universität
Marchioninistraße 15
D-81366 München, Germany

Round Table

Quality Control and Standardization

Quality control and standardization of tumor marker assays

A. Maurer

Roche Diagnostic Systems, a Division of F. Hoffmann-La Roche Ltd. Basel, Switzerland

Quality control, standardization and automation have become key elements for the performance and reliability of immunoassays (1). Immunoassays should be easy to perform with minimal hands-on time and results obtained with different quantitative tests should be comparable. The three issues quality control, standardization and automation are linked together and they all serve to improve the reliability of the results.

Quality control starts at the beginning of the design and manufacturing of an assay. Quality control of an assay can be divided into several areas: quality control of the raw materials, single kit components, whole kit.

The raw materials are very important for the immunoassays as the antibodies really determine the quality of an immunoassay. If the antibodies change their properties, a standardization becomes obsolete. The choice of an antibody should be influenced by the following factors:

Polyclonal or monoclonal antibody? Specificity of antibody (what epitope is recognized?); affinity and avidity of the antibody (which influences assay time and range); reproducibility and rate of production of the antibodies; subclass of monoclonal antibody.

The choice of the assay format and of the antibodies has an influence on standardization. The following formats can be selected:

1-step, 2 different monoclonal antibodies,
1-step, 1 mono-/ polyclonal ab,
2-step, 2 monoclonals,
2-step, 1 monoclonal,
2-step, 1 monoclonal/ 1 polyclonal.

In most countries the 1-step formats are covered by patents depending on the label employed (2). Therefore, alternative test formats and polyclonal tracer antibodies are often chosen to avoid royalty payments.

If monoclonal antibodies are chosen, the question of the subclasses becomes an important issue. Whenever possible, IgGs of subclass I should be chosen. Tests that employ IgMs show rather high CVs and suffer from poor reproducibility.

The monoclonal antibodies can be made available in almost unlimited quantities and (if the right analytical tests are performed) at a constant quality level. These antibodies are either produced in mice as ascitic fluid or they are produced in Bioreactors. In both cases, they are produced in batches and subsequently the IgG-fraction is purified. To secure the supply on a long term base, the quality of these antibodies needs to be specified and checked.

In a first step the hybridoma clone has to be stabilized and secured: It is recloned at least twice and a subclone is used for the master cell bank. The master cell bank is stored at two different locations. From the master cell bank a working cell bank is estasblished. This material is then used for the production. The procedure is shown in figure 1.

The antibodies produced are then purified by standard procedures and they are analyzed in parallel with a reference lot on a routine base with the following criteria:

Isoelectric focusing (3), SDS – PAGE (4), chromatographic methods, functional tests which include a relative titer test, stress tests.

The stress tests consist of storing the antibodies at elevated temperature for prolonged periods of time. The activitiy of the antibodies is measured before and after the storage at elevated temperature.

Concerning the chromatography, the following methods are applied: gel filtration, ion exchange, hydrophobic interaction chromatography.

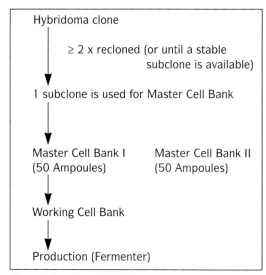

Figure 1. Securing of Hybridoma clones.

All the data obtained in these analytical checks are compared to the masterlot analyzed in parallel. If the requirements specified are fulfilled the batch is released for production. In this way the uniformity and quality of the antibodies can be guaranteed. Together with the quality control undertaken during the production of the kit a good lot to lot reproducibility can be ensured. Monoclonal antibodies, whether produced in-house or bought from a supplier, are subjected to such quality control measures. Especially antibodies obtained from external sources need to be checked carefully, because there is no control over the manufacturing process.

The assay CA 125 II demonstrates that if all things to be considered are done the proper way, chances for a correct standardization are good. The enzyme immunoassay Cobas Core CA 125 II EIA correlates well to the radioimmunoassay method of Centocor (5). Both kits employ the antibody M 11 as catcher and OC 125 as tracer as required for a CA 125 II assay (6, 7). The slope is almost 1 and the coefficient of correlation r is better than 0.987 (see figure 2).

Nevertheless, there is one CA 125 assay available that employs the monoclonal antibody OC 125 as tracer and polyclonal antibodies instead of the antibody M11 as catcher. As mentioned before it is clear that granted patents and non scientific reasons are the reason for the choice of the additional polyclonal antibody. Such an assay can no longer be called CA 125 or CA 125 II because one of the antibodies (the catcher antibody M 11)

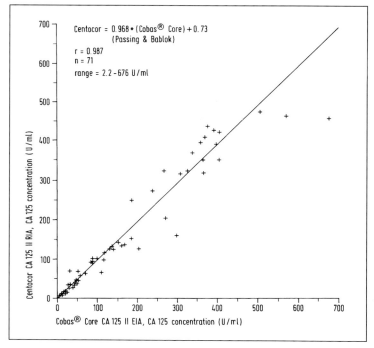

Figure 2. Correlation of Cobas Core CA 125 II with the Centocor CA 125 II RIA assay (n = 71). Sera were compared.

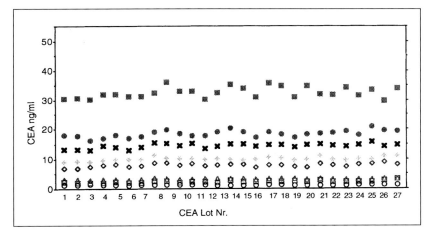

Figure 3. Roche CEA Lot: Lot reproducibility observed on 27 lots. With each lot eight reference sera were measured in triplicates as part of the final analysis before release.

Table I. A. Inter-lot precision of Cobas Core CA 125 II EIA and B. Cobas Core PSA EIA assay. For both assays the three lyophilized samples were reconstituted prior to use and then analyzed on 13 consecutive days on Cobas Core.

A. Cobas Core CA 125 II EIA

Level	Laboratory 1			Laboratory 2		
	n/ml	SD	% CV	ng/ml	SD	% CV
1	17.72	0.94	5.3	16.77	0.64	3.8
2	47.38	1.61	3.4	46.62	1.36	2.86
3	167.54	4.4	2.6	166.29	4.09	2.5

B. Cobas Core PSA EIA

Level	Laboratory 1			Laboratory 2		
	n/ml	SD	% CV	ng/ml	SD	% CV
1	3.24	0.16	4.8	3.08	0.09	3.13
2	6.37	0.25	3.9	6.30	0.12	2.03
3	32.01	1.45	4.5	32.30	0.91	2.82

that defines one of the epitopes of the analyte is not employed.

Another important factor is the use of the correct configuration of the catcher and tracer antibody: If tracer and catcher are exchanged as seen in the CA 72-4 assay, no correlation can be found with the assays that employ the antibodies in the original configuration: It is very important to use the antibody cc 49 as catcher and the antibody B 72.3 as tracer.

The careful choice of the raw materials and the constant surveillance of their quality provides continuous high quality and a good lot-to-lot reproducibility. Figure 3 exhibits the lot-to-lot reproducibility of the Cobas Core CEA EIA assay over the past 27 lots as measured with reference sera. The lots analyzed include the CEA Duomab assay as well as the new Cobas Core assay using tetramethylbenzidine (TMB) instead of orthophenylendiamin (oPD) as substrate. The first assays are used without shaking in a manual method, the latter are on the immunoassay analyzer Cobas® Core with shaking. As can be seen, the individual lots correlate well to each other and enable the user to detect small changes in the follow-up of the CEA level of a patient.

Automation of the immunoassays is another step toward improving the reliability (8). Table 1A demonstrates inter-assay CVs of the Cobas Core CA 125 II EIA test as measured on Cobas Core in two different laboratories. Both labs received lyophilized samples and reconstituted them before performing the measurements over 13 consecutive days on Cobas Core. In both labs very good CVs are obtained and the results are almost identical even in the very low range. For the Cobas Core PSA EIA assay the interassay CVs were determined in the same way and the results obtained in two laboratories are also very good (see table 1B).

Conclusion

It can be said that for an immunoassay all raw materials need to be investigated to ensure maximum quality. In particular the antibodies need to be checked with several analytical methods and additional measures need to be taken to secure a supply of the antibodies that fulfil the specifications. Only with such raw materials the lot-to-lot reproducibility of a kit can be maintained and a chosen standardization can be upheld. The test format and the choice of the antibodies are important for standardization. And finally, automation helps to improve the reliability and precision of the immunoassay with less hands-on time.

References

1. Nyfeler F (1991) Quality control and standardization. In: Klapdor R (ed) 6th Symposium on tumor markers. Hamburg, Zuckschwerdt, München, pp 313–314
2. Gallati H (1982) Interferon: wesentlich vereinfachte, enzym-immunologische Bestimmung mit zwei monoklonalen Antikörpern. J Clin Chem Clin Biochem 20:907
3. Righetti PG (1983) Isoelectric focusing: Theory, methodology and applications. Elsevier Biomedical Press, Amsterdam
4. Lämmli UK Cleavage of structural proteins during the assembly of the head bacteriophage T4. Nature (Lond) 227, 680–685
5. Girardin P (1991) Cobas Core CA 125 II EIA: Improved CA 125 determinations using a second monoclonal antibody. In: Klapdor R (ed) 6th Symposium on tumor markers. Hamburg, Zuckschwerdt, München, pp 248–252.
6. Bast RC, Feeney M, Lazarus H, Nadler LM, Covin RB, Knapp RC (1981) Reactivity of a monoclonal antibody with human ovarian carcinoma. J Cl Invest 68, 1331–1337
7. Hardadottir H, Parmley TH, Quirk JG, Sanders MM, Miller, FC, O'Brien TJ (1990) Distribution of CA 125 in embryonic tissues and adult derivates of the fetal periderm. Am J Obstet Gynecol 163, 1925–1931
8. Caravatti M (1991) Automation of heterogeneous immunoassays. In: Klapdor R (ed) 6th Symposium on tumor markers. Hamburg, Zuckschwerdt, München, pp 331–333

Address for correspondence:
Dr. A. Maurer
Roche Diagnostic Systems
a Division of F. Hoffmann-La Roche Ltd.
CH-4002 Basel, Switzerland

In: R. Klapdor (ed)
Current Tumor Diagnosis: Applications, Clinical Relevance, Research, Trends
Cancer of the Lung – State and Trends in Diagnosis and Therapy
© 1994 W. Zuckschwerdt Verlag München · Bern · Wien · New York

Sensitivity profiles and normalized dot plots

Tools for the clinical evaluation of new methods and comparison of methods

H.-M. Jansen, Petra Stieber, A. Fateh-Moghadam†
Institute for Clinical Chemistry, Klinikum Großhadern,
Ludwig-Maximilians-University, Munich, Germany

Introduction

Correlations, histograms, cross tabs, dot plots (1) and ROC curves (2) are mainly used for the statistical evaluation of the clinical relevance of new tumor markers and the comparison with other methods. Because of sometimes very different ranges of the values the comparison of methods in a dot plot is nearly impossible. The interpretation of the clinical interesting part of the ROC-curves between 80 and 100% specificity is very difficult. We want to demonstrate two graphical methods for a better comparison and evaluation of new markers.

Normalized dot plot

One condition for the comparison of new methods is, to fix one variable and compare all methods at the same value of the fixed variable. For our evaluations we decided to use the specificity against a collective of benign diseases, being interesting in differential diagnosis as the fixed variable. All calculations of sensitivity are done with a specificity of 95% against this population of benign diseases. Since two years this procedure is also recommended by the standardisation commitee of tumor markers (3).
For the normalized dot plot all values of one marker are divided by the cut-off, calculated for this subset at 95% specificity. In this way every value will be presented independent of the method used as multiples of the cut-off. The line with the equation y = 1 represents the cut-off. In this manner a comparative evaluation of the single values in a dot plot is possible, independent of the different value ranges. An example for this kind of presentation will be shown in figure 1. The left graph shows a not normalized dot plot of two different markers in three different subsets. Because of the very different cut-off values to obtain a specificity of 95% a direct comparison of the two markers is not possible. Only when all points are normalized it becomes evident, that the distribution of values looks almost the same, but more dots of marker 1 are clearly above the cut-off at 95% specificity.

Sensitivity profile

In most of the cases the clinical relevance of new markers is evaluated in comparison to other established methods. In the sensitivity profiles described in this paper the sensitivities of a new marker as comparative marker on the y-axis are plotted against the sensitivities of the established marker as reference marker on the x-axis at the same specificity for the two methods. Discrimination criterion is the 45°-line which represents the reference marker and describes the same sensitivity of two methods at the same specificity. A better marker than the reference marker shows points above this line, if the points are under the 45°-line the new marker is poor in comparison to the reference marker. Especially the range between 80–100% specificity can be jugded very easily in this kind of presentation.
Examples are shown in figure 2 and 3. On the left side ROC-curves are demonstrated and on the right side the corresponding sensitivity profile for the methods investigated. In figure 2 all four markers are plotted nearly as one curve, but the overall performance is not very well because the curves are very close to the 45° line. The sensitivity profile shows the same picture. All sensitivities are very close to the 45°-line, which represents the marker 4 choosen as reference marker. The overall performance of the method is

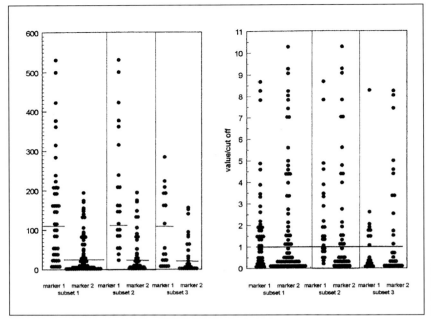

Figure 1. An example for a dot plot (left) and its normalized form (right).

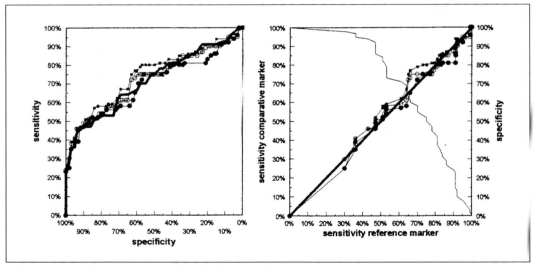

Figure 2. ROC-curve (left) and sensitivity profile (right); four different CA 125 II-assays for primary diagnosis of ovarian cancer.

shown by the plotted specificity curve of the reference marker.

Figure 3 shows a different situation. Whereas the ROC-curve on the left side shows, that TPS is inappropiate for primary diagnosis of squamous cell carcinoma of the lung, you can only see in the sensitivity profile that this is the same for TPA.

Conclusion

For the clinical evaluation of new tumor marker methods one variable should be fixed and then compared to the other methods at the same value of this variable. According to the standardization commitee (3) for tumor markers we recommend

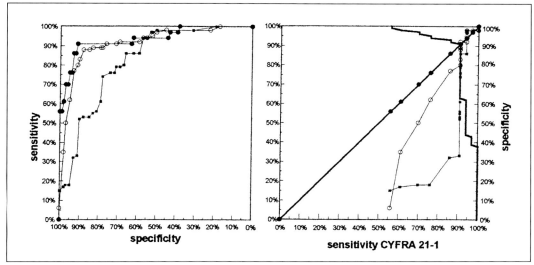

Figure 3. ROC-curve (left) and sensitivity profile (right); four different markers for primary diagnosis of squamous cell carcinoma of the lung. (—●—, CYFRA 21-1; —○— TPA, —■— TPS).

to fix the specificity for all evaluations, then to compare all sensitivities at 95% specificity against a well defined collective of benign diseases and to search the cut-off point for this value. Therefore it is very useful to present dot plots in the normalized form described here as multiples of this cut-off because of an easier judgement on the value-distribution of a method. Also the sensitivity profiles described in this paper show better than the normally used ROC-curves the "diagnostic correlation" of two or more different markers. Especially the range between 80–100% specificity can be jugded very easily in this kind of presentation.

As graphical tools the two described methods, sensitivity profile and normalized dot plot, allow an easier and better judgement of the clinical relevance of new tumor markers in comparison to established methods.

References

1. Krieg AF, Beck JR, Bongiovanni MB (1988) The dot plot – a starting point for evaluating test performance. JAMA 22(260):3309–3312
2. Zweig MH, Cambell G, (1993) Receiver-operating characteristics (ROC) plots: A fundamental evaluation tool in clinical medicine. Clin Chem 39(4): 561–577
3. Klapdor R (1992) Arbeitsgruppe Qualitätskontrolle und Standardisierung von Tumormarkertests im Rahmen der Hamburger Symposien über Tumormarker. Tumordiagn u Ther 13:XIX–XXII

Address for correspondence:
Dr. Petra Stieber
Institut für Klinische Chemie
Klinikum Großhadern
Ludwig-Maximilians-Universität
Marchioninistraße 15
D-81366 München, Germany

The analysis of variance as a statistical procedure for assessing tumor marker tests

H. Scheurlen[a], A Fateh-Moghadam[b], H. Fiedler[c], A. Klapdor[d], R. Kreienberg[e], V. Möbus[c],
R. Spitzer[f], Petra Stieber[b], P. Diziol[f], R. Ziergöbel[f], E. Spanuth[f]

[a] Institut für medizinische Biometrie und Informatik, Universität Heidelberg;
[b] Klinikum Großhadern, Munich; [c] Klinikum Suhl; [d] Universitätskliniken, Hamburg;
[e] Universitäts-Frauenklinik Ulm; [f] Boehringer Mannheim, Germany

Introduction

Studies on patients with gastric carcinoma show a higher diagnostic sensitivity for the tumor marker CA 72-4 than for the established markers CEA and CA 19-9. In addition, there are signs that CA 72-4 also has high sensitivity for mucinous ovarian carcinoma and can therefore be used as a suitable second marker alongside CA 125.

Methods

Clinical multicentre study

The clinical value of the tumor marker CA72-4 is to be investigated in a multicentre longitudinal study on patients with gastric and ovarian carcinoma and to be compared with that of the markers CEA, CA 19-9 and CA 125.
Included in the study are patients with gastric carcinoma who have had operations at least two months previously as well as patients with ovarian carcinoma who had undergone operations at least six months ago. The tumor markers CA 72-4, CEA, CA 19-9 and CA 125 are each to be determined four times at constant (4-week) intervals. These studies should yield further findings on the clinical value of the above-mentioned tumor markers in monitoring during post-operative tumor follow-up. The measurement data from a series are to be condensed to a measurement figure for the rise in the marker during the observation period of three months. In a follow-up study (with a deadline about one year after the commencement of the study), these measurement figures are to be related to relapse-free survival time.

Performance evaluation

In order to permit a common evaluation of the data from all participating centres, all laboratories should uniformly use the Enzymun-Test® method for determining the tumor markers. At the same time, various methods of determination should be compared with each other. For this purpose, parallel determinations using the laboratories' established routine methods should be carried out. A corresponding preliminary study (performance evaluation) has been carried out in the meantime. This is reported below[1].

---

[1] Participants in the multicentre study: Klinikum Karlsruhe; Laborgemeinschaft Westmecklenburg; Diagnostisches Zentrum Berlin; Klinikum der Albert-Ludwigs-Universität, Freiburg; Evangelisches Diakoniekrankenhaus, Freiburg Stadtkrankenhaus Neuwied; Städtisches Oststadt-Krankenhaus, Hannover; Zentralkrankenhaus "Links der Weser" Bremen; Evangelische Diakonissenanstalt, Bremen Universitätsklinik Hamburg-Eppendorf, Hamburg; Medizinische Akademie Magdeburg; St. Salvator-Krankenhaus, Halberstadt; Klinikum Jena; Medizinische Hochschule, Hannover; Institut Dr. Salinger, Dr. Löbel, Offenburg; Carl-Thiem-Kliniken, Cottbus; Klinikum Chemnitz; Medizinische Akademie Dresden; Universitätsfrauenklinik, Mainz; Städtisches Krankenhaus St. Georg, Leipzig; Frauenklinik der Universitätsklinik, Tübingen; Evangelisches Krankenhaus, Oberhausen; St. Josef-Hospital, Bochum; Laborfacharzt Prof. Röcker, Berlin; Klinikum Großhadern; Klinikum Neubrandenburg; Städtischen Krankenhaus Harlaching; Sonnenbergklinik, Bad Sooden-Allendorf; Westfälische Wilhelms-Universität, Münster; Medizinische Universitätsklinik, Würzburg; Vogtland-Kliniken, Plauen; Klinikum der Stadt Gera; St. Markus-Krankenhaus, Frankfurt/Main.

Implementation of the performance evaluation

Three lyophilized pooled sera based on human sera were prepared having tumor marker concentrations in the vicinity of the decision range/cut-off value (pooled serum A), in the low pathological range (pooled serum B) and in the highly pathological range (pooled serum C). On ten successive days, each laboratory carried out two determinations per day on each of the pooled sera for the tumor markers CA 72-4, CEA, CA 19-9 and CA 125 using the Enzymun-Test® system in parallel with the established routine method.

Mathematical model for the evaluation

Of every good measuring method it is demanded that it should be sensitive in its reaction to concentration changes of the substrate measured while at the same time keeping the random error as low as possible. The latter is generally characterized by the standard deviation s of replicate measurements on the same substrate. It is also usual to state a relative and non-dimensional measure of dispersion, with the mean, $\bar{x}$ given as the measuring unit. One considers a measure of this kind, e.g. the coefficient of variation $CV = s/\bar{x}$, as a criterion for the precision of a measuring method. In doing so, one assumes that there is a relationship between the two parameters of position and dispersion. It would be desirable to have a method-specific measure of precision that is constant from one substrate to another. If measurements from a defined and relative homogeneous population of independent items are normally distributed, then one can assume that the means and standard deviations of replicate measurements are independent of each other and that the coefficients of variation show a tendency to decrease as the substrate concentration increases.

Experience has shown, however, that measurements of marker concentrations are not normally distributed. If the data to be evaluated originate from a relatively homogeneous group of patients, then they often show an approximately log-normal distribution. This can be recognized by, among other things, the fact that a linear relationship exists between the means and standard deviations of replicate measurements: as the means increase so do also the standard deviations of the replicate measurements. For the simple proportionality $s = b\bar{x}$, the coefficient of variation remains constant when the marker concentration changes: $CV = s/\bar{x} = b$. In this case, b is hence a method-specific constant. If one compares two methods with each other, then, provided the means of the repeat measurements lie in roughly the same range, the CV can be applied as a measure of the method's precision. However, even with a comparatively small span in the measuring range a test with high precision (small CV) can react less sensitively to existing concentration changes than a less "precise" method. If both parameters follow the (linear) relationship $s = a + b\bar{x}$, then the CV becomes a concentrationdependent variable: $CV = s/\bar{x} = a/\bar{x} + b_1$ decreases or increases with increasing $\bar{x}$ (a > 0 or a < 0, respectively).

It is hence quite possible for a situation to arise in which the coefficients of variation are difficult to interpret. In this situation one can attempt to resolve the total variance s_T^2 of all n measurements (n = number of pooled sera multiplied by the number of repeated measurements) into two components with the aid of a hierarchical analysis of variance: the variance s_A^2 between the concentrations and the variance s_E^2 within a series of measurements. The quotient $\hat{Q} = s_A^2/s_E^2$ then represents a measure of the resolution power of the method.

A pre-requisite for the use of this procedure is a normal distribution of the data X. If a log-normal distribution is present, this can be achieved by a logarithmic transformation $Y = \log X$. In the typical experimental set-up for inter-laboratory studies described here – a small number of sera with excessive concentration differences and a large number of repeated measurements mixed distributions must be expected which cannot be "normalized" by log transformation. Log transformation does, however, enable the most important pre-requisite for the use of variance analysis methods to be fulfilled: relative variance stability.

There is yet another reason why the usual inter-laboratory studies are poorly suited for comparing measuring methods: they lead to a quite avoidable enlargement of the confidence intervals for the parameter Q to be estimated.

As a rule of thumb it can be said: increase the number of sera used in the inter-laboratory studies at the cost of the number of repeated measurements! At the same time the concentration differences should be drastically reduced. In our case this means roughly: 12 sera with 5 replicate measurements instead of 3 sera with 20 repetitions. It is more difficult to show that quite obvious differences are better "recognized" by one method than by the comparison method than it is to show that one method more reliably shows slight differences – as can occur in intra-individual pathological courses – than does another.

Results

Inter-assay variation

Results from 30 laboratories were included in the evaluation. For Enzymun-Test®, coefficients of variation of between 4% and 8% were yielded via 20 determinations on 10 days; the coefficients of variation for the comparison methods investigated were between 5% and 14% (table I).

Analysis of variance

Data

At the time of the final evaluation following conclusion of the performance evaluation, the following data structure exists: a relatively homogeneous group of six laboratories can be identified which in parallel to the Enzymun-Test® carried out at least 18 of the envisaged 20 replicate measurements on the three pooled sera (A, B and C) with a uniform routine method. On this group the following report of our statistical evaluation is based. In addition, we have defined a "reference laboratory" which fulfilled all of the points given in the protocol and used a radioimmunoassay (E-RIA) parallel to the Enzymun-Test®.

Distribution of the data

Replicate measurements carried out with a particular measuring method on a particular pooled serum are adequately normally distributed (distribution of measuring errors). As would be

Table I. Inter-assay coefficients of variation (CV%) for the samples A, B and C (medians).

CA 72-4	Enzymun-Test	B/LIA	C/RIA
Sample A	4.8	11.0	14.1
Sample B	4.0	11.9	9.0
Sample C	4.0	14.5	9.1
Laboratories (n)	28	3	7

CA 19-9	Enzymun-Test	B/LIA	A/MEIA
Sample A	4.8	8.0	6.9
Sample B	4.4	7.3	8.8
Sample C	3.9	12.8	7.3
Laboratories (n)	25	4	7

CEA	Enzymun-Test	F/RIA	A/MEIA
Sample A	5.9	8.9	6.2
Sample B	5.7	8.9	5.8
Sample C	4.9	8.7	4.9
Laboratories (n)	30	3	11

CA125	Enzymun-Test	C/RIA	A/MEIA
Sample A	7.6	8.5	5.2
Sample B	7.2	8.7	6.4
Sample C	6.9	4.3	6.2
Laboratories (n)	24	3	6

expected, for both measuring methods the standard deviations increase almost linearly with the means. Due to the experimental set-up, in which the concentration differences between the pooled sera A, B and C were in the ratio 1:2:5, there is – as an artefact – a trimodal distribution of the 3 x 20 data points. The variances can be adequately stabilized by log transformation of the data; they are then only slightly dependent upon the magnitude of the mean.

The discriminance problem

Figure I summarizes the measurements obtained in the reference laboratory. The standard deviations are plotted (as ordinates) against the means (abscissa) of the non-transformed original data as points in a right-angled co-ordinate system, with one point for each of the three pooled sera fo-

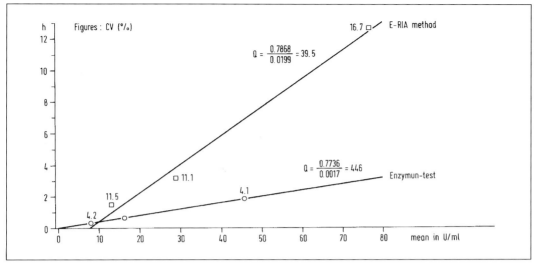

Figure 1. Multicentre study. Performance evaluation of the reference laboratory for CA 72-4.

each measuring method. One can see the more or less perfect linear relationship which is also manifested in the almost constant (method-specific) coefficient of variation: approx. 4% for the Enzymun-Test® and over 11% for the E-RIA. Figure 2 shows the same procedure carried out on pooled data from the six laboratories of the C-RIA group. According to this it would appear that the Enzymun-Test® is indeed superior to the RIA test. At all events, the absolute intervals between the means in the E-RIA are clearly greater than with the Enzymun-Test®. We therefore calculate the measure of resolution, Q,

$$Q = \frac{\text{Variance component between the concentrations } S_A^2}{\text{Variance component within the measurement series } S_E^2}$$

In the case of our "reference laboratory" this goes in favor of the Enzymun-Test®. However, the 90% confidence intervals of the two quotients show considerable overlap for the Enzymun-Test® and the laboratory method, it is hence not possible to speak of greater than random differences between the quotients in individual cases. (The poor resolution power of the estimating procedure is – as described above – due to the irrational structure of the inter-laboratory study.) This experience should be taken into account in future studies.
Figure 3 shows the quotients for all laboratories taking part in the performance study and for all methods relating to the parameter CA 72-4. Apart from one exception, the quality criterion for the Enzymun-Test® is consistently above that of the laboratory methods wherever parallel measurements were carried out; this was the case in eleven laboratories. This bias in favor of the Enzymun-Test® is highly significant ($P < 0.01$, sign test).

Inter-laboratory reliability

How good is the between-laboratory agreement of the measurements?

Here, too, the procedure of additive analysis of the total variance suggests itself here: the laboratory effect on the one hand (between-laboratory variance component) and a component due to measuring errors on the other. For simplicity's sake and to facilitate the integratability, we consider the relationships for the three pooled sera separately.
In each case we can assume that the data are adequately normally distributed. Again, only data from the C-RIA group were used in the evaluation. The criterion for quality used was again the quotient

$$Q = \frac{\text{Variance component between the laboratories}}{\text{Variance component within the measurement series}}$$

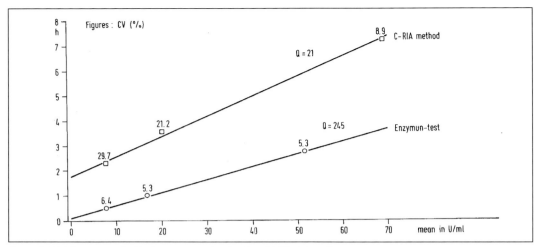

Figure 2. Multicentre study. Performance evaluation for CA 72-4 (n = 6).

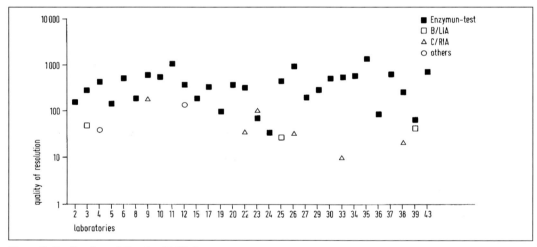

Figure 3. Quality of resolution for CA 72-4.

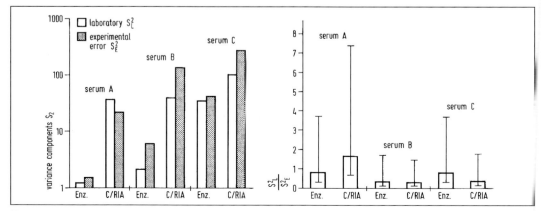

Figure 4. Multicentre study. CA 72-4, inter-laboratory reliability for CA 72-4 (n = 6); lower part, 90% confidence limits

Quality Control and Standardization 469

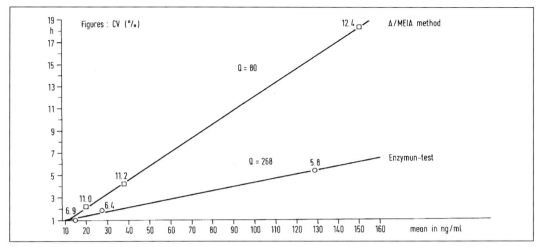

Figure 5. Multicentre study. CA 72-4, performance evaluation for CEA (n = 9).

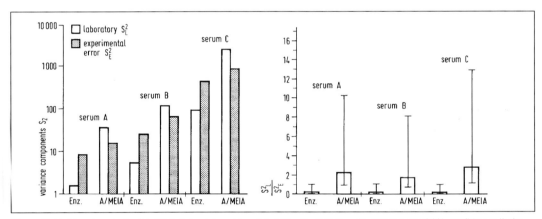

Figure 6. Multicentre study. CA 72-4, inter-laboratory reliability for CEA (n = 9); lower part, 90% confidence limits.

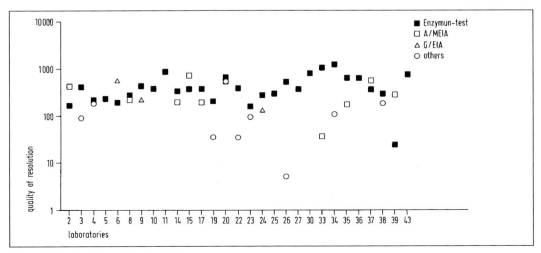

Figure 7. Quality of resolution for CEA.

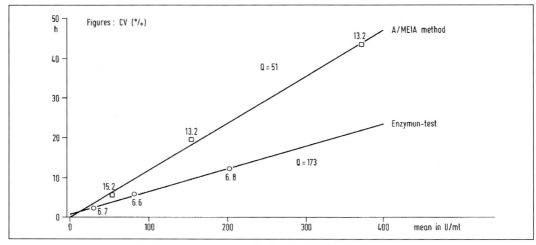

Figure 8. Multicentre study. CA 72-4, performance evaluation for CA 19-9 (n = 7).

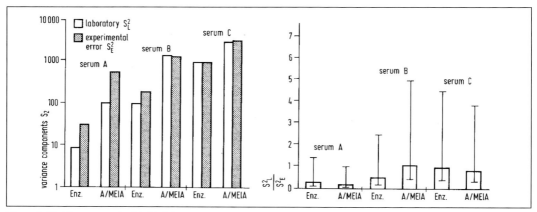

Figure 9. Multicentre study. CA 72-4, inter-laboratory reliability for CA 19-9 (n = 7); lower part, 90% confidence limits.

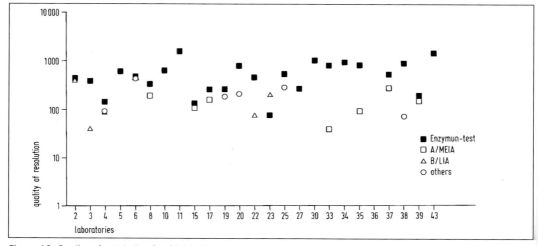

Figure 10. Quality of resolution for CA 19-9.

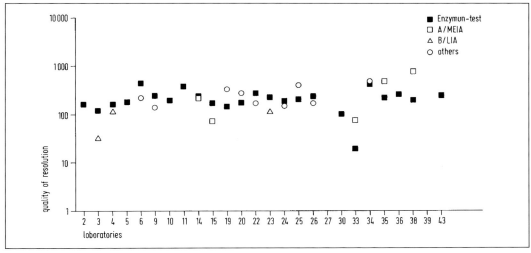

Figure 11. Quality of resolution for CA 125.

In contrast to the assessment of the quotients with the discriminance problem, reliability is, however, synonymous with low quotient values. It should, if possible, not exceed 1 (laboratory error = measurement error).

The upper part of figure 4 shows the two components of the total variance. In the lower part of figure 4 the quotients together with the 90% confidence intervals are shown. It can be seen that there are no significant differences between the measuring methods with regard to inter-laboratory reliability.

Measurements for the markers CA 19-9, CA 125 and CEA analyzed in the same way are given in figures 5–11.

Conclusions

According to our preliminary study on performance evaluation, there are clear differences in the discriminating power of the various tests. It remains to be seen whether such differences have an effect on the prognosis of the course of an illness, particularly with regard to the early recognition of relapse. Also still to be clarified is whether a combination of various markers increases the prognostic power. We expect to obtain answers to these questions from our currently running multicentre longitudinal study.

References

1. Scheffé H (1958) The analysis of variance. John Willy & Sons, New York
2. Ahrens H (1968) Varianzanalyse. Akademie-Verlag, Berlin
3. Klapdor R (1992) Arbeitsgruppe Qualitätskontrolle und Standardisierung von Tumormarkertests im Rahmen der Hamburger Symposien über Tumormarker. Tumordiag u Therapie 13
4. Stieber P et al (1993) CA 72-4: Ein sinnvoller Tumormarker beim Magenkarzinom. Lab med 17:441
5. Guadagni F (1992) CA 72-4 Measurement of tumor-associated glycoprotein 72 (TAG-72) as a serum marker in the management of gastric carcinoma. Cancer Res 52:1222–1227
6. Kreienberg R, Möbus V (1992) Tumormarker in der Gynäkologie. Lab med 16:21–26

Address for correspondence:
Dr. E. Spanuth
Boehringer Mannheim
Sandhoferstraße 116
D-68305 Mannheim, Germany

Long-term quality control exemplified by laboratory radioimmunoassays for AFP and CEA

R. Lamerz, A. Brandt, E. Segura

Medical Department II, Klinikum Großhadern, University of Munich, Germany

Introduction

Among the multiple indications for tumor marker (TM) use the follow-up control of course of disease and therapy is acknowledged as the most realistic one (1) dependent on the quality of statistical parameters (sensitivity, specificity, positive/negative predictive value) and the reliability and reproducibility of serial measurements (intra-, inter-assay-variability, internal/external quality control) (2). A further critical factor is the fact that multiple commercially available tests made by different manufacturers are offered for many tumor markers whose actual marker values may differ considerably by means of the various antigen and antibody charges as well as different methods of detection (ionic strength, pH, matrix effects etc.). Therefore for follow-up a change of tests of different manufacturers is not advisable and at least should always be indicated together with the result. For reduction of the differences and an improvement of tumor marker measurements, during the last years many efforts have been undertaken like for the chemical identification of marker epitopes, preparation of international standards for antigens (e.g. for AFP, CEA) as well as the performance of comparative investigations and agreements as to the composition of study and control groups (3).

In the following a demonstration is presented for the successful use of internal and external quality control on the example of two conventional laboratory radioimmunoassays for AFP and CEA used for more than 17 years.

Material and methods

AFP (4, 6)

The antigen was extracted and purified from ascites of patients with hepatocellular (HCC) or germ cell tumors (GST) by cartridge electrophoresis, gelfiltration on Sephadex G100 and immunoaffinity gel filtration (CNBr-activated Sepharose 6B with fixed anti-AFP-IgG from a rabbit) and used as tracer as well as in semipurified form as standard. The tracer antigen (4–5 µg) was labeled by ^{125}I according to the chloramin T method (250–500 µCi/9.3–18.5 MBq) during 20–45" at room temperature and purified on Sephadex G50 and G100 by gel filtration. As first antibody an own anti-AFP-IgG from a rabbit or commercial rabbit anti-AFP-antiserum (Behringwerke, working dilution 1/8,000–1/10,000) and as second antibody an own and a commercial goat anti-rabbit-immunoglobulin-antiserum (Behringwerke, working dilution 1/20) were used for the assay. In addition, quite recently commercial AFP antigen and antiserum preparations (Biogenes, Berlin) were used comparatively.

CEA (5, 7)

The antigen was extracted by perchloric acid from different primary or liver-involved tumors (colonic, pancreatic, breast, ovarian, lung cancer) and purified by gel chromatography on Sepharose 6B, Sephadex G200 and by affinity chromatography (CNBr-activated Sepharose 4B with fixed anti-CEA-IgG from a rabbit) and used as tracer as well as in a semipurified form as standard. As tracer 2–6 µg of the CEA preparation was labeled by ^{125}I according to the chloramin T method for 20–45" at room temperature and the tracer then purified by gel filtration on Sephadex G50 and G200 for use in the assay. As first antibody rabbit anti-CEA serum exhaustively absorbed by PCA extracts from normal lung, liver or gall bladder bile extracts and then purified (DEAE cellulose, Protein A Sepharose) as anti-CEA-IgG was used (working dilution 1/6,000–1/60,000). In addition, quite recently commercial CEA antigen and antiserum preparations (Biogenes, Berlin) were used comparatively. For 2nd antibody see AFP.

For both assays the same test buffer (PBS +1% BSA + EDTA, pH 8.2) was used for standard curves with 100 µl/tube, with 100 (AFP) or 200 µl (CEA) of patient's serum (total incubation volume 500/600 µl) with 3 incubation steps of 4h (cold preincubation) and 2 overnight incubations, one centrifugation step at 2000 g, 15' at room temperature. Serum determinations were done in duplicate.

The evaluation of the count rates for AFP and CEA standard curves and tests was performed according to the logit-log procedure in the past and more recently according to the spline function method computer-integrated in the gamma-counter (LKB/Pharmacia-Wallac).

Results and discussion

From 1976 to 1993 regular AFP and CEA measurements were done in > 900 AFP/CEA single tests from 67/77 consecutive ^{125}I labelings accounting for more than 100,000 double determinations as single or serial follow-up serum measurements of patients with different tumor diseases.

For the 67 AFP and 77 CEA labelings a mean specific activity of 123.3 ± 51.5 (AFP) or 131.4 ± 85.5 (CEA) µCi/µg protein was found. The RIA tests showed a mean unspecific binding rate (Bn/T) of 2.4 ± 0.6% (AFP, n = 733) or of 2.4 ± 1.3% (CEA, n = 765) in contrast to a mean specific binding rate (Bo/T) of 32.4 ± 4.1% (AFP) or 33.4 ± 4.8% (CEA).

The AFP-test showed a lower sensitivity of 1.5 ng/ml at a working range up to 200 ng/ml, the CEA test a sensitivity of about 2 ng/ml at a working range up to 160 ng/ml.

The intra-assay-variation (IAV) was calculated according to 20fold measurements of control sera between 5.3 ($\bar{x}$ = 17.3 ng/ml) and 9.6% ($\bar{x}$ = 138 ng/ml; AFP) or between 5.0–5.5% ($\bar{x}$ between 38 and 141 ng/ml) or 11.9% ($\bar{x}$ = 13 ng/ml; CEA).

As internal quality control 4–6 single control sera from different consecutive charges prepared from pooled serum, amniotic fluid (AFP) or ascites partially diluted by RIA buffer (PBS + 1% albumin) to a concentration range between 19–180 ng/ml (AFP) or 8–160 ng/ml (CEA) were used and stored as frozen aliquots at –80° C. In total 4 to 5 different charges were used over the 17 years. For these controls coefficients of variation (inter-assay-variation, IEV) between 7.4 ($\bar{x}$ = 35 ng/ml) and 15% ($\bar{x}$ = 183 ng/ml) (AFP; figure 1) or 7.6 ($\bar{x}$ = 156 ng/ml) and 16.2% ($\bar{x}$ = 7 ng/ml) (CEA; figure 2) were obtained. These values were obviously higher than those for IAV.

As external quality control our laboratory participated since 1980 in 2–3 yearly tumor marker ring trials (control cycles, n = 33) of the German Society of Clinical Chemistry covering a range of 5–250 ng/ml (AFP) or of 5–60 ng/ml (CEA). In comparison with the median of a larger group of participants using the same commercial assay (Abbott IRMA/EIA), a mean transforming factor between laboratory and comparative test of 1.07 ± 0.15 (laboratory-AFP ng/ml into Abbott-AFP IU/ml, CV = 14.5%, n = 58; figure 3) or of 1.93 ± 0.43 (laboratory-CEA into Abbott-CEA, CV = 22.5%, n = 52; figure 4) as well as a linear coefficient of correlation of r = 0.96 (AFP, $S_{y.x}$ = 14.6, n = 66) or 0.93 (CEA, $S_{y.x}$ = 2.79, n = 66) were found.

As additional proof of comparability between laboratory and commercial test results, the coefficient of correlation between laboratory and commercial test measurements in tumor patients yielded a value for AFP (laboratory-AFP versus AFP III enzyme test or ESCO enzyme test of Boehringer Mannheim) of 1.00 in patients with germ cell tumors (n = 105) or of 0.99 in hepatocellular cancer (n = 62) and of r = 0.96 for CEA (laboratory-CEA versus CEA-Liamat, Byk-Sangtec; n = 125) in patients with different tumors (lung, breast, ovarian, pancreatic, stomach, colorectal cancer). In addition, AFP follow-up curves for different patients were nearly identical for the laboratory and comparative assays, whereas CEA follow-up curves – according to the mean transforming factor of about 2 – were less steep for the laboratory assay but cor-

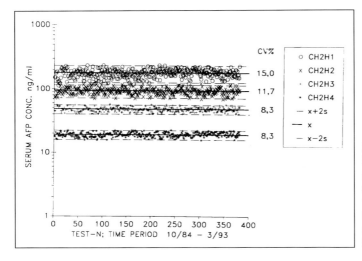

Figure 1. Inter-assay variation of the laboratory AFP-RIA from internal controls of one charge (CH2) for four different concentrations (median H1 = 183 ng/ml; H2 = 94 ng/ml; H3 = 48 ng/ml; H4 = 19 ng/ml) during about nine years yielding CV values between 8.3 and 15.0%.

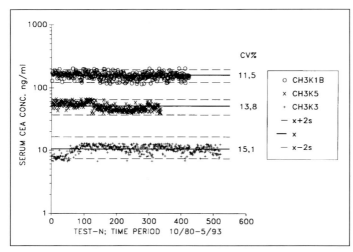

Figure 2. Inter-assay variation of the laboratory CEA-RIA from internal controls of one charge (CH3) for three different concentrations (median K1B = 160 ng/ml; K3 = 10.7 ng/ml; K5 = 50 ng/ml) during about 11 years yielding CV values between 11.5 and 15.1%.

responded exactly concerning the marker increases and decreases.

When comparing IAV and IEV values for AFP and CEA it is remarkable that CV values for both IAV and IEV are lowest for AFP in the lower and nearly normal range (5–9%) and higher in the upper range > 50 ng/ml (8–15%) in contrast to the CEA test with higher IAV and IEV values in the lower range (12–16%) and decreasing CV values with higher control concentrations (5–12%). This means for the AFP test that it can be used for normal AFP distribution curves and a broader normal range between 2 and 15 ng/ml (1–10 IU/ml) in contrast to the CEA test with the narrower normal range between < 1 and 3 ng/ml which is only partially covered by our CEA-RIA.

Concerning the transformation factors for AFP (figure 3) and CEA (figure 4) between the laboratory test and the comparative larger study group within the external quality control program, the mean factor for AFP was about 1 yielding nearly identical AFP values by both tests. In contrast for CEA the mean factor between laboratory and comparative CEA test was nearly 2 yielding about 50% of values of the control test, however, a good coefficient of correlation of

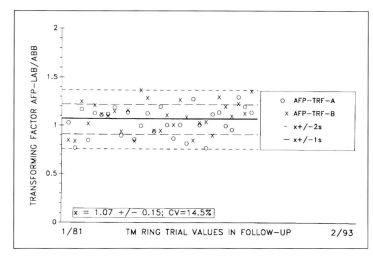

Figure 3. Transforming factor AFP laboratory RIA versus commercial comparative AFP-IRMA/EIA calculated from serial tumor marker ring trials using two different controls (A, B) per trial (n = 58).

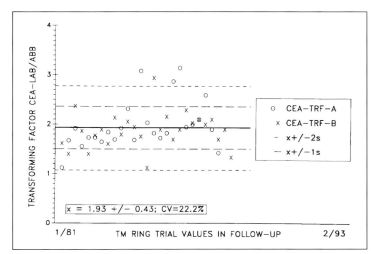

Figure 4. Transforming factor CEA laboratory RIA versus commercial comparative CEA-IRMA/EIA calculated from serial tumor marker ring trials using two different controls (A, B) per trial (n = 52).

r = 0.93. Because of the long-term use of our test and serial serum CEA measurements in tumor patients over 5–10 years of follow-up, we did not see the need for adapting our standard to the comparative Abbott standard appreciating more the maintenance of the same standard for better comparability in follow-up.

Our internal quality control values for AFP and CEA are consistent with the values reported by *Pilo* et al. (8) for the external quality assessment program in Italy with a total variability seen in 1990 of 17.3 CV% subdivided into a within-kit variability of 15.2% and between-kit values of 8.1% (CEA: total 20.6%, within-kit 14.0%, between-kit 15.2%) with better values obtained versus 1986 (AFP: 22.6, 20.5, 9.6%; CEA: 35.6, 18.4, 30.5%). Yet between-laboratory and between-kit precision variability versus the consensus mean in the lower range (AFP < 20 ng/ml, CEA < 10 ng/ml) was higher for CEA (20–30%) than for AFP (17–25%).

In conclusion the data presented strengthen the need for internal as well as external quality control for a long-term application of tumor marker assays in serial serum measurements of tumor patients.

References

1. Lamerz R (1992) Allgemeine Kriterien zur Bestimmung von Tumormarkern im Labor und Anwendung in der Klinik. Lab med 16:13–20
2. Bonfrer JMG (1990) Working group on tumor marker criteria (WGTMC) Letter to the Editor. Tumor Biol 11:287–288
3. Klapdor R (1992) Arbeitsgruppe Qualitätskontrolle und Standardisierung von Tumormarkertests im Rahmen der Hamburger Symposien über Tumormarker. Tumordiagn u Ther 13:19–22
4. Lamerz R, Rjosk H, Schmalhorst U, Fateh-Moghadam A (1976) Alpha-Fetoprotein: Methodik und klinische Erfahrungen mit einem neuen Radioimmunoassay. Z Anal Chem 279:120
5. Lamerz R, Ruider H (1976) Zur Bestimmung des carcinoembryonalen Antigens (CEA): Erfahrungen mit einem neuen Radioimmunoassay. Z Anal Chem 279:105
6. Lamerz R, Staehler G, Hiermeyer L, von Lieven H (1977) Radioimmunologische Serumbestimmungen von Alpha-Fetoprotein bei Patienten mit Hodentumoren. Urologe A 16:213–218
7. Lamerz R, Ruider H (1976) Bestimmungen von karzinoembryonalem Antigen bei Patienten mit Dickdarmtumoren. Erfahrungen mit einem neuen Radioimmunoassay. Münch med Wschr 118:377–380
8. Pilo A, Zucchelli GC, Masini S, Torre GC, Ballesta AM (1990) Progress report on an external quality assessment program for immunoassays of tumor markers. J Nucl Med Allied Sci 34 (Suppl to No.3):75–82

Address for correspondence:
Prof. Dr. med. R. Lamerz
Medizinische Klinik II, Klinikum Großhadern
Marchioninistraße 15
D-81377 München, Germany

Long-term standardization of tumor marker tests

N. Dahlmann

Central Laboratory, General Hospital Harburg, Hamburg, Germany

Introduction

Tumor markers are defined as substances produced by tumor cells in larger quantities than by normal cells and measurable in body fluids. They have gained increasing importance in the follow-up of cancer patients during and after therapy. To fullfill these medical requirements the demands on quality assurance should be the same as those that apply to all parameters in clinical chemistry. However, the lack of international reference preparations and of reference methods for most turmor maker tests are the main reasons for problems in these assays.

Results of interlaboratory surveys reveal that there is a considerable scatter of results between different kits. This ist not caused by inaccuracy of measurement of the individual participants but by the varying degrees of calibration of the individual test. Namely, if the whole number of results is differentiated according to individual manufacturers, differences of between 200 and 300% between the medians of the individual manufacturers are produced, whereas the precision is adequate. This phenomenon is often described (1, 2) and gives an explanation why interlaboratory results so often differ in results.

Another aspect of quality control and standardization is the question, how stable are assays over time as a main aspect of tumor patient survey. The present study contributes to the question of long time stability of tumor marker kit calibration.

Materials and methods

Basis of the study were the ring trials of the German Society for Clinical Chemistry (DGKCh) of the years 1988 till 1993. Sample material was prepared of pooled human sera spiked with commercial preparations and/or pooled patient sera of high elevated tumor markers. For details see (3). Two different probes were prepared (A and B). The results are presented in a Youden-diagramm with presentation of all single values and labeling of the distinguished values of each participant. For details see the survey of *Kruse* et al. (3). The following tumor markers were analyzed: CEA, CA 15-3, CA 19-9.

The codes of companies are as indicated: 04 Abbott, 28 Boehringer Mannheim, 30 CIS Isotopen Diagnostik, 32 Byk Sangtec Diagnostik, 74 Roche.

The methods used are indicated as follows: (1) radioimmunoassay, (2) enzyme immunoassay. N represents the number of participants. Only the results of kits used by ten or more laboratories were taken into account. The medians of the individual kits were compared with the total median and the deviations were calculated in percent. The results for different kits are depicted over time.

Results

An example of the kind of analysis can be seen in figure 1. In this figure the results for the tumor marker CEA are presented. The bars correspond to the median of all measurements for ring trial sample A. In addition the medians for kits 04 and 74 are depicted. This allows direct reading of the absolute deviations from the total median. In order to examine the quality of the analysis the percentual deviations for the ring trial samples A and B were compared with each other.

For kit 04 absolutely congruent courses with a slight deviation from the total median were seen

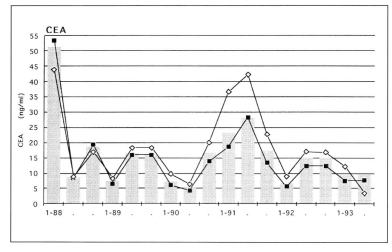

Figure 1. Ring trials of the years 1988 to 1993 for the tumor marker CEA. Depicted are the medians for the following kits (methods) of the ring trial sample A: ■ kit 04 (2) and ◇ kit 74 (2). The bars indicate the median of all data.

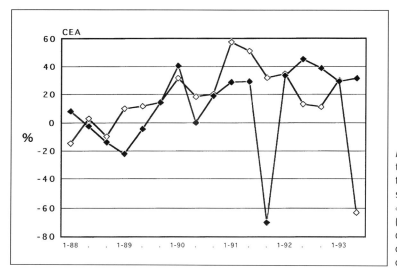

Figure 2. Ring trial results for the tumor marker CEA for the following kits (methods; samples), respectively: ◇ kit 74 (2; A) and ◆ kit 74 (2; B). Depicted are the deviations from the medians of individual kits in percent of the total median.

(not shown). Parallel curves were also seen with kit 74 for samples A and B. Concerning this kit it is evident, however, that over years there is an upward trend with a deviation from the total median of approximately 40% for the period 1991 to 1993. Furthermore, two outliers predominate for sample A as well as sample B.

The same kind of analysis was undertaken for tumor marker CA 15-3 (figure 3). The results for kits 28, 30 or 32 are presented. On the whole all three kits showed a largely stabile course. Only kit 32 demonstrated a sudden rise from −15% to +15% within one year.

For tumor marker CA 19-9 kits 04, 28 and 74 were evaluated (figure 4). A stabile course was seen for kit 28 and 04 (not shown). For kit 74 the values oscillated from 100% to −60% in the year 1989 followed by a continual decrease in amplitude before finally stabilizing around 40%.

Discussion

Tumor patients are often cared for at different locations over a long period. Tumor markers must allow for this fact to ensure an optimal follow-up.

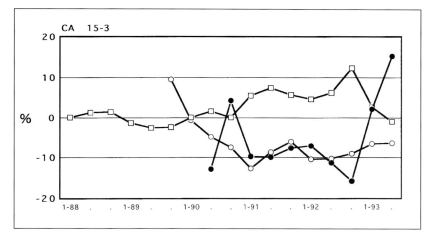

Figure 3. Ring trial results for the tumor marker CA 15-3 for the following kits (methods) of sample A: ○ kit 28 (2), □ kit 30 (1), ● kit 32 (1). Depicted are the deviations from the medians of individual kits in percent of the total median.

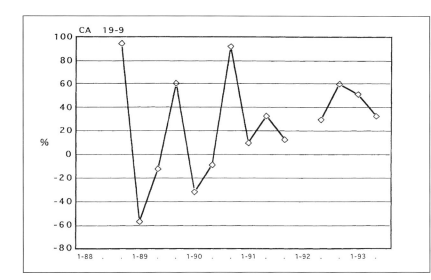

Figure 4. Ring trial results for the tumor marker CA 19-9 for the following kits (methods) of sample A: ◇ kit 74 (2). Depicted is the deviation from median of the individual kit in percent of the total median.

With respect to this requirement it is essential for tumor marker tests to possess a high accuracy and precision. The criteria are examined by means of ring trial using reference materials and reference methods at authorized institutions. These conditions cannot be met for tumor markers, however, as there are neither reference methods nor reference materials. As already elaborated at another location, this means that measurements obtained using different kits vary considerably (4).

In order to gain information on this point, the medians of the individual kits were compared with the total median. This comparison serves as a methodical aid since reference material is missing for most tumor markers. The results with ring trial samples A and B were compared with each other for one kit and one method to appraise the value of this method. For the most part the curves were parallel to each other, allowing the exclusion of gross methodical uncertainties. Therefore, on the whole the method assumes to be reliable.

For the tumor marker CEA there is nothing striking for the investigated kits 04, 28 and 74, with the exception of single outliers which are at least in part attributable to the low sample concentrations. Kit 74 showed a continual upward trend from 1988 to 1992. A longer term trend is not observable for tumor marker CA 15-3. In contrast, short term trend alterations are seen for kit 28 in the period from 1990 to 1991 and kit 32 from 1992 to 1993. The deviations range over an acceptable margin from ± 10%, however.

The results from kit 74 for the tumor marker CA 19-9 were grotesque. During the years 1989 to 1993 the values oscillated between 100% and – 60% while the kits 04 and 28 demonstrated stable courses. For kit 74 the results reflect the attempt of the manufacturer to focus the standardization on the total median.

In all, the results underline the problem that there is no reference material for tumor markers. While some kits demonstrate a high constancy of charges, by other kits adjustments in "running operations" are carried out by alterations of the master calibrator. This is not to be tolerated from a clinical or economical standpoint. It is therefore imperative to demand that the industry agrees on reference preparations such as are already realized by the WHO for some tumor markers.

Acknowledgment

I would like to thank *Professor G. Röhle* for ring trial data.

References

1. Dahlmann N (1992) Progress and problems in the quality assurance of tumor marker tests. In: Klapdor R (ed) Tumor associated antigens, oncogenes, receptors, cytokines in tumor diagnosis and therapy at the beginning of the nineties. Zuckschwerdt, München Bern Wien New York, pp 291–293
2. Dahlmann N (1991) Qualitätssicherung bei der Bestimmung von Tumormarkern: Darstellung und Diskussion eines Ringversuches. Lab Med 15:344–346
3. Kruse R, Geilenkeuser WJ, Röhle G (1993) Interlaboratory surveys of the determination of tumor markers scatter and repeatability of the results. Eur J Clin Chem Clin Biochem 31:139–146
4. Zwirner M (1992) Longitudinal quality control of tumor marker assays: Results of an international proficiency study with CEA. In: Klapdor R (ed) Tumor associated antigenes, oncogenes, receptors, cytogenes in tumor diagnosis and therapy at the beginning the nineties. Zuckschwerdt, München Bern Wien New York, pp 283–290

Address for correspondence:
Prof. Dr. med. N. Dahlmann
Allgemeines Krankenhaus Harburg
Eißendorfer Pferdeweg 52
D-21075 Hamburg, Germany

Determination of CA 19-9 with various commercial assays

Results of an international proficiency study

M. Zwirner, Th. Risse[a], R. Benz[b], G. D. Birkmeyer[c], W. Buchterkirche[b], U. Baum[e], B. Brandt[f], A. van Dalen[g], R. Förster[h], W. Hubl[i], S. Kapp[j], R. Klapdor[k], J. Spitz[l], N. Wieser[m]

[a]Department of Obstetrics and Gynecology, University of Tübingen, [b]Department of Obstetrics and Gynecology, University of Ulm, Germany; [c]Labor for Bioanalytic, Wien, Austria; [d]Institute of Laboratory Medicine, Bremen, [e]Department of Nuclear Medicine, [f]University of Frankfurt, [g]Department of Clinical Chemistry, University of Münster, Germany; [h]Department of Nuclear Medicine, Bleuland Hospital, Gouda, The Netherlands; [i]Medical Clinic Essen, [j]Institute of Laboratory Medicine, Mainz, [k]Medical Clinic, University of Hamburg, [l]Department of Nuclear Medicine, Clinic Wiesbaden, [m]bioscientia, Ingelheim (Mainz), Germany

Indroduction

Nowadays the domain of the tumor marker tests is the survey of cancer patients in long term follow-up. For this task an adequate quality control for the tumor marker tests applied is required to reliably interpret any fluctuations of individual patients results. An unresolved problem still is the between test comparability of test results if the tumor markers are measured in different laboratories using different test kits as well as variations when using the same test kit. The present study was carried out to review the current performance of five different commercial test kits over a period of approximately one year in a 12 center international proficiency study. This is the second study following results of a first international proficiency study performed in the year 1983 which showed considerable problems of reliability.

Material and methods

The CA 19-9 reference materials were supplied by BIOREF Ltd., Mömbris, Germany. The test material consisted of human serum containing CA 19-9 from a human stomach carcinoma. Due to a special way of production the CA 19-9 antigen must not be biochemically treated and therefore is present in its native form in a physiological serum matrix so that the samples can be looked upon as patients' serum samples (2). Using this way of production the materials can be offered in large quantities of identical quality, being ideal for a long-term use reference material as stability has been confirmed in various investigations over a period of more than two years (3). The CA 19-9 was estimated using commercially available immunoassays. As listed in table I, five different test systems were applicated from the participating laboratories including RIA-methods as well as EIA-methods. A total number of 12 laboratories participated in the study. For the data of entry a pc-cream application (4) was used. The statistical analysis was performed on an AT-personal computer using SAS statistical package.

Experimental design

The reference materials were sent out unfrozen as bulk material of the same lot in three different concentration ranges (high, medium, low). Upon receipt each laboratory divided these bulk materials into aliquots and stored them frozen below –20 °C until final testing. All measurements were done in duplicates and ran along in each routine assay. The results were reported monthly together with additional information about the

Table I. List of tests.

Code	Manufacturer
1	Centocor RIA
2	CIS ELSA
3	Roche EIA
4	Boehringer ES 300/600 EIA
5	Abbott MEIA/IMX

test kit and test-batch and the date of performance to the coordinating center for data evaluation. Descriptive statistics were performed for all laboratories as well as in respect of the various kits.

Results

The current results are derived from a one year period of testing. During this time a total number of 253 assays were performed by the participating laboratories. The individual laboratory test frequencies ranged from 4 to 42 runs. Descriptive statistics were performed for all laboratories as well as in respect of the various test kits. The individual means per center calculated for the low reference sample ranged from 0.5 to 15.3 units/ml. The overall average CA 19-9 concentrations calculated from all laboratories was 10.3 units/ml (range ND to 28.3 units/ml). The corresponding average values for the medium and high reference were 25.4 units/ml and 69.0 units/ml, respectively. The individual mean ranged from 10.1 units/ml to 33.1 units/ml for the medium, and from 33.3 units/ml to 86.5 units/ml for the high CA 19-9 reference. Summaries of all statistical parameters are listed in tables II to V. To correct for between laboratory variances in frequency of tests an additional statistical approach was performed producing "weighted" parameters for average, median, range and coefficient of variation. Such weighted averages were 7.8 units/ml, 14.4 units/ml and 66.4 units/ml for the low, medium and high reference. The individual laboratory inter-assay imprecision expressed as coefficient of variation ranged from 13.3% to 62.4% for the low, from 5.9% to 33.3% for the medium, and from 4.8% to 41.1% for the high level CA 19-9-reference. The overall weighted coefficient of variations were 17.9%, 7.8% and 8.3% for the low, medium and high references respectively. Summary statistics were also performed for each of the five methods used. These between test comparability data are listed in tables 5–7. Combining data of all laboratories the test dependent averages of the low reference ranged from 2.0 units/ml to 12.6 units/ml, the test dependent coefficient of variation ranged from 0.1 to 70.0%. Corresponding averages for the medium reference ranged from 10.1 to 29.4 units/ml and from 33.3 to 84.6 units/ml for the high reference (figure 1). The coefficient of variation for the medium control ranged from 5.9% to 27.4% and from 4.8% to 41.9% for the high reference (figure 2). Some testkits were associated with batch dependent drifts. For one test, which was used in five laboratories, the average values oscillated batch dependent between 61 units/ml and 100 units/ml in the high reference control. Comparable drifts are observed in both low and medium controls. Another test exhibits similar batch dependent fluctuation. These effects are illustrated in figure 3.

Discussion

Compared with similar proficiency studies in the past (1, 4, 5, 6) a wide range of values between different laboratories became evident in all three references. The problem can be discussed exemplarily in the data for the medium reference, which is near cut-off value for the CA 19-9 test. In eight laboratories the overall average ranged from 26 U/ml to 33 U/ml derived from three different testkits manufacturer including two immunoradiometric tests (test 1, 2) and one enzymetric test (test 5). In the remaining four laboratories which used two different enzymatic test systems significant lower average concentrations for the same control material were measured. In these laboratories the average values ranged betweeen 10 U/ml and 18 U/ml. The same problems occurred in parallel for the high control serum. Thus between laboratory comparability becomes poor expressed by a between laboratory coefficient of variation of 31.2% and 27.4%, respectively, in both the medium and high control serum. These discrepancies may result from a different test calibration or may be related to interferences of the enzymatic tests with the preservative sodium azid, which was used in the reference materials. One of the fully automated test systems exhibited excellent perfomance characteristics with overall period CVs of 6% in all concentration ranges, whereas in the other fully automated test a concentration dependend precision profile was found. The CVs decreased from 25% in low control to 4.8 % in the high control. The CVs in the manual test systems ranged from 70% to 13% in the low control, from

Quality Control and Standardization 483

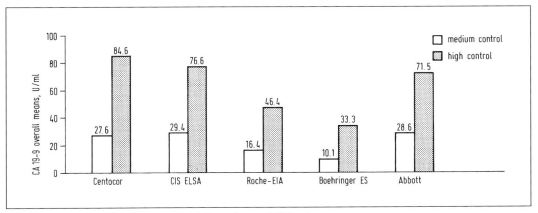

Figure 1. Between test comparability; BIOREF-medium and high references.

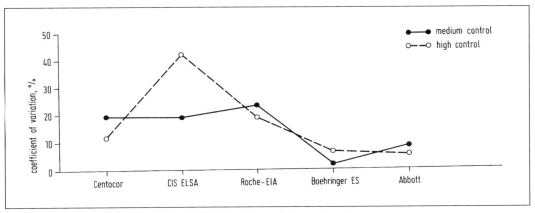

Figure 2. Test performance characterics; BIOREF-medium and high reference.

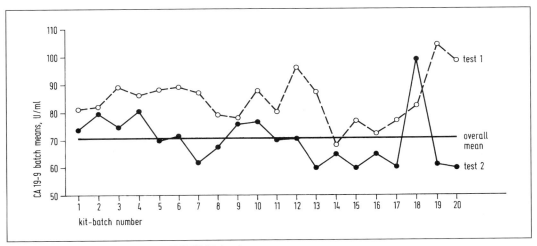

Figure 3. Batch to batch variations; BIOREF-high reference.

Table II. Descriptive statistics for each laboratory stratified by test code and overall statistics, range 1 (low).

Lab	Test#	No.	Mean	SD	VK	Max.	Med.	Min.
1	2	42	8.3	1.1	13.3	15	8.0	8.0
2	3	32	10.3	4.3	41.7	20.5	9.3	6.0
3	4	1	0.8	–	–	0.8	0.8	0.8
5	3	32	14.5	2.6	17.9	18.5	14.9	9.5
6	4	1	0.5	–	–	0.5	0.5	0.5
7	1	4	7.7	3.5	45.5	10.0	9.2	2.5
8	4	12	2.3	1.3	56.5	3.8	2.1	0.1
9	3	11	9.3	5.8	62.4	18.0	5.5	3.0
10	3	23	15.3	4.7	30.7	28.3	15.0	2.5
11	3	18	12.0	1.6	13.3	14.0	12.5	8.4
12	6	24	7.8	1.9	24.3	12.2	7.1	5.0
13	5	1	5.1	–	–	5.1	5.1	5.1
All		201	10.3	4.7	45.6	28.3	9.5	0.1
Weighted		12	7.8	1.4	17.9	28.3	9.5	0.1

Table III. Descriptive statistics for each laboratory stratified by test code and overall statistics, range 2 (medium).

Lab	Test	No.	Mean	SD	VK	Max.	Med.	Min.
1	2	42	27.6	6.5	23.6	48.0	28.0	14.0
2	3	32	26.2	6.1	23.3	38.6	24.6	15.2
3	4	20	16.1	3.2	19.9	20.8	15.3	11.7
5	3	32	33.1	6.2	18.7	44.1	34.5	22.2
6	4	11	18.0	4.5	25.5	27.6	17.3	11.0
7	1	4	32.7	5.0	15.3	39.5	32.0	27.5
8	4	24	15.9	5.3	33.3	27.0	14.0	8.5
9	3	11	25.3	6.1	24.1	33.5	23.0	17.0
10	3	23	32.9	7.2	21.9	49.8	32.8	15.2
11	3	18	26.4	3.4	12.9	31.2	26.8	19.6
12	6	24	28.6	3.5	12.2	34.8	27.8	23.5
13	5	12	10.1	0.6	5.9	11.0	10.1	9.3
All		253	25.4	8.6	33.8	49.8	26.1	8.5
Weighted		12	24.4	1.9	7.8	49.8	–	8.5

Table IV. Descriptive statistics for each laboratory stratified by test code and overall statistics, range 3 (high).

Lab	Test	No.	Mean	SD	VK	Max.	Med.	Min.
1	2	42	84.6	9.3	11.0	106.0	82.5	65.0
2	3	32	82.1	58.0	7.1	395.0	70.6	47.8
3	4	20	51.2	7.4	14.4	60.6	54.1	39.1
5	3	32	71.1	13.6	19.1	97.9	69.2	44.0
6	4	11	47.8	6.5	13.6	59.0	46.6	37.0
7	1	4	86.5	8.1	9.4	94.0	86.7	78.5
8	4	24	41.8	8.8	21.1	55.7	42.0	30.5
9	3	12	69.3	8.6	12.4	88.5	67.0	61.5
10	3	23	80.1	14.9	18.6	117.0	78.6	32.2
11	3	17	76.6	4.8	6.3	84.3	77.0	66.8
12	6	24	71.5	3.4	4.8	77.7	71.3	64.4
13	5	12	33.3	1.9	5.7	37.0	33.5	30.4
All		253	69.0	27.4	39.7	395.0	71.0	30.4
Weighted		12	66.4	5.5	8.3	395.0	–	30.4

Table V. Descriptive statistics stratified by test, range 1 (low).

Test	No.	Mean	SD	VK	Max.	Med.	Min.
1	46	8.3	1.1	13.3	15.0	8.0	2.5
2	116	12.6	4.4	34.9	28.3	13.0	2.5
3	14	2.0	1.4	70.0	3.8	2.0	0.1
4	12	5.1	0.1	0.1	5.1	5.1	5.1
5	24	7.8	2.0	25.6	12.2	7.1	5.0

Table VI. Descriptive statistics stratified by test, range 2 (medium).

Test	No.	Mean	SD	VK	Max.	Med.	Min.
1	46	27.6	6.5	23.6	48.0	28.0	14.0
2	116	29.4	6.8	23.1	49.8	29.3	15.2
3	55	16.4	4.5	27.4	27.6	16.6	8.5
4	12	10.1	0.6	5.9	11.0	10.1	9.3
5	24	28.6	3.5	12.2	34.8	27.8	23.5

Table VII. Descriptive statistics stratified by test, range 3 (high).

Test	No.	Mean	SD	VK	Max.	Med.	Min.
1	46	84.6	9.3	11.0	106.0	82.5	65.0
2	116	76.5	32.1	41.9	395.0	74.9	37.2
3	55	46.4	8.8	19.0	60.6	47.3	30.5
4	12	33.3	1.9	5.7	37.0	33.5	30.4
5	24	71.5	3.4	4.8	77.7	71.3	64.4

23% to 27% in medium and from 41% to 11% in the high control indicating poor reliability at distinct concentration levels. In one test which exhibited the poorest perfomance characteristics data considerable batch to batch drifts became evident. These batch to batch drifts were most distinct in the isotopic tests. For example the individual test results of test 2 stratified by batch oszillated between 68 U/ml and 104 U/ml in the high reference with comparable patterns also in the medium or low control (figure 3). Similar pattern could be objected in the other radiometric test (batch to bach range from 61 U/ml to 100 U/ml). This effect could only be detected using the external reference materials which were used in the study. The poor performance data in the low reference (CV 70%) of the manual enzymatic test depend to the low concentration, which was measured beyond first standard of the calibration curve of this test. Tolerable perfomance data with this test were got in the medium and high reference material. On the other hand one of the fully automated test in which the low control was also measured below the lowest standard of the calibration curve had an excellent performance characteristics.

Conclusion

The study showed, that aside from other checks of routinely used immunoassay runs, e.g. tracer binding, calibration curves, an adequate quality assurance including a kit manufacturer independent control materials of human matrix is an important factor in the quality control of tumor marker tests. Due to the discrepancies of the between test comparabilities such external reference materials with biochemically untreated antigens can be used as internal standards to correct for high batch to batch drifts. In addition, drifts of the baseline in individual patient's follow-up e.g. switching over from other test kits can be detected better. Thus the interpretation of long-term tumor marker courses becomes more accurate.

References

1. Risse TH, Wolf S (1992) Einsatz von PC-CREAM im Krankenhaus – ein Werkzeug für Medizinsche Dokumentation, Berichtswesen und klinische Studien. In: Rathgeber A, Fleischer S, Prote U (Hrsg) Einsatzmöglichkeiten medizinischer Dokumentation. 3. Fachtagung des Deutschen Verbands Medizinischer Dokumentare, Hannover, pwd Verlag, pp 130–139
2. Patentschrift Bioref de 39 37 660 C2 (1994)
3. Zwirner M, Staab HJ, Brümmendorf T, Schindler AE (1985) Proficiency studies with tumor marker tests: Results of multicentric investigations. Tumor Biology 6:420–422
4. Zwirner M, Bieglmayer CH, Kreienberg R, Klapdor R, Lüthgens M (1987) Ergebnisse einer internationalen Ringstudie zur Qualitätssicherung des tumorassoziierten antigens CA 125 Tumor Diagn Ther 8:150–156
5. Zwirner M, Bieglmayer CH, De Bruijn HW, Crombach G, Ebert G, Kreienberg R, Kißing F, Lietmann W, Schmid L, Schindler AE, Sturm G, Wieser N, Wiebecke K, Würz H (†) (1990) Results of an international proficiency study with the SCC tumor marker. In: Klapdor R (ed) Recent results in tumor diagnosis and therapy. Zuckschwerdt, München, pp 285–289
6. Zwirner M (1992) Longitudinal quality control of tumor marker assays: Results of an international proficiency study with CEA. In: Klapdor R (ed) Tumor associated antigens, oncogens, receptors, cytokines in tumor diagnosis and therapy at the beginning of the nineties. Zuckschwerdt, München pp 283–289

Address for correspondence:
Dr. med. M. Zwirner
Abteilung für Geburtshilfe und Gynäkologie
Universitätsfrauenklinik
Schleichstraße 4
D-72076 Tübingen, Germany

Quality control and standardization of tumor marker tests in Finland

C. Haglund

Fourth Department of Surgery, Helsinki University Central Hospital, Helsinki, Finland

In 1993, tumor marker tests were performed in about 25 laboratories in Finland. The laboratories are recommended to take part in external interlaboratory quality assessment programs, but there are no obligations to participate in quality control programs, and there are no national quality control standards. Each laboratory is responsible for its own internal and external quality control.

In Finland, tumor marker tests are performed almost exclusively using commercially available kits. In addition to kit controls, most laboratories use commercially available quality control sera, e.g. Lymphochek Tumor Marker Control® (Bio-Rad Laboratories, California), to monitor the accuracy and precision of tumor marker tests. A few laboratories use internal control sera of their own.

Most Finnish laboratories performing tumor marker tests take part in the Murex Diagnostics Immunoassay Quality Assessment Programme. The results of the control samples are reported to Murex Diagnostics Limited® (Dartford, England) every second week. The laboratories attending the program get reports on the results every six months.

In 1992, 21 laboratories, i.e. practically all laboratories performing tumor marker tests, attended a tumor marker test program by Labquality®, a Finnish company specialized on quality control programs for clinical laboratories. The next test round by Labquality® will be performed in 1994.

In Finland, like in many countries, a large number of different assay kits by various manufacturers are used for individual tumor markers. According to the report of Labquality®, the carcinoembryonic antigen (CEA) concentration was measured by seven different kits, CA 19-9 by three, CA 125 by five, alpha-fetoprotein (AFP) by three, human chorionic gonadotrophin (HCG) by five and prostate specific antigen (PSA) by five kits. In some cases there was a considerable difference between the results of different kits.

In conclusion, Finnish laboratories quite well take care of their internal and external quality control of tumor marker tests. Still, national and international quality control stipulations and standards would be needed.

Address for correspondence:
C. Haglund, M.D.
Fourth Department of Surgery
Helsinki University Central Hospital
Kasarmikatu 11-13
SF-00130 Helsinki, Finland

Tumor markers: Quality control and standardization in Italy

G.C. Zucchelli[a], A. Pilo[a], R. Cohen[b], A. Cianetti[c], G.C. Torre[d]

[a]Istituto di Fisiologia Clinica, CNR, Pisa, Italy;
[b]Service de Radiopharmacie et Radioanalyse, Université de Lyon, France;
[c]Laboratorio Centrale, Ospedale S. Camillo, Roma, Italy;
[d]Divisione Ostetricia e Ginecologia, Ospedale S. Corona, Pietra Ligure, Italy

Introduction

In recent years, an increasing number of clinical laboratories, which routinely carry out immunoassay for tumor markers, participate in external quality assessment (EQA) schemes organized by various agency. It is well accepted, in fact, that participating in EQA programs contributes to the improvement of the analytical performance of the laboratories involved through the comparison of their results with those produced by others; moreover, by assessing the periodic EQA reports, laboratories obtain useful information on the reliability of the method/kits used in the survey. Update of the performance of the methods, which is easily and reliably obtained from the large amount of data collected during the EQA is a major tool for improving the quality of the assays: the laboratories gain some quantitative basis for choosing among the commercially available kits and the manufacturers are prompted to provide more reliable products.

With these aims we organized an external quality assessment program for tumor markers immunoassay (1–6). The scheme, sponsored by National Research Council (CNR), is in operation for CEA and AFP since 1984, and for CA 19-9, CA 125 and CA 15-3 since 1989. Starting from December 1991 the CNR EQA program joined with Service de Radiopharmacie et Radioanalyse, Université de Lyon (France) to carry out the international EQA program "Oncocheck" for tumor markers. At present time, Oncocheck includes AFP, CEA, CA 19-9, CA 15-3, CA 125 and PSA and involves more than 250 European laboratories.

The main results collected during the last cycles of this EQA scheme are reported in this paper.

Outline of the EQA scheme

The survey for tumor markers does not substantially differ from other EQAs (7–9); participants are supplied with the control material (24 samples every year) and are asked to perform the assay routinely and to return results indicating the method/kit used. The samples (freeze-dried) are prepared from human sera of normals added with sera of patients containing high concentration of the analytes.

The collected results are computer processed and a periodic report containing statistics for each quality control sample are printed and sent back to the laboratories; all data accumulated during a EQA cycle are used to prepare an "end-of-period" or cumulative report. The aim of the periodic report is to allow the comparison between the result of the laboratory on a single EQA sample, with those produced by all the other participants and in particular by the users of the same method/kit. The aim of the cumulative report is to provide the participant with an estimate of the average bias (accuracy) and the average precision achieved in assaying all the samples despatched in the control cycle. In addition, the report contains estimates of the analytical performance of the kits more widely used in the survey based on data accumulated in the whole cycle.

Results and comments

Figure 1 depicts the trends of the total variability (also refered as between-laboratory agreement and estimate as average CV of all control samples assay in a EQA cycle) over time for CEA and AFP

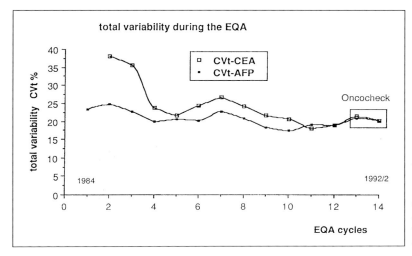

Figure 1. Total variability (CVt, also refered as between-laboratory agreement) of CEA and AFP assays observed in the cycles of EQA carried out since 1984.

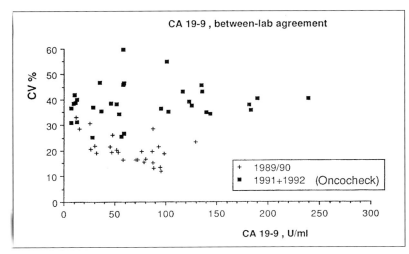

Figure 2. EQA of CA 19-9: Variability observed in the control samples sent in the 1989–1990 cycle (cross) and in the control samples assayed from the second half of 1991 (closed squares); a significant worsening of the between-laboratory agreement in these last EQA samples is evident.

assays; the last two cycles refer to Oncocheck program. The variability of AFP assay slightly decreased from 25% to 18–20%. In the case of CEA we observed a marked decrease of the variability from 1987 on: this improvement is mainly attributable to a better alignment of the calibrators supplied with the different kits in respect to the international reference standard (WHO preparation 73/601) (10). In the last cycles also CEA assay achieved a total variability of about 20%. Worth noting, however, that in CEA assay the between-kit differences still play an important role, in respect to AFP, in determining the total variability.

The total variability (or between-lab agreement) of CA 19-9 observed during the EQA, is reported in figure 2. We found a CV of about 20% for the control samples distributed during 1989 and 1990, successively (from the second half of 1991) we observed a consistent worsening of the variability (CV 25–50%). This wider dispersion is mainly attributable to systematic between-kit differences, as demonstrated by the break-down of the variability into its components by ANOVA (11): the between-kit component accounted for 53% of the total variability in the last EQA period but only 20% in the 1989–1990 cycle.

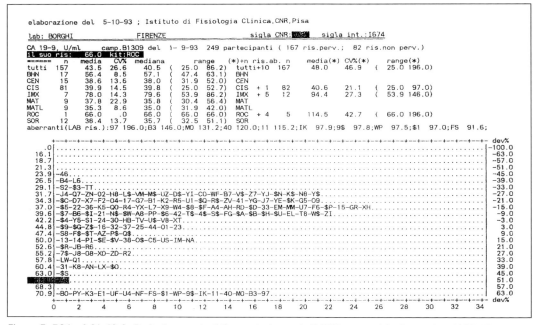

Figure 3. EQA of CA 19-9: Periodic report of the control sample B1309 assayed in September 1993. The report contains all results (identified by the laboratory code) collected for the sample together with the main statistical variables both of all data and of data grouped according to kits (identified by the kit codes). The report prepared for the participant coded A3 (I674) also contains the result obtained by the laboratory and the method/kit used.
Kit codes: BHN = Enzymun Test Boehringer Mannheim; CEN = IRMA Centocor; CIS = IRMA CIS; IMX = IMX Abbott; MAT = IRMA Byk-Sangtec; MATL = LIA-mat Byk-Sangtec; ROC = IEMA Roche; SOR = IRMA Sorin.

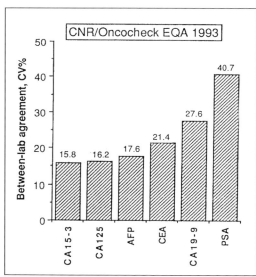

Figure 4. Mean between-laboratory agreement exibited by the six tumor markers (CEA, AFP, CA 19-9, CA 15-3, CA 125, PSA) during the 1993 cycle of Oncocheck EQA program.

The report of CA 19-9 results of a control sample distributed during the Oncocheck program (September 1993) is shown, as an example, in figure 3. In this sample, the users of IRMA Centocor, IRMA Cis, IRMA Byk-Sangtec and IRMA Sorin found very similar values (mean values ranging from 37.8 to 39.9 U/ml), while the users of the new non-radioactive immunoassays Enzymun Test Boehringer, IMx Abbott and IEMA Roche obtained results (from 56.4 to 115 U/ml) different from each others and remarkably higher than those produced by IRMAs; values reported by the users of the luminescent technique Byk-Gulden are close to IRMAs.

The increasing use in the survey of the new techniques represents the major cause of the sudden worsening of the between-lab agreement of CA 19-9 determinations (12).

The reasons for these discrepancies are unclear at present time; it is, however, conceivable that different methods/kits for CA 19-9, even if based on the same monoclonal antibody (1116-NS 19-9, from Centocor) and the same antigen for standard preparation (also from Centocor), show a different degree of specificity against the CA 19-9 determinant due to differences in the tracer and in the solid-phase preparation and/or in the experimental assay conditions (pH, time and temperature of the antigen/antibody reaction). In addition the presence in serum of different molecular forms of CA 19-9 which may be differently recognized by the method/kits can contribute to the discrepancies observed.

Figure 4 reports the mean between-laboratory agreement observed in the 1993 cycle of the CNR/Oncocheck program. It can be seen that CA 15-3 and CA 125 assays exhibit a total variability (CA 15-3 = 15.8 CV%; CA 125 = 16.2 CV%) comparable or better than that achieved by CEA and AFP (21.4 and 17.6 CV% respectively). The between-laboratory variabilities of CA 19-9 and PSA were found to be remarkably higher (27.6 and 40.7CV% respectively).

The large dispersion of PSA results is mainly attributable to systematic between-kit differences due to the use of local kit standards calibrated versus different preparations. It is therefore advisable that either the kit producers refer their kits to the same calibrators or, at least, indicate the conversion factors against a common standard. This would certainly produce a consistent decrease of the total variability as previously observed for CEA assay.

Conclusions

The performance achieved for CEA, AFP, CA 125 and CA 15-3 are satisfactory and not different from that observed, in the EQA of proteic hormones.

Concerning the results reported for CA 19-9 and PSA, we observed a higher between-laboratory variability due to larger systematic between-kit differences. In particular for CA 19-9, the new non-isotopic methods produce results generally higher than those found by traditional IRMAs; for PSA assay the use of different local kit standards is responsible of the large variability observed.

References

1. Pilo A, Zucchelli GC, Masini S, Torre GC, Ballesta AM (1990) Progress report on an external quality assessment program for immunoassays of tumor markers. J Nucl Med All Sci 34 (suppl):75–82
2. Zucchelli GC, Pilo A, Chiesa MR, Masini S, Prontera C, Cianetti A (1993) The CNR External Quality Assessment program for tumor markers. In: Up dating on tumor markers in tissues and in biological fluids. Edizioni Minerva Medica, Torino, pp 129–140
3. Pilo A, Zucchelli GC, Chiesa MR, Masini S, Ferdeghini M (1987) Anomalous between-laboratory variability in a collaborative study of CEA immunoassay. Clin Chem 33:1694–169
4. Albertini A, Zucchelli GC, Pilo A, Bolelli GF, Signorini C, Malvano R (1985) The quality of RIA in Italy as observed trough an interlaboratory survey. J Clin Immunoassay 8:117–124
5. Zucchelli GC, Pilo A, Ferdeghini M, Chiesa MR, Masini S, Clerico A (1989) External quality control survey for AFP assay. J Nucl Med All Sci 33:30–34
6. Zucchelli GC, Pilo A, Malvano R, Signorini C, Bolelli GF, Albertini A (1991) External quality assessment of the assays for hormones and tumor markers in Italian laboratories. Ann Ist Super Sanità 27:479–486
7. Seth J, Sturgeon CM, Al Sadie R, Hanning I, Ellis AR (1991) External quality assessment of immunoassay of peptide hormones and tumor markers: principles and practice. Ann Ist Super Sanità 27:443–452
8. Sufi SB, Goncharov N (1984) Standardization of radioimmunoassays for use in WHO collaborative studies. In: Albertini A, Ekins RP, Galen RS (eds) Cost/benefit and predictive value of radioimmunoassay. Elsevier, Amsterdam, pp 39–48
9. Cohen R, Bizollon Ch A (1991) Immunoassay external quality assessment schemes in France. Ann Ist Super Sanità 27:503–510
10. Zucchelli GC, Pilo A, Chiesa MR, Masini S, Baccini C (1986) Minimizing between-kit variability in immunoassay of CEA by use of a common standard. Clin Chem 32:1942–1944
11. Pilo A, Zucchelli GC, Chiesa MR, Bolelli GF, Albertini A (1986) Components of variance analysis of data produced in a national quality control survey of radioimmunoassay of T3,T4, TSH, prolactin and progesterone. Clin Chem 32:171–175
12. Zucchelli GC, Pilo A, Chiesa MR, Cohen R, Bizollon CA (1993) Growing use of nonisotopic CA 19-9 immunoassays increases between-laboratory variability. Clin Chem 39:909–911

Address for correspondence:
Dr. G. C. Zucchelli
Istituto di Fisiologia
Clinica del CNR
Via Savi, 8
I-56100 Pisa, Italy

Tumor marker determinations: How should they be reported?

L. N Fischer
Sangtec Medical, Bromma, Sweden

Quality in clinical determinations is quality in a long sequence of steps: sampling and sample handling, transport of the sample to the laboratory, manufacture of reagents, transport of reagents to the laboratory, the performance of the assay in the laboratory, the data reduction, the report of the results and the action of the physician on the basis of the results. When quality is discussed, the interest is, however, mostly focused on the performance of the assay in the laboratory. It must, however, be kept in mind that this is only one step, and it is usually the step in the sequence introducing least loss of quality. In a previous communication (1), the earlier steps in this sequence were discussed, and in this communication the last step will therefore be scrutinized. The report is the basis for the clinicians' treatment of the patient. Just to report the serum concentration is therefore not adequate, particularly in a situation where many laboratory parameters are involved.

A first step is to include in the report also previous values from the same patient, so that the development can be followed. Particularly if the samples have been taken with short time intervals, such diagrams are very informative. If several parameters are included, it may take time to analyze them, and the treating physician with a very heavy work load therefore may miss important informations. One attempt to overcome this is to calculate an index of the relevant marker values, based on their relative importance for the clinical situation. Some attempts have been made to develop such indices. The relative weights of the marker values (and of other clinical information available) should be derived by multivariate analysis or some related statistical method (for instance neural networks)[1].

With the aid of such statistical methods, it would also be possible to make an evaluation of the time sequences of markers, and to include not only the marker values but also their development with time (trend analysis) in the calculations. This would make it possible to calculate the probability for given clinically relevant questions quantitatively, such as the probability of disease dissemination, the prognosis or the probability of the patient responding to a given treatment.

The report should therefore ideally include the relevant conclusions about the patient. This is only possible if very large clinical studies with the relevant parameters have been performed and evaluated in such a way that the probability for the relevant clinical distinction is given. Modern statistical methods, including multivariate analysis and its refinement neural network are capable of analyzing the large amount of data to yield as much information as possible. This can be made available to the physician by an expert system. Only if the probability for a given condition (for instance metastatic spread) is given numerically from a well validated program it will be possible to make medical decisions rationally (4) on the basis of tumor markers, and possibly to replace more expensive and invasive diagnostic methods.

---

[1]Multivariate analysis, factor analysis, cluster analysis are old statistical techniques, described in all basic text-books on biostatistics. – Neural networks were developed as a branch in "Artificial Intelligence". Neural networks that can be used practically in biostatistics, in practice statistical techniques related to multivariate analysis are now available commercially for personal computers.

The large clinical studies required and their statistical evaluation should not be left entirely to one interested party, for instance a manufacturer or a reference laboratory, as this will create a suspicion that the system may be biased. Therefore an independent body must administer this development. An international committee should be responsible for the administration of the project, giving specialized institutes the task of running the clinical investigations for a given localization, or even for a given clinical question. Only by such an approach it will be possible to make comparative data for the fairly large number of potentially interesting markers available for the large number of samples form normal subjects, patients with benign conditions and malignancies in different stages.

Considering the economic crisis that medicine is experiencing in many countries, even relatively inexpensive diagnostic techniques, such as tumor marker determinations, must demonstrate their efficacy and clinical and economic value to remain on the agenda. It is therefore very urgent that a program of this kind is carried out, to prove the value of markers, and to make them more useful in the management of cancer patients.

References

1. Fischer L (1993) Quality in tumor marker assay: what is important for the physicians judgement of the patient. 10th International conference on human tumor markers. Bonn, Sept 8–11
2. Lahousen M, Stettner H, Pürstner P (1989) A tumour marker combination versus second look surgery in ovarian cancer. I. Clinical experience. Ballières Clin Obstet Gynaecol 31:201–208
3. Lahousen M, Stettner, H, Pickel H, Urdl W, Pürstner P (1987) The predictive value of a combination of tumour markers in monitoring patients with ovarial cancer. Cancer 60:2228–2232
4. Sox HC, Blatt MA, Higgins MC, Marton KI (1988) Medical decision making. Butterworth, Boston, p406

Address for correspondence:
Dr. L. N. Fischer
AB Sangtec Medical
Box 20045
S-16102 Bromma, Sweden

Quality control in immunohistology: Evaluation of the interpretation instead of technique and reagents

M. Nap, W. W. Wilhelm
Institute of Public Health, Department of Pathology, Leeuwarden, Friesland,
SIG, Institute for Healthcare Informatics, Utrecht, The Netherlands

Introduction

Quality and quantity are related to each other in a complex way. If either of them runs out of control, the consequences for the other follow shortly thereafter. Mostly a quantitative overload has a negative effect on the quality of the product that is generated. However, if there is too little quantity, the quality will also be difficult to maintain. Since an equilibrium between all the factors that play a role often does not occur spontaneously, control procedures to warrant the quality of the product have been developed at all levels of industry but also in healthcare. In the determination of tumor markers, both in blood and tissues, combined groups of technicians, clinicians, industrials and scientists collaborate in various forms to achieve and maintain good quality. The control of quality is often directed towards reagents and the performance of tests compared to control samples with known expression of the antigen(s).

We think, quality control in immunohistology (I.H.) lacks the aspect of interpretation of a given staining result by the pathologist in relation to the final diagnosis. Because we were interested in the possible relationship between staining results of multiple antigens, either alone or in combination, and the final diagnosis, we started some years ago to collect data and investigated how quality of this combined product of staining and interpretation could be monitored, but also what approaches could be made to learn about patterns of staining.

Materials and methods

Data from routine I.H. have been collected systematically in a database application in a personal computer since 1989. This database was linked with the administrative database PALGA, which contains the full histology reports of the department including the final diagnosis in terms that follow the SNOP terminology. SNOP stands for systematic nomenclature of pathology and the terms correspond to codes build up out of one alphabetic character followed by four digits. Each diagnosis must contain at least a topographical term, a functional term and a morphological term. This combination indicates the site of the body involved, the way the sample was obtained and the disorder. The Dutch abbreviation PALGA stands for National pathology database. All institutes of pathology in the Netherlands send their daily production results by data communication to the central computer in Amsterdam. Here translation of semantical terms into SNOP codes, and more recently into SNOMED codes, takes place. Also maintenance of the thesaurus, containing all authorized terms, takes place. Based on the encoded diagnosis from the central computer we have carried out the analysis.

Before the actual analysis, we have applied some form of datareduction by grouping both diagnosis and markers in hierarchical levels. For the markers this resulted roughly in epithelial (EP), mesenchymal (ME) and lymphoid (LY) groups. Within these groups further specifications can be made, down to the individual marker. Apart from grouping markers with common characteristics, it is also possible to define combinations of positive or negative staining results of markers from different groups as new tests and analyse their contribution to diagnosis.

Figure 1 illustrates the hierarchical ranking of the diagnosis down to the level of individual SNOP or SNOMED codes. We decided to use the sensitivity and specificity of test results, either positive or

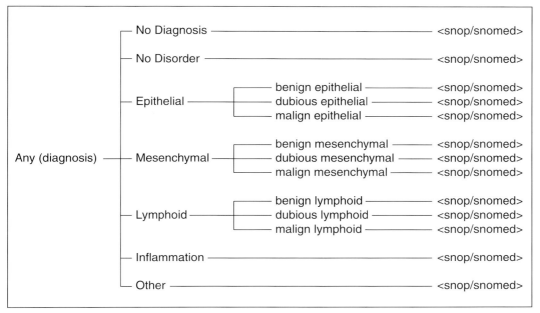

Figure 1. Hierarchical concept arrangement. In this figure the hierarchical ranking of the various diagnostic classes is shown as a tree like structure.

negative, to learn about the relation between diagnosis and tests. In the period from 1989 until 1992 that was analysed, we collected approximately 1600 cases where tumor markers had been applied in I.H. Using a simple 2*2 matrix sensitivity and specificity can be calculated as well as the prevalence of the diagnosis within the test group and the level of positive results in this group, Q-level (1) that could be reached. Furthermore the size of the data set in combination with the datareduction allowed us to split the data set in four years and compare the variations of the items mentioned above over the years. For visualisation of the data we displayed the test points with coordinates of sensitivity and specificity in graphs in relation to the prevalence and Q-level. The graph in figure 2 illustrates how the different items can be read.

Results

From the analysis of our data at the level of epithelial, mesenchymal and lymphoid malignant tumors it becomes evident that the test points, defined by the sensitivity and specificity of the different markers can be used to illustrate the variations in time. In figure 2 this is visualised for malignant epithelial tumors, stained in the years 1989 until 1993. The prevalence of this subgroup varied from 0.39 to 0.49 (mean 0.45) within the test group. In 1989 the sensitivity and specificity of a positive reaction for an epithelial marker in this group were 0.80 and 0.69 respectively. For the positive reactions of lymphoid or mesenchymal markers in this subgroup the values were low. However, if we use the reversed values, which means that we consider the presence of a negative stain as a positive observation, we reached 0.93 and 0.71 for the lymphoid markers and 0.83 and 0.72 for mesenchymal markers. If a combination of a positive epithelial marker (E P) with a negative lymphoid marker (L N) and a negative mesenchymal marker (M N) is defined as a separate test, this test is positive if the condition is fulfilled and negative if not. The sensitivity of this specific example becomes 0.67 with 100% specificity.

Table I shows how these values can change over the years for the various test combinations. If we look at this combination in the following years, the values of sensitivity show a slight increase with

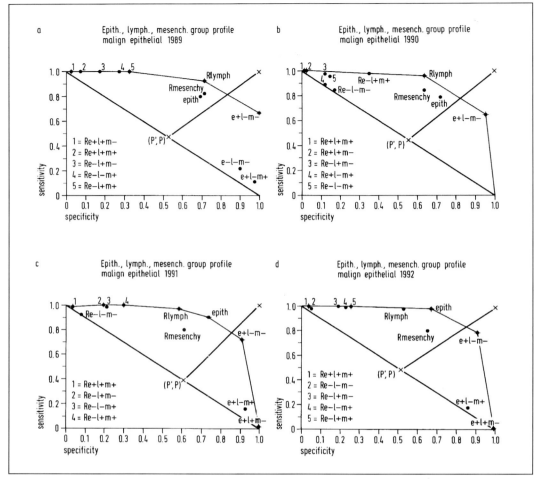

Figure 2. Graphic representation of sensitivity and specificity. The diagonal represents the line on which random testpoints can be found. If this occurs the test result does not contribute to the diagnosis and could evenly well have been reached by tossing a coin. Reading the graphs it is important to note the variation in distance of the test points to the random line and the line of diagnosis. Throughout the years the points in the graphs a, b, c and d with the same names obtain slightly different positions. The extend of these alterations gives a visual impression of the quality of interpretation from one year to another.

0.12 and the specificity comes down from 1 to 0.91. In the malignant mesenchymal tumors there is a 10% variation in sensitivity for a positive mesenchymal marker whereas the specificity only varies between 0.59 and 0.64. The reversed values of epithelial and lymphoid markers showed similar variations in time. The combined test of E N; L N; M P started with a very high sensitivity in 1989 and a good specificity but in the second year of registration the sensitivity of this combination dropped to 0.45 and did not increase above 0.50. The specificity of this combination remained constant around 0.90. For lymphoid malignant tumors it is remarkable how close the positive staining for lymphoid markers and the reversed value of a negative epithelial marker approach each other. Sensitivities of positive lymphoid markers were constantly 10% lower during three years but in 1992 they both were calculated at 0.91. Specificity of a positive lymphoid marker remained constantly 10% above that of the reversed epithelial data. The values for

Table I. Marker group results. This table shows the values of prevalence (P), Q-level, sensitivity and specificity of the various combinations of marker results as they were calculated for the malignant epithelial tumors. The names of the tests, marker combinations, are build up out of epithelial (E) mesenchymal (M), and lymphoid (L), each in combination with either a P for positive or an N for negative results. If the first digit is an R, this means that we have used the reversed value of the test.

Malignant epithelial 1989

	P	Q	Sen	Spec
REPLPMN	0.47	0.99	1.00	0.03
REPLPMP	0.47	0.96	1.00	0.08
RENLPMN	0.47	0.91	1.00	0.18
RENLNMP	0.47	0.86	1.00	0.28
RENLPMP	0.47	0.83	1.00	0.33
Epith	0.47	0.54	0.80	0.69
RLymph	0.47	0.59	0.93	0.71
RMesench	0.47	0.54	0.83	0.72
ENLNMN	0.47	0.16	0.22	0.90
EPLNMP	0.47	0.07	0.11	0.98
EPLNMN	0.47	0.32	0.67	1.00

Malignant epithelial 1991

	P	Q	Sen	Spec
REPLPMP	0.39	0.97	0.99	0.04
RENLNMN	0.39	0.92	0.92	0.08
RENLPMN	0.39	0.88	1.00	0.20
RENLNMP	0.39	0.86	0.99	0.21
RENLPMP	0.39	0.82	1.00	0.30
RLymph	0.39	0.63	0.97	0.59
RMesench	0.39	0.55	0.80	0.61
Epith	0.39	0.51	0.91	0.74
EPLNMN	0.39	0.34	0.72	0.91
EPLNMP	0.39	0.11	0.16	0.93
EPLPMN	0.39	0.01	0.01	1.00

Malignant epithelial 1990

	P	Q	Sen	Spec
REPLPMP	0.45	0.99	1.00	0.01
REPLPMN	0.45	0.99	1.00	0.02
RENLPMN	0.45	0.92	0.98	0.12
REPLNMP	0.45	0.88	0.89	0.12
RENLNMP	0.45	0.90	0.96	0.15
RENLNMN	0.45	0.84	0.85	0.17
RENLPMP	0.45	0.79	0.98	0.35
RMesench	0.45	0.58	0.85	0.64
RLymph	0.45	0.63	0.96	0.64
Epith	0.45	0.51	0.79	0.72
EPLNMN	0.45	0.32	0.65	0.95

Malignant epithelial 1992

	P	Q	Sen	Spec
REPLPMP	0.49	0.98	1.00	0.04
RENLNMN	0.49	0.97	0.98	0.05
RENLPMN	0.49	0.90	1.00	0.20
RENLNMP	0.49	0.88	0.99	0.23
RENLPMP	0.49	0.87	1.00	0.25
RLymph	0.49	0.72	0.98	0.53
RMesench	0.49	0.57	0.80	0.65
Epith	0.49	0.65	0.98	0.67
EPLNMP	0.49	0.16	0.18	0.86
EPLNMN	0.49	0.43	0.79	0.91
EPLPMN	0.49	0.01	0.01	0.99

the various combinations of marker group results can be seen in table I. In this table the column with Q-values shows the percentage of positive tests for any marker in one of the subgroups. Q may vary between zero and 1, and represents the quotient of the true positives plus false positives and the total number of tested specimens. As an example we can see that the Q-level for a positive epithelial marker in malignant epithelial tumors was more or less constant in the first three years but in the last year it changed from 0.50 to 0.65.

Discussion

From what is shown above it should be clear that this approach has to be seen as an additional aspect of quality control in I.H. If the basic principles of quality control at the level of reagents, tissue preservation and immunohistochemical techniques are not fulfilled, then the analyses of the aspects aimed at in this paper are without meaning.

In the literature on QC in I.H. over the last ten years most papers deal with the basic principles. Some are especially directed to the comparison of steroid receptor status of breastcarcinoma determined by I.H. or biochemical assay (2, 3). Others deal with external QC in a broader sense (4, 5, 6, 7, 8). In the present approach the individual pathologist is offered a mirror in which he can see whether his interpretation of the same observations leads to a constant pattern. At this level it is not important what the exact values of sensitivity and specificity of a given marker result for a diagnosis will be, but the variation in time is an indication of the reproducibility of the decision.

On the other hand the exact data on sensitivity and specificity from the analysis of these marker results give insight into their mutual relation and contribution in the process of diagnosis.

Not only the sensitivity and specificity deserve attention but also the Q-value of a test. The change in Q-level for instance, gives insight in the composition of the test group. In the situation described in the last part of results, the change in Q-level, in combination with a constant prevalence, an increased sensitivity and a slightly decreased specificity, may be the effect of both decreased true negatives and increased true positives. The point with the x; y coordinates (1-Q); Q, is a point at the random line, the line that connects the maximum sensitivity with maximum specificity as a diagonal in the graphs in figure 2. If the Q-level equals the sensitivity, the test point falls on this line. If Q is smaller than sensitivity the distance between the random line and test point increases. The position of the test point will than shift upwards and to the right where the ideal situation of 100% specificity and sensitivity is waiting.

Another important point at this line is the point (1-P); P which represents the prevalence of the diagnosis of interest within the test population. The line between this point and the right upper corner is called the line of diagnosis. It appears that tests with the same Q-level have test points in the graph with the same distance to this line of diagnosis. In this way there will be a line through all points with the same Q-level, parallel to the line of diagnosis. A test carrying the same Q-level as P-value will show a test point that falls exactly on the line of diagnosis. The difference between sensitivity and Q-level will than determine the position towards the hypothetical maximum. A difference in Q-level between tests will influence the distance between a test point and the line of diagnosis and by that inform the user about the weigth of the test points in relation to each other and the diagnosis.

Conclusions

Using this approach it becomes possible to formulate and analyse concepts at different hierarchical levels of diagnosis and markers, from rough data collections until very detailed described cases. A tool has become available for QC at the level of interpretation by the person who is responsible for the final diagnosis. In addition to this, validation of the data takes place that makes it possible to use the outcome of the analysis to build a knowledge domain that can be used in decision support systems.

References

1 Kraemer HC (1992) Evaluating medical tests. SAGE publications, Newbury Park, London, New Delhi
2 Chapman JA, Mobbs BG, Hanna WM, Sawka CA, Pritchard KI, Lickley HL, Trudeau ME, Ryan ED, Ooi TC, Sutherland DJ et al (1993) The standardization of estrogen receptors. J Steroid Biochem Mol Biol 45 (5):367–373
3 Vermousek I, Szamel I, Goerlich M, Brdar B, Cvtila D, Graf D, Padovan R, Paszko Z, Safarcik K (1992) Quality control program of steroid receptor assays: an international study. Neoplasma 39:65–69
4 Elias JM, Gown AM, Nakamura RM, Wilbur DC, Herman GE, Jaffe ES, Battifora H, Brigatti DJ (1989) Quality control in immunohistochemistry. Report of a workshop sponsored by the biological stain commission. Am J Clin Pathol 92:836–843
5 Reynolds GJ (1989) External quality assurance and assessment in immunocytochemistry. Histopathol 15:627–633
6 Rickert RR, Maliniak RM (1989) Intralaboratory quality assurance of immunohistochemical procedures. Recommended practices for daily application. Arch Pathol Lab Med 113:673–679
7 Sheibani K, Tubbs RR (1984) Enzyme immunohistochemistry: technical aspects. Semin Diagn Pathol 1 235–250
8 Battifora H (1986) The multitumor (sausage) tissue-block: novel method for immunohistochemical antibody testing. Lab Invest 55:244–248

Address for correspondence:
Dr. M. Nap
Institute of Public Health
Department of Pathology
Jelsumerstraat 6
NL-8917 En Leeuwarden, The Netherlands

Oncogenes – Receptors – Cytokines

Serum levels of a c-*erb*B-2 oncogene product in ovarian cancer patients

H. Meden[a], D. Marx[b], A. Fattahi[a], W. Rath[a], M. Krohn[c], W. Wuttke[a], A. Schauer[b], W. Kuhn[a]

[a]Department of Obstetrics and Gynecology, [b]Department of Pathology,
[c]Department of Medical Statistics, University of Göttingen, Germany

Introduction

Amplification of the c-*erb*B-2 oncogene has been reported to be a prognostic factor in ovarian cancer (1, 9, 10, 12, 13, 17).

The human neu oncogene encodes a glycoprotein of 185 000 D (p185) which is closely related to, but distinct from, human epidermal growth factor receptor (EGFR). Several groups have reported that it is possible to detect this oncoprotein fragment in sera from a subset of breast cancer patients (3, 5, 7, 8, 19).

The present study was conducted to determine whether the p185 oncoprotein fragment can be detected in sera from ovarian cancer patients. We further examined the relationship between p185 oncoprotein fragment serum levels and immunohistochemical p185 findings in ovarian cancer tissue samples. In addition, we analysed serum samples from a healthy control group.

Patients and methods

Ovarian cancer patients

Material for the present study was obtained from 57 ovarian cancer patients admitted to the Department of Obstetrics and Gynecology, University of Göttingen. These patients underwent exploratory laparotomy and surgical treatment between 1989 and 1992. All serum samples were taken before initial surgery, all histological material was obtained at initial surgery and reviewed by a single pathologist (A.S.) using the WHO criteria (16) for the histological type. The histological grade was determined according to the Broders classification (2).

Control group

Reference values were based on the sera of 80 healthy women who attended our out-patient clinic for routine examinations.

Serum determination of the p185 oncoprotein fragment

All serum samples were divided into aliquots and frozen at −70° Celsius. The amount of c-*erb*B-2 oncoprotein fragment was quantified by ELISA using the Human neu Oncoprotein ELISA kit (Oncogene Science, provided by Dianova, Hamburg). All measurements are means of duplicate determinations.

Immunohistochemistry

Sections (1–2 μm) from formalin-fixed, paraffin-embedded tumor tissue were air-dried over night at 37° Celsius. C-*erb*B-2 overexpression was determined using a monoclonal antibody directed against the extracellular domain of p185 protein and a polyclonal antibody directed against the kinase domain (9G6 and c-neu, Oncogene Science, Dianova Hamburg). Immune complexes were detected using the avidin-biotin-peroxidase technique (6, 14, 18).

Results

Ovarian cancer patients

Among the 57 patients with ovarian cancer, 22 patients had serous tumors, 13 patients had mucinous tumors, 12 patients had undifferentiated tumors, and 9 patients had endometroid tumors. There was one Brenner tumor, one granulosa cell tumor and one yolc sac tumor. The histological grade of these tumors was: G1 (n = 3), G2 (n = 16), G3 (n = 22), G4 (n = 28). Tumor stages (FIGO): stage I (n = 8), stage II (n = 10), stage III (n = 29), stage IV (n = 10). Eight of these 57 cases (14%) were found to be immunohistochemically positive for the c-erbB-2 encoded protein p185.

The ovarian cancer patients' serum values ranged from 526 to 16 332 HNU/ml. In the sera from the 49 cancer patients without overexpression the values were distributed in the range of 526 to 2 892 HNU/ml (mean 1 120 HNU/ml, standard deviation (SD) 411 HNU/ml). The oncoprotein fragment levels in the sera from the eight patients with overexpression in their tumors ranged from 878 to 16 332 HNU/ml (mean 3 384 HNU/ml, S.D. 5 247 HNU/ml). Four individuals in this group showed serum levels within the normal range, the other four showed elevated levels (1 802, 1 914, 2 110 and 16 332 HNU/ml). The highest level was found in a patient with both ovarian and simultaneously diagnosed endometrial cancer. The histological specimens of both malignancies showed intensive staining for immuno histochemically detectable c-erbB-2 encoded protein. Two of the 49 patients without overexpression in their tumor showed increased serum levels of p185 oncoprotein fragment. There was no association between serum oncoprotein fragment levels and tumor stage, histological type or grading.

Serum concentrations of the p185 fragment in the control group

The mean serum value for the normal controls (n = 80) was 1.203 HNU/ml with a standard deviation of 279 HNU/ml and a range of 595 to 1 947 HNU/ml. We choose a level of 1 761 HNU/ml (two SD above the mean) as a cut-off to distinguish individuals with elevated levels. Using this cut-off, only four out of the 80 healthy controls had elevated levels (1 765, 1 773, 1 899 and 1 947 HNU/ml).

Discussion

In a previous study of our group, immunohistochemically detected p185 has been found to be an important independent prognostic factor for survival time in ovarian cancer (13). Several investigators described the detection of a p185 oncoprotein fragment in sera of breast cancer patients (3, 5, 7, 8, 19). The determination of a p185 oncoprotein fragment serum level might be useful as a diagnostic tool for patients with c-erbB-2 positive tumors. The frequency of the immunohistochemically detected c-erbB-2 gene amplification in the present study (8 out of 57 ovarian cancers) corresponds to the results of previous studies (4, 9, 10, 12, 15). Not all cases with immunopathological c-erbB-2 positive tumors had elevated serum levels of the p185 oncoprotein fragment. The fact that elevated levels of the p185 oncoprotein fragment were only found in four out of eight patients who had overexpression in their tumors may indicate that the afore mentioned ELISA is yet not of sufficient sensitivity to distinguish between elevated serum levels and the background measured in the sera of the control group.

On the other hand, recent work by *Slamon* et al. (17) indicates, that fixation of the tumor decreases the sensitivity of the immunohistochemical detection of p185 as compared to fresh frozen specimens. Therefore, the lack of immunohistochemical staining may underestimate the level of expression in these tumors. This could be the explanation for elevated serum levels in cases with negative immunohistochemistry.

We found that serum levels of p185 oncoprotein fragment in the control female population were approximately normally distributed with a mean of 1203 HNU/ml and a SD of 279 HNU/ml. Elevated serum levels of four individuals above the cut-off level (1761 HNU/ml) may be due to inherent biological variation, or the result of a yet not identified neoplasm.

The fact that all of the 137 individuals studied showed some reactivity in the ELISA suggests that the epitope of the c-erbB-2 encoded protein detected in the ELISA is commonly found in the population. Efforts to isolate and sequence this shed antigen from serum are necessary.

In most studies, overexpression of p185 has been determined by either immunohistochemical or

Western blot procedures (1, 9–13, 17). Unfortunately, both these procedures are limited by their capacity and lack of standardization between laboratories.

Conclusions

Our findings suggest that p185-overexpressing tumors may shed a truncated extracellular derivative of this oncoprotein fragment. Measuring circulating shed protein levels in addition to immunohistochemistry may be helpful for quantification and standardization and provide insights into the mechanisms of cell transformation.
Furthermore, the assay might be a useful test for early diagnosis of ovarian cancer and monitoring therapy. Before possible clinical use of this ELISA system as a diagnostic tool or for monitoring ovarian cancer patients, more studies are necessary to determine the limits of detection.

References

1. Berchuck A, Kamel A, Whitaker R, Kerns B, Olt G, Kinney R, Soper JT, Dogde R, Clarke-Pearson DL, Marks P, McKenzie S, Yin S, Bast RC (1990) Overexpression of HER-2/neu is associated with poor survival in advanced epithelial ovarian cancer. Cancer Res 50: 4087–4091
2. Broders AC (1926) Carcinoma: Grading and practical application. Archs Pathol 2:76–381
3. Carney WP, Hamer PJ, Petit D, Retos C, Greene R, Zabrecky JR, McKenzie S, Hayes S, Kufe D, DeLellis R, Naber R, Wolfe H (1991) Detection and quantification of the human neu protein. J Tumor Marker Oncol 6:53–72
4. Haldane JS, Hird V, Hughes CM, Gullick JW (1990) c-erbB-2 oncogene expression in ovarian cancer. J Pathol 162:231–237
5. Hayes DF, Carney W, Tondini C, Petit D, Henderson IC, Kufe DW (1989) Elevated circulating c-neu oncogene product in patients with breast cancer (abstract). 12th Annual San Antonio Breast Cancer Symposium
6. Hsu SM, Raine L, Fanger H (1981) Use of avidin-biotin-peroxidase complex (ABC) in immunoperoxidase techniques: A comparison between ABC and unlabeled antibody (PAP) procedures. J Histochem Cytochem 29(4):577–580
7. Kynast B, Binder L, Marx D, Zoll B, Schmoll HJ, Oellerich M, Schauer A (1993) Determination of a fragment of the c-erbB-2 translational product p185 in serum of breast cancer patients. J Cancer Res Clin Oncol 119:249–252
8. Mori S, Mori Y, Mukaiyama T, Yamada Y, Sonobe Y, Matsushita H, Sakamoto G, Akiyama T, Ogawa M, Shiraishi M, Toyshima K, Yamamoto T (1990) In vitro and in vivo release of soluble erbB-2 protein from human carcinoma cells. Jpn J Cancer Res 81:489–494
9. Meden, H., D. Marx, H. Hammadi, A. Schauer, W. Kuhn (1991) C-erbB-2- Onkogenüberexpression beim Ovarialkarzinom – Prognostische Bedeutung und Korrelation mit klinischen Befunden bei 119 Patientinnen. Verh Dtsch Ges Path 75:341
10. Meden H, Marx D, Hammadi H, Reles A, Rath W, Schauer A, Kuhn W (1992) Immunohistochemically detected oncoprotein p185/NEU in ovarian cancer: a new prognostic factor? In: Klapdor R (ed) Tumor associated antigens, oncogenes, receptors, cytokines in tumor diagnosis and therapy at the beginning of the nineties. Zuckschwerdt, München, pp 431–432
11. Meden H, Rath W, Marx D, Tsikuras P, Kuhn W, Schauer A (1992) Mammakarzinom in der Schwangerschaft. Klinische, histologische und immunhistochemische Befunde. Zentralbl Chir 117:216–219
12. Meden H, Marx D, Rath W, Kuhn W, Hinney B, Schauer A (1992) c-erb-B-2-Onkogenüberexpression bei primären Ovarialkarzinomen: Häufigkeit und prognostische Bedeutung bei 243 Patientinnen. Geburtsh u Frauenheilk 52:667–673
13. Meden H, Marx D, Rath W, Kron M, Fattahi-Meibodi A, Hinney B, Kuhn W, Schauer A (1994) Overexpression of the oncogene c-erbB-2 in primary ovarian cancer: evaluation of the prognostic value in a Cox proportional hazards multiple regression. Intern J Gynecol Pathol 13:45–53
14. Nadji JD, Morales AR (1984) Immunoperoxidase: Part II, Practical applications. Lab Med 15(1) 33–37
15. Rubin SC, Finstad CL, Wong GY, Almadrones L, Plante M, Lloyd O (1993) Prognostic significance of HER-2/neu expression in advanced epithelial ovarian cancer: a multivariate analysis. Am J Obstet Gynecol 168 162–169
16. Serov SF, Scully RE, Sobin LH (1973) Histological typing of ovarian tumors. In: International histological classification of tumors, No 9, Geneva, Switzerland, WHO, pp 37–42
17. Slamon DJ, Godolphin W, Jones LA, Holt JA, Wong SG, Keith DE, Levin WJ, Stuart SG, Udove J, Ullrich A, Press MF (1989) Studies of the HER-2/neu protooncogene in human breast and ovarian cancer. Science (Wash DC) 244:707712
18. Sternberger LA, Hardy PH, Cuculis JJ, Meyer HG (1970) The unlabeled antibody-enzyme method of

immunohistochemistry. Preparation and properties of soluble antigen-antibody complex (horseradish peroxidase-anti-peroxidase) and its use in identification of spirochetes. J Histochem Cytochem 18. 315-333

19 Teramoto Y, Wallingford S, Mauceri J, Sampson E (1991) Serum enzyme imunnoassay kit for the detection of c-erbB-2 oncoprotein (abstract). Eighty-third Annual Meeting of the American Association for Cancer Research, Houston

Address for correspondence:
Dr. med. H. Meden
Abteilung für Geburtshilfe und Gynäkologie
Universität Göttingen
Robert-Koch-Straße 40
D-37077 Göttingen, Germany

Detection of p185^(HER-2) fragments in sera of breast cancer patients – A new prognostic factor and tumor marker?

B. Kynast[a], J. Isola[b], L. Binder[c], Y. Teramoto[d], D. Marx[e], M. Oellerich[c], C. Bokemeyer[a], H. Poliwoda[a], H. J. Schmoll[a], A. Schauer[e]

[a]Hematology and Oncology, Medical University Center Hannover, [b]Biomedical Science, University of Tampere, Tampere, Finnland, [c]Clinical Chemistry, University Göttingen, [d]Triton Laboratories, Ciba Corning Diagnostics Corp, Alameda CA, USA, [e]Pathological Department, University of Göttingen, Germany

Introduction

Members of the ERBB oncogenes and their translational products (EGFR, p185[HER-2], p160[HER-3]) were described as important factors in oncogenesis in subgroups of human breast cancer (1–3). The c-erbB-2 gene, also called HER-2, was independently isolated by different groups by screening a DNA library with c-erbB probes (4). This gene is localized on chromosome 17 q21–22 (5) and codes a transmembrane glycolosylised phosphoprotein of 185 kD with tyrosine kinase activity (6). p185 is a member of the EGFR related subctass of class I growth factor receptors with an extracellular domain for which are several suggested binding ligands (7, 8), a small transmembrane domain and an internal domain with tyrosinase activity. Amplification of the HER-2 gene and p185 overexpression were described as activating mechanisms to an oncogene in breast cancer (2). In many studies HER-2 gene amplification and p185 overexpression have been found to correlate with poor prognosis in node positive and node negative (9, 10) mammary carcinomas. On the other hand, one study has not found such a correlation between HER-2 gene amplification and short survival even with a long period of follow-up (11). However, in a recently published study with a 30 years follow-up of breast cancer patients there was p185 overexpression in breast cancer tumor tissue a highly significant parameter for short survival and early recurrence (12). In supernatants of breast cancer cell lines a shed fragment of the p185 protein, with molecular weight of approximately 105 kD was detected by Westem blot and ELISA (13–17). Proteolytic cleavage of the extracellular domain of the p185 receptor (18) and its secreted form produced by alternative RNA processing (19) were supposed as causal mechanisms. Elevated p105 serum concentrations have also been measured in breast cancer patients (20–27). An association between elevated p105 serum concentrations in breast cancer patients and poor prognosis and worse response to therapy have also been demonstrated (28–31). So we have initiated a study to evaluate the role of quantitation of the p185 receptor fragment p105 in sera of breast cancer patients in order to define a clinically relevant cut-off.

Material and methods

Tumor tissues and serum samples

151 paraffin embedded tumor tissue, serum samples taken from 184 breast cancer patients (with partly known moleculargenetic results (HER-2 gene amplification, RNA-overexpression and point mutation), 69 healthy persons, 50 patients with benigne breast lesions, 18 pregnant woman were provided from Medical, Surgical and Pathological Departments of University Göttingen and the University of Tampere, Tampere, Finnland.

Concentration of the p185 shedding fragment p105 in serum

Aliquoted, deep frozen serum samples were stored at –70° Celsius. Commercial avaiable monoclonal antibody based immunoenzymetric assays (Ciba Corning, Alameda, CA, USA) were used – as scheduled from CCD – for determination of p105 serum concentrations.

Immunohistochemical analysis (ICA) of p185 expression

Paraffin-embedded tumor tissues were investigated by ICA with monoclonal antibodies 9G6 against the extracellular domain, in part moAb3B5 (Dianova, Hamburg, FRG) and a polyclonal antibody (Ciba Corning, Alameda, CA, USA) against the internal domain.

Results

In an early phase of our study (20) we found 9/70 (13%) breast cancer patients elevated p105 serum concentrations (figure 1). All of the patients (9/35, 26%) with increased p105 serum concentration greater than 30 kU/l had evident metastatic disease (figure 1). Every breast cancer patient with a p185 overexpression in her primary tumor and metastatic disease (3/3, 100%) had also elevated p105 serum concentrations (figure 1). No patient with negative c-erbB2 status of the primary tumor were found to have p105 serum levels greater than 40 kU/l. In five patients without p185 overexpression of their we measured p105 serum concentrations between 30 kU/l and 40 kU/l. In a later phase of our study we measured serum p105 in 114 serum samples obtained preoperatively from breast cancer patients – in 11/114 seras elevated p105 levels were determined. In 10/11 cases with preoperatively elevated p105 levels in serum we detected a p185 overexpression of their primary tumor (figure 2). Elevated p105 serum concentrations were found in 10/47 patients (21%) with "c-erb-2 positive" and in 1/67 (1.5%) with "c-erbB-2 negative" primary tumors (figure 3). Most of the patients with stage III/IV-disease (3/5, 60%) were found to have elevated p105 concentrations in serum. 68/69 healthy persons and all 18 pregnant women had p105 serum concentrations below 30 kU/l (figure 4). One male blood donor had – controlled – serum concentrations higher than 100 kU/l (118 kU/l). Clinical data of this person were not available – with respect to the anonymity of the blood donor.

Discussion

Like other investigators we found in nearly 15% elevated p105 serum concentrations in breast cancer patients, in 26% of the breast cancer patients with metastatic disease and in nearly 10% of preoperatively obtained serum samples. Previous results of four small studies in preoperative patients and in patients prior to

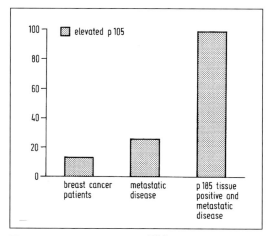

Figure 1. Elevated serum p105^{HER-2} levels (sensitivity, %) in breast cancer patients.

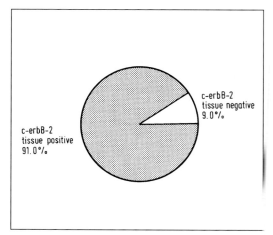

Figure 2. Preoperatively elevated p105^{HER-2} levels (n = 11) in breast cancer patients depending on the "c-erbB-2 - status" of their primary tumor.

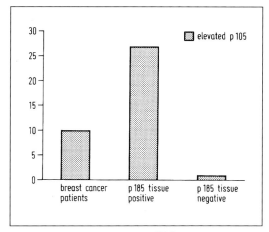

Figure 3. Sensitivity of p105^HER-2 in preoperatively obtained serum from breast cancer patients (n = 118).

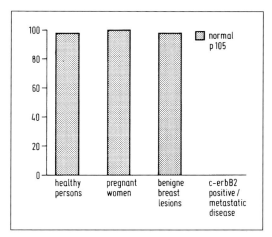

Figure 4. Specifity (%) of p105^HER-2 in breast cancer patients.

chemotherapy suggested that elevated levels of serum p105 predicted a poorer prognosis (29, 30) and a poorer response to therapy (28, 31). In our collectives elevated p105 serum concentrations were associated with p185 overexpression of the primary tumor. These results were confirmed by some studies (20, 22, 29), which found also such a correlation for breast and ovarian cancer patients. Only in two smaller studies of breast and ovarian cancer patients there were no correlation between these two c-erbB-2 parameters (19, 32). No prognostic value regarding survival (19) or therapeutic outcome (35) has been found in two smaller clinical trials for breast cancer and in one study for ovarian cancer patients (34). However, all of our breast cancer patients with p185 overexpression of their primary tumor and elevated p105 serum concentrations were found to have metastatic disease. Thus, a very high specificity (> 95%) and only in breast cancer primary tumors with p185 overexpression either with preoperatively elevated p105 levels (depending on the pTNM stage up to 60%) or with metastatic disease (up to 100%) a higher sensitivity was obtained in our own investigations and in other published studies. Further ongoing prospective multicentric studies are needed to establish a clinically relevant cut-off for determination of p105 in serum. This should improve the value of increased p105 serum concentration as a new biological prognostic parameter with potential clinical relevance in human breast cancer, may be ovarian, urinary bladder and gastric cancer – maligninacies with an important subgroup of primary tumor tissues with p185 receptor overexpression.

Conclusions

Since more than two years we have used an EIA for the quantitation of an approx. 105 kD fragment of the c-erbB-2/HER-2 translational product, p185, found shed in the sera of breast cancer patients. We initiated a study to evaluate the performance and significance of the available testkit and the determination of p105 in sera as a new, potential biological parameter in human breast cancer. We investigated sera from breast cancer patients (n = 184), healthy persons (n = 69), pregnant women (n = 8) and patients with benign lesion of the breast (n = 50) for the presence of the 105 kD p185 fragment, using a monoclonal antibody based heterogeneous immunoenzymetric assay. In all the pregnant women (18/18), in 68/69 of the healthy persons and in 49/49 of the patients with benign lesions of the breast serum p105 concentrations were below 30 kU/l. One of the healthy persons - an anonymous male blood donor – had a reproducible p105 serum concentration of 118 kU/l. All of the 70 patients, who were evaluable for clinical status, without metastatic disease (35/70) had serum p105 concentrations below 30 kU/l. There was no breast cancer patient with an elevated serum p105 that did not have metastatic disease. The highest serum p105 concentration (578 kU/l) was obtained in a breast cancer patient who also had high level of p185 expressed in the primary tumor but lacked any evidence of HER-2 gene amplification. In this tumor we discovered a somatic point mutation in the region of the HER-2 sequence which encodes for the transmembrane domain of the p185 receptor (data not shown). Upon completion of this part of the study, we next measured p105 in 114 serum samples taken preoperatively from breast cancer patients using the same test kit. Preoperatively elevated p105 serum concentrations were found in 9.6% (11/114) of the breast cancer patients. 91% (10/11) of the patients with preoperative elevated p105 serum concentrations had a p185 overexpression in the primary tumor. Only in one patient with preoperatively elevated serum p105 a p185 overexpression of its primary tumor was not detected (1/67), vice versa had 21% (10/47) of the p185 overexpressing tumors preoperatively elevated serum p105 concentrations, most of these cases had Stage III/IV tumors. p185 tumor tissue expression was measured by ICA with two monoclonal antibodies – 9G6 directed against the extracellular domain, one polyclonal antibody (Ciba Corning) and MoAb against the internal domain – and in part with the help of an EIA. Further, ongoing studies will be carried out to obtain relevant cut-offs for serum p105 and p185 in tumor tissue of breast cancer patients. Determination of cut-offs will help in the assessment of p185/p105 as new prognostic parameters in breast cancer.

References

1. Toi M, Osaki A, Yamada H, Toge T (1991) Epidermal growth factor expression as prognostic indicator in breast cancer. Eur J Cancer 27:977–980
2. Pierce JH, Arnstein P, DiMarco E, Artrip J, Kraus MH, Lonardo F, Di Fiore PP, Aaronson SA (1991) Oncogenic potential of erbB-2 in human mammary epithelial cells. Oncogene 6:1189–1194
3. Lemoine NR, Barnes DM, Hollywood DP, Hughes CM, Smith P, Dublin E, Prigent SA, Gullick WJ, Hurst HC (1992) Expression of the ERBB3 gene product in breast cancer. Br J Cancer 66:1116–1121
4. Coussens L, Yang-Feng TL, Liao YC, Chen E, Gray A, McGrath J, Seeburg PH, Liberman TA, Schlessinger J, Francke U, Levinson A, Ullrich A (1985) Tyrosine kinase receptor with extensive homology to EGF receptor shares chromosomal location with neu oncogene. Science 230:1132–1139
5. Fukushige SI, Matsubara KL, Yoshida M, Sasaki M, Suzuki T, Semba K, Toyoshima K, Yamamoto T (1986) Localisation of a novel v-erbB -related gene, c-erbB-2, on human chromosome 17 and its amplification in a gastric cancer cell line. Mol Cell Biol 6:955–958
6. Akiyama T, Sudo CH, Ogawara H, Toyoshima K, Yamamoto T (1986) The product of the human c-erb B2 gene: a 185 kilodalton glycoprotein with tyrosine kinase activity. Science 232:1644–1646
7. Lupu R, Colomer R, Kannan B, Lippman ME (1992) Charaterisation of a growth factor that binds exclusively to the erbB-2 receptor and induces cellular responses. Proc Natl Acad Sci USA 89:2287–2291
8. Peles E, Bacus SS, Koski RA, Lu HS, Wen D, Ogden SG, Levy RB, Yarden Y (1992) Isolation of the neu/Her-2 stimulatory ligand: a 44 kd glycoprotein that induces differentiation of mammary tumor cells. Cell 69:205–216
9. Allred DC, Clark GM, Tandon AK, Molina R, Tormey DC, Osborne CK, Gilchrist KW, Mansour EG, Abeloff M, Eudey L, McGuire WL (1992) Overexpression of HER-2/neu and its relationship with other prognostic factors change during the progression of in situ to invasive breast cancer. J Clin Oncol 10:599–605
10. Slamon DJ, Clark GM, Wong SG, Levin WL, Ullrich, A, McGuire WL (1987) Human breast cancer: Correlation of relapse and survival with amplification of the HER-2/neu oncogene. Science 235:177–182
11. Clark GM, McGuire WL (1991) Follow-study of TIER-2/neu amplification in primary breast cancer. Cancer Res 51:944–948
12. Toikkanen S, Helin H, Isola J, Joensuu H (1992) Prognostic significance of HER-2 oncoprotein expression in breast cancer: a 30-year follow-up. J Clin Oncol 10:1044–8
13. Alper N, Yamaguchi K, Hitomi J, Honda S, Matsushima T, Abe K (1990) The presence of c-erbB-2 gene product-related protein in culture medium conditioned by breast cancer cell line SK-BR-3. Cell Growth Differentiation 1:591–599
14. Zabrecky JR, Lam T, McKenzie SJ, Carney W (1991) The extracellular domain of p185/neu is released from the surface of human breast carcinoma cells, SK-BR-3. J Biol Chem 266:1716–1720
15. Mori S, Mori Y, Mukaiyama T, Yamada Y, Sonobe V, Matsushima H, Sakamoto G, Akiyama T, Ogawa M,

15 Shiraishi M, Toyoshima K, Yamamoto T (1990) In vitro and in vivo release of soluble erbB-2 protein from human carcinoma cells. Jpn J Cancer Res 81:489–494
16 Lin YZ, Clinton GM (1991) A soluble protein related to the TIER-2 proto-oncogene product is released from human breast carcinoma cells. Oncogene 6:639–643
17 Langton BC, Crenshaw MC, Chao LA, Stuart SG, Akita RW, Jackson JE (1991) An antigen immunologically related to the external domain of p185 is shed from nude mouse tumors overexpressing the c-erbB-2 (HER-2/neu) oncogene. Cancer Res 51:2593–2598
18 Pupa SM, Menard S, Morelli D, Pozzi B, De Paolo G, Colnaghi MT (1993) The extracellular domain from the c-erbB-2 oncoprotein is released from tumor cells by proteolytic cleavage. Oncogene 11:2917–2923
19 Scott GK, Robles R, Park JW, Montgomery PA, Daniel J, Holmes WE, Lee J, Keller GA, Li WL, Fendly BM, Wood WI, Shepard HM, Benz CC (1993) A truncated intracellular HER2 NEU receptor produced by alternative RNA processing affects growth of human carcinoma cells. Mol Cell Biol 13:2247–2257
20 Kynast B, Binder L, Marx D, Zoll B, Schmoll HJ, Oellerich M, Schauer A (1993) Determination of a fragment of the c-erbB-2 translational product p185 in serum of breast cancer patients. J Cancer Res Clin Oncol 119:249–252
21 Hayden CL, Brower ST, Tartter PI (1992) Circulating HER-2/NEU levels in primary benign and malignant breast disease. Abstract. Proc Annu Meet Am Soc Clin Oncol 11:A163
22 Konrad K, Teramoto Y (1993) Measurement of the extracellular domain of the c-erbB-2 oncoprotein in sera of breast cancer patients. J Tumor Marker Oncol 8:33(9)
23 Narita T, Funashi H, Satoh, Takagi H (1992) c-erbB-2 protein in the sera of breast cancer patients. Gan To Kagaku Ryoho 19:909–911
24 Breuer B, Luo JC, Devico I, Pincus M, Tatum AH, Daucher J, Minick R, Osborne M, Miller D, Nowak E, Cody H Caeney WP, Brandtrauf PW (1993) Detection of elevated c-erbB-2 oncoprotein in the serum and tissue in breast cancer. Med Sci Res 21:383–384
25 Leitzel K, Teramoto Y, Sampson E, Mauceri J, Langton BC, Demers L, Podczaski E, Harvey H, Shambaugh S, Volas G, Weaver S, Lipton A (1992) Elevated soluble c-erbB-2 antigen levels in the serum and; effusions of a proportion of breast cancer patients. J Clin Oncol 10:1436–1443
26 Sias PE, Kotts CE, Vetterlein D, Shepard M, Wong WLT (1990) ELISA for quantitation of the extracellular domain of p185HER2 in biological fluids. J Immunol Methods 132:73–80
27 Wu JT, Astill ME, Zhang P (1993) Detection of the extracellular domain of c-erbB-2 oncoprotein in sera from patients with various carcinomas: correlation with tumor markers. J Clin Lab Anal 7:31–40
28 Kath R, Höffken K, Otte C, Metz K, Scheulen ME, Hulskamp F, Seeber S (1993) The neu-oncogene product in serum and tissue of patients with breast carcinoma. Ann Oncol 4:585–590
29 Isola J, Kallioniemi O-P, Mauceri J, Sampson E, Teramoto Y (1992) Elevated preoperative serum levels of c-erbB-2 antigen in a small group of breast cancer patients with poor survival. Abstract. Eighty-third Annual Meeting of the American Association for Cancer Research, San Diego
30 Mitze N, Kreienberg R (1993) Serum c-erbB-2 levels correlated to prognosis of breast cancer. Eighty-fourth Annual Meeting American Association for Cancer Research 34:1339
31 Classen S, Possinger K, Flath B, Wilmanns W (1993) c-erb-B2 Onkoprotein im Serum von Mamma-karzinompatientinnen. Acta Chirurgica Austriaca (suppl 103) 25:26 (abstract)
32 Meden H, Marx D, Fattahi A, Rath W, Wuttke W, Schauer A, Kuhn W (1993) Serologischer Nachweis eines p185- Onkoprotein- Fragments (cerbB-2) bei Patientinnen mit Ovarialkarzinom. Abstract. In: Klapdor R (ed) 7. Hamburger Symposium über Tumormarker. Zuckschwerdt, München, pp 162
33 McKenzie SJ, Desombre KA, Bast BS, Hollis DR, Whitaker RS, Berchuck A, Boyer M, Bast RC (1993) Serum levels of HER-2 neu (c-erbB-2) correlate with overexpression of p185 neu in human ovarian cancer. Cancer 71:3942–3946
34 Fisken J, Roulston JE, Beattie G, Hayes DF, Leonard RCF (1992) Investigation ofthe c-neu protooncogene related protein, p185, in the serum of primary epitheial ovarian-cancer patients. Int J Gyn Cancer 2:134–140
35 Volas G, Leitzel D, Teramoto Y, Sampson EL, Mauceri J, Demers L, Santen R, Harvey H, Mulagha M, Lipton A (1992) Serial serum c-erbB-2 levels and response in breast cancer patients. Abstract. Eighty-third Annual Meeting of the American Association for Cancer Research, San Diego

Address for correspondence:
Dr. med. B. Kynast
Abteilung für Hämatologie und Onkologie
Medizinische Hochschule Hannover
Konstanty-Gutschow-Straße 6
D-30625 Hannover, Germany

Quantitation of c-*erb*B-2 oncoprotein in human breast tissue

Ellen Sampson, Y. Teramoto
Ciba Corning Diagnostics Corp., Alameda, California, USA

Introduction

The c-*erb*B-2 oncogene, also referred to as HER-2 or neu, was independently identified in DNA studies from chemically induced rat neuroblastomas (1) and in cross-hybridisation studies with v-*erb*B and human epidermal growth factor receptor (EGFR) DNAs (2, 3, 4). The c-*erb*B-2 oncogene encodes for a 185 kD glycoprotein with extensive homology to EGFR (2, 3, 4, 5, 6) and is found on q21 of chromosome 17 in humans (2). The gene product has an intracellular domain with tyrosine kinase activity (7), a transmembrane domain and a cysteine-rich extracellular domain. The c-*erb*B-2 molecule is believed to be a cellular receptor for recently identified specific ligands (8, 9).

c-*erb*B-2 gene amplification and protein overexpression have been shown to occur in 10–46% of primary human breast cancers (10–24). When approximately 3000 breast cancer patients were analysed as a combined total population an average amplification or protein overexpression rate of 20% was found (24). The prognostic significance of c-*erb*B-2 in breast cancer has been the focus of numerous studies. Some reports have found a correlation between c-*erb*B-2 gene amplification or protein overexpression and poor survival for lymph node positive breast cancer patients (18, 23, 25). Other findings suggest that there is no direct correlation (24, 26–28). Similarly, for lymph node negative breast cancer, some investigations report that c-*erb*B-2 amplification or protein overexpression is an indicator of a poorer prognosis (21, 29) while other studies do not support these findings (16, 18, 23). Amplification or protein overexpression of c-*erb*B-2 has also been shown to occur in other human malignancies including ovarian (16, 30), lung (31), gastric carcinoma (32, 33), and bladder (34). Some of these findings suggest that c-*erb*B-2 may be useful as a prognostic indicator in these other cancers, in addition to breast cancer (16, 30, 33). An enzyme immunoassay (EIA) utilizing two monoclonal antibodies to the extracellular domain of the c-*erb*B-2 protein in extracts prepared from human breast tissue has been developed (Triton c-*erb*B-2 Tissue Extract EIA Kit; Ciba Corning Diagnostics Corp., Alameda, CA). In this study, we evaluate the performance of the EIA and then demonstrate the ability to detect and quantitate the c-*erb*B-2 protein in tissue extracts obtained from breast cancer patients. EIA results are correlated with immunohistochemical (IHC) and Western blot (WB) testing of selected breast carcinomas.

Materials and methods

Specimens

Tissue samples were obtained from 201 patients diagnosed with histologically confirmed breast cancer (infiltrating ductal carcinoma, infiltrating lobular carcinoma, comedo carcinoma, lobular carcinoma in situ, invasive lobular carcinoma, and mucinous carcinoma) and 41 patients with benign breast disease (fibroadenoma, fibrocystic disease, intraductal papilloma, fibrosis or inflammatory disease).

Preparation of specimen tissue extracts

Specimen tissue extracts were prepared by first pulverizing tissue followed by homogenization of tissue in cold TEN buffer (0.05M Tris, pH 7.4;

0.15M NaCl; 0.001 EDTA) at a ratio of 10:1 (v:w). Tissue homogenates were then centrifuged at 13,000 to 14,000 x g for 15 minutes at 2–8 °C. Following centrifugation, the supernatant fluid was removed. Chilled TEN buffer containing 1.0% Triton X-100 (extraction solution) was added to the residual pellet. The pelleted material, which was enriched for tissue membranes, was resuspended in the extraction solution and incubated for 15 minutes on ice with occasional vortexing. This was followed by a centrifugation step (13,000–14,000 x g, 15 minutes, 2–8 °C). The resultant supernatant fraction was the tissue membrane extract and contained most of the c-erbB-2 activity. A protein determination was done (Pierce BCA Protein Assay; Pierce Chemical Company) on the tissue extract. Tissue extracts were diluted to 0.1 mg/ml prior to performing the assay for c-erbB-2 antigen.

Enzyme immunoassay

The c-erbB-2 antigen was measured in the tissue extracts with a monoclonal antibody-based enzyme immunoassay (EIA) (Ciba Corning Diagnostics Corp.; Alameda, CA) according to the manufacturer's instructions. Briefly, an anti-c-erbB-2 conjugate is incubated with specimen tissue extracts as well as with manufacturer supplied kit control and calibrators. During this incubation the antigen contained within the specimen, control and calibrators is bound by the two monoclonal antibodies specific to c-erbB-2. One of the monoclonal antibodies is also conjugated to horseradish peroxidase. The immune complexes formed are contained within the liquid phase. In the next step, the resulting immune complexes are bound onto a coated polystyrene tube by a linking solution. Any unbound reactants are removed by a washing step. Next, the tubes with the bound immune complexes are incubated with a substrate-chromogen solution (3, 3', 5, 5'-tetramethylbenzidine and hydrogen peroxide) to develop a color. The intensity of the color formed by the enzyme reaction is proportional to the concentration of the c-erbB-2 antigen contained within the specimen. The color development step is stopped by the addition of acid (1 M phosphoric acid). The intensity of color developed is read spectrophotometrically at 450 nm.

Immunohistochemical analysis of breast carcinomas for c-erbB-2 antigen

Formalin-fixed, paraffin-embedded tissue sections (4–6 microns) were placed on poly-L-lysine coated slides. The slides were deparaffinized with xylene and rehydrated stepwise with absolute, 95%, 70% ethanol and finally, water. Sections were then stained with a rabbit polyclonal antibody that was generated to a specific peptide sequence, corresponding to a cytoplasmic epitope of the c-erbB-2 protein (PAb-1, Ciba Corning Diagnostics Corp.; Alameda, CA). An avidin-biotin based immunoperoxidase system (Vectastain, Vector Labs; Burlingame, CA) was used as the detection system. Sections prepared from NIH 3T3 cells transfected with the c-erbB-2 gene and stained with PAb-1 were used as a positive control. An adjacent tissue section prepared for each of the breast carcinomas examined was also stained with normal rabbit serum to serve as a negative control. Staining was scored as positive if distinct plasma membrane staining was evident. The presence of cytoplasmic staining in the absence of any specific plasma membrane staining was interpreted as non-specfic and as a negative result.

Western blot analysis of breast carcinomas for p185 c-erbB-2 antigen

Sample buffer (62.5 mmol/l Tris, 5% SDS, 10% glycerol, 0.001% bromophenol blue, and 2% dithiothreitol, pH 6.75) was added to each of the specimen tissue extracts (20 mg total protein) and boiled for five minutes. The sample was then loaded onto a 10% polyacrylamide gel and electrophoresed at 60 mA. Proteins were transfered to nitrocellulose (70 V for 2 h at 2–8 °C). The blot was blocked with PBS containing 5% nonfat dry milk and 0.05% Tween-20 (30 minutes at room temperature). After rinsing the blot in PBS containing 0.05% Tween-20 (PBS-TW20), the blot was incubated with PAb-1 (diluted 1:30 in PBS-TW20 containing 1.0% BSA) for 1 hour at room temperature. Next the blot was rinsed with PBS-TW20 and then incubated with an avidin-biotin based immunoperoxidase system (Vectastain, Vector Labs; Burlingame, CA) as per the manufacturer's instructions. After another rinse step, the blot was developed with 3, 3', 5, 5'-tetramethylbenzidine (TMB) and hydrogen peroxide with membrane enhancer (Kirkegaard and Perry Laboratories, Gaithersburg, MD). After five minutes incubation time the reaction was stopped by rinsing the blot in distilled water.

Results

EIA performance characteristics

The calibration curve for the Triton c-erbB-2 Tissue Extract EIA Kit ranged from 0 units/ml to 100 units/ml and was relatively linear with a correlation coefficient of 0.99946 (figure 1). Within run and between-run reproducibility were each measured with two specimens and found to range from 6.5% to 8.6% (with-in run) and 8.5% to 9.2% (between-run) (table I). The linearity of the EIA was determined by performing duplicate determinations of two different tissue extract specimens. Specimens were adjusted to 100 µg/ml and then serially (twofold) diluted. Linear regression analysis yielded correlation coefficients of 0.9999 and 0.9989 for the two specimens evaluated (table II). Recovery was determined by the addition of known amounts of c-erbB-2

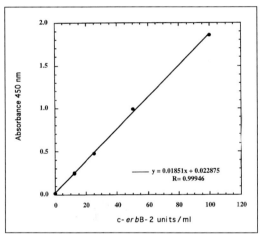

Figure 1. Calibration curve for c-erbB-2 Tissue Extract EIA Kit.

Table I. Imprecision of the c-erbB-2 Tissue Extract EIA Kit.

1. Within-run reproducibility of the c-erbB-2 Tissue Extract EIA Kit was measured by performing 20 replicate determinations of two different specimens in one assay.

Specimen	Mean c-erbB-2 (units/ml)	Standard deviation	Within-run (%) CV
A	36.8	2.4	6.5%
B	83.3	7.2	8.6%

2. Between-run reproducibility of the c-erbB-2 tissue extract EIA kit was determined by replicate measurements of two specimens in 15 individually calibrated assays.

Specimen	Mean c-erbB-2 (units/ml)	Standard deviation	Between-run (%) CV
A	33.1	2.8	8.5%
B	72.9	6.7	9.2%

Table II. Linearity of specimen tissue extracts in the c-erbB-2 Tissue Extract EIA Kit. Linearity was determined by performing duplicate determinations of two different tissue extract specimens. Specimens were adjusted to 100 µg/ml and serially diluted. Linear regression yielded correlation coefficients of 0.9999 (Specimen A) and 0.9989 (Specimen B).

	Dilution	Value expected (units/ml)	Value obtained (units/ml)	Expected (percent)	Observed (percent)
Specimen A	1	70.15	70.15	100	100
	1:2	35.08	38.40	50	55
	1:4	17.54	19.95	25	28
	1:8	8.77	9.95	12.5	14
Specimen B	1	49.15	49.15	100	100
	1:2	24.58	22.25	50	45
	1:4	12.29	11.70	25	24
	1:8	6.14	4.70	12.5	10

Table III. Recovery of c-*erb*B-2 in the c-*erb*B-2 Tissue Extract EIA Kit.

c-*erb*B-2 added (units/ml)	Assay value (units/ml)	Recovery (%)
100	94.8	94.8%
50	45.4	90.8%
25	22.7	90.8%
12.5	12.3	98.4%

Known amounts of c-*erb*B-2 antigen were added to a c-*erb*B-2 negative tumor tissue extract and then assayed in the c-*erb*B-2 Tissue Extract EIA Kit.

Table IV. Comparison of c-*erb*B-2 expression by Western blot and Tissue Extract EIA Kit (EIA).

		Western Blot	
		positive	negative
TE EIA	positive	11	2
	negative	2	45

Concordance: 56 of 60 = 93%

Table V. Comparison of c-*erb*B-2 expression by immunohistochemical staining and c-*erb*B-2 Tissue Extract EIA Kit (EIA).

		IHC staining	
		positive	negative
TE EIA	positive	17	11
	negative	4	75

Concordance: 92 of 107 = 86%

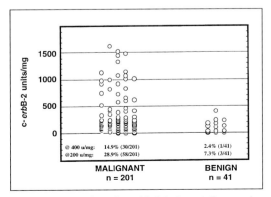

Figure 2. Expression of c-*erb*B-2 in breast tissue using the c-*erb*B-2 Tissue Extract EIA Kit.

antigen to a c-*erb*B-2 negative tumor tissue extract. The recovery ranged from about 91% to 98% (table III).

Expression of c-erbB-2 in breast tissue

Extracts prepared from tissues obtained from patients with either breast carcinomas (n = 201) or benign breast disease (n = 41) were analysed in the EIA.
c-*erb*B-2 values ranged from 0 units/ml to greater than 1500 units/ml for tissue obtained from carcinomas and 0 units/ml to about 400 units/ml when tissue was analysed from benign tissues. When 200 units/ml was utilized as a cut-off value, 58 of 201 (28.9%) cancers and 3 of 41 (7.3%) benigns were considered to overexpress c-*erb*B-2. When the cut-off value was raised to 400 units/ml, 30 of 201 (14.9%) cancers and 1 of 41 (2.4%) benigns were considered to overexpress c-*erb*B-2 (figure 2).

Comparison of c-erbB-2 expression by WB and EIA

Sixty specimens were analysed by both WB and EIA. Fifty six of 60 (93%) of these specimens were in agreement between the two methods. However, there were two specimens that were negative by EIA and positive by WB as well as two specimens that were positive by EIA and negative by WB (table IV). For the purpose of this comparison, a cut-off value of 400 units/ml was used.

Comparison of c-erbB-2 expression by IHC and EIA

One hundred and seven (107) specimens were analyzed by both IHC and EIA for comparative purposes (table V). The concordance was 86% (92/107). There were eleven specimens that were negative by IHC but positive by EIA (> 400 units/ml). In addition, there were four specimens negative by EIA (< 400 units/ml) but positive by IHC.

Conclusions

The performance of the Triton c-erbB-2 Tissue Extract EIA Kit has been evaluated and been shown to be reliable for the quantiation of c-erbB-2 in extracts prepared from tissues obtained from patients with breast cancer. Measurement of the c-erbB-2 antigen in specimens was confirmed by both WB and IHC for selected specimens. Concordance between the EIA and WB or IHC was 93% and 86%, respectively. This level of agreement between the EIA and these more standard methodologies suggests that the EIA can be used reliably in place of WB and/or IHC. From a technical perspective, this option offers greater ease in performing an analysis for c-erbB-2 in tissue extracts. In addition, the EIA offers the advantage of quantitatively determining the c-erbB-2 expression level as opposed to IHC and WB methods which tend to be more subjective measures of c-erbB-2 expression. The discordance between EIA and IHC may be explained by either the loss of antigenicity due to fixation of tissue for IHC or the fact that different pieces of tissue from a tumor are utilized for the separate methodologies. Similarly for WB, heterogeneity of tissue specimens may contribute to the low level of discordance seen in this study.

From a research perspective, this EIA has the potential to serve as a tool to further study c-erbB-2 amplification and overexpression in breast cancer, as well as other human malignancies which, in turn, may help to elucidate the biological significance of c-erbB-2 in cancer. Such studies could result in additional information with therapeutic implications. In particular, the ability to quantitatively measure c-erbB-2 in tissues could be of great interest and value since c-erbB-2, as a prognostic indicator for node negative breast cancer patients, would have the potential to identify a subset of patients who would otherwise be classified as having a good prognosis based upon their nodal status.

References

1 Schechter AL, Stern DF, Vaidyanathan L, Decker SJ, Drebin JA, Greene MI, Weinberg RA (1984) The neu oncogene: an erbB-related gene encoding a 185,000-Mr tumor antigen. Nature 312:513–516

2 Coussens L, Yang-Fen TL, Liao Y-C, Chen E, Gray A, McGrath J, Seeburg PH, Libermann TA, Schlessinger J, Francke U, Levinson A, Ullrich A (1985) Tyrosine kinase receptor with extensive homology to EGF receptor shares chromosomal location with neu oncogene. Science 230:1132–1139

3 King CR, Kraus MH, Aaronson SA (1985) Amplification of a novel v-erbB-related gene in human mammary carcinoma. Science 229:974–976

4 Semba K, Kamata N, Toyoshima K, Yamamoto T (1985) A v-erbB-related proto-oncogene, c-erbB-2 is distinct from c-erbB-1/epidermal growth factor receptor gene and is amplified in a human salivary gland adenocarcinoma. Proc Natl Acad Sci USA 82:6497–6501

5 Schechter AL, Hung M-C, Vaidyanathan L, Weinberg RA, Yang-Fen TL, Francke U, Ullrich A, Coussens L (1985) The neu-gene: an erbB homologous gene distinct from and unlinked to the gene encoding the EGF receptor. Science 229:976–978

6 Yamamoto T, Ikawa S, Akiyama T, Semba K, Nomura N, Miyajama N, Saito T, Toyoshima K (1986) Similarity of protein encoded by the human c-erbB-2 gene to epidermal growth factor receptor. Nature 319:230–234

7 Akiyama T, Sudo C, Ogawara H, Toyoshima K, Yamamoto T (1986) The product of the human c-erbB-2 gene: a 185-kilodalton glycoprotein with tyrosine kinase activity. Science 232:1644–1646

8 Lupu R, Colomer R, Kannan B, Lippman ME (1992) Characterization of a growth factor that binds exclusively to the erbB-2 receptor and induces cellular responses. Proc Natl Acad Sci USA 89:2287–2291

9 Holmes WE, Sliwkowski MX, Akita RW, Henzel WJ, Lee J, Park JW, Yansura D, Abadi N, Raab H, Lewis GD, Sheperd M, Kuang W-J, Wood WI, Goeddel DV, Vandlen RL (1992) Identification of Heregulin, a specific activator of p185erbB2. Science 256:1205–1210

10 Zhou D, Battifora H, Cline MJ (1987) Association of multiple copies of the c-erbB-2 oncogene with spread of breast cancer. Cancer Res 47:6123–6125

11 Fontaine J, Tesseraux M, Klein V, Bastert G, Blin N (1988) Gene amplification and expression of the neu (c-erbB-2) sequence in human mammary carcinoma. Oncology 45:360–363

12 van de Vijver MJ, Peterse JL, Mooi WJ, Wisman F, Lomans J, Dalesio O, Nusse R (1988) Neu-protein overexpression in breast cancer. N Eng J Med 319:1239–1245

13 Lacroix H, Iglehart JD, Skinner MA, Kraus MH (1989) Overexpression of erbB-2 or EGF receptor proteins present in early stage mammary carcinoma is detected simultaneously in matched primary tumors and regional metastases. Oncogene 4:145–151

14. Ro J, El-Naggar A, Ro JY, Blick M, Frye D, Fraschini G, Fritsche H, Hortobagyi G (1989) c-erbB-2 amplification in node-negative human breast cancer. Cancer Res 49:6941–6944
15. Seshadri R, Matthews C, Dobrovic A, Horsfall DJ (1989) The significance of oncogene amplification in primary breast cancer. Int J Cancer 43:270–272
16. Slamon DJ, Godolphin W, Jones LA, Holt JA, Wong SG, Keith DE, Levin WJ, Stuart SG, Udove J, Ullrich A, Press MF (1989) Studies of the HER-2/neu proto-oncogene in human breast and ovarian cancer. Science 244:707–712
17. Spandidos DA, Yiagnisis M, Papdimitriou K, Field JK (1989) Ras c-myc, and c-erbB-2 oncoproteins in human breast cancer. Anticancer Res 9:1385–1394
18. Tandon AK, Clark GM, Chamness GC, Ullrich A, McGuire WL (1989) HER-2/neu oncogene protein and prognosis in breast cancer. J Clin Oncol 7:1120–1128
19. Wright C, Angus B, Nicholson S, Sainsbury JRC, Cairns J, Gullick WJ, Kelly P, Harris AL, Horne CHW (1989) Expression of c-erbB-2 oncoprotein: a prognostic indicator in human breast cancer. Cancer Res 49:2087–2090
20. McCann A, Dervan PA, Johnston PA, Gullick WJ, Carney DN (1990) c-erbB-2 oncoprotein expression in primary human tumors. Cancer 65:88–92
21. Paik S, Hazan R, Fisher ER, Sass RE, Fisher B, Redmond C, Schlessinger J, Lippman ME, King CR (1990) Pathologic findings from the national surgical adjuvant breast and bowel project: prognostic significance of erbB-2 protein overexpression in primary breast cancer. J Clin Oncol 8:103–112
22. Uehara T, Kaneko Y, Kanda N, Yamamoto T, Higashi Y, Nomoto C, Izumo T, Takayama S, Sakurai M (1990) c-erbB-2 and c-erbA-1 (ear-1) gene amplification and c-erbB-2 protein expression in Japanese breast cancers: their relationship to the histology and other disease parameters. Jpn J Cancer Res 81:620–624
23. Borg A, Baldetorp B, Ferno M, Killander D, Olsson H, Siggurdsson H (1991) ERBB2 amplification in breast cancer with a high rate of proliferation. Oncogene 6:137–143
24. Clark GM, McGuire WL (1991) Follow-up study of HER-2/neu amplification in primary breast cancer. Cancer Res 51:944–948
25. Slamon DJ, Clark GM, Won SG, Levin WJ, Ullrich A, McGuire WL (1987) Human breast cancer: correlation of relapse and survival with amplification of the HER-2/neu oncogene. Science 235:177–182
26. Barnes DM, Lammie GA, Millis RR, Gullick WL, Allen DS, Altman DG (1988) An immunohistochemical evaluation of c-erbB-2 expression in human breast carcinoma. Br J Cancer 58:448–452
27. Gusterson BA, Machin LG, Gullick WL, Gibbs NM, Powles TJ, Elliott C, Ashley S, Monaghan P, Harrison S (1988) c-erbB-2 expression in benign and malignant breast disease. Br J Cancer 58:453–457
28. Zhou D-J, Ahuja H, Cline MJ (1989) Proto-oncogene abnormalities in human breast cancer: c-ERBB-2 amplification does not correlate with recurrence of disease. Oncogene 4:105–108
29. Paterson MC, Dietrich KD, Danyluk J, Paterson AHG, Lees AW, Jamil N, Hanson J, Jenkins H, Krause BE, McBlain WA Slamon DJ, Fourney RM (1991) Correlation between c-erbB-2 amplification and risk of recurrent disease in node-negative breast cancer. Cancer Res 51:556–567
30. Berchuk A, Kamel A, Whitaker R, Kerns B, Olt G, Kinney R, Soper JT, Dodge R, Clarke-Pearson DL, Marks P, McKenzie S, Yin S, Bast RC (1990) Overexpression of HER-2/neu is associated with poor survival in advanced epithelial ovarian cancer. Cancer Res 50:4087–4091
31. Weiner DB, Nordberg J, Robinson R, Nowell PC, Gadzar A, Greene MI, Williams WV, Cohen JA, Kern JA (1990) Expression of the neu gene-encoded protein (p185neu) in human non-small cell carcinomas of the lung. Cancer Res 50:421–425
32. Kameda T, Yasui W, Yoshida K, Tsujino T, Nakayama H, Ito M, Ito H, Tahara E (1990) Expression of ERBB2 in human gastric carcinomas: relationship between p185ERBB2 expression and the gene amplification. Cancer Res 50:8002–8009
33. Yonemura Y, Ninomiya I, Yamaguchi A, Fushida S, Kimura H, Ohoyama S, Miyazaki I, Endou Y, Tanaka M, Sasaki T (1991) Evaluation of immunoreactivity for erbB-2 as a marker of poor short-term prognosis in gastric cancer. Cancer Res 51:1034–1038
34. Zhau HE, Zhang X, von Eschenbach AC, Scorsone K, Babaian RJ, Ro JY, Hung M-C (1990) Amplification and expression of the c-erbB-2/neu proto-oncogene in human bladder cancer. Molecular Carcinogenesis 3:254–257

Address for correspondence:
Dr. Ellen Sampson
Ciba Corning Diagnostics Corp.
1401 Harbor Bay Parkway
Alameda, California, 94502 USA

Measurement of the extracellular domain of the c-*erb*B-2 oncoprotein in sera of breast cancer patients

Y. Teramoto, Kristine Konrad

Triton Laboratories, Ciba Corning Diagnostics Corp., Alameda, CA, USA

Introduction

The c-*erb*B-2 oncogene, also referred to as HER-2 or neu, was independently identified in DNA studies from chemically induced rat neuroblastomas (1) and in cross-hybridisation studies with v-*erb*B and human epidermal growth factor receptor (EGFR) DNAs (2–4). The c-*erb*B-2 oncogene is found on band q21 of chromosome 17 in humans (2) and encodes a 185 kD glycoprotein with extensive homology to EGFR (2–6). The c-*erb*B-2 gene product has an intracellular domain, a transmembrane region and cysteine-rich extracellular domain, and, like EGFR, the c-*erb*B-2 protein has tyrosine kinase activity (7). The c-*erb*B-2 protein is believed to be a cellular receptor for a newly described growth factor (8, 9).

Amplification of the c-*erb*B-2 gene or c-*erb*B-2 protein overexpression has been shown to occur in 10–46% of primary human breast cancers (10). The average amplification or overexpression rate was 20% when almost 3,000 breast cancer patients were considered as a combined total population for analysis. The prognostic significance of c-*erb*B-2 amplification in breast cancer has been the focus of numerous studies. Although the results are still somewhat controversial, more evidence is accumulating suggesting that c-*erb*B-2 is a significant prognostic indicator in node negative and node positive breast cancer.

The extracellular domain of the c-*erb*B-2 protein has been found to be released into culture supernatants from cell lines, such as SK-BR-3, MKN7, and ZR-75-1, known to overexpress the c-*erb*B-2 protein (11, 12). The extracellular c-*erb*B-2 protein has been shown to have a molecular weight of 105–110 kD, a value that is in agreement with the predicted size of the extracellular domain of the full-length gp185 protein. It has also been demonstrated that immunisation of concentrated SK-BR-3 culture fluid into mice resulted in the generation of antibodies that were immunoreactive with the full-length c-*erb*B-2 protein (11). This finding suggests that the extracellular c-*erb*B-2 protein found in the SK-BR-3 culture fluid is immunologically similar to the full-length c-*erb*B-2 gene product, gp185.

Detection of the extracellular domain of the c-*erb*B-2 protein has potential diagnostic and prognostic utility in those human malignancies that overexpress this gene product. In recent investigations, EIAs specific for c-*erb*B-2 have been used to detect the extracellular domain of c-*erb*B-2 in mouse and monkey sera (13) and in sera from human metastatic breast cancer patients (12). In the present study, we describe the measurement of the extracellular domain of the c-*erb*B-2 oncoprotein in the sera of breast cancer patients by use of the Triton Laboratories c-*erb*B-2 serum EIA kit.

Methods

Preoperative serum samples were collected 1–2 days before surgery and were frozen at –70 °C until assayed. Serum samples were also taken during follow-up visits to the Department of Oncology and Radiotherapy, University of Tampere, Tampere, Finland. Clinical status and follow-up data for the cancer patients were derived retrospectively from medical records without knowledge of the assay results. Serum samples were also obtained from randomly selected patients with malignant or benign breast disease or from healthy females. All human serum samples were obtained in accordance with standard patient consent procedures. Sera were maintained at −70 °C until tested.

Serum c-erbB-2 was measured using the serum c-erbB-2 EIA kit developed by Triton Laboratories, Ciba Corning Diagnostics Corp. All reagents necessary to perform the assay are included in the kit. Briefly, undiluted serum (50 µl) was added to duplicate streptavidin coated tubes containing 200 µl of serum sample diluent. The diluted sample was mixed and 200 µl of combined monoclonal antibody (MAb) conjugates were added to each tube. The combined MAb solution contains a horseradish peroxidase labeled MAb (TAb 257) and a fluorescein isothiocyanate (FITC) labeled MAb (TAb 259) both specific for the c-erbB-2 oncoprotein. After a 2 h incubation at room temperature, immune complexes were linked to the coated tube by the addition of 200 µl of biotinylated anti-FITC MAb and the incubation continued for another 2 h. The tubes were then washed three times with wash buffer included in the kit and allowed to drain briefly. The colorimetric reaction was initiated by the addition of 3, 3' 5, 5' tetramethylbenzidine and H_2O_2. After 25 min the reaction was stopped by the addition of 1 M phosphoric acid. The absorbance was measured with a Chem-Stat spectrophotometer (Source Scientific Instruments) using dual wavelengths of 450 nm and 650 nm. Unit per ml values for the test samples were determined from a curve generated with reference calibrators included in the kit.

Results

Assay performance

The calibration curve for the immunoassay was linear from 0 µ/ml to 240 µ/ml with an r-value equal to 0.99995. Imprecision measured at three different µ/ml levels gave within run CV% ranging from 4.04% to 5.99% and between run CV% ranging from 4.12% to 5.39%. The total CV% ranged from 5.83% to 8.06%. Interoperator CV% ranged from 4.70% to 6.40%. Assay linearity as determined by sample dilution showed less than 2% deviation from expected values and recovery ranged from 93.5% to 108.9%. The minimum detectable concentration for the assay was 2.4 µml

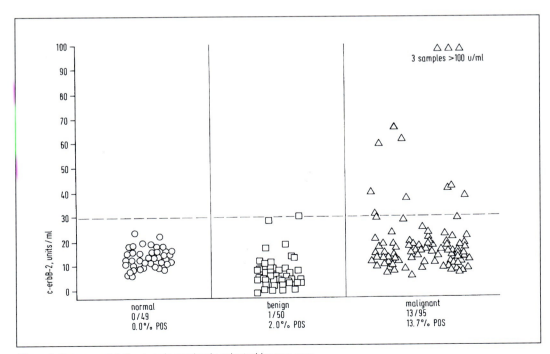

Figure 1. Serum c-erbB-2 values in randomly selected human sera.

Table I. Elevated c-*erb*B-2 in preoperative serum of breast cancer patients. Serum expression (%) with elevated levels (no. elevated/no. tested).

Tissue expression	Stage I	Stage II	Stage III	All stages
c-*erb*B-2 negative	2.5% (1/40)	0% (0/26)	0% (0/1)	1.5% (1/67)
c-*erb*B-2 positive	5.3% (1/19)	26% (6/23)	60% (3/5)	21% (10/47)
All tumors	3.4% (2/59)	12% (6/49)	50% (3/6)	9.6% (11/114)

and there was no hook effect observed with samples spiked with greater than 2500 µ/ml of c-*erb*B-2. The assay was specific for c-*erb*B-2 and showed no reactivity to EGFR, HMFG, TAG-72, CEA, or ras and myc oncoproteins. Additionally, sera that had elevated levels of CA 15-3 or CEA, or increased quantities of bilirubin or hemoglobin did not react in the assay unless they also contained elevated levels of c-*erb*B-2. Immunoreactivity of certain sera were confirmed by Western blotting (data not shown).

Serum samples

Randomly selected sera from patients with breast cancer or benign breast disease or from normal women of either pre- or post menopausal status were assayed in the serum EIA (figure 1). At a cut-off value of 30 units/ml none of 49 (0%) normal sera and only 1 of 50 (2%) sera from benign breast cancer patients were positive, while 13 of 95 (13.7%) malignant breast cancer patients were positive. Lowering the cut-off value to 20 units/ml increased the positive rate for the malignant breast cancer patients to 24% (23 of 95), and the rates for the normal and benign groups increased to 4% (2 of 49) and 4% (2 of 50), respectively.

Preoperative serum samples from breast cancer patients showed similar levels of positivity (table I). The overall positive rate for this group was 9.6% (11 of 114). Most of the serum c-*erb*B-2 positive patients had an advanced disease stage. In addition, all but one of the serum positive patients were also tissue positive for c-*erb*B-2. Serum c-*erb*B-2 levels were measured in 339 samples taken during follow-up of 225 breast cancer patients (figure 2). A total of 63 samples (19%) showed elevated values. Only 9% (17 of 189) of samples from patients without recurrent

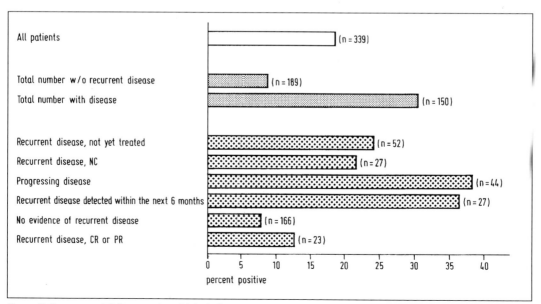

Figure 2. Serum c-*erb*B-2 percent positivity in breast cancer patients with and without recurrent desease.

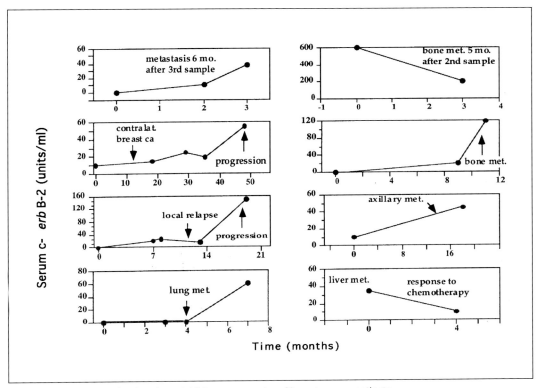

Figure 3. Serum c-erbB-2 values in serial follow-up samples of breast cancer patients.

disease showed elevated serum c-erbB-2, however, 31% (46 of 150) of patients with recurrent disease were elevated for c-erbB-2. Elevated serum c-erbB-2 was most prevalent (14 of 44; 39%) in patients who had progressing disease despite treatment. Patients with recurrent disease either not yet treated (13 of 52; 25%) or with no change (6 of 27; 22%) or whose recurrent disease was detected within the next six months (10 of 27; 37%) had the next highest prevalence of serum c-erbB-2 positivity. Only 3 of 23 (13%) patients samples with complete or partial response to therapy had elevated values.

Changes in serum c-erbB-2 values during the disease course were studied in detail in patients from whom multiple follow-up samples were available (figure 3). Elevated serum c-erbB-2 levels were associated with recurrent disease that was either evident at the time the sample was taken or appeared later. In one case, a decrease in serum c-erbB-2 was found after a partial response to chemotherapy.

Conclusions

Elevated levels of c-erbB-2 can be measured in the sera of breast cancer patients with an immunoassay kit developed by Triton Laboratories, Ciba Corning Diagnostics Corp. The assay is highly specific and sensitive and can be used to reliably measure the »shed« external domain portion of the c-erbB-2 oncoprotein. Approximately 10–15% of breast cancer patients show elevated values of c-erbB-2. It is important to keep in mind, that unlike previously described tumor markers, c-erbB-2 is a prognostic indicator which may be useful in the management of disease for a subset of all breast cancer patients. Elevated values of serum c-erbB-2 may indicate a higher probability of recurrent disease or metastases (14) or resistance or sensitivity to endocrine therapy (15). Further clinical studies need to be undertaken in order to validate the utility of measuring c-erbB-2 in the serum of breast cancer patients.

References

1. Schechter AL, Stern DF, Vaidyanathan L, Decker SJ, Drebin JA, Greene MI, Weinberg RA (1984) The neu oncogene: an erbB-related gene encoding a 185,000-Mr tumor antigen. Nature 312:513–516
2. Coussens L, Yang-Fen TL, Liao Y-C, Chen E, Gray A, McGrath J, Seeburg PH, Libermann TA, Schlessinger J, Francke U, Levinson A, Ullrich A (1985) Tyrosine kinase receptor with extensive homology to EGF receptor shares chromosomal location with neu oncogene. Science 230:1132–1139
3. King CR, Kraus MH, Aaronson SA (1985) Amplification of a novel v-erbB-related gene in human mammary carcinoma. Science 229:974–976
4. Semba K, Kamata N, Toyoshima K, Yamamoto T (1985) A v-erbB-related proto-oncogene, c-erbB-2 is distinct from c-erbB-1/epidermal growth factor receptor gene and is amplified in a human salivary gland adenocarcinoma. Proc Natl Acad Sci USA 82:6497–6501
5. Schechter AL, Hung M-C, Vaidyanathan L, Weinberg RA, Yang-Fen TL, Francke U, Ullrich A, Coussens L (1985) The neu-gene: an erbB homologous gene distinct from and unlinked to the gene encoding the EGF receptor. Science 229:976–978
6. Yamamoto T, Ikawa S, Akiyama T, Semba K, Nomura N, Miyajima N, Saito T, Toyoshima K (1986) Similarity of protein encoded by the human c-erbB-2 gene to epidermal growth factor receptor. Nature 319:230–234
7. Akiyama T, Sudo C, Ogawara H, Toyoshima K, Yamamoto T (1986) The product of the human c-erbB-2 gene: a 185-kilodalton glycoprotein with tyrosine kinase activity. Science 232:1644–1646
8. Lupu R, Colomer R, Kannan B, Lippman ME (1992) Characterisation of a growth factor that binds exclusively to the erbB-2 receptor and induces cellular responses. Proc Natl Acad Sci USA 89: 2287–2291
9. Holmes WE, Sliwkowski MX, Akita RW, Henzel WJ, Lee J, Park JW, Yansura D, Abadi N, Raab H, Lewis GD, Shepard HM, Kuang W, Wood WI, Goeddel DV, Vandlen RL (1992) Identification of Heregulin, a specific activator of p185 erbB2. Science 256: 1205–1210
10. Clark GM, McGuire WL (1991) Follow-up study of HER-2/neu amplification in primary breast cancer. Cancer Res 51:944–948
11. Alper O, Yamaguchi K, Hitomi J, Honda S, Matsushima T, Abe K (1990) The presence of c-erbB-2 gene product-related protein in culture medium conditioned by breast cancer cell line SK-BR-3. Cell Growth and Differentiation 1:591–599
12. Mori S, Mori Y, Mukaiyama T, Yamada Y, Sonobe Y, Matsushita H, Sakamoto G, Akiyama T, Ogawa M, Shiraishi M, Toyoshima K, Yamamoto T (1990) In vitro and in vivo release of soluble erbB-2 protein from human carcinoma cells. Jpn J Cancer Res 81: 489–494
13. Sias PE, Kotts CE, Vetterlein D, Shepar M, Wong WLT (1990) ELISA for quantitation of the extracellular domain of p185HER2 in biological fluids. J Immunol Meth 132:73–80
14. Narita T, Funahishi H, Satoh F, Takagi H (1992) C-erbB-2 protein in the sera of breast cancer patients. Breast Cancer Res and Treat 24:97–102
15. Wright C, Nicholson S, Angus B, Sainsbury JRC, Farndon J, Cairns J, Harris AL, Horne CHW (1992) Relationship between c-erbB-2 protein product expression and response to endocrine therapy in advanced breast cancer. Br J Cancer 65:118–121

Address for correspondence:
Dr. Y. Teramoto
Ciba Corning Diagnostics Corp.
1401 Harbor Bay Parkway
Alameda, California, 94502, USA

In: R. Klapdor (ed)
Current Tumor Diagnosis: Applications, Clinical Relevance, Research, Trends
Cancer of the Lung – State and Trends in Diagnosis and Therapy
© 1994 W. Zuckschwerdt Verlag München · Bern · Wien · New York

Comparision of the epidermal growth factor receptor (EGF-R) and of Her-2/neu protein ($p^{185/Her2}$) expression in breast cancer

M. W. Beckmann [1,a], A. Scharl [b], B. Tutschek [a], U. J. Göhring [b], G. Schenko [a], A. Beckmann [a], D. Niederacher [a], H. G. Schnürch [2,b]

[a] Women's Clinic, Heinrich-Heine-University, Düsseldorf,
[b] Women's Clinic, University of Cologne, Germany

Introduction

The decision for adjuvant therapy of breast cancer patients is mainly based on histomorphologic criteria (1–4), but functional tumor characteristics including steroid receptor status (estrogen (ER) and progesterone receptor (PgR)) proved to have prognostic significance and relevance for therapeutic decisions (2–5). Other functional tumor characteristics, including factors involved in tumor invasion and promotion of tumor growth, are currently under investigation (3, 6). These factors include the family of epidermal growth factor receptors, c-erbB, which consists of four members (7–9) (table I). Analyses of the level of expression of the epidermal growth factor receptor (EGF-R) and the Her-2/neu protein ($p^{185/Her2}$) in breast cancer tumors may add information about the prognosis of individual patients. Furthermore, the use of monoclonal antibodies directed against EGF-R or $p^{185/Her2}$ as therapeutic tools (e.g., MAb 425 or 4D5) require reliable evaluation of the EGF-R or $p^{185/Her2}$ content. Different routine analytical methods have been published, including 1. biochemical detection of EGF-R using ^{125}I EGF or, 2. immunohistochemical EGF-R or $p^{185/Her2}$ detection on frozen sections. Various studies evaluating $p^{185/Her2}$ expression in formalin-fixed and paraffin-embedded tissues are published, but evaluation of EGF-R expression as well as comparative studies in the same material are rare (10). We therefore analyzed EGF-R and $p^{185/Her2}$ expression in 142 formalin-fixed and paraffin-embedded breast cancer specimens and 12 benign breast samples by immunohistochemistry. Simultaneously, estrogen (ER) and progesteron (PgR) immunohistochemistry was performed on sections of the same tumors. Various cell lines and normal skin tissue samples served as positive or negative controls. Results of the two expression analyses were compared with other biological characteristics of the tumors including histological grade, tumor size, lymphnode metastases and menopause. In this study, the determination of EGF-R or $p^{185/Her2}$ in formalin-fixed, paraffin-embedded tumor samples proved to be feasable.

Materials and methods

Paraffin-embedded, formalin-fixed sections from 142 patients treated with surgery for primary breast cancer and 12 patients with benign breast tumors (January 1980 until December 1985) were analyzed. In case of axillary dissection, the number of lymph node metastasis was determined. Hematoxylin-eosin staining was performed for routine pathological evaluation (diameter, margins, grading, histologic typing). EGF-R and $p^{185/Her2}$ expression was correlated with menopausal status, tumor size, number of lymph node metastases, histological grading, and immunohistochemical determined ER or PgR expression.

---
[1] Grant (Be 1215/6-1) from Deutsche Forschungsgemeinschaft, Bonn, Germany.
[2] Grant (Be 1068/2-1) from Deutsche Forschungsgemeinschaft, Bonn, and MERCK Inc., Darmstadt, Germany.

Table I. Molecular characteristics of the *erb*B-family.

Gene	c-*erb*B1	c-*erb*B2	c-*erb*B3	c-*erb*B4
Chromosom location	7p12	17q21	12q13	?
Open reading frame	3558 bp	3768 bp	4026 bp	3712 bp
Protein	EGFR	HER2/neu	HER3	HER4
Aminoacids	1186	1256	1342	1247
Molecular weight	133.000 D	138.000 D	148.000 D	144.000 D
App. molecular weight	170.000 D	185.000 D	?	180.000 D
Autophosphorylation	Tyrosin 1173	Tyrosin 1248	?	?
Homology in tyrosin kinase domain	100%	83%	60%	79 %
ligand(s)	EGF TGFα amphiregulin	gp30.000 heregulin	cripto (?) amphiregulin (?)	heparin-binding factor
Transform. potence	dominant	dominant	dominant	dominant
Overexpression	16–30%	10–33%	30%	?
Gene amplification	4%	> 90%	?	?

Cell cultures of A431, BT 20 and MCF-7 cell lines

Human vulvar carcinoma cell line A431 (high EGF-R expression), breast cancer cell lines SKBR3 (high $p^{185/Her2}$ expression), and MCF-7 (no EGF-R or $p^{185/Her2}$ overexpression), were cultured as previously described (8, 11, 12). For immunohistochemical determinations, different cell lines were cultured on sterile culture slides.

Steroid receptor (ER, PgR) analyses

ER- and PgR-status were determined by immunohistochemistry as described previously by *Scharl* et al. (13). The peroxidase–anti-peroxidase (PAP)-method using either 1. ER antibody from the ER-ICA Monoclonalkit (Abbott) as primary antibody with rabbit–anti-rat IgG-Ab as secondary antibody (Vector Laboratories) or 2. PgR mPR (Dianova) as primary antibody with sheep–anti-mouse IgG-Ab (Vector Laboratories) as secondary antibody. For staining procedure, the PAP-Kit Komplex (ABC Elite-Kit Vectastain, Vector Laboratories) was used, counter staining was performed with hematoxylin. Immunohistochemical reaction was scored according to the recommendations of *Remmele* and *Stegner* (16), the immunoreactive score ranged from 0 to 12.

Immunohistochemical detection of EGF-R

EGF-R expression was determined by immunohistochemistry as described previously by *Beckmann* et al. (14). Primary antibody was MAb E30, detection was performed by the streptavidin-peroxidase-method using the TissuGnost® Uni-Pak-Detektion systems (Firma Merck). Semiquantitative scoring was applied according to *Lewis* et al. (15) modified by *Beckmann* et al. (14).

Immunohistochemical detection of $p^{185/Her2}$

$p^{185/Her2}$ expression was determined by immunohistochemistry as described previously by *Göhring* et al. (17). The peroxidase–anti-peroxidase (PAP)-method was applied using c-*erb*B-2 mAb (Triton Diagnostics) as primary antibody, pig–anti-rabbit IgG-Ab as secondary antibody (DAKO). Semiquantitative scoring was applied according to *Göhring* et al. (17).

Statistics

Qualitative analyses of ER, PgR, EGF-R, $p^{185/He2}$, and other prognostic factors were performed by chi-square contingency table or exact Fisher's test; quantitative analyses between EGF-R or $p^{185/Her2}$ and ER or PgR expression were performed with a rank correlation test.

Table II. Relationship between ER-, PgR-, EFG-R, and $p^{185/Her2}$ measured by immunohistochemical analyses in human breast cancer specimens (n = 142).

Number total (n = 142)		$p^{185/Her2}$ negative (113/142)	$p^{185/Her2}$ positive (29/142)	Statistics: chi-square test
ER				
negative	61	46	15	
positive	81	67	14	n.s.
PgR				
negative	72	56	16	
positive	70	57	13	n.s.
Number total (n=142)		EGF-R negative (90/142)	EGF-R positive (52/142)	Statistics: chi-square test
ER				
negative	61	38	23	
positive	81	52	29	n.s.
PgR				
negative	72	51	21	
positive	70	39	31	n.s.
EGF-R				
negative	90	73	17	
positive	52	40	12	n.s.
		ER negative (61/142)	ER positive (81/142)	
PgR				
negative	72	44	28	
positive	70	17	53	$p < 0,001$

n.s. = $p > 0.05$

Results

Our study group included 53 women aged below 50 years (premenopausal) and 89 women ≥ 50 years (postmenopausal). Age rage was 31 to 76 years.
Twelve benign tumors of the breast including fibroadenomas and mastophatic lesions were evaluated for EGF-R or $p^{185/Her2}$. Stromal cells and ductal epithelium were EGF-R or $p^{185/Her2}$ negative in nearly all cases, only the myoepithelial cells showed faint EGF-R staining in five cases. EGF-R immunostaining of EGF-R positive carcinoma was not restricted to tumor cells, but also myoepithelial cells, fibroblasts and epithelium cells of normal ducts were highly positive in a few cases. The staining was mainly restricted to the membrane, but in some tumors a perinuclear or nuclear staining could be seen.
EGF-R and $p^{185/Her2}$ expression determined by immunohistochemistry were compared with various characteristics of the patients. There were no significant correlations between EGF-R and patients' age or $p^{185/Her2}$ expression and menopause, number of positive lymph nodes, and tumor grade. EGF-R expression was significantly correlated with increasing tumor size, lymph node metastases and higher histological grade; $p^{185/Her2}$ was significantly correlated with tumor size, only.
Table II demonstrates the correlations between EGF-R, $p^{185/Her2}$, ER, and PgR. Correlations between EGF-R or $p^{185/Her2}$ and ER or PgR were not significant. The relation between ER and PgR was significant ($p < 0.001$).

Discussion

Members of the erbB-family have been proposed to have relevance for patients with breast cancer. Klijn et al. (10) tried to summarize the results of the EGF-R analyses of more than 40 individual groups of investigators. The clinical impact of EGF-R was critically reviewed, but still it has been proposed as being a prognostic factor (18–20), an indicator of response to hormonal therapy (21), and, possibly, a target for blocking or cytotoxic agents (22). In node positive breast cancer patients, Her-2/neu overexpression indicates decreased disease free and overall survival (23–25), and is thought to be correlated with resistance to hormonal and chemotherapy (26, 27).

Overexpression of the two proteins have been reported to vary between 14–38%. These values are consistent with our own data as well as the distribution of different patients' characteristics including tumor size, number of patients with lymph node metastases, histological grade. It has been established that there is an inverse relationship between expression of the sex steroid receptor proteins and EGF-R or $p^{185/Her2}$ (11, 23–27). Patients with positive steroid receptor status are considered to have an improved prognosis (2, 5), whereas overexpression of EGF-R or $p^{185/Her2}$ is associated with a poor prognosis (15, 18, 19, 26, 27). We were able to confirm the previously described relationship of the presence of EGF-R and negative ER and PgR expression in the A431 cell-line (12) or $p^{185/Her2}$ and negative ER and PgR expression in the SKBR3 cell-line analyzed (11). In human tumors from our clinical study group, the inverse relationship could not be confirmed, even though ER and PgR correlated significantly. Positive EGF-R or $p^{185/Her2}$ staining showed no significant difference in disease free and overall survival.

In accordance with other groups (28, 29), EGF-R and $p^{185/Her2}$ staining was not restricted to tumor cells, but occasionally found in myoepithelial and stromal cells. Furthermore, in malignant cells as well as the reference cell-line BT20 EGF-R was partially localized in the cytoplasm (28, 29). This could reflect intracellular production of the receptor protein or internalization of the receptor via receptor mediated endocytosis. During the later process, both, the EGF and the receptor are found in coated vesicles with the ultimate destination directed towards the lysosome for degradation. $p^{185/Her2}$ could not be demonstrated in the cytoplasm. EGF-R and $p^{185/Her2}$ expression within a tumor can be heterogenic reflecting the influence of various exogenous growth factors, and autocrine, juxtacrine, or paracrine mechanisms, which are involved in the induction and maintenance of malignant transformation and growth control (30). Molecular interactions among the various cell-regulatory and biological mechanisms of growth factors and steroid receptor expression are still unclear. Dickson et al. (31) showed that physiological proliferation is under endocrine control by induction of autocrine growth factors. With the malignant differentiation of the tumor this regulatory mechanism is abolished, proliferation is now independent of endocrine control and is directed mainly by mechanisms mediated by growth factor receptors (including EGF-R or $p^{185/Her2}$).

References

1 Scarff RW, Torloni H (1968) Histological typing of breast tumors. International Histological Classification of Tumors No. 2, World Health Organization, Geneva
2 Early Breast Cancer Trialists' Collaborative Group (1992) Systemic treatment of early breast cancer by hormonal, cytotoxic, or immune therapy. Lancet 329:1–15
3 McGuire WL, Clark GM (1992) Prognostic factors factors and treatment decisions in axillary node-negative breast cancer. N Engl J Med 326: 1756–1761
4 Harris JR, Lippman ME, Veronesi U, Willett W (1992) Breast cancer (First of three parts). N Engl J Med 327:319–328
5 Pertschuk LP, Kim DS, Nayer K et al (1990) Immunocytochemical estrogen and progestin receptor assays in breast cancer with monoclonal antibodies. Cancer 66:1663–1670
6 Harris JR, Lippman ME, Veronesi U, Willett W (1992) Breast cancer (Third of three parts). N Engl J Med 327:473–480
7 Downward J, Yarden Y, Mayes E et al (1984) Close similarity of epidermal growth factor receptor and v-erb-B oncogene protein sequence. Nature 307:521–527
8 Niederacher D, Beckmann MW, Scharl A, Picard F, Schnürch HG, Bender HG (1993) Biochemische und molekulargenetische Analyse von Onkogenen der c-erb-Familie in Mammakarzinomen. Tumorimmunologie in der Gynäkologie. In: Koldovsky U, Kreienberg R (eds) Aktuelle Onkologie (D). Zuckschwerdt, München (D) 79:73–78
9 Kraus MH, Issing W, Miki T et al (1989) Isolation and characterization of ERBB3, a third member of the ERBB/epidermal growth factor receptor family: evidence for overexpression in a subset of human mammary tumors. Proc Natl Acad Sci USA 86:9193–9197
10 Klijn JGM, Berns PMJJ, Schmitz PIM, Foekens JA (1992) The clinical significance of epidermal growth factor receptor (EGF-R) in human breast cancer: a review on 5232 patients. Endocrine Rev 13:3–17

11 Beckmann MW, Toney LJ, Scharl A (1992) Detection of the HER-2/neu proto-oncogene protein $p^{185erbB2}$ by a novel monoclonal antibody (MAB-145ww) in breast cancer membranes from estrogen and progesterone receptor assays. Eur J Cancer 28:322–326

12 Beckmann MW, Stegmüller M, Niederacher D et al (1993) Modifications of the routine biochemical analysis of the epidermal growth factor receptor (EGF-R) on breast tumor specimens. Tumordiagn u Ther 14:41–48

13 Scharl A, Vierbuchen M, Würz H (1989) Immunohistochemischer Nachweis von Östrogen- und Progesteronrezeptoren mit Hilfe monoklonaler Antikörper in Mammakarzinomgeweben. Vergleich mit der biochemischen Rezeptoranalyse. Pathologe 10:31–38

14 Beckmann MW, Tutschek B, Göhring UJ et al (1994) Immunhistochemischer Nachweis des 'epidermal growth factor receptor (EGF-R)' in Paraffin-eingebetteten Mammakarzinomgeweben: Korrelation und klinische Wertigkeit. Geburtsh Frauenheilk, in press.

15 Lewis S, Locker A, Todd JH et al (1990) Expression of epidermal growth factor receptor in breast carcinoma. J Clin Pathol 43:385–389

16 Remmele W, Stegner HG (1986) Immunohistochemischer Nachweis von Östrogenrezeptoren (ER-ICA) im Mammakarzinomgewebe: Vorschlag zur einheitlichen Formulierung des Untersuchungsbefundes. Deutsches Ärzteblatt 48:3362–3364

17 Göhring UJ, Vierbuchen M, Scharl A (1993) Der immunhistochemische Nachweis des Onkoproteins $p^{185erbB2}$ – Marker einer ungünstigen Prognose beim primären Mammakarzinom. Tumordiagn Ther 14, in press.

18 Sainsbury JRC, Malcolm AJ, Appleton DR et al (1985) Presence of epidermal growth factor receptors as an indicator for poor prognosis in patients with breast cancer. J Clin Pathol 38:1225–1231

19 Sainsbury JRC, Farndon JR, Needham GK et al (1987) Epidermal growth factor receptor status as a predictor of relapse and death from breast cancer. Lancet 1:1398–1402

20 Scharl A, Göhring UJ, Vierbuchen M et al (1990) Epidermal growth factor receptor (EGF-R) – a marker for morphological and functional anaplasia in human breast carcinoma. Geburtsh Frauenheilk 50:877–882

21 Nicholson S, Sainsbury JRC, Needham GK et al (1988) Quantitative assays of epidermal growth factor receptor in human breast cancer: cut-off points of clinical relevance. Int J Cancer 42:36-41

22 Schnürch HG, Beckmann MW, Stegmüller M, Bender HG (1992) Growth inhibiton of human female genital and breast cancer tissues transplanted in nude mice by a monoclonal antibody (Mab 425) directed against the epidermal growth factor receptor. In: Klapdor R (ed) Tumor associated anigens, oncogenes, receptors, cytokines in tumor diagnosis and therapy at the beginning of the 90th. Zuckschwerdt, München, pp 621–624

23 Slamon DJ, Godolphin W, Jones LA, Holt JA et al (1989) Studies of the HER-2/neu protooncogene in human breast and ovarian cancer. Science 244:707–712

24 Wright C, Angus B, Nicholson S et al (1989) Expression of c-erbB-2 oncoprotein: a prognostic indicator in human breast cancer. Cancer Res 49:2087-2090

25 Zeilinger R, Kury F, Czerwenka K, Kubista E et al (1989) Her-2 amplification, steroid receptors and epidermal growth factor receptor in primary breast cancer. Oncogene 4:109–114

26 Berger MS, Locher GW, Saurer S, Gullick WJ et al (1988) Correlation of c-erbB2 gene amplification and protein expression in human breast carcinoma with nodal status and nuclear grading. Cancer Res 48:1238–1243

27 Roux-Dosseto M, Romain S, Dussault N (1989) $p^{185/Her2}$ and pS2 protein overexpression in breast cancer specimens: improvement for prediction of response to endocrine therapy? Biomed Pharmacother 43:641–649

28 Möller P, Mechertsheimer G et al (1989) Expression of epidermal growth factor receptor in benign and malignant primary tumors of the breast. Virchows Archiv A Pathol Anat 141:157–164

29 Umekita Y, Enokizono N et al (1992) Immunohistochemical studies on oncogene products (EGF-R, c-erbB-2) and growth factors (EGF, TGF-a) in human breast cancer: their relationship to oestrogen receptor status, histological grade, mitotic index and nodal status. Virchows Archiv A Pathol Anat 420:345–351

30 Beckmann MW, Niederacher D et al (1993) Die erbB-Gen-Familie: Bedeutung für die Tumorentwicklung, Prognose und für neue Therapiemodalitäten. Geburtsh Frauenheilk 11:742–753

31 Dickson RB, McManaway ME, Lippman ME (1986) Estrogen included factors of breast cancer cells partially replace estrogen to promote tumor growth. Science 232:1540–1543

Address for correspondence:
M. W. Beckmann, M.D.
Universitätsfrauenklinik
Heinrich-Heine-Universität
Moorenstraße 5
D-40225 Düsseldorf, Germany

Prognostic impact of c-*erb*B-2 oncoprotein overexpression in adenocarcinoma of the esophagus

H. Nekarda[a], T. Nakamura[a,c], A. H. Hoelscher[a], K. Becker[b], E. Bollschweiler[a], J.R. Siewert[a]

[a]Department of Surgery, [b]Institute of Pathology, Klinikum rechts der Isar, Technical University of Munich, Germany; [c]Department of Surgery, Institute of Gastroenterology, Tokyo Women's Medical College, Tokyo, Japan

Introduction

During the last two decades, a rising incidence of adenocarcinomas of the esophagus has been observed (1–3). In general, the prognosis for survival is poor, because most of these patients already have an advanced carcinoma at the time of diagnosis (4–7). However, patients with early carcinomas show a quite favorable long-term survival rate after surgery (6–9). Thus, depth of wall penetration and lymph node spread are the most relevant prognostic factors for overall survival (4, 6, 7). Recently, interest has focused on "tumor-biological" prognostic factors like "growth factors" in order to detect subgroups of differing prognosis.

The *cerb*B2 (or HER2/neu) gene encodes a transmembrane cell receptor protein, p185*erb*B-2, which is highly homologous to the epidermal growth factor (EGF) receptor and to c-*erb*B-3, a newly identified member of the growth factor receptor family with tyrosine kinase activity (10, 11). Recently, two ligands (gp3, p75) have been identified that induce receptor phosphorylation and clonogenetic growth of receptor overexpressing cells (12). C-*erb*B-2 gene amplification is found in various adenocarcinomas; it is associated with oncoprotein overexpression, resulting in a typical cell-membrane-associated immunohistochemical staining (13–18). C-*erb*B-2 alterations and prognostic impact were first investigated intensively in breast cancer (19, 20). In gastric carcinomas, c-*erb*B-2 overexpression has been linked to poor prognosis in advanced cancer (21, 22), but not in early cancer (23). Interestingly, there are two reports of c-*erb*B-2 overexpression associated with better prognosis (24, 25).

To our knowledge, the prognostic value of c-*erb*B-2 overexpression has not yet been reported in adenocarcinoma of the esophagus.

Patients, material and methods

Patients

The restrospective study (7/1982–12/1991) included 80 patients (73 men (91%) and 7 women; mean age 60.4 years (range : 38 to 76 years])) who underwent subtotal esophagectomy with regional lymphadenectomy for adenocarcinoma of the esophagus. None of the patients had adjuvant therapy. In 64 patients (80%), the tumor was removed by transmediastinal esophagectomy, whereas in 16 patients with tumor location in the distal part of the thoracic esophagus, an en-bloc esophagectomy was performed by a transthoracic approach (6, 7).
Specialized columnar metaplasia (Barrett's esophagus) was documented histologically in the resected specimens of 58 patients (72.5%). The other 22 patients, endoscopically and macroscopically suspected columnar metaplasia was not detected by microscopical examination. In nearly all of these cases, microscopic examination of those areas revealed carcinoma in situ of superficially spreading primary tumor (9). Depth of tumor invasion (pT), node involvement (pN), distant metastasis (pM), tumor stage, grading, and residual tumor (R) were determined according to the TNM classification system of esophageal cancer (UICC 1987) (26). In addition, each tumor was classified according to the types of Laurén (27) and WHO (28).

Survival was analyzed for those 62 patients who had an R0 resection (UICC) and survived at least three months after the operation. 16 patients (26%) were classified as stage I, 17 patients (27.5%) as stage II (IIa: n = 9 (14.5%); IIb: n = 8(13%)), 20 patients (32%) as stage III and 9 patients (14.5%) as stage IV. At present, 31 patients (50%) died due to tumor recurrence (median survival time: 15 months). One patient died by cardiac arrest with no implication for tumor relapse. Thirty patients (48%) are still alive. The follow-up period was 4 to 109 months (median 39 months). The median survival time of the 62 patients who had a complete resection (R0-UICC) was 43 months.

Immunohistochemical staining of c-erbB-2

The stored tumor material was reinvestigated and 3 μm sections were stained with the mouse monoclonal antibody NCL-CB11 (Boehringer Mannheim Biochemica, Mannheim/Germany) (29). This antibody recognizes a site near the C-terminus of the internal domain of the c-erbB-2 receptor protein. A slight modification of the alkaline phosphatase and anti-alkaline phosphatase (APAAP) method (30) was employed (31). Briefly, the sections were dewaxed, rehydrated, and washed in phosphate-buffered saline (PBS). The first antibody, diluted 1:20 (45μg / ml protein (32) (BCA-protein assay, Pierce Chemical Company, USA)), was applied at room temperature for two hours. Another section was incubated with the isotypic monoclonal antibody MOPC-21, diluted 1:200 (Sigma) to detect unspecific staining. After washing in PBS, sections were incubated with rabbit anti-mouse immunoglobulin (DAKO Patts, Copenhagen, Denmark) diluted 1:20, followed by incubation with APAAP complex (DAKO) at a dilution of 1:80. The slides were then incubated in an alkaline phosphatase substrate solution for 30 minutes. Negative controls in which PBS replaced the primary antibody were performed for every specimen to detect endogenous alkaline phosphatase activity. A previously identified, intensively stained tumor was used as a positive control. Only tumors showing intensive membrane staining (++) were designated positive for overexpression of the c-erbB-2 oncoprotein (17,29). No staining (-) or weak staining (+) were denoted "negative" or "normal" for expression of the c-erbB-2 oncoprotein. The percentage of tumor cells with positive staining was then estimated.

Statistics

Comparison of frequency in the two groups was performed using the Exact Fisher chi-square test. Continous variables were compared using the Mann-Whitney rank-sum test. The probability of survival was calculated for the different subgroups by the Kaplan-Meier method (33). Statistical differences in survival were evaluated by the Mantel-Cox test (34). The prognostic factors were evaluated by Cox's proportional hazard model with a log-linear risk function (35). The maximum-partial-likelihood ratio test (MPLR) was used in assessing the significant probability of each variable to enter or exit the model. All evaluations were carried out using BMDP Statistical Software, Cork, Ireland.

Results

C-erbB-2 oncoprotein overexpression

In 57 of 80 patients (71%), c-erbB-2 oncoprotein was detectable in immunohistochemical staining of the primary tumor. In 42 of 57 patients (74%), there was only a weak homogenous staining pattern (+) of the cytoplasm. In 15 of 80 patients (19%), c-erbB-2 oncoprotein was much more highly expressed in the cell membrane (++ = overexpression) (figure 1). Six of these 15 patients (40%) had a patchy staining pattern, but in general more than 40% of the tumor cells of the primary tumor were strongly positive. For subsequent statistical analysis, the weak protein expression (n = 42) and negative staining (n = 23) groups were combined, because their overall survival rates were indistinguishable according to Kaplan-Meier product limit survival analysis. Therefore, they were designated negative.

C-erbB-2 oncoprotein overexpression was significantly correlated with depth of tumor invasion (pT), lymph node involvement (pN), distant metastases (pM [Lym]) and tumor stage (table I). There was also a significant positive correlation between c-erbB-2 oncoprotein overexpression

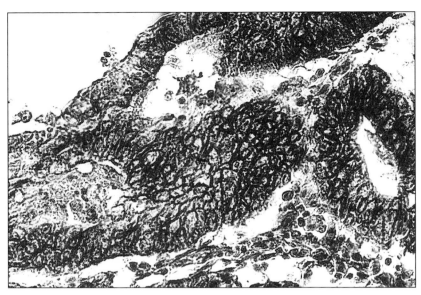

Figure 1.
Adenocarcinoma of Barrett's esophagus with intensive membrane staining of c-erbB-2 protein by MCA NCL-CB 11 (APAAP-staining, 100x).

and residual tumor status. Only 8 of 65 patients (12%) with R0-resection had c-erbB-2 oncoprotein overexpression, in contrast to 7 of 15 (47%) with residual tumor following resection. Only one of the early Barrett's carcinomas had an overexpression of c-erbB-2 oncoprotein, but this tumor demonstrated node involvement. No significant correlation was seen between c-erbB-2 oncoprotein overexpression and tumor grading, Laurén-classification, size or Barrett-metaplasia.

Survival analysis

Survival analysis was performed in those 62 patients who had a R0-resection and survived more than three months after operation. Size of tumor, depth of invasion (pT), node status (pN), distant lymphatic node metastases (pM[lym]) and c-erbB-2 oncoprotein overexpression were significant prognostic variables in univariate survival analysis (table II). The survival curves according to c-erbB-2 overexpression are shown in figure 2. All but one of the patients with c-erbB-2 oncoprotein overexpression died within two years. The median survival time of the patients with weak or negative c-erbB-2 oncoprotein expression was 48 months. In multivariate survival analyses, depth of tumor invasion (pT1,2/T3,4), distant metastases (pM [lym]) and c-erbB-2 overexpression were independent prognostic parameters. The relative risk computed by the Cox regression model was 7.3-fold for distant lymphatic node metastases, 5,9-fold for cancer invasion below the muscularis layer and 3.3-fold for overexpression of c-erbB-2 (Table II). In the subgroup of the 53 pM0-R0 resected patients (85%) depth of tumor invasion (pT1,2/T3,4) (RR: 5.7-fold) and c-erbB2 overexpression (RR: 3.1-fold) were the only independent prognostic factors, whereas in the subgroup of the 26 node negative patients (42%) non of these factors were significantly associated with survival.

Discussion

It is well known that gene amplification of c-erbB-2 in adenocarcinoma is associated with an overexpressed protein content in the cell membrane, which can easily be detected immunohistochemically using monoclonal antibodies (17, 19, 29). Most experiments concerning the significance of c-erbB-2 are available from studies in breast cancer. At present, prognostic relevance of gene amplification and oncoprotein overexpression is confined to node-positive and subsets of node-negative breast carcinomas (19, 20, 36).
The rate of patients with an amplified c-erbB-2 gene is lower in gastric cancer, ranging from 6% (37,38) to 12% (13), than in breast cancer, with a mean of 20% and a range 10% – 46% (review of

Table I. c-erbB-2 protein overexpression in relation to the criteria of staging (UICC, 1987) and histomorphological criteria in adenocarcinoma the esophagus (n = 80).

Variables (Categories)	Patients n (%)	c-erbB-2 positive n = 15 (19%)	c-erbB-2 negative n = 65 (81%)	p-value[a]
Primary tumor (pT)				
T1	19 (24)	1	18	
T2	13 (16)	1	12	
T3	31 (39)	6	25	
T4	17 (21)	7	10	<0.05
Nodal status (pN)				
N0	28 (35)	0	28	
N1	52 (65)	15	37	<0.05
Distant metastasis (pM)				
M0	59 (74)	6	53	
M1(Lym)	21 (26)	9	12	<0.05
Stage-UICC				
I	16 (20)	0	16	
II	20 (25)	2	18	
III	23 (29)	4	19	
IV	21 (26)	9	12	<0.05
Residual tumor				
R0	65 (81)	8	57	
R1	10 (13)	4	6	
R2	5 (6)	3	2	<0.05
Size				
4 cm	33 (41)	5	28	
> 4 cm	47 (59)	10	37	n.s.
Lymphangiosis carcinomatosa				
no	37 (46)	2	35	
yes	43 (54)	13	30	< 0.05
Grading				
G1	7 (9)	0	7	
G2	35 (44)	6	29	
G3	38 (47)	9	29	n.s.
Laurén classification				
intestinal type	69 (86)	11	58	
diffuse type	3 (4)	2	1	
mixed type	8 (10)	2	6	n.s.

[a]Contingency table analysis: chi-square statistics with one tailed test, < 0.2; n.s. = p > 0.05

2992 patients by Clark et al. in 1991 (20). The rate of overexpression of c-erbB-2 detectable by immunohistochemistry ranges in gastric cancer from 9% (24) to 38% (22). In breast cancer, a rate of about 20% has been reported (19). In gastric cancer, the c-erbB-2 overexpression is positively correlated with better differentiated cancer (22, 25), tubulary type of cancer (13, 22), node involvement (13, 21, 23) and advanced tumor stages (13, 21). For Barrett's carcinoma, we found a rate of 19% (12% in the R0-group) overexpressed c-erbB-2 receptor protein, which is much lower than the previously reported (39) result of 73% in a small number of esophageal

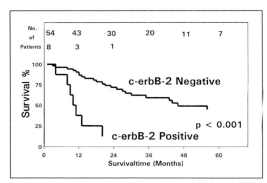

Figure 2. Kaplan-Meier product limit overall survival curves of 62 patients with R0-resection according to c-erbB-2 oncoprotein expression (log-rank p < 0.001).

adenocarcinomas. Significant correlations were evident between c-erbB2 overexpression and depth of tumor invasion, node involvement and distant lymph node metastases, but no correlation was seen to the histological types of Laurén-classification. Interestingly, we observed a significant correlation between c-erbB-2 overexpression and residual tumor stage. Only 53% of the patients with an overexpressed c-erbB-2 receptor experienced a complete macroscopic and microscopic resection (R0-category, UICC 1987). In contrast, in the group without c-erbB-2 overexpression, the R0-resection rate was 88%. Therefore, the R0-category should be taken into account in all studies dealing with survival analysis for c-erbB-2, because gastrointestinal cancer patients with incomplete resection margins generally have a significantly worse prognosis than R0-resected patients, independent of tumor-biological factors (40).

The prognostic value of c-erbB-2 overexpression in gastric cancer is still controversial. Two studies (21, 22) reported a significantly shorter survival for patients with overexpressed c-erbB-2 receptor, while two other studies (24, 25) reported that c-erbB-2 overexpression is associated with better overall survival. In a multivariate analysis by Yonemura et al. in 1991 (21), c-erbB-2 was an independent prognostic factor for overall survival in addition to depth of tumor invasion (pT), node involvement and peritoneal metastases. In the study of Jaehne in 1992 (22), c-erbB-2 failed to be an independent prognostic factor in contrast to residual tumor category and TNM stage. Further studies are necessary to define the prognostic relevance of c-erbB-2 overexpression for gastric cancer.

If our multivariate analysis is restricted to R0-resected patients, the independent prognostic factors were depth of local tumor invasion (pT), node involvement of the celiac lymph nodes and c-erbB-2 overexpression. The relative risk for death was 3.3-fold higher in the case of c-erbB-2 overexpression.

Table II. Calculated relative risk of survival and 95% confidence intervall according to univariate and multivariate Cox regression analysis in 62 patients with complete resected Barrett's carcinoma.

Variable	Category	Univariate analysis	Multivariate analysis		
		p-value[a]	p-value[a]	relative risk	confidence intervall
Primary tumor (pT)	T1,2/T3,4	0.0002	0.0002	5.9	2.3–15
Nodal status (pN)	N0/N1,2	0.001	n.s.	–	
Distant metastasis (pM)	M0/M1 (Lym)	< 0.0001	< 0.0001	7.3	2.8–19
Grading	G1,2/G3,4	0.05	n.s.	–	
Lymphangiosis carcinomatosa	no/yes	0.03	n.s.	–	
Laurén classification	intestinal/mixed/diffus type	n.s.	n.s.	–	
Size	continous	0.009	n.s.	–	
c-erbB-2 overexpression	no/yes	0.0001	0.02	3.3	1.2–8.7

[a] n.s. : p > 0.05

These first results on the prognostic impact of c-*erb*B-2 in adenocarcinoma of the esophagus should be validated by further studies. Nonetheless, our results indicate that c-*erb*B-2 overexpression implies a high risk of death due to tumor recurrence. For node-negative patients, c-*erb*B-2 overexpression is not a relevant prognostic factor.

Summary

In a retrospective study of 80 patients with adenocarcinoma of the esophagus, the prognostic impact of overexpression of c-*erb*B-2 oncoprotein was studied by immunohistochemical APAAP-staining of formalin-fixed, paraffin-embedded tissue sections of the primary tumor. c-*erb*B-2 oncoprotein overexpression of the primary tumor was detected in 15 patients (19%). A significant correlation was seen between c-*erb*B-2 overexpression and depth of tumor invasion (pT), node involvement (pN), distant metastases (pM[Lym]) and status of residual tumor after resection (R-category, UICC 1987). In a multivariate Cox regression analysis for survival of those 62 patients (78%) whose tumor resection (R0-UICC) was macroscopically and microscopically complete, depth of tumor invasion (pT1,2/T3,4), distant metastases (pM1[Lym]) and c-*erb*B-2 overexpression were independent prognostic factors. The relative risk of death due to recurrence were 5.9-fold, 7.3-fold and 3.3-fold, repectively. In the subgroup of the 53 "absolutely" complete resected patients (pM0-R0) depth of tumor invasion and c-*erb*B2 overexpression were the only independent prognostic factors, whereas in node-negative patients (n = 26) non of these factors were associated with survival.
These findings demonstrate that c-*erb*B-2 oncoprotein overexpression is a valuable prognostic factor in patients with adenocarcinoma of the esophagus after complete tumor resection.

Acknowledgement

Supported by grant no. 91.027.1 of the Wilhelm-Sander-Stiftung, Munich. The expert technical assistance of *A. Habermann, C. Seidl* and *R. Frimberger* is gratefully acknowledged.

References

1. Blot WJ, Devesa SS, Kneller RW, Fraumeni JF (1991) Rising incidence of adenocarcinoma of the esophagus and gastric cardia. JAMA 265: 1287–89
2. Kalish RJ, Clancy PE, Orringer MB, Appelman HD (1984) Clinical epidemiologic and morphologic comparison between adenocarcinomas arising in Barrett's esophageal mucosa and in the gastric cardia. Gastroenterol 86:461–7
3. Hesketh PJ, Clapp RW, Doos WG, Spechler SJ (1989) The increasing frequency of adenocarcinoma of the esophagus. Cancer 64:526–30
4. Mahoney JL, Condon RE (1987) Adenocarcinoma of the esophagus. Ann Surg 557–62
5. Streitz JM, Ellis FH, Gibb SP, Balogh K, Watkins E (1991) Adenocarcinoma in Barrett's esophagus. Ann Surg 213(2):122–5
6. Hoelscher AH, Schueler M, Siewert JR (1988) Surgical treatment of adenocarcinamas of the gastro-esophageal junction. Dis Esoph I(1):35–49
7. Siewert JR, Hoelscher AH, Bollschweiler E (1992) Surgical therapy of cancer in Barrett's esophagus. Dis Esoph V(1):57–62
8. Hoelscher AH, Bollschweiler E, Schueler M, Tachibana M, Nakamura T, Siewert JR (1992) Early esophageal cancer: prognostic advantage of adenocarcinoma compared to squamous cell carcinoma. 5th World Congress of the ISDE, August 5–8, Kyoto/Japan. Book of Abstracts, p 95
9. Nishimaki T, Hoelscher AH, Schueler M, Bollschweiler E, Becker K, Siewert JR (1991) Histopathologic characteristics of early adenocarcinoma in Barrett's esophagus. Cancer 68(8):1731–6
10. Semba K, Kamata N, Toyoshima K, Yamamoto T (1985) v-erb-related protooncogene, c-erbB-2, is distinct from the c-erbB-1/epidermal growth factor receptor gene and is amplified in a human salivary gland adenocarcinoma. Proc Natl Acad Sci 82: 6497-501
11. Kraus M, Issing W, Miki T, Popescu N, Aaronson S (1989) Isolation and characterization of erbB3, a third member of the erbB epidermal growth factor receptor family: evidence for overexpression in a subset of human mammary tumors. Proc Natl Acad Sci 186:9193–7
12. Lupu R, Dickson RB, Lippman ME (1992) The role of erbB-2 and its ligands in growth control of malignant breast epithelium. J Steroid Biochem Molec Biol 43(1–3):229–36
13. Yokota J, Yamamoto T, Miyajima N et al (1988) Genetic alterations of the c-erbB-2 oncogene occur frequently in tubular adenocarcinoma of the stomach and are often accompanied by amplification of the v-erbA homologue. Oncogene 2:283–7

14. McCann A, Dervan PA, Johnston PA, Gullick WJ, Carney DN (1990) c-erbB-2 oncoprotein expression in primary human tumors. Cancer 65:88–92
15. Tal M, Wetzer M, Josephsberg Z, Deutch A, Gutman M, Assaf D, Kris R, Givol Y, Schlessinger J (1988) Sporadic amplification of the HER/neu proto-oncogene in adeno-carcinomas of various tissues. Cancer Res 48:1517–20
16. Slamon DJ, Clark GM, Wong SG, Levin WJ, Ullrich A, McGuire WL (1987) Human breast cancer: correlation of relapse and survival with amplification of the HE-2/neu oncogene. Science 235:177–82
17. Paik SM, Simpson S, King CR, Lippmann ME (1991) Quantification of erbB-2/neu levels in tissue. Methods Enzymol 198:290–302
18. Mori S, Akiyama T, Morishita Y et al (1987) Light and electron microscopical demonstration of c-erbB-2 gene product-like immunoreactivity in human malignant tumors. Virchows Arch B 54:8–15
19. Perren TJ (1991) c-erbB-2 oncogene as a prognostic marker in breast cancer. Br J Cancer 63:328–32
20. Clark GM, McGuire WL (1991) Follow-up study of HER-2/neu amplification in primary breast cancer. Cancer Res 51:944–8
21. Yonemura Y, Ninomiya I, Yamaguchi A et al (1991) Evaluation of immunoreactivity for erbB-2 protein as a marker of poor short term prognosis in gastric cancer. Cancer Res 51:1034–8
22. Jaehne J, Urmacher C, Thaler HT, Friedlander-Klar H, Cordon-Cardo C. Meyer HJ (1992) Expression of Her2/neu oncogene product p185 in correlation to clinicopathological and prognostic factors of gastric carcinoma. J Cancer Res Clin Oncol 118:474–9
23. Yonemura Y, Ninomiya I, Ohoyama S, Fushida S, Kimura H, Tsugawa K et al (1992) Correlation of c-erbB-2 protein expression and lymph node status in early gastric cancer. Oncology 49:363–7
24. Hilton DA, West KP (1992) c-erbB-2 oncogene product expression and prognosis in gastric carcinoma. J Clin Pathol 45:454–6
25. Jain S, Filipe MI, Gullick WJ, Linehan J, Morris RW (1991) c-erbB-2 proto-oncogene expression and its relationship to survival in gastric carcinoma: an immunohistochemical study on archival material. Int J Cancer 48:668–71
26. Hermanek P, Sobin LH (1992) UICC TNM Classification of malignant tumors. 4th ed. 2nd rev. Springer, Berlin, p 402
27. Laurén P (1965) The two histological main types of gastric carcinoma: diffuse type and so-called intestinal-type carcinoma. Acta Pathol Microbiol Scand 64:31–49
28. Oota,K., and Sobin, L.H (1977) Histological typing of gastric and esophageal tumours. International histological classification of tumours. No.18, WHO, Geneva
29. Corbett IP, Henry JA, Angus B, Watchorn CJ, Wilkinson L, Hennessy C et al (1990) NCL-CB11, a new monoclonal antibody recognizing the internal domain of the c-erbB-2 oncongene protein effective for use on formalin-fixed, paraffin-embedded tisue. J Pathol 161:15–25
30. Cordell JL, Falini B, Erber WN, Ghosh AK, Abdulaziz Z, MacDonald S et al (1984) Immunoenzymatic labeling of monoclonal antibodies using immune complexes of alkaline phosphatase and monoclonal anti-alkaline phosphatase (APAAP complexes). J Histochem Cytochem 32:219–29.
31. Latza U, Niedobitek G, Schwarting R, Nekarda H, Stein H (1990) Ber-Ep4: new monoclonal antibody which distinguishes epithelia from mesothelia. J Clin Pathol 43:213–9
32. Smith PK, Krohn RI, Hermanson GT, Mallia AK, Gartner FH, Provenzano MD, Fujimoto EK, Goeke NM, Olson BJ, Klenk DC (1985) Measurement of protein using bicinchoninic acid. Anal Biochem 150:76–85
33. Kaplan EL, Meier P (1958) Nonparametric estimation from incomplete observations. J Amer Statist Asoc 53:457–81
34. Mantel N (1966) Evaluation of survival data and two new rank order statistics arising in its consideration Cancer Chemother Reports 50:163–70
35. Kalbfleisch JD, Prentice RL (1980) The statistical analysis of failure time data. Wiley, New York, p 84–92
36. McGuire WL, Clark GM. Prognostic factors and treatment decisions in axillary-node-negative breast cancer. New Engl J Med 326:1756–61
37. Ranzani GN, Pellegata NS, Previdere C et al (1990) Heterogenous protooncogene amplification correlates with tumor progression and presence of metastases in gastric cancer patients. Cancer Res 50:7811–14
38. Tsujino T, Yoshida K, Nakamaya H, Ito H, Shimosato T, Tahara E (1990) Alterations of oncogenes in metastatic tumors of human gastric carcinomas. Br J Cancer 62:226–30
39. Jankowski J, Coghill G, Hopwood D, Wormsley KG (1992) Oncogenes and onco-suppressor gene in adenocarcinoma of the esophagus. Gut 33:1033–3
40. Siewert JR, Fink U (1992) Multimodale Therapieprinzipien bei Tumoren des Gastrointestinaltraktes. Chirurg 63:242–50

Address for correspondence:
Dr. med. H. Nekarda
Chirurgische Klinik der Technischen Universität
Klinikum rechts der Isar
Ismaninger Straße 22
D-81675 München, Germany

An enzyme immunoassay for the detection of epidermal growth factor receptor in tissue extracts of breast cancer specimens

J. Harvey, V. Crebbin, G. Gorrin, S. Hammond, J. Mauceri, Y. Teramoto, R. Walker

Triton Laboratories, Ciba Corning Diagnostics Corp., Alameda, California, USA

Introduction

Epidermal growth factor receptor (EGFR) is a 170 kilodalton transmembrane glycoprotein that is found in many mammalian cells. It consists of three domains: A cytoplasmic domain that contains tyrosine kinase, a transmembrane region, and a cysteine-rich extracellular domain that contains the binding site for epidermal growth factor (EGF) and transforming growth factor alpha (TGF-a). The v-erbB oncoprotein of the acute transforming avian erythroblastosis virus is highly homologous with the trans-membrane and tyrosine kinase domains of EGFR; however, it does not encode the extracellular ligand-binding domain or a short c-terminal region that contains the main sites of auto-phosphorylation (1). EGFR has also been shown to have a high degree of homology with both c-*erb*B-2 and *erb*B-3 (2, 3).

Although many normal cells express EGFR, overexpression of EGFR has been shown for several types of human tumors, including gliomas (4), squamous carcinomas of lung (5), ovarian (6), bladder (7), and head and neck (8) carcinomas. In both bladder (7) and ovarian cancers (6), elevated levels of EGFR have been shown to correlate with poor outcome. The most extensive correlations of EGFR expression with clinical data have been carried out in studies with breast cancer patients. In early studies, *Sainsbury* et al. (9, 10) demonstrated that EGFR is a highly significant marker of poor prognosis for breast cancer. One study suggests that it may be the most important variable in predicting relapse-free and overall survival in lymph node negative patients, and to be the second most important variable, after nodal status, in lymph node-negative patients (11). Additionally, EGFR has been shown to be as good an indicator as the estrogen receptor (ER) for predicting the response to endocrine therapy (12). Although a number of reports in the literature have supported these initial results (13–16), others have been unable to find a significant relationship between status and poor prognosis (17).

The expression of EGFR has been investigated in tumor samples using either immunohistochemistry or radiolabeled ligand-binding methodologies. Immunohistochemistry analyses are qualitative and give information about only a small portion of tumors that are typically quite heterogeneous. Although radiolabeled ligand-binding assays are quantitative, they are not standardized and suffer from high variability both within and especially between laboratories (18). An enzyme immunoassay was developed at Triton Laboratories, Ciba Corning Diagnostics Corp. to provide a standardized method for determining EGFR values in tissue extracts. A simple and reproducible assay is a prerequisite for defining the prognostic value of EGFR in prospective clinical studies.

Methods

One hundred and seventeen tumor samples from patients with breast cancer were obtained from Nichols Institute, San Juan Capistrano, CA, as frozen tissue powders. All samples had been shown to be ER/PR negative and had associated EGFR values determined by radiolabeled binding assay done at Nichols Laboratories. If the sample was of sufficient size (n = 98), a portion was fixed in neutral buffered formalin and embedded in paraffin using standard techniques. Immunohistochemical staining was done using the EGFR MAb research reagent (Triton Laboratories, Ciba Corning Diagnostics Corp.) using the conditions described in the product insert. A set of 201 tissue pellets, residue from ER/PR cytosol testing, were kindly provided by Dr. Craig Jordan of the University of Wisconsin.

EGFR values were determined using the EGFR tissue extract EIA kit developed by Triton Laboratories, Ciba Corning Diagnostics Corp. All reagents required, as well as a detailed protocol, were included in the kit. Tissue extracts were prepared from pelleted, membrane-enriched tissue homogenates by solubilization in 1% Triton X-100. Protein determinations were made using a BCA assay (Pierce). Two hundred ml of the sample (at 0.1 mg/ml) and 200 µl of combined monoclonal antibody (MAb) conjugates were added to each tube. The combined MAb solution contains a horseradish peroxidase labeled MAb (MAb 4C7) and a fluorescein isothiocyanate (FITC) labeled MAb (MAb 31G7) both specific for EGFR. After a 2 h incubation at room temperature, immune complexes were linked to the coated tube by the addition of 200 µl of biotinylated anti-FITC MAb and the incubation continued for another 2 h After three washes, the tubes were allowed to drain briefly. The colorimetric reaction was initiated by the addition of 3,3'5,5 -tetramethyl benzidine and H_2O_2 and stopped after 15 min by the addition of 1 M phosphoric acid. Absorbance was measured with a Chem-Stat spectrophotometer (Source Scientific Instruments) using dual wavelengths of 450 nm and 650 nm. Milligram per ml values for the test samples were determined from a curve generated with reference calibrators included in the kit.

The 201 pellets obtained from the University of Wisconsin were assayed both in the EGFR EIA and in a c-erbB-2 tissue extract kit (Triton Diagnostics, CCD Corp.). For the c-erbB-2 assay, the protocol provided in the product insert was followed. Basically, it is the same as that for the EGFR kit, except for having conjugated MAbs reactive to the ectodomain of c-erbB-2 forming the immune complexes that are linked to the coated tube. Twenty-five tissue extracts were also assayed using the procedure detailed in Grimaux et al. (13).

Results

Assay performance

Imprecision was measured by performing five replicate determinations of three different specimens in ten assays. Within-run reproducibility had CV% values of 6.00, 6.15 and 5.91%; between-run reproducibility had CV% values of 7.18, 6.8, and 5.19%. Assay linearity as determined by dilution of two different tissue extract specimens showed less than 2% deviation from expected values. Recoveries of known amounts of EGFR antigen added to a EGFR-negative tumor tissue extract for seven samples ranged from 92% to 104%. The minimum detectable concentration for the assay was 0.042 fmol/ml. This was calculated as the concentration that is two standard deviations above the mean value of 20 replicates of a pool of tissue extracts with EGFR values near zero. The assay was specific for EGFR and showed no reactivity to c-erbB-2 or erbB-3 oncoproteins. Immunoreactivity of certain samples was confirmed by Western blotting (data not shown).

Clinical samples

The EGFR values obtained using radiolabeled ligand binding methodology were compared to those obtained with the EIA. For values less than 10 this comparison was problematic, as the binding assay values were reported at < 10 fmol/mg with no differentiation given for values under the cut-off. Nonetheless, when all 117 samples were included in the comparison, the correlation coefficient was 0.84. For samples with less than 300 fmol/mg EGFR (n = 108), the correlation fell to 0.78. Finally, for samples with less than 50 fmol/mg (n = 91), the correlation was 0.54 (figures 1A, B and C).

The EGFR values given by the Triton EIA were compared to those given by another immunoassay described by Grimaux et al. (16) that utilized R1 and 528 monoclonal antibodies. For the 25 samples assayed, the correlation coefficient was 0.97 (figure 2).

The EGFR values obtained by immunohistochemistry were compared to those from the EIA. A cut-off of 10 fmol/mg was used for the EIA. Staining was designated as positive using both

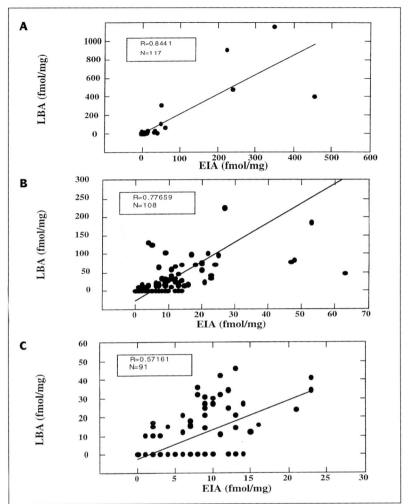

Figures 1A, B, and C. Correlation between EGFR values from radioligand binding assay and EIA.

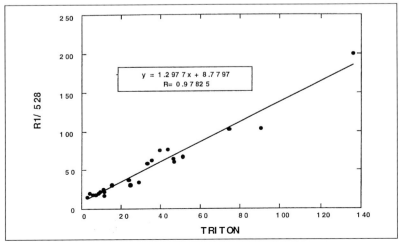

Figure 2. Comparison of 25 breast cancer samples tested in two EIAs.

Table I. Comparison of 98 samples assayed for EGFR by EIA and by immunohistochemistry.

	positive	negative
IHC		
positive	38	6
negative	15	39

Table II. Comparison of 201 breast cancer pellets assayed for EGFR and c-*erb*B-2 by.

	positive	negative
c-*erb*B EIA		
positive	8	22
negative	31	140

intensity and percentage of cells stained data. Only membrane staining was scored as positive. Of the 98 samples examined, there was a concordance of 79% (table I).

The set of 201 samples from the University of Wisconsin was tested in both EGFR EIA and c-*erb*B-2 EIA (table II). A cut-off of 10 fmol/mg was used for EGFR and a cut-off of 400 U/mg was used for c-*erb*B-2. Only 4.0% of the tumor samples expressed both c-*erb*B-2 and EGFR; the majority of samples were negative for both.

Conclusion

A standardized sandwich immunoassay was developed for the measurement of EGFR in tissue extract samples. Assay performance characteristics (imprecision, recovery, linearity and minimum detectable concentration) were determined. EGFR values obtained from the EIA were compared to values obtained with one radioligand binding assay, immunohistochemisty, and another EIA that had been described in the literature using breast cancer tissue sample. As would be expected, the correlation between the two EIAs was very high. These immunoassays would be measuring the same entities in the samples, that is both functional and non-functional receptors. The concordance seen between the EIA and immunohistochemistry was relatively high. Again, both functional and non-functional receptors are measured, but immunohistochemistry examines only a small slice of the tumor in fine detail, whereas the EIA averages the EGFR value over a large portion of the specimen. For the one variety of radioligand binding assay that was compared with the EIA, the correlation was not strong and was weakest for EGFR values below 50 fmol/mg, the level in which the majority of samples will occur. Evaluations of the EIA with comparisons done to other radiolabeled ligand binding assays have given inconsistent results (data not shown). Correlations range from high to very low. This result is not unexpected due to the failure of binding assays to correlate between laboratories. Additionally, binding assays measure only functional, unoccupied receptors. Further studies have been initiated to establish the clinical utility of EGFR values obtained using immunoassay methodology.

References

1. Downward J, Yarden Y, Mayes E, Scrace G, Totty N, Stockwell P, Ullrich A, Schlessinger J, Waterfield MD (1984) Close similarity of epidermal growth factor receptor and v-erb-B oncogene protein sequences. Nature 307:521–527
2. Carpenter G (1987) Receptors for epidermal growth factor and other polypeptide mitogens. Ann Rev Biochem 56:881–914
3. Kraus MH, Issing W, Miki T, Popescu NC, Aaronson SA (1989) Isolation and characterization of erbB3, a third member of the ERBB/epidermal growth factor receptor family: evidence for overexpression in a subset of human mammary tumors. Proc Natl Acad Sci USA 86:9193–9197
4. Liberman TA, Nusbaum HR, Rason N (1985) Amplification enhances expression and possible rearrangement of EGF receptors in primary human brain tumors. Nature 313:144–147
5. Berger MS, Gullick WJ, Greenfield C, Evans S, Addis BJ, Waterfield MD (1987) Epidermal growth factor receptors in lung tumours. J Pathol 152(4):297–307
6. Scambia G, Panici PB, Battaglia F, Ferrandina C, Baiocchi G, Greggi S, De Vincenzo R, Mancuso S (1992) Significance of epidermal growth factor receptor in advanced ovarian cancer. J Clin Oncol 10(4):529–535
7. Smith K, Fennelly JA, Neal DE, Hall RR, Harris AL (1989) Characterization of quantitation of the epidermal growth factor receptor in invasive and superficial bladder tumors. Cancer Res 49:5810–5815
8. Ishitoya J, Toriyama M, Oguchi N, Kitamura K, Ohshima M, Asano K, Yamamoto T (1989) Gene

amplification and overexpression of EGF receptor in squamous cell carcinomas of the head and neck. Br J Cancer 59:559–562
9. Sainsbury JRC, Farndon JR, Needham GK, Malcolm AJ, Harris AL (1987) Epidermal-growth-factor receptor status as predictor of early recurrence of and death from breast cancer. Lancet 1:1398–1402
10. Nicholson S, Halcrow P, Farndon JR, Sainsbury JRC, Chambers P, Harris AL (1989). Expression of epidermal growth factor receptors associated with lack of response to endocrine therapy in recurrent breast cancer. Lancet 1:182–184
11. Nicholson S, Richard J, Sainsbury C, Halcrow P, Kelly P, Angus B, Wright C, Henry J, Farndon JR, Harris AL (1991) Epidermal growth factor receptor (EGFr); results of a 6 year follow-up study in operable breast cancer with emphasis on the node negative subgroup. Br J Cancer 63:146–150
12. Nicholson S, Wright C, Sainsbury JRC, Halcrow P, Kelly P, Angus B, Farndon JR, Harris AL (1990) Epidermal growth factor receptor (EGFr) as a marker for poor prognosis in node-negative breast cancer patients: neu and tamoxifen failure. J Steroid Biochem Molec Biol 36(6):811–814
13. Rios MA, Macias R, Perez A, Lage A, Skoog L (1988) Receptors for epidermal growth factor and estrogen as predictors of relapse in patients with mammary carcinoma. Anticancer Res 8:173–176
14. Toi M, Osaki A, Yamada H, Toge T (1991) Epidermal growth factor receptor expression as a prognostic indicator in breast cancer. Eur J Cancer 27(8):977–980
15. Hainsworth PJ, Henderson RG, Stillwell RG, Bennett RC (1991) Comparison of EGFR, c-erbB-2 product and ras p21 immunohistochemistry as prognostic markers in primary breast cancer. Eur J Cancer 27(8):977–980
16. Grimaux M, Mady E, Remvikos Y, Laine-Bidron C, Magdelenat H. (1990) A simplified immuno-enzymetric assay of the epidermal growth factor receptor in breast tumors: evaluation of 282 cases. Int J Cancer 45:255–262
17. Klijn JGM, Berns P, Schmitz PIM, Foekens JA (1992) The clinical significance of epidermal growth factor (EGF-R) in human breast cancer a review of 5232 patients. Endocr Rev 13:3–17
18. Koenders PG, Faverly D, Beex LVAM, Bruggink EDM, Kienhuis CBM, Benraad TJ (1992) Epidermal growth factor receptors in human breast cancer: a plea for standardisation of assay methodology. Eur J Cancer 28:693–697

Address for correspondence:
Dr. J. Harvey
Ciba Corning Diagnostics Corp.
1401 Harbor Bay Parkway
Alameda, California, 94502, USA

Expression and function of GM-CSF receptors in solid tumor cell lines

E.-M. Suciu[a], S. Singh[a], C. Stocking[b], I. Meybohm[a], H.W. Goedde[a]

[a]Institute of Human Genetics, [b]Heinrich-Pette-Institute, University of Hamburg, Germany

Introduction

Granulocyte-macrophage colony-stimulating factor (GM-CSF) is a cytokine which stimulates the proliferation, differentiation and functional activation of granulocytes and macrophages in vitro and in vivo. The therapeutic use of the recombinant human GM-CSF (rhGM-CSF) is being studied clinically in patients with solid tumors to accelerate bone marrow recovery after myelotoxic anticancer therapy and/or bone marrow transplantation.

GM-CSF exerts its biologic actions via specific cell-surface receptors (GMR) (figure 1). In view of the clinical use of rhGM-CSF, it should be considered that both high- and low-affinity GMR occur also on non-hematopoietic cells, including certain tumor cells (1, 2). Recently, it was demonstrated that the human high-affinity GMR, expressed ectopically in non-hematopoietic cells, has ligand-dependent oncogenic activity and can transduce mitogenic signals in vitro (3, 4). A growth stimulatory effect of rhGM-CSF on certain solid tumor cells in vitro was reported (5, 6).

To study the role of GMR in non-hematopoietic tumor cells, we characterized GMR subunit expression in solid tumor cell lines by RNA analysis and investigated the biological activity of rhGM-CSF on receptor-positive cell lines.

Materials and methods

Cell lines and culture

MCF7, T-47D and Hs578T human breast carcinoma, A549 human lung carcinoma, HT-1080 human fibrosarcoma and HL-60 human promyelocytic leukemic cell lines were obtained from the ATCC (American Type Culture Collection, Rockville) and cultured according to the suppliers recommendation. The human erythroleukemic cell line TF-1 was kindly provided by *Dr. T. Kitamura*, Palo Alto, Carlifornia.

For analysis of the induction of proto-oncogenes, HT-1080 cells were cultured under reduced serum conditions (2% FCS). The cells were then incubated for 24 h in serum-free culture medium after which rhGM-CSF was added. HL-60 cells were stimulated with TPA (12-O-tetradecanoyl-phorbolacetate).

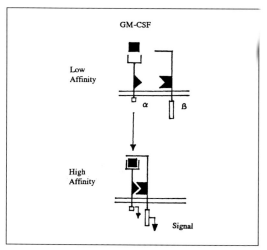

Figure 1. The human GM-CSF receptor (GMR). The high-affinity GMR results from a heterotypic dimerization of the low-affinity α-chain (GMRα) with a non-ligand binding β-chain (GMRβ). It was shown, that the cytoplasmic domain of the GMRβ is essential for signaling and the α-subunit is involved in, but not essential for growth signal transduction. However, the cytoplasmic domain of the GMRα has been reported to possibly play an important role in mediating cytokine specific signals (7).

Clonal culture of cells in methylcellulose: $1 \cdot 10^4$ cells/ml were cultured in RPMI 1640 medium containing 5% FCS, 0.6% PSN antibiotic solution, 0.2% bovine serum albumine and 0.9% methylcellulose. Each culture was performed in triplicate. On day 7 of incubation cell aggregates consisting of > 20 cells were scored as colonies. In stimulation or neutralization assays, rhGM-CSF or neutralizing monoclonal anti-hGM-CSF antibody were preincubated with cells for 30 min at room temperature.

RNA studies

Total cellular RNA was prepared by the guanidine/cesium chloride method and poly A^+-RNA was selected with oligo (dT) cellulose columns.
Northern blot analysis: RNA was glyoxylated, separated by agarose gel electrophoresis and blotted onto nylon membranes. To confirm integrity and equal loading of total RNA, aliquots were separated on agarose gels and stained with ethidium bromide and the blots were rehybridized with a c-raf cDNA probe. cDNA probes were labeled by the random primer method and hybridization was carried out under high stringency conditions.
RT-PCR: Total RNA (2 µg) was subjected to first strand cDNA synthesis with Mo-MuLV reverse transcriptase using oligo (dT)$_{15}$ primers. Aliquots of the RT reaction were used in PCR amplification with Taq polymerase. Primers for GMRβ RT-PCR were nt2115–2135 and nt2872–2853 of the cDNA sequence. As an internal control, primers for GAPDH (glyceraldehyde-3-phosphate dehydrogenase) were used in duplex PCR technique. PCR products were separated on agarose gels, blotted and hybridized with a ^{32}P-marked GMRβ specific cDNA probe. GAPDH PCR products were visiualized by staining the gel with ethidium bromide.

Results

Northern blot analysis revealed that the HT-1080 fibrosarcoma, A549 lung carcinoma and T-47D breast carcinoma cell lines express specific mRNA for the GMRα subunit, whereas in breast carcinoma cell lines MCF7 and Hs578T no GMRα transcripts could be detected (figure 2). Expression of GMRβ was found in Northern blot analysis only in the hematopoietic cell line HL-60, known to express high-affinity GMR. All cell lines, except Hs578T, produced GM-CSF mRNA suggesting autocrine mechanisms in GMR positive cells.
In RT-PCR analysis GMRβ specific PCR products were detectable in the solid tumor cell lines A549, HT-1080, T-47D and MCF7 (figure 3). If these low levels GMRβ are sufficient for signal transduction still remains to be clarified. RNA of the hematopoietic cell lines TF-1 and HL-60 were used as positive controls.
Stimulation of GM-CSF responsive cells normally results in the activation of nuclear protooncogenes such as c-fos and c-myc (8). However, no induction of c-fos and c-myc was observed after stimulation of the fibrosarcoma cell line HT-1080 with rhGM-CSF (figure 4).

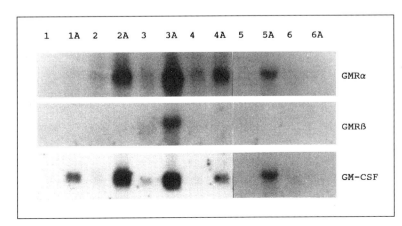

Figure 2. Northern blot analysis of GMRα, GMRβ and GM-CSF expression. Total RNA (20 µg) and Poly A^+-RNA (10µg) from MCF7 (lanes 1/1A), HT-1080 (lanes 2/2A), HL-60 (lanes 3/3A), A549 (lanes 4/4A), T-47D (lanes 5/5A) and Hs578 (lanes 6/6A) cells was analysed as described in: Materials and methods.

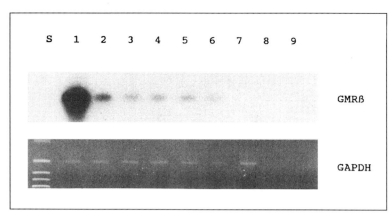

Figure 3. PCR analysis of the GMRβ mRNA expression in tumor cell lines. RNA from TF-1 (lane 1), HL-60 (lane 2), A549 (lane 3), HT-1080 (lane 4), T-47D (lane 5), MCF7 (lane 6) and Hs578T (lane 7) cells was reverse transcribed; aliquots were used in PCR reactions with primers for GMRβ and GAPDH. Negative controls: no RNA (lane 8) and HL-60 RNA not subjected to cDNA synthesis (lane 9). Standard (lane S).

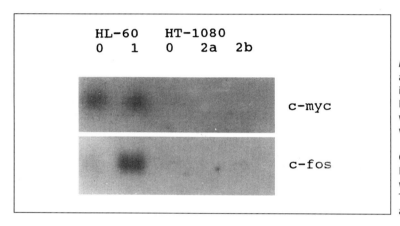

Figure 4. Northern blot analysis of c-myc and c-fos induction. Serum-starved HT-1080 cells were incubated without (lane 0) or stimulated with 100 U/ml (lane 2a) and 1000 U/ml (lane 2b) rhGM-CSF for 30 min at 37 °C. HL-60 cells were stimulated with $5 \cdot 10^{-7}$ M TPA (lane 1). Total RNA (20 µg) was analysed as described above.

Table I. Effect of rhGM-CSF and neutralizing monoclonal anti-hGM-CSF antibody (anti hGM-CSF mAb) on clonal growth of cell lines. One representative experiment is shown. Colony numbers are the mean of three cultures.

Cell line	rhGM-CSF	anti hGM-CSF MAb	No. of colonies
HT-1080	–	–	37
	1000 U/ml	–	38
	–	20 µg/ml	40
A549	–	–	12
	1000 U/ml	–	10
	–	20 µg/ml	9

In a methylcellulose assay for clonal growth the GMR positive human solid tumor cell lines HT-1080 and A549 showed no responsiveness to exogenously added rhGM-CSF (table I). Furthermore, neutralizing monoclonal anti-hGM-CSF antibody had no influence on proliferation of these cell lines at the cell densities used, suggesting that an autocrine growth modulation by endogenous GM-CSF is unlikely. However, intracellular autocrine loops cannot be excluded

Discussion

In three solid tumor cell lines examined, GMRα mRNA expression and minor amounts of GMRβ transcripts were found. We were not able to demonstrate functional activity of these receptors either in growth stimulation assays nor by analysis of induction of immediate early response genes. Our preliminary results may be interpreted to support reports that certain human non-hemato-poietic tumor cells express low-affinity GMR which do not appear to transduce growth signals (2). However, the cytoplasmic domain of the GMRα chain has been reported to possibly play an important role in mediating cytokine-specific signals (7). Thus, the role of low-affinity GMR on human malignant non-hematopoietic cells, especially that for non-mitogenic responses, still remains to be elucidated. Additionally, it may be possible that overexpressed GMRα chains are physiological modulators of GM-CSF, comparable to soluble forms of cytokine receptors.

In hematopoietic cells the expression of GMRβ chain is upregulated by the cytokines IL-1 and TNF-α (8). Since it was recently demonstrated that the human high-affinity GMR, composed of α and β chains, is functionally active in non-hematopoietic cells (4), the question if GMRβ subunits may be upregulated by cytokines and drugs in solid tumor cells too, is of special interest. We are currently investigating this possibility.

The clinical significance of GMR expression on the surface of tumor cells is still unknown, and needs further in vitro and in vivo experiments for its clear understanding.

References

1. Baldwin GC, Gasson JC, Kaufman SE, Quan SG, Williams RE, Avalos BR, Gazdar AF, Golde DW, DiPersio JF (1989) Non-hematopoietic tumor cells express functional GM-CSF receptors. Blood 73:1033–1037
2. Baldwin GC, Golde DW, Widhopf GF, Economou J, Gasson JC (1991) Identification and characterization of a low-affinity granulocyte-macrophage colony-stimulating factor on primary and cultured human melanoma cells. Blood 78:609–615
3. Areces LB, Jücker M, San Miguel JA, Mui A, Miyajima A, Feldman RA (1993) Ligand-dependent transformation by the receptor for human granulocyte/macrophage colony-stimulating factor and tyrosine phosphorylation of the reception of the receptor β subunit. Proc Natl Acad Sci USA 90:3963–3967
4. Yokota T, Watanabe S, Mui AL-F, Muto A, Arai K-I (1993) Reconstitution of functional human GM-CSF receptor in mouse NIH3T3 fibroblasts and BA/F3 proB cells. Leukemia 7:101–107
5. Berdel WE, Danhauser-Riedl S, Doll M, Herrmann F (1990) Effect of hematopoietic growth factors on the growth of nonhematopietic tumor cell lines. In: Mertelsmann M, Herrmann F (eds) Hematological growth factors in clinical applications. Mercel Dekker, New York
6. Joraschkewitz M, Depenbrock H, Freund M, Erdmann G, Meyer H-J, De Riese W, Neukam D, Hanouske U, Krumwieh M, Poliwoda H, Hanauske A-R (1990) Effects of cytokines on in vitro colony formation of primary human tumor specimens. Eur J Cancer 26:1070-1074
7. Sakamaki K, Miyajima I, Kitamura T, Miyajima A (1992) Critical cytoplasmic domains of the common β subunit of the human GM-CSF, IL-2 and IL-5 receptors for growth signal transduction and tyrosine phosphorylation. EMBO J 11:3541-3549
8. Watanabe Y, Kitamura T, Hayahida K, Miyajima A (1992) Monoclonal antibody against the common β subunit (β) of the human interleukin-3 (IL-3), IL-5, and granulocyte-macrophage colony-stimulating factor receptors shows upregulation of β by IL-1 and tumor necrosis factor-α. Blood 80:2215–2220

Address for correspondence:
Dr. rer. nat. E.-M. Suciu
Institut für Humangenetik
Universität Hamburg
Martinistraβe 52
D-20246 Hamburg, Germany

Interleukin-6 (IL-6) expression in breast cancer and correlation with pathological prognostic factors

Carmen Minguillon[a], D. Judith[b], T. Heinze[b], A. Schäfer[b], B. Köppen[c], W. Lichtenegger[b]

[a]Department of Gynecological Pathology, [b]Department of Gynecology, UKVR,
Free University, Berlin, [c]Dianova-Immunotech, Hamburg, Germany

Introduction

The histological demonstration of lymphocytic infiltration in breast carcinomas is interpreted as a reaction of the immunosystem to resist tumor growth. Some authors were able to relate a more favorable clinical course of carcinomas with lymphoid infiltrates (3) others could not confirm this (2, 4, 9). Moreover *Wintzer* (10) found that the prognosis of tumors is not influenced by the type of lymphocytic subpopulations. In all cases the lymphocytic infiltration does not exclude the possibility of tumor growth and the development of metastasis. Cytokines likes IL-6 constitute a class of soluble small proteins, they represent a complex pleiotropic network and intercellular signalling system for immune reactions, hematopoiesis, and inflammatory response. Cytokine IL-6 is synthetized by many types of cells including T-cells, monocytes, fibroblasts as well as numerous tumor cell lines (8). High IL-6 concentrations were found in body fluids from patients with autoimmune diseases and also in serum of patients with sepsis (5, 7, 8). The aim of our study was to determine the IL-6 concentration quantitatively in tumor tissue of primary breast cancer patients and to evaluate the clinical significance of IL-6 as a prognostic factor. We describe in this paper the first experiences to measure IL-6 in cytosol by 181 patients and the correlation between IL-6 values and established pathological prognostic factors.

Materials and methods

IL-6 concentrations were measured retrospectively in 181 cytosol samples of primary breast cancer tissue. Tumor stage, degree of differentiation and mononuclear cell reaction (MCR) were determined in the course of the routine pathological assessment. The tumors were immunostained with monoclonal antibodies (MoAb) in frozen and paraffin embedded tissue. Bound antibodies were visualized with APAAP Method according to *Cordell* (1).

We used MoAb: for the estrogen receptor (ER-ICA/Abbott GmbH Wiesbaden, Germany), for the progesteron receptor (PR/Dianova Germany), for the growth fraction Ki67 (Ki67/Dako Germany), for the Proliferating Cell Nuclear Antigen (PCNA = PCIO/Dako Germany), for the T-cells (CD45RO/ Dako Germany) and for the macrophages (CD68/Dako Germany). The results were expressed in percent of positive nuclear immunostained cells for hormon receptors and growth fractions. The degree of mononoclear cell infiltration, T-cells and macrophages was classified semiquantitatively in two groups: slight/moderate and strong. No negative tissue was found. The tumor cytosol fraction was prepared according to DCC method and the values of IL-6 were correlated to the cytosol protein concentration according to *Lowry* (5). The IL-6 immunoassay used in this study was distributed by Dianova (sensitivity 0.5 pg/ 1), 100 µl cytosol were used for the ultrasensitive procedure. For the statistical analysis we used the SPSS package and the chi-square test, a value of $p < 0.05$ was considered statistically significant.

Results

The clinical-pathological data of the patients at the time of surgery are listed in table I, IL-6 concentrations ranged from 0.33 to 193 pg/mg protein (figure 1), the median value was 1.87

Table I. Characteristics (n) of 181 patients with primary breast cancer.

Tumor size	
T1	68
T2	66
T3	12
T4	29
Nodal status	
N0	80
N1	67
N2	10
Grading	
1	39
2	106
3	35
Patient's age	
≤ 50 years	52
> 50 years	125

Table II. Correlation of IL-6 status with established prognostic factors in primary breast cancer.

Prognostic factor	No.	p-Value
Tumor size	175	n.s.
Nodal status	157	n.s.
Grading	180	< 0.008
ER status	179	< 0.001
PR status	179	< 0.006
Ki-67	152	< 0.001
PCNA (PC-10)	179	< 0.001
Patient's age	177	n.s.

Table III. Correlation of IL-6 status with mononuclear cell reaction (MCR), T-cell- and macrophage infiltration (MAC) in the stroma of primary breast cancer.

	No.	p-Value
MCR	76	0.047
T-cell infiltration	76	0.008
MAC infiltration	76	0.025

pg/mg protein. These results were correlated with histological and immunhistochemical parameters (table II). Significant correlations between IL-6 values and grading (p < 0.008), Ki67 (p < 0.001), PCNA (p < 0.001), T-cells (p < 0.008) MCR (p < 0.047) and macrophages (p < 0.025) were found. A high value of IL-6 correlated with an unfavourable histological grading, with a high index of proliferation (Ki 67 and PCNA) and with a stronger mononuclear cell reaction (Table III). An inverse correlation between IL-6 and hormon receptor status was observed (ER-ICA p < 0.001, PRG p < 0.006). Tumor size and nodal status showed no correlation to IL-6 values.

Discussion

We used a quantitative method for the measurement of IL-6 in tumor cytosol. Our method is not related to the anatomical substratum of the production of IL-6. A significant correlation between IL-6 concentration and mononuclear cell reaction, T-cells and macrophages in the tumor were found. These results suggest that the mononuclear cells may be involved in the production of IL-6. A high concentration of IL-6 correlates

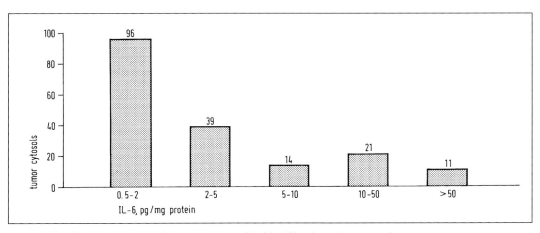

Figure 1. Distribution of the cytosol concentrations of IL-6 in 181 primary breast carcinomas.

significantly with a high index of tumor proliferation (Grading, Ki67, PCNA). This may underline the role of IL-6 as tumor growth factor. In vitro experiences have shown that IL-6 is the major growth factor for human myeloma cells (10). IL-6 does not correlate with tumor size and nodal status. These results suggest that IL-6 does not probably influence the tumor progression. At this point our results are rather complex and controversial. Further studies will be necessary to investigate the prognostical outcome of IL-6 in the behavior of breast cancer patients.

References

1. Cordell JL, Falini B, Erber WN, Ghosh AK, Abdulaziz Z, Macdonald S, Pulford KAF, Stein H, Mason DY (1984) Immunoenzymatic labeling of monoclonal antibodies using immune complexes of alkaline phosphatase and monoclonal anti-alkaline phosphatase (APAAP Complexes). Histochem Cytochem 32:219–229
2. Dawson PJ, Karrison T, Ferguson DJ (1986) Histological features asociated with longterm surviva in breast cancer. Hum Pathol 17:1015–1021
3. Elston CW, Greshman GA, Rao GS, Zebro T, Haybittle JL, Houghton J, Kearney G (1982) The cancer research campaign (King's/Cambridge) trial for early breast cancer: clinicopathological aspects. Br J Cancer 45:655–669
4. Fisher ER, Kotwal N, Hermann C, Fisher B (1983) Types of tumor lymphoid response and s nus histiocytosis. Arch Pathol Lab Med 107:222–227
5. Gallati H (1992) Cytokines as diagnostic parameters? In: Klapdor R (ed) Tumor associated antigens, oncogens, receptors, cytokines in tumor diagnosis and therapy at the beginning of the nineties. Zuckschwerdt, München, Bern, Wien, New York, pp 466–468
6. Lowry OH, Rosebrough AL, Farr AL, Randall RJ (1951) Protein measurement with folin phenol reagent. J Biol Chem 193:265–268
7. Munoz C, Misset B, Fitting C, Bleriot JP, Carlet JC, Cavaillon JM (1991) Dissociation between plasma and monocyte associated cytokines during sepsis. Eur J Immunol 21:2177–2184
8. O'Garra A (1989) Interleukins and the immune system 1. The Lancet 29:943–946
9. Roses DF, Bell DA, Flotte TJ, Taylor R, Ratech H, Dubin N (1982) Pathologic predictors of recurrence in stage I (TINOMO) breast carcinoma. Ann Surg 193:15–25
10. Wintzer HO, Bohle W, von Kleist S (1991) Study of the relationship between immunohistologically demonstrated lymphocytes infiltrating human breast carcinomas and patients survival. J Cancer Res Clin Oncol 117:163–167
11. Zhang XG, Bataille R, Widjenes J, Klein B (1991) Interleukin-6 dependence of advanced malignant plasma cell dyscrasias. Cancer 69:1373–1376

Address for correspondence:
Dr. med. Carmen Minguillon
Abteilung für gynäkologische Pathologie
UKRV, Freie Universität, Berlin
Pulsstraße 4-14
D-14059 Berlin, Germany

Steroid hormone receptors (SR) in normal (NTT) and pathological (PTT) thyroid tissue samples – New tumor markers?

*I. Vainas, K. Dimitriadis, K. Pasaitu, I. Stergiou, I. Tsirintanis,
D. Kapetanos, E. Zakapas, D. Delopoulos*

Endocrinological – Oncological Unit, 2nd Medical Oncology and 2nd Surgical Department, Research and Pathology Departments "Theagenion" Cancer Center, Thessaloniki, Macedonia, Greece

Introduction

It is well known that thyroid nodules appear more often in women (6-fold) than in men. On the other hand cold solitary nodules are more often malignant in men than in women (1). Differentiated thyroid carcinomas in women, and especially in a younger productive age (< 40 years) have better prognosis (2, 3).

Male rats also develop more often (2-fold) thyroid cancer either spontaneously or after the application of carcinogens, but after being orchidectomized they either show regression of their tumors, or the incidence of thyroid cancer becomes equal to that of female rats (4). Finally in a few sporadic studies estrogen (ER) and androgen (AR) receptors have been found in normal and pathological thyroid tissue. Some high ER and AR concentrations have been found in thyroid cancer (1, 5, 6, 7).

It seems logical to assume that the steroid hormones must play a role in the growth and proliferation of the thyroid cell, either as promoters or as suppressors (1, 8, 9). The purpose of this study is to detect and measure the ER, PgR and AR concentrations in thyroid tissue samples of patients with benign (BTD) and malignant (MTD) thyroid disease and their eventual significance for diagnosis, staging, prognosis and treatment of thyroid cancer.

Material and methods

From March 1990 till September 1993, 69 patients with BTD or MTD underwent surgical excision. In all 69 surgical specimens we

Table I. Material (thyroid tissue samples).

Tissue samples	Total number	Female	Male
Pathological	69	60	9
nodular goiter (BND)	39	35	4
toxic adenomas (TA)	18	15	3
thyroid cancer (MTD)	12	10	2
Normal thyroid tissue	21	20	1

measured the three sex hormone receptors. In 21 of these specimens we took probes of apparently normal thyroid tissue from sites away from the pathological lesions (table I). The mean age was 48 years for BTD (21–67) and 50.5 years for MTD (31–81). Twentyseven women were premenopausal (PRM) and 33 postmenopausal (POM). All measurements have been made according to the DDC (Dextran coated charcoal) method. As positive we saw concentrations of SR > 1 fmole/mg of cytoplasma protein.

Results

We found SR positivity in 25% for ER, 50% for Pgr and 58% for AR in thyroid cancer tissue samples. For normal tissue samples positivity was 13% for ER, 17% for PgR and 32% for AR. The further analysis showed that for BTD the positivity for benign nodular goiter (BND) was 18% for ER, 18% for PgR and 41% for AR while for toxic adenomas (TA) it was 17% for ER, 39% for PgR and 72% for AR. Table II shows the mean concentration in fmoles/mg in the examined samples. Table III shows the SR concentrations found in pathological thyroid tissue (BND, TA and MTD). It shows higher SR concentrations in malignant

Table II. Mean SR values (fmoles/mg) in normal thyroid tissue (NTT), benign (BTD) and malignant (MTD) thyroid disease.

SR	NTT n = 21	BTD n = 57	MTD n = 12
ER	4.3	12	7
femal	4.3	12	15
male	0	0	4.5
PgR	16	36	19
femal	16	35.5	0
male	0	4.3	20.5
AR	10.5	17	18
femal	11	17	18
male	7	26.5	13

Table III. SR % positivity in pathological thyroid tissue (BND, TA, MTD).

SR	BND n = 39	TA n = 18	MTD n = 12
ER	18	17	25
PGR	18	39	50
AR	41	72	58

Table IV. SR % positivity combination in pathological thyroid tissue.

SR pairs	BND	TA	MTD
ER/PgR	17	0	33
ER/AR	34	66	100
PgR/AR	71	71	50

samples and somehow unexpected much higher AR concentrations in TA samples. Combinations of SR pairs showed again higher ER/PgR and ER/AR concentrations in malignant and higher PgR/AR concentrations in non malignant thyroid disease (table IV).

The pathological samples of men are few (9) and can not allow any conclusions, still they were all ER negativ while four out of nine were PgR/AR positiv. Finally the pathological tissue samples of PRM-women with 19% positivity for ER, 26% for PgR and 56% for AR as compared to those of POM-women with 21% for ER, 27% PgR and 48% for AR showed no differences between the two groups while there was a distinct difference to the much lower SR concentrations in normal tissue samples of the same groups of women.

Conclusions

Pathological tissue samples from thyroid cancer show higher concentrations of ER and PgR than those of normal thyroid tissue. AR concentrations are higher in TA and MTD than in BND an MTD. PRM-women have higher ER and AR concentrations in PTT than in NTT. POM-women have higher PgR and AR concentrations, respectively. There are no significant SR positivity differences in PTT between PRM- and POM-women. PTT have higher mean SR concentration values as compared to NTT. The elevations in TA and MTD are comparable. Men with TA show the highest mean concentration values of PgR and AR. SR pair combinations have been found more often in MTD (ER/PgR 33%, ER/AR 100% and PgR/AR 50%). Toxic adenomas showed an even higher occurence (ER/AR 66% and PgR/AR 71%).

This study shows that "bad prognosis" SR (i.e. combinations of PgR/AR or ER/AR) may play a role in the appearance of benign and malignant proliferative thyroid disease. They may also play a role in the developement of more malignant and aggressive thyroid cancer in postmenopausal women and especially in men. In these two groups there exists higher activity of androgens of testicular and adrenal origin which act upon the thyroid cells through AR and PgR. On the other hand, the appearance of more benign thyroid diseases and of differentiated thyroid cancer in PRM-women, may be due to the combination of ER and PgR which may be considered as "good prognosis" tumor markers and are connected to the higher production of estrogens and progesterons of ovarian origin.

References

1 Clark OH, Gerend PL, Davis M, Goretzki PE, Hoffman PG JR (1985) Estrogen and thyroid-stimulating hormone (TSH) receptors in neoplastic and nonneoplastic human thyroid tissue. J Surg Res 38:89–96
2 Duh QY, Clark OH (1987) Factors influencing the growth of normal and neoplastic thyroid tissue. Surg Clin N Am 67:281–298

3. Crile G (1966) Endocrine dependency of papillary carcinoma of the thyroid. J Am Med Ass 195:721–724
4. Paloyan A, Hoffman X, Prinz RA, Oslapas R, Shoch KH, Ku WW, Ernst K, Smith M, Lawrence F (1982) Castration induces a marked reduction in the incidence of thyroid cancers. Surgery 92 (5) 839–848
5. Molteni A, Warpeha RL, Britzio-Molteni L, Fors EM (1981) Estradiol receptors binding protein in head and neck neoplastic and normal tissue. Arch Surg 116:207–210
6. Mizukami Y, Michigishi T, Nonomura A, Hashimoto T, Noguchi M, Matsubara F (1991) Estrogen and estrogen receptors in thyroid carcinomas. J Surg Oncol 47:165–169
7. Prinz RA, Sandberg L, Chaudhuri PK (1984) Androgen receptors in human thyroid tissue. Surgery 96 (6), 996–1000
8. Mc Tiernan A, Weiss NS, Daling JR (1984) Incidence of thyroid cancer in women in relation to reproductive and hormonal factors. Am J Epidem, 120:423–435
9. Vainas I, Pasaitou K, Antonoglou O, Apostolakis G, Sahpasidou D, Stergiou I, Nikokyrakis A, Tsirintanis I, Dimitriadis K (1993) Steroid hormone receptors (SR) in normal (NTT) and pathological (PTT) thyroid tissue samples. Abstracts of the 7th Panhellenic Oncology Congress, Athens 4–7 November 1993, (in greek)

Address for correspondence:
Dr. K. Dimitriadis
2nd Medical Oncology Department
Theagenion Cancer Center
Al Symeonidis Street 2
GR-Thessaloniki, Greece

Expression of p53 in gastric cancer

W. Müller, F. Borchard

Department of Pathology, University of Düsseldorf, Germany

Introduction

Mutations of the tumor suppressor gene p53 frequently occur during the development of various human malignancies (1). These mutations lead to a more stable gene product which has a longer half-life and can easily be detected by immunohistochemical methods. The p53 protein has been implicated in the control of the cell cycle, DNA repair and programmed cell death (2, 3), whereas mutant forms can act as dominant oncogenes (4). Overexpression of p53 protein has been demonstrated in a variety of human tumors (5) and seems to be associated with malignant progression in colon tumors (6) or correlated with markers of poor prognosis in breast carcinomas (7) and more advanced stages in lung tumors (8). On the other hand, there are only a few studies dealing with p53 expression in gastric cancer (9). In the present study p53 expression was investigated by immunohistochemistry in a series of 120 consecutive gastric carcinomas. The staining results were correlated with clinico-pathological parameters and survival rates in order to verify a possible influence of p53 on progress and prognosis of gastric cancer.

Material and methods

We studied a series of 120 consecutive gastric carcinomas investigated at the Department of Pathology, University of Düsseldorf, Germany, from 1986 to 1988. Specimen were fixed in formalin 10% and embedded in paraffin. All tumors were classified and graded according to the International Union Against Cancer (UICC) as well as Laurén and Ming classifications. The tumor specimen were stained immunohistochemically for p53 using the avidin-biotin-complex-technique with a monoclonal antibody (AB-6, Dianova) after incubating in a microwave oven 3 times for 5 minutes at 750 W. The primary antibody was diluted 1:100. The immunoreactive tumor cells were estimated in percent in relation to all tumor cells. Tumors expressing p53 were divided into two groups of carcinomas: 1. those with immunoreactivity for p53 in less than 35% of tumor cells and 2. those with immunoreactivity for p53 in more than 35% of tumor cells. The staining results were compared with the evaluated clinico-pathological parameters (table I) and the survival time of each patient.

Results

We found p53 expression in 42.5% (n = 51) of all gastric carcinomas tested, in 32.1% (n = 9) of early cancers (pT1), and in 45.7% (n = 42) of all advanced carcinomas (pT2-pT4). Immunoreactivity

Table I. Investigated clinico-pathological parameters in a series of 120 consecutive gastric carcinomas.

Age	Ming classification
Sex	Laurén classification
Tumor site	postoperative survival
Tumor size	Kaplan Meier analysis
UICC-stage (pTNM)	p53 protein expression
Grading	(AB-6, Dianova, ABC-method)

Table II. p53 immunoreactivity in 120 consecutive gastric carcinomas.

p53-Positive	42.5% (n = 51)
< 35% of tumor cells	22.5% (n = 27)
> 35% of tumor cells	20.0% (n = 24)
p53-Negative	57.5% (n = 69)

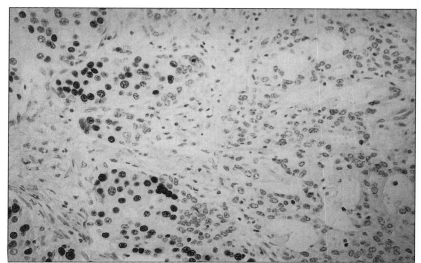

Figure 1. Advanced gastric carcinoma with heterogenous p53 expression only in the nuclei of the tumor cells. ABC-method; original magnification 160fold.

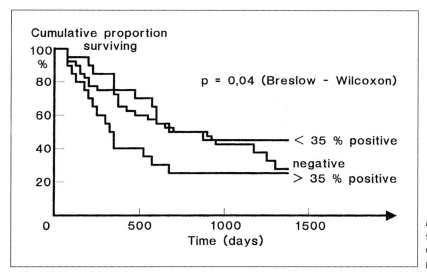

Figure 2. Kaplan-Meier survival analysis of p53 expression in 120 gastric carcinomas.

Table III. Statistical correlation between p53 expression and clinico-pathological findings in 120 gastric carcinomas.

	p-Value		p-Value
Age	0.55	tumor site	0.31
Sex	0.53	tumor size	0.48
Grading	0.21	pT-state	0.59
Ming	0.84	pN-state	0.29
Laurén	0.12	pTNM-stage	0.57

was only observed in the nuclei of tumor cells with a heterogenous staining pattern from 1% up to 95% of p53-positive tumor cells (figure 1). In the tumor-associated non-neoplastic gastric mucosa or tumor stromal cells no immunoreactivity was present. There was no significant correlation between the Ming or Laurén classifications and p53 expression by the tumor cells. Additional analysis showed that carcinomas with p53 expression did not differ from those without in terms of age and sex of the patients. The same was true for tumor site, size, grading and pTNM-stage (table III). However, we found a statistically significant shorter overall survival for patients whose tumors had more than 35% of p53-positive tumor cells in comparison with those with p53-negative tumors or with less than 35% of p53-positive tumor cells (figure 2). In a finally performed multivariate Cox regression analysis these differences concerning the postoperative survival did not gain statistical significance ($p = 0.45$).

Discussion

It has been shown that overexpression of the p53 protein as determined by immunohistochemistry is closely related to the presence of mutations of the p53 gene in different human tumors and cell lines (10, 11). In our study 42.5% of the tumors showed immunoreactivity for p53 which was strictly restricted to tumor tissue and not to the tumor-associated non-neoplastic mucosa. Comparison of p53-positive and p53-negative tumors revealed no differences in terms of tumor histology or established prognostic factors such as pTNM-stage, nodal-state or wall invasion. Nevertheless, by univariate analysis, the present study demonstrates a statistically significant correlation between strong p53 expression of the tumors and shorter postoperative survival. p53 expression could be shown to have prognostic influence in gastric cancer (9), however, in our series p53 expression could not be proofed as an independant prognostic marker by a multivariate analysis, which might depend on the number of tumors of our series. Although the role of mutated p53 protein in tumor development and tumor progression is still unclear, it might have prognostic influence in gastric cancer. However, further studies on a larger number of tumors including investigations on DNA-level are necessary to establish mutations of the p53 gene and their role for development and progress of gastric carcinomas. It still has to be shown whether p53 is a new independent prognostic marker in gastric cancer that can easily be detected in routine formalin-fixed specimen.

References

1 Levine AJ, Momand J, Finlay CA (1991) The p53 tumor suppressor gene. Science 253:453–6
2 Hollstein M, Sidransky D, Vogelstein B, Harris CC (1991) p53 mutations in human cancers. Science 253:49–53
3 Vogelstein B, Kinzler KW (1992) p53 function and dysfunction. Cell 70:523–6
4 Lane DP, Benchimol S (1990) p53: Oncogene or anti-oncogene? Genes Dev 4:1–8
5 Porter PL, Gown AM, Kramp SG, Coltrera MC (1992) Widespread p53 overexpression in human malignant tumors. Am J Pathol 140:145–153
6 Purdie CA, O'Grady J, Piris J, Wyllie AH, Bird CC (1991) p53 expression in colorectal tumors. Am J Pathol 138:807–813
7 Cattoretti G, Rilke F, Andreola S, D'Amato L, Domenico D (1988) p53 expression in breast cancer. Int J Cancer 41:178–183
8 Caamano J, Ruggeri B, Momiki S, Sickler A, Zhang SY, Klein-Szanto AJP (1991) Detection of p53 in primary lung tumors and nonsmall cell lung carcinoma cell lines. Am J Pathol 139:839–845
9 Martin HM, Filipe MI, Morris RW, Lane DP, Silvestre F (1992) p53 expression and prognosis in gastric carcinoma. Int J Cancer 50:859–862
10 Bartek J, Iggo R, Gannon J, Lane DP (1990) Genetic and immunochemical analysis of mutant p53 in human breast cancer cell lines. Oncogene 5:893–899
11 Iggo R, Gatter K, Bartek J, Lane DP, Harris A (1990) Increased expression of mutant forms of p53 oncogene in primary lung cancer. Lancet 335:675–679

Address for correspondence:
Dr. med. W. Müller
Abteilung für Pathologie
Universität Düsseldorf
Moorenstraße 5
D-40001 Düsseldorf, Germany

Immunohistochemical p53 protein expression and its correlation with proliferative activity in clinical stage I non-seminomatous germ cell tumors of the testis (NSGCT)

C.W. Biermann[a], W. de Riese[a], T.M. Ulbright[b], O. Orazi[b], A. Hinkel[a], R.S. Foster[c], Th. Senge[a]

[a]Department of Urology, Ruhr University Bochum, Herne, Germany;
[b]Department of Pathology, [c]Department of Urology, Indiana University, Indianapolis, Indiana, USA

Introduction

Immunohistochemical detection of the protein product of the p53 tumor suppressor gene has been found to correlate with mutations in the p53 gene, the wild-type protein having too short a half life and therefore existing in too small a concentration to be detected by ordinary immunohistochemical techniques (2, 3). Mutations in the p53 gene, assessed either by DNA analysis or the immunohistochemical overexpression of p53 protein, have been implicated in the evolution of a number of different human malignancies (3, 12). Several studies have shown that those cancers which have p53 mutations are associated with more aggressive behaviors or poor prognostic features compared to similar neoplasms lacking such mutations (9, 12, 14). Relatively little is known, however, concerning the possible role of p53 mutations in testicular germ cell tumors (1, 11), despite the recent suggestion that testicular malignancies may be involved by mutations of the p53 gene (1). For these reasons, we elected to study a series of 84 non-seminomatous germ cell tumors of the testis (NSGCT) by immunohistochemistry for expression of p53 protein and to correlate p53 expression with proliferative parameters obtained by flow cytometry (FC).

Material and methods

Eighty-four cases of NSGCT having one or more non-seminomatous components were identified in a database of 464 patients who had retroperitoneal lymph node dissections performed at Indiana University Hospital between 1965 and 1989 for clinical stage I disease. Most of these orchiectomy specimens were processed at hospitals other than University Hospital, with the paraffin blocks kindly provided by the pathologists at the refering institution. For the immunostaining of p53, we used a microwave based with hydrogen peroxide, slides were placed in a coplin jar filled with 0.1 M citrate buffer (pH = 6.0) and heated twice for five minutes in a microwave oven at 700 watts. After cooling for 15 minutes at room temperature, the slides were rinsed in phosphate buffered saline, covered with goat serum for 20 minutesl blotted, and incubated overnight at 4 °C with mouse monoclonal antibodies directed against either p53 (PAb 1801, Oncogene Science, Manhasset, NY, USA; dilution 1:10). The primary antibodies were localized with a biotin-streptavidin system (Kirkegaard and Perry Laboratories, Gaithersburg, MD, USA). The immunohistochemical staining for p53 was scored in a semiquantitative fashion depending upon the percentage of positively stained tumor nuclei assessed in ten random high-power (x40 objective) fields, as follows: +: 0–5%; ++: 6–30%; +++: > 30%. Nuclei from 50 micron thick paraffin sections of the same blocks that were analyzed by immunohistochemistry were prepared for flow cytometry (FC) according to the method of *Hedley* and his co-workers (6). Approximately $2 \cdot 10^6$ nuclei from each block were stained with propidium iodide according to the method of *Vindelov* et al. (15). A hematoxylin and eosin stained section from each block taken subsequent to the

50 micron section were examined to ensure the continued presence of neoplasm. Flow cytometry was performed on a Coulter Profile II flow cytometer (Coulter Electronics, Hialeah, FL, USA) equipped with a water cooled argon laser set at 488 nm excitation wavelength for propidium iodide and calibrated with "DNA check beads" (Coulter). Approximately 25,000 to 50,000 events were collected per sample by the use of two parameter gating. Doublets were excluded by gating on peak versus linear propidium iodide fluorescence. The first peak in all the DNA histograms was assumed to represent the 2c G0/G1 peak of the non-neoplastic cells present in the sample. DNA histograms that contained peaks with a full peak coefficient of variation (CV) > 10%, aneuploid peaks < 10%, and closely overlapping peaks with CVs > 10% were classified as non-interpretable and excluded from the study. S-phase data were determined from DNA histograms by MODFIT software (Verity Software, Topshaw, ME, USA).

Results

Expression of p53 protein was demonstrated in 37 of 84 (44.0%) clinical stage I non-seminomatous germ cell tumors of the testis (table I). In 16 cases (43.2%), the p53 expression was scored as +, in 13 (35.1%) as ++, and in 8 cases (21.6%) as +++. p53 expression usually occured as focal intranuclear positivity. Cytoplasmic staining was not observed. As shown in table II, the percentage of cells in S-phase was significantly higher in the p53-positive cases compared to the p53-negative cases (Student's test). p53 expression was observed in 14 pathological stage I and in 23 pathological stage II cases. This tumor biological parameter did not correlate to pathological stage of the patients. However, p53 protein expression exhibited a strong correlation to the proliferative behavior of the tumors (S-phase fraction measured by flow cytometry, see table II) as analyzed in this study.

Discussion

According to the data obtained in this study there is a significant correlation between p53 expres-

Table I. p53 expression of 84 NSGCT tumors of pathological stage I (n = 29) and II (n = 55).

p53-positive cells	Path. stage I		Path. stage II	
	n	(%)	n	(%)
0%	15	(51.7)	32	(58.2)
1–5%	7	(24.1)	9	(16.4)
6–30%	4	(13.8)	9	(16.4)
> 30 %	3	(10.3)	5	(9.1)

Table II. Correlation of p53 expression in clinical stage I non-seminomatous germ cell tumors of testis with S-phase fraction measured by flow cytometry.

	p53+ cases (n = 37)	p53– cases (n = 47)	p-Value
S-phase (mean)	27.8%	17.6%	<.025
± SD	11.6%	11.7%	

sion and high S-phase values measured by flow cytometry. The results suggest that, as in other malignancies, the presence of p53 protein (correlating with mutations in the p53 gene) is positively associated with markers of increased tumor aggressiveness. The identification of a parameter which correlates with increased tumor aggressiveness is of particular relevance in testicular germ cell neoplasia. The best management for patients with clinical stage I non-seminomatous germ cell tumors (NSGCT) of the testis is controversial. About 35% of NSGCT clinical stage I patients develop recurrence after tumor orchiectomy, most of them within two years during follow-up. Current clinical staging fails to identify those patients at high risk for recurrent disease. Some authors recommend retroperitoneal lymph node dissection (RPLND) for such patients (4, 7, 8), whereas others suggest that careful follow-up with no additional therapy, unless recurrence develpos, is the proper approach, at least in selected patients (10, 13). Since only about 30% of clinical stage I patients have occult retroperitoneal metastases (4), RPLND represents overtreatment for most patients. However, "surveillance alone" results in recurrence in about 35 to 40% of the patients (10, 13), most of whom would have had occult retroperitoneal metastases identified by RPLND. It would obviously be useful, therefore, to stratify this group of patients into two subgroups which have increased and decreased risks for occult metastases compared to the group as a whole. The correlation of p53 expression with high proliferative indices suggests that p53 immunostaining may be useful in helping to make this kind of stratification. We are, therefore, currently studying this issue in our laboratory. The identification of p53 expression in a significant proportion of testicular germ cell tumors in our study and in other studies (1, 11) argues that mutations in the p53 gene may represent a fundamental and early step in testicular oncogenesis. Such expression in the malignant cells of intratubular germ cell neoplasia (so called "carcinoma-in-situ" of the testis) provides additional support for the early phase of p53 mutations in the genesis of testicular germ cell neoplasia (1). Our experience with p53 expression in early stage NSGCT reinforces the evidence that such mutations are associated with a more aggressive subset of neoplasms compared to cases lacking such mutations, as judged by the immunohistochemical expression of the p53 protein.

References

1. Bartkova J, Bartek J, Lukas J et al (l991) p53 protein alterations in human testicular cancer including pre-invasive intratubular germ-cell neoplasia. Int J Cancer 49:196-199
2. Bodner SM, Minna JD, Jensen SM et al (1992) Expression of mutant p53 proteins in lung cancer correlates with the class of p53 gene mutation. Oncogene 7:743-747
3. Cunningham J, Lust JA, Schaid W et al (1992) Expression of p53 and 17p allelic loss in colorectal carcinoma. Cancer Res 52:1974-1979
4. Donohue JP, Thornhill JA, Foster RS (1993) Primary retroperitoneal lymph node dissection in clinical stage A nonseminomatous germ cell testis cancer. Brit J Urol 71:326-331
5. Gerdes J, Becker MHG, Key G, Cattoretti G (1992) Immunohistochemical detection of tumour growth fraction (Ki-67) antigen in formalin-fixed and routinely processed tissues. J Pathol 168:85-91
6. Hedley DW, Friedlander ML, Taylor IW, Rugg CA, Musgrove EA (1983) Method for analysis of cellular DNA content of paraffin embedded pathological material using flow cytometry. J Histochem Cytochem 31:1333–1338
7. McLeod DG, Weiss RB, Stablein DM et al (1991) Staging relationship and outcome in early stage testicular cancer: a report from the Testicular Cancer Intergroup Study. J Urol 145:1178
8. Pizocarro G, Nicolai N, Salvioni R (1992) Comparison between clinical and pathological staging in low stage nonseminomatous germ cell testicular tumorfi. J Urol 148:76–81
9. Quinlan DC, Davidson AG, Summers CL, Warden HE, Doshi HM (1992) Accumulation of p53 protein correlates with a poor prognosis in human lung cancer. Cancer Res 52:4828
10. Read G, Stenning SP, Horvich A (1992) Medical Research Council (URfMRC) prospective study of surveillance for stage I testicular teratoma. J Clin Oncol 10 (11):1762-1768
11. Schultz DS, Linden MD, Korman HJ (1993) Immunohistologic characterization of tumor proliferation and p53 expression in non-seminomatous germ cell tumors. Mod Pathol 6:69A (abstract)
12. Soini Y, Paakko P, Nuorva K, Kamel D, Lane DP, Vahakangas K (1992) Comparative analysis of p53 protein immunoreactivity in prostatic, lung and breast carcinomas. Virch Arch (A) 421:223–229
13. Stephenson RA (1991) Surveillance for clinical stage I nonseminomatous testis carcinoma: rationale and results. Urol Int 46:290–296
14. Thor AD, Moore DH, Edgerton SM et al (1992) Accumulation of pS3 tumor suppressor gene protein: an independent marker of prognosis in breast cancers. J Natl Cancer Inst 84:845–849
15. Vindelov LL, Christensen IJ, Nissen NI (1983) A detergent trypsin method for preparation of nuclei for flow cytometric DNA analysis. Cytometry 3:323–331

Address for correspondence:
Dr. med. C. W. Biermann
Urologische Klinik
Ruhr-Universität Bochum,
D-44627 Herne, Germany

p 53 immunohistochemistry as a new prognostic factor for bladder cancer

M.A. Kuczyk[a], J. Serth[a], E.P. Allhoff[b], K. Höfner[a], W.F. Thon[a], U. Jonas[a]
[a]Department of Urology, Hannover Medical School, Hannover,
[b]Department of Urology, Hospital of the Federal Miner's Society, Würselen, Germany

Introduction

Mutations of the p53 tumor suppressor gene resulting in an accumulation of the gene product, the p53 oncoprotein, have been identified in a variety of human malignancies (1, 2, 3). It has been shown that the p53 protein can also be detected in patients with urological tumors such as prostate cancer and testicular germ cell tumors by immunohistochemical staining (4, 3). For patients with transitional cell carcinoma of the bladder a correlation between a strong immunohistochemical staining reaction for p53 and an invasive behavior of the tumors has been postulated (5, 6).

Until now comparable results of p53 immunostaining between fresh-frozen and paraffin-embedded tissue have been described for the monoclonal antibody pAb 1801 in different epithelial tumors such as esophageal cancer (7). However, no investigations concerning urological tumors have been published so far. Therefore, one of the first aims of the present study was to determine if the monoclonal antibody 1801 the most commonly used commercially available antibody for the detection of p53, would be able to yield comparable results in paraffin-embedded tissue and in fresh-frozen material from urological tumors.

Furthermore, for tumor biopsies of bladder cancer, the possible correlation between the immunohistochemical reactivity for p53 and the grade of tumor invasion and differentiation was investigated.

For selected cases, it was tested if the specificity of the immunohistochemical reaction could possibly replace a genetic evaluation of the results.

Material and methods

To investigate the correlation between the immunohistochemical detection of the p53 protein expression and the invasiveness and differentiation in tumor specimens of bladder cancer, fresh-frozen tissue from 58 bladder tumors of different tumor stages and histological grading was stained for the p53 protein. p53 immunoreactivity was also studied in seven biopsy specimens from normal bladder epithelium and in biopsies of six patients presenting with an inflammatory reaction of the bladder.

To determine the effects of formalin fixation on p53 immunoreactivity, one piece of tissue from nine bladder tumors was kept fresh-frozen and another piece of the same tumor was embedded in paraffin following formalin fixation. The number of specimens tested and the histological types of tumors, as well as the number of normal tissue specimens, are listed in Table I.

Following deparaffinization the paraffin-embedded specimens were, as well as the fresh-frozen tissue, cut serially at 8 µm and stained by an absolutely identical immunohistochemical procedure, as described below.

Positive controls were represented by sections from bladder tumors with a mutational inactiva-

Table I. Method of fixation, number, origin and histological type of tissue specimens and tumors investigated.

Tumor histology	Tumors investigated (fresh-frozen)	Normal tissue	Paraffin-embedded
Transitional cell carcinoma (TCC)	58	7	9

tion of the p53 gene, as detected by sequence analysis.

Loss of heterozygosity (LOH) was examined by PCR directed analysis of the Msp I (8), Apa I (9) and BsTU I (10) restriction fragment length polymorphisms and one variable number of tandem repeats polymorphisms (VNTR) (11). Such allelic loss is often accompanied by mutational inactivation of the remaining allele, as it was shown for p53 tumor suppressor gene in colorectal cancer, for example (12).

Immunohistochemistry for p53 protein was performed as follows: Tumor carrying slides were first incubated with normal human serum in a dilution of 1:100 in Tris-buffered saline (TBS; 0.05 M, pH 7.6) to prevent unspecific binding of the first antisera. Then the specific primary antisera for the detection of p53 (Dianova, Hamburg, FRG, clone pAb 1801) (13) was added for the immohistochemical analysis of the tumors. This monoclonal mouse antibody recognizes a denaturation-resistant epitope in both mutant and wild-type p53 proteins and enables the detection of altered p53 proteins within the cell nucleus due to their prolonged half life (25). pAb 1801 antibodies were applied in a dilution of 1:50 in TBS at room temperature for one hour in a moist chamber. After rinsing with TBS/0.1% Tween 20 for 10 minutes the sections were incubated with a second monoclonal antibody of rabbit-anti-mouse specificity (Dako, Hamburg, FRG, Z 259). This antibody was applied in a mixture of human serum and TBS (1:25) in a dilution of 1:25 for 30 minutes. After a third rinsing with Tween 20/TBS the APAAP-complex (Dako) was added in a dilution of 1:50 in TBS for 30 minutes. After a final rinsing with Tween 20/TBS the red reaction product was obtained following the typical chemical reaction procedure. Finally the slides were stained by hematoxylin.

The immunohistochemical reaction was considered to be positive only in case of nuclear staining.

Results

In 25 informative bladder tumors the results of the immunohistochemical detection of p53 mutant protein were controlled using the polymerase chain reaction for the detection of an eventually occurring loss of heterozygosity. In 87% of cases the immunohistochemical results could be verified by genetic evaluations demonstrating an allelic loss of heterozygosity at the p53 gene locus by PCR-directed RFLP-technique. Therefore, in cases of bladder cancer, the immunohistochemical staining localized within the cell nucleus was considered as specific for p53.

In nine cases we were able to compare the immunohistochemical reaction in fresh-frozen and paraffin-embedded tissue. In comparison with the fresh-frozen tumor samples all paraffin-embedded tissue sections exhibited an identical immunohistochemical reaction and in seven cases (77.8%) we observed an even stronger staining intensity in sections of paraffin-embedded tissue.

The intensity of the immunohistochemical staining reaction increased in advanced tumor stages, but even in 14 (48.3%) low stage tumors (Ta/T1) a positive reaction was observed (table II). However, p53 detectability correlated to the tumor stage, with 38.5%–56.2% of tumors positive at Ta–T2 and it was enhanced to 81.8% –83.3% of T3/T4 tumors.

Seven tumors (46.7 %) graded as G1 and 12 G3-tumors (75%) exhibited a positive staining reaction (table III).

All seven cases of normal tissue were negative for the p53 protein, whereas one of six biopsy specimens with an inflammatory reaction of the epithelium exhibited a positive staining reaction. Moreover, the normal mesenchymal cells in all 58 bladder tumors did not exhibit any nuclear reactivity.

Discussion

Tumor suppressor genes represent cellular control mechanisms regulating cell growth and proliferation. Considering the existence of tumor suppressor genes tumorigenesis may not only result from the activation of genes with the ability of cellular transformation, so called "oncogenes", but also from the inactivation of tumor suppressor genes (14).

To understand the role of these genes it is important to know that in most tumors related to a dysfunction of a tumor suppressor gene, the gene loci on both alleles are affected. As demonstrated for the retinoblastoma (Rb) gene,

Table II. Relation between positive staining reaction for p53 and tumor invasion of bladder cancer specimens.

	pTa	pT1	pT2	pT3	pT4	Inflammatory tissue	Normal tissue
Number of patients	13	16	12	11	6	6	7
Negative	8 (61.5%)	7 (43.8%)	6 (50%)	2 (18.2%)	1 (16.7%)	5 (83.3%)	7 (100%)
Positive	5 (38.5%)	9 (56.2%)	6 (50%)	9 (81.8%)	5 (83.3%)	1 (16.7%)	0

Table III. Positive staining reaction for p53 related to the histological grading of the bladder tumors.

	G1	G2	G3
Number of patients	15	27	16
Negative	8 (53.3%)	10 (37%)	4 (25%)
Positive	7 (46.7%)	17 (63%)	12 (75%)

this genetic loss is homozygous (15, 16). Consequently, homozygosity of genetic alterations in regulatory gene loci can indicate a defect or the inactivation of tumor suppressor genes.

The p53 gene was identified as a suppressor gene located on chromosome 17. The loss of an allele on the short arm of chromosome 17, indicating a loss of heterozygosity (LOH) that in most cases includes the p53 locus (17), is very frequent in a variety of human malignancies (4). In many cases the allelic loss is accompanied by single base substitutions and, as a result, mutational inactivation of the remaining allele (14). Although some genetic experiments showed characteristics and a pattern of activity similar to an oncogene (18, 19) it became evident that the p53 gene mainly functions as a tumor suppressor gene (20).

Although mutations of the p53 gene can be found in a variety of cancers they do probably not represent an obligate step in cancerogenesis. Furthermore, the type of p53 mutation may differ between tumors (21). The non-mutated, unaffected wild-type p53 tumor suppressor gene codes for a nuclear protein which is assumed to be closely involved in the regulation of the cell cycle (20, 22), since it arrests tumor cells in the G1-phase (19). The mutant p53 gene codes for a protein with an altered configuration. Mutant p53 proteins, characterized by single aminoacid substitutions, have a longer half life, which results in an accumulation of the protein and a higher intracellular level as compared to the wild type protein (23). This results in the unique situation in which the immunohistochemical detection of a protein due to increased intracellular levels gives indirect evidence of a mutated gene. Although the importance of p53 gene alteration for different types of tumors has not been clearly defined, the accumulation and immunohistochemical detection of the p53 protein, as described for carcinoma of the breast (2, 24, 25), colorectal carcinoma (1, 26) and primary lung cancer (27, 28), has been correlated to their malignant potential and a poor prognostic outcome. Moreover, accumulation of the p53 protein was found in bladder cancer (4, 16), in testicular germ cell tumors (4), and in prostate cancer (3) it was partially correlated with an unfavorable clinical outcome.

The use of paraffin-embedded material for the immunohistochemical staining of p53 has been described for different epithelial tumors, e.g. for esophageal cancer (7). One objective of our study was to compare the immunohistochemical staining results for p53 obtained in fresh-frozen tissue to those in paraffin-embedded tissue sections of bladder cancer. The method applied including the use of the monoclonal antibody pAb 1801 proved valuable for both types of tumor material, since a good correlation between the staining results was observed.

In order to demonstrate the specifity of the staining procedure for p53 protein, the immunohistochemical results were in accordance with the loss of heterozygosity, as detected by PCR. This demonstrates that the monoclonal antibody pAb 1801 is suitable for retrospective studies of formalin fixed and paraffin-embedded material. Although a higher percentage of p53 positive tumors with a more intensive staining reaction was seen in more undifferentiated tumors (G3), bladder tumors of low grading (G1/G2) and low stage (Ta/T2) also exhibited an accumulation of p53 protein in up to 56.2% and 63% of cases. The correlation of p53 in low stage bladder cancer with the clinical behavior of the tumors will show, whether the detectability of p53 is of clinically prognostic value. However, a recently published study has already described a higher probability of disease progression for superficially infiltrating transitional cell bladder carcinomas (T1), when a nuclear accumulation and immunohistochemical detectability of the p53 protein was detected (29). The importance of our observations for the prognosis of patients with bladder cancer will have to be investigated in a larger series.

References

1. Starzynska T, Bromley M, Ghosh A, Stern PL (1992) Prognostic significance of p53 overexpression in gastric and colorectal carcinoma. Br J Cancer 66:558–562
2. Thor AD, Moore DH II, Edgerton SM, Kawasaki ES, Reihsaus E, Lynch HT, Marcus JN, Schwartz L, Chen LC, Mayall BH, Smith HS (1992) Accumulation of p53 tumor suppressor gene protein: an independent marker of prognosis in breast cancers. J Natl Cancer Inst 84:845–854
3. Visakorpi T, Kallioniemi OP, Heikkinen A, Koivula T, Isola J (1992) Small subgroup of aggressive, highly proliferative prostatic carcinomas defined by p53 accumulation. J Natl Cancer Inst 84:883–887
4. Bartek J, Bartkova J, Vojtesek B, Staskova Z, Lukas J, Rejthar A, Kovarik J, Midgley CA, Gannon JV, Lane DP (1991) Aberrant expression of the p53 oncoprotein is a common feature of a wide spectrum of human malignancies. Oncogene 6:1699–1703
5. Wright C, Mellon K, Johnston P, Lane DP, Harris AL, Horne CH, Neal DE (1991) Expression of mutant p53, c-erbB-2 and the epidermal growth factor receptor in transitional cell carcinoma of the human urinary bladder. Br J Cancer, 63:967–970
6. Sidransky D, Von Eschenbach A, Tsai YC, Jones P, Summerhayes I, Marshall F, Paul M, Green P, Hamilton SR, Frost P (1991) Identification of p53 gene mutations in bladder cancers and urine samples. Science 252:706–709
7. Bennett WP, Hollstein MC, He A, Zhu SM, Resau JH, Trump BF, Metcalf RA, Welsh JA, Midgley C, Lane DP (1991) Archival analysis of p53 genetic and protein alterations in Chinese esophageal cancer. Oncogene 6:1779–1784
8. Mc Daniel T, Carbone D, Takahashi T, Chumakov P, Chang EH, Pirollo KF, Yin J, Huang Y, Meltzer SJ (1991) The Msp I polymorphism in intron 6 of p53 (TP 53) detected by digestion of PCR products. Nucleic Acids Res 19:4796
9. Prosser J, Condie A (1991) Biallelic Apa I polymorphism of the human p53 gene (TP 53). Nucleic Acids Res 19:4799
10. Merlo GR, Cropp CS, Callahan R, Takahashi T (1991) Detection of loss of heterozygosity in human DNA samples by PCR. Biofeedback 11:166-168
11. Hahn M, Serth J, Fislage R, Wolfes H, Allhoff E, Jonas U, Pingoud A. Detection of a highly polymorphic VNTR segment in intron 1 of the human p53 gene. Clin Chem (in press)
12. Nigro JM, Baker SJ, Preisinger AC, Jessup JM, Hostetter R, Cleary K, Bigner SH, Davidson N, Baylin S, Devilee P, Glover T, Collins FS, Weston A, Modali R, Harris CC, Vogelstein B (1989) Mutations in the p53 gene occurr in diverse human tumor types. Nature 342:705–708
13. Banks L, Matlashewski G, Crawford L (1986) Isolation of human-p53-specific monoclonal antibodies and their use in the studies of human p53 expression. Eur J Biochem 159:529–534
14. Marshall CJ (1991) Tumor suppressor genes. Cell 64:331–326.
15. Knudson AG (1971) Mutation and cancer statistical study of retinoblastoma. Proc Natl Acad Sci USA 68:820–823
16. Brewster SF, Gingell JC, Brown KW (1992) Tumor suppressor genes in urinary tract oncology. Br J Urol 70:585–590
17. O'Rourke RW, Miller CW, Kato GJ, Simon KJ, Chen D-L, Dang CV, Koeffler HP (1990) A potential transcriptional activation element in the p53 protein. Oncogene 5:1829–1832
18. Parada LF, Land H, Weinberg, RA, Wolf D, Rotter V (1984) Cooperation between gene encoding p53 tumour antigen and ras in cellular transformation. Nature 312:649–651
19. Jenkins JR, Rudge K, Currie GA (1984) Cellular immortalisation by a cDNA clone encoding the transformation associated phosphoprotein p53. Nature 312:651–654
20. Bischoff JR, Friedman PN, Marshak DR, Prives C, Beach D (1990) Human p53 is phosphorylated by p60-cdc2 and cyclin B-cdc2. Proc Natl Acad Sci USA 87:4766–4770
21. Eliyahu D, Michalowitz D, Eliyahu S, Pinhasi, Kimhi O, Oren M (1989) Wild-type p53 can inhibit oncogene-mediated focus formation. Proc Natl Acad Sci USA 86:8763–8767
22. Finlay, C.A., Hinds PW, Levine AJ (1989) The p53 proto-oncogene can act as a suppressor of transformation. Cell 57:1083–1093

23 Finlay CA, Hinds PW, Tan TH, Eliyahu D, Oren M, Levine AJ (1988) Activating mutations for transformation by p53 produce a gene product that forms an hsc-70-p53 complex with an altered half life. Mol Cell Biol 8:531–539
24 Horak E, Smith K, Bromley L, Le Jeune S, Greenall M, Lane D, Harris AL (1991) Mutant p53, EGF receptor and c-erbB-2 expression in human breast cancer. Oncogene 6:2277–2284
25 Harris AL (1992) p53 expression in human breast cancer. Adv Cancer Res 59:69–88
26 Hamilton SR (1992) Molecular genetics of colorectal cancer. Cancer 70:1216–1221
27 Gazdar AF (1992) Molecular markers for the diagnosis and prognosis of lung cancer. Cancer 69:1592–1599
28 Quinlan DC, Davidson AG, Summers CL, Warden HE, Doshi HM (1992) Accumulation of p53 protein correlates with a poor prognosis in human lung cancer. Cancer Res 52:4828–4831
29 Sarkis AS, Dalbagni G, Cordon-Cardo C, Zhang ZF, Sheinfeld J, Fair WR, Herr HW, Reuter VE (1993) Nuclear overexpression of p53 protein in transitional cell bladder carcinoma: a marker for disease progression. J Natl Cancer Inst 85:53–59

Address for correspondence:
Dr. med. M. Kuczyk
Abteilung für Urologie
Medizinische Hochschule Hannover
Postfach 61 01 80
D-30625 Hannover, Germany

Expression of the nuclear oncogene p53 in human breast cancer in relation to prognostic factors

Carmen Minguillon[a], I. Schönborn[b], W. Friedmann[b], D. Judith[b], U. Bartel[b], W. Lichtenegger[b]

[a]Department of Gynecological Pathology, [b]Department of Gynecology,
UKRV Free University, Berlin, Germany

Introduction

The oncogene p53 is a nuclear phosphoprotein of 53 kilodaltons first described in 1979 by Lane and Crawford. The function of p53 in normal cells is not well known, it has been suggested to be a cell cycle protein playing a regulatory role in the control of cell proliferation. It has been demonstrated that active p53 expression is an essential component in the malignant transformation of tumor cells (7). An overexpression of p53 in primary breast carcinomas was found in 25% to 54% of tumors (1, 2, 4). The aim of this study was to determine the predictive value of p53 in a large series of 211 breast tumors by immunohistochemistry and to investigate its correlation with stage-related parameters. Our results suggest that overexpression of p53 is associated with more aggressive carcinomas.

Patients and methods

The tumors for this study were obtained from 211 operable breast cancer patients who had undergone surgery at the Universitätsfrauenklinik Charlottenburg in Berlin. Mastectomy and lumpectomy specimens were received fresh immediately following surgery and a tissue block selected from the tumor was snap-frozen. The rest tumor was fixed in buffered formalin. Frozen material was stored at –80 °C until required. Histological tumor type, tumor size, lymph node status and tumor grade were determined in the course of the routine pathological assessment (table I). Staining was carried out using monoclonal antibodies (MoAb) for the p53-protein (BP53-12/Bio Genex Hamburg, Germany), for the proliferating associated antigens Ki67 (Ki67/Dako Diagnostika, Germany) and Proliferating Cell Nuclear Antigen (PCNA = PC10/Dako Diagnostika, Germany), for steroid receptors (ER-ICA/Abbot GmbH Wiesbaden, Germany and anti progesteron/Dianova Germany). Frozen tissue was sectioned in five-micron sections and collected on poly-L-lysine coated glass slides, air-dried, and fixed for 10 min in aceton at room temperature. Formalin-fixed and paraffin-embedded tumor tissue was cut in two micron-sections and stored at 37 °C. Primary antibody was used in a 1:20 dilution in phosphate buffered saline (PBS), only ER-ICA was applied undiluted. The endogenous peroxidase activity was inhibited with 3% H_2O_2 for 5 min before the

Table I. Patient characteristics.

Total number of patients	211
Histological type	
invasive ductal	137
invasive lobular	45
special types	29
Grading	
G1	52
G2	125
G3	34
Tumor size	
ca. in situ	10
T1	101
T2	54
T3	10
T4	24
missing[a]	12
Nodal status	
negative	103
positive	75
missing[a]	33

[a] Not determined

primary antibody incubation step. Binding of the BP53-12 was visualized with the avidin biotinilated HRP complex (ABC-HRP) according to the recommendations of the supplier. For Ki67, PCNA and steroid receptors the APAAP-method according to Cordell (3) was used (APAAP/Dako Diagnostika GmbH, Germany). The slides were counterstained with Harris hematoxylin. For Ki67, PCNA and steroid receptors, the results were expressed as the percentage of tumor cells with positively stained nuclear area, for p53 only samples with intense nuclear staining were considered positive. For the statistical analysis the SPSS program package was used. Chi-square test was performed to determine the relationships between the variables, a value of $p < 0.05$ was considered statistically significant.

Results

A high level of p53 expression was detected in 79 (37.4%) of the 211 primary breast carcinomas. The remaining tumors had no detectable p53. Our study showed no significant differences in the frequency of p53 overexpression with respect to histological type, grading, tumor size and nodal status (table II).
A significant correlation between p53 overexpression and Ki67 ($p = 0.002$) or PCNA ($p = 0.001$) were found (figures 1 and 2). A low receptor status correlated significantly with a high value of p53. This inverse correlation was significant for both estrogen receptor (ER-ICA) and progesteron receptor (PgR) (ER-ICA $p = 0.05$, PgR $p = 0.02$).

Table II. Relationship between p53 and morphological features.

Parameters	p53 negative	p53 positive	p-Value
	n (%)	n (%)	
Histological type			
invasive ductale	84 (61.3)	53 (38.7)	
invasive lobular	26 (57.8)	19 (42.2)	
special types	22 (75.9)	7 (24.1)	0.2
Grading			
G1	39 (75.0)	13 (25.0)	
G2	74 (59.2)	51 (40.8)	
G3	19 (55.9)	15 (44.1)	0.7
Tumor size			
ca. in situ	9 (7.1)	1 (1.4)	
T1	61 (48.4)	40 (54.8)	
T2	33 (26.2)	21 (28.8)	
T3	6 (4.8)	4 (5.5)	
T4	17 (13.5)	7 (9.6)	0.3
missing[a] (12)			
Nodal status			
negative	68 (66.0)	35 (34.0)	
positive	48 (41.3)	27 (43.5)	0.4
missing[a] (33)			
Estrogen receptor			
≤ 20% positive	54 (55.7)	43 (44.3)	
> 20% positive	78 (68.4)	36 (31.6)	0.05
Progesteron receptor			
≤ 20% positive	67 (55.8)	53 (44.2)	
> 20% positive	65 (71.4)	26 (28.6)	0.02

[a] Not determined

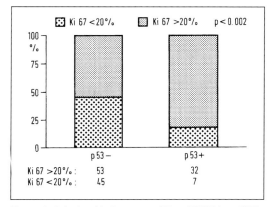

Figure 1. Relationship between p53 and Ki67 (n = 137).

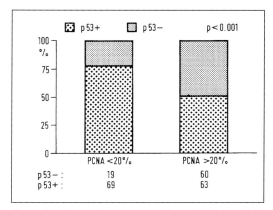

Figure 2. Relationship between p53 and PCNA (n = 211).

Discussion

In the present study 36.7% (73/211) tumors showed a positive nuclear staining for the MoAb p53 (BP53-120). Several authors reported dissenting results on p53 staining from 10% to 50% (1, 2, 4, 6). Reasons may be the variety of different MoAb to p53 and variations in epitope availability. Tumor cells positively stained for p53 showed a fairly uniform nuclear staining and the nuclear protein appeared to be restricted to the neoplastic tissue and was undetectable in both normal epithelia and mesenchymal cells. In the present study we found a good correlation between p53 and the proliferation associated antigens Ki67 and PCNA. The nuclear phosphoprotein p53 appears to play a role in the regulation of cell proliferation. Failure to regulate p53 expression appropriately may lead to uncontrolled cell growth. In agreement with *Cattoretti* (2) we observed in our study that p53 positive tumors had a negative or low receptor status. No correlation was observed between p53 expression and tumor size or lymph node status. These results suggest that p53 is not related to local tumor progression. Our results show that p53 is associated with predictive factors of more agressive carcinomas and might provide additive prognostic information in breast cancer.

References

1. Bártek J, Bártková J, Vojtesek B, Staskova Z, Rejthar A, Kovarik J, Lane DP (1990) Patterns of expression of the p53 tumour suppressor in human breast tissues and tumours in situ and in vitro. Int J Cancer 46:839–844
2. Cattoretti G, Rilke F, Andreola S, D'Amato L, Delia D (1988) P53 expression in breast cancer. Int J Cancer 41:178–183
3. Cordell JL, Falini B, Erber WN, Ghosh AK, Abdulaziz Z, Macdonald S, Pulford KAF, Stein H, Mason DY (1984) Immunoenzymatic labeling of monoclonal antibodies using immune complexes of alkaline phosphatase and monoclonal anti-alkaline phosphatase (APAAP Complexes). Histochem Cytochem 32:219–229
4. Davidoff AM, Herndon JE, Glover NS, Kerns B-JM, Pence JC Iglehart D, Marks JR, Durham NC (1991) Relation between p53 overexpression and established prognostic factors in breast cancer. Surgery 110/2:259–264
5. Lane DP, Crawford LV (1979) T antigen is bound to a host protein in SV-40 transformed cells. Nature 278:261–263
6. Ostrowski JL, Sawan A, Henry L, Wright C, Henry A, Hennessy C, Lennard TJW, Angus B, Horne CHW (1991) p53 expression in human breast cancer related to survival and prognostic factors: an immunohistochemical study. J Pathol 164:75–81
7. Wolf D, Harris N, Rotter V (1984) Reconstitution of p53 expression in a non-producer Ab-MuLV-transformed cell line by transfection of a functional p53 gene. Cell 38:651–653

Address for correspondence:
Dr. med. Carmen Minguillon
Abteilung für Gynäkologische Pathologie
UKRV, Freie Universität Berlin
Pulsstraße 4-14
D-14059 Berlin, Germany

Detection of p53-antibodies by immunoblot and ELISA in various human malignancies[1] – A new serological test?

P. R. Galle[a], Martina Müller[a], H. Zentgraf[b], M. Volkmann[a]

[a] Department of Internal Medicine, University of Heidelberg, Gastroenterology Unit (PRG, MM, MV),
[b] Applied Tumor Virology, German Cancer Research Center, Heidelberg, Germany

Introduction

Alterations of the 53 gene are the commonest genetic change detected in human cancer (8). The most frequent alterations (about 80%) are single point mutations in one p53 allele and subsequent amino acid substitutions, usually in the evolutionary conserved regions of the gene (1, 11). The resulting mutant p53 proteins display a prolonged half life accounting for the increased nuclear levels of p53 protein frequently detected in tumors (5, 11).

Mutant p53 proteins may induce a humoral immune response in tumor patients. In an initial study the presence of antibodies against p53 (anti-p53) had been demonstrated in patients with breast carcinomas (3). Several other publications have confirmed and extended these data (2, 4, 7, 9, 10, 13, 14), describing anti-p53 as an ubiquitous serological marker for malignancy, present in up to 30% of the tumor patients. Here we present data on more than 500 patients with different tumor entities using a newly developed immmunoblot assay based on recombinant p53. Furthermore, to facilitate large scale analysis we have developed an anti-p53 ELISA.

In addition to molecular analysis of the p53 gene or detection of its gene product, testing for anti-p53 provides another experimental approach for assessment of the involvement of p53 in human cancer.

Methods

Immunoblot (Western blot)

We have used a cDNA fragment of wild type p53 comprising all of the 393 codons of the protein (kindly provided by L. Crawford, London). The recombinant protein was expressed in a T7 RNA polymerase directed vector system after induction with 2 mM isopropyl-b-D-thiogalactopyranoside. Recombinant p53 was then purified by urea extraction and electroelution as described previously (13). For detection of anti-p53 antibodies, 100 ng recombinant p53 per lane were electrophoretically separated by SDS-PAGE in a 10% gel and subsequently transferred to nitrocellulose filters. Patient sera were used at a 1:100 dilution.

ELISA

To facilitate large scale analysis we have developed an ELISA based on recombinant p53 antigen which is licensed and distributed by Dianova, Hamburg, FRG (Volkmann, Zentgraf, Galle, in preparation).

Results

532 sera from tumor patients (cancer of: liver (n = 80), esophagus (n = 47), stomach (n = 128), colon (n = 182), rectum (n = 35), pancreas

---

[1]This project is supported by grant I.1.2. from the Tumorzentrum Heidelberg/Mannheim.

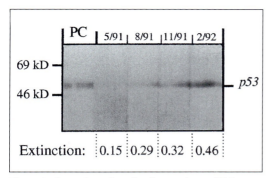

Figure 1. Detection of antibodies against p53 in sera (dilution 1:50) of a patient with colon cancer during clinical progression. Top: Immunoblot; bottom: ELISA. PC: positive control (rabbit antiserum HZp53R, raised against recombinant p53); kD:kilodalton.

(n = 17), breast (n = 24) or urogenital tract (n = 19)) were tested by immunoblotting and in part by ELISA. 379 patients free of malignancies served as controls. Overall, anti-p53 could be demonstrated in 116 of 532 (21.8%) (range 6–33%) of the patients with malignant disease but not in the controls. The association of anti-p53 with malignancy was highly significant ($p < 0.0003$; Fisher's exact test, 2-tail). Individual sera displayed high anti-p53 titers, showing reactivity up to a dilution of 1:130,000 in a patient with metastasizing breast cancer. Furthermore, anti-p53 can be detected in about 25% of the patients negative for conventional tumor markers. Figure 1 gives the example of a patient with cancer of the colon who developed metastases of the liver and, during the course of clinical progression, became positive for anti-p53 (8/91) and six months later for CEA (2/92). In general, anti-p53 seroconversion could be shown for 40% (10 of 25) of the patients with progressive disease during a 12 year follow-up. Vice versa, in some patients, a postoperative decline of anti-p53 reactivity was observed.

Discussion

Mutations in the p53 gene have been demonstrated for a variety of different tumors (6, 8). Typically, they give rise to a mutant p53 protein with increased biological half life and subsequent nuclear accumulation. Several studies demonstrated that this may result in a humoral immune response against p53 (2, 3, 4, 7, 9, 10, 12, 13, 14).

Our data confirm the specificity of anti-p53 as a serological marker of malignancy. Anti-p53 serum antibodies can be readily detected in a significant proportion of tumor patients by immunoblotting or ELISA procedures. Both tests can easily be integrated in a clinical laboratory set-up and provide an additional diagnostic tool in the follow-up and management of oncological patients. Serologically otherwise negative tumors of different entities can be identified and disease progression and response to treatment can be monitored.

The small number of studies investigating the relation of anti-p53 to clinical data found no correlation of anti-p53 positivity with tumor stage, presence of extrahepatic metastases, underlying disease or patients' sex or age. Our data demonstrate the appearance of anti-p53 during disease progression. Moreover, analysis of sera from patients with breast cancer revealed a correlation with the presence of anti-p53 and high grading and negative hormone receptor status, respectively (12). However, further studies in a prospective setting will be needed to fully assess the clinical potential of anti-p53.

References

1 Baker SJ, Fearon ER, Nigro JM, Hamilton SR, Preisinger AC Jessup JM, van Tuinen P et al (1989) Chromosome 17 deletions and p53 gene mutations in colorectal carcinomas. Science 244:217–21

2 Caron de Fromentel C, May-Levin F, Mouriesse H, Lemerle J, Chandrasekeran K, May P (1987) Presence of circulating antibodies against cellular protein p53 in a notable proportion of children with B-cell lymphoma. Int J Cancer 39:185–9

3 Crawford LV, Pim DC, Bulbrook RD (1982) Detection of antibodies against cellular protein p53 in sera from patients with breast cancer. Int J Cancer 30:403–408

4 Davidoff AM, Iglehart JD, Marks JR (1992) Immune response to p53 is dependent upon p53/HSP70 complexes in breast cancer. Proc Natl Acad Sci USA 89:3439–42

5 Hinds P, Finlay C, Levine AJ (1989) Mutation is required to activate the p53 gene for cooperation with the ras oncogene and transformation. J Virol 63:739–46

6. Hollstein M, Sidransky D, Vogelstein B, Harris CC (1991) P53 mutations in human cancer. Science 253:49-53
7. Labrecque S, Naor N, Thomson D, Matlashewski G (1993) Analysis of the anti-p53 antibody response in cancer patients. Cancer Res 53:3468-3471
8. Levine AJ, Momand J, Finlay CA (1991) The p53 tumor suppressor gene. Nature 351:453-6
9. Lubin R, Schlichtholz B, Bengoufa D et al (1993) Analysis of p53 antibodies in patients with various cancers define B-cell epitopes of human p53: distribution on primary structure and exposure on protein surface. Cancer Res 53:5872-5876
10. Müller M, Volkmann M, Zentgraf H, Galle PR (1994) Clinical implications of the p53 tumor suppressor gene. New Engl J Med (letter) 330: 864-865
11. Nigro JM, Baker SJ, Preisinger AC, Jessup JM, Hostetter R, Cleary K, Bigner SH et al (1989) Mutations in the p53 gene occur in diverse human tumor types. Nature 342:705-8
12. Schlichtholz B, Legros Y, Gaillard C et al (1992) The immune response to p53 in breast cancer patients is directed against immunodominant epitopes unrelated to the mutational hot spot. Cancer Res 52:6380-6384
13. Volkmann M, Müller M, Hofmann WJ, Meyer M, Hagelstein J, Räth U, Kommerell B, Zentgraf H, Galle PR (1993) The humoral immune response to p53 in patients with hepatocellular carcinoma is specific for malignancy and independent of the alpha-fetoprotein status. Hepatol 18:559-565
14. Winter SF, Minna JD, Johnson BE, Takahashi T, Gazdar AF, Carbone DP (1992) Development of antibodies against p53 in lung cancer patients appears to be dependent on the type of p53 mutation. Cancer Res 52:4168-4174

Address for correspondence:
Priv.-Doz. Dr. P. R. Galle
Medizinische Universitätsklinik
Abteilung Gastroenterologie
Bergheimerstraße 58
D-69115 Heidelberg, Germany

Immunohistochemistry

＃ Basement membrane expression as a marker for the differentiation of squamous cell carcinomas of the larynx

H. Hagedorn[a], M. Schreiner[b], I. Wiest[a], E. Schleicher[c], A. Nerlich[a]

[a] Institute for Pathology, [b] ENT-Clinic, Klinikum Großhadern, University of Munich,
[c] Institute for Diabetes Research, Municipal Hospital Schwabing, Munich, Germany

Introduction

The continuity of the epithelial basement membrane (BM) is widely accepted as a criterium for a benign biological behavior of tumors, while the loss of an intact BM has been regarded as a sign for malignant growth (1, 5). Until now, there exist, however, only few studies dealing with the correlation of BM-expression and the biological behavior of malignant tumors (4, 6, 7, 11). These studies have mainly been performed on bladder, colon and hepatocellular carcinomas showing a positive correlation between the loss of BM material and the aggressivity of tumor growth. Isolated studies provide additonal evidence that the degree of BM expression is correlated with the degree of tumor differentiation (6).

Since squamous cell carcinomas have not yet been the subject of an extensive analysis, we decided to investigate the qualitative and (semi-)quantitative expression of various BM components in a series of squamous cell carcinomas of the larynx. To obtain insight into the interaction between tumor differentiation and BM expression, the resulting immunohistochemical observations were correlated with the histopathologically estimated degree of tumor differentiation. In this analysis, we furthermore applied antibodies against BM components that have not, or only very rarely been analysed in malignant squamous cell neoplasms – particularly collagen VII and the BM associated heparan sulfate proteoglycan (HSPG) – so that their potential role in tumor cell invasion and tumor aggressivity is elucidated by this study.

Materials and methods

The present study was conducted on specimens from 44 patients that had undergone laryngectomy due to squamous cell carcinoma. 41 patients were males, while only three patients were females. The patients' ages ranged between 41 and 81 years. In all instances, we used representative formalin-fixed and paraffin-embedded tissue blocs of the carcinoma (tumor center) for the preparation of routine histology staining (hematoxyline and eosin) (H/E) and subsequent immunohistological staining procedures. The H/E stained slides were subsequently used for the estimation of the degree of tumor differentation. Furthermore, we simultaneously analyzed laryngeal tissue specimens that showed either hyperplasia or dysplastic epithelial changes (n = 14).

For the immunohistochemical analysis we used type specific antibodies against the major BM components collagen IV and VII, laminin, heparan sulfate proteoglycan (HSPG) and fibronectin which had been obtained from the following sources: Collagen IV and laminin antibodies had been purchased from Eurodiagnostics, Apeldoorn, NL, the fibronectin antibody from Dako, Hamburg, FRG. The anti-HSPG antibodies had been prepared as described previously (12). The anti-collagen VII antibodies had been greatfully supplied by *Dr. R. Burgeson*, Portland, Oregon, USA. Appropriate tissue sections were then stained by use either of the avidin-biotin-peroxidase complexe method (ABC-method) (8) or the alkaline phosphatase anti-alkaline phosphatase method (APAAP-method) (3) using the procedure previously described (9, 10).

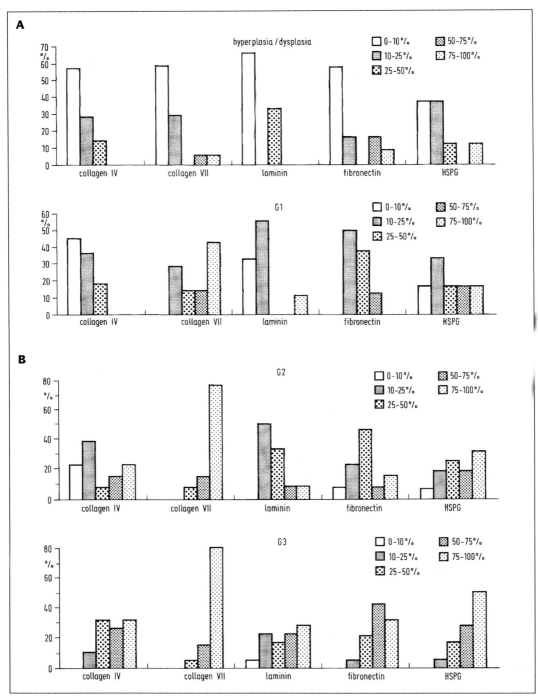

Figure 1. Graphic evaluation of the tumor BM disruption. This graph shows the percentage of gaps for the different BM components. Therefore, the amount of gaps in random fields of the tumor-stroma interface was morphometrically estimated and ranked into five categories ranging between 0–10% gaps and 100% gaps. The relative values are given (A) for dysplastic/hyperplastic epithelium and grade 1 carcinomas, as well as (B) for grade 2 and 3 carcinomas.

Results

The immunohistochemical analysis revealed in all carcinomas a discontinuous BM as evidenced by a focal loss of BM material. This loss in BM expression, however, was variable with respect to the various BM components, as well as concerning the different degrees of tumor differentiation (see figure 1).

Thus, we found in well differentiated carcinomas (grade 1) in most cases a peritumoral BM that showed only minor fragmentation and small gaps. In these tumors, the expression of collagen IV and laminin was accordingly mostly preserved, while collagen VII was affected much more extensively resulting in only small fragments of collagen VII that remained (figure 1). The expression of HSPG and that of fibronectin was interindividually variable providing no major trend of changes.

In moderately differentiated carcinomas (grade 2) the extent of BM loss was more extensive than in grade 1 carcinomas. Again, collagen VII was much more affected than the other components which again seemed to be discoordinately expressed since the observed gaps comprised not all BM components tested simultaneously. In the tumor stroma often an overexpression of fibronectin occured.

In poorly differentiated carcinomas, a further loss in BM expression was obvious. The BM defects resulted in most cases in only small fragments of BM material that were deposited around tumor cell nests. Likewise collagen VII was present as only minor fragments adjacent to tumor cell complexes. Again, a disorganization of the remaining BM material deposition could be found and in isolated areas spot-like and small drop-like inclusions of BM material in tumor cell nests were evident.

The analysis of hyperplastic and dysplastic epithelium revealed in these instances a BM that was occasionally interrupted. Here again, various components were involved in this fragmentation phenomenon. In contrast to the invasive growth pattern, however, in dysplastic as well as in non-dysplastic, but hyperplastic epithelium a nearly continuous collagen VII staining could be found. Mostly, the gap formation of this non-invasive epithelium was associated with an inflammatory stromal infiltrate, mostly by lymphocytes.

Discussion

In the present study, we analyzed the expression of major BM components in a series of squamous cell carcinomas of the larynx. Our study was designed to prove whether previous results on other types of carcinomas can be transferred to squamous cell carcinomas. These previous studies had indicated a correlation between the degree of BM expression and the biological behavior of a tumor (4, 6, 7, 11). Furthermore this study seemed to be necessary, since former analyses had reported on the intactness of the subepithelial BM in well differentiated squamous cell carcinomas of the head and neck (2). These results were in contrast to previous preliminary own observations (10), as well as to the findings in squamous cell carcinomas of other origin or localization, like at the uterine cervix (13), where the formation of gaps even in highly differentiated tumor areas had been observed. Our present results may explain these differences (14), since we observed a disorganized expression of the various BM components analyzed. This may result in an apparent intact BM around tumor cell complexes when only one or two components are tested. To this regard our analysis provides clear evidence that the loss of collagen VII is the "earliest" morphological BM change that is associated with stromal invasion. Furthermore, we confirmed the previous observation (13) that inflammatory infiltrates underneath an otherwise non-neoplastic epithelium may be associated with a disruption of the BM. This observations indicates that the loss of a continuos BM staining is not an absolute criterium for malignant growth.

Conclusions

The present analysis provides the following major conclusions:
The amount of BM material expression correlates with the degree of tumor differentiation, i.e. the more BM material is expressed by tumor cells, the higher is the degree of tumor differentiation.
The various BM components are qualiatively and quantitatively differently expressed at the tumor-stroma interface indicating a disbalance in the usually coordinate expression of various BM components.

The "earliest" loss in BM material comprises the collagen VII which shows significant gaps even in well differentiated carcinomas whereas the expression of the other components may still be preserved.

Dysplastic and hyperplastic epithelia may also show a BM disruption, mostly associated with an inflammatory infiltrate in the stroma.

Therefore, a loss of BM expression is not an absolute criterion for malignant epithelial growth. Nevertheless, a major loss in the BM specific component collagen VII seems to be indicative for malignant infiltrative growth.

References

1 Barsky SH, Siegal GP, Jannotta F, Liotta LA (1983) Loss of basement membrane components by invasive tumors but not by their benign counterparts. Lab Invest 49:140–147
2 Cam Y, Caulet T, Bellon G, Poulin G, Legros M, Pytlinska M (1984) Immunohistochemical localization of macromolecules of the basement membrane and the peritumoral stroma in human laryngeal carcinomas. J Pathol 144:35–44
3 Cordell JL, Falini B, Erber WN, Ghosh AK, Abdulaziz Z, MacDonald S, Pulford AF, Stein H, Mason DY (1984) Immunoenzymatic labeling of monoclonal antibodies using immune complexes of alkaline phosphatase and monoclonal antialkaline phosphatase. J Histochem Cytochem 32:219–225
4 Daher N, Abourachid H, Bove N, Petit J, Burtin P (1987) Collagen IV staining pattern in bladder carcinomas: relationship to prognosis. Br J Cancer 55:665–671
5 D'Ardenne AJ (1989) Use of basement membrane markers in tumor diagnosis. J Clin Pathol 42: 449–457
6 Fuchs ME, Brawer MK, Rennels MA, Nagle RB (1989) The relationship of basement membrane to histologic grade of human prostatic carcinoma. Mod Pathol 2:105–111
7 Grigioni WF, Garbisa S, D'Errico A, Baccarini P, Stetler-Stevenson WG, Liotta L, Mancini AM (1981) Evaluation of hepatocellular carcinoma aggressiveness by a panel of extracellular matrix antigens. Am J Pathol 138:647–654
8 Hsu SM, Raine L, Fanger H (1981) A comparative study on the peroxidase-antiperoxidase method and an avidin-biotin- complex method for studying polypeptide hormones with radioimmunoassay antibodies. Am J Clin Pathol 75:734–739
9 Nerlich A, Schleicher E (1991) Immunohistochemical localization of extracellular matrix components in human diabetic glomerular lesions. Am J Pathol 139:889–899
10 Nerlich A (1992) Basalmembran und assoziierte Matrixproteine in normalem und pathologischem Gewebe. Immunhistochemische und molekularbiologische Untersuchungen. Habilitationsschrift, München
11 Offerhaus GJA, Giardiello FM, Bruijn JA, Stijnen T, Molyvas EN, Fleuren GJ (1991) The value of immunohistochemistry for collagen IV expression in colorectal carcinomas. Cancer 67:99–105
12 Schleicher ED, Wagner EM, Olgemöller B, Nerlich A, Gerbitz KD (1989) Characterization and localization of basement membrane associated heparan sulfate proteoglycan in human tissues. Lab Invest 61: 323–332
13 Stewart CJR, McNicol AM (1992) Distribution of type IV collagen immunoreactivity to assess questionable early stromal invasion. J Pathol 45:9–15
14 Visser R, van Beek JMH, Havenith MG, Cleutjens JPM, Bosman FT (1986) Immunocytochemical detection of basement membrane antigens in the histopathological evalution of laryngeal dysplasia and neoplasia. Histopathol 10:171–180

Address for correspondence:
Priv.-Doz. Dr. A. Nerlich
Pathologisches Institut der Universität
Thalkirchnerstraße 36
D-80337 München, Germany

Detection of keratins in microvascularized jejunal autografts to the oral cavity and adjacent oral mucosa

R. E. Friedrich[a], D. Hellner[a], H. Arps[b]

[a] Oral and Maxillofacial Surgery (Nordwestdeutsche Kieferklinik), Eppendorf University Hospital, University of Hamburg, [b] Institute of Pathology, Municipial Hospital, Fulda, Germany

Introduction

Jejunal autografts

The microvascularized jejunal autograft is a valuable surgical tool in head and neck surgery especially in the therapy of patients who had been subjected to a preoperative percutaneous radiotherapy leading to a xerostomia (12). However, the functional benefit to irradiated patients in replacing the oral mucosa by a jejunal segment secreting a new saliva seems to be limited. Indeed, in some cases with a perfect ingrowth to the resection site the clinical aspect reveals a reduction of the transplants size, a rarefication of the surface corresponding to a reduced saliva production. The intestinal mucosa seems to become pale during the time of ectopical use, sometimes making it difficult to distinguish oral and transplanted mucosa by clinical inspection. Previous morphological investigations in experimental animals have presented a flattening and compression of the jejunal villis and a partial replacement of simple by squamous epithelia (10, 12, 13, 14, 17). On the other hand, a marginal overgrowth of residual squamous cells on to the jejunal epithelia was noticed (10, 12). In microvascularised jejunal oral autografts a new formation (12) or an increase of the number of desmosomes (17) due to altered function and scary fixation to the recipient connective tissue can be observed. The healthy jejunal epithelia are characterised by the expression of keratins no. 8, 18, 19 and 20 (4-6) characterizing simple epithelia. An alteration of intestinal keratin expression is a rare phenomenon but within the range of differentiation detectable by immunocytochemistry (6). Immunocytochemical typings of keratins in microvascularized jejunal autografts and adjacent oral mucosa have shown a persistence of entodermal keratins in the jejunal transplant and of ectodermal keratins in the oral mucosa (16), but occasionally a reduction of keratins characterizing simple epihelia in the microvascularized jejunal transplant is noticed (7). Temporary ulcerations of the jejunal mucosa (10) are not followed by an inflammatory degradation of the subepithelial connective tissue or an inflammatory proliferation of the transplant vessels (10, 12) and even a reduction of the marginal squamous cells metaplasia of the jejunal transplants mucosa was noticed (11).

Oral mucosa

The oral mucosa at the recipient site seems to hyperproliferate according to an increase of TPA-positivity in epithelia of the oral mucosa located close to the transplant (10). The patterns of TPA expression have been correlated to that of keratin 19 and homology or even identity of both proteins has been suggested (5).

Material and methods

Nineteen biopsies of the transplants and adjacent oral mucosa in seven patients with microvascularized jejunal autografts to the oral cavity were excised (preoperative percutaneous radiotherapy: 60–75 Gy, initial staging: > T2). The percutaneous application of the radiotherapy was carried out about three months before ablative surgery and reconstruction using a microvascularized jejunal autograft. The biopsies were taken

10 to 12 month after transplantation. All the patients had a history of alcohol and nicotine abuse for years. The tissue samples were gained from marginal and central parts of the transplants, immediately shock frozen in liquid nitrogene and stocked at −70 °C up to the time of immunocytochemical investigation. For detection of keratins monoclonal antibodies to keratins no. 13/16 (clone K8.12, Sigma), 4 (clone 215 B8, Boehringer Mannheim), no. 10/11/1 (clone K8.60, ICN Immunobiologicals), 18 (clone CK 5, Sigma), 19 (clone 4.62, ICN Immunobiologicals) and a broad spectrum of keratins decorating antibody (K8.13, Sigma) were applied using the APAAP-technique (1). Control reactions were explored for each antibody by omitting the primary antibody. Two specimens of native jejunum gained at the time of reconstructive surgery were used as controls, too.

Results

Immunocytochemically the cytoplasmas of the jejunal epithelial cells homogeneously were decorated after incubation with keratin 18 resp. 19 specific antibodies (clones: CK5 resp. 4.62) both in native and transplant specimens (figure 1) but not in squamous cells of the recipient oral mucosa. The suprabasal cell layers of the adjacent oral mucosa is marked by the keratin 4 specific antibody (clone 215B8). Neither basal squamous cells (oral mucosa) nor the epithelial cells of the

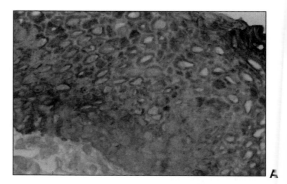

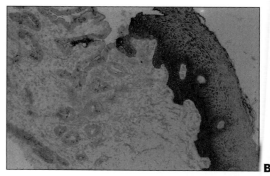

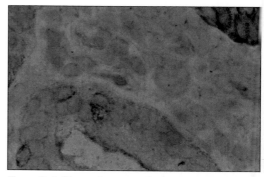

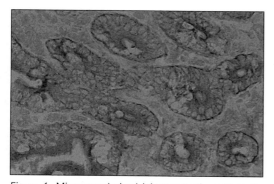

Figure 1. Microvascularized jejunum to the oral cavity (transplantation one year ago): the cytoplasmas of jejunal epithelia are entirely decorated by the antibody identifying keratin no. 19 (clone: 4.62), APAAP. (magnification x 67).

Figure 2. A. The oral mucosa close to the jejunal transplant. All layers are decorated by the immunological reaction including basal cells (magnification x 124). B. Predominantly basal reaction of the antibody in oral squamous epithelia (arrow, top), sharp demarcation of oral and jejunal tissues (arrow, left), and decoration of secretory products of the jejunum (arrow, bottom) (magnification x 25). C. Immunoreactivity of enterocytes (arrow, left) and of oral basal sqamous epithelia (arrowhead, right) for K8.12 (magnification x 268). (Clone: K8.12, keratins no. 13 and 16, APAAP).

Table I. Immunocytochemical detection of keratins in microvascularised jejunal autografts to the oral cavity.

Clones / target antigens	Normal jejunal enterocytes	Oral mucosa	Jejunal transplant enterocytes
CK5/18	4/4	0/6	19/19
4.62/19	4/4	0/6	19/19
215B/4	0/4	6/6a	0/19
K8.12/13, 16	0/4	6/6b	10/9
K8.13/1, 5, 6, 7, 8, 10, 11, 18	4/4	6/6	19/19
K8.60/1, 10, 11	0/4	3/6	11/19

a Suprabasal oral epithelia cells;
b Basal and suprabasal oral epithelia cells

intestine were keratin 4 positive. In some cases the keratin 13 and 16 identifying antibody (clone K8.12) marked both suprabasal and basal layers of oral squamous epithelia and enterocytes (figure 2). Besides a cytoplasmatic reaction product of basal and to a greater extent of suprabasal cell layers also some enterocytes were K8.60 positive, too (keratins 1, 10, 11) (table I).

Discussion

Keratins no. 8, 18 and 19 and 20 are typical for simple epithelia of the gastrointestinal tract (4, 5). The expression of keratin no. 19 in normal oral mucosa seems to be restricted to the basal and a few suprabasal cell layers (16) or might even be absent (15). The presence of keratin no. 19 in oral mucosa was found in normal oral epithelia (8), inflammation (9), epithelial dysplasia (3, 15) and carcinomas (15) and was not detected in the specimens investigated in this study. TPA has been detected in basal cells of the normal oral mucosa and an increase of amount and suprabasal decoration of oral mucosa adjacent to jejunal autografts with a TPA-antibody has been correlated to a hyperproliferative status of the marginal oral mucosa (10). The assumption of a hyperproliferative status of the oral mucosa is supported by a decoration of basal cell layers after incubation with the antibody reacting with keratins 13 and 16 (K8.12; (2)). The hypothesis of a keratin 16 expression in basal cells adjacent to the jejunal autograft is supported by the pattern of epithelia decoration with a keratin 4 specific antibody (clone 215B8): This antibody marked suprabasal cell layers of stratified epithelia only and was completely negative in jejunal epithelia and basal cell layers of marginal oral mucosa. There usually is an expression of keratin pairs in vivo and the association of keratin 4 and 13 is typical for non-keratinizing epithelia of the upper aerodigestive tract (4). The cytoplasmic decoration of enterocytes after incubation with the antibody specific for keratins (K8.60, keratins no. 1, 10, 11) has been not reported so far. A cytoplasmic keratinization of intestinal epithelia is a rare phenomenon but within the range of differentiation of intestinal epithelia (6). This result is supporting former reports of an initiation of squamous cell metaplasia in jejunal transplants (12) despite the micromorphological aspect of an intact jejunal structure at least in the crypts of the transplants in transmission electron microphotographs (17).

References

1. Cordell JL, Falini B, Erber WN, Ghosh A, Abdulaziz Z, Macdonald S, Pulford KAF, Stein H, Mason D (1984) Immunoenzymatic labeling of monoclonal antibodies using complexes of alkaline phosphatase and monoclonal anti-alkalinephosphatase (APAAP-Complexes). J Histochem Cytochem 32:219
2. de Mare S, van Erp P, van de Kerkhof PCM (1989) Epidermal hyperproliferation assessed by the monoclonal antibody Ks 8.12 in frozen sections. J Invest Dermatol 92:130
3. Lindberg EK, Reinwald JG (1989) Suprabasal 40 kd keratin (K19) an immunohistologic marker of premalignancy in oral epithelium. Am J Pathol 134:89
4. Moll R, Franke WW, Schiller DL (1982) The catalog of human cytokeratins: patterns of expression in normal epithelia, tumors and cultured cells. Cell 31:11

5. Moll R (1987) Epithelial tumor markers: Cytokeratins and tissue polypeptide antigen (TPA). Curr Top Pathol 77:71
6. Moll R (1988) Differenzierungsprogramme des Epithels und ihre Änderungen. Verh Dtsch Ges Pathol 72:102
7. Nielsen IM, Riis A, Clausen P (1990) Morphological and histological studies of human jejunal grafts transplanted to the oral cavity. Joint Meeting Deutschsprachige Arbeitsgemeinschaft für Mikrochirurgie and Scandivian Work Group for Reconstructive Microsurgery. Hansaari, Espoo, Finland, pp 51
8. Ouhayoun JP, Gosselin F, Forest N, Winter N, Franke WW (1985) Cytokeratin patterns of human oral epithelia: differences in cytokeratin synthesis in gingival epithelium and the adjacent alveolar mucosa. Differentiation 30:123
9. Ouhayoun JP, Goffaux JC, Sawaf MH, Shabana AHM, Collin C, Forest N (1990) Changes in cytokeratin expression in gingiva during inflammation. J Periodont Res 25:283
10. Reichart P, Löning Th, Hausamen J-E, Becker J (1984) Morphologic study on jejunal mucosal transplants for the replacement of oral mucosa. J Oral Pathol 13:595
11. Reichart P, van den Berghe P, Becker J, Schuppan J, Hausamen J-E (1990) Zur Bedeutung epithelialmesenchymaler Interaktionen in mikrovaskulär gestielten Dünndarmtransplantaten zum Ersatz oraler Mukosa. In: Schwenzer N, Pfeifer G (eds) Mikrochirurgie in der Mund-, Kiefer- und Gesichts-Chirurgie, Fortschritte der Kiefer- und Gesichts-Chirurgie, Bd. XXXV, Thieme, Stuttgart, pp 63
12. Reuther JF, Steinau HU, Wagner R (1984) Reconstruction of large defects in the oropharynx with a revascularised intestinal graft: an experimental and clinical study. Plastic Recontruct Surg 73:345
13. Reuther J (1989) Microsurgical small bowel transfer for intraoral reconstruction. In: Riediger D, Ehrenfeld M (eds) Microsurgical tissue transplantation. Quintessence, Chicago, pp 95
14. Robinson D W (1984) Discussion remark on the publication of Reuther et al (1984) Plastic Reconstruct Surg 73:359
15. Schulz J, Ermich T, Kasper M, Raabe G, Schumann D (1992) Cytokeratin pattern of clinically intact and pathologically changed oral mucosa. Int J Oral Maxillofac Surg 21:35
16. Shabana AHM, Ouhayoun JP, Sawaf MH, Forest N (1989) A comparative biochemical and immunological analysis of cytokeratin patterns in the oral epithelium of the miniature pig and man. Archs Oral Biol 34:249
17. Vollrath M, Reiss G (1989) Submikroskopische Veränderungen des Jejunums an ektopischer Lokalisation. HNO 37:133

Address for correspondence:
Dr. med. Dr. med. dent. R. E. Friedrich
Klinik für Mund-, Kiefer- und Gesichtschirurgie
(Nordwestdeutsche Kieferklinik)
Martinistraße 52
D-20246 Hamburg, Germany

Undifferentiated carcinomas of the nasopharyngeal type (UCNT) – Correlation of EBV-genome detection by ^{35}S-labeled plasmids and detection of keratin, vimentin and EMA

R.E. Friedrich[a], S. Bartel-Friedrich[b], G. Niedobitek[c], H. Herbst[c], H. Lobeck[d]

[a]Department of Oral and Maxillofacial Surgery, Eppendorf University Hospital, University of Hamburg,
[b]Department of Otorhinolaryngology, [c]Institute of Pathology, Steglitz University Hospital,
[d]Institute of Pathology, Rudolf Virchow University Hospital, Free University of Berlin, Germany

Introduction

According to the WHO classification presently revised nasopharyngeal carcinomas (NPC) are typed as keratinizing squamous cell carcinomas and non-keratinizing carcinomas (NKC). In NKC subtypes are identified: differentiated or undifferentiated (UCNT) types (14). NKC are highly associated with the presence of Epstein-Barr-Virus (EBV) (17). This association was demonstrated by serological investigations, nucleic acid and in situ hybridization (ISH) (10, 17). In a recent ISH study a specific association of EBV and lymphoepithelioma like carcinomas outside the nasopharynx was suggested (12). However, as far as carcinomas of the head and neck are concerned, results of another current investigation (6) supports the hypothesis of a unique association of EBV with undifferentiated and non-keratinizing carcinomas (16). According to immunocytochemical analysis the expression of intermediate filaments in primary and metastatic neoplastic carcinomas is well preserved and can be used as a powerful diagnostic tool for characterization of tumor histogenesis and localization in cases of unknown primary lesions (1). In this study the evidence of EBV genomes in undifferentiated carcinomas of the head and neck region by ISH of ^{35}S-labeled genomes and its correlation to the expression of keratin, vimentin and EMA in regions where autoradiographical signals of EBV could be demonstrated.

Materials and methods

Tissues

Routinely processed biopsy specimens (formalin-fixed, paraffin-embedded) of 20 epithelial tumors collected over a period of five years were included in this study. All specimens were reclassified and UCNT was diagnosed according to the revised WHO classification (14) on routinely processed HE-slides (3).

In situ hybridization (ISH)

As previously described ISH was carried out on paraffin sections (8) using ^{35}S-labeled plasmids pBa-W (3.1 kb BamHI EBV interneal repeat fragment (11)) and pM961-20 (6.4 kb HindIII/SalI fragment from the right end of the linear EBV genome). ISH with a cytomegalovirus (CMV) probe (13) served as control. In brief, rehydrated paraffin sections were pretreated with 0.2 N HCl for ten minutes at room temperature (RT), 0.1% Triton X-100 for 1.5 minutes (RT), and 0.1 mg/ml pronase (Boehringer, Mannheim, FRG) for 30 minutes (37 °C), followed by acetylation with 0.1 M triethanolamine/0.25% acetic anhydride for ten minutes (RT). Slides were washed in 2 x SSC (0.3 M NaCl, 0.03 M sodium citrate, pH 7.6) between the incubation steps. After pretreatment slides were dehydrated through graded ethanols and 25 µl hybridization mixture (50% deionised formamide/2 x SSC/10% dextran sulphate/0.1 mg/ml herring sperm DNA/20 to 40 ng/ml of labeled probe) were applied. Simultaneous denaturation of probe and tissue DNA was performed by heating the slides to 90 °C for three minutes, followed by incubation of slides in a humide chamber at 37 °C for 12 hours. On the next day slides were washed in several changes of 50% formamide/0.1 x SSC at 37 °C for four hours and rinsing in 0.1 x SSC for 30 minutes (RT). The hybridization mixture and all washing solutions contained 10 mM dithiothreitol (Sigma, St.Louis). The slides were then dehydrated through graded ethanols and dipped into Ilford-G5 emulsion. Simultaneous ISH of parallel sections of each specimen was used for variant exposure times of three to eight days. Then the slides were developed with Kodak D19 Developer and Kodak Rapid Fixer, followed by counterstaining with hematoxylin and eosin. Sections of oral hairy leukoplakias (immunocompromised patients) served as positive control tissue for EBV-DNA. Positive results were accepted only in the case of negative hybridization results with the CMV probe on simultaneously processed slides. Negative results required a strong labeling of sections of oral hairy leukoplakias with the EBV probe in synchronous positive control experiments for approval. The specifity of the labeled CMV probe was tested on sections of tissues showing evidence of CMV infection by immunocytochemistry in agree to clinical and autoptic data of CMV-sepsis (7).

Immunocytochemistry

Specimens were dewaxed, rehydrated, buffered in TRIS-buffer, followed by incubation either with KL-1 (1:300, Dianova, Hamburg, FRG), vimentin (V9,1:80, Dako, Hamburg, FRG), Epithelial Membrane Antigen (EMA, E29, 1:50, Dako) or LCA (PD7/26, 1:50, Dako) for 30 minutes (RT) in a humide chamber. Then the slides were incubated with second antibody (1:40, rabbit-antimouse, dianova) and APAAP-complex for 30 minutes each (RT) and repeated for 15 minutes. Antigen binding was detected by substrate of alkaline phosphatase as previously described (4). Then the slides were counterstained with hemealaune.

Results

In situ hybridization

Of a total of 20 cases a virus related positive nuclear staining after EBVISH was recognized in 14 (70%) and correlated to cases which were classified as UCNT there was an association to EBV detection of 86%. Two tissues (one patient with follow-up biopsies) of UCNT could not be classified as EBV positive. Further negative staining results could be related to morphology: partially low differentiated squamous cell carcinomas (n = 3), one of them non-keratinizing.

Immunocytochemistry

All NPC could be identified by the broad spectrum keratin antibody KL-1. The immunoreactivity varied in a wide range. Vimentin positive carcinoma cells appeared in nine cases. There was no correlation of the rate of decorations of carcinoma cells in KL-1 and V9 positive tissues. Lack of EMA expression was found in nine cases and immunoreactivity for LCA was restricted to lymphocytes adjacent to the carcinoma cells (table I).

Table I. Correlation of EMA expression and EBV detection in UCNT.

EBV	EMA (E29)	
	positive	negative
Positive	5	8
Negative	6[a]	1

[a]Predominantly a lack of immunoreactivity for EMA in the majority of carcinoma cells and focal staining pattern in three cases

Correlation of ISH with intermediate filament expression

A positive correlation of EBV genome detection and immunoreactivity for V9 was found in nine cases (45%). EBV positive cases which failed to be vimentin positive were five cases (25%). There was no tissue of NPC negative after EBVISH but decorated by the vimentin antibody. The remaining six cases (30%) were negative for EBV and vimentin. These results are summarized in table II.

Table II. Correlation of vimentin expression and EBV detection in UCNT.

EBV	Vimentin (V9)	
	positive	negative
Positive	9	5
Negative	0	6

Discussion

The aim of this investigation was to prove the hypothesis of an virus-associated alteration of keratin, vimentin and EMA expression in UCNT. Indeed, herpes simplex virus induced changes of keratin type intermediate filament expression in rat epithelial cells have been reported (9). On the other hand in early mouse embryo a co-expression of vimentin and keratins in parietal endoderm was found and it was concluded vimentin expression to be specifically related to a reduced cell-to-cell contact in tissues (5). So, this hypothesis fits well to other reports: The same phenomenon was found in human keratinocytes in cell culture lacking a close cell-to-cell contact (3) and is supposed to be a common event in invasive carcinomas of the upper aerodigestive tract (*Friedrich* et al., in preparation). Recently it was stated the evidence of morphological transformation of human keratinocytes expressing the late membrane protein (LMP) gen of EBV (2). The EBV encoded LMP induces phenotypic changes in epithelial cells: A down regulation of EMA expression was found in a human keratinocyte cell line (RHEK-1) (10). In normal epithelia of the nasopharynx vimentin is not expressed. It was concluded any expression of keratin synthesis in NPC to be lacking (12). However, there are several reports on cytoplasmatic keratin synthesis in NPC (15). The presented alteration of pattern of keratin expression in UCNT compared to normal nasopharyngeal epithelia might be related to EBV induced genetic changes of the cytoskeleton and antigenicity, e. g. EMA expression, or a common phenomenon of highly undifferentiated carcinomas.

References

1. Altmannsberger M (1988) Intermediärfilamente als Marker in der Tumordiagnostik / Tumor diagnosis by intermediate filament typing. Veröffentlichungen aus der Pathologie/Progress in Pathology. Bd/Vol 127, Fischer, Stuttgart
2. Fahraeus R, Rymo L, Rhim JS, Klein G (1990) Morphological transformation of human keratinocytes expressing the LMP gene of Epstein-Barr virus. Nature 345:447-449
3. Franke WW, Schmid E, Schiller DL, Winter S, Jarasch ED, Moll R, Denk H, Ackson BW, Illmensee K (1982) Differentiation patterns of expression of proteins of intermediate sized filaments in tissues and cultured cells. Cold Spring Harbor Symp Quant Biol 46:431-435
4. Friedrich RE, Lobeck H, Wild G, Mischke D, Friedrich KH, Bartel-Friedrich S (1992) Immunohistochemical investigations of patterns of cytokeratin-expression in undifferentiated nasopharyngeal carcinomas. In: Klapdor R (ed) Tumor associated antigens, oncogenes, receptors, cytokines in tumor dignosis and therapy at the beginning of the nineties. Zuckschwerdt, München, pp 486-489
5. Lane EB, Hogan BLM, Kurkinen M, Garrels JI (1983) Co-expression of vimentin and cytokeratins in parietal endoderm cells of early mouse embryo. Nature 303: 701-704
6. Lobeck H (1990) Orthologie und Pathologie der Zytokeratine. Habilitationsschrift, Universität Berlin
7. Niedobitek G, Hansmann ML, Herbst H, Young LS, Dienemann D, Hartmann CA, Finn T, Pitteroff S, Welt A, Anagnostopoulos I, Friedrich R, Lobeck H, Sam CK, Araujo I, Rickinson AB, Stein H (1991) Epstein-Barr virus and carcinomas: undifferentiated carcinomas but not squamous cell carcinomas of the nasopharynx are regularly associated with the virus. J Pathol 165:17-24
8. Niedobitek G, Fahraeus R, Herbst H, Latza U, Ferszt A, Klein G, Stein H (1992) The Epstein-Barr virus encoded membrane protein (LMP) induces phenotypic changes in epithelial cells. Virchows Arch B Cell Pathol 62:55-59
9. Nielsen LN, Forchhammer J, Dabelsteen E, Jepsen A, Teglbjaerg CS, Norrild B (1987) Herpes simplex virus-induced changes of the keratin type intermediate filament in rat epithelial cells. J Gen Virol 68:737-748
10. Pearson GR, Weiland LF, Neel III HB, Taylor W, Goepfert H, Huang A, Hyams V, Lanier A, Levine P, Pilch B, Henle G, Henle W (1981) Evaluation of antibodies to the Epstein-Barr virus (EBV) in the diagnosis of american nasopharyngeal carcinoma. In: Grundmann G, Krueger GRF, Ablashi DV (eds) Nasopharyngeal carcinoma. Cancer Campaign Vol 5, Fischer, Stuttgart, pp 231-236

11. Polack A, Hartl G, Zimber U, Freese UK, Laux G, Takaki K, Hohn B, Gissmann L, Bornkamm GW (1984) A complete set of overlapping cosmid clones of M-ABA virus derived from nasopharyngeal carcinoma and its similarity to other Epstein-Barr virus isolates. Gene 27: 279–288
12. Raab-Traub N (1992) Epstein-Barr virus and nasopharyngeal carcinoma. Sem Cancer Biol 3: 297–307
13. Rüger R, Bornkamm GW, Fleckenstein B (1984) Human cytomegalovirus DNA sequences with homology to the nuclear genome. J Gen Virol 65:1351–1364
14. Shanmugaratnam K, Sobin LH (1991) Histological typing of tumors of the upper respiratory tract and ear. Springer, Berlin, Heidelberg, New York, pp 32–33
15. Shi SR, Goodman ML, Bhan AK, Pilch, BZ, Chen LB, Sun TT (1984) Immunohistochemical study of nasopharyngeal carcinoma using monoclonal keratin antibodies. Am J Pathol 117:53–63
16. Weiss LM, Mohaved LA, Butler AE, Swanson AE, Frierson HF, Cooper PH, Colby TV, Mills SE (1989) Analysis of lymphoepithelioma and lymphoepithelioma-like carcinomas for Epstein-Barr virus by in situ hybridization. Am J Surg Pathol 13:625–631
17. zur Hausen H, Schulte-Holthausen H, Klein G, Henle W, Henle G, Clifford P, Santesson L (1970) EBV DNA in biopsies of Burkitt's tumors and anaplastic carcinomas of the nasopharynx. Nature 228:1056–1058

Address for correspondence:
Dr. med. Dr. med. dent. R. E. Friedrich
Klinik für Mund-, Kiefer- und Gesichtschirurgie
(Nordwestdeutsche Kieferklinik)
Martinistraße 52
D-20246 Hamburg, Germany

Detection of keratins in lymph node metastases of poorly differentiated carcinomas in the head and neck region

Comparison of patterns of expression to primary sites of lesions

R. E. Friedrich[a], S. Bartel-Friedrich[b], H. Lobeck[c]

[a]Department of Oral and Maxillofacial Surgery, Eppendorf University Hospital, University of Hamburg,
[b]Department of Otorhinolaryngology, Steglitz University Hospital,
[c]Institute of Pathology, Rudolf Virchow University Hospital, Free University of Berlin, Germany

Introduction

The diagnosis and therapy of patients with poorly differentiated lymph node metastases (LNM) of the neck (adenocarcinomas and squamous cell carcinomas) and an unknown primary site still is an important clinical problem. Despite improvements of diagnostic techniques sometimes the localization of the primary lesions cannot be found. Especially in poorly differentiated carcinomas any indication might be missing using conventional techniques and electron microscopy of tumor specimens needs some time for preparation and evaluation. Among others predominantly carcinomas of the naso-, oro- and hypopharynx, tonsils, thyroid gland and bronchus have to be taken into account as a locus of the first lesions. Immunocytochemical techniques, e.g. detection of keratins in the cytoplasmas of carcinomas, might support the histological diagnosis and give additional informations concerning the primary site of LNM with poorly differentiated carcinomas.

Material and methods

We investigated the patterns of keratin expressions in LNM of poorly differentiated carcinomas (grading 2-3 (1)) in a variety of known or suspected primaries (nasopharynx = 10 (undifferentiated carcinomas of nasopharyngeal type (UCNT)); oro-/hypopharynx and tonsils = 8; thyroid gland = 2; bronchus = 6; basaloid = 3; sebaceous = 1, breast = 4) using a panel of monoclonal keratin antibodies with defined specifity (clones: KL-1, CAM5.2, 4.62, K8.12, K8.60) in routinely fixed tissues (formalin-fixed, paraffin-embedded). The pattern of antigens identified by the antibodies used in this study is presented elsewhere (3). The APAAP-technique was used to visualize antigen-antibody reactions.

Results

Basaloid and thyreoideal LNM were all negative for the antibodies applied with the exception of a weak positive 4.62 (2/3) staining and an immunoreactivity for KL-1 in all biopsies. Keratinizing LNM of the oropharyngeal region were characterized by a positive cytoplasmatic reaction of carcinoma cells after application of the clones K8.12 and K8.60 (figure 1). These carcinomas reacted CAM5.2-negative in 7/8 cases. On the other hand, all adenocarcinomas were K8.12 negative and just 2/6 bronchial carcinoma were decorated by this antibody. In bronchial LNM there was a partial positive staining for several keratins (CAM5.2, 4.62, K8.60) and a co-expression of vimentin in 50%. Breast LNM were all positive after application of antibodies marking keratins characteristic for simple type of epithelia (CAM5.2, 4.62) (figure 2), a pattern of keratin expression which was shared with the LNM of a sebaceous carcinoma (figure 3). The majority of nasopharyngeal LNM were immunoreactive for K8.12 (keratins no. 12, 16) in carcinoma cells. The results are summarized in table I.

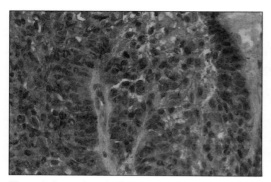

Figure 1. Detection of K8.12 positive carcinoma cells in a lymph node metastasis of the neck (primary: oropharyngeal carcinoma; basaloid feature).

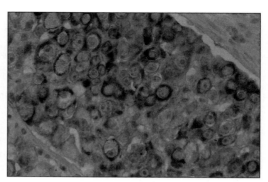

Figure 3. Detection of immunoreactivity for CAM5.2 in a lymph node metastasis of the neck (primary: sebaceous carcinoma of the head).

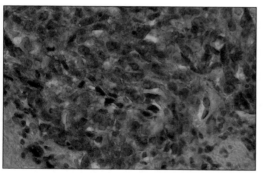

Figure 2. Detection of immunoreactivity for CAM5.2 in a lymph node metastasis of the neck (primary: medullary carcinoma of thyroid gland).

Discussion

The expression of keratins in neoplasms is highly preserved even in poorly differentiated carcinomas. Additionally to the keratins typical for squamous cell carcinomas the keratins 18 and 19 are expressed (4). On the other hand in a recent report, only 19% (n = 9) of squamous cell carcinomas of different origins were immunoreactive for CAM5.2 and poorly differentiated carcinomas did not express keratins no. 6, 18 (8). It is suggested CAM5.2 to identify predominantly keratins 8 and 18 in routinely fixed tissues (4, 5) and a different spectrum of keratins identified by this antibody in frozen sections might be possible (7). Our own results support the hypothesis of a facultative expression of keratins no. 18 and 19 just in a few LNM of squamous cell carcinomas as the LNM of adenocarcinomas are all decorated by

Table I. The identification of keratins in lymph node metastases of the neck (poorly differentiated carcinomas) by monoclonal keratin antibodies with defined specifity.

LNM (history of the primary site)	n	Keratin antibodies					
		KL-1	CAM5.2	K8.12	K8.60	4.62	V9
UCNT	10	10/10	1/10	6/10	2/10	2/10	3/10
Oro-/hypopharynx, tonsils	8	8/8	0/8	7/8	6/8	3/8	2/8
Basaloid	3	3/3	0/3	2/3	0/3	2/3	1/3
Bronchus	6	6/6	2/6	2/6	3/6	4/6	3/6
Breast	4	4/4	4/4	2/4	0/4	3/4	1/4
Thyroid[a]	2	2/2	0/2	0/2	0/2	1/2	1/2
Sebaceous	1	1/1	1/1	0/1	0/1	0/1	0/1

[a]Thyreoglobulin and calcitonin: negative

CAM5.2 and 4.62. Surprisingly, immunoreactivity of oro- and nasopharyngeal carcinomas for K8.12 is high. In G-2-carcinomas the detection of keratin no. 13 is optional (6) and the identification of hyperproliferation associated expression of keratin 16 has to be taken into account when interpreting the reaction of this antibody (1). On the other hand, the LNM of poorly differentiated carcinomas seem to be frequently immunoreactive for another keratin no. 13 identifying antibody (clone 13.1, unpublished results). Concerning a clinical application CAM5.2 immunoreactivity in routinely fixed LNM of poorly differentiated carcinomas supports a primary of glandular origin; K8.12-stained carcinoma cell are in the majority of cases correlated to non-keratinizing epithelia of the upper aerodigestive tract and are preserved in a lot of squamous cell carcinomas in LNM of the neck. K8.60 immunoreactivity indicating cytoplasmatic keratinization is found in a subset of all LNM and is not recommended to add further information to the topography of the primary. A co-expression of vimentin is found in almost all LNM indicating the loss of epithelial differentiation and junction (8). Although a de-novo expression of keratins has to be considered in neoplastic cells it is concluded, keratin patterns of LNM of the neck in poorly differentiated carcinomas can give additional information about the primary lesions in some cases.

References

1 de Mare S, van Erp P, van de Kerkhof PCM (1989) Epidermal hyperproliferation assessed by the monoclonal antibody Ks 8.12 in frozen sections. J Invest Dermatol 92:130

2 Diamandopoulos GT, Meisner WA (1985) Neoplasia. In: Kissane JM (ed) Anderson's Pathology. 8th ed, Mosby, St. Louis, pp 514–559

3 Friedrich RE (1993) Immunhistochemische und autoradiographische Untersuchungen zum anaplastischen Karzinom der Kopf- und Halsregion. Med Diss (Thesis), Free University of Berlin

4 Lobeck H (1990) Orthologie und Pathologie der Zytokeratine. Habilitationsschrift, Free University of Berlin

5 Makin CA, Bobrow LG, Bodmer WF (1984) Monoclonal antibody to cytokeratin for use in routine histopathology. J Clin Pathol 37:975–983

6 Mischke D, Lobeck H, Wild AG, et al (1991) Neue monoklonale Antikörper gegen Keratine: Immunoblot und immunhistochemische Ergebnisse an normalem und malignem transformiertem Plattenepithel des Kopf-Hals-Bereiches. Arch Oto-Rhino-Laryngol Suppl 1991/1, Teil II:67–68

7 Ogden GR, Lane EB, Hopwood DC, Chisholm DM (1993) Evidence for field change in oral cancer based on cytokeratin expression. Br J Cancer 67:1324–30

8 Suo Z, Holm R, Nesland JM (1992) Squamous cell carcinomas, an immunohistochemical and ultrastructural study. Anticancer Res 12:2025–31

Address for correspondence:
Dr. med. Dr. med. dent. R. E. Friedrich
Klinik für Mund-, Kiefer- und Gesichtschirurgie
(Nordwestdeutsche Kieferklinik)
Martinistraße 52
D-20246 Hamburg, Germany

Correlation of the immunocytochemical demonstration of keratin phenotypes in undifferentiated carcinomas of the nasopharyngeal type (UCNT) to the hypotheses of its histogenesis

R. E. Friedrich[a], S. Bartel-Friedrich[b], H. Lobeck[c], K.H. Friedrich[c], D. Hellner[a],

[a]Department of Oral and Maxillofacial Surgery, Eppendorf University Hospital, University of Hamburg, [b]Department of Otorhinolaryngology, Steglitz University Hospital, [c]Institute of Pathology, Rudolf Virchow University Hospital, Free University of Berlin, Germany

Introduction

Undifferentiated carcinomas of the nasopharynx (UCNT) are characterized by tumor cells arranged in irregular or moderately well defined masses or as loosely connected cells in a lymphoid stroma. The tumor cell margins are indistinct giving the impression of a syncytium, the nuclei are oval or round and nucleoli are prominent. Occasionally spindle shaped tumor cells might be present (16). This fairly characteristic histological feature facilitates morphological diagnosis but any hints to the origin of the neoplasia are missing in the vast majority of cases judging routinely processed tissues. Despite a crucial desription of the differences of nasopharyngeal carcinomas (NPC) the essential unity of the diverse neoplasmas was emphasied summarizing them as variants of squamous cell carcinoma (15). There is evidence of carcinomas arising from any of the normal epithelial types of the nasopharynx (15): squamous, respiratoray and transitional epithelia (1), and it was suspected that any of the normal epithelia can give rise to both squamous and undifferentiated forms of NPC (15). On the other hand a squamous metaplasia as a prerequisite to the development of NPC was described by *Prasad* (14). Indeed, in the same untreated patient the histological appearance of the tumor may be both squamous in one area and quite undifferentiated a few millimeters distant (15) making it difficult or even imposssible to estimate the origin of the neoplasia. There have been proposed several classifications of NPC and actually there are two entities of NPC accepted by WHO: squamous versus non-keratinizing carcinomas (NKC) (16). The UCNT is a subtype of NKC. The identification of intermediate filaments specific for differentiations of epithelial cells (keratins) and the persistence of their expression in a lot of dys- and neoplastic diseases make keratin-antibodies with defined specifty a valuable tool to assess the histogenesis of this entity (12, 17). Immunocytochemical detections of keratins in NPC according to data presented in the literature were reviewed and are presented in table I. The expression of keratins in NPC by means of monoclonal antibodies was investigated and interpreted with special reference to the histogenetical relation of keratins in epithelia.

Materials and methods

The techniques of immunocytochemical detection of keratins in undifferentiated carcinomas used in this study are described in detail elsewhere (7). In brief, routinely processed formalin-fixed, paraffin-embedded and hematoxylin-eosin stained sections of primary and metastatic lesions of NPC were re-evaluated according to the revised WHO-classification (16) and tissue preservation. Wel preserved undifferentiated carcinomas (grading G III (5)) were selected and thin sections (5 μm were fixed on poly-L-lysine covered slides. The pretreatment of sections with pronase was recommended for some antibodies and the detection of antigen-antibody reaction was visualised using the APAAP-technique (4). The antbodies applied are listed in table II. KL-1 and

Table I. Results of keratin detections in undifferentiated carcinomas of the nasopharyneal type (UCNT) (review of the literature).

Author	Cases[a]	Clone	Specificity[c] no.[d]/MW	Keratin-positve[b]
Espinoza, Azar (1982)	108	n.m. (pc)	?/?	3/6
Madri, Barwick (1982)	9	n.m. (pc)	?/?	9/9
Miettinen et al. (1982)	12	n.m. (pc)	?/?	8/8
Gusterson et al. (1983)	14	n.m. (pc)	?/?	14/14
Shi et al. (1984)	121	RAK (pc)	?/?	117/119
		AE1	40; 50; 56.5	119/119
		AE2	56.5; 65–67	2/117
		AE3	46; 52; 58; 65–67	22/118
Vollrath et al. (1984)	7	n.m. (pc)	18/?	3/3
Ziegels-Weissman et al. (1984)	6	n.m. (pc)	(anti-56kD-keratin-serum)	7/7
Taxy et al. (1985)	18	AE1	40; 50; 56,5	17/17
Bosq et al. (1985)	35	CAM5.2	8/18(19)	33/35
		KL-1	broad	35/35
Nakai et al. (1986)	115	TK (pc)	41–65	3/3
		KL-1	55–57	3/3
		PKK1	41–56	3/3
Terry et al. (1986)	140	CAM5.2	40; 45; 52	11/13
Ben-Cheng et al. (1988)	38	n.m. ("K")		11/12
Kamino et al. (1988)	40	EAB902	54	6/28
		EAB903	57; 66	25/28
		EAB904	57; 66	27/28

n.m. = Not mentioned; kD = kilo Dalton; pc = polyclonal; [a]number of cases with carcinomas; [b]number of solid undifferentiated and non-keratinizing carcinomas of the nasopharynx; [c]specifity: no. of keratins and/or molecular weight of keratin(s) (original data); [d]no. of keratins according to Moll et al. (1982)

PD7/26 (common leukocyte antigen) were used as a control for detecting epithelial cells resp. lymphocytes in the undifferentiated tumors.

Results

Keratin typical for the terminal differentiated non-keratinizing mucosa of the upper aerodigestive tract (no. 4) was not detectable by monospecific keratin antibody (215B8). K8.12 positive stained cytoplasmas of UCNT were found in 17/24 cases (70%). Surprisingly, the preservation of simple epithelia specific keratins (8, 18) was demonstrated by the oligospecific keratin antibody CAM5.2 only in a few cases (n = 2, 8.3%). The expression of keratin no.19 (4.62) was weak and a predominantly focal one in eight cases. The immunocytochemical detection of keratins in routinely processed biopsies of undifferentiated carcinomas of the nasopharynx is summerized in table III. The signs of a cytoplasmatic keratinization were not found by routine histological investigations. A few UCNT were immunoreactive for K8.60 in a predominantly focal staining pattern (n = 5/24, 20.8%).

Discussion

Using oligospecific keratin antibodies (AE1-3) in UCNT resulting in different patterns of staining an origin of this entitiy of respiratory epithelia was supposed. However, some squamous morphological ultrastructural features were considered to be present in UCNT (17). In another study a

Table II. Keratin antibodies: clones, species, specifity and supplier; keratin classification according to *Moll* et al. (1982).

Clones	Species	Target antigen(s)	Source
215B8	Mouse	4 (5)	Boehringer Mannheim
K8.60	Mouse	1, 10, 11	ICN
K8.12	Mouse	13, 15	ICN
CAM5.2	Mouse	8, 18, 19	Becton & Dickinson
4.62	Mouse	19	ICN
KL-1	Mouse	8, 6 [1, 4, 10)	Dianova

Table III. Results of keratin detection in undifferentiated carcinomas of the nasopharynx (UCNT) using monoclonal antibodies with defined anti-keratin specifity.

Clone	No. of positively reacting UCNT/ total no. of cases
215B8	0/24
K8.60	5/24
K8.12	17/24
CAM5.2	2/24
4.62	8/24
KL-1	24/24

significant larger proportion of low molecular weight keratins in poorly differentiated carcinomas was reported (CAM5.2) but it was not possible to differentiate between squamous carcinomas derived from different sites including UCNT (19). Refering to our own results a cytoplasmatic keratinization (K8.60) is rarely detected in UCNT both in primaries and lymph node metastases. Simple type epithelia are to be expexted in UCNT. Just a few UCNT are immunoreactive for 4.62 indicating the lack of sensitivity of this marker in routinely processed tissues On the other hand, the small amount of CAM5.2 positive UCNT might be explained by a reduced antigen spectrum recognised by this antibody. Keratins typical for a regular differentiation of non-keratinizing epithelia of the upper aerodigestive tract, e.g. no. 4, are not expressed in G-III carcinomas. It is supposed immunoreactivity of UCNT for K8.12 to be related to hyperproliferative carcinoma cells at least in a subgroup of cases.

References

1 Ali MY (1967) Distribution and character of the squamous epithelium in the human nasopharynx. In: Muir CS, Shanmugaratnam K (eds) Cancer of the nasopharynx. UICC Monograph Series, Vol 1, Munksgaard, Copenhagen, pp 138–146
2 Ben-cheng F, Yi-ran D, Zhen-de X (1988). Practical value of immunohistochemistry in histopathological diagnosis of nasopharyngeal carcinoma. Chin Med J 101: 745–747
3 Bosq J, Gatter KC, Micheau C, Mason DY (1985) Role of immunohistochemistry in diagnosis of nasopharyngeal tumors. J Clin Pathol 38: 845–848
4 Cordell JL, Falini B, Erber WN, Gnosh AK, Abduklaziz, Macdonald S, Preford KAF, Stein H, Mason DY (1984) Immunoenzymatic labelling of monoclonal antibodies using immune complexes of alkaline phosphatase and monoclonal anti-alkaline phosphatase (APAAP-complexes). Histochem Cytochem 32: 219–229
5 Diamandopoulos GT, Meissner WA (1985) Neoplasia. In: Kissane JM (ed) Anderson's Pathology. 8th ed., Mosby, St. Louis, pp 514–559
6 Espinoza CG, Azar HA (1982) Immunohistochemical localisation of keratin-type proteins in epithelia neoplasms. Correlation with electron microscopic findings. Am J Clin Pathol 78: 500–507
7 Friedrich RE, Lobeck H, Wild G, Mischke D, Friedrich KH, Bartel-Friedrich S (1992) Immunohistochemical investigations of patterns of cytokeratin-expression in undifferentiated nasopharyngeal carcinomas. In: Klapdor R (ed) Tumor associated antigens, oncogenes, receptors, cytokines in tumor diagnosis and therapy at the beginning of the nineties. Zuckschwerdt, München, pp 486–489
8 Gusterson BA, Mitchell DP, Warburton MJ, Carter RL (1983) Epithelial markers in the diagnosis of nasopharyngeal carcinoma: an immunocytochemical study. J Clin Pathol 36:628-631
9 Kamino H, Huang SJ, Fu YS (1988) Keratin and involucrin immunohistochemistry of nasopharyngeal carcinoma. Cancer 61:1142–1148
10 Madri JA, Barwick KW (1982) An immunohistochemical study of nasopharyngeal neoplasms using keratin antibodies. Am J Surg Pathol 6:143–149
11 Miettinen M, Lehto V-P, Virtanen I (1982) Nasopharyngeal lymphoepithelioma. Virchows Arch (Cell Pathol) 40:163–169

12 Moll R, Franke WW, Schiller DL, Geiger R, Krepler R (1982) The catalogue of human cytokeratins. Patterns of expression in normal epithelia, tumors and cultured cells. Cell 31:11–24
13 Nakai M, Mori M (1986) Immunohistochemical distribution of monoclonal antibodies against keratin in papillomas and carcinomas from oral and nasopharyngeal regions. Oral Surg Oral Med Oral Pathol 62: 292-302
14 Prasad U (1981) Significance of metaplastic transformation in the pathogenesis of nasopharyngeal carcinoma. Clinical, histopathological, and ultrastructural studies. In: Grundmann E, Krueger GRF, Ablashi DV (eds) Nasopharyngeal carcinoma. Cancer Campaign Vol 5, Fischer, Stuttgart, pp 31–40
15 Shanmugaratnam K, Muir CS (1967) Nasopharyngeal carcinoma: origin and structure. In: Muir CS, Shanmugaratnam K (eds) Cancer of the nasopharynx. UICC Monograph Series, Vol 1, Munksgaard, Copenhagen, pp 153–162
16 Shanmugaratnam K, Sobin LH (1991) Histological typing of tumors of the upper aerodigestive tract and ear. Springer, Berlin, Heidelberg, New York, p 32–33
17 Shi S-R, Goodman ML, Bhan AK, Pilch BZ, Chen LB, Sun TT (1984) Immunohistochemical study of nasopharyngeal carcinoma using monoclonal keratin antibodies. Am J Pathol 117:53–63
18 Taxy JB, Hidvegi DF, Battifora H (1985) Nasopharyngeal carcinoma: antikeratin immunohistochemistry and electron microscopy. Am J Clin Pathol 83:320–325
19 Terry RM, Gray C, Bird CC (1986) Aberrent expression of low molecular weight cytokeratins in primary and secondary carcinoma of the head and neck. J Laryngol Otol 100:1283–1287
20 Vollrath M, Altmannsberger M, Debus E, Osborn M (1984) Differential-Diagnose von Tumoren des Kopf-Hals-Bereiches mit Hilfe immunhistologischer und elektronenoptischer Untersuchungen. Laryngol Rhinol Otol 63:475–482
21 Ziegels-Weissman J, Nadji M, Penneys NS, Morales AR (1984) Prekeratin immunohistochemistry in the diagnosis of undifferentiated carcinoma of the nasopharyngeal type. Arch Pathol Lab Med 108:588–589

Address for correspondence:
Dr. med. Dr. med. dent. R. E. Friedrich
Klinik für Mund-, Kiefer- und Gesichtschirurgie
(Nordwestdeutsche Kieferklinik)
Martinistraße 52
D-20246 Hamburg, Germany

Expression of tenascin in gastric carcinoma – An immunohistochemical investigation

R. Broll[a], K. Kayser[a], G. Vollmer[b], H.-P. Bruch[a]
[a]Surgical Clinic and [b]Institute of Biochemical Endocrinology, Medical University of Lübeck, Germany

Introduction

Tenascin, an oligomeric glycoprotein of the extracellular matrix of mesenchymal tissue components, is involved in the proliferation, differentiation and migration of cells in the epithelial tissue during prenatal development (2, 8). In adults, however, it can only be detected in certain tissue areas, e.g. along the basal membrane of colonic and esophageal mucosa, and also along the epidermis and smooth muscles (8). Furthermore, it also plays an important role in proliferative processes such as wound healing (7) and, particularly, in tumor growth, where it is also expressed increasingly. Furthermore, it seems to constitute a molecular factor of epithelial-mesenchymal interactions (3).

By means of electron microscopy, this protein could be visualized as hexamer, i.e. a six-armed molecule (figure 1) (4).

Numerous investigations have convincingly detected the expression of tenascin in various tumors, particularly in endometrial carcinoma (11), carcinoma of the breast (5), colonic carcinoma (10), lung tumors (9) and many other tumors (8).

The principal aims of our investigations were, first, to detect tenascin immunohistochemically in the tissue of gastric adenocarcinoma and also in regional lymph nodes and, secondly, to correlate tenascin expression, particularly in the surroundings of the basal membrane, with the tumor grades, the classification according to Laurén and the tumor stages.

Material and methods

We investigated sections from paraffin-embedded material of 25 patients (12 men and 13 women; mean age 67.3 years, range 46–84) who underwent surgery for gastric carcinoma at the Surgical Clinic, Medical University of Lübeck. Tumor staging, tumor grading and the classification according to Laurén are presented in table I.

The paraffin blocks were provided by the Institute of Pathology, Medical University of Lübeck, FRG (Director: *Prof. Dr. A. C. Feller*). Generally, investigations were performed on sections taken from the centers of tumors, the bordering areas between tumor tissue and normal tissue and from the regional lymph nodes.

The tissue samples had been fixed in formalin and embedded in paraffin prior to cutting in 5 μm-thick sections. After this, the samples were deparaffinised and prepared with 0.1% pronase to evoke the release of antigen determinants.

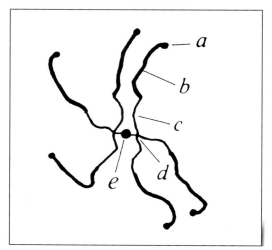

Figure 1. Tenascin model; a: terminal knob, b: thick distal segment, c: thin proximal segment, d: T-junction (3 arms = trimer), e: central globular particle (2 trimers = hexamer), from (4).

Table I. Tumor staging, grading and Laurén-classification.

Staging	n
St. I A	1
St. I B	3
St. II	4
St. III A	11
St. III B	2
St. IV	4

Grading	n
G 1-3	1
G 2	4
G 2-3	3
G 3	17

Laurén-Classification	n
Intestinal Type	14
Diffuse Type	11

On the first series of sections, a polyclonal rabbit antibody (AB) against human tenascin (provided by Dr. H. P. Erickson, Department of Cell Biology, Duke University Medical Center, Durham, North Carolina/USA) was used. After dilution of this primary AB with the antibody buffer in a proportion of 1 to 1000, the sections were incubated for 1 h. In order to detect tenascin, the sections were incubated for another hour with a goat anti-rabbit IgG antibody, labeled with alkaline phosphatase and, too, this AB was diluted with the antibody buffer in a proportion of 1 to 250. The red reaction product of the alkaline phosphatase was visualized with the new fuchsin method using 40 mg levamisol to inhibit the endogenous alkaline phosphatase. After contrast staining of the nuclei by adding hemalum solution for 5 sec, the staining procedure was finished by embedding the material into aquatex.
On another series of sections monoclonal mouse-AB against human tenascin (Dako, Hamburg) was used. Deparaffinisation and the release of antigens on adding pronase was performed as described above. To reduce endogenous peroxidase activity, the material was overlaid with 7.5% hydrogen peroxide. Then the primary AB diluted with tris-buffer in a proportion of 1 to 70 was added prior to incubation for 30 min. Furthermore, a biotinylised secondary AB (reagent C; Dako, Hamburg) was diluted with tris-buffer in a proportion of 1 to 1000 and also incubated for 30 min. Finally, a peroxidase-conjugated avidin-biotin-complex (reagent A + B; Dako, Hamburg) diluted in a proportion of 1 to 1000 was used for another incubation of 30 min. The staining for a brown reaction product of the peroxidase was performed using 3-amino-9-ethylcarbazole solution (AEC; Merck, Darmstadt). Contrast staining of the nuclei was performed using hemalum solution. For the embedding of the sections, aquatex was used as described previously.
Sections incubated with IgG normal serum instead of primary AB and the respective secondary AB served as controls.

Results

A positive staining reaction was detectable in all normal tissue samples and tumor tissue samples, but solely in the mesenchymal tissue components. Staining of the epithelium or tumor epithelium was not observed at all.
In normal gastric sections, the muscularis mucosae clearly stained tenascin-positive as a narrow smooth band. The muscularis propia was also homogenously stained as well as the smooth musculature of vessels well supplied with muscles in the submucosa.
In the normal lymph nodes examined, clear staining of the fibrous capsule as well as the trabeculae coursing to the medullary space was clearly detectable.
In the tumor area, however, the lamina muscularis was thickened and loosened, partially also thin and completely disintegrated in zones where a tumor cell invasion was in the state of progression to the submucosa. In the forefront of the invading tumor cell clusters intensive staining was found, possibly indicating directional growth of the tumor.
In highly differentiated tumors and in the intestinal type according to Laurén fibrillary staining of the stroma was found in the periphery of the glandular structures. Tenascin could be detected to be associated with the basal membrane, even though staining was always discontinuous there (figure 2).
In undifferentiated tumors and in the diffuse type according to Laurén, the tumor cell clusters or the individual tumor cells were surrounded by a thick

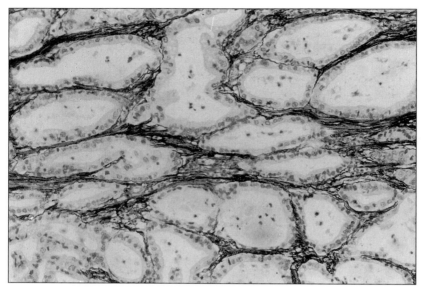

Figure 2. Tenascin-positive staining, even though discontinuous, along the basal membrane of a highly differentiated tumor (G1-2, intestinal type), (x200 magnification, monoclonal AB).

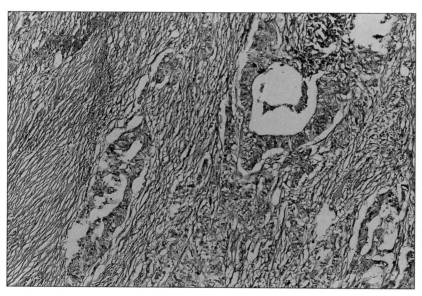

Figure 3. Network-like staining of the tumor stroma between the tumor cell clusters without "basal membrane-like" staining (G3, diffuse type) (x100 magnification, polyclonal AB).

network of fibrillary connective tissue with positive staining (figure 3). In 94% of the G 3 tumors and in 100% of the tumors of the diffuse type according to Laurén, tenascin could not be demonstrated along the basal membrane.

Tumor cell clusters in metastatic lymph nodes were detectable due to the tenascin-positive reaction of the surrounding stroma. Thus, even small tumor cell nests could easily be detected. Like in the primary tumor, a positive reaction surrounding the glandular tumor structures was found in lymphatic node metastases of well differentiated tumors along the discontinuous basal membrane. No correlation could be recognised between tumor stages and the expression of tenascin.

Discussion

Our investigations on normal gastric tissue confirmed the fact that both smooth muscles of the gastric wall and vessels rich in musculature show a positive reaction.

In the tumor samples, it was mainly the stroma which stained clearly positive in the area of invasive growth. This seems to indicate directional interactions from the epithelium towards the mesenchyma which are possibly responsible for directional growth of the tumor as well.

Tenascin-positive staining in the area along the basal membrane was mostly found in well differentiated tumors (G1–2) and in the intestinal type. In contrast, almost all badly differentiated tumors (G3) and all tumors of the diffuse type according to Laurén did not show any staining related to the basal membrane. Consistent with the findings of *Riedl* et al. (10), the staining along the basal membrane was discontinuous. The most likely explanations for this are a partial break down of the basal membrane by proteases or decreased production (1, 6).

In contrast to previous observations in colonic carcinoma by *Riedl* et al. (10), we could not see any relationship between tenascin expression and tumor stages, indicated by a graded intensity of staining (-/+/++/+++). As a rule, tenascin was distributed rather diffusely in the stroma at various intensities within the tumor. We also frequently found areas without staining although they partially consisted of stroma. This seems to be an indicator of the various proliferative activities within a tumor.

These findings suggest that tenascin also plays an important role in tumor cell invasion into regional lymph nodes. Thus, we have found a clear staining of the stroma surrounding the invading tumor cells within the metastatic lymph nodes. Consequently, even small tumor cell nests were detectable. Here, too, well differentiated tumors could be demonstrated by staining alongside the basal membrane. This suggests that these differentiated tumors are able to produce another, even though incomplete, basal membrane in metastatic lymph nodes, as described in previous reports on colorectal tumors by *Burtin* et al. (1).

Our investigations have shown that tenascin is of major importance for tumor growth and the development of metastases in lymph nodes in gastric carcinoma, too. Demonstration of tenascin along the basal membrane is an indicator for well differentiated tumors and, therefore, may well be used as parameter in tumor grading.

References

1. Burtin P, Chavanel G, Foidart JM et al (1983) Alterations of the basement membrane and connective tissue in human metastatic lymph nodes. Int J Cancer 31:719–726
2. Chiquet-Ehrismann R, Mackie EJ, Pearson C A et al (1986) Tenascin: an extracellular matrix protein involved in tissue interactions during fetal development and oncogenesis. Cell 47:131–139
3. Ekblom P, Aufderheide E (1989) Stimulation of tenascin expression in mesenchyme by epithelial-mesenchymal interactions. Int J Dev Biol 33:71–79
4. Erickson HP, Bourdon MA (1989) Tenascin: an extracellular matrix protein prominent in specialized embryonic tissue and tumors. Annu Rev Cell Biol 5:71–92
5. Gould VE, Koukoulis GK, Vitanen I (1984) Extracellular matrix proteins and their receptors in the normal, hyperplastic and neoplastic breast membrane. Am J Pathol 117:339–348
6. Mackie EJ, Halfter W, Liverani D (1988) Induction of tenascin in healing wounds. J Cell Biol 107:2757–2767
7. Natali PG, Nicotra MR, Bigotti A et al (1991) Comparative analysis of the expression of the extracellular matrix protein tenascin in normal human fetal, adult and tumor tissues. Int J Cancer 47:811–816
8. Oyama F, Hirohashi S, Shimosato Y et al (1991) Qualitative and quantitative changes of human tenascin expression in transformed lung fibroblast and lung tumor tissues: comparison with fibronectin. Cancer Res 51:4876–488
9. Riedl SE, Faissner A, Schlag P et al (1992) Altered content and distribution of tenascin in colitis, colon adenoma, and colorectal carcinoma. Gastroenterol 103:400–406
10. Vollmer G, Siegal GP, Chiquet-Ehrismann R et al (1990) Tenascin expression in the human endometrium and in endometrial adenocarcinomas. Lab Invest 62:725–730

Address for correspondence:
Dr. med. R. Broll
Chirurgische Klinik
Medizinische Universität
Ratzeburger Allee 160
D-23538 Lübeck

Different growth patterns in primary colorectal carcinomas and their lymph node metastases

B. Dippe[a], M. Lorenz[a], H. Petrowsky[a], F. Engels[a], S. Krüger[b], M. Schneider[c]

[a] Departments of Surgery and [c] Pathology, University of Frankfurt, Medical Centre, Frankfurt
[b] Institute of Pathology, Medical University of Lübeck, Germany

Introduction

In order to assess the prognosis of colorectal carcinomas and reach decisions concerning adjuvant therapeutic procedures such as chemotherapy and radiatio, morphometrical and proliferation kinetic investigations could be helpful. Since chemotherapy mainly affects actively dividing cells, this should be more successful in rapidly proliferating tissues.

Numerous studies have been performed on the histopathological characteristics of colorectal carcinomas using morphometrical (1, 11), histochemical (10, 13), or immunohistochemical techniques (2, 7, 8, 14). However, these methods have not been studied simultaneously on the same tissue specimens. In this study, a combination of nuclear area morphometry, silver staining of nucleolar organizer regions (AgNORs) and expression of Ki67 antigen and proliferative cell nuclear antigen (PCNA) were analyzed in the same tissue specimens of both colorectal adenocarcinomas and their lymph node metastases.

Materials and methods

32 colorectal adenocarcinomas (G2; T2N1M0) and their lymphatic metastases together with ten biopsies of normal colonic mucosa were included in the study. Tissue material was fixed in buffered formalin (10%, pH = 7.0) and embedded in paraffin.

Morphometry was carried out using histological sections of 5 µm, stained with hematoxylin and eosin. A semiautomatic analyzing system (ELAS, Leitz/Germany) with thousendfold magnification was used. The mean nuclear area of 200 representative tumor cells was determined per section.

The visualization of nucleolar organizer regions was performed on 5 µm paraffin sections using the histochemical silver staining method described by *Ploton* et al. (12). In 200 representative tumor cells, all silver stained NORs were counted per nucleus according to the recommendations of *Crocker* et al. (4).

Immunhistochemical staining of the Ki67 antigen was performend using the MIB1 antibody (Dianova, Germany) and the avidin-biotin complex method. PCNA or cyclin was recognized by the PCNA human antibody (Dianova) and the avidin-biotin complex method. To improve antigen detection, the sections were pretreated in a microwave (700W for 30 min). The ratio of positively stained cells per 200 tumor cells was given as Ki67 and PCNA index, respectively.

All data are presented as mean plus standard deviation. Differences and correlations were analyzed statistically using the Wilcoxon-Mann-Whitney test and the least squares method of linear regression, respectively. Results were considered significant if $p < 0.05$ unless otherwise indicated.

Results

The results of mean nuclear area determination, mean number of AgNORs per tumor cell, and indices of Ki67 and PCNA are presented in figures 1–4. All parameters examined revealed significant differences ($p < 0.001$) between the carcinoma (nuclear area: 42.8 ± 5.9 µm^2; AgNORs: 7.0 ± 0.5; Ki67: $44.0 \pm 4.8\%$; PCNA: $48.8 \pm 4.7\%$) and normal mucosa tissue (nuclear area: 28.8 ± 2.0

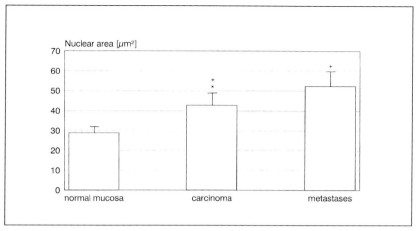

Figure 1. Mean nuclear area; significance (p > 0.001) versus normal mucosa (+), p < 0.01 versus metastases (x).

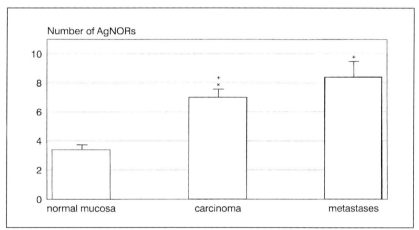

Figure 2. Mean number of AgNORs (compare to figure 1).

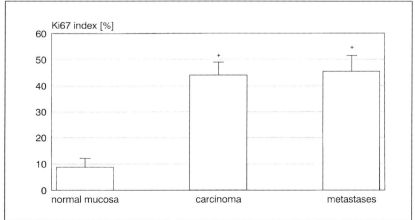

Figure 3. Ki67 index (compare to figure 1).

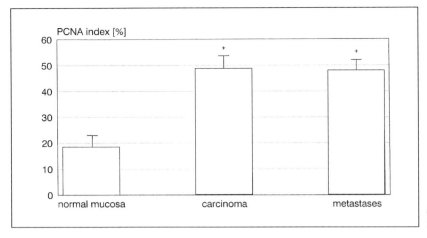

Figure 4. PCNA index (compare to figure 1).

μm^2; AgNORs: 3.4 ± 0.3; Ki67: 8.8 ± 3.2%; PCNA: 18.5 ± 4.0%).
Tumor cells in lymph node metastases had a larger mean nuclear area (52.3 ± 7.4 μm^2 to 46.9 ± 5.9 μm^2; p < 0.01) and a higher AgNOR number (8.4 ± 1.0 to 7.0 ± 0.5; p < 0.001) than cells in the primary tumors, but they did not differ significantly in their Ki67 and PCNA indices. A strong correlation (p < 0.01) was found between primary tumor and lymph node metastases for all parameters, but there was no interparametric correlation between these markers for the carcinomas and their lymph node metastases (data not shown).

Discussion

The nuclear area does not generally show a strong correlation with growth rate, since it not only depends on the tumor cell's DNA, but also on physical factors (e.g. nuclear shrinkage during fixation) and nuclear shape factor (10). However, morphometrical investigations enable a further differential characterization of the biological behavior of colorectal carcinomas in addition to the conventional histopathological tumor diagnosis.
There are considerable differences in the validity and practicability of the different proliferative parameters. NORs – non-histonic regulator proteins of ribosomal DNA – are found in increased numbers in tissue with high proliferative activity (4), but a correlation between AgNOR number and proliferation exists only in interphase nuclei (5) and therefore can not be found in all tumor cells. The Ki67 antigen – a nuclear antigen expressed in all cell cycle phases except G0 – is strongly associated with growth fraction (3) and has been shown to correlate significantly with the autoradiographic 3H-thymidine labeling index (6). In contrast to the Ki67 antigen, the proliferating cell nuclear antigen (PCNA) is also expressed under non-proliferative conditions, e.g. under cytokine influence (9).
Correlation between different parameters can therefore not generally be expected in all tumors. This hypothesis is confirmed by this study where no significant correlations between nuclear area, AgNOR number, Ki67 and PCNA index could be found within the same tumor specimens (data not shown).
The increased nuclear area and AgNOR number in primary tumors suggest that the metastazing subpopulation of the tumor has a higher proliferative potential than the main bulk of the primary tumor. It remains unclear whether this is the result of a selection within the tumor, or the result of a different growth pattern within the lymph node. Markers of proliferation such as AgNOR number, Ki67 and PCNA index represent different cellular functions, as does nuclear size. Therefore, AgNOR numbers may well provide valuable additional information to nuclear area determinations in assessing the prospective treatment plan of patients with colorectal carcinomas.

References

1. Ambros RA, Pawel BR, Mashcheryakow I, Kotrotsios J, Lamber W, Trost RC (1990) Nuclear morphometry as a prognostic indicator in colorectal carcinomas resected for cure. Anal Quant Cytol Histol 12:172–176
2. Benetti A, Berenzi A, Grigolato P (1992) Growth fraction of colorectal carcinoma (Ki67); a comparative study. Int J Biol Markers 7:93–96
3. Brown DC, Gatter KC (1990) Monoclonal antibody Ki67; its use in histopathology. Histopathology 17:489–503
4. Crocker J, Boldy DAR, Egan MJ (1989) How should we count AgNORs? Proposals for a standardized approach. J Pathol 158:185–188
5. Derenzini M, Pession A, Farabegoli F, Trere D, Budiac M, Dehan P (1989) Relationship between interphasic nucleolar organizer regions and growth rate in two neuroblastoma. Am J Pathol 134:925–932
6. Horny HP, Horst HA (1988) Proliferation of invasive breast carcinomas and colorectal carcinomas; an immunhistochemical in situ investigation with the monoclonal antibody Ki-67. Zentralbl Allg Pathol 134:547–554
7. Kubota Y, Petras RE, Easley KA, Bauer TW, Tubbs RR, Fazio VW (1992) Ki-67-determined growth fraction versus standard staging and grading parameters in colorectal carcinoma. A multivariante analysis. Cancer 70:2602–2609
8. Mayer A, Takimoto M, Fritz E, Schellander G, Kofler K, Ludwig H (1993) The prognostic significance of proliferating cell nuclear antigen, epidermal growth factor receptor, and mdr gene expression in colorectal cancer. Cancer 71: 2454-2460
9. McCormick D, Hall PA (1992) The complexities of proliferating cell nuclear antigen. Histopathology 21:591–594
10. Mitmaker B, Begin LR, Gordon PH (1991) Nuclear shape as a prognostic discriminant in colorectal carcinoma. Dis Colon Rectum 34:249–259
11. Moran K, Cooke T, Forster G, Gillen P, Sheehan S, Dervan P, Fitzpatrick JM (1989) Prognostic value of nucleolar organizer regions and ploidy values in advanced colorectal cancer. Br J Surg 76:1152–1155
12. Ploton D, Menager M, Jeannesson P, Himber G, Pigeon F, Adnet JJ (1986) Improvement in the staining and in the visualization of the argyrophilic proteins of the nucleolar organizer region at the optical level. Histochem J 18:5–14
13. Rüschoff J, Bittinger A, Neumann K, Schmitz-Moormann P (1990) Prognostic significance of nucleolar organizer regions (NORs) in carcinomas of the sigmoid colon and rectum. Path Res Pract 186:85–91
14. Shepherd NA, Richman PI, England J (1988) Ki-67 derived proliferative activity in colorectal adenocarcinoma with prognostic correlations. J Pathol 155:213–219

Address for correspondence:
Dr. med. B. Dippe
Klinik für Allgemeinchirurgie
Klinikum der J.W. Goethe-Universität
Theodor-Stern-Kai 7
D-60590 Frankfurt am Main, Germany

Concanavalin A affinity pattern of CA 19-9

An in vitro and in vivo study

D. Basso[a], M. Plebani[a], G. Del Giudice[a], M. P. Panozzo[a], R. Venturini[a],
T. Meggiato[b], M.D. Carbone[a], G. Del Favero[b], A. Del Mistro[c], A. Burlina[a]

[a]Institute of Laboratory Medicine, [b]Department of Gastroenterology,
[c]Institute of Oncology, University of Padova, Italy

Introduction

CA 19-9 is one of the most sensitive and specific serum markers available for pancreatic neoplasia, and it is widely used in clinical practice (1–4). However, CA 19-9 serum determination has some drawbacks in the diagnosis of pancreatic cancer: 1. As its sensitivity is low in the early stages, it is not useful for screening (2, 4, 5); 2. blood group Lewis a-/b-subjects (5% of the total population) never have high CA 19-9 levels (6, 7) since the biosynthesis of the CA 19-9 antigen depends on the activity of a fucosyltransferase which is also involved in the biosynthesis of the Lewis blood group antigen; 3. cholestasis, frequently associated with tumors of the head of the pancreas, can affect CA 19-9 serum levels, probably by reducing its metabolism in the liver (8–10).

Some of the factors above limiting the diagnostic utility of CA 19-9 depend on the properties of the CA 19-9 molecule, which is a high molecular weight (> 5 x 10 kD) mucin-type glycoprotein with a large glucidic moiety (11, 12). Glycoproteins are mainly catabolized by the liver, after sugar determinants have been specifically recognized by membrane receptors (e.g. glycoprotein receptor) (13, 14). The circulating levels of CA 19-9 in patients with pancreatic cancer or cholestasis are therefore probably the result of an enhanced production and of a reduced catabolism, while in patients with benign cholestasis they are probably the result of a reduced catabolism (10). The glucidic pattern of CA 19-9 circulating molecule may differ in patients with benign and malignant cholestasis, despite similar circulating values.

The aims of this study were therefore to assess the Concanavalin A affinity pattern of CA 19-9 in human pancreatic cancer cell line culture media and the in sera of patients with malignant or benign cholestasis.

Materials and methods

Cell culture

Human pancreatic carcinoma cell line MIA PaCa-2 were cultured in Dulbecco's modified Eagle's medium (DMEM from Gibco) supplemented with 10% fetal calf serum, 2% glutamine and 0.1% gentamycin (Gibco). Cells ($\approx$ 15,000 per flask) were plated in 25 flasks (Falcon, No. 3013E, 25 cm^2 growth area; Becton Dickinson Labware, Lincoln Park, N.J.) each containing 4 ml of DMEM. Cells were incubated in quintuplicate for 1, 2, 3, 4 and 7 days. The experiments were ended by removing the medium; the cells were then treated with 0.25% trypsin solution containing 0.1 mol/l EDTA for the subsequent count, which was performed using phase contrast microscopy (x 10).

The supernatants were stored at –20 °C until affinity chromatography and CA 19-9 determination.

Patients

We studied 19 cholestatic patients. Thirteen (eight males, five females, age range 40–73) had pancreatic cancer of duct cell origin histologically confirmed by means of surgical or autoptic specimens (15). Six (three males, three females, age range 45–75) had benign extra-hepatic cholestasis due to choledocholithiasis. From each patient, a serum sample was obtained after overnight fasting, and stored at −20 °C until affinity chromatography and CA 19-9 determination. The sera from four pancreatic cancer patients and from three patients with choledocholithiasis were pooled separately.

Concanavalin A affinity chromatography

We used a column of 1 x 10 cm, which was packed with Concanavalin A Sepharose 4B (Pharmacia Fine Chemicals, Piscataway, NJ). The resin was equilibrated with 50 mmol/l Tris HCl buffer pH 7.5 containing 1 mmol/l NaCl, 1 mmol/l $CaCl_2$ and 1 mmol/l $MgCl_2$. A sample volume of 200 µl was applied and eluted first with the equilibrating buffer and then with the same buffer with the addition with of 0.5 mol/l methyl-alpha-D-glucopyranoside. The flow rate was 1 ml/min. We collected frations of 2 ml after the chromatography of the cell culture supernatant and of the serum pools. When chromatography was performed for each serum sample, two fractions were collected, one (non-reactive) before and the other (reactive) after the eluting sugar has been applied. The fractions were lyophilized and resuspended in saline solution before CA 19-9 assay.
CA 19-9 was determinated in the single patient's sera, in patients' pools, in cell culture media and in the eluates, using an ILMA procedure (Byk Gulden). CA 19-9 recovery after Concanavalin A affinity chromatography ranged from 70 to 95%.

Results

Figure 1 shows the number of MIA PaCa-2 cells in relation to the culture period, as well as corresponding levels of CA 19-9 recorded in the culture media. Affinity chromatography of the cell culture media showed two peaks, one non-reactive and another reactive with Concanavalin A. The ratio between these two peaks was about 10:1.
Figure 2 shows CA 19-9 chromatographic profile after Concanavalin A affinity chromatography of two serum pools, one obtained from four patients with pancreatic cancer and the other from three patients with benign cholestasis. This profile was overlapped to that obtained from cell culture media chromatography.

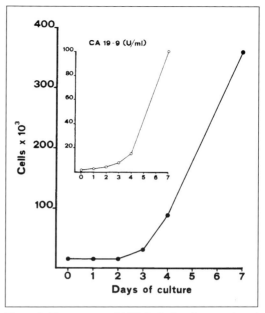

Figure 1. Time course of MIA PaCa-2 cells growth and CA 19-9 levels detected in culture media. Each value was determined in quintuplicate, and this experiment is representative of four others.

Table I illustrates the results of serum CA 19-9 levels found in the 12 patients singly studied and the corresponding percentages of Concanavalin A reactive fractions of CA 19-9 antigen. In these patients, we found significant correlations between total serum CA 19-9 and the corresponding non-reactive (r = 0.999, p < 0.001) and reactive (r = 0.997, p < 0.001) Concanavalin A CA 19-9 fractions. The two CA 19-9 fractions were not found to be correlated with any of the following serum indices: total bilirubin, ALP, GGT, AST, glucose or albumin. The ratio between the non-reactive and reactive Concanavalin A CA 19-9 ranged from 10 to 30 and it was not correlated with any of the above serum indices.

Discussion

It is believed that in cancer patients the circulating levels of CA 19-9, a syalosyl Le-a antigen present on glycolipids, glycoproteins and on mucin-like glycoproteins, derive mainly from tumor cells (11, 12). In vitro, we found this antigen

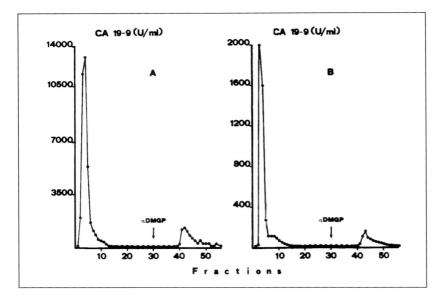

Figure 2. CA 19-9 chromatographic profile after Concanavalin A affinity chromatography of two serum pools, one obtained from four patients with pancreatic cancer (A) and the other from three patients with benign cholestasis (B). DMGP = methyl-alpha-D-glucopyranoside.

Table I. Individual values of serum CA 19-9 and of the percentage of CA 19-9 reacting with Concanavalin A (Con A) in the 12 patients singly studied. PC = pancreatic cancer; EHC = benign extra-hepatic cholestasis.

Patients	Diagnosis	Serum CA 19-9 U/ml	Con A reactive CA 19-9 (%)
1	PC	610000	6
2	PC	103000	7
3	PC	3350	7
4	PC	33900	7
5	PC	3600	4
6	PC	24000	3
7	PC	7100	8
8	PC	245	5
9	PC	102	3
10	EHC	15000	9
11	EHC	340	6
12	EHC	1200	3

was directly produced by pancreatic tumor cell line MIA PaCa-2 as already reported for the line SUIT-2 (16). This suggests that tumor cell CA 19-9 production and release determines the circulating levels of this substance. In cancer patients, the glucidic moiety of CA 19-9 may be modified, since oncogenesis is associated with several biochemical aberrations, including a modified protein glycosylation (17, 18).

To study the glucidic pattern of CA 19-9 bearing molecules, we performed Concanvalin A affinity chromatography, since the lectin Concanavalin A binds terminal and some internal mannose and glucose structures onto N-linked oligosaccharides. Cell culture media after Concavalin A chromatography showed two distinct peaks: The first, larger, represents the non-reactive material and the second the reactive material. The ratio between these two peaks was about 10:1. A similar profile was observed after pancreatic cancer sera chromatography. The circulating CA 19-9 bearing molecule is therefore a heterogeneous glycoprotein, probably released directly by tumor cells and this disagrees with the results of Wu and Chang, who did not find Concanavalin A reactive CA 19-9 in pancreatic cancer patients sera (19).

In vivo, together with direct tumor release, other factors are probably involved in determining increased CA 19-9 levels. Firstly, cholestasis is often claimed to significantly influence this serum marker, probably by reducing its liver catabolism (8–10). Cholestasis might interfere not only with the total CA 19-9 circulating levels, but also with its Con A profile, as occurs for other glycoproteins after liver injury (20). In patients with benign bile duct obstruction we found that the chromatographic CA 19-9 pattern was almost equal to that of neoplastic patients. Furthermore, none of the cholestatic indices, such as total bilirubin, ALP and GGT, were correlated with the non-reactive or with the reactive CA 19-9 fractions.

On the basis of our observations, we may conclude that CA 19-9 antigen is produced by tumor cells and released into the circulation in two fractions, one reacting and the other not reacting with Concanavalin A. The ratio between these two fractions, about 10:1, is independent of the presence of cholestasis or of its severity. Unlike findings made for other tumor markers, like alpha-fetoprotein or HCG (18), our findings suggest that Concanavalin A affinity chromatography is not useful for discriminating pancreatic cancer patients from patients with benign jaundice.

References

1 Steinberg WM, Gelfand R, Anderson KK et al (1986) Comparison of the sensitivity and specificity of the CAI9-9 and carcinoembryonic antigen assays in detecting cancer of the pancreas. Gastroenterol 90:343–349
2 Del Favero G, Fabris C, Plebani M et al (1986) CA 19-9 and carcinoembryonic antigen in pancreatic cancer diagnosis. Cancer 57:1576–1579
3 Safi F, Roscher R, Beger HG (1989) Tumor markers in pancreatic cancer. Sensitivity and specificity of CA 19-9. Hepatogastroenterol 36:419–423
4 Steinberg W (1990) The clinical utility of the CA 19-9 tumorassociated antigen. Am J Gastroenterol 85: 350–355
5 Frebourg T, Bercoff E, Manchon N et al (1988) The evaluation of CA 19-9 antigen level in the early detection of pancreatic cancer. A prospective study of 866 patients. Cancer 62:2287–2290
6 Uhlenbruck G, Holler U, Heising J, van Mil A, Dienst C (1985) Sialylated Le a blood group substances detected by the monoclonal antibody CA 19-9 in human seminal plasma and other organs. Urol Res 13:223–226
7 Pour PM, Tempero MM, Takasaki H et al (1988) Expression of blood group-related antigens ABH, Lewis A, Lewis B, Lewis X, Lewis Y, and CA 19-9 in pancreatic cancer cells in comparison with the patient's blood group type. Cancer Res 48:5422–5426
8 Del Favero G, Fabris C, Panucci A et al (1986) Carbohydrate antigen 19-9 (CA 19-9) and carcinoembryonic antigen (CEA) in pancreatic cancer. Role of age and liver dysfunction. Bull Cancer 73:251–255
9 Ohshio G, Manabe T, Watanabe Y et al (1990) Comparative studies of DU-PAN-2, carcinoembryonic antigen, and CA 19-9 in the serum and bile of patients with pancreatic and biliary tract diseases: evaluation of the influence of obstructive jaundice. Am J Gastroenterol 85:1370–1376
10 Basso D, Meggiato T, Fabris C et al (1992) Extrahepatic cholestasis determines a reversible increase of glycoproteic tumour markers in benign and malignant diseases. Eur J Clin Invest 22:800–804
11 Magnani JL, Steplewski Z, Koprowski H, Ginsburg V (1983) Identification of the gastrointestinal and pancreatic cancer-associated antigen detected by monoclonal antibody 19-9 in the sera of patients as a mucin. Cancer Res 43:5489–5492
12 Lan MS, Bast RC, Colnaghi MI et al (1987) Co-expression of human cancer-associated epitopes on mucin molecules. Int J Cancer 39:68–72
13 Ashwell G, Harford J (1982) Carbohydrate-specific receptors of the liver. Ann Rev Biochem 51:531–554
14 McFarlane IG (1983) Hepatic clearance of serum glycoproteins. Clin Sci 64:127–135
15 Cubilla AL, Fitzgerald PJ (1978) Pancreas cancer. 1. Duct adenocarcinoma. Pathol Annu 13:241–289
16 Iwamura T, Katsuki T (1987) Kinetics of carcinoembryonic antigen and carbohydrate antigen 19-9 production in a human pancreatic cancer cell line (SUIT-2). Gastroenterol Jpn 22:640–646
17 Hakomori SI (1985) Aberrant glycosylation in cancer cell membranes as focused on glycolipids: overview and perspectives. Cancer Res 45:2405–2414
18 Kobata A (1988) Structural changes induced in the sugar chains of glycoproteins by malignant transformation of producing cells and their clinical application. Biochimie 70:1575–1585
19 Wu JT, Chang J (1992) Chromatographic characterization of CA 19-9 molecules from cystic fibrosis and pancreatic carcinoma. J Clin Lab Anal 6:209–215
20 Jezequel M, Seta NS, Corbic MM, Feger JM, Durand GM (1988) Modifications of concanavalin A patterns of 1-acid glycoprotein and 2-HS glycoprotein in alcoholic liver disease. Clin Chim Acta 176:49–57

Address for correspondence:
Dr. M. Plebani
Istituto di Medicina di Laboratorio
c/o Laboratorio Centrale
Via Giustiniani 2
I-35128 Padova, Italy

A high fraction of proliferating cell nuclear antigen (PCNA) in breast cancer indicates poor prognosis

U.-J. Göhring, A. Scharl, M. Stoffl, U. Thelen, G. Crombach

Department of Obstetrics and Gynecology, University of Cologne, Germany

Introduction

The proliferating cell nuclear antigen (PCNA; synonym "cyclin") is a 36 kD nuclear polypeptide, which acts as a co-factor of DNA-polymerase δ (4). It causes metabolic stimulation of resting cells during the late G1- and the following S-phase. PCNA is needed for DNA replication and synthesis (3, 9). Its expression in a cell nucleus indicates proliferation activity of the cell (2, 3, 4, 7, 9). The prognostic significance of this proliferation marker for breast cancer is debated controversially (1, 5, 10, 12, 13, 14). To assess, whether PCNA detection may be useful as a prognostic factor in breast cancer, we tested 208 breast carcinoma tissues for PCNA expression immunohistochemically and correlated the results to established prognostic markers and to the clinical outcome.

Material and methods

PCNA was tested immunohistochemically using a monoclonal antibody (Mouse antibody Ab1 NA03; Dianova, Hamburg) in 208 formalin-fixed and paraffin-embedded tissues of primary breast cancer (T1–4 N0–2 M0) using a modified 11-step avidin-biotin-method. PCNA expression was evaluated through a semiquantitative threepoint score: PCNA low < 10%, PCNA moderate 10–50%, PCNA high > 50% positive tumor cells.
The results were correlated to clinical parameters (age, menopausal status, tumor size, nodal status, histological differentiation) and to the immunohistochemical detection of steroid hormone receptors (11). In 202 patients the clinical follow-up was complete for at least five years (mediane observation time 72 month). Chi-square test and Kaplan-Meier survival analyses (log-rank test) were used for statistical evaluation of data with a niveau of significance of 0.05.

Results

PCNA was missed or only weekly expressed in 36.5% of breast cancer tissues. In 63.5% of carcinomas a moderate or strong expression of PCNA was observed in the nucleus of tumor cells (PCNA moderate: 36.1%; PCNA high: 27.4%) (figure 1). In tumors staining was heterogeneous. Staining intensity and distribution of positive tumor cells varied. The mean percentage of positive tumor cells was 20.4% (range 0–95%; SD 8.7). PCNA detection increased with increasing tumor size ($p = 0.028$) and dedifferentiation of tumors ($p = 0.012$). No significant correlation was observed to age, menopausal status, node involvement or steroid hormone receptor status (table I). Clinical follow-up was known in 202 patients over 5–10 years. 120 of the 202 patients (61.2%) had no evidence of disease after the primary therapy. 76 patients (38.8%) developed tumor relapse. Of these latter patients seven are still alive, whereas 69 patients died from the tumor. Six patients died from other causes with no evidence of disease.
In node negative patients (n = 84) survival analysis showed no correlation between a low or moderate PCNA expression and relapse free survival or overall survival. However, high PCNA expression correlated significantly to early relapse (figure 2) and death. In node positive patients (n = 118) the level of PCNA expression correlated significantly to the clinical course of disease (figure 3).

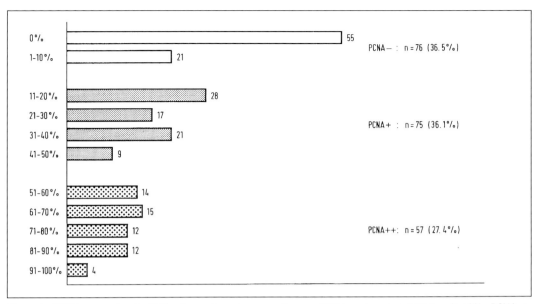

Figure 1. PCNA-expression in 208 primary breast cancer tissues. PCNA –: low expression = 0–10%; PCNA +: moderate = 11–50%; PCNA ++: high => 50% positive tumor cells.

Table I. PCNA-expression and clinical and morphological parameters in 208 tissues of primary breast cancer (chi-square test).

	n	PCNA 0–10%	PCNA 11–50%	PCNA 51–100%	p
Age					
≤ 50 years	77	24 (31%)	31 (40%)	22 (29%)	
> 50 years	131	52 (40%)	44 (34%)	35 (27%)	0.444
Menopausal status					
prae	61	19 (31%)	23 (38%)	19 (31%)	
peri	23	8 (35%)	11 (48%)	4 (17%)	
post	124	49 (40%)	41 (33%)	34 (27%)	0.526
Tumor size					
≤ 2cm	69	28 (41%)	26 (38%)	15 (22%)	
2–5cm	99	40 (40%)	33 (33%)	26 (26%)	
> 5cm	36	5 (14%)	15 (42%)	16 (44%)	0.028
Lymph node involvement[a]					
0	84	31 (37%)	32 (38%)	21 (25%)	
1–3	65	24 (37%)	23 (35%)	18 (28%)	
≥ 4	53	19 (36%)	16 (30%)	18 (34%)	0.822
Tumor grade (*Bloom* and *Richardson*)					
I	30	11 (37%)	17 (57%)	2 (7%)	
II	117	46 (39%)	40 (34%)	31 (26%)	
III	61	19 (31%)	18 (30%)	24 (39%)	0.012
Steroid hormone receptor status[b]					
ER/PR –	60	20 (33%)	22 (37%)	18 (30%)	
ER/PR +	128	44 (34%)	49 (38%)	35 (27%)	0.931

[a]202 Patients with a lymphonodectomy;
[b]immunohistochemically detected estrogen- (er) and progesterone-receptor (pr) in 188 tissues of breast carcinomas

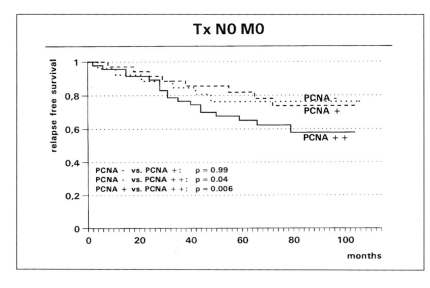

Figure 2. Relapse free survival and PCNA-expression (PCNA -: 0–10%; PCNA +: 11–50%; PCNA ++: > 50% positive tumor cells) in 84 patients without lymph node involvement (Tx N0 M0).

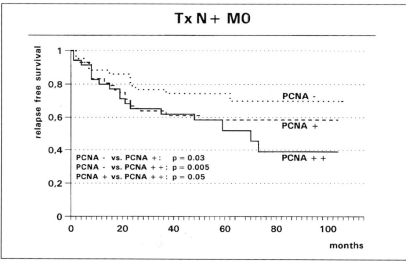

Figure 3. Relapse free survival and PCNA-expression (PCNA -: 0–10%; PCNA +: 11–50%; PCNA ++: > 50% positive tumor cells) in 118 patients with lymph node involvement (Tx N+ M0).

Discussion

Hitherto Ki-67, an antibody against proliferating cells was used for immunohistochemical detection of proliferation activity (6). This antibody, however, requires fresh tissue, wheras proliferating cell nuclear antigen works in fixed material. The results correlate to those obtained with Ki-67 in a linear fashion (5, 7). In our study PCNA detection was reliably and reproducibly performed in formalin-fixed and paraffin-embedded tissues of primary breast cancer. Within a single tumor percentage of positive tumor cells varied considerably, mirroring the heterogenity of a tumor (2, 13). Our positivity rate is in accordance with those of other authors (1, 5, 10, 14), although the use of different antibodies, the way and duration of fixation, or the thickness of the tissue block, as well as interperson variations in the assessment of staining may cause different results (7, 8, 10). In computer based picture analysis systems Shrestha et al. (12) and Siitoner et al. (13) found a mean of 12.3% and 14.4% positive tumor cells, respectively.

In studies published on breast cancer, the results concerning the correlation of PCNA expression and clinical and histological or histochemical parameters showed some variation. This variation may in part be due to differences in the techniques used and to differences in the population investigated. A correlation of PCNA detection to tumor size was found by *Leonardi* et al. (10), but missed by *Aaltomaa* et al. (1), *Shresta* et al. (12) and *Visscher* et al. (14). A correlation to tumor grade was reported unanimously (1, 5, 12, 13, 14). In discordance to our results *Leonardi* et al. (10) reported a significant correlation of PCNA detection to nodal and receptor status.

PCNA only detects proliferating cells, no resting G0-phase cells (3). Thus PCNA mirrors the fraction of duplicating tumor cells within a tumor and thereby the proliferation activity of a tumor. This fact may explain the results of the survival analyses: High PCNA detection correlates to a short relapse free and overall survival. This observation confirms the results of other studies (1, 12). In our group of patients PCNA detection is of prognostic sigificance in node positive and also in node negative patients. The latter group is of special importance because it presents special problems in whether to apply adjuvant systemic therapy. According to these results PCNA detection may have some use in clinical management of breast cancer patients. However, multivariance analysis still has to show whether PCNA is an independent factor.

References

1. Aaltomaa S, Lipponen P, Syrjänen K (1992) Prognostic value of cell proliferation in breast cancer as determined by proliferating cell nuclear antigen (PCNA) immunostaining. Anticancer Res 12:1281–1286
2. Beerman H, Smit VTHBM, Kluin PM (1991) Flow cytometric analyses of DNA stemline heterogenity in primary and metastatic breast cancer. Cytometry 12:147–154
3. Bravo R, Macdonald-Bravo H (1985) Changes in the nuclear distribution of cyclin (PCNA) but not its synthesis depend on DNA replication. EMBO J 349:655–661
4. Bravo R, Frank R, Blindell PA, Macdonald-Bravo H (1987) Cyclin/PCNA is the axillary protein to DNA polymerase-delta. Nature 326:515–520
5. Dawson AE, Norton JA, Weinberg DS (1990) Comparative assessment of proliferation and DNA content in breast carcinoma by image analysis and flow cytometry. Am J Pathol 136:1115–1124
6. Gerdes J, Schwab U, Lemke H, Stein H (1983) Production of a mouse monoclonal antibody reactive with a human nuclear antigen associated with cell proliferation. Int J Cancer 31:13–20
7. Hall PA, Levison DA, Woods AL, Yu CCW, Kellock DB, Watkins JA, Barnes DM, Gillett CE, Camplejohn R, Dover R, Waseem NH, Lane DP (1990) Proliferating cell nuclear antigen (PCNA) immunolocalization in paraffin sections: an index of cell proliferation with evidence of deregulated expression in some neoplasms. J Pathol 162:285–294
8. Huff JP, Roos G, Peeblees CL, Hougten R, Sullivan KE, Tan EM (1990) Insights into native epitopes of proliferating cell nuclear antigen using recombinant DNA protein products. J Exp Med 172:419–429
9. Jasulski D, de Riel JK, Mercher WE, Calabretta B, Baserga R (1988) Inhibition of cellular proliferation by antisense oligodeoxynucleotides to PCNA cyclin. Science 240:1544–1546
10. Leonardi E, Girlando S, Serio G, Mauri FA, Perrone G, Scampini S, Dalla Palma P, Barbareschi M (1992) PCNA and Ki67 expression in breast carcinoma: Correlation with clinical and biological variables. J Clin Pathol 45:416–419
11. Scharl A, Vierbuchen M, Würz H (1989) Immunhistochemischer Nachweis von Östrogen- und Progesteronrezeptoren mit Hilfe monoklonaler Antikörper in Mammakarzinomgeweben. Vergleich mit der biochemischen Rezeptoranalyse. Pathologe 10:31–38
12. Shrestha P, Yamada K, Wada T, Maeda S, Watatani M, Yasutomi M, Takagi H, Mori M (1992) Proliferating nuclear cell antigen in breast lesions: correlation of c-erb B2 oncoprotein and EGF receptor and its clinicopathological significance in breast cancer. Virchows Archiv A Pathol Anat 421:193–202
13. Siitonen SM, Isola JJ, Rantala IS, Helin HJ (1993) Intratumor variation in cell proliferation in breast carcinoma as determined by antiproliferating cell nuclear, antigen monoclonal antibody and automated image analysis. Am J Clin Pathol 99:226–231
14. Visscher DW, Wykes S, Kubus J, Crissman JD (1992) Comparison of PCNA/cyclin immunohistochemistry with flow cytometric S-phase fraction in breast cancer. Breast Cancer Res Treat 22:111–118

Address for correspondence:
Dr. med. U.-J. Göhring
Abteilung für Geburtshilfe und Gynäkologie
Universität Köln
Kerpener Straße 34
D-50931 Köln, Germany

Immunhistochemical detection of cathepsin D (Cath D) in formalin-fixed, paraffin-embedded breast cancer samples[1]

M. W. Beckmann[a], B. Tutschek[a], U.J. Göhring[b], A. Scharl[b],
K. Loaiciga[a], Meike Bracht[a], Anne Beinlich[a], H.G. Schnürch[a]
[a]Women's Clinic of the Heinrich-Heine-University, Düsseldorf
[b]Womens Clinic of the University of Cologne, Germany

Introduction

Functional tumor characteristics including factors involved in tumor invasion and promotion of tumor growth are currently under investigation as prognostic factors for decision of adjuvant therapy of breast cancer patients (1–3). The mechanism of proteolysis is a prerequisite of tumor invasion and metastasis. Collagenases, plasmin, plasminogen activator and cathepsin D (Cath D) are all associated with tumor cell spreading (4–6). Cathepsin D is a lysosomal protease that exists intracellular as a precursor form (procathepsin D, 52 kD), intermediate active enzyme (48 kD), and a mature active enzyme (34 kD and 14 kD dimer) that normally functions in the lysosomes at acidic pH. In estrogen-dependent breast cancer cell lines the synthesis of procathepsin D is regulated by estrogens (7, 8). In normal mammary cells, most of procathepsin D is processed into the active form in lysosomes and only small amounts of procathepsin D are secreted. In cell culture proteolytic activity on various substrates including the basement membrane and proteoglycans after autoactivation at acidic pH, and an autocrine mitogenic activity could be demonstrated (8). The most published method of Cath D detection is the immunobiochemical assay performed on tumor lysates. Immunohistochemical studies are rare as well as comparative studies between both methods. Furthermore, a detailed scoring system including differentiation between Cath D positive tumor cells and surrounding interstitial cells and stroma has been published only recently (9). We analyzed Cath D expression in 142 formalin-fixed and paraffin-embedded breast cancer specimens and 12 benign breast samples by immunohistochemistry. Simultaneously estrogen (ER) and progesteron (PgR) receptor immunohistochemistry were performed on sections of the same tumors. Various cell lines and normal skin tissue samples served as sections of the same tumors. Various cell lines and normal skin tissue samples served as positive or negative controls. Results of the expression analyses were compared with other biological characteristics of the tumors including histological grade, tumor size, lymph node metastases and menopause.

Materials and methods

Paraffin-embedded, formalin-fixed sections (January 1980 until December 1985) from 142 patients treated with surgery for primary breast cancer and 12 patients with benign breast tumors were analyzed. In case of axillary dissection, the number of lymph node metastases was determined. Hematoxylin-eosin staining was performed for routine pathologic evaluation (diameter, margins, grading, histological typing). Cath D expression was correlated with menopausal status, tumor size, number of lymph node metastasis, histological grading, and immunohistochemical determined ER or PgR expression.

Cell cultures of T47D, MCF-7 and CHO cell lines

Human breast cancer cell lines T47D and MCF-7 (both expressing Cath D), and ovarian cell line

---
[1]Grant (Be 1215/6-1) from Deutsche Forschungsgemeinschaft, Bonn, Germany.

CHO were cultured as previously described (10, 11). For immunohistochemical determinations, different cell lines were cultured on sterile culture slides.

Steroid receptor (ER, PgR) analyses

ER- and PgR-status were determined by immunohistochemistry as described previously by *Scharl* et al. (12). The peroxidase-anti-peroxidase (PAP-method used either ER antibody from the ER-ICA monoclonal kit (Abbott) as primary antibody with rabbit-anti-rat IgG-Ab as secondary antibody (Vector Laboratories) or PgR mPR (Dianova) as primary antibody with sheep-anti-mouse IgG-Ab (Vector Laboratories) as secondary antibody. For staining procedure, the PAP-Kit complex (ABC Elite-kit Vectastain, Vector Laboratories) was used, counter staining was performed with hematoxylin. Immunohistochemical reaction was scored according to the recommondations of *Remmele* and *Stegner* (16), the immunoreactive score ranged from 0 to 12.

Immunohistochemical detection of Cath D

Cath D expression was determined by immunohistochemistry as described previously by *Göhring* et al. (9). Primary antibody was His-Cath-Ab1, which detects the 52 kD precursor as both secreted forms (48 kD and 34 kD). Detection was performed with avidin-biotin-complex (Vectastain Eliten ABC-Kit). The differentiating score system used was identical to that published by *Göhring* et al. (9).

Statistics

Qualitative analyses of ER, PgR, Cath D and other prognostic factors were performed by chi-square contigency table or extact Fisher's test; quantitative analyses between Cath D and ER or PgR expression were performed with a rank correlation test.

Results

Our study group included 53 women aged below 50 years (premenopausal) and 89 women $\geq$ 50 years (postmenopausal). The rage was 31 to 76 years.
Twelve benign tumors of the breast including fibroadenomas and mastophatic lesions were evaluated for Cath D. In some cases stromal cells and macrophages were slightly positive. Immunostaining of Cath D positive carcinoma was not restricted to tumor cells. The surrounding connective tissue as well as tumor infiltrating and surrounding macrophages and histocytes also showed positive staining. Therefore the scoring system was divided and scored as described (table I).
Cath D expression determined by immunohistochemistry was compared with various characteristics of the patients. There were no significant correlations between Cath D expression and menopause, number of lymph nodes, tumor grade, or tumor size.
Table II demonstrates correlations between Cath D, ER and PgR. Correlation between Cath D and PgR was inverse ($p < 0.01$), between ER and Cath D not significant; ER and PgR correlated significantly ($p < 0.001$).

Table I. Application of the scoring system for Cath D immunohistochemistry.

A. Tumor cells

PP (percent positive cells)	SI (staining intensity)
0 = 0	0
1–10 = 1	1
11–50 = 2	2
51–80 = 3	3
< 80 = 4	

Score ≥ 2 is considered to be positive staining: 44/142

B. Stroma cells/macrophages/interstitial tissue

SI (staining intensity)

0
1
2
3

Score ≥ 1 is considered to be positive staining: 34/142

Total number of positive tumors   64/142

Table II. Relationship between ER-, PgR- and Cath D protein measured by immunohistochemical analyses in human breast cancer specimens (n = 142).

Total number (%) (142 = 100%)	Cath D negative (78/142)	Cath D positive (64/142)	Statistics chi-square test
ER			
negative 61	28	33	
positive 81	50	31	n.s.[a]
PgR			
negative 72	33	39	
positive 70	45	25	$p < 0.01$
		ER negative (61/142)	ER poitive (81/142)
PgR			
negative 72	44	28	
positive 70	17	53	$p < 0.001$

[a] n.s. = $p > 0.05$

Discussion

In this study the detection of Cath D expression proved feasible in formalin-fixed, paraffin-embedded section of breast cancer tumors. Using the scoring system published by *Göhring* et al. (9) 32% of tumor cells and 25% of the surrounding tissue were Cath D positive. The overall positivity rate was 45%. This percentage is slightly below rates published by *Garcia* et al. (64%) (14), *Henry* et al. (66%) (7), *Maudelonde* et al. (48%) (15, 16) and *Göhring* et al. (63%) (9). Prolonged storage of tumor tissue or differences in primary tissue fixation may be responsible for this discrepancy. Cath D distribution in tumor tissue was heterogenous as described for other factors of tumor invasion, i.e. urokinase plasminogenic activator (17).

Comparision of Cath D expression with distribution of different patients' characteristics including tumor size, number of patients with lymph node metastasis, histologic grade, or tumor size did not show any significant correlation. This supports results from most other research groups stating the lack of correlations between these parameters, even though some of them used a biochemical assay (4, 15, 16, 18, 19). Cath D is supposed to be an estrogen-regulated protein, suggesting a correlation between ER or PgR and Cath D expression. In our study no correlation could be seen between ER and Cath D expression. This confirms results of *Göhring* et al. (9), but is contradictory to studies of *Thorpe* et al. (20) or *Maudelande* et al. (15, 16). PgR and Cath D showed an inverse correlation, what is also contradictory to other studies (5, 14, 18). Supposing estrogen-dependent regulation of Cath D expression and knowing the interpendence of PgR and ER epression this finding is astonishing. In our study group no statistical hints could be found to explain this finding. In accordance with other groups, Cath D staining was not restricted to tumor cells, but occasionally found in stromal cells and macrophages (3, 9). This Cath D expression pattern could reflect influence of various exogenous growth factors of precursor proteases, and autocrine, juxtacrine, or paracrine mechanisms, which are involved in the induction and maintenance of malignant transformation, growth control, and invasion. Molecular interactions among the various cell-regulatory and biological mechanisms of tumor proteases, growth factors, and steroid receptor expression are still unclear. With malignant transformation regulatory mechanisms are abolished, proliferation and invasion are now independent of endocrine control.

References

1. Early Breast Cancer Trialists' Collaborative Group: Systemic treatment of early breast cancer by hormonal, cytotoxic, or immune therapy (1992) Lancet 329:1–15
2. Mc Guire WL, Clark GM (1992) Prognostic factors and treatment decisions in axillary-node-negative breast cancer. N Engl J Med 326:1756–1761
3. Beckmann MW, Niederacher D, Schnürch H-G, Bender HG (1993) Significance of members of the erbB-gene family for tumour development as prognostic factors and for novel therapeutic options. Geburtsh Frauenheilk 11:742–753
4. Crombach G, Ingenhorst A, Göhring UJ, Möbus V, Peters D, Schaeffer HJ, Bolte A (1992) Cathepsin D concentrations in the cytosol of benign and malignant tumors of the breast and the female genital tract. Tumordiagn u Ther 3:14–18
5. Tandon AK, Clark GM, Chamness GC, Chirgwin JM, McGuire WL (1990) Cathepsin D and prognosis in breast cancer. N Engl J Med 322:297–302
6. Rempen A, Caffier H (1991) Kathepsin D beim primären Mammakarzinom in Korrelation zu verschiedenen Prognosefaktoren. Geburtsh Frauenheilk 51:943–949
7. Henry JA, McCarthy AL, Angus B (1990) Prognostic significance of the estrogen-regulated protein, cath D in breast cancer. Cancer 65:265–271
8. Rochefort H, Capony F, Garcia M (1990) Cathepsin D in breast cancer: from molecular and cellular biology to clinical application. Cancer Cells 2:383–388
9. Göhring UJ, Ingenhorst A, Crombach G, Scharl A (1993) Kathepsin D Expression im primären Mammakarzinom. Der Pathologe 14:313–317
10. Beckman MW, Toney LJ, Scharl A, Fuchs-Young R, Greene GL, Holt JA (1992) Detection of the HER-2/neu proto-oncogene protein p185^{erbB2} by a novel monoclonal antibody (MAB-145ww) in breast cancer membranes from estrogen and progesterone receptor assays. Eur J Cancer 28:322–326
11. Niederacher D, Beckmann MW, Scharl A, Picard F, Schnürch HG, Bender HG (1994) Biochemische und molekulargenetische Analyse von Onkogenen der c-erbB-Familie in Mammakarzinomen. Tumorimmunologie in der Gynäkologie. In: Koldovsky U, Kreienberg R (eds) Aktuelle Onkologie 79. Zuckschwerdt, München, pp 73–78
12. Scharl A, Vierbuchen M, Würz H (1989) Immunhistochemischer Nachweis von Östrogen- und Progesteronrezptoren beim Mammakarzinom mit Hilfe monoclonaler Antikörper: Vergleich mit der biochemischen Rezeptoranalyse. Pathologe 10:31–38
13. Remmele W, Stegner HG (1986) Immunhistochemischer Nachweis von Östrogenrezeptoren (ER-ICA) in Mammakarzinomgewebe. Deutsches Ärzteblatt 48:3362–3364
14. Garcia M, Lacombe MJ, Duplay H, Cavailles V, Rochefort H (1987) Immunohistochemical distribution of the 52-kDa protein in mammary tumors: a marker associated with cell proliferation rather than with hormone responsivness. J Steroid Biochem 27:439–445
15. Maudelonde T, Khalaf S, Garcia M, Freiss G, Duporte J, Benatia M, Rogler H, Paolucci F, Simony J, Pujol H, Pau B, Rochefort H (1988) Immunoenzymatic assay of M52,000 cathepsin D in 182 breast cancer cytosols: low correlation with other prognostic parameters: Cancer Res 48:462–466
16. Maudelonde T, Brouillet JP, Roger P, Giraudier V, Pages A, Rochefort H (1992) Immunostaining of cathepsin D in breast cancer: quantification by computerised image analysis and correlation with cytosolic assay. Eur J Cancer 28A10:1686–1691
17. Ruppert C, Ehrenforth S, Tutschek B, Vering A, Beckmann MW, Scharrer I, Bender HG (1994) Proteases associated with gynecological tumours. Int J Oncol 4:717–721
18. Duffy MJD, Reilly D, Brouillet JP, McDermott EW, Faul C, O'Higgins N, Fennelly JJ, Maudelonde T, Rochefort H (1992) Correlation with disease-free interval and overall survival. Clin Chem 38/10:2114–2116
19. Kute TE, Shao ZM, Sugg NK, Long RT, Russell GB, Case LD (1992) Cathepsin D as a prognostic indicator for node-negative breast cancer patients using both immunoassay and enzymatic assays. Cancer Res 52:5198–5203
20. Thorpe SM, Rochfort H, Garcia M, Freiss G, Christensen I, Khalaf S, Paolucci F, Pau B, Rasmussen BB, Rose C (1989) Association between high concentrations af M 52,000 cathepsin D and poor prognosis in primary human breast cancer. Cancer Res 49:6008–6014

Address for correspondence:
Dr. med. M. W. Beckmann
Universitätsfrauenklinik
Heinrich-Heine-Universität
Moorenstraße 5
D-40225 Düsseldorf, Germany

Cathepsin D tissue cytosol enzyme immunoassay (EIA) and immunohistochemical (IHC) reagent in breast cancer prognosis

S. Weitz, N. Khabbaz, L. Carne, J. Harvey

Ciba Corning, Triton Laboratories, Alameda, California, USA

Introduction

Cathepsin D is a lysosomal aspartate protease that is generally expressed in liver, spleen, lung, brain, activated macrophages (1), and lactating breast epithelial cells with little or no expression in normal non-lactating breast epithelial cells (in-house data). The connection of Cathepsin D with breast cancer was first shown by *Rochefort* using a human breast cancer cell line (2–4). This early work was followed by many clinical studies showing that tumor tissue cytosol Cathepsin D levels correlated with poor prognosis in node negative breast cancer patients (5–12).

Reports on the prognostic use of Cathepsin D by immunohistochemical (IHC) detection have been mixed. Some investigators have suggested a lack of prognostic value for Cathepsin D by IHC (13, 14), whereas we have reported a clear prognostic value for Cathepsin D by IHC using our 1C11 monoclonal antibody with formalin-fixed, paraffin-embedded tissue sections (15). In addition to our clinical agreement between IHC and published quantitative tissue extract assays in terms of prognostic value, *Rochefort* has reported analytical correlation between IHC and tissue extract values (16).

Two immunological methods may be used for the detection of Cathepsin D in breast tumors. The quantitative tissue cytosol and the immunohistochemical methods are discussed separately. This paper describes the characteristics of the triton tissue extract immunochemical kit and IHC reagent.

Tissue assay characteristics

The Cathepsin D tissue extract EIA kit is an antibody-based immunoenzymetric assay. Specimen tissue cytosols are prepared by the homogenization procedure used for routine preparation of cytosol estrogen (ER) and progesterone (PgR) receptor assays. A monoclonal antibody and a rabbit polyclonal antibody, both specific for CD, are simultaneously incubated with specimen tissue cytosols, calibrators and control. During this incubation, the CD present in the specimen, calibrators and control is bound by the two anti-CD antibodies. The monoclonal antibody within this reagent is conjugated to biotin causing the formed immunecomplexes to be bound onto the streptavidin-coated tube. Unbound materials present in the specimen are removed by washing of the tubes. In the second incubation, an anti-rabbit antibody conjugated with horseradish peroxidase (conjugate) is added to the tube. If CD is present in the specimen, it complexes with the polyclonal rabbit-anti-CD contained within the anti-CD solution. The conjugate is then bound to this complex. Unbound conjugate is removed by a second tube washing step. The tubes are next incubated with TMB substrate solution (hydrogen peroxide and 3,3',5,5'-tetramethylbenzidine) to develop a color. The intensity of the color formed by the enzyme reaction is proportional to the concentration of CD in the specimen, within the working range of the assay. Stopping solution (phosphoric acid) is then added to the tubes to stop the enzyme reaction. The intensity of the color developed is read with a spectrophotometer set at 450 nm. A calibration curve is obtained by plotting the CD concentration of the calibrators versus the absorbance. The CD concentration of

Table I. Comparison of CIS and triton kit performance characteristics.

	Triton	CIS
Sensitivity	20 fmoles/ml	20 fmoles/ml
Linearity	90% over assay range	not stated
Imprecision	5% (n = 20 x 5)	4% (n = 30)
Recovery	< 10% deviation	< 12% deviation
X-reactivity	Cathepsin B,G,H: none	not stated
	Renin: neg. at plasma conc.	not stated

the specimen and control, run concurrently with the calibrators, can be determined from this calibration curve.

The Triton EIA requires only 10 µl of the tissue cytosol per result (including repeats) thus permitting its use with small tumor specimens. The high calibrator is 2 picomoles/ml and from our experience only ~1% of samples are above this level when the kit protocol is followed. The assay has no high dose hook effect at 8 picomoles/ml, far above any reported specimens concentrations. The triton EIA performance characteristics (table I) compare favorably with the CIS monoclonal/monoclonal immuno-radiometric assay (CIS data from kit insert). Correlation results between the two assays are shown in figure 1.

Immunohistochemical characteristics

An immunohistochemical (IHC) reagent provided by Triton Laboratories uses a specific monoclonal antibody intended for use as an immunopathology research reagent to further understand the role of Cathepsin D as a potential prognostic factor for breast cancer. Purified Cathepsin D derived from human liver was used as immunogen for this monoclonal antibody (MAb 1C11). The reagent is provided as an HPLC purified MAb (from ascites) in a liquid of 1% BSA in PBS buffer and preservatives. The staining protocol involves incubation at a suggested concentration of 0.5 µg/ml for 1 hour or 50 ng/ml over night which stains routine formalin-fixed, paraffin-embedded tissue sections. Titration of the MAb concentration should be performed by each laboratory in order to fit with existing fixation and signal amplification parameters.

The specificity of MAb 1C11 includes the 52 kD, 48 kD, and 34 kD forms of Cathepsin D from human breast cancer tissues and placenta. Characteristic granular cytoplasmic lysosomal staining may be seen with breast cancer cells as well as with activated macrophages. Western blot intensity, tissue extract levels, and tissue staining intensity roughly correlated with each other when compared from the same frozen tissue powders. This IHC reagent has been shown to have significant prognostic value in node-negative breast cancer (J. Clin. Oncol. 11:36, 1993).

Conclusion

The above data suggest that the Ciba Corning (Triton Laboratories) Cathepsin D EIA and IHC reagent are effective in detecting Cathepsin D in breast tumor tissue cytosol and in routine formalin-fixed, paraffin-embedded tissue sections.

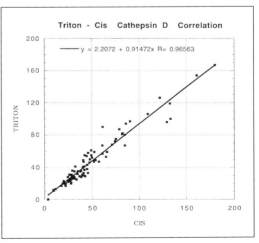

Figure 1. CIS and Triton Cathepsin D assay correlation. Units are picomoles Cathepsin D per mg total protein (n = 85; range = 0–180 pmoles/mg protein).

References

1. Reid WA, M Valler, J Kay (1986) Immunolocalisation of Cathepsin D in normal and neoplastic human tissues. J Clin Pathol 39:1323–1330.
2. Westley B, Rochefort H (1980) A secreted glycoprotein induced by estrogen in human breast cancer cell lines. Cell 20: 352–362
3. Capony F, Rougeot C, Barrett AJ, Capony JP et al (1987) Phosphorylation, glycosylation and proteolytic activity of the 52-kDa estrogen-induced protein secreted by MCF-7 Cells. J Cell Biol 104: 253–262
4. Garcia M, Capony F, Derocq D, Simon D, Pau B, Rochefort H (1985) Monoclonal antibodies to the estrogen-regulated Mr 52,000 glycoprotein: characterization and immunodetection in MCF-7 cells. Cancer Res 45: 709–716
5. Maudelonde T, Khalaf S, Garcia M, Freiss G, Duporte J, Benatia M, Rogier H, Paolucci F, Simony J, Pujol H, Pau B, Rochefort H. 1988. Immunoenzymatic assay for Mr 52,000 Cathepsin-D in 1982 breast cancer cytosols. Low correlation with other prognostic parameters. Cancer Res 48: 462–466
6. Thorpe SM, Rochefort H, Garcia M, Freiss G, Christensen IJ, Khalaf S, Paolucci F, Pau B, Rasmussen BB, Rose C (1989). Association between high concentrations of 52K Cathepsin-D and poor prognosis in primary breast cancer. Cancer Res 49: 6008–6014
7. Spyratos F, Maudelonde T, Brouillet JP, Brunet M, Defrenne A, Andrieu C, Hacene K, Desplaces A, Rochefort H (1989) An important marker predicting metastasis in primary breast cancer. Lancet II: 1115–1118
8. Tandon A, Clark G, Chamness G, Chirgwin J, McGuire WL (1990) Cathepsin D and prognosis in breast cancer. N Engl J Med 322:297–302
9. Brouillet JP, Theillet C, Maudelonde T, Defrenne A, Simony-Lafontaine J, Sertour J, Pujol H, Jeanteur P, Rochefort H (1990) Cathepsin D assay in primary breast cancer and lymph nodes: relationship with c-myc, c-erb-B-2 and int-2 oncogene amplification and node invasiveness. Eur J Cancer (in press)
10. Duffy MJ, O'Grady P, O'Siorain L (1988) Plasminogen activator. A new marker in breast cancer. In: Bresciani T, King RJB, Lippman ME, Raunaud JP (eds) Progress in cancer research and therapy, hormones and cancer. Raven Press, New York Vol 35, pp 300–303
11. Kute TE, Shao ZM, Sugg NK, Long RT, Russell GB, Case LD (1992) Cathepsin D as a prognostic indicator for node-negative breast cancer patients using both immunoassays and enzymatic assays. Cancer Res 52: 5198–5203
12. Pujol P, Maudelonde T, Daures JP, Rouanet P, Brouillet JP, Pujol H, Rochefort H (1993) A prospective study of the prognostic value of Cathepsin D levels in breast cancer cytosol. Cancer 71: 2006–2012
13. Domagala W, Striker G, Szadowska A, Dukowicz A, Weber K, Osborn M (1992) Cathepsin D in invasive ductal NOS breast carcinoma as defined by immunohistochemistry. Amer J Pathol 141:1003–1012
14. Kandalaft PL, Chang KL, Ahn CW, Traveek ST, Mehta M, Battifora H (1993) Prognostic significance of immunohistochemical analysis of Cathepsin D in low-stage breast cancer. Cancer 71:2756–2762
15. Isola J, Weitz S, Visakorpi T, Holli K, Shea R, Khabbaz N, Kallioniemi OP (1993) Cathepsin D expression detected by immunohistochemistry has independent prognostic value in axillary node-negative breast cancer. J Clin Oncol 11:36–43
16. Maudelonde T, Brouillet JP, Roger P, Giraudier A, Pages A, Rochefort H (1992) Immunostaining of Cathepsin D in breast cancer: Quantification by computerized image analysis and correlation with cytosolic assay. Eur J Cancer 28:1686–1691

Address for correspondence:
Dr. J. Harvey
Triton Laboratories, Ciba Corning Diagnostics
1401 Harbor Bay Parkway
94502 Alameda, CA, USA

Relationship between tumor labeling index, serum markers of cell proliferation and CA 125

Michaela Paganuzzi[a], M. Onetto[a], P. Marroni[a], M. Bruzzone[a], A. Alama[a], E. Catsafados[a], G. Reggiardo[a], N. Ragni[b], G.C. Torre[c], F. Boccardo[a]

[a]National Institute for Cancer Research of Genoa, [b]Obstetric and Gynecological Clinic, University of Genoa, [c]Department Obstetrics and Gynecology, Pietra Ligure Hospital, Italy

Introduction

TLI or thymidine labeling index is the percentage of cells in DNA synthesis wich reflects proliferative activity within biological systems (10, 11).

Its clinical relevance in human tumors can be 1. as prognostic factor (TLI can give important informations about the biological aggressiveness of the tumor) and 2. as parameter to optimize the drug administration scheduling, in the attempt to overcome cell kinetic based drug resistance.

As for the first clinical aspect, TLI has been reported to be a prognostsic factor in different tumors, hematological or solid tumors (16, 8, 6, 1, 5). In breast cancer TLI was demonstrated to be an independent prognostic factor, capable of defining subgroups of node negative patients, at risk for early relapse, eligible for adjuvant chemotherapy (12). Limited and controversial are instead the data on the prognostic value of TLI in ovarian carcinoma (14, 15, 1).

As for the second clinical aspect, TLI could be helpful overall to the cancer therapist as guide to treatment in several respect: a) to identify rapidly growing tumors that might be quite sensitive to cell cycle specific drugs, b) to monitor the tumoral response to specific chemotherapy and c) to test whether synchronization or recruitment has been achieved within a tumor population by drug manipulation.

The use of TLI for the last two clinical applications requires serial determinations of TLI on multiple tumor sampling. This factor limits the clinical application of this methodology, besides two other drawbacks: 1. the method is complicated and tedious, 2. the length of the time required to develop autoradiographs.

Aim of this work was to evaluate the correlation of TLI with some alternative serum cell proliferation markers, the thymidine kinase (TK) and the TPS. We also wanted to verify whether these proliferative markers are correlated with tumor marker CA 125.

TK is an essential enzyme involved in the DNA synthesis (13), activated during the G1/S phase of the cell cycle. It is present in eukaryotic cells as at least two isoenzymes (Kit), of wich the fetal type, also called TK1, represents the 95% of the serum TK. High levels of TK were found in the sera of patients with different tumors or associated to non-tumor related causes, such as virus infections (7). TPS is an immunoradiometric assay that ulilizes a monoclonal antibody specific for the M3 epitope of TPA. TPA is made during late S and G2 phase of the cell cycle and released during and immediately after mitosis (2). The levels of TPS are not correlated to the stage (size and distribution) of the tumor but measures the proliferation rate or growth activity (3).

To compare TLI, TK and TPS we measured the cell proliferation markers in the sera of patients with pathologically confirmed ovarian carcinoma on which TLI was previously evaluated.

Patients and methods

We measured TLI, TK, TPS and CA 125 in 35 women with ovarian carcinoma, 25 of them at initial surgery and ten at relapse.

TLI

Cell kinetics, considered as the percentage of thymidine-labeled cells in DNA synthesis over all the tumor population, were evaluated on tumor samples obtained at the time of staging laparotomy and/or on ascitic fluid samples using the tritiated thymidine incorporation method (4). Single cell suspension was incubated at 37° C in 5% CO_2 for 30 minutes in RPMI-1640 with 10% fetal calf serum (FCS) and 10 µCi/ml of tritiated thymidine (^{3}HdThd) (specific activity 5 Ci/mmol/l, Amersham). The cells were washed in cold saline, cytocentrifuged onto acid-cleaned slides and fixed with methanol-acetic acid (3:1).

For autoradiographic study, the slides were dipped in Kodak NTB2 nuclear track emulsion (Eastern Kodack, Rochester, NY) and kept at 4° C for 24 hours. Labeling indices were blindly counted on at least 1000 tumoral cells by two researchers. We used as median TLI the 2% value.

TK, TPS and CA 125

We measured TK, TPS and CA 125 with commercially available kits: TK-REA kit (Prolifigen Sangtec, Sweden), TPS-IRMA kit (Beki Diagnostics, Sweden), CA-125 RIA (Abbott, USA).

The blood samples were collected synchronously with the tumor samples, centrifuged at 3000 rpm and stored at –80° C until tested.

TK, TPS and CA 125 determinations were performed on sera in duplicate, using 6 U/l, 100 U/l and 35 U/ml respectively as cut-off values.

Statistical analysis

The statistical significance of the correlations between cell proliferation and tumoral markers and TLI were evaluated by likelihood ratio chi-square (P < 0.05).

Results

Table I shows the results obtained comparing TLI, TPS, TK and CA 125. A very high correlation (0.0067) was found between TLI and TK, whereas a negative relationship (0.16) was found between TLI and TPS.

The correlation between TK and TPS was equally negative, even if near to the statistical significance (0.08). None correletation was found between the tumor marker CA 125 and the cell proliferation markers.

Table I. Correlation between TLI and cell proliferation markers and between CA 125 and cell proliferation markers.

	chi-Square	p-Value
TLI-TK	7.35	0.0067
TLI-TPS	1.89	0.17
TK-TPS	2.96	0.085
CA 125-TLI	0.39	0.052
CA 125-TK	0.004	0.95
CA 125-TPS	0.64	0.42

Discussion

Few studies have investigated the possible role of TLI as prognostic variable in ovarian carcinoma and the results are sometimes controversial. *Sevin* and coworkers (14) for example found no correlation between pretreatment TLI value and survival, whereas other authors (15) reported that a high TLI has a negative influence on survival.

Conte et al. (4) demonstrated that 1. a high TLI loses its prognostic significance following aggressive first line chemotherapeutic treatment, 2. TLI is a significant prognostic factor for survival in chemotherapeutic resistant ovarian carcinoma, since these tumors are not longer affected by second line treatments.

These are the TLI clinical applications so far studied in the ovarian carcinoma. However, a more stimulating and promising application of TLI could be seen in the modulation of cytokinetic therapy to evaluate the best time of cell recruitment. This clinical study has been until now only theoretical because the bone marrow depression during drug administration or because repetition of TLI measurements is often impossible. This project now seems to be more feasible with the availability of the granulocites-colony stimulating factor (G-CSF). Furthermore, the possibility to use serum cell proliferation markers, alternatively to TLI, could reinforce the expectations from this clinical study.

Our preliminary results seem to confirm this hypothesis. In particular TLI seems to be better correlated with TK than TPS, but none conclusion can be done considering the low number of clinical cases. We did not find any relationship between cell proliferation markers and CA 125, that is a tumor mass marker.

Additional data on larger series are needed before a routinely use of these markers in alternative to TLI might be considered.

References

1. Alama A, Merlo F, Chiara S et al (1992) Prediction of survival by thymidine labeling index in patients with resistant ovarian carcinoma. Eur J Cancer 28A: 1079-1080
2. Björklund B (1992) Tumor markers TPA,TPA-S and cytokeratins. A working hypothesis. Tumor Diagn Ther 13:78-80
3. Björklund B (1980) On the nature and clinical use of tissue polypeptide antigen (TPA). Tumor Diagnostik I:9-20
4. Conte PF, Alama A, Rubagotti A et al (1989) Relationship to clinicopathologic features, responsiveness to chemotherapy and survival. Cancer 64: 1188-1191
5. Costa A, Bonadonna G, Villa E, Valagussa P, Silvestrini R (1981) Labeling index as a prognostic marker in non Hodgkin lymphomas. J Natl Cancer Inst 66:1-5
6. Gentili C, Sanfilippo O, Silvestrini R (1981) Cell proliferation and its relationship to clinical features and relapse in breast cancer. Cancer 48:974-979
7. Gronowitz JS, Kallander CFR, Diderholm H, Hagberg H, Petterson U (1984) Application of an in vitro assay for serum thymidine kinase: results on viral disease and malignancies in humans. Int J Cancer 33:5-12
8. Hiddemann W, Buchner T, Andreeff M, Wormann B, Melamed MR, Clarckson BD (1982) Cell kinetics in acute leukemia. Cancer 50:250-258
9. Kit S, Leung WC, Jorgensen GN, Trikula D, Dubbs DR (1973) Viral-induced thymidine kinase isozymes. Prog Med Virol 21:13-34
10. Livingstonn RB, Ambus U, George SL, Freireich EJ, Hakt JS (1974) In vitro determination of thymidine 3H labeling index in human solid tumors. Cancer Res 34:1376-1380
11. Meyer JS (1982) Cell kinetic measurements of human tumors. Human Pathol 13:874-877
12. Meyer JS, Friedman E, McCrate MM, Bauer WC (1983) Prediction of early course of breast carcinoma by thymidine labeling. Cancer 51:1879-1886
13. Reichard P, Estborn B (1951) Utilization of deoxyribosides in the synthesis of polyynucleotides. J Biol Chem 188:839-846.
14. Sevin BU, Ramon R, Averette E (1983) The potential use of cell kinetics in the treatment of ovarian malignancy. In: Grundmann E (ed) Cancer Compaign: Carcinoma of the ovary. Vol 7, Springer, New York pp 23-38
15. Silvestrini R, Daidone MG, Bolis G et al (1989) Cell kinetics: a prognostic marker in epithelial ovarian cancer. Gynecol Oncol 35:15-19
16. Tubiana M, Pejovic MH, Contesso G, Malaise EP (1984) The long term prognostic significance of the thymidine labeling index in breast cancer. Int J Cancer 33:441-445

Address for correspondence:
Dr. Michela Paganuzzi
Laboratorio di Patologia Clinica
Istituto Nationale per la Recerca sul Cancro
Viale Benedetto XV, n. 10
I-16132 Genova, Italia

Epithelial percentage in breast cancer sections obtained by true color image analysis – Correction factor for quantitative data on cytosolic tumor extracts?

F. Willemse[a], M. Nap[b], J. A. Foekens[c], S.C. Henzen-Logmans[d]

[a]Department of Pathology, University Hospital Groningen, [b]Department of Pathology, Laboratory for Public Health, Leeuwarden, [c]Division of Endocrine Oncology, [d]Department of Pathology, Dr. Daniël den Hoed Cancer Center, Rotterdam, The Netherlands

Introduction

Image analysis systems (IAS) may be used for quantification of oncogene products stained by routine immunohistochemistry. With this method it is possible to evaluate factors as errors of sampling and heterogeneity in staining (3, 5). Nevertheless when compared with results of immunochemical assays on cytosolic extracts there remains a considerable amount of discordance in agreement (1). This may be a consequence of field selection when IAS quantification of immunohistochemistry is concerned, which makes this method less reliable. Another reason for the discordance may be the fact that in immunochemical assays the epithelial percentage (EP%) of a tumor is not taken into account (2, 7, 10, 11). Consequently tumors with low cellularity containing cells with a high concentration of the cell constituent of interest or, vice versa, highly cellular tumors containing cells with a low concentration might be incorrectly classified as negative or positive respectively. As *van Netten* et al. suggested more than ten years ago, EP% of a carcinoma may be used as correction factor for data obtained by immunochemical assays to overcome this problem (11). At that time this quantification was performed subjectively by visual estimation. One may wonder if it would be more appropriate to use the knowledge obtained by image analysis quantification of immunohistochemistry in such a way that a parameter is quantified which is less susceptible to effects of field selection, avoids duplicature of expensive immunotechniques and may provide additional information for data of immunochemical assays.

In this study we evaluated a relatively simple and low-cost method to quantify the EP% in breast cancer sections by using true color image analysis. This percentage was evaluated as possible correction factor for cytosolic data on tumor extracts.

Material and methods

We used a set of 49 formalin-fixed, paraffin-embedded breast carcinoma samples of 49 patients. For quantification of the EP% in the tissue samples we used an inexpensive connective tissue stain, known as Heidenhain's Azan, in which collagen stains blue, chromatin, muscle tissue and erythrocytes red (9). In the breast carcinoma samples the epithelial parts stained red and the stromal parts, containing merely collagen, blue. Parts containing fat tissue remained unstained. For quantification of the EP% image analysis was performed using the Vidas IAS. The hardware of this system consists of an Axioplan microscope with halogen illuminator (Carl Zeiss, Oberkochen, Germany) fed by a stabilized power source, a low cost, single chip charge coupled device (CCD) color camera (WV-CD130, Panasonic, Matshushita Communication Co. Ltd., Yokohama, Japan), and a personal computer based on a 286 AT processor equipped with a frame grabber and expanded with a 287 mathematic co-processor (Kontron Elektronik, Eching, Germany). The software used for quantification is VIDAS 2.0, capable of processing true color images, which are formed by a red, green and blue (RGB) image partition respectively. The quantification procedure of the

EP% was designed in a similar way as one for quantification of immunohistochemical staining, described previously (14, 15).

In brief, in the quantification procedure the epithelial (red staining) and stromal (respectively blue and white staining) area percentages (Area%s) were quantified by application of three sets of predefined, fixed threshold levels. Quantification was performed in maximal ten image fields per specimen. Using an objective with a magnification of 2.5x, this corresponded to a total measured surface of 47.5 mm^2 on specimen level. If the mean sum of the EP% and the stromal Area%s did not exceed 100% ± 10% the measurement of an image field was accepted. As a control for the IAS method, interactive morphometry (IM) was performed on 15 specimens by point counting. This was done by placing a grid over the imagefield and by, subsequently, counting points overlying epithelial parts manually.

The IM EP% was obtained by multiplication of the ratio of counted points and total points by hundred. To evaluate reproducibility, which may be especially influenced by field selection, the image processing procedure was applied a second time for ten breast carcinoma samples in which the surface of the tumor exceeded 47.5 mm^2.

To evaluate the possible effect of the EP% as correction factor for results of an immunochemical assay we used data on pS2, an estrogen regulated protein (13). These data were obtained with a radiometric immunoassay (ELSA-pS2, CIS-Bio International, Gif-sur-Yvette, France) and were from those reported before (4). In the assay the monoclonal antibody BC4 anti-pS2 was coated on the solid phase. The initial ELSA-pS2 values were corrected according to the equation: corrected pS2 = (100/EP%) · pS2.

Results

The EP%s obtained by the true color IAS ranged from 18.42% to 85.56% (mean = 53.87%; standard deviation = 14.47%). Evaluation of the IAS procedure by IM, performed on fifteen specimens showed a high correlation coefficient: r = 0.94, p < 0.001 (figure 1). Moreover, there appeared to be no significant systematic differences between both methods (Friedman test; p = 0.8). Evaluation of reproducibility, which was performed by repeating the IAS quantification on ten of the breast carcinoma samples in which the surface of the tumor exceeded 47.5 mm^2, also showed a high correlation coefficient: r = 0.91, p < 0.001 (figure 2.). There were no significant systematic differences between the two successive quantifications (Friedman test; p = 0.2). Evaluation of the effect of the EP% as correction factor for data of an immunochemical assay is shown in figure 3. The x-axis displays the EP%s obtained by true color image analysis. On the y-axis the data of the ELSA-pS2 are displayed on a logarithmic scale. The open squares represent

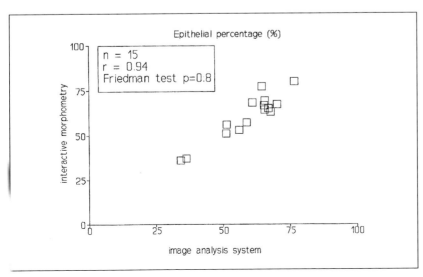

Figure 1. Comparison of results of quantification of EP% in Azan stained breast carcinoma samples obtained by true color image analysis (x-axis) and interactive morphometry (y-axis).

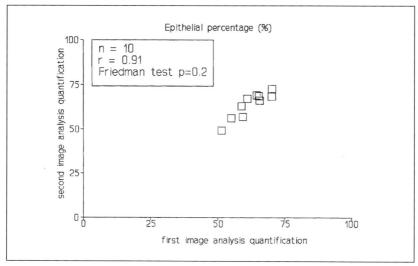

Figure 2. Evaluation of reproducibility of IAS quantification. First (x-axis) and second (y-axis) quantification of EP% in Azan stained breast carcinoma samples.

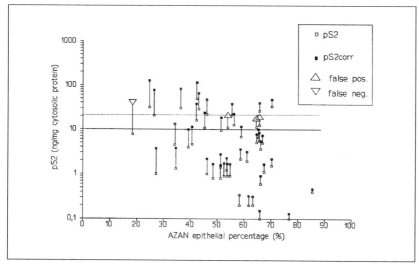

Figure 3. Evaluation of the effect of EP% (x-axis) as correction factor for data on cytosolic tumor extracts obtained by ELSA-pS2 (y-axis). See text for explanation.

the initial pS2 values, whereas the closed squares and the triangles represent the corrected values. To visualize where they position after correction, the initial and corrected values were connected by a line. According to the above mentioned equation the smaller the EP% the larger the effect of correction. When comparing the initial values to a hypothetical cut-off line, placed at 10 ng/mg cytosolic protein (solid horizontal line), a distinction in negative and positive may be made. However, when comparing the corrected pS2 values to a corrected cut-off line (dashed horizontal line), which was obtained by multiplica- tion of the initial cut-off value by 2.1, the mean correction factor overall, one tumor changes from negative to positive (triangle point down), whereas three change from positive to negative (triangles point up).

Discussion

When comparing quantitative data of immuno-histochemical staining obtained by image analysis with those of a immunochemical assay on cytosolic tumor extraxts there remains a considerable amount of discordance in agreement (1). This may be due to a relatively small area used for IAS quantification in tissue sections of notoriously heterogeneous tumors, which may introduce effects of field selection (3, 5, 10). But also the fact that in immunochemical assays the cellularity of a tumor is not taken into account may play a role (2, 7, 10, 11). Based on this we developed a method to quantify the EP% in breast carcinoma samples and evaluated this percentage as possible correction factor for data on cytosolic tumor extracts. A prerequisite for this approach is that the cell constituent of interest is exclusively present within tumor cells. For the IAS quantification of EP% we used a true color IAS, with which it is possible, although with some restrictions, to reproduce colors from (immuno-) histological sections and to separate and quantify structures based on color information (6, 8, 12). We used an inexpensive, routine connective tissue stain (Heidenhain's Azan) which provides contrasting colors (9) and allows to separate epithelial and stromal parts in breast carcinoma samples. The advantage of using a stain providing such contrasting colors is that a relatively low magnification may be used. As a consequence, within an acceptable period of time, quantification may be performed in a large area of tumor, thus making the measurement procedure less susceptible to effects of field selection.

In our method we used an objective with a magnification of 2.5x and quantified a maximum of ten image fields per specimen, resulting in a total measured area of 47.5 mm^2 maximally on specimen level. The results provided by this method proved to be reliable: Comparison with results obtained by IM, which may be considered as "gold standard", showed a high correlation coefficient ($r = 0.94$; $p < 0.001$) and analysis of variance did not show significant systematic differences (Friedman test; $p = 0.8$). The IAS quantification also proved to be reproducible: Repeating the quantification on ten specimens with tumors larger than 47.5 mm^2 showed a correlation coefficient of 0.91 ($p < 0.001$). Moreover, there were no significant systematic differences (Friedman test; $p = 0.2$) or in other words – the method lacks effects of field selection. It must be noted that, especially concerning possible effects of field selection, it is important to perform additional statistical tests such as the Friedman test; high correlation coefficients alone do not rule out the possibility of systematic differences.

The effect of EP% as correction factor in our population was restricted to a total of four cases which changed category. However, as stated before, this evaluation was hypothetical and merely meant to visualize possible effects. The extent to which this correction factor may influence patient selection for therapy in the clinic remains to be determined.

We conclude that quantification of EP% by using a true color IAS on breast carcinoma samples stained by a relatively inexpensive connective tissue stain can be performed reliably and reproducibly. Furthermore, this study shows that it is possibile to use this relatively low cost method to obtain additive information for the interpretation of data from cytosols. This may be important for the individual patient who is otherwise incorrectly considered negative or positive for a specific cell constituent and makes both methods in combination more valuable than when used separately.

References

1 Allred DC (1993) Should immunohistochemical examination replace biochemical hormone receptor assays in breast cancer? Am J Clin Pathol 99:1–3
2 Colley M, Kommoss F, Bibbo M, Dytch HE, Franklin WA, Holt JA, Wied GL (1989) Assessment of hormone receptors in breast carcinoma by immunocytochemistry and image analysis. II Estrogen receptors. Analyt Quant Cytol Histol 11:307–314
3 Esteban JM, Battifora H, Warsi Z, Bailey A, Bacus S (1991) Quantification of estrogen receptors on paraffin embedded tumors by image analysis. Mod Pathol 4:53–57
4 Foekens JA, Rio MC, Seguin P, Putten WLJ, Fauque J, Nap M (1990) Prediction of relapse and survival in breast cancer patients by pS2 protein status. Cancer Res 50:3832–3837
5 Helin HJ, Helle MJ, Kallioniemi OP, Isola JJ (1989) Immunohistochemical determination of estrogen and progesterone receptors in human breast carcinoma. Correlation with histopathology and DNA flow cytometry. Cancer 63:1761–1767
6 Julis I, Mikes J (1992) True colour image analysis and histopathology. Eur Micr Anal 7:11–13
7 Parham DM, Baker PR, Robertson AJ, Vasishta A, Baker PG, Smith G (1989) Breast carcinoma

cellularity and its relation to oestrogen receptor. J Clin Pathol 42:1166–1168
8 Ramm P (1990) Image analyzers for bioscience applications. Comp Med Im Graph 14:287–306
9 Romeis B, Denk H, Künzle H, Plenk H, Rüschoff J, Sellner W (1989) Mikroskopische Technik. Urban & Schwarzenberg, München, Wien, Baltimore
10 Underwood JCE, Dangerfield VJM, Parsons MA (1983) Estrogen receptor assay of cryostat sections of human breast carcinomas with simultaneous quantitative histology. J Clin Pathol 36:399–405
11 van Netten JP, Algard FT, Coy P, Carlyle SJ, Brigden ML, Thornton KR, To MP (1982) Estrogen receptor assay on breast cancer microsamples. Implications of percent carcinoma estimation. Cancer 49:2383–2388
12 Wells WA, Rainer RO, Memoli VA (1993) Equipment, standardization and applications of image processing. Am J Clin Pathol 99:48–56
13 Westley B, Rochefort H (1979) Estradiol induced proteins in the MCF 7 human breast cancer cell line. Biochem Biophys Res Commun 90:410–416
14 Willemse F, Nap M, de Kok LB, Eggink HF (1993) Image analysis in immunohistochemistry: Factors with possible influence on the performance of VIDAS 2.0, a commercially available true color image analysis system. Analyt Quant Cytol Histol 15:136–143
15 Willemse F, Nap M, Henzen–Logmans SC, Eggink HF (1994) Quantification of area percentage of (immunohistochmical) staining by true color image analysis with application of fixed thresholds. Analyt Quant Cytol Histol, in press

Address for correspondence:
F. Willemse
Department of Pathology
University Hospital Groningen
PO Box 30001
NL-9700 RB Groningen, The Netherlands

Prognostic significance of elevated levels of urokinase in breast cancer cytosols – A novel quantitative luminometric assay applicable on steroid receptor cytosols

M. Fernö[a], Å. Borg[a], D. Killander[a], L. Hischberg[b], J. Brundell[b]

[a]Department of Oncology, University Hospital, Lund, [b]AB Sangtec Medical, Bromma, Sweden

Introduction

The identification of breast cancer patients at high risk of relapse is currently one of the most important issues in breast cancer research. Hitherto, histopathological variables including lymph node involvement, tumor size and morphological pattern, and biological variables such as steroid receptor status and DNA content in individual breast cancer cells have shown to be useful for prognostic purposes in the clinical management of breast cancer. However, we still need better prognostic instruments than those used today. Oncogenes, tumor suppressor genes, proteases and plasminogen activators have also shown to provide prognostic information. Their role in the clinical managment of breast cancer needs further studies. Plasminogen activators includes enzymes such as urokinase plasminogen activator (uPA), which degrade the extracellular matrix, and are reported to play significant roles in tumor invasion and in the development of distant metastasis (1). The uPA participates in this degradation by activating plasminogen to plasmin. Its prognostic importance in breast cancer has been demonstrated previously in some studies (2-4).

The aim of the present study was to investigate the prognostic importance of uPA with a new luminometric immunoassay, applicable in cytosol samples routinely used for steroid receptor determinations.

Material and methods

Patients

The series comprised 400 breast cancer samples, 250 from postmenopausal and 150 from premenopausal patients. Information about tumor size was available in all cases: 153 (38%) < 20 mm; 247 (62%) > 20 mm. Histopathological axillary node status was known for 398 patients; 157 (39%) were node negative, 241 (61%) were node positive. With a median follow-up time of 50 months 314 (75%) had no sign of recurrences, while 86 (21%) had developed recurrences.

Local treatment was given in accordance with guidelines adopted by the South Sweden Breast Cancer Group. Surgery consisted either of modified radical mastectomy with axillary dissection, or of conservative segmental resection with axillary dissection in some patients with tumors less than 20 mm in diameter, combined with postoperative radiation of the remaining breast tissue. In general, patients with metastasis to the axillary lymph nodes received postoperative radiation.

Analysis of uPA

A newly developed quantitative luminometric assay (LIA), a sandwich type immuno assay, has been used to measure uPA content in cytosol samples, stored at −80 °C after routine ER and PgR determination as outlined in the following. Briefly, 100 µl sample is added to a tube coated with monoclonal antibodies to uPA. The detection reagent (200 µl of monoclonal antiodies labeled with isoluminol derivate) is also added to the tube which then is incubated for two hours at room temperature under moderate shaking. The tube is washed three times with 2 ml 0.9% NaCl and read in a luminometer. The assay detects uPA in the proenzyme form, the active two-chain form, uPA bound to its receptor and also uPA bound to the inhibitor PAI-I. The detection limit is about 5 pg uPA/ml sample, and the range of detection is up to 40 ng/ml. The concentrations of uPA was expressed as ng uPA per mg cytosol protein, and the protein concentration of the sample were 1–2 mg/ml.

Table I. Correlations between urokinase plasminogen activator (uPA) and other prognostic factors in breast cancer. Cut-off value: 0.80 ng uPA/mg cytosol protein.

Factor	n	uPA+	(%)	p-Value
All	400	86	22	
Age				
< 50 years	150	40	27	
≥ 50	250	46	18	0.051
Tumor size				
≤ 2cm	153	29	19	
> 2 cm	247	57	23	0.33
Lymph node status				
negative	157	38	24	
1–3 positive	148	26	18	
4+ positive	93	22	24	0.32
Estrogen receptor				
< 10 fmol	134	46	34	
10–200	210	37	18	
≥ 2200	56	3	5.4	< 0.00001
Progesterone receptor				
< 10 fmol	171	49	29	
10–200	171	30	18	
≥ 2200	58	7	12	0.0073
Cathepsin D				
< 50 pmol	85	13	15	
≥ 250	121	29	24	0.13
p53				
< 0.2 ng	184	27	15	
≥ 20.2	26	13	50	0.00002
DNA ploidy				
diploid	98	10	10	
non-diploid	189	54	29	0.0003
S-phase fraction				
< 7%	101	6	5.9	
7-12	58	15	26	
≥ 212	107	39	36	< 0.00001
erbB-2				
single copy	100	16	16	
amplified	27	7	26	0.42

Results and discussion

With a cut-off value of 0.80 ng uPA/mg protein, 86 samples (22%) of totally 400 were classified as high uPA tumors and 314 (78%) as low uPA tumors. Tumors with a high uPA content manifested with chi-squared analysis a positive correlation with high S-phase fraction and DNA-non-diploidy (flow cytometric DNA analysis), high p53 expression, and a negative correlation with estrogen and progesterone receptor status (table I).

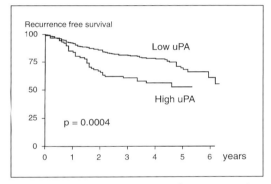

Figure 1. The prognostic importance for recurrence free survival of tumor urokinase plasminogen activator content (µPA, low versus high).

No statistically significant correlation was found between uPA (low versus high content) and lymph node status, tumor size, patient age, cathepsin D and erbB-2 amplification.

The level of uPA (low versus high) was found to correlate strongly to short recurrence free survival (log-rank test; p = 0.004) (figure 1), and short overall survival (p < 0.0001). The recurrence rate was 25% in the low uPA subgroup and 43% in the high uPA subgroup. The multivariate analysis (Cox's proportional hazards model with stepwise covariate selection) showed uPA to be an independent prognostic factor (together with lymph node status, tumor size and progesterone receptor status) for both shorter recurrence free survival (table II) and shorter overall survival.

Summarizing, the prognostic value of tumor associated proteases has been demonstrated by an increasing number of reports (5). Our results support the findings that high levels of uPA in breast cancer cytosols correlate strongly to both recurrence free survival and overall survival. The new luminometric assay (LIA) is a single step and easy to use method, and is well suited for routine measurement of uPA in cytosols. To further evaluate the prognostic value in subgroups of patients, the study group needs to be increased with a few hundred of cases.

Table II. Recurrence free survival, according to univariate and multivariate analysis (Cox's proportional hazards model) of prognostic covariates (n = 398).

Covariate	Univariate	Multivariate		
	p-value	p-value	RR[1]	95% confidence interval
Axillary lymph nodes 0, 1–3, 4+	< 0.0001	< 0.0001	2.0	1.6–2.5
Tumor size ≤ 20 mm versus > 20mm	0.0015	0.0034	1.8	1.2–2.8
PgR status negative versus positive	0.0005	0.011	1.6	1.1–2.4
ER status negative versus positive	0.0115	n.s.		
uPA low versus high	0.0010	0.0025	1.9	1.3–2.9
Menopausal status pre- versus post-menopausal	n.s.	n.s.		

[1]RR = relative risk

References

1. Schmitt M, Jänicke F, Graeff H (1992) Tumor associated proteases. Fibrinolysis 6 suppl 4:3–26
2. Foekens JA, Schmitt M, van Putten WLJ, Peters HA, Bontenbal M, Jänicke F, Klijn JGM (1992) Prognostic value of urokinase-type plasminogen activator in 671 primary breast cancer patients. Cancer Res 52:6101–6105
3. Gröndahl-Hansen J, Christensen IJ, Rosenquist C, Brunner N, Mouridsen HT, Danö K, Blichert-Toft M (1993) High levels of urokinase plasminogen activator and its inhibitor PAI-I in cytosolic extracts of breast carcinomas are associated with poor prognosis. Cancer Res 53:1–9
4. Jänicke F, Schmitt M, Pache L, Ulm K, Harbeck N, Höfler H, Graeff H (1993) Urokinase (uPA) and its inhibitor PAI-I are strong and independent prognostic factors in node-negative breast cancer. Breast Cancer Res Treatm 24:195–208
5. Graeff H, Harbeck N, Pache L, Wilhelm O, Jänicke F, Schmitt M (1992) Prognostic impact and clinical relevance of tumors-associated proteases in breast cancer. Fibrinolysis 6 suppl 4:45-53

Address for correspondence:
M. Fernö, M. D.
Department of Oncology
University Hospital
S-22185 Lund, Sweden

OKT9 as a tumor marker in endometrial and uterine cervical carcinoma

A. Abdel Salam[a], A. Mangoud[b], M. Ramadan[b], A. Khalifa[c], O. El-Ahmady[d]

[a] Department of Obstetrics and Gynecology, [b] Department of Pathology and the Oncology Unit, Zagazig, [c] Ain Shams and [d] El-Azhar Universities, Cairo, Egypt

Introduction

In the past, malignant neoplasms were distinguished from normal tissue mainly by the application of the classical morphological criteria observed with the light microscope. In the last decade immunohistological analysis of biopsy materials using monoclonal or polyclonal antibodies has gained the status of a routine diagnostic procedure (5, 6). Some of these antibodies react with neoplastic tissues but do not react with normal tissues so that they can be used as tumor markers in histological sections (10).

Various antibodies have been applied to uterine cervical tissue, for example antibodies to alpha fetoprotein, human chorionic gonadotrophin, MCG HLA, ABC, CEA (carcinoembryonic antigen), Ca 1 antigen, HMFG 1 and 2 antigen and the monoclonal antibody OKT9. Of these only OKT9 appeared of value in distinguishing between normal and abnormal cervical tissues (5, 9, 11). These results encouraged us to investigate the distribution of the monoclonal antibody OKT9 in human uterine cervix and endometrium using the immunoperoxidase technique.

Material and methods

Tissue samples: Specimens of tissue were obtained at surgery or biopsy from 117 women. Paraffin embedded blocks were prepared. The blocks were selected on hematoxylin and eosin stained, and were found to include 14 cases of invasive cervical carcinoma. 25 cases of cervical intra-epithelial neoplasia (CIN), nine cases of which were CIN I (mild dysplasia), eight cases were CIN II (moderate dysplasia) and eight cases were CIN III (severe dysplasia and/or carcinoma in situ), nine cases of endometrial carcinoma, 22 cases of endometrial cystic hyperplasia, seven cases of atypical hyperplasia.

Normal cervix (16 cases) and normal proliferative endometrium (24 cases) were also collected.

Immunoperoxidase staining: The immunoperoxidase procedure used in this work was based on that used by *McGee* et al. (10) and *Jha* et al. (5). The monoclonal antibody OKT9 was obtained from Ortho Diagnostic System Ltd. (OKT9 recognizes the transferrin receptor.)

Results

The results of immunoperoxidase staining of 55 cervical preparations with OKT9 are summarized in table I (figures 1–3). All malignant and CIN III lesions showed positive reactions. CIN II lesions showed positive reaction in most of cases (75%), while CIN I lesions and normal cervical epithelium showed positive reactions in 33.3% and 31.3%, respectively.

The 62 endometrial preparations studied showed similar results (table II), all cases of endometrial carcinoma and most cases of atypical hyperplasia (71.4%) showed positive reaction with OKT9. Cystic hyperplasia and normal proliferating endometrium showed positive reaction in 27.37 and 25%, respectivley.

This pattern of staining suggests positive correlation between the severity of cellular abnormality and the incidence of OKT9 positive reaction.

Immunohistochemistry

Table I. OKTA9 reaction in cervical epithelium.

Histological diagnosis	No. of cases	OKT9 reaction			
		positive		negative	
		no.	(%)	no.	(%)
Normal cervix	16	5	31.3	11	68.7
CIN I	9	3	33.3	6	66.7
CIN II	8	6	75	2	25
CIN III	8	8	100	–	–
Invasive carcinoma	14	14	100	–	–

Table II. OKT9 reaction in endometrial lesions.

Histological diagnosis	No. of cases	OKT9 reaction			
		positive		negative	
		no.	(%)	no.	(%)
Proliferative endometrium	24	6	25	18	75
Cystic endometrial hyperplasia	22	6	27.3	16	72.7
Atypical hyperplasia	7	5	71.4	2	28.6
Endometrial adenocarcinoma	9	9	100	–	–

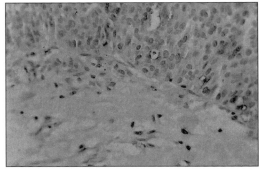

Figure 1. OKT9 positive reaction in cervical CIN I, PAP technique, X 60.

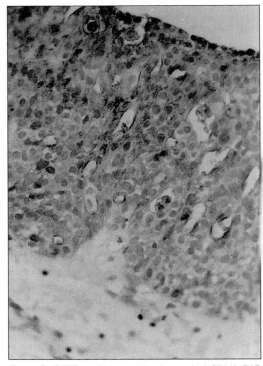

Figure 2. OKT9 positive reaction in cervical CIN II, PAP technique, X 600.

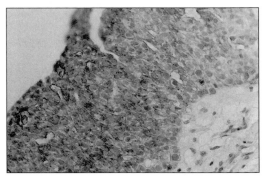

Figure 3. OKT9 positive reaction in cervical CIN III, PAP technique, X 600.

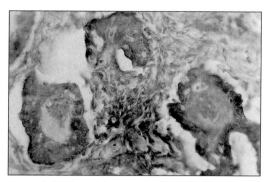

Figure 4. OKT9 positive reaction in cervical carcinoma, PAP technique, X 600.

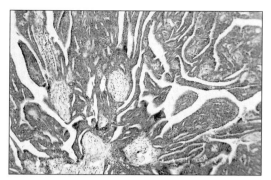

Figure 5. OKT9 positive reaction in endometrium carcinoma, PAP technique, X 600.

Discussion

The monoclonal antibody OKT9 raised against human leukemia cells recognises an epitope of the transferrin receptor (TFR) (1, 8). This receptor seems to have an essential role in the transport of iron across the cell membrane and has been detected on cells which have large iron requirements such as reticulocytes and placental syncytiotrophoblasts (4). In addition, this receptor has an association with cell proliferation and activation, and has been found in breast cancer (2, 3, 7, 17). The association of transferrin receptor (TFR) with cell proliferation and cancer encouraged us to investigate its distribution in human uterine cervix and endometrium using the monoclonal anti-TFR antibody (OKT9) in immunoperoxidase technique.

In our study, all cases of cervical and endometrial carcinoma showed positive reaction with OKT9. Cases of cervical intra-epithelial neoplasia (CIN) showed positive reaction which increased in intensity and incidence with the increase of the degree of aggressiveness of the lesion. The same findings were observed for endometrial hyperplasia where the incidence and intensity of the staining reaction increased in atypical compared with cystic hyperplasia.

This relation between OKT9 staining reaction and both neoplastic and preneoplastic changes was not reported with other antibodies. Staining with Ca 1 antibody showed positive reaction in 25 out of 27 normal cervical transformation zones (9). Similar results were obtained with a panel of monoclonal antibodies including HMFG I and 2, Ca 1, 8.30% and 77.1 (5), all of which failed to distinguish between benign and neoplastic conditions. On the other hand Lloyd et al. (8, 9) found widespread immunohistochemical staining with OKT9 in all sections of malignant epithelia and in most sections of severely dysplastic epithelium. Normal epithelium showed positive reaction in only 36% of the cases and this was mild and limited to basal layer. This positive reaction in normal epithelium was reported in our study in 31.2% and in 25% of normal cervical and endometrial tissue respectively. Gatter et al. (4) have reported positive staining with OKT9 in the basal layer of the cervix and epidermis. This positive OKT9 reaction in non-malignant condition suggests that OKT9 antibody is not a specific marker for malignancy. However, our results together with those of others may suggest a place for OKT9 as borderline of a screening method for cervical and endometrial carcinoma. More important, immunohistochemical staining for OKT9 can help in diagnosis of borderline cases and can be used as an objective diagnostic test where the diagnosis of malignancy or dysplasia is in doubt and subjective. Positive staining for OKT9 may indicate a more aggressive potentiality of the lesion and this may signify a role of this marker in prediction of malignancy in both cervical and endometrial CIN lesions.

Follow-up of cases of normal and CIN lesions with positive OKT9 staining is needed to verify its role in prediction of cellular behavior.

In conclusion, immunohistochemical staining for OKT9 appears to distinguish between normal and abnormal epithelium. It may have a role in diagnosing borderline lesions and in predicting the probability for malignancy in cervical and endometrial CIN lesions. Prolonged follow-up of cases of normal tissue and of CIN lesions with positive OKT9 reaction is needed to cofirm these findings.

References

1. Chitambar CR, Masscey E, Seligmann P (1983) Regulation of transferrin receptor expression on human leukemic cells during proliferation and induction of differentiation. J Clin Invest 72:1314
2. Falkenburg J, Koning F, Duinkerken N, Fibbe W, Voogt P, Jansen J (1986) Expression of CDII, CD 5 and TRF antigens on human hemopoetic progenitor cells. Exper Haematol 14:90–96
3. Paulk WP, Hsi BL, and Stevens BJ (1980) Transferrin and transferrin receptors in carcinoma of the hreast. Lancet 11:390–392
4. Gatter KC, Brown G, Trowbridg I, Woodston R, Mason DY (1983) Transferrin receptors in human tissues: Their distribution and possible clinical significance. J Clin Pathol 36:539
5. Jha RS, Wickensden C, Anderson MC, Coleman DV (1984) Monoclonal antihodies for histopathological diagnosis of cervical neoplasia. Br J Obstet Gynecol 91:483–488
6. Klavins J V (1983) Advances in hiological markers in cancer. Clin and Lab Sci 13:275–280
7. Kozlowski R, Reilly AG, Sowter D, Robins RA, Pussell NH (1988) Transferrin receptor expression on AML blasts is related to their proliferative potential. Br J Hematol 69:275-280
8. Lloyd JM, O'Dowd T, Driver M, Tee DEH (1984) Immunohistochemical detection of Ca antigen in normal, dysplastic and neoplastic squamous epithelia. J Clin Pathol, 37:14–19
9. Lloyd JM, O'Down T, Driver M, Tee DEH (1984) Demonstration of an epitope of the transferrin receptor in human cervical eptihelium: a potentially useful cell marker. J Clin Pathol, 37:131–135
10. McGee JOD, Woods JC, Ashall F, Bramwell ME, Harris HA (1982) New marker for human cancer cells, immunohistochemical detection of Ca antigen in human tissues with the Ca antibody. Lancet 11: 7–10
11. Omary MB, Trowbridge IS, Minowada J (1980) Human cell surface glycoprotein with unusual properties. Nature 216:888–891

Address for correspondence:
Prof. Dr. O. El-Ahmady
Tumor Marker Oncology Research Center
Al-Azhar University
2 Roshdy Street, Safeer Spuare
ET-Heliopolis, Cairo, Egypt

Epithelial antigens in normal ovary and ovarian mixed mesodermal tumors

A. Abdel Salam[a], A. Mangoud[b], M. Ramadan[b], A. Khalifa[c], O. El-Ahmady[d]

[a]Departments of Obstetrics and Gynecology, [b]Department of Pathology and the Oncology Unit, Zagazig, [c]Ain-Shams and [d]El-Azhar Universities, Cairo, Egypt

Introduction

Mixed mesodermal tumor (MMT) of the ovary is a rare tumor which shows a characteristic histological appearance composed of carcinomatous and sarcomatous elements (2). Mixed mesodermal tumors are classified into homologous and heterologours types, depending on the characteristics of the mesenchymal elements. While the mesenchymal elements are composed of non-specific spindle shaped sarcomatous cells in the homologous type, sarcomatous cells show special differentiation such as cartilage, oestoid tissue and straited muscles in the heterologous tumors (10).

The histogenetic origin of such tumors has been discussed by several authors (1, 3–6), but no definite origin has been reached so far and it is unknown whether these tumors arise by intermingling of two originally independent tumors, one a carcinoma and the other a sarcoma, or if they result from the transformation of a single multipotent mesenchymal stem cell which gives rise to a clone of malignant cells some of which differentiate as epithelial and some as stromal cells (8).

Endometrium and ovary are unusual in that both their epithelial and stromal elements are derived from mesoderm and this may account for the tendency of mixed tumors with malignant epithelium and stroma to occur at these sites. It has recently been shown that immunohistochemical staining with the monoclonal antibodies E29 (anti-epithelial membrane antigen) and CAM 5.2 (anti-cytokeratin MW 39,000–50,000 daltons) effectively distinguishes epithelium (antigen positive) from stroma (antigen negative) in normal endometrium but not in endometrial mixed Mullerian tumors whose epithelium and stroma give abnormal reactions in some cases (9). This paper reports a similar study carried out on ovarian tissue. While the staining properties of the ovarian mixed mesodermal tumors were similar to those of the endometrium, selective staining of the various components of normal ovary did not allow a simple distinction between epithelium and stroma.

Material and methods

The study was carried out on formalin-fixed 5 μm paraffin sections from two groups of cases.

Normal ovary

These were obtained from the files of the Pathology Department at Zagazig University. 20 of the cases were aged between 18 and 50 years.

Malignant mixed mesodermal tumors of ovary

Unstained paraffin sections were obtained from colleagues in Sharkia Hospitals. There were eight cases with typical morphological changes of malignancy both in epithelial components and stromal spindle cells, but one was excluded because of diffuse CAM 5.2 staining attributed to fixation artifact. Special histological features of the remaining seven cases are shown in table I. In every case a section was stained with phosphotungstic acid hematoxylin to demonstrate striated muscle.

Table I. Staining of malignant mixed mesodermal tumors of ovary with E29 and CAM 5.2.

Case no.	Special histological features	Epithelial staining		Stromal staining	
		E29	CAM 5.2	E29	CAM 5.2
1	multinucleate stromal giant cells; areas of myxoid stroma	some++	–	+	–
2	areas of myxoid stroma very anaplastic areas	few++	few–	many++	–
3	areas of cartilage	++	++	–	–
4	areas of bone	–	+	–	(type 1 and 2) endothelium+
5	areas of straited muscles	++	++	plasma cells+	++ (near necrotic area)
6	small cell carcinoma	–	–	++ (near necrotic area)	
7	multinucleate stromal giant cells; areas of myxoid stroma; anaplatic epithelium	–	–	–	–

Immunohistochemical staining

Following removal of endogenous peroxidase with 0.5 percent H_2O_2 in ascending grade of methanol, an indirect immunoperoxidase technique was used. The primary antibodies were the mouse monoclonals E29 (anti-human milk fat globule membrane, Dako, EMA) (11) diluted 1/10 and CAM 5.2 (Becton Dickinson) diluted 1/10. The second layer was horse-radish peroxidase conjugated rabbit anti-mouse serum (Dako) (7) diluted 1/50; the primary antibody is omitted in negative control sections of each block. Diaminobenzidine dihydrochloride was used as chromogen and the sections were counterstained with hematoxylin.

Results

Normal ovary

The staining reactions obtained in normal ovary were as follows: When present, surface epithelium and the flat pregranulosa cells surrounding the oocytes of primitive follicles were consistently positive with CAM 5.2 (figure 1) and negative with E29. Granulosa cells gave a negative reaction with E29 but in some cases were positive or weakly positive with CAM 5.2. As a rule some lutein cells were weakly positive with both antibodies. Positive E29 staining of varying intensity was encountered in some stromal cells in most cases; it was often restricted to one site e.g. beneath the tunica albuginea or around a Graffian follicle. In 20 of the ovaries CAM 5.2 staining was observed beneath the tunica. Fibroblasts organizing the plugs within corpora lutea were often strongly positive with CAM 5.2. Groups of stromal cells reacting both with E29 and CAM 5.2 were never encountered. Inclusion cysts lined with flat or columnar-epithelium stained heavily with CAM 5.2 and in a few instances, with E29.

Malignant MMT

A summary of the results is shown in table I. In two cases most of the neoplastic epithelial cells stained with both antibodies; three tumors with poorly differentiated epithelium most or all of the epithelial cells did not react with either antibody. Of the remaining two tumors the epithelium of one reacted only with E29 and of the other only with CAM 5.2.
E29 staining of stromal cells was encountered in three cases and CAM 5.2 in two; one of these both antibodies gave a strong reaction restricted to strap-like and tadpole-shaped cells at the edge of necrotic areas. Case 5 contained CAM 5.2 stained cells which appeared to line vascular spaces; E29 positive plasma cells were also present in this specimen.

Figure 1. Normal ovary from a woman aged 30 years. Staining of surface epithelium and granulosa cells of early follicle. CAM 5.2 counterstained with hematoxylin, x 250.

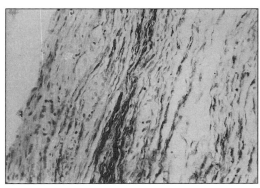

Figure 4. Normal ovary from a woman aged 30 years. Staining of spindle cells near ovarian surface. E29 counterstained with hematoxylin, x 100.

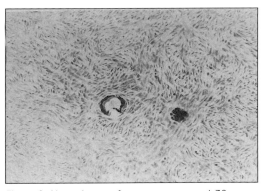

Figure 2. Normal ovary from a woman aged 30 years. Staining of pre-granulosa cells of primitive follicle. CAM 5.2 counterstained with hematoxylin, x 250.

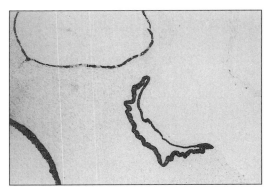

Figure 5. Normal ovary from a woman aged 30 years. Inclusion cyst lined with columnar epithelium. CAM 5.2 counterstained with hematoxylin, x 250.

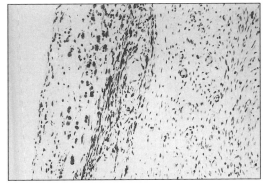

Figure 3. Normal ovary from a woman aged 35 years. Staining of lutein cells; the paraluteal cells are unstained. CAM 5.2 counterstained with hematoxylin, x 250.

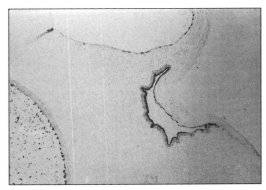

Figure 6. The same case as figure 5 stained with E29, counterstained with hematoxylin, x 250.

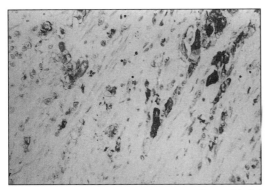

Figure 7. MMT of ovary (case 6, table I). The epithelial masses are stained as spindle cells in the hyaline stroma. CAM 5.2 counterstained with hematoxylin, x 250.

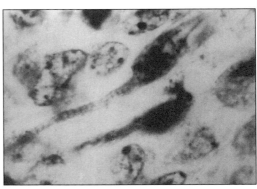

Figure 10. MMT of ovary (case 5, table I) showing areas of straited muscles (PTAH x 650).

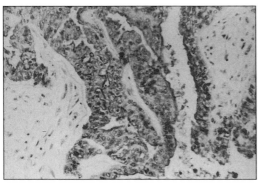

Figure 8. MMT of ovary (case 7, table I). Staining of luminal margin of neoplastic epithelium and spindle cells in myxoid stroma. E29 counterstained with hematoxylin, x 250.

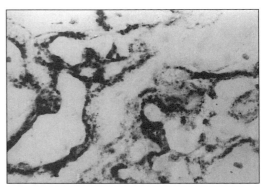

Figure 11. MMT of ovary (case 4, table I) showing E29 positive oestoid tissue. (E29 counterstained with hematoxylin x 250).

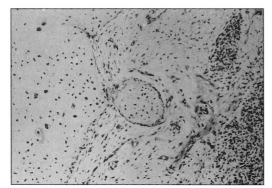

Figure 9. MMT of ovary (case 3, table I) showing areas of cartilage (H and E, x 250).

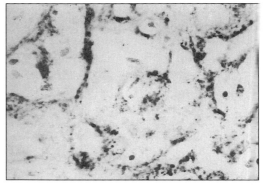

Figure 12. MMT of ovary (case 4, table I) showing CAM 5.2 positive oestoid tissue with few positively stained spindle stromal cells. (CAM 5.2 counterstained with hematoxylin, x 250).

Discussion

Unlike the epithelium of normal endometrium which is CAM 5.2 positive and for the most part E29 positive, the epithelial components of normal ovary (other than a minority of inclusion cysts and some weakly stained lutein cells) do not react with E29. The epithelial reactions of CAM 5.2 are complex and appear to be related to the developmental history of the Graffian follicle. The flattened pregranulosa cells surrounding the primary oocytes are strongly positive as is the surface epithelium from which they are thought to be derived. The change from pregranulosa to granulosa is marked by diminution or loss of CAM 5.2 staining, especially in atretic follicles. Cells of the functioning corpus luteum gave a weak reaction with CAM 5.2 which became negative, following the next menstrual period. It is of interest that most of so-called ("inclusion cysts") react strongly with CAM 5.2 but only the minority with E29. The latter are lined with columnar cells with morphological features of endometrial or tubal epithelium. The occurrence of some CAM 5.2 and E29 positive stromal cells in normal ovary contrasts with the absence of staining in normal endometrial stroma. A reaction with CAM 5.2 was most constantly observed in fibroblasts in the fibrous plugs of the corpus luteum, a finding suggesting antigen induction in responsive cells by a local environmental factor. Given the normal ovarian stroma may express E29 and CAM 5.2, it is not surprising that a similar phenomenon is seen in ovarian MMT. In a previous paper on mixed Mullerian tumors of endometrium two possible explanations were given for the finding of epithelial antigens in cells in the neoplastic stromal invasion by isolated epithelial tumor cells or commencing epithelial differentiation in mesenchymal epithelial precursor cells. A third possibility should now be added, while metaplasia of endometrial stroma to that of ovarian type, in which case mixed Mullerian tumors of endometrium containing stromal cells with epithelial markers would properly be classified as heterologous.

References

1. Cooper P (1978) Mixed mesodermal tumor and clear cell carcinoma arising in ovarian endometriosis. Cancer 42: 2827–2831
2. Czernobilsky B (1982) Primary epithelial tumors of the ovary. In: Blaustein A (ed) Pathology of the female genital tract. 2nd ed. Springer New York, pp 511–560
3. Decker JP, Hirsch NB, Garnet JD (1968) Mixed mesodermal (Mullerian) tumor of the ovary. Report of two cases. Cancer 12:920–932
4. Dehner LP, Norris HJ, Taylor HB (1971) Carcinosarcoma and mixed mesodermal tumor of the ovary. Cancer 27:207–216
5. Edghill AR, Gardiner J, Hayes JA (1967) Mixed mesodermal tumors of the ovary. Am J Obstet Gynecol 97:578–579
6. Fathala MF (1967) Primary mesodermal mixed tumors of the ovary. A report of two cases. J Obstet Gynecol Br Common Wealth 74:605–607
7. Makin CA, Bobrow LG, Bodmer WF (1984) Monoclonal antibody to cytokeratin for use in routine histopathology. J Clin Pathol 37:475–983
8. Norris HJ, Taylor HB (1966) Mesenchymal tumors of the uterus III. A clinical and pathologic study of 31 carcinosarcomas. Cancer 19:1459–1465
9. Ramadan M, Goudie RB (1986) Epithelial antigens in malignant mixed mullerian tumors of endometrium. J Pathol 148:13–18
10. Takeda A, Matsuyama M, Kuzuya K, Tsubonchi S, Takeuchi S (1984) Mixed mesodermal tumor of the ovary with carcinoembryonic antigen and alkaline phosphatase production. Cancer 53:103–112
11. Wells CA, Heryet A, Gatter KC, Mason DY (1984) The immunohistochemical detection of axillary micro-metastases in breast cancer. Br J Cancer 50:193–197

Address for correspondence:
Prof. Dr. O. El-Ahmady
Tumor Marker Oncology Research Center
Al Azhar University
2 Roshdy Street, Safeer Spuare
ET-Heliopolis, Cairo, Egypt

Immunohistochemistry in prostatic pathology – Diagnostic value of PSA, PSAP and high molecular weight cytokeratin

Evaluation of 650 fine needle biopsies

S. Ardoino[a], P. Durante[a], M.A. Ferro[a], F. Li Causi[a], C. Parodi[a], P. Puppo[b], G. Sanguineti[a], A. Vitali[a]

[a]Servizio di Anatomia Patologica, [b]Divisione di Urologia, Ospedale S. Corona, Pietra Ligure, Italia

Introduction

At present more and more suspicious cases of prostatic pathology have been discovered in the population by wide seric tumor marker screenings (PSA-PSAP).
Pathologists are required to make early and correct histological diagnosis on prostatic biopsies. The results are sometimes doubtful because the samples are very small and fragmented. Routine diagnostic immunohistochemical techniques can aid in revealing and confirming small, isolated cancer foci, expecially in fine needle biopsies.
Prostatic adenocarcinoma as normal prostatic luminar cells shows a similar immunohistochemical pattern: PSA, PSAP and low molecular weight cytokeratin are positive, while high m.w. cytokeratin is negative. Basal epithelial cells on the contrary show positivity for high m.w. cytokeratins.
Prostate-specific antigen (PSA) is a 33 kD glycoprotein produced only by the benign and malignant prostatic glandular epithelium cells. It has been identified as a kallicrein like serine protease.
Acid phosphatases are a heterogeneous group of enzymes present in a variety of normal and abnormal tissues. However, prostate-specific acid phosphatase (PSAP) has been isolated as a sialoglycoprotein with molecular weight of approximately 100 kD, distinct from non-prostatic acid phosphatase. It is produced by benign and malignant prostatic epithelial cells regulated by androgen.
High molecular weight cytokeratin (34betaE12) identifies a panel of cytokeratins of 56, 56.5, 58 and 68 kD. It is a pool of cytoskeleton proteins of epithelial cells expressed by the human stratum corneum. Cytokeratin 34beta E12 in particular marks basal cells in prostatic glands.

Material and methods

We tested n = 650 prostatic biopsies taken for diagnostic purposes from patients with clinical suspicion of cancer in our Urology Department in the years 1991–1993.
10% buffered formalin-fixed, paraffin-embedded samples were stained with hematoxylin-eosin and Van Gieson for histological examination.
Immunohistochemical studies were performed on the same cases using MoAb PSA (Dako, 1:20 dilution), rabbit PSAP (Ortho, 1:5 dilution), MoAb high m.w. cytokeratin 34betaE12 (Enzo, 1:100 dilution), over night incubation and stained with streptavidin-biotin-peroxidase method for monoclonal antibodies and PAP method for polyclonal antibodies. Sections stained with cytokeratin were pretreated with pronase.
We observed 168 cases of adenocarcinoma (ADK), one case of basal cell carcinoma (BCC) 399 cases of benign hyperplasia (BH), 16 cases of basal cell hyperplasia (BCH), 102 cases of displasia (D), 25 cases of atrophy (A), six cases of squamous metaplasia (SM) and 178 cases of prostatitis (P). Different lesions eventually present in the same biopsy were evaluated separately.
When possible we classified ADK according to Gleason grading. In every case we considered the tissue expression of PSA, PSAP and high molecular weight cytokeratin; in particular, with regard to PSA and PSAP we observed the positivity of the markers, the number of positive cells (percentage of all cells), the intensity and the distribution of staining. With regard to high molecular

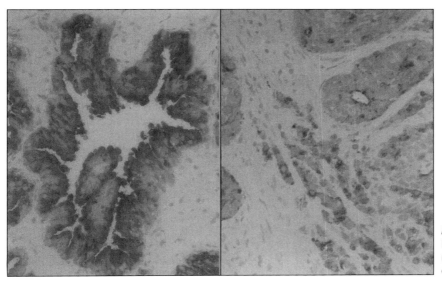

Figure 1. PSA: Benign hyperplasia (left) and adenocarcinoma (right).

weight cytokeratin we observed the positivity and the negativity of the marker and the distribution of staining (focal, discontinous or continuous). Every case was examined by two pathologists.

Results

We observed a positivity of PSA and PSAP in the luminal epithelial layer of almost all the lesions we examined. We found a variety of differences.
In the ADK and BH we noted a similar immunohistochemical pattern. In both lesions we found a high percentage of positive cells with moderate or intense staining. In particular we saw that 49% of ADK had more than 80% of PSA positive cells, 29% had a positivity between 50% and 80%, 21% had less than 50% of positive cells and only 1% of cases was negative. In cases of BH we observed that 69% had more than 80% of positive cells, 22% had a positivity between 50% and 80%, 8% had less than 50% of positive cells and only 1% of cases was negative. We found similar results with PSAP, however, this marker was generally expressed by higher number of cells showing a more intense staining than PSA. Both markers did not show any different expression between the various Gleason grading in ADK. The staining pattern was fairly homogenous in the same gland, independent of the kind of lesion. The stain distribution was cytoplasmatic.

In BH we observed a more uniform staining pattern, generally with apical predominance.
The cases of D and A, on the contrary, showed a lower expression of both markers. In particular we found that with PSA only 13% of D had more than 80% of positive cells, 8% had a positivity beween 50% and 80%, 32% had less than 50% of positive cells while 47% of cases were negative. We observed similar aspects in cases of A: only 3% of cases had more than 80% of positive cells, 2% had a positivity between 50% and 80%, 52% had less than 50% of positive cells and 43% of cases are negative.
Also in cases of D and A PSAP was expressed in a higher number of cells showing a more intense staining than PSA. Both these markers had no homogeneous pattern of staining in foci of D and A. The only case of BCC resulted negative. All cases of squamous metaplasia resulted completely negative with PSA and PSAP staining.
The pattern and the intensity of staining in different lesions is not modified by the presence of other in the same biopsy. Only in P, in particular in glands with a leucocytic infiltration we did not find any PSA and PSAP staining.
With regard to HMWC we observed that this marker resulted negative in all cases of ADK out of 2, which showed a discontinuous basal layer positivity in foci of in situ ADK. In 98% of all other lesions we found a positivity of this marker with different expression. In BH, SM and P we noted

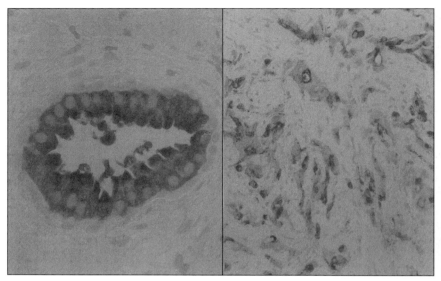

Figure 2. PSAP; Benign hyperplasia (left) and adenocarcinoma (right).

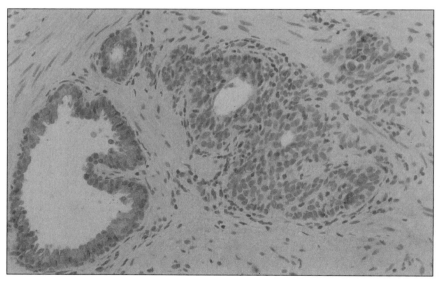

Figure 3. PSA negativity of epithelial cells in prostatitis with leukocytic infiltration.

that there was a general continuous staining of the basal layer of glands. In D and A the staining resulted continuous (40% of D cases and 50% of A cases) or focal (17% of D cases and 10% of A cases). In BBC and BCH we saw a strong staining of all cells.

Discussion

Prostatic fine needle biopsy is an important diagnostic instrument that together with PSA and PSAP serum value, ultrasound and digital rectal examination, permits a diagnosis of prostatic cancer, also in the initial phases.

However, the histological evaluation of these biopsies is often difficult because the samples are small, sometimes they are poor or fragmented and the diagnosis is based on evaluation of small and isolated foci. In these cases employment of IIC techniques with PSA, PSAP and HMWC can give additional very useful informations in differential diagnosis between neoplastic and non-neoplastic lesions.

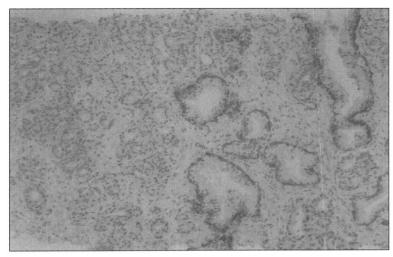

Figure 4. 34betaE12 negative in well differentiated adenocarcinoma; positivity of the marker in normal glands.

In particular PSA and PSAP cells positivity, besides confirming prostatic orign of the neoplasia, is useful in identifying very small foci of cancer, often constituted of single cells or lines of cells difficult to recognize or to distinguish from fibroblast and endothelial cells in prostatic fibrous tissue. The negativity of PSA or PSAP and the positivity of HMWC in a neoplastic infiltration can indicate a secondary prostatic neoplasia or can identify the cases of BCC.

Moreover, because it was only in ADK we observed the disappearance of basal layer of prostatic glands, the use of a basal marker, like HMWC, can help to distinguish basal cells from fibroblasts or from a double layer of cells in ADK, when conventional histochemical staining is not sufficient.

Therefore in the evaluation of suspicious foci the basal layer absence can indicate a correct diagnosis of ADK, while basal cell identification can help us to define dysplastic or atrophic glands. PSA and PSAP tissue expression in cases of D or A reduced with respect to normal, hyperplastic or neoplastic glands and the discrepancy between the elevated seric values and PSA and PSAP tissue lack in P are two further important fields to be explored.

References

1. Devaraj LT et al (1993) Atypical basal cell hyperplasia of the prostate. Am J Surg Pathol 17(7):645–659
2. Allsbrook WC et al (1993) Histochemistry of the prostate. Hum Pathol 23:297–305
3. Nagle RB et al (1991) Phenotypic relationships of prostatic intreaepithelial neoplasia to invasive prostatic carcinoma. Am J Pathol 138:119–128
4. Brawer MK (1991) Prostate specific antigen. Acta Oncologica 30(2):161–168
5. Gleason DF (1992) Histologic grading of prostate cancer. Hum Pathol 23:273–299
6. Mostofi FK et al (1992) Prostatic carcinoma. Hum Pathol 23:223–241
7. Brawer MK (1992) Prostatic inraepithelial neoplasia. Hum Pathol 23:242–248
8. Tomasino RM et al (1989) Ruolo dell' antigene prostatico specifico nel carcinoma prostatico. Pathologica 81:109–126
9. Di Sant'Agnese PA (1992) Neuroendocrine differentiaton in human prostatic carcinoma. Hum Pathol 23:287–296
10. Grignon DJ et al (1988) Basal cell hyperplasia, adenoid basal cell tumor, and adenoid cystic carcinoma of the prostate gland: an immunohistochemical study. Hum Pathol 19:1425–1433
11. Dhom G et al (1988) Histology and immunohistochemistry studies in prostate cancer. Am J Clin Oncol 11(Suppl 2):S37–S42
12. Hedrick L et al (1989) Use of keratin 903 as an adjunct in the diagnosis of prostate carcinoma. Am J Surg Pathol 13(5):389–396

Address for correspondence:
Dr. S. Ardoino
Servizio di Anatomia Patologica
Ospedale S. Corona
Via Aprile
I-Pietra Ligure, Italy

DNA cytophotometry of human bladder carcinomas – A comparative study of scanning cytophotometry and flow cytophotometry

S. Götze, J. Caselitz

Department of Pathology, General Hospital of Altona, Hamburg, Germany

Introduction

Human bladder cancer presents about 3% of malignant tumors of man. The ratio male/female is about 3:1 or 6:1 according to data of the literature. Out of a collective of 800 cases, 142 human bladder carcinomas were collected in the files of the Department of Pathology of the General Hospital of Altona during the years 1985–1990 (figure 1, age distribution). The aim of this study was the comparison of conventional grading, DNA measurement on the scanning level and DNA flow cytophotometry.

Methods

All theses 142 cases were graded by two independent investigators and were analysed by DNA cytophotometry, on the level of scanning cytophotometry and flow cytophotometry.
For scanning cytophotometry, slides with a thickness of 8 µ were stained by the Feulgen technique. Using the same paraffin block additional slides with a thickness of 20 µ to 40 µ were prepared for flow cytophotometry.
Flow cytophotometry was done according to the modified Hedley method. The material of the paraffin blocks was mechanically and enzymatically dispersed and the cell suspension was stained by Hoechst 33 258. The cells were measured by a conventional flow cytophotometer. Scanning cytophotometry was done as follows: The Feulgen reaction is a selective and quantitative reaction with the DNA of the nucleus. Using a computer system (Ahrens) 100 nuclei were measured concerning to their quantitative DNA content.

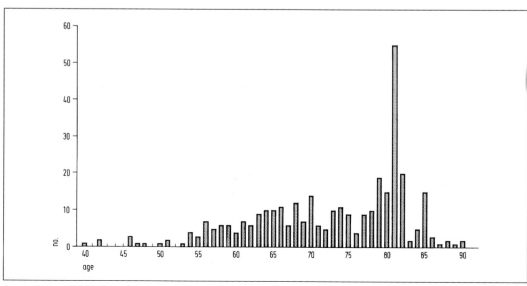

Figure 1. Age distribution of the patients.

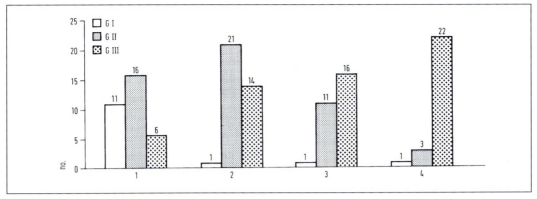

Figure 2. Data of scanning cytophotometry. The four Auer groups are presented together with the different grades of bladder carcinoma (n = 123).

The DNA content of cells reflects the cell cycle. The G1-phase is the postmitotic phase with a diploid content of chromosomes. The next phase, the S-phase, is characterized by a doubling of the chromosomal material. The content of chromosomal material is between diploid and tetraploid. The G2-phase is characterised by a tetraploid content of chromosomal material and is followed by mitosis. Tissue with proliferative activity displays an augmentation of the part between 2 c (diploid) and 4 c (tetraploid). If there is an augmentation of DNA beyond the 4 c level, this is generally regarded as "aneuploidy".

The DNA histograms in our material were classified in a modified manner according to the features of Stockholm group (Auer). The histograms were classified in to four groups.

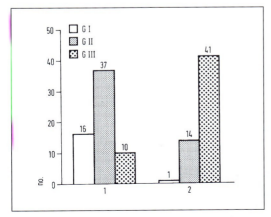

Figure 3. Flow cytophotometry of human bladder carcinomas (n = 142).

The histogram typing was compared to the grading to the tumors.

Results and discussion

Almost all grade 1 tumors had diploid histograms (Auer 1). Grade 2 tumors displayed histograms of type Auer 1 and 2 in 37 cases, whereas 14 grade 2 tumors showed histograms of type Auer 3 and 4. Most of the grade 3 tumors showed a histogram of type Auer 3 oder 4 (figure 1).

The results of flow cytophotometry were interpreted by two categories, diploid tumors and aneuploid tumors. Due to the artifact, a further analysis of these data was not possible. The date for flow cytophotometry correlated to those of scanning cytophotometry.

Summarizing, cytophotometry is a valuable tool for diagnostic interpretation of bladder carcinomas. Especially in grad II tumors of the human bladder, further informations are presented by cytophotometry, since parts of the tumors were diploid and parts were aneuploid. The biological behavior of aneuploid grade II tumors was similar to grade II tumors. In paraffin material scanning cytophotometry appears to give more relevant data than flow cytophotometry.

Address for correspondence:
Prof. Dr. med. Caselitz
Abteilung für Pathologie
Allgem. Krankenhaus Altona
Paul-Ehrlich-Straße 1
D-22763 Hamburg, Germany

Expression of CEA in normal and malignant tissues of Egyptian bladder cancer patients

O. El-Ahmady[a], A. G. El-Din[d], S. Eissa[b], T. Helal[c], I. Khalaf[d]

[a]Tumor Marker Oncology Research Center and [d]Urology Department, Faculty of Medicine, Al-Azhar University; Oncology Diagnostic Unit, [b]Biochemistry and [c]Pathology Departments, Faculty of Medicine, Ain Shams University, Cairo, Egypt

Introduction

Schistosomiasis is considered as one of the major public health problems in Egypt since about 21 millions rural inhabitants are at risk of acquiring the infestation. Bilharziasis is considered as one of the most predisposing factors for bladder cancer which is the most common malignant tumor among Egyptians. Patients usually present in an advanced stage; 25% were considered inoperable and 81% of the cases at operation were at advanced stages (1). CEA is the most widely used tumor marker in clinical medicine (2). CEA could be detected in normal, neoplastic and pre-neoplastic urothelium as well as tumor tissue. CEA was mainly localized on cell membrane, but with increasing tumor malignancy and infiltration a shift to cytoplasmic localized CEA was noted (3). The immunohistochemical expression of CEA in formalin-fixed paraffin sections in urinary bladder carcinomas (transitional and squamous cell carcinomas) indicated that both, TCC and SCC were positive for CEA and the degree of staining was markedly dependent on the grade of malignancy in TCC (4). Also, two cases of signet-ring cell adenocarcinoma of the urinary bladder were CEA positives (5). The expression of CEA in the tissues may reflect the prognosis and invasion stage (6, 7). Serum and urinary CEA can be used as a prognostic value since higher serum CEA levels were reported in bilharzial than in non-bilharzial bladder cancer patients (8). Also, serum CEA can be used for monitoring of the patients during chemotherapy and radiotherapy (9).

There are no findings in the literatures concerning the quantitative estimation of CEA in bladder cancer by the biochemical method. The aim of this work is to study the expression of CEA marker in both normal and malignant tissues of bladder cancer patients and its correlation with serum and 24 h urine levels of the same patients.

Material and methods

This study was done on 226 individuals. They were classified into three group: apparently healthy control group (n = 45), bilharzial patients group (n = 45) and bladder cancer patients group (n = 136).

Tissue samples from tumor and from normal tissue of the same bladder with safety margin at least 5 cm distant from the tumor were obtained directly at the operating theatre, chilled on ice, necrotic tissue and fat were dissected away, washed with cold saline, then frozen quickly and stored at −80° C in a deep freezer. Histopathological examination was done on a part of each tissue sample which was saved in 10% formaline solution. 24 h urine and blood samples were taken from the patients three days before radical cystectomy. Sera obtained by centrifugation of clotted blood samples and urine samples after centrifugation and adjusting of pH at 7.3 were stored at −20° C untill assayed.

Subcellular fractionations of cytosol and membrane

The tumor or normal tissue was weighed and finely chopped. The minced tissues were homogenized in 10 volumes of ice cold phosphate buffer. The tissue was homogenized for 10–15 sec at medium speed with 45–60 sec, elapsing between pulses. Ultracentrifugation was done for tissue homogenate at 800 g for 10 min at 4° C.

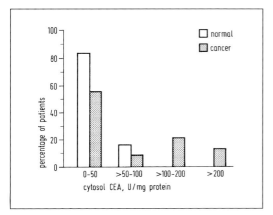

Figure 1. Frequency distribution of cytosol CEA values in normal and malignant bladder tissues.

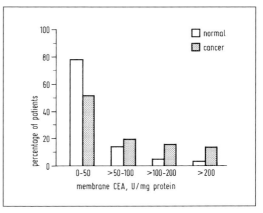

Figure 2. Frequency distribution of membrane CEA values in normal and malignant bladder tissues.

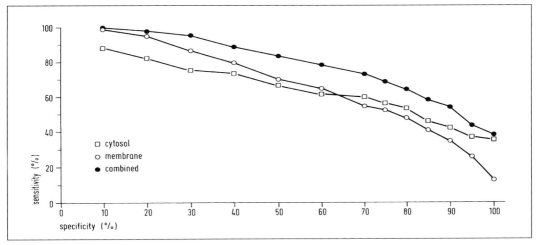

Figure 3. ROC curve for tissue CEA of bladder cancer patients.

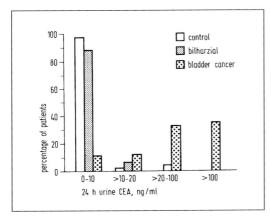

Figure 4. Frequency distribution of 24 h urine CEA values in normal, bilharzial and bladder cancer groups.

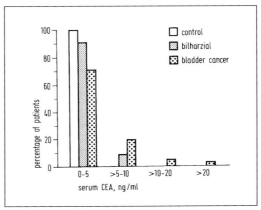

Figure 5. Frequency distribution of serum CEA values in normal, bilharzial and bladder cancer groups.

Table I. CEA ng/mg protein (M ± SE) in normal and malignant tissues of bladder cancer patients.

	Cytosol		Membrane	
	M ± SE	range	M ± SE	range
Normal bladder tissue	24.6 ± 1.9	2.6 – 93	33.5 ± 3.5	0 – 216
Malignant bladder tissue	82.8[a] ± 8.4	2 – 550	163.6[a] ± 36	0 – 3411

[a]Significant from normal tissue at $p < 0.01$

Table II. 24 h urine CEA (M ± SE) in control, bilharzial and bladder cancer patients.

Urine CEA	Control group	Bilharzial group	Bladder cancer group
M ± SE (ng/ml)	1.6 ± 0.36	3.77 ± 0.86	146.8[a] ± 19.5
Range	0.1 – 16	0 – 26	2.9 – 1627

[a]Significant from both normal and bilharzial groups at $p < 0.01$

Table III. Serum CEA (M ± SE) in control, bilharzial and bladder cancer patients.

Serum CEA	Control group	Bilharzial group	Bladder cancer group
M ± SE (ng/ml)	1.55 ± 0.16	2.4 ± .25	8.11[a] ± 2.8
Range	0 – 4.3	0 – 7.8	0 – 326

[a]Significant from both normal and bilharzial group at $p < 0.01$

The supernatant was separated and ultracentrifuged at 100,000 g for 30 min at 4° C. The supernatant contained cytosol fraction while the pellet represented the membrane fraction. The membrane pellet was resuspended by sonication in 1 ml phosphate buffer, then, ultracentrifugation for the membrane suspension was done at 100,000 g for 30 min. The supernatant containing membrane enriched fraction in addion to the cytosol fraction were divided into aliquotes which were stored at −80° C untill assayed.

Proteins were estimated using Bradford method (1976). Serum, 24 h urine, cytosol and membrane levels of CEA were determined using the reagents supplied by Roche Diagnostica, Basel, Switzerland (CEA EIA < Roche>).

Discussion

CEA is the most widely investigated and frequently used tumor marker in clinical oncology. A significant elevation was found in cytosol CEA of malignant tissue (82.8 ± 8.4 ng/mg protein) than that of normal tissue (24.6 ± 1.9 ng/mg protein).

Regarding membrane CEA, its expression in malignant tissue showed marked elevation (165.3 ± 36.1 ng/mg protein) compared to normal tissue (33.5 ± 3.5 ng/mg protein). The scattering distribution of CEA showed that about 35% of cytosol values of malignant tissue were above highest value in normal tissue. The results are in accordance with that of *Fujioka* et al. (6) who reported that about 25% of bladder cancer tumors had CEA positive tumor cells using immunohistochemical techniques. *Nap* et al. (11) reported that CEA is not present in normal tissue of the bladder using immunohistochemical techniques; this controversy with our results may be attributed to the higher sensitivity and accuracy of biochemical method in comparison with the semi-quantitative immunohistochemical method. When using the highest normal value as a cut-off, cytosol CEA sensitivity was 35.3% at 100% specificity which is in concordance with *Fujioka* et al. (6). On the other hand, membrane CEA of malignant tissue showed a lower sensitivity (12.5%) at 100% specificity. In relation to the histological type of bladder cancer, cytosol CEA showed highest sensitivity (44.1%) in squamous cell carcinoma followed by adenocarcinoma (28.6%), then transitional cell carcinoma (20.5%). *Asamoto* et al. (4) found no difference in CEA expression in Sq.C.C. or T.C.C. using immunohistochemical techniques. On the other hand, membrane CEA sensitivity increased with advancement of disease (P2 = 0%, P3 = 11.3% and 26.7% respectively). This is in accordance with *Fujioka* et al. (6) who reported lower sensitivity of CEA in lower stages of the disease by immunohistochemical techniques.

Both 24 h urine and serum CEA levels in bladder cancer patients (146.8 ± 19.5, 8.11 ± 2.8 U/l) were significantly higher than those of either normal or bilharzial groups. When using cut-off values calculated from the normal group, 24 h urine sensitivity was 81.1% at 100% specificity which is in agreement with those of *Fraser* et al. (12) and *Hall* (13). Serum CEA sensitivity was 33.8% at 100% specificity. There is no correlation between serum and 24 h urine CEA.

Zimmerman et al. (15) attributed the high levels of 24 urine CEA of bladder cancer to the production from carcinoma cells lysis or cell desquamation.

References

1. EL-Bolkainy MN, Mokhtar NM, Ghoneim MA, Hussein MH (1981) The impact of schistosomiasis on the pathology of bladder carcinoma. Cancer 48:2643
2. Klee GG, Go VLW (1987) CEA and its role in clinical practice. In: Ghosh BC, Ghosh L (eds) Tumor marker and tumor associated antigens. Mc Graw-Hill Book Company, New York, London, pp 22–43
3. Jakes G, Rauschmeier H, Rosmanith P, Hofstadter F (1983) Determination of CEA in tissue, serum and urine in patients with transitional cell carcinoma of the urinary bladder. Urol Int 38(3):121
4. Asamoto M, Fukushima S, Tatemoto Y, Yamada K, Yoloa R, Mori M (1989) Immunohistochemical evaluation of non specific cross reactive antigen and CEA in urinary bladder carcinoma. Anticancer Res 9(2):319
5. Azadeh B, Vijayan P, Chej Fec G (1989) Linitis plastica-like carcinoma of the urinary bladder. Br J Urol 63(5):479
6. Fujioka T, Tanji S, Koike H, Kubo T, Ohhori T (1985) Immunohistochemical demonstration of CEA and ABo(H) blood group antigens on tissue sections of urinary bladder tumors. Hinyo Kikia, Kiyo 31(10): 1709
7. Fujioka T, Ohhori T, Lovrekovich L, Dekernion JB (1986) Investigation of blood group antigens and CEA in urinary bladder carcinoma. Urol Int 41(6):397
8. EL-Ahmady O, Khalifa A, Eissa S, Ibrahim MT (1988) Certain tumor markers in bilharzial patients in relation to bladder cancer. J Tumor Marker Oncol 3:227
9. Maklin NV, Strotskii AV, Ryneiskaia ES (1989) The control of CEA in the blood serum of patients with bladder tumors at various stages of combined treatment in relation to the disease stage. Urol Nefrol (Mosk) 1:49 (english abstract)
10. Bradford MM (1976) A rapid and sensitive method for the quantitation of microgram quantities of protein utilizing the principle of protein dye binding. Analyt Biochem 72:248
11. Nap M, Mollgard K, Burtin P, Fleuren GJ (1988) Immunochemistry of CEA in the embryo, fetus and adult. Tumor Biol 9(2–3):145
12. Fraser RA, Ravry MJ, Segura JW, Go V L W (1975) Clinical evaluation of urinary and serum CEA in bladder cancer. J Urol 114:226
13. Hall RR (1980) Carcinoembryonic antigen and urological carcinoma. A review after 7 years. Br J Urol 52:166
14. Tailly G, Cornelissen M, Vereecken RL, Verduyn H, Devos P, De Roo M (1983) Urinary carcinoembryonic antigen (CEA) in the diagnosis and follow up of bladder carcinoma. Br J Urol 55:501
15. Zimmerman R, Wahren B, Edsmyr F (1980) Assessment of serial CEA determinations in urine of patients with bladder carcinoma. Cancer 46:1802

Address for correspondence:
Prof. Dr. O. El-Ahmady
Tumor Marker Oncology Research Center
Al-Azhar University
2 Roshdy Street, Safeer Square
ET-Heliopolis, Cairo, Egypt

The role of motility, adhesion and migration factors in bladder carcinomas

T. Otto[a], K.-H. Heider[b], M. Goepel[a], F. Noll[a], A. Raz[c], H. Rübben[a]

[a]Department of Urology, University of Essen Medical School, Essen, [b]KfK, Institute for Genetics, Karlsruhe, [c]Metastasis Research Program, Michigan Cancer Foundation, Detroit, Michigan, USA

Introduction

In order to define a high-risk bladder cancer group and to improve the diagnosis and treatment decision in each individual patient we examined factors of tumor cell adhesion, i.e. E-cadherin, tumor cell motility factor receptor, i.e. gp78-hAMFR and migration factors, i.e. CD44v, in 43 patients. We correlated these findings to the histopathological result of the same tissue specimen.

Adhesion factors

It has been shown in several in vitro studies that the disturbance or loss of E-cadherin, a specific epithelial cell-cell adhesion molecule, induces new behavior in cells, i.e. the cells change their morphology from an epitheloid to a fibroblastoid phenotype and the in vitro invasiveness increases for collagen and heart tissue (1, 2, 3). We recently determined the expression of E-cadherin in prostatic carcinoma, normal prostate and BPH. We found strong E-cadherin expression in all specimens of normal prostate, benign prostatic hyperplasia and well differentiated prostatic carcinoma. E-cadherin was reduced in 89% of poorly differentiated and in 93% of locally advanced prostatic carcinomas (11, 12).

Motility factors

The group of *A. Raz* (8, 9) identified by recombinant techniques the human autocrine motility factor receptor, a 78 kD protein. This protein was used to prepare antibodies to human autocrine motility factor receptor. The monoclonal antibody was found to mimic the physiological effect of AMF and the enhanced motility induced by anti-gp78mAB was mediated by a pertussis/toxine sensitive G-protein pathway as has been described for other motility factors (14). We found different expression pattern of gp78-hAMFR in various bladder cancer cell lines. The poorly differentiated, highly motile cell line EJ 28 expressed high amount gp78-hAMFR measured by immunofluorescence technique. On the other hand the well differentiated bladder papilloma cell-line RT4 and the normal fetal urothelial cell-line HTBFS160 have shown a decreased expression pattern for gp78-hAMFR. On motile cells, i.e. EJ28 cell line, gp78-hAMFR was localized by immunofluorescence to the leading lamella as well as to the trailing edge, suggesting shuffling of gp78-hAMFR during cell migration (9, 14).

Migration factors

In a similar context the function of certain variants of the surface glycoprotein CD44 can be seen. The expression of CD44 variants was recently demonstrated to be necessary and sufficient to transfer so-called spontaneous metastatic behavior onto a non-metastatic rat pancreatic adenocarcinoma cell-line, as well as onto a nonmetastatic rat fibrosarcoma cell line (4, 6). These findings indicate that variant forms of CD44 play an important, but yet unknown role in tumor development and progression. Due to knowledge of the multifactorial process of tumorigenesis we investigated in this study if there is a relationship between the expression of the earlier described molecules E-cadherin and hAMFR and the expression of variant CD44 in bladder tumors.

Materials and methods

After clinical staging, transitional cell carcinoma of the urinary bladder was surgically removed by transurethral resection or radical cystectomy. The material was immediately frozen in liquid nitrogen. Frozen tissue sections were prepared in a Frigocut 2800-E microtome (Reichert-Jung, Germany). Serial sections of 5 µm were cut and stained with hematoxylin/eosin to determine the histopathological grading and staging according to the criteria of the UICC. Immuno-fluorescence staining was performed with the anti-E-cadherin monoclonal antibody 6F9 and the anti-human autocrine motility factor receptor antibody gp78-hAMFR (3, 8). Immunohistochemical staining was performed with antibodies directed against the variant regions of the CD44 molecule (anti-CD44v, Anti-DI, anti-DIII, VFF7, VFF8) (5).

Results

We examined the specimens of 43 caucasian patients, 45–81 years of age, with normal bladder tissue (n = 16) and bladder carcinoma (n = 27). The bladder tissue was surgically removed by transurethral resection (n = 24) and radical cystectomy (n = 19). The normal epithelial cells of the urothelium were highly positive for E-cadherin while negative for hAMFR expression. 63% and 44% of the non-invasive carcinoma were negative for E-cadherin and positive for hAMFR, respectively. Invasive carcinomas have shown a further departure from the normal labeling; 100% and 85% of the specimens were negative for E-cadherin and positive for hAMFR, respectively. All tested antibodies directed against the variant region of CD44 showed a positive reaction both on normal bladder tissue and on bladder carcinomas. The expression in carcinomas, however, was enhanced i.e. a higher percentage of positively stained samples was observed (table I). In contrast to the findings with the anti variant-CD44 antibodies, immunofluorescence staining with anti E-cadherin and anti hAMFR antibodies revealed a clear difference between normal bladder tissue and tumors. Expression of E-cadherin was dramatically reduced in the carcinomas, whereas hAMFR expression was clearly increased in comparison to normal tissue.

Discussion

Until now depth of infiltration and differentiation grade are the most important prognostic parameters concerning tumor progression and survival. However, these parameters fail in up to 36% even in patients with superficial bladder carcinoma (10, 13). The major problem is to select those patients who are at risk for tumor recurrence and progression and who may benefit from adjuvant treatment modalities. In order to define a high risk group we examined factors which are known to be involved in steps necessary for tumor progression and metastasis formation. Here we investigated the expression pattern of the cell adhesion molecules E-cadherin and variant CD44 and the human autocrine motility factor receptor hAMFR in 43 specimens of bladder carcinomas and normal bladder tissue. Bladder tumors show a similar high expression of variant CD44 as it was observed in other types of carcinomas, i.e. in adenocarcinomas of the colon, the stomach and the breast (5). In contrast to the

Table I. Expression of E-cadherin, human autocrine motility factor receptor and migration factors in human bladder specimens.

Results	n	E-cad. (%)	hAMFR (%)	CD44v (%)	DI (%)	DIII (%)	VFF7 (%)	VFF (%)
Normal bladder Tissue	16	100	7	66	31	36	47	33
Bladder Carcinoma	27	11	79	89	70	73	81	78
non-invasive	11	37	44	100	82	100	100	100
invasive	16	0	85	81	63	57	71	65

results obtained with normal colon and breast tissue, normal bladder epithelium shows a clear reaction with the antibodies directed against the variant portion of the CD44 molecule, indicating that normal urothelium belongs to the group of CD44v positive tissues. The reaction pattern with the different variant CD44 specific antibodies leads to the conclusion that the variant CD44 exons v3, v5 and v6 are expressed, both in normal tissue and in the tumors. Thus, the CD44 variants expressed in bladder tissue might be similar to those found on normal skin keratinocytes but differ markedly from the variants detected in colon, stomach and in breast tumors (5, 7, Heider et al. sumitted and unpublished data). Interestingly, non-invasive tumors show a higher CD44v expression than invasive specimens. We determined an inverse correlation between gp78-hAMFR and E-cadherin. Poorly differentiated, invasive bladder carcinomas were characterized by an increased gp78-hAMFR staining (85%) and an decreased E-cadherin expression pattern (89%).

There was a clear distinction between superficial non-invasive and invasive tumors. 100% respectively 85% of the invasive tumors were found to be E-cadherin reduced and hAMFR increased. On the other hand 37% of the superficial non-invasive bladder cancers expressed E-cadherin strongly and have shown a reduced, i.e. normal hAMFR expression (56%).

Furthermore we determined in 51 patients after a median follow-up of 24 months a correlation of decreased E-cadherin and increased gp78 hAMFR expression to progression and survival (11, 12). Clearly, we need a longer follow-up and more patients, but the different expression of cell adhesion molecules and motility factors give us an answer for some of these perplexing questions about the biology of bladder tumors.

References

1. Behrens J, Birchmeier W, Goodman SL, Imhof BA (1985) Dissociation of madin-darby canine kidney epithelial cells by the monoclonal antibody anti-arc-1: Mechanistic aspects and identification of the antigen as a component related to uvomorulin. J Cell Biol 1001:1307
2. Behrens J, Birchmeier W (1990) Specific activity of the arc-1/uvomorulin promoter in epithelial cells. J Cell Biol 111:157a
3. Frixen UH, Behrens J, Sacks M, Eberle G, Voss B, Warda A, Lachner D, Birchmeier W (1991) E-cadherin mediated cell-cell adhesion prevents invasiveness of human carcinoma cells. J Cell Biol 113:173
4. Günthert U, Hofmann M, Rudy W, Reber S, Zöller M, Haußmann I, Mazku S, Wenzel A, Ponta H, Herrlich P (1991) A new variant of glycoprotein CD44 confers metastatic potential to rat carcinoma cells. Cell 65:13–24
5. Heider KH, Hofmann M, Horst E, van den Berg F, Ponta H, Herrlich P, Pals ST (1993) A human homologue of the rat metastasis-associated variant of CD44 is expressed in colorectal carcinomas and adenomatous polyps. J Cell Biol 120:227–233
6. Herrlich P, Pals ST, Zöller M, Ponta H (1993) CD44 splice variants: Metastases mett lymphocytes. Immunol. Today, submitted
7. Koopman G, Heider KH, Horst E, Adolf GR, van den Berg F, Ponta H, Herrlich P, Pals ST (1993) Activated human lymphocytes and aggressive Non-Hodgkin lymphomas express a homologue of the rat metastasis-associated variant of CD44. J Exp Med; (in press)
8. Nabi IR, Watanabe H, Raz A (1990) Identification of B16-F1 melanoma autocrine motility – like factor receptor. Cancer Res 50:409
9. Nabi IR, Watanabe H, Silletti S, Raz A (1991) Tumor cell autocrine motility factor receptor In: Goldberg ID (ed) Cell motility factors. Birkhäuser, Basel, pp 164
10. Otto T, Rübben H (1992) Risikoorientierte Klassifikation oberflächlicher Harnblasenkarzinome. Urol [A] 31:199–200
11. Otto T, Goepel M, Rembrink K, Rübben H (1993) E-cadherin: Parameter for differentiation and invasiveness in prostatic carcinoma. Urol Res 21 (5):359–362
12. Otto T, Raz A, Birchmeier W, Schmidt U, Rembrink K, Rübben H (1993) E-cadherin and autocrine motility factor receptor: Progression associated parameters in bladder carcinoma. J Urol 149 (4), 458 A:981
13. Rutt (Registry for Urinary Tract Tumors): Harnwegstumorregister, Jahresbericht (1985) Verh Dtsch Ges Urol 37:665
14. Silletti S, Yao J, Sanford J, Mohammed, AN, Otto T, Wolman SR, Raz A (1993) Autocrine motility factor receptor in human bladder carcinoma: Gene expression, loss of cell-contact regulation, and chromosomal mapping. Int J Oncol 3:801–807

Address for correspondence:
Dr. med. T. Otto
Urologische Klinik der Universität – GHS – Essen
Hufelandstraße 55
D-45122 Essen, Germany

Ki-67 immunostaining as a new prognosticator in non-metastatic renal cell carcinoma

W. de Riese[a], C.W. Biermann[a], W.N. Crabtree[b], T.M. Ulbright[b],
A. Hinkel[a], E.P. Allhoff[c], Th. Senge[a]

[a]Urological Clinic of the Ruhr-University, Bochum, Herne, Germany,
[b]Department of Pathology, Indiana University, Indianapolis, USA,
[c]Hospital of the Bundesknappschaft, Urological Clinic, Würselen, Germany

Introduction

About 40% of the RCC patients with no evidence of metastatic disease at time of nephrectomy will develop recurrence within five years and die of disease (1, 11). Therefore efforts have to be focused on defining this subset of high risk patients. Tumor grade and tumor stage are currently considered as the most reliable prognosticators in non-metastatic RCC (8, 11, 14). However, this has to be improved for discriminating patients at high and low risk, especially in those cases of identical staging and grading. Investigators dealing with oncological issues have the opinion that the individual proliferation (synoyma: growth rate, growth fraction) is an important, independent parameter concerning relapse rate and prognosis in human solid neoplasms. The proliferation rate of a tumor is defined by the proportion of cycling cells in the total cell population.

Direct clinical evaluation of proliferation rates is impossible. Proliferation rates have been determined by thymidine labeling (16), bromodeoxyuridine incorporation (15) or flow cytometric measurement (6, 13). However, because each of these methods is either costly, time consuming or requires a special laboratory set-up, there is considerable interest in Ki-67 immunostaining as an alternative approach.

In 1983, Gerdes and his co-workers first isolated and characterised the monoclonal antibody Ki-67, which reacts with a human nuclear antigen associated with cell proliferation (3). Cell cycle analysis demonstrated that the nuclear antigen detected by Ki-67 is expressed only in the G1-, S-, G2-, and M-phases of proliferating cells but is absent in G0- (resting) cells (4).

In the prospective study described in this report Ki-67 immunostaining was performed on frozen sections of histologically proved node-negative RCC from 58 patients operated on between 1986 and 1988 in order to examine its prognostic value and its association with other clinicopathologic parameters.

Patients and methods

Patients

Fifty-eight patients with pathologically proved node-negative renal cell carcinoma entered this prospective study. The patients were 21 (36.2%) women and 37 (63.8%) men, ranging in age from 21 to 83 years (median, 59 years). All patients underwent tumor nephrectomy between 1986 and 1988 and were clinically free of distant metastasis at time of surgery. None of these patients received adjuvant therapy postoperatively. All 58 patients were followed according to a standard protocol.

The histopathological characteristics of the 58 RCCs are shown in table I. Pathological tumor staging and grading were performed according to the UICC classification (7). Histological evaluation of the specimens was done by a pathologist, who had no previous knowledge of the proliferation rates.

Specimens

Depending on the individual tumor size several random biopsies were taken from each tumor (table II). The highest proliferation rate of all biopsies taken from one individual tumor was considered as representative for the entire tumor. As outlined in another report, it is necessary to analyze several biopsies in order to receive representative data for the entire tumor ("sampling error") (12). The fresh tumor samples were stored at –70 °C until immunostaining.

Antibodies and staining

Ki-67 immunostaining was performed on cryostat sections approximately 5 micron in thickness, using the APAAP complex technique (APAAP = alkaline phosphatase anti-alkaline phosphatase) (2). In brief, the frozen sections were air-dried and fixed in acetone for 10 minutes, and then washed three times for 5 minutes each in phosphate-buffered saline (PBS, pH 7.4). Subsequent procedures were carried out in a humid chamber. The slides were incubated with the primary monoclonal antibody Ki-67 (1:20; Dianova, Hamburg, Germany) for 30 minutes. Then the slides were washed twice with PBS, each for 5 minutes, before the APAAP complex technique was performed as described by other investigators (2, 5). After the addition of fast red as a substrate for the peroxidase, positively reacting cells had red nuclei. After washing in deionized water for 2 minutes, the sections were counterstained with hemalum (12). Ki-67 positive cells were red, negativ cells were stained blue. Negative control staining was performed by replacing the primary monoclonal antibody (Ki-67) with non-immune mouse serum. Sections of a strongly Ki-67 positive lymphoma as well as of normal renal tissue (proliferation rate of about 1%) were used as positive controls.

Quantification of staining results, statistical analysis

Ki-67 positive (red) and Ki-67 negative (blue) nuclei were counted at a magnification of X 250 on a Zeiss microscope. Microscopic fields in the sections were chosen randomly from left to right and up to down. Cells were considered Ki-67 positive regardless of the intensity or location of nuclear Ki-67 staining. In each case the Ki-67 immunostained slides were evaluated by counting an average number of 200 cells in four different fields. A minimum of 800 cells were evaluated. The Ki-67 proliferation rate was defined by the proportion of Ki-67 positive cells. The highest proliferation rate of different sections obtained from one tumor was considered as representative for the entire tumor.

The results were computed by dBASE III+ program. The chi-square, log-rank, Kruskal-Wallis and Mann-Whitney tests served to check for significant differences. The significance level was set to a p-value of 0.05 (10). The worst level of significance among the tests is cited. These tests were applied to correlate the proliferation rate (PR) to pathologic stage (pT), grading and tumor size. Disease free survival curves of the RCC patients were estimated according to Kaplan-Meier.

Results

All samples analyzed in this study were histologically proven renal cell carcinomas. Three tumors were < 2 cm, twenty-two were ranging between 2 and 5 cm, and thirty-three were more than 5 cm in diameter. All the tumors showed immunoreactivity with Ki-67 antibody. The clinicopathologic parameters are shown in table I. The percentage of Ki-67 positive cells (= proliferation rate) of all RCC tumors analyzed in this study ranged between 2 and 23%, while normal renal tissue exhibited proliferation rates up to 2% only. In almost all cases, the highest proliferation rates (PR) were observed in the peripheral zone of malignant tissue close to the normal renal tissue.

No correlation between individual proliferation rates (PR) and tumor stage (pT) (figure 1) was found. In low stage tumors (pT1-2), a 5-fold variation in PR was measured. Several small

Table I. Pathological characteristics of 58 RCC patients analyzed in this study.

Tumor stage (pT)	Number (%)
pT 1–2	31 (53.4%)
pT 3–4	27 (46.6%)
Grade	
G 1	17 (29.3%)
G 2	22 (37.9%)
G 3	19 (32.8%)

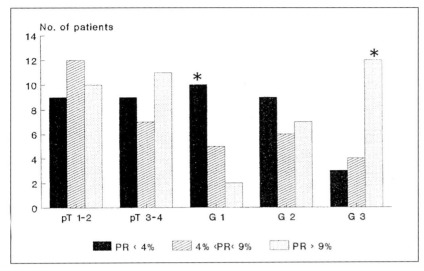

Figure 1. Distribution of PRs in 58 non-metastatic RCCs of different tumor stages and grades $p < 0.05^*$ (chi-square).

Table II. Number of specimens according to tumor size for representative measurement of proliferation rates (PR).

Tumor size in diameter	Number of specimens	
	peripheral zone	central zone
< 3 cm	2	1
3–6 cm	4	2
> 6 cm	6	2

Table III. Combination of pT stage, grading (G) and proliferation rate (PR) as prognosticators for tumor recurrence.

Combined parameters	p-Value
pT stage + grading	0.042
pT stage + PR	0.0059
Grading + PR	0.002
pT + grading + PR	0.0009

tumors (< 3 cm in diameter) had proliferation rates over 9%, whereas some large tumors (> 9 cm in diameter) showed low proliferation rates (< 4%). In contrast, a strong correlation between Ki-67 staining percentage (= proliferation rate) and low grade (G1) as well as high grade (G3) RCC tumors was observed (figure 1).
The median follow-up of the patients described in this study was 62 months (range 46 to 71). 35 (60.4%) had no evidence of disease, whereas 23 (39.6%) developed relapse after nephrectomy.

No correlation between pT stage, tumor size and tumor recurrence was found, whereas tumor grade (G) (p = 0.03) and PR (p = 0.0075) showed each a strong correlation to recurrence. Patients with low PRs (< 4%) had a significant (p < 0.0001) lower risk for relapse compared to patients with high PRs (> 9%). In a multivariat analysis tumor grade and proliferation rate were independent parameters. Table III shows the statistical results for the combination of pT stage, tumor grade (G), and PR as prognosticators. The combination of the two conventional histological parameters (pT stage, tumor grade (G)) with the proliferation rate as a new tumor biologic parameter were statistically more predictive (p = 0.0009) compared to the predictive value of the two histopathological parameters alone (p = 0.042) (see table III).
In conclusion, the conventional histopathological parameters (pT, G) were less predictive for tumor recurrence as the combination of pT, G and proliferation rate (PR).

Discussion

According to the data presented in this study individual proliferation rates (PRs) show a strong correlation to tumor grade (G), but not to tumor stage (pT). Similar results were found in another RCC study recently published (9). Therefore, the individual tumor stage cannot be deduced from an individual proliferation rate, as tumor stage is a function of individual cell proliferation as well as of individual age of a given tumor, which is not measureable at time of diagnosis. These results correspond with data in breast cancer recently published: A positive correlation between histological grading and proliferation rate was observed (13, 17).

Investigators assumed a correlation between Ki-67 labeling and prognosis in RCC patients (9). Up to this moment, however, there has been no data available concerning this issue. The results presented in this study show that the presence of high proliferation rates (> 9%) worsens the prognosis significantly independent of other risk factors. Regarding all findings we suggest that the proliferation rate obtained by Ki-67 immunostaning is a relevant marker for the biological behavior of individual RCC tumors. This study should help to define subgroups of patients at high risk for recurrent disease who will then be targets for adjuvant therapeutic procedures.

References

1 Buzaid AC, Todd MB (1989) Therapeutic options in renal cell carcinoma. Sem Oncol suppl 1, 16:12
2 Cordell JL, Falini B, Erber NW (1985) Immunoenzymatic labeling of monoclonal antibodies using immune complexes of alkaline phosphatase and monoclonal anti-alkaline phosphatase (APAAP complexes). J Histochem Cytochem 32:219–229
3 Gerdes J, Schwab U, Lemke H, Stein H (1983) Production of a mouse monoclonal antibody reactive with a human nuclear antigen associated with cell proliferation. Int J Cancer 31:13–20
4 Gerdes J, Lemke H, Baisch H, Wacker HH, Schwab U, Stein H (1984) Cell cycle analysis of a cell proliferation-associated human nuclear antigen defined by the monoclonal antibody Ki67. J Immunol 133:1710–1715
5 Gerdes J, Dallenbach F, Lennert K (1984) Growth fractions in malignant non-Hodgkin's lymphomas (NHL) as determined in situ with the monoclonal antibody Ki-67. Hematol Oncol 2:365–371
6 Gerdes J (1990) Ki-67 and other proliferation markers useful for immunohistological diagnostic and prognostic evaluation in human malignancies. Sem Cancer Biol 1 (3):199–200
7 Hedley DW (1989) Flow cytometry using paraffin-embedded tissue: Five years on. Cytometry 10:229–241
8 Hermanek P, Sobin LH (1987) TNM classification of malignant tumors. 4th ed, Springer, Berlin
9 Hermanek P, Schrott KM (1990) Evaluation of the new tumor, nodes and metastases classification of renal cell carcinoma. J Urol 144:238
10 Kaiser U, Hansmann ML, Papadopulos I (1991) Does the immunophenotype of renal cell carcinoma correlate with its clinical stage? Urol Int 47(4): 194–198
11 Lew RA, Menon M (1991) A user's guide to statistical analysis. J Urol 146:199–205
12 Mrstik C, Salamon J, Weber R, Stögermayer F (1992) Predictors of relapse in renal cell carcinoma. J Urol 148:271–274
13 de Riese W, Allhoff E, Werner M, Atzpodien J, Kirchner H, Stief CG (1991) Proliferative behavior and cytogenetic changes in human renal cell carcinoma. W J Urol 9:79–85
14 Stenfert-Kroese MC, Rutgers DH, Wils IS, Van Unnik JAM, Roholl PJM (1990) The relevance if DNA index and proliferation rate in the grading of benign and malignant soft tissue tumors. Cancer 65:1782–88
15 Strohmeyer T, Ackermann R (1991) Classic and modern prognostic indicators in renal cell carcinoma, review of the literature. Urol Int 47:203–212
16 Tsujihasha H, Nakanishi A, Matasuda H, Uejima S Kurita T (1991) Cell proliferation of human tumors determined by BrdUrd and Ki-67 immunostaining. J Urol 145 (4):846–849
17 Verhoeven D, Buyssens N, Van Marck C (1991) Comparison of Ki-67 and tritiated thymidine in measuring tumor proliferation. Am J Clin Pathol 95 (4):602
18 Wintzer HO, Zipfel I, Schulte-Möning J, Hellerich, U, von Kleist S (1991) Ki-67 immunostaining in human breast tumors and its relationship to prognosis. Cancer 67:421–428

Address for correspondence
Priv.-Doz. Dr. med. W. de Riese
Urologische Klinik
Marienhospital
Ruhr-Universität Bochum
Widumerstraße 8
D-44627 Herne, Germany

Comparative immunohistochemical examinations on the corpora amylacea in the brain, lung and prostatic gland

J. Makovitzky, P. Gyürüs

Department of Pathology, Martin-Luther-University, Halle Wittenberg, Germany,
Department of Pathology, University Medical School of Pecs, Hungary

Introduction

The corpora amylacea (c.a.) are considered to be degenerative products. Their most common localisations are the prostatic gland, the lung and the brain. According to the literature c.a. in the brain are a degenerative product of astrocytes (3, 4, 10). In the prostatic gland the congestion of secretion products seems to play a dominant role (5, 6). In the lung they appear in ill ventilated areas along with macrophages and alveolar cells (2, 9).

The c.a. present in these organs showed an amyloid like behavior in jodine + sulphuric acid reaction. The histological and histochemical properties, however, do not stand for amyloidal similarity (5). *Marx* et al. (7) could show by electronmicroscopical examinations, that there are some differences between the c.a. and their filamented structures. These filaments are ordered in the lung and prostatic gland in a concentric way, and in the brain in a radial way, on the contrary.

It is known from the immunohistochemical literature and from our own previous examinations, that the bronchial- and prostatic secretions and the secreting gland epithel show immunohistochemical positive reaction with the anti-CA 19-9. We have examined the c.a. in the upper stated localizations with monoclonal carbohydrate antibodies, with cytokeratines, GFAP and with two further Alzheimer antibodies to look for the differences.

Methods

Paraffin-embedded tissue blocks from human prostata, lung and brain were examined with various immunohistochemical procedures. We used commercially available monoclonal antibodies against CA 19-9 (Isotopendiagnostik CIS Gmbh, Dreieich, Germany), CA 50 and CA 242 (kindly provided by *O. Nilsson*; Pharmacia CanAg, Gothenburg, Sweden) and cytokeratins (Dako, Hamburg, and Boehringer, Mannheim), GFAP and two antibodies, (anti-Alzheimer precursor protein A4 (monoclonal) and anti-β-amyloid-Alzheimer (polyclonal).

The ABC method of immunoperoxidase histochemistry and the method of APAAP-Dual-System (Dianova, Hamburg) was performed. Negative controls were performed by substituting PBS buffer for specific antibodies.

Results

1. The corpora amylacea (c.a.) in the brain produce a negative immunohistochemical reaction with GFAP, anti-CA 19-9, anti-CA 50 and anti-CA 242. So there was no immunohistochemical reaction in the lung with the first three antibodies. On the contrary, the c.a., macrophages and

Table I. Reaction of corporea amylacea in brain, lung, prostate with the antibodies tested.

	GFAP	CA 19-9	CA 50	CA 242
Brain	–	–	–	–
Lung	–	–	–	+++
Prostata	–	+	++	+++

alveolar cells brought a distinct positiv result. In the prostatic gland the c.a. reacted (except GFAP) with the three monoclonal carbohydrate antibodies in a positive way (table I, figure 1 and 2).

2. With the cytokeratines the c.a. showed a negativ immunohistochemical reaction in the lung and in the brain. In the prostatic gland we registered (except cytokeratin 7) a negativ reaction with the cytokeratines used (Pancytokeratin, CK4, CK5/6, CK8/18, CK13, CK19 and CK20). CK7 showed a clear cut positive reaction (centrally and marginally).

3. The c.a. in the brain were positiv with the both Alzheimer antibodies. In contrast there were negative results in the prostatic gland and the lung (table II).

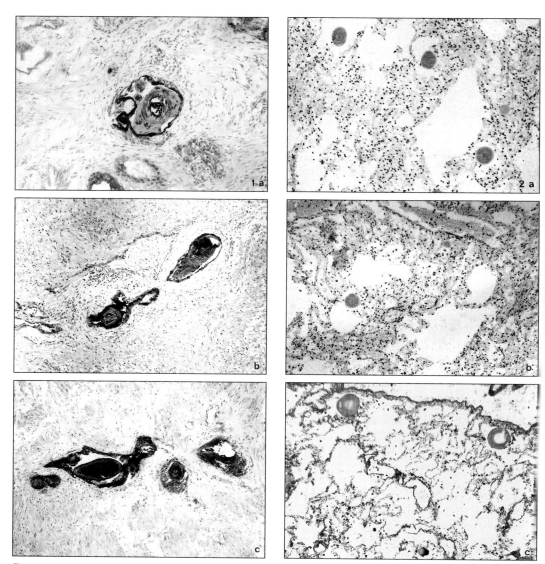

Figure 1. Corpora amylacea in the prostatic gland. a) Immunohistocemical reaction with anti CA 19-9 (185x); b) with CA 50 (100x); c) with CA 242 (100x).

Figure 2. Corpora amylacea in the lung. a) Immunohistochemical reaction with anti CA 19-9 (100x); b) with CA 50 (100x); c) with CA 242 (100x).

Table II. Reaction of the c.a. in brain, lung, prostate, with the Alzheimer antibodies.

	Alzh. precursor protein A4	Anti-β-amyloid Alzheimer
Brain	++	++
Lung	–	–
Prostate	–	–

Discussion

The c.a. in the brain show an imminent PAS reaction. In the prostatic gland and the lung a weaker discrete reaction resulted accordingly anisotrope PAS-(ABT)-reaction at pH 1-2 was positiv (preparations by *Makovitzky*, 11). C.a. showed strong increased birefrigence in the form of positive spheroids after ABT reaction, and indicated a radially oriented, spheroid filamentous polysaccharide structure (11). The unstained c.a. had a very weak birefringence (8). The optical polarization measurements hint to the submicroscopic structure of the c.a. It is interesting, that all the three c.a. can be stained with Congo red and toluidine blue, with a definitive anisotropic effect (as in case of amyloids). According to *Romhanyi* and *Deak* c.a. in the brain are constituted from hexoglycose (87%), protein (4.7%) and phosphate (2.2%). The c.a. of the brain are resistent to a $KMnO_4$-oxidation combined with the pepsin- and/or trypsin digestion. In contrast, c.a. of the lung and prostatic gland were sensitive.

Some authors found a GFAP- positivity of c.a. in the brain (3, 4). This refers to their astrocytic origin. *Cross* et al. have found amyloid components in c.a. of prostatic gland with β-2-microglobuline antibody.

Our results with monoclonal carbohydrate antibodies in the prostatic gland and the lung suggest a glycoprotein nature of our c.a. This result confirms optical polarization measurements.

The negative GFAP reaction in the brain does not suggest the astrocytary origin of the c.a. The positive reaction with both Alzheimer antibodies hints to a amyloid similarity and clearly to a degenerative product. The positive reaction with cytokeratin 7 agrees with that of *Schrodt* and *Murray*. It should be created next from kreatin like material and a cross reaction should be discussed eventually.

These examinations confirm the inhomogeneity of the c.a. of the lung, the prostatic gland and brain.

References

1 Cross PA, Bartley CJ, McClure J (1992) Amyloid in prostatic corpora amylacea. J Clin Pathol 45:894–897
2 Deak G, Karlinger K (1972) Submicroscopic structure of the corpora amylacea of the central nervous system. Acta Morph Acad Sci Hung 20:77–84
3 Leel-össy L (1981) The origin and the pathological significance of the corpus amylaceum. Acta Neuropathol, Springer, Berlin, suppl VII:396–399
4 Leel-össy L (1991) Patological significance and characteristics of corpus amylaceum. Neuropathol 11:105–114
5 Makovitzky (in prepatation)
6 Marx AJ, Gueft B, Moskal JE (1965) Prostatic corpora amylacea. Arch Path 80:487–594
7 Marx aJ, Gueft B, Kikkawa Y (1965) The cellular origin and fibrous structure of prostatic corpora amylacea: An electron microscopic and electron probe study. Lab Invest 14:593–594
8 Molnar J (1951) Corpora amylacea in the central nervous system. Nature (London) 168:39
9 Rahn J (1964) Häufigkeit und Verteilung der Corpora amylacea pulmonum. Frankf Z Pathol 73:598–601
10 Ramsey HI (1965) Ultrastructure of corpora amylacea. J Neuropathol Exp Neurol 24:25–39
11 Romhanyi G, Deak G (1975) Topo-optical studies on age pigment, corpora amylacea and senile amyloid-like substances of the brain. In: Könyey S, Tariska ST, Gosztonyi G (eds) Proc. VIIth Intern Congr Neuropathol. Exc Med Amsterdam, Akademiai Kiado, Budapest, pp 123–126
12 Schrodt RG, Murray M (1966) The keratin structure of corpora amylacea. Arch Pathol 82:518–525

Address for correspondence:
Prof. Dr. med. J. Makovitzky
Abteilung für Pathologie
Martin-Luther Universität
Halle-Wittenberg
Magdeburger Straße 14
D-06097 Halle (Saale), Germany

DNA synthesis in human osteosarcoma (HOS) cells treated with lead chromate[1]

M. S. Latif

Department of Chemistry, Faculty of Science, Al-Azhar University, Nasr City, Cairo, Egypt

Introduction

DNA is a double helix and each strand of this helix acts as a template for the synthesis of a new, complementary strand. DNA replication is a semi conservative process since only one strand of the parental duplex is conserved in each new duplex formed (1). Chromium salts are known to be highly toxic. In vitro cell studies done on chromium show that the hexavalent form of chromium, rather than the trivalent form, is the relevant toxic and carcinogenic species. In addition, Cr^{6+} is highly clastogenic and mutagenic to cultured mammalian cells and its soluble forms induce dose-dependent cytotoxicity and base substitution mutations (2).

Materials and methods

Cell and culture conditions

American type culture collection book (ATCC) CRL 1543 human osteogenic sarcoma (HOS) TE85. The source of cancer tissue: A biopsy was obtained before x-ray or chemotherapy from an osteosarcoma of the distal right femur of a 13 year old caucasian girl. The cell lines were propagated at 37 °C in Dulbecco's modified Eagle's medium supplemented with 10% fetal bovine serum in an atmosphere of 5% CO_2. The cells were routinely passaged using trypsin-EDTA (3). Lead(II) chromate ($PbCrO_4$): 98% A.C.S. reagent, from Aldrich Chemical Company. Thymidine, (methyl-3H) lot no. 2561003; specific activity: 3226.4 GBq/mmol, 87.2 Ci/mmol; concentration: 37.0 MBq/ml, 1.0 mCi/ml, 0.012 µmol/ml, 0.0028 mg/ml. Sodium hydroxide (NaOH) 19.1 M, purchased from fisher. Hydrochloric acid (HCl) 12.1 N, trichloroacetic acid (TCA), sodium pyrophosphate, potassium hydroxide, sodium chloride, 3-, 5-diaminobenzoic acid (DABA) and activated charcoal, all from Sigma.

DNA assay

After the cells began to grow, the media was aspirated off and the plates were then washed once with phosphate buffered saline (PBS). The plates were treated for either 1 hour, 4 hours, or 18 hours with 1 µg/ml lead chromate in media (1.25 ml lead chromate to 23.75 ml media, 3 ml/plate). After incubation with lead chromate, the plates were removed from the incubator washed twice with PBS and tritiated thymidine 2 µCi/plate, in serum free media (42 µl tritiated thymidine to 21 ml media, 3 ml/plate) was added to each set of plates. The plates were then incubated over a time course of 30 minutes, 1 hour, and 2 hours. The control set of plates received only the tritiated thymidine. The amount of DNA synthesis was determined using the fluorescence methods of Kissane and Robins (4) and Hinegardner (5). The cell monolayer was washed twice with 3 ml of ice cold 0.9% NaCl washed once with 2 ml 10% TCA, 5% pyrophosphate to remove unincorporated thymidine and the monolayer was solubilized with 1 ml of 0.33 N KOH. The plate was incubated for 1 hour at 37 °C and

---

[1] This work was conducted at the Biochemistry and Molecular Biology, UMDNJ, New Jersey Medical School, under an Egyptian Commission Fellowship grant on leave from Al-Azhar University.

transferred to a plastic tube. The plate was washed with 1 ml 20% TCA, 10% pyrophosphate, this was added to the tube. The tube was placed in an ice bath and then refrigerated overnight to pellet, DNA and protein. The tube was centrifuged at 2000 rpm for 10 minutes to pellet DNA. The supernatant, which contains ribonucleotides from RNA, was decanted and the pellet was washed with 4 ml 10% TCA, 5% pyrophosphate. The tube was centrifuged again, the supernatant decanted, the sides of the tube dried with cotton tip applicators, and 1.5 ml 5% TCA was incubated with the pellet at 37 °C in a water bath for 20 minutes to extract DNA. The DNA is in the supernatant. A 2 M DABA solution was prepared and added to tubes containing 0.5 ml of the DNA supernatant. DABA also was added to a blank, 10 µl, 20 µl, 30 µl, and 40 µl (done in duplicate) of salmon sperm DNA in a 0.1 µg/µl concentration, so a standard curve could be prepared. The tubes were incubated in a water bath at 60 °C for 45 minutes which allowed the complex to form. A 0.8 ml aliquot of the prepared 0.1 N HCl solution was then added to the tubes to stop the reaction and the amount of DNA present was determined using a fluorometer set at wave lengths of 405 nm for excitation and 525 nm for emission. The amount of radioactivity was determined by adding the DNA supernatant (0.5 ml) to 5 ml of ecoscint contained in a scintillation vial. The total amount of radioactivity per total amount µg DNA was calculated for each set of plates

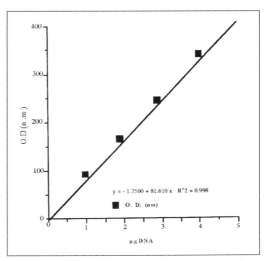

Figure 1. Standard curve using salmon sperm DNA for 4 hours and 18 hours treatments with lead chromate.

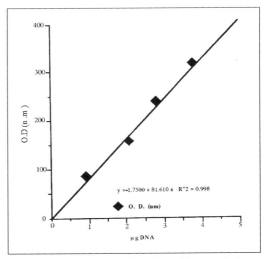

Figure 2. Standard curve using 0.1 µg/µl conc of salmon sperm DNA for 4 hours and 18 hours treatments with lead chromate.

Results

To test the ability of lead chromate in altering the rate of DNA synthesis, HOS cells were treated for short and long periods of time with a 1 µg/ml concentration of the carcinogen. After treatment periods with lead chromate, the 3H-thymidine incorporation was performed after a time course of 30 minutes, 1 hour, and 2 hours. As indicated by the figure 9, the CPMs were similar for control and 1 hour treatment, decreased for 4 hours treatment, and increased for 18 hours treatment with lead chromate. Two standard curves were then prepared using salmon sperm DNA in a 0.1 µg/µl concentration. This concentration was multiplied by various volumes of the salmon sperm DNA, 10 µl, 20 µl, 30 µl, and 40 µl, to give µg DNA. The respective O.D. readings for each volume were subtracted from the blank and the slope of the line was calculated. The O.D. reading obtained for each lead chromate treatment was divided by the slope of the standard curve to give µg DNA. The µg DNA increased from control to one hour treatment, decreased for four hours treatment, and increased for 18 hours treatment with lead chromate, as shown in the figure 8. The

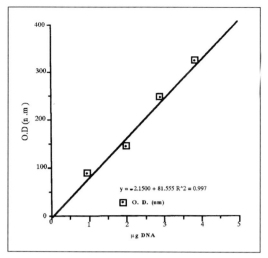

Figure 3. Standard curve using 0.1 µg/µl conc. of salmon sperm DNA for control and 1 hour treatments with lead chromate.

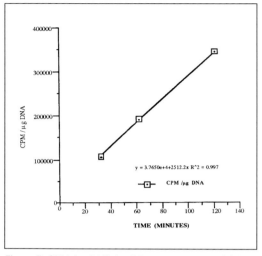

Figure 5. CPM /µg DNA for 1 hour treatments with lead chromate.

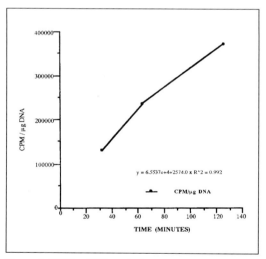

Figure 4. CMP/µg DNA control.

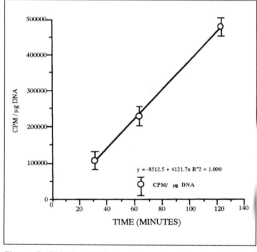

Figure 6. CPM/µg DNA for 4 hour treatments with lead chromate.

CPMs then were divided by the µg DNA to give CPM/µg DNA. As shown in the figures 4–8, there was a decrease from control to 1 hour treatment, increase for 4 hours treatment, and decrease for 18 hours treatment in the CPM/µg DNA after exposure to lead chromate. As indicated by the graphs for CMP/µg DNA versus time, the slope of the line was 2574.0 for the control, close to the 1 hour treatment slope of 2512.5. After four hours treatment, the slope increased to 4121.7, and decreased to 2104.6 after 18 hours treatment with lead chromate.

Discussion

The biological activity of chromium compounds is a function of valence and solubility. The most insoluble hexavalent compound, for example, lead chromate, is the most carcinogenic compound. In

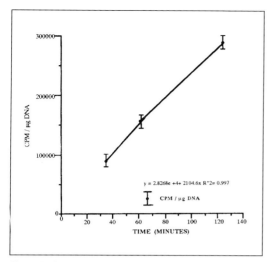

Figure 7. CPM /µg DNA for 18 hour treatments with lead chromate.

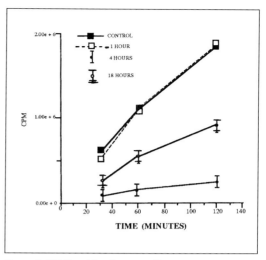

Figure 9. 3H-thymidine incorporation.

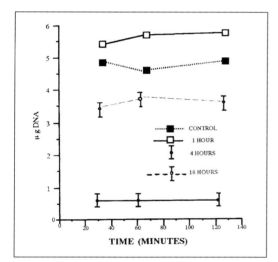

Figure 8. µg DNA for control, 1 hour, 4 hours and 18 hours.

this investigation, I treated HOS cells with a 1 µg/ml concentration of lead chromate to see if the rate of DNA synthesis was altered after short and long periods of time.

The nucleus is the major site of DNA synthesis. Tritiated thymidine was the radioisotope used in this study because it is the only radioisotope which just labels DNA (6). In this quantitative assay, the cells were labeled in vitro with 3H-thymidine in serum-free media (media with serum contains thymidine, and if 3H-thymidine is added to this media, it will dilute out and the CPMs will be lower) and their constituents were isolated and purified. The amount of radioactivity then was measured using a scintillation counter, which counts the flashes of light generated by mixing the radioactive sample with scintillation liquid. This scintillation liquid fluoresces after absorbing the energy of a particle resulting from the decay of the nucleus of the radioactive atom.

The DNA assay was performed next. This revealed that the 4 hours treatment with lead chromate gave the lowest amount of DNA. This does not mean that there was less DNA present for this treatment but that an experimental error occured. It is possible that the DNA was sheared and the particles which broke off did not solublize in the TCA. This would account for the decreased µg amounts obtained in the DNA assay. Next, the slopes of the line were used to compare the CMP/µg DNA for control, one hour, 4 hours, and 18 hours treatments with lead chromate. There was little change between the slope of the control group and the 1 hour treatment group. It is belived that at 1 hour, lead chromate has not yet penetrated the cell's plasma membrane, so DNA synthesis is not affected. However, it is known that lead chromate does not enter the cell after 4 hours and it is suggested that the compound induces single strand breaks in DNA. The slope of the line for the 4 hour treatment group increased and a possible explanation is that DNA synthesis was carried out at the same time as DNA repair. However, most of the cells are still alive after 18 hours treatment because the slope of the line, although decreased, is still linear. This is important because it has been shown that cells can still be transformed after an 18 hours treatment with lead chromate. If the cells were dead, this transformation could not take place.

References

1. Avers C (1986) Molecular cell biology. Addison – Wesley Publishing Company Inc, Massachusetts, p 479–486
2. Patierno SR, Banh D, Landolph JR (1988) Transformation of C3H/IOT1/2 mouse embryo cells to focus formation and anchorage independence by insoluble lead chromate but not soluble calcium chromate: Relationship to mutagenesis and internalization of lead chromate particles. Cancer Res 48:5280–5288
3. BR, Forrester FT (1971) Basic Laboratory Techniques in Cell Culture. U.S. Department of Health And Human Services
4. Kissans JM, Robins E (1958) The fluorometric measurement of deoxyribnucleic acid in animal tissues with special reference to the central neruous system. J Biol Chem 223:184–188
5. Hinegardner RT (1971) An improved fluorometric assay for DNA. Anal Biocchem 39:197–201
6. Darnell J, Lodish H, Baltimore D (1990) Molecular cell biology. Scientific America Books Inc. New York p 190–194

Address for correspondence:
Dr. M. S. Latif
Department of Chemistry
Faculty of Science
Al-Azhar University
ET-Nasr City, Cairo, Egypt

Expression of endogenous sugar-binding proteins (endogenous lectins) in tumors of peripheral nerves in correlation to the growth pattern[1]

H.-J. Holzhausen[a], J. Knolle[a], H. Bahn[a], F.-W. Rath[a], H.-J. Gabius[b]

[a] Institute of Pathology, Martin-Luther-University, Halle, [b] Institute of Physiological Chemistry, Veterinary Medical School, Ludwig-Maximilians-University, Munich, Germany

Introduction

The determination of expression of certain sugar structures in cellular glycoconjugates by antibodies or lectins and of sugar-binding sites like endogenous lectins (EL) by neoglycoconjugates is supposed to enhance our understanding of molecular determinants with supposed importance in cell-cell and cell-substrate interactions (1–3). Malignant transformation is already known to be accompanied by defined changes in the structure of the carbohydrate part of cellular glycoconjugates (3–5). Notably, these alterations, detected by means of laboratory tools as monoclonal antibodies or plant lectins (6, 7) deserve attention with regard to their potential functional significance as ligand in recognizable protein-carbohydrate interactions. This type of molecular recognition involving endogenous lectins as physiological receptors is believed to participate in the mediation of a variety of biological processes relevant to tumor growth and spread, like cell adhesion or immunomodulation with potential antitumoral response (1, 3). By using synthetic carrier immobilized carbohydrate ligands the receptor side of this interaction can be readily evaluated by common histochemical techniques (1–3).

The following glycohistochemical study of benign and malignant tumors of the periphere nerve system focused on the questions:

1. Do qualitative and/or quantitative differences exist in the expression of EL in correlation to the growth pattern and malignancy?

2. What can the potential biological significance of protein-carbohydrate interactions be, discerned by application of neoglycoproteins on section?

Material and methods

Formalin-fixed, paraffin-embedded specimens of tumors (table I) were used. Glutaraldehyde fixed tissue of all tumors was investigated ultrastructurally (Tesla, BS 500). Neoglycoproteins (sugar-bovine serum albumin conjugates) were obtained by diazo coupling of respective derivatives of p-aminophenylglycosides.

For glycohistochemical procedure see (1, 2). 5 µm sections were dewaxed and dehydrated. Blocking of endogenous peroxidase activity as well as unspecific binding sites of proteins was performed. The incubation of biotinylated neoglycoprotein was done with 50 µg/ml for 90 min

Table I. Investigated tumors (n = 26).

Type of tumor	n
Benign tumors	14
neurinoma	7
neurofibroma	2
traumatic neuroma	4
Abrikosoff tumor	1
Malignant tumors	12
neurogenic sarcomas	7
epitheloid schwannoma	3
melanotic schwannoma	1
myxoid schwannoma	1

---

[1] Dedicated to *Prof. Dr. Jürgen Knolle*, Flensburg, on the occasion of his 60th birthday.

at room temperature. Visualization of the specific binding sites with ABC kit reagents and DAB/H_2O_2 or AEC/H_2O_2 as chromogenic substrates; controls ascertained specificity (lack of binding of the labeled carrier, competitive inhibition).

Carbohydrate structures as part of the neoglycoproteins were as follows:
lactose (lac), α-N-acetylgalactosamine (α-galNAc), β-N-acetylgalactosamine (β-galNAc), β-N-acetylglucosamine (β-glcNAc), mannose (man), fucose (fuc), maltose (mal).

Results and discussion

Different expression patterns of endogenous lectins occur in benign (figure 1) and malignant (figure 2, table II) tumors of peripheral nervous system. The binding pattern of neoglycoproteins clearly depends on the nature of the individual carbohydrate component. It is noteworthy that the pattern is also dependent on the growth pattern and the cellular subpopulation (figure 3, 4) in the tumor. Ultrastructurally all types of peripheral nerve sheath tumors show long small cytoplasmic processes with tendency for infoldings, surrounding each other and arranged in a complex manner. This tendency to cover neighbouring surfaces with cytoplasmic processes is called "flächenumhüllendes Wachstum" (surface wrapping growth) and believed to be a characteristic of Schwann cells' nature (8). In malignant types of nerve sheath tumors a comparatively lower density of cell processes as in benign counterparts exists.

With respect to the extent of binding of the synthetic probes it was shown that a change of the extent of presence of neoglycoprotein binding sites appears to be related to the principle of so called "flächenumhüllendes Wachstum" and to malignancy of the tumors investigated: In correlation to Antoni A- or Antoni B-pattern benign tumors exhibit a uniform binding of neoglycoproteins; malignant tumors show a great intra- and intertumoral heterogeneity of the detectable endogenous lectins.

The pattern of endogenous sugar-binding proteins can have significance (1–3, 9, 10–12) for: tumor

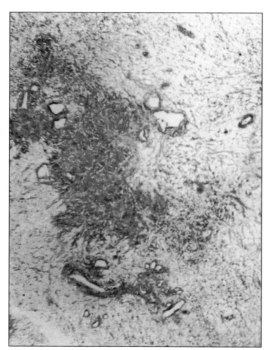

Figure 1. Binding pattern in solid and myxoid areas of neurinomas. High perivascular intensity of neoglycoprotein binding (Lac-BSA-biotin, x 40).

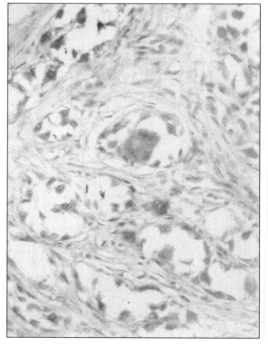

Figure 2. Moderate neoglycoprotein binding in an epitheloid malignant schwannoma (α-galNAc-BSA-biotin, x 250).

Table II. Binding pattern of EL in benign and malignant human nerve sheath neoplasms.

Tumor	Sugar						
	α-galNAc	fuc	mal	lac	β-glcNAc	man	β-galNAc
Schwannoma (n = 7)							
Antoni A	+/++	+	(+)	(+)	+	++	+
Antoni B	+/++	++	+/++	+++	+/++	+/++	+/++
interstitial	−	−	−	−	−	−	−
perivascular	+++	+++	+++	+++	+++	+++	+++
Neurofibroma (n = 2)	++	++	+	(+)/+	(+)/+	+	(+)/++
Traumatic neuroma (n = 4)	++	+	++	++	(+)/+	++	(+)/+
Neurogenic sarcoma (n = 7)	+/+++	(+)	(+)/++	++	(+)/++	+/++	(+)/+
epitheloid type (n = 3)	(+)/++	−/+	−/+++	−/++	−/++	+/++	−/++
melanotic type (n = 1)	++	++	+	+	+	++	++
myxoid type (n = 1)	−/(+)	−/(+)	−/(+)	−/(+)	−/(+)	−/(+)	−/(+)
Abrikosoff tumor (n = 1)	++	++	(+)	(+)	+	++	(+)

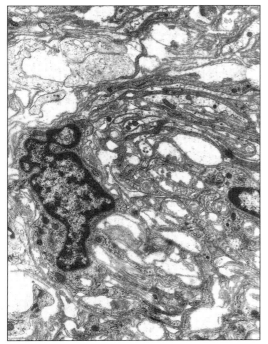

Figure 3. Benign schwannoma: complex aggregates of this long cytoplasmic processes with spiral arrangements (x 9000).

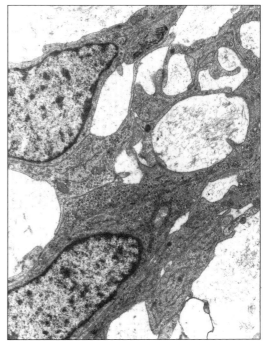

Figure 4. Malignant schwannoma: reduction in complexity of behavior of cytoplasmic processes, tendency for spiral like arrangements (x 6 000).

cell-stroma cell interactions, intratumoral immune response, modulation of the morphological behavior, tumor progression and prognosis.

The variability could be of importance for tumor cell invasion and metastasis and therefore for prognosis.

In answering the initially raised questions at present it is reasonable to give the following statements:

1. Malignant lesions show intra-tumoral and inter-tumoral heterogeneity of neoglycoprotein-binding capacity in neoplastic elements. Benign lesions show a uniform pattern.
2. There is a possible modulation of interaction between neoplastic and non-neoplastic cells with potential for the modulation of intra- and peri-tumoral immune response.

The prognostic significance of the binding pattern of endogenous lectins thus deserves further attention in subsequent studies.

References

1 Gabius HJ, Gabius S (eds) (1993) Lectins and glycobiology. Springer, Berlin, New York
2 Gabius HJ, Bardosi A (1991) Neoglycoproteins as tools in glycohistochemistry. Progr Histochem Cytochem 22:1-63
3 Gabius HJ, Gabius S (1990) Tumorlektinologie – Status und Perspektiven klinischer Anwendung. Naturwissenschaften 77:505-514
4 Alhadeff JA (1989) Malignant cell glycoproteins and glycolipids. CRC Crit Rev Oncol/Hematol 9:37-107
5 Cervos-Navarro J, Matakas F (1968) Elektronenmikroskopischer Beitrag zur Histogenese der Neurinome. Verh Dtsch Ges Path 52:391-393
6 Hakamori SI (1989) Aberrant glycosylation in tumors and tumor-associated carbohydrate antigens. Adv Cancer Res 52:257-331
7 Allison RT (1986) Lectins in diagnostic histopathology, a review. Med Lab Sci 43:369-376
8 Knolle J, Bahn H, Holzhausen HJ, Stiller O, Gabius HJ (1992) Glycohistochemical approach to unravel grade-dependent alterations by application of synthetic markers. In: Klapdor R (ed) Tumor associated antigens, oncogenes, receptors, cytokines in tumor diagnosis and therapy at the beginning of the nineties. Cancer of the breast – state and trends in diagnosis and therapy. Zuckschwerdt, München, pp 413-416
9 Gabius HJ (1991) Detection and functions of mammalian lectins-with emphasis on membrane lectins. Biochim Biophys Acta 1071:1-18
10 Gabius HJ, Gabius S (1993) Animal lectins: their contribution to the software of biocommunication, Bioregulators 1:18-26
11 Gabius S, Wawotzky R, Wilhelm S, Martin U, Wörmann B, Gabius HJ (1993) Adhesion of human lymphoid cell lines to immobilized carbohydrates and to bone marrow stromal cell layers by surface sugar receptors. Int J Cancer 54:1017-1021
12 Kayser K, Bovin NV, Korchagina EY, Zeilinger C, Zeng FY, Gabius HJ (1994) Correlation of expression of binding sites ror synthetic blood group A-, B-, and H-trisaccharides and for sarcolectin with survival of patients with bronchial carcinoma. Eur J Cancer. 30A:653-657

Address for correspondence:
Dr. med. J. Knolle
Institut für Pathologische Anatomie
Martin-Luther-Universität
Magdeburger Straße 14
D-06097 Halle/Saale, Germany

Patterns of endogenous sugar-binding proteins in benign and malignant soft tissue tumors[1]

J. Knolle[a], H. Bahn[a], H.-J. Holzhausen[a], F.-W. Rath[a], H.-J. Gabius[b]

[a] Institute of Pathology, Martin-Luther-University, Halle
[b] Institute of Physiological Chemistry, Veterinary Medical School, Ludwig-Maximilians-University, Munich, Germany

Introduction

Carbohydrate structures are increasingly considered as signals within tumor progression, metastasis formation and prognosis (1, 2). Assuming that recognitive protein-carbohydrate interactions are involved to mediate the biological effects of such epitopes, the concomitant localization of endogenous sugar binding sites like lectins is clearly warranted. By chemically conjugating suitable carbohydrate ligands to a histochemically inert carrier, neoglycoconjugates are produced for this purpose, already being tested in histology (3–7). Here, we report on initial studies of the application of labeled neoglycoproteins with respect to different benign and malignant soft tissue tumors.

Material and methods

Formalin-fixed, paraffin-embedded specimens of the soft tissue tumors (table I) were used. For details of the glycohistochemical procedure see (3–6).
Neoglycoproteins were obtained by diazo coupling of respective derivatives of p-aminophenyl-glycosides. 5 µm sections were dewaxed and dehydrated. Blocking of endogenous peroxidase activity as well as of unspecific binding sites of proteins was performed. The incubation with biotinylated neoglycoproteins was done with 50 µg/ml, for 90 min at room temperature. Visualization of specific binding sites was obtained with ABC kit reagents and DAB H_2O_2 or AEC/H_2O_2 as chromogenic substrates. Control reaction as given in detail in (5) were negative. In the majority of cases material was fixed in glutaraldehyde for electronmicroscopic investigations.

Results

Application of a panel of neoglycoproteins with various types of ligand structures yielded a positive reaction in most cases. A striking difference of expression of binding sites was seen in the different benign and malignant soft tissue tumors (table II). The extent of specific staining revealed a non-uniform distribution, in relation to the growth texture and also to the various cellular subpopulations (figures 1–4) in the tumors. Benign tumors exhibited a relative homogenous staining by labeled neoglycoproteins, whereas malignant soft tissue tumors had a great intra- and inter-tumoral heterogeneity of expression of endogenous lectins. With an increasing degree of cellular atypia the heterogeneity of cytoplasmic staining is enhanced. Nuclear staining was not detectable in the sarcomas.

Table I. Investigated tumors.

Type of tumor	n
Lipomas	4
Liposarcomas	5
Rhabdomyoma	1
Rhabdomyosarcomas	7
Fibrosarcomas	2
Benign fibrohistiocytic tumors	18
Malignant fibrous histiocytomas	12

---

[1] Dedicated to *Prof. Dr. Jürgen Knolle*, Flensburg, on the occasion of his 60th birthday.

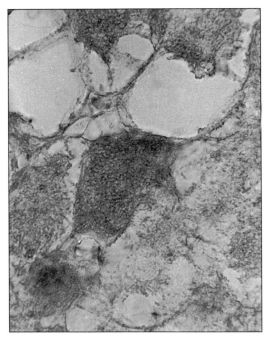

Figure 1. Embryonal rhabdomyosarcoma. Neoglycoprotein binding in well differentiated neoplastic cells (mal-BSA-biotin, 1000 x).

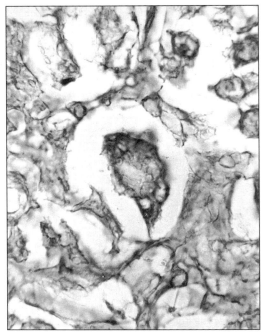

Figure 2. Alveolar rhabdomyosarcoma. Staining in mononuclear and multinuclear non-cohesive tumor cells (lac-BSA-biotin, 1000 x).

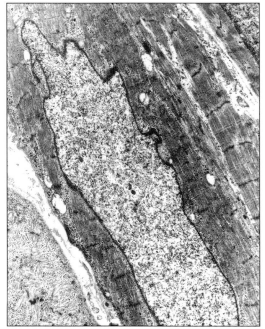

Figure 3. Embryonal rhabdomyosarcoma. Well differentiated myotube-like rhabdomyoblasts with typical myofibrillar organization (6000 x).

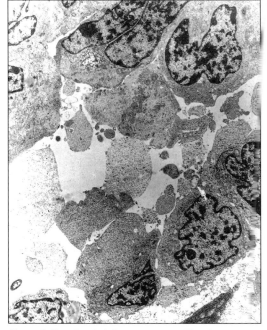

Figure 4. Alveolar rhabdomyosarcoma. Alveolar arrangement of primitive mesenchymal tumor cells with loss of cohesivity at the luminal surface (3000 x).

Table II. Neoglycoprotein binding in neoplastic cells in rhabdomyosarcomas and embryonal and alveolar rhabdomyosarcomas.

	Sugar						
	lac	α-galNAc	β-galNAc	β-glcNAc	α-man	α-fuc	mal
Tumor type							
Rhabdomyoma (genitial) (n = 1)							
Neoplastic cells	–	–	–	–	–	–	–
Embryonal rhabdomyosarcoma (n = 5)							
Neoplastic cells	(+)/++	(+)/+	(+)/++	(+)/++	(+)/++	–/++	(+)/++
Alveolar rhabdomyosarcoma (n = 2)							
Mononuclear giant cells	+/++	++	–/+	(+)/+	–/++	–/(+)	–/++

Discussion

Our initial results indicate that the binding of neoglycoproteins to the mesenchymal cells can correlate to the entity, the growth pattern and the cellular subpopulation. The nature of the carbohydrate ligand is responsible for the specific protein-carbohydrate interaction, warranting further synthetic efforts to extent the panel.

In contrast to the sarcomas, the benign tumors have a uniform pattern. Since the presence of such activities can influence various intracellular processes as well as tumor-cell-tumor-cell interaction, tumor-stroma cell (tumor cell-macrophage) interaction, and the tumor-cell-matrix interaction the results presented are also considered as guidelines for ensuing biochemical and cell biological research that may have benefit for therapeutical approaches. It is also noteworthy that lectin-carbohydrate interactions are relevant for immunomodulation, as currently discussed for a plant lectin and its potential oncological application (8). A comprehensive analysis of the sugar-binding proteins within sarcomas thus seems to offer aspects for further research.

Acknowledgement

The gererous financial support of the Dr. M. Scheel Stiftung für Krebsforschung is gratefully acknowledged.

References

1 Hakomori SI (1991) Possible functions of tumor-associated carbohydrate antigens. Curr Opinion Immunol 3:546–653
2 Muramatsu T (1993) Carbohydrate signals in metastasis and prognosis of human carcinomas. Glycobiol 3:291–296
3 Gabius HJ, Nagel GA (eds) (1988) Lectins and glycoconjugates in oncology. Springer, Berlin
4 Gabius HJ, Gabius S (eds) (1991) Lectins and cancer. Springer, Berlin
5 Gabius HJ, Bardosi A (1991) Neoglycoproteins as tool in glycohistochemistry. Progr Histochem Cytochem 22:1–66
6 Gabius HJ, Gabius S (eds) (1993) Lectins and glycobiology. Springer-Berlin
7 Danguy A, Akif F, Pajak B, Gabius HJ (1994) Contribution of carbohydrate histochemistry to glycobiology. Histol Histopathol 9:155–171
8 Gabius HJ, Gabius S, Joski SS, Koch B, Schröder M, Manzke WM, Westerhausen M (1994) From ill-defined extracts to the immunomodulatory lectin: will there be a reason for oncological application of mistletoe? Planta med 60:2–7

Address for correspondence:
Dr. med. J. Knolle
Institut für Pathologische Anatomie
Martin-Luther-Universität
Magdeburger Straße 14
D-06097 Halle/Saale, Germany

Immunohistochemical analysis of various basement membrane components in dermal cylindromas

A. Nerlich[a], R. Berndt[b], I. Wiest[b], E. Schleicher[c]

[a]Institute for Pathology of the University of Munich, [b]Institute for Pathology of the Municipal Hospital, Worms, [c]Institute for Research on Diabetes, Municipal Hospital, Munich, Germany

Introduction

Cylindromas are rare tumors of the dermis which are presumed to be derived from cells of skin appendeges, most obviously from the sweat gland duct epithelium (2). Their characteristic histomorphological feature is the deposition of excessive amounts of a basement membrane material around and between the tumor cell nests (2, 13). Dermal cylindromas usually show a locally invasive, but not otherwise aggressive or metastatic biological growth pattern. In rare instances, however, a malignant course of the tumor growth has been observed. Thus, up to now approximately 16 cases of malignant dermal cylindromas have been reported in the literature (5). These are characterized by a locally aggressive growth pattern as well as the occurence of a systemic metastatic spread has also been described (5).

Previous immunohistochemical analyses demonstrated that the cylindromas share an overexpression of the basement membrane components analyzed up to now (2, 6, 8, 10, 12, 13). There exists, however, until now no comprehensive analysis on the expression and distribution of major BM-components in the tumor center in comparison to the marginal tumor front where the local stroma invasion takes place. Furthermore, no immunohistochemical analysis has yet been performed on cylindroma tissue from a malignant cylindroma. Such an analysis, however, seems to be useful for the interpretation of the biological tumor behavior, since it is presumed that the usually benign growth pattern is linked to the excessive BM expression.

Material and methods

In the present study, we used tumor tissue from eleven patients with histologically proven cylindroma all of which showed a benign clinical course, as well as tumor material from one case with a clearly malignant and locally aggressive dermal cylindroma (5). The detailed patient data, the tumor localization and the tumor size are given in table I.

The tumor tissue specimens had been routinely processed for histological examination. For the immunohistochemical analysis we used monospecific antibodies against the major BM-components collagen IV and VII, laminin, heparan sulfate proteoglycan (HSPG) and fibronectin which had been obtained from the following sources: collagen IV and laminin antibodies had been purchased from Eurodiagnostics, Apeldoorn, NL, the fibronectin antibody from Dako, Hamburg, FRG. The anti-HSPG antibodies had been

Table I. Clinical data of the cylindroma patients.

No.	Age	Sex	Localization	Size
1	50	m	head	1.5 cm
2	36	f	back	1.5 cm
3	77	m	hand	1 cm
4	57	f	shoulder	0.5 cm
5	67	f	retroauricular	0.8 cm
6	80	m	head	0.8 cm
7	62	f	fore head	0.7 cm
8	86	f	shoulder	4 cm
9	49	f	head	0.5 cm
10	66	m	ear concha	1 cm
11	72	m	head	1.5 cm
12[a]	69	f	head	3 cm

[a]Malignant cylindroma

prepared as described previously (11). The anti-collagen VII antibodies had been greatfully supplied by Dr. R. Burgeson, Portland, Oregon, USA. Appropriate tissue sections were then stained by use either of the avidin-biotin-peroxidase complexe method (ABC-method) (7) or the alkaline phosphatase-anti-alkaline phosphatase method (APAAP-method) (3) using the previously described procedure (9).

Results

All eleven benign dermal cylindromas showed cytomorphologically a monomorphic cellular aspect. These tumors were rather circumscribed with some finger-like tumor cell nests extending into the adjacent stroma providing a locally infiltrative growth pattern. Most of these tumor cell nests were surrounded by variably broad bands of a hyaline PAS-positive material. Occasionally, droplet-like inclusions of a similar material were seen within tumor nests. In the malignant case, focally the typical features of cylindroma were preserved. In addition, major parts of this tumor showed enhanced cellular pleomorphism and a disseminated tumor cell growth into the stroma, including invasion of peripheral nerves and skin adnexal structures.

In all cytomorphologically benign tumors we observed an excessive expression of BM-components which was most prominent in the tumor center and occasionally at the tumor border. This BM material consisted mainly of collagen IV, collagen VII and HSPG and in most cases to a slightly lesser extent of laminin (table II). Fibronectin in contrast was only weakly positive in most cases and there were only few tumors analyzed where the band-like hyaline mass was intensely fibronectin positive (table II). A similar staining pattern was also seen in the BM-droplets within tumor cell nests. In contrast to this extensive BM-deposition, we found at the "invasion front" in all specimens tumor nests which showed a very weak and often fragmented BM. Here again the afore mentioned BM-components were affected.

In the malignant dermal cylindroma, those areas of typical cylindroma aspect showed a BM pattern as indicated before. In the "less differentiated" infiltrating areas, however, only fragments of BM-material around individual cells or small cell nests could be found as reported.

Discussion

The excessive production and deposition of BM material around or within tumor cell nests of dermal cylindromas has repeatedly been described (2, 6, 8, 10, 12, 13). None of these previous studies, however, analyzed the expression of BM-components in different areas of the tumor tissue. Since it is widely believed that an expression of BM-material is associated with a benign tumor growth (4), such an analysis seems to be useful to find out whether there exists an intratumoral heterogeneity in the BM-expression which may explain the locally expansive and invasive tumor growth. We observed indeed a marked variability in the deposition of BM-material around tumor cell nests with particular reference to a focal lack of BM at the "invasion front". Our observations are furthermore supported by the findings in the malignant dermal cylindroma which shows an extensive fragmentation of the BM-material in the "less differentiated" and obviously aggressively infiltrating tumor parts. This observation explains the (mostly limited) infiltrative tumor behavior. It is thus

Table II. Immunohistochemical staining results in cylindroma tissue.

No.	Coll IV	Coll VII	Laminin	HSPG	Fibronectin
1	+/++	+	(+)	+	(+)
2	++	++	+/++	++	(+)
3	+++	++	++	+++	+
4	+	+	+	+	(+)
5	+++	++	++	++	+
6	+++	++	++	+	-
7	++	++	++	++	-
8	+++	++	+++	+++	+/++
9	++	+	+	++	(+)
10	++	++	+	+	(+)
11	++	++	++	+	(+)
12[a]	(+)/++[b]	(+)/++[b]	(+)/++[b]	(+)/+[b]	(+)[b]

[a]Malignant cylindroma, [b]staining intensity depending on the degree of tissue invasion; - = not detectable, (+) = weakly/focally detectable; +-+++ = detection with increasing intensity

conceivable that isolated tumor cells or small tumor cell groups (temporarily?) loose their BM-synthetic capacity which may lead to a local tumor invasion into the surrounding stroma. It is furthermore assumable that invasive tumor growth stops with regain of the BM-production "control" by these cells. In very rare instances, malignant transformation occurs which is associated with an at least partial loss in BM-production. This feature has been shown in this study where for the first time the BM-pattern of a malignant cylindroma was analyzed. The phenomenon of BM-loss is quite well known from invasive carcinomas (1). It is thus fair to assume that the analysis of BM-material in cylindromas allows an estimation of its invasive growth potential.

References

1. Barsky SH, Siegal GP, Jannotta F, Liotta LA (1983) Loss of basement membrane components by invasive tumors but not by their benign counterparts. Lab Invest 49:140–147
2. Bruckner-Tuderman L, Pfaltz M, Schnyder UW (1991) Cylindroma overexpress collagen VII, the major anchoring fibril protein. J Invest Dermatol 96:729–734
3. Cordell JL, Falini B, Erber WN, Ghosh AK, Abdulaziz Z, MacDonald S, Pulford AF, Stein H, Mason DY (1984) Immunoenzymatic labeling of monoclonal antibodies using immune complexes of alkaline phosphatase and monoclonal antialkaline phosphatase. J Histochem Cytochem 32:219–225
4. D'Ardenne AJ (1989) Use of basement membrane markers in tumor diagnosis. J Clin Pathol 42:449–457
5. Grouls V, Iwaszkiewicz J, Berndt R (1991) Malignes dermales Zylindrom. Pathologe 12:157–160
6. Haustein UF, Wichmann K, Herrmann K. (1986) Basalmembrankomponenten beim Basaliom, Zylindrom und Plattenepithelcarcinom. Dermatol Mnschr 172:648–656
7. Hsu SM, Raine L, Fanger H (1981) A comparative study on the peroxidase-antiperoxidase method and an avidin-biotin- complex method for studying polypeptide hormones with radioimmunoassay antibodies. Am J Clin Pathol 75:734–739
8. Kallioninen M (1985) Immunelectronmicroscopic demonstration of the basement membrane components laminin and type IV collagen in the dermal cylindroma. J Pathol 147:97–102
9. Nerlich A, Schleicher E (1991) Immunohistochemical localization of extracellular matrix components in human diabetic glomerular lesions. Am J Pathol 139:889–899
10. Pfaltz M, Bruckner-Tuderman L, Schnyder UW (1989) Type VII collagen is a component of cylindroma basement membrane zone. J Cutan Pathol 16:388–395
11. Schleicher ED, Wagner EM, Olgemöller B, Nerlich A, Gerbitz KD. Characterization and localization of basement membrane associated heparan sulfate proteoglycan in human tissues. Lab Invest 61:323–332
12. Stanley JR, Beckwith JB, Fuller RP, Katz SI (1982) A specific antigen defect of the basement membrane found in basal cell carcinoma but not in other epidermal tumors. Cancer 50:1486–1490
13. Weber L, Wick G, Gebhart W, Krieg T, Timpl R (1984) Basement membrane components outline tumour islands in cylindroma. Br J Dermatol 111:45–51

Address for correspondence:
Priv.-Doz. Dr. med. A. Nerlich
Pathologisches Institut der Universität
Thalkirchnerstraße 36
D-80337 München, Germany

Characterization of LDL receptor-binding and LDL internalization with various human tumor cell lines

Sylvia Egert, Reingard Senekowitsch
Nuclearmedical Clinic, Technical University, Munich, Germany

Introduction

Rapidly growing tumor cells require a high amount of cholesterin for membrane synthesis and therefore take up low density lipoprotein (LDL), the main cholesterol carrier in blood, via LDL receptor mediated endocytosis (1, 2). Dividing cells have higher receptor-mediated uptake of LDL than non-dividing cells. With scintigraphic methods, it has been shown in previous studies that certain types of tumors have higher LDL receptor activity than the corresponding normal tissue (3, 4). Hence, LDL receptors may possibly be used in distinguishing between tumor tissue and normal tissue, which may give further advantages in diagnosis and prognosis. In regard to LDL as a carrier for antineoplastic drugs and radionuclides (5, 6) characterization of LDL internalization efficacy may determine tumor therapy.

The aim of this study was to establish an in vitro LDL radioreceptor assay with ^{125}I-LDL as a ligand to determine the LDL receptor density (Bmax), the dissociation constant (k_D) of the ligand-receptor complex and the ability to internalise surface-bound LDL among different tumor cell lines. Stimulation of LDL receptors and LDL internalisation with lipoprotein deficient medium compared to normal medium was investigated and, also, the effect of chloroquine (an inhibitor of lysosomal LDL-degradation) on receptor density and LDL internalization.

Material and methods

LDL was prepared by sequential KBr-density-gradient ultracentrifugation (7) with subsequent extensive dialysis and iodinated with ^{125}I by the N-bromosuccinimide-method (8). Lipoprotein deficient serum (LPDS) was obtained by ultracentrifugation of human serum at a density of 1.215 g/ml followed by 72 hours of dialysis (9).

Five human cell lines were investigated: Hep G2, a hepatocellular carcinoma, A 431, an epidermoid cell carcinoma of the vulva, Hela, a cervix carcinoma, J 82, a bladder transitional cell carcinoma and SW 707, a colon adenocarcinoma.

Radioligand binding assays were carried out with adherent cell monolayer in culture (9). 48 h LPDS-stimulated and non-stimulated cells were incubated with 10 µg/ml ^{125}I-LDL (total binding) and various concentrations (0–500 µg/ml) of non-radiolabeled LDL (3 h of incubation). Non-specific binding was determined with the 50-fold excess of unlabeled LDL (500 µg/ml). The specific binding was calculated from the difference between total binding and non-specific binding. To differentiate surface-bound LDL from internalised LDL, cells were incubated with a heparin containing buffer, which leads to a release of surface-bound LDL. The cellular LDL-uptake was measured with cells homogenized in 0.1 n NaOH.

Maximal receptor binding (Bmax), maximal LDL internalization/3 hours and the dissociation constant (k_D) were achieved by "Scatchard"-plot analysis of binding data (10).

Results

All cell lines investigated show LDL-displacable specific binding indicating the existence of specific LDL receptors (figure 1). Nearly 100% of ^{125}I-LDL is internalised via LDL receptor mediated endocytosis, (figure 2). Scatchard-plot analysis of the data represented yield saturable, high affinity binding of LDL to its receptor. The cell lines show the following characteristic k_D (µg LDL-prot./ml): SW 707 (11), A 431 (13), Hela (27), Hep G2 (29),

J 82 (32). 48 h LPDS stimulated cells express a high amount of LDL receptors. Among the cell lines used, Bmax varies over a wide range (ng LDL-prot./mg cell-prot.), (figure 3a): SW 707 (40) < Hela (81) < Hep G2 (101) < J 82 (119) < A 431 (156). For LDL internalization, Scatchard-plot analysis results in following maximal concentrations (ng LDL-prot./mg cell-prot./3h), (figure 3b): SW 707 (380) < Hep G2 (580) < A 431 (600) < J 82 (850) < Hela (940).

Represented data are indicating, that maximal internalization of surface-bound LDL not only depends on Bmax, which is typical for a cell line, but also on the cell line-specific internalization efficiency.

The stimulation of lipoprotein deficient medium versus lipoprotein containing medium and the effect of chloroquine (100 µM chloroquine was added to the incubation medium as an inhibitor of lysosomal LDL degradation (9, 11) on receptor density and internalization were investigated.

Stimulation of LDL binding and internalization were SW 707 (18%) < Hep G2 (22%) < J 82 (180%) (figure 4 a, b).

The addition of chloroquine to the incubation medium shows no negative effect on SW 707 and J 82 cells but with Hep G2 cells, a 50%-reduction of LDL-binding and internalization could be found (figure 5 a, b).

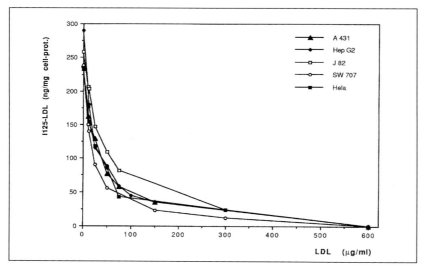

Figure 1. Specific binding of ^{125}I-LDL to different cell lines with increasing concentrations of unlabeled LDL.

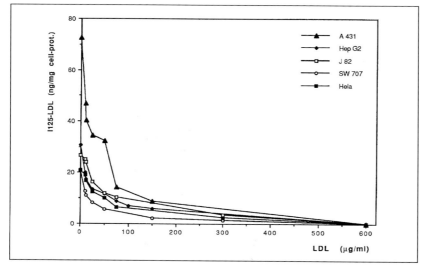

Figure 2. Specific internalization of ^{125}I-LDL in different cell lines with increasing concentrations of unlabeled LDL.

Immunohistochemistry 667

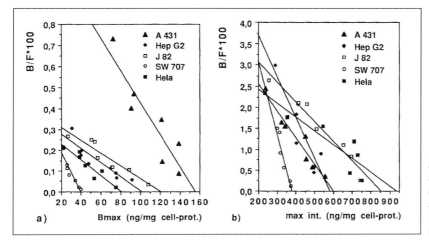

Figure 3. Scatchard plot analysis of LDL binding and internalization; a) LDL binding, B_{max} b) LDL internalization, max intern/3 h.

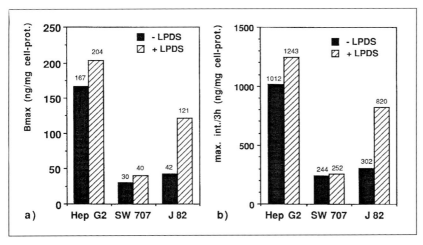

Figure 4. a) LDL binding and b) LDL internalization depending on LPDS stimulation.

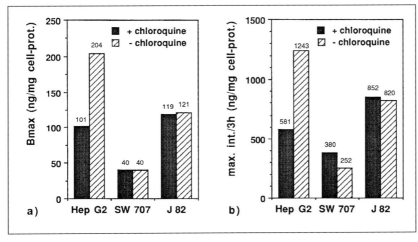

Figure 5. a) LDL binding and b) LDL internalization of LPDS stimulated cells depending on chloroquine.

Discussion

This study compared five cell lines with different tissue origin in regard to their ability to bind and to internalize LDL in a specific receptor-dependent mechanism.

The results show, that the amount of specifically internalized LDL does not only correlate with the amount of LDL bound to the LDL receptor but also with the efficiency of LDL internalization, which differs among the investigated cell lines. Hela cells, which internalize an 11.6-fold amount of LDL (per 3 h) to LDL-surface binding, appear to have the best internalization efficacy with respect to their surface-bound receptors. The corresponding factor for SW 707 is 9.5, for J 82 it is 7.2, for Hep G2 5.8 and A 431 cells only internalize a 3.9-fold amount of LDL in respect to their LDL surface binding.

A probable explanation for the large differences in LDL internalization efficacy is a various LDL-distribution at the membrane surface of each cell line. Of importance, for the most effective LDL uptake, is the amount of receptors localized in the so called "coated pits" (12, 13). In our opinion, the efficacy of tumor LDL internalization is decisive for possible tumor therapy with LDL conjugates (radioisotopes or drugs).

The newly characterised LDL receptor systems of J 82 and SW 707 possess all properties of the well-known LDL receptor system of Hep G2 cells. Receptor binding shows high affinity, specificity, saturation and the capacity for LPDS stimulation. Fast proliferation, easy handling and chloroquine-resistance are properties suggesting further use in studies with LDL as a carrier of cytotoxic drugs.

Furthermore, the established in vitro LDL receptor assay gives application possibilities for tumor diagnosis and prognosis. This is especially valuable in combination with noninvasive scintigraphic imaging since tumor tissue has higher LDL receptor density than corresponding normal tissue.

References

1. Vitols S, Gahrton G, Öst A, Peterson C (1984) Elevated low density lipoprotein receptor activity in leucemic cells with monocytic differentiation, Blood, Vol 63:1186–1193
2. Peterson C, Vitols S, Rudling M, Blomgren H, Edsmyr F, Skoog L (1985) Hypocholesterolemia in cancer patients may be caused by elevated LDL receptor activities in malignant cells. Med Oncol Tumor Pharmacother 2:143–147
3. Friedrich E, Dresel HA, Sinn HJ, Schettler G (1985) Visualisation of the hepatic low density lipoprotein receptor in rats by sequential scintiscans. FEBS 184: 134–138
4. Vitols S, Söderberg-Reid K, Masquelier M, Sjöstrom B, Peterson C (1990) Low density lipoprotein for delivery of a water-insoluble alkylating agent to malignant cells. In vitro and in vivo studies of a drug-lipoprotein complex. Br J Cancer 62: 724–729
5. Lestavel-Delattre S, Martin-Nizard F, Clavey V, Testard, P, Favre G, Doualin G, Houssaini H, Bard J, Duriez P, Delbart C, Soula G, Lesieur D, Lesieur I, Cazin JC M, Fruchard J, (1992) Low density lipoprotein for delivery of an acrylophenone antineoplastic molecule into neoplastic cells. Cancer Res 52:3629–3635
6. Filipowska D, Filipowski T, Morelowska B, Kazanowska W, Laudanski T, Lapinjoki S, Akerlund M, Breeze A (1992) Treatment of cancer patients with a low density lipoprotein delivery vehicle containing a cytotoxic drug. Cancer Chemother Pharmacol 29:396–400
7. Havel R, Eder H, Bragdon J (1955) The distribution and chemical composition of ultracentrifugally separated lipoproteins in human serum. J Clin Invest 34:1345–1353
8. Sinn HJ, Schrenck HH, Friedrich EA, Via DP, Dresel HA (1988) Radioiodination of proteins and lipoproteins using N-bromosuccinimide as oxidizing agent. Anal Biochem 170:186–192
9. Goldstein JL, Basu SK, Brown MS (1983) Receptor mediated endocytosis of low density lipoprotein in cultured cells. Meth Enzymol 98:241–260
10. Repke H, Liebmann C (1986) Membranrezeptoren und ihre Effektorsysteme. VHC-Verlagsgesellschaft mbH, Weinheim p 1–101
11. Anderson RG, Brown MS, Goldstein JL (1981) Inefficient internalization of receptor bound low density lipoprotein in human carcinoma A-431 cells. J Cell Biol 88:441–452
12. Goldstein B, Wiegel FW (1988) The distribution of cell surface proteins on spreading cells. Comparison of theory with experiment. Biophys J 53 (2): 175–185
13. Goldstein JL, Anderson RG, Brown MS (1979) Coated pits, coated vesicles and receptor-mediated endocytosis. Nature 279: 679–684

Address for correspondence:
Prof. Dr. Dr. Reingard Senekowitsch
Nuklearmedizinische Klinik
Technische Universität München
Ismaninger Straße 22
D-81675 München, Germany

Immunoscintigraphy

Radioimmunoscintigraphy of head and neck squamous cell cancer with 99mTc-labeled antibody SQ 174 – First results in 10 patients

L. Fritsche[a], B. Grünert[a], E. Heissler[b], G. Barzen[a], M. Cordes[a], R. Felix[a]

[a]Clinic for Radiology and Policlinic, Department of Nuclear Medicine,
[b]Clinic for Maxillofacial Surgery, Klinikum Rudolf Virchow, Free University, Berlin, Germany

Introduction

Squamous cell carcinomas (SCC) rank high in the global incidence figures for human cancers and their frequency in both men and women is rising again in several western countries (1). It is generally accepted that the status of the cervical lymph nodes is the single most important prognostic factor in head and neck SCC (5). But although high resolution computed tomography (CT) and magnetic resonance imaging (MRI) have improved the clinical assessment, the staging of lymph nodes is still a problem (2). Radioimmunoscintigraphy (RIS) as the only non-invasive diagnostic tool depending on histological dignity instead of morphological criteria may have the potential to fill this gap. In this study, the new 99mTc-labeled antibody SQ 174 has been evaluated for its safety and diagnostic accuracy in patients with histologically proven head and neck SCC.

Patients and methods

Antibody SQ 174

SQ 174 is a murine monoclonal antibody of the IgG1 subclass. The antigen recognized by SQ 174 is situated in the proliferative compartment of mammalian stratified squamous epithelium and SCC. It was characterized as a cytoskeletal protein with a molecular weight of 57.000, is soluble in SDS but not in Nonidet P-40. Histopathological studies of the frozen tissue sections (n = 201) demonstrated selective binding of SQ 174 to SCCs of human (49/49), bovine, canine, feline and murine origin. Tumors of other histological types did not show reactivity with the antibody. Studies on normal human tissue showed selective binding of the antibody to the basal layer of stratified squamous epithelia, thymic epithelial cells and myoepithelial cells around breast ducts. No antibody binding was observed for the suprabasal layers of stratified epithelia, simple epithelia or tissues of non–epithelial origin (3). Attempts to detect the antigen in the serum of SCC-patients were not successful.

Preparation

All radiolabeling procedures were performed under aseptic conditions using sterile and pyrogen free glassware, plastics and solutions. SQ 174 is supplied by Biomira Inc., Edmonton, Canada, as a deep frozen one-vial-kit (Tru-Scint SQ). The antibody was labeled with 99mTc from a Behring Tc Gen Generator applying the reduction mediated technique developed by *Schwarz* and *Steinsträsser* (4). Binding of the 99mTc by the antibody preparation was assessed by chromatography on ITLC-SG strips (Gelman Sciences, Ann Arbor, MI) and always found to be over 92% (mean 96%).

Patient study

We investigated ten patients with histologically proven SCC aged 51 to 73 (median = 64) presurgically staged according to the UICC-classification as T1 in two cases, T3 in one and T4 in seven patients. Six patients were staged as neck node negative (N0), the other four patients as stage N2. The primary lesions were situated in the tongue (n = 2), palate (n = 1), lower jaw (n = 3), pharynx (n = 2). Two cases showed recurrences (lower jaw, orbita). Histological grading ranged from I to IV (I: n = 1, II: n = 7, III: n = 1, IV: n = 1). None of the patients had recieved radiotherapy before investigation in this study. Written informed consent was obtained from each patient. CT, MRI and ultrasound (US) imaging was performed prior to RIS. MRI and CT were performed in native and contrast technique (Magnetovist®, Isovist®) using a Somatom Plus or DR3 (Siemens) for CT and a 1,5-Tesla-Magnetom (Siemens) for MRI. A linear-array-head at 7.5 MHz was used for US. Blood chemistry and full blood count were acquired before and after antibody application and evaluated for significant changes using the Wilcoxon test for paired values. Serum samples for monitoring HAMA formation were drawn before, two and four weeks after RIS. Vital parameters (heart rate, blood pressure and respiration frequency) were controlled in narrow intervals (15, 30, 60, 120, 180 min) during the first three hours after application.

Each patient received 2 mg SQ 174 radiolabeled with 1 to 1.7 GBq 99mTc by injection into the cubital vein. Imaging was performed in planar and single photon emission computed tomography (SPECT) technique 3-4 and 22-25 hours post injection using a large field of view single head gamma camera (Apex SP 415, Elscint, Haifa). Additional early planar images for visualizing the blood pool were acquired within the first 30 minutes. A general purpose low energy parallel hole collimator was used. Planar images were acquired with a matrix size of 256 x 256 (= 2.21 mm/pixel) until a total of 1 million counts had been registered. Images were obtained in anterior and posterior views of head and chest. SPECT was performed in step-and shoot mode (6°, 10-45 s/step) with a matrix size of 64 x 64 (= 8.84 mm/pixel). The acquired data were processed by filtered backprojection applying a ramp- and a metz-filter-algorithm. All images were interpreted by three clinicians experienced in the field of CT, MRI and scintigraphy. The evaluation of locations with increased activity in RIS was based on comparison between early and late images and on asymmetries of activity distribution. For optimal topographical comparability of findings by the different investigations and histopathological results the lymph nodes were classified as topographic levels (figure I) according to recommendations by the DÖSAK (German Austrian Swiss working group on tumors in the maxillo-facial region) and ADT (association of German tumor centres). Thus eight lymph node levels were evaluated per patient (level I-IV right/left).

After the investigation five patients (TI = I, T4 = 4, N0 = 4, N2 = 1) recieved radical surgery with neck dissection within six days after RIS. In the other five patients surgery was not performed with regard to the advanced stage of disease. These patients were controlled by repeated routine investigations during a follow-up period of at least six months and all data was retrospectively integrated into a concordant result.

Results

No adverse reactions were observed after antibody application. The blood investigations showed a significant rise (p < 0.05) in the leukocyte count. All other parameters did not show significant changes (Wilcoxon test for paired values). Nine out of ten primary sites were detected by SQ 174 immunoscintigraphy (figure 2). The tumor which could not be detected by RIS was a T1/G I lesion in the aryepiglottic fold and was seen in CT and MRI. The tumor/non-tumor activity ratio ranged between 1.3 and 1.7 as determined by region of interest (ROI)-technique in planar images. In eight

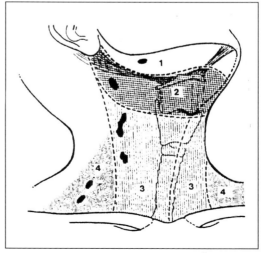

Figure 1. Topographic lymph node levels (DÖSAK classification).

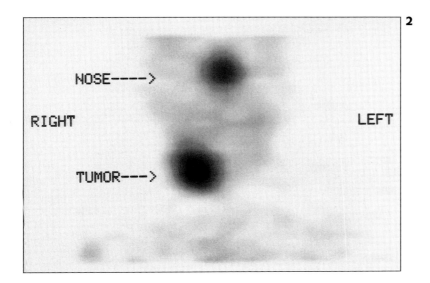

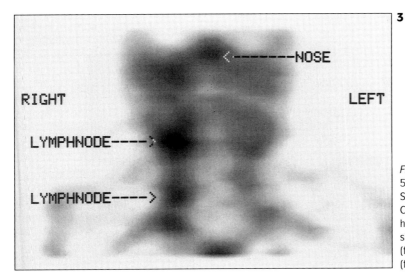

Figures 2 and 3. Patient 8, age 58, with right paramandibular SCC (T4 N2c, Grade II). Coronar SPECT images 24 hours after application showing the primary lesion (figure 2) and lymph node (figure 3).

patients the ratio in the 24 hour images exceeded the 4 hour ratio. No non-lymphatic metastases were found by any diagnostic means. In RIS-imaging 14 lymph node levels were visualized as positive (figure 3, table I). Of the five patients who recieved neck dissection one had a histopathologically proven positive lymph node in level 2 (left side) which was visualized by RIS, CT and MRI. In these patients CT, MRI and US showed several false positive lymph nodes. The group of patients not surgically evaluated shows a higher incidence of lymph node involvement in accordance to the advanced stage of disease.

Under the assumption that the concordant follow-up results are applicable as a standard, SQ 174 RIS showed a sensitivity of 78% (CT = 70%, MRI = 90% and US = 47%) and specificity of 87% (CT = 83%, MRI = 100% and US = 30%) for all investigated sites.

Conclusions

In the patients investigated the application of SQ 174 appeared to be safe. The primary lesion was visualized in nine out of ten cases. Both recur-

Table I. Presence of metastases per lymph node level (1, 2, 3, 4) as assessed by SQ 174 radioimmunoscintigraphy and conventional investigations (+: true positive; –: true negative; 0: false positive; #: false negative; /: not done).

Patient	CT	MR	US	RIS	Histology
1 right	# # – –	/	# – – –	– – – –	– – – –
left	– – – –	/	– – – –	– – – –	– – – –
2 right	– – – –	– – – –	– – – –	– – – –	– – – –
left	– – – –	– – – –	– – – –	– – – –	– – – –
3 right	– – – –	– – – –	– – – –	– – – –	– – – –
left	– – – –	– – – –	– – – –	– – – –	– – – –
4 right	# # – –	# – – –	/	– – – –	– – – –
left	# + – –	– + – –	/	– + – –	– + – –
5 right	– – + –	– – – –	– # # –	– – – –	– – – –
left	– – – –	– – – –	# – # –	– – – –	– – – –
6 right	+ + + +	+ + + +	+ + + +	+ + + +	+ + + +
left	+ + – –	+ + – –	+ + – –	+ 0 – –	+ + – –
7 right	– – – –	– – – –	– – – –	– – – –	– – – –
left	– – – –	– – – –	– – – –	– – # –	– – – –
8 right	+ + – –	+ + # –	+ + # –	+ + # #	+ + – –
left	0 – – –	+ – – –	0 # – –	+ – – –	+ – – –
9 right	– – – –	– – – –	– – – –	– – – –	– – – –
left	– – – –	– – – –	– – – –	– – – –	– – – –
10 right	– – – –	/	– # # –	– – # –	– – – –
left	# – # –	/	# # # –	– – # –	– – – –

In most cases the best images were produced by 24 hour SPECT. The image quality suffered from the low signal noise ratio and low count rates 24 hours after application.

rences investigated were visualized. The majority of the investigated lymph node metastases could be detected by RIS using SQ 174. In this group of patients MRI was the superior diagnostic tool. With regard to the small number of patients and the unrandomized study design, our findings suggest that SQ 174 RIS may contribute to the diagnostics of recurrences and lymph node metastases in SCC of head and neck in selected cases. Studies with larger patient numbers are underway to evaluate the potential of SQ 174 for general clinical application.

References

1 Carter RL, (1993) Pathology of squamous carcinomas of the head and neck. Curr Opin Oncol 5(3):491–495
2 Hillsamer PJ, Schuller DE, McGhee RB, Chakeres D, Young DC (1990) Improving diagnostic accuracy of cervical metastases with computed tomography and magnetic resonance imaging. Arch Otolaryngol Head Neck Surg 119:1297–1301
3 Samuel J, Noujaim AA, Willans DJ et al (1989) A novel marker for basal (stem) cells of mammalian stratified squamous epithelia and squamous cell carcinomas. Cancer Res 49:2465–2470
4 Schwarz A, Steinsträsser A (1987) A novel approach to Tc99m labelled Mab. J Nucl Med 28:721
5 Snow GB, Patel P, Leemans CR, Tiwari R (1992) Management of cervical lympnodes in patients with head and neck cancer. Eur Arch Otorhinolaryngol 249:187–194

Address for correspondence:
Dr. med. Dr. med. dent. E. Heissler
Klinik für Mund-, Kiefer- und Gesichtschirurgie
Universitätsklinikum Rudolf Virchow
Augustenburger Platz 1
D-13353 Berlin, Germany

Urine 5-HIAA excretion alone or in combination with ^{123}I-MIBG scintigraphy in patients with carcinoids?

Th. Behr[a], M. Pavel[b], W. Becker[a], J. Hensen[b], F. Wolf[a]
[a]Departments of Nuclear Medicine, [b]Medicine I, Friedrich-Alexander-University,
Erlangen-Nuremberg, Germany

Introduction

Carcinoid tumors are defined as neuroendocrine tumors originating from the enterochromeaffine cells, i.e. the disseminated endocrine cells of the primitive gut (1). Depending on their localization (foregut, midgut, hindgut), they express a different frequency of endocrine activity and clinical symptomatology, e.g. the carcinoid syndrome, which is associated with the serotonin production together with several additional hormones (histamine and other) (2).

For nuclear medical diagnosis and localization of carcinoids and their metastases, there are two major radiopharmaceutics in use: The first, used since almost ten years, is ^{123}I-metaiodobenzylguanidine (MIBG) (3), the second ^{111}In-DTPA-octreotide as the successor of ^{123}I-Tyr$_3$-octreotide. MIBG was developed as chemical derivative of guanethidine, which is taken up by sympathetic postganglionic neurons, the adrenal medulla and last but not least also neuroendocrine cells of the gut. Octreotide was developed as somatostatin analogue, binding specifically to several somatostatin receptor subtypes with high affinity.

The aim of the present study was to examin, whether there is a correlation between the endocrine activity of carcinoids especially concerning the serotonin metabolism and the uptake of ^{123}I-MIBG, assuming that a related type 1 uptake mechanism (i.e. the ATP-dependent active one in contrast to the passive diffusion type 2) exists for both, serotonin or its precursors and the radiopharmaceutical (4). The urine excretion of 5-hydroxyindoleacetic acid (5-HIAA) was used as metabolic marker for activity in the serotonin metabolism. A short view on this metabolic pathway: The amino acid tryptophan is taken up by the carcinoid cells, hydroxylated and decarboxylated to form 5-hydroxytryptamine (serotonin). Serotonin is excreted and metabolized by the monoamine-oxidase (MAO) to form finally 5-HIAA, which is renally excreted and can be measured in the patient's urine.

Patients and methods

We investigated eleven patients sequentially with ^{111}In-octreotide for diagnosis and localization of carcinoid tumors and the assessment of somatostatin receptor status, and ^{123}I-MIBG for evaluation of MIBG uptake and elegibility for a possible palliative ^{131}I-MIBG therapy. For somatostatin receptor scintigraphy, 111–148 MBq ^{111}In-octreotide were injected intravenously. After 2–4 hours planar scans, whole body scans and single photon emission computed tomography (SPECT) of the abdomen and additional regions depending on the clinical problem were performed. After 18–24 h, in special cases, e.g. search for a primary in the gut after 48 h, again planar scans were performed. MIBG scintigraphy was performed similarly: After thyroid blocking with perchlorate, 185–260 MBq of ^{123}I-MIBG were injected. After 4–6 h planar scans and SPECT of the critical regions was performed, after 18–24 h additional planar scanning was done.

Of the eleven patients examined, eight had a metastasized carcinoid with carcinoid syndrome, two had gastrinoma, one an endocrine inactive neuroendocrine tumor metastasized into the liver.

Results and discussion

Some typical cases in octreotide and MIBG scintigraphy are demonstrated.
The first one is the case of a fourty years old male with the typical clinical anamnesis and appearance of a carcinoid syndrome. He suffered from diarrhea and flushing, and its urine 5-HIAA was elevated up to 154 mg/24 h, but no primary could be detected although multiple liver metastases were seen in computed tomography or ultrasonography. Somatostatin receptor imaging was performed: The multiple liver metastases could be seen very well after four hours; after 24 hours, and even better after 48 h, a tiny tracer accumulation could be visualized in the right lower abdomen. The barium enema could reveal the primary then in the terminal ileum. Additionally, by somatostatin receptor scintigraphy, previously unknown mediastinal metastases could be revealed. The patient was also investigated with MIBG, and good tracer accumulation occured. In this case, high 5-HIAA excretion and good MIBG uptake coincided.
The second case is a 55 years old woman, also presenting with a carcinoid syndrome. Her 5-HIAA values were elevated (39 mg/24 h). Somatostatin receptor imaging showed multiple liver metastases, which did not take up the radiopharmaceutical in MIBG imaging.
The third case is a 66 year old woman with the clinical feature of Zollinger-Ellison's syndrome. No gastrinoma could be detected despite every effort including ultrasound, CT and even endosonography. Somatostatin receptor scintigraphy revealed the primary to be situated in the gallbladder with multiple liver metastases (it is the 22nd case of a gallbladder carcinoid known in literature and was published just recently (5). Despite her normal 5-HIAA levels (5 mg/24 h), clear MIBG uptake was seen in the primary and its metastases.
Summarizing, somatostatin receptor scintigraphy could detect the tumors and their metastases in 10 from the 11 investigated cases, whereas MIBG could only detect 7. The sensitivities reported here are therefore in good accordance to values reported in the literature (table I).
In 7/11 cases reported here, urine 5-HIAA measurements showed elevated values for this metabolic product of the serotonin metabolism. The mean 5-HIAA excretion for these seven patients was 148 mg/24h (normal range until 10mg/24 h). There could not be detected any stronger correlation between the MIBG uptake and the urine 5-HIAA excretion (table II).
The observed values shown are close to those expected for complete independence of both, MIBG uptake and hormone release.
We conclude from these data, that for diagnosis and localization of neuroendocrine tumors, ^{111}In-octreotide scintigraphy is the procedure of choice because of its excellent sensitivity. There is almost no correlation between the MIBG-uptake and the serotonin metabolism (measured as 5-HIAA excretion). Therefore the active transporter systems must be different for both. These results are in accordance to in vitro studies on the rat serotonin uptake system, as was published just recently by Glowniak and coworkers (8). They could demonstrate that MIBG is selectively taken up by the adrenergic uptake mechanism, not by the serotonin uptake system. Therefore ^{123}I-MIBG scintigraphy cannot replace 5-HIAA measurements for assessment of endocrine activity of malignant carcinoid tumors and vice versa. Nevertheless, MIBG scintigraphy should be routinely performed in malignant carcinoid patients. First, some additional tumor sites which do not express (enough) somatostatin receptors to be detected by octreotide scintigraphy can be revealed, second, it offers the chance for evaluation of a possible palliative ^{131}I-MIBG therapy (9).

Table I. Sensitivities of ^{111}In-octreotide and ^{123}I-MIBG.

	Own results	Literature (6, 7)
[111]In-octreotide	90.9%	85–100%
^{123}I-MIBG	63.6%	55–65%

Table II. MIBG uptake and urine 5-HIAA excretion.

5-HIAA	MIBG found		MIBG theoretically for independence[a]	
	+	−	+	−
+	45.5%	18.2%	40.5%	23.2%
−	18.2%	18.2%	23.1%	13.2%

[a]For an empirical sensitivity of MIBG-scintigraphy of 63.6% and a frequency of 63.7% for elevated 5-HIAA excretion.

References

1 Creutzfeldt W, Stöckmann F (1987) Carcinoid and carcinoid syndrome. Am J Med 82 suppl 5B:4–13
2 Gardner B, Dollinger M, Silen W, Bach N, O'Reilly S (1967) Studies on the carcinoid syndrome: its relationship to serotonin, bradykinin, and histamine. Surgery 61:846–852
3 Bomanji J, Ur E, Mather S, Moyes J, Ellison D, Grossman A, Britton KE, Besser GM (1991) A scintigraphic comparison of iodine-123-metaiodobenzylguanidine and an iodine-labeled somatostatin analog (Tyr-3-octreotide) in metastastic carcinoid tumors. J Nucl Med 39:1121–1124
4 Jaques S, Tobes MC, Sisson JC, Baker JA, Wieland DM (1984) Comparison of the sodium dependency of uptake of meta-iodobenzylguanidine and norepinephrine into cultured bovine adrenomedullary cells. Mol Pharmacol 26:539–546
5 Behr Th, Becker W, Koch W, Grebmeier J, Wolf F (1994) Somatostatin-Rezeptor-Szintigraphie bei neuroendokrinen Tumoren am Beispiel einer Patientin mit hepatisch metastasiertem Gastrinom. Z Gastroenterol 32:100–104
6 Kwekkeboom DJ, Krenning EP, Bakker WH, Yoe Oei H, Kooij PPM, Lamberts SWJ (1993) Somatostatin analogue scintigraphy in carcinoid tumours. Eur J Nucl Med 20:1025–1028
7 Joseph K, Stapp J, Reinecke J, Höffken H, Benning R, Neukam C, Trautmann ME, Schwerk WB, Arnold R (1992) Rezeptorszintigraphie bei endokrinen gastroenteropankreatischen Tumoren. Dtsch med Wschr 117:1025–1028
8 Glowniak JV, Kilty JE, Amara SG, Hoffmann BJ, Turner FE (1993) Evaluation of metaiodobenzylguanidine uptake by norepinephrine, dopamine, and serotonin transporters. J Nucl Med 34:1140–1146
9 Bomanji J, Britton KE, Ur E, Hawkins L, Grossman AB, Besser GM (1993) Treatment of malignant phaeochromocytoma, paraganglioma and carcinoid tumours with 131I-metaiodobenzylguanidine. Nucl Med Comm 14:856–861

Address for correspondence:
Dr. med. Th. Behr
Nuklearmedizinische Klinik mit Poliklinik
Universität Erlangen-Nürnberg
Krankenhausstraße 12
D-91054 Erlangen, Germany

Clinical value of ^{111}In-pentetreotide SPECT in the assessment of gastro-entero-pancreatic (GEP) tumors and medullary thyroid cancer (MTC)

D. Platz, K.F. Gratz, M. Luebeck

Department of Nuclear Medicine, University of Hamburg, Germany

Introduction

The ^{111}In-pentetreotide (SMS) whole body scintigraphy and SPECT is a well established method in detecting 50–90% of the GEP tumors and metastases (i.e. carcinoid) (1, 2) and related tumors like MTC (3). However, it is not well examined to what extend the SMS scan will produce additional relevant information for the clinicians and their therapeutic decision. The highest probability of a benefit can be expected in the problematic patient group with high certainty of tumor and still unknown localization after non-diagnostic conventional evaluation.

Patients and methods

In a group of 14 patients with primary tumor or recurrence proven by pathological hormon levels and non-conclusive findings in abdominal or thoracic CT, MRI or ultrasound (US), we evaluated the additional gain of the SMS scan and the inferable consequences on therapy and prognosis. In particular, seven patients with MTC and pathological pentagastrin stimulation test after thyroidectomy and seven patients with suspected GEP tumor (three primaries, four recurrent tumors) and elevated hormon levels. We used 110 MBq ^{111}In-pentetreotide. The gamma-camera images were performed 4 h and 24 h p.i using a HEAP-collimator. Whole body planar views as well as SPECT analyses (360°, 64 steps, each 40 s) were done. The therapeutic results were re-evaluated 2–6 months after the initial treatment.

Results

1. In the seven patients with MTC, tumor was detected in four patients. Three of them were aggressivly resected, but in the later follow-up the pathological pentagastrin-test persisted, thus demonstrating the incurability of their disease. One of the SMS-negative patients got a mediastinal and neck-lymphadenectomy, with temporary normalization of the test. The other two SMS-negative patients had a follow-up only.

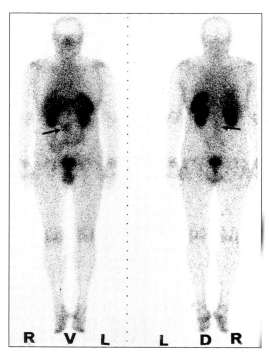

Figure 1. Whole body scan of a patient with local recurrence of a carcinoid.

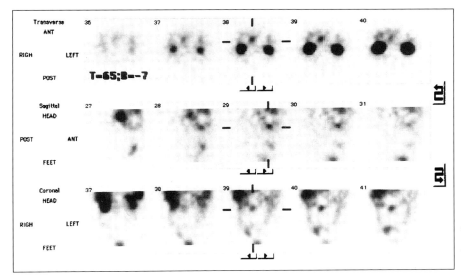

Figure 2. SPECT sequence of the same patient (1).

2. In the seven patients with suspected GEP tumor SMS scintigraphy detected tumor in 3/3 carcinoids, 1/3 gastrinomas and 0/1 insulinoma (figures 1–4). In the further course 3/4 SMS-positive symptomatic patients with diffuse metastases were treated with octreotide. The last one of the SMS-positive patients showed local recurrence only, and a curative resection was done. In one patient with insulinoma and negative SMS-scan a curative resection could be done after explorative laparatomy. The remaining two SMS scan negative patients had a follow-up only.

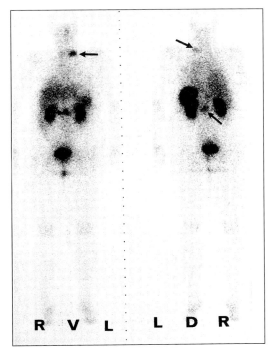

Figure 3. Whole body scan of a patient with local recurrence and lymph node metastases of a carcinoid.

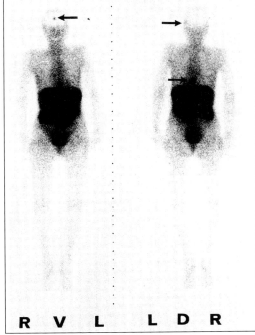

Figure 4. Whole body scan of a patient with liver and bone metastases of a carcinoid.

Discussion and conclusion

In patients with MTC and persisting pathologic calcitonin levels after thyreoidectomy the SMS whole body scintigraphy detected in about 55% foci not found by abdominal and thoracic CT, MR or US. This is a lower rate than reported by *Dörr* (3), but surprisingly high in this problematic group with rather low calcitonin levels reflecting the small tumor mass. Nevertheless it is dissapointing that the following resection was non-curative in all cases. So there was a diagnostical but no therapeutic benefit. In patients with clinically high suspicion of GEP tumor not detected by CT, MRI or US, SMS scintigraphy showed tumor localization in approximately 50%. This is a lower rate than generally reported in patient groups with GEP tumors (1, 2). This is explained by the fact that in more than half of these reported patients the tumor and the metastases were detectable with conventional methods too, reflecting a greater tumor bulk which will be easier detectable with SMS scintigraphy as well. The result compares nicely with those reported by *Joseph* et al. (4) who reported tumor localization in 34% of the patients with negative conventional diagnostic results. In one case the resection of a local recurrence was possible, in three other SMS-postive symptomatic patients palliative treatment with octreotide was initiated. So there was a diagnostical and therapeutic benefit.

References

1   Lamberts WJ, Krenning EP, Reubi J-C (1991) The role of somatostatin and its analogs in the diagnosis and treatment of tumors. Endocr Rev 12:450–482
2   Lamberts WJ, Bakker WH, Reubi J-C, Krenning EP (1990) Somatostatin-receptor imaging in the localisation of endocrine tumors. N Engl J Med 323:1246–1249
3   Dörr U et al (1993) Somatostatin receptor scintigraphy and magnetic resonance imaging in recurrent medullary thyroid carcinoma: a comparative study. Hormone Met Res Suppl 27:48–35
4   Joseph K et al (1993) Rezeptorszintigraphie mit 111-In-Pentetreotid bei endokrinen gastroenteropankreatischen Tumoren. Nuklear Med 32:299–306

Address for correspondence:
Dr. med. D. Platz
Abteilung für Nuklearmedizin
Universitätskrankenhaus Eppendorf
Martinistraße 52
D-20246 Hamburg, Germany

Somatostatin receptor imaging of intracranial tumors

K. Scheidhauer[a], G. Hildebrandt[b], C. Luyken[b], K. Schomäcker[a], N. Klug[b], H. Schicha[a]

[a] Department of Nuclear Medicine, [b] Department of Neurosurgery,
University of Cologne, Cologne, Germany

Introduction

Receptors of the peptide hormone somatostatin are located on the cell membrane of tumors of neuroendocrine origin, but also others including intracranial tumors (9). Endocrine functions of somatostatin, mainly inhibition of metabolic processes, are not known for all tissues of intracranial tumors. In pituitary adenomas (3) unlabeled octreotide is used for treatment to control hormone production and tumor growth in acromegaly (10). The significance of the receptors in meningiomas and gliomas is unknown. Development of long-acting somatostatin analogues like octreotide and the recent availability of radiolabeling with ^{123}I or ^{111}In made the in vivo detection of somatostatin receptors possible (4).

Meningiomas as well as pituitary adenomas, although generally benign and non-metastasizing tumors, may pose serious problems due to recurrences after primary therapy and local invasiveness in areas such as clivus or cavernous sinus. Despite advances in skull-base surgery treatment of tumors in this area remain often unsolved. In an attempt to establish different modes of non-surgical treatment the concept of hormonal manipulation of meningiomas was suggested (2). Somatostatin receptor presence in gliomas is correlated to tumor grading: low malignant gliomas (WHO grade I and II) are known to express receptors, while gliomas of higher grade (WHO grade III and IV) do not have measurable contents of them (6).

Knowledge about receptor status and function could provide new insights into tumor biology and reaction as already known in pituitary tumors and may have predictive or palliative input to therapeutic approaches. Purpose of the present study was to evaluate the value of somatostatin receptor scintigraphy using ^{111}Indium labeled octreotide in the diagnostic work-up of patients suffering from intracranial tumors.

Patients, material and methods

92 patients suffering from newly diagnosed, residual or recurrent intracranial tumors were studied. All tumors were documented by computer tomography (CT) or magnetic resonance imaging (MR). ^{111}In labeled octreotide, a DTPA bearing analogue of somatostatin (Octreo Scan® 111, provided by Mallinckrodt Diagnostica, Petten, Holland), was injected i.v. as a 10 mg bolus, respectively, corresponding to 110 MBq (3 mCi) ^{111}In. ^{111}In octreotide binds specifically to somatostatin receptors (1).

Gamma camera images of the head were performed 4–6 hours p.i.; digital planar images (128 x 128 matrix, four views) were taken as well as single photon emisson computed tomography (SPECT) images (64 x 64 matrix). Acquisition parameters for planar images were 5 minutes per planar view, and 64 projections of 20 seconds each for the SPECT studies. Scintigrams were judged independently without knowledge of the results of other imaging modalities (CT, MR) by two observers. All tumors were evaluated histologically or could be classified by the conventional imaging methods (CT or MR). In ten patients, the scintigraphic results could be correlated to the somatostatin receptor content of tumor specimens determined by a gold-ligand technique in vitro.

Results

The tumors studied consisted of meningiomas I-III (WHO): n = 40; gliomas WHO-stage II, III, IV: n = 20; pituitary adenomas: n = 18; neurofibromatosis: n = 6; others (metastases, lymphoma, abscess): n = 8. Tumor size ranged from 1.5 to 10 cm in diameter.

Meningioma

All patients but one with meningiomatous lesions showed a high focal tracer uptake (n = 39/40; sensitivity: 98 %). Somatostatin receptor containing tumor tissue could be visualized in multifocal, intraosseous or intraorbital lesions. One small lesion (1.5 cm) of the skull base was missed.

Pituitary adenoma

Nine out of 18 patients with pituitary tumors showed focal uptake of the radiopharmacon. The uptake was lower compared with that in meningiomatous lesions. Due to the spatial resolution of gamma cameras, a differentiation between tumor and non-tumoral tissue of the pituitary gland was not possible. A correlation with the endocrine activity was not found.

Glioma

Low malignant gliomas (WHO grade II) with an intact blood-brain barrier (n = 10) presented no uptake of ^{111}In octreotide, while gliomas with WHO-grade III and IV and disrupted blood-brain-barrier (n = 10) showed focal uptake of the radiopharmacon.

Others

A cranial metastasis of an adeno carcinoma was visualized by receptor scintigraphy in vivo and had also a positive somatostatin receptor prove in vitro.
In general, the target to non-target signal ratios (tumor to brain) were highest in meningiomas (up to 8 : 1) and higher in images obtained 24 hours after injection of the radiopharmacon than in the earlier images after 3 to 6 hours. No side effects were noted during or after application of ^{111}In-octreotide.

Discussion

Scintigraphy reveals no increased uptake of the normal leptomeninx, although containing somatostatin receptors as proven in vitro (13), because ^{111}In-octreotide does not cross the intact blood-brain-barrier. Meningiomas are devoid of a blood-brain-barrier (7). Thus, irrespective of meningioma location, histology or WHO grade, in all but one patients with meningioma, a high uptake of ^{111}In-octreotide was found, indicating a high density of somatostatin receptors. Only one false negative result was observed in this group. These data are consistent with published in vitro data (12), demonstrating a high density of somatostatin receptors in all of the investigated meningiomas by in vitro binding assays and receptor autoradiography. The function of these somatostatin receptors, however, is yet not clear (14).
Pituitary tumors displayed only a moderate receptor density in 50% of patients, independent from the endocrine activity. This is in agreement with findings of other investigators, who found nearly 50% positive scans in growth hormone secreting tumors with ^{123}I-labeled octreotide (5).

On the other hand, gliomas with an intact blood-brain-barrier (WHO grade II) showed no enhanced uptake in vivo, while gliomas with damaged blood-brain-barrier (WHO grade III-IV) had a moderate uptake of the radiopharmacon. This is contrasted by in vitro studies, where somatostatin receptors were shown to be present in low malignant gliomas (WHO grade I, II), but not in high malignant gliomas (8). Preliminary results of in vitro tests of our tumor specimens confirm this findings. Unspecific mechanisms of tracer accumulation have to be discussed and investigated in further studies.
All scintigraphically receptor-positive tumors could be detected already by planar images, but the tomographic technique (SPECT) could provide a better anatomical orientation and did improve comparison with other tomographic techniques and seems therefore to be mandatory. Images

after 24 hours showed a higher contrast than those after 4-6 hours. Quantification of activity accumulation or correlation with growth hormone secretion (in pituitary tumors) was not possible due to relatively low count rates.

In conclusion, somatostatin receptor scintigraphy with ^{111}In-octreotide is able to image intracranial tumors and can provide some additional non-invasive, pre-operative informations important for therapeutical decisions. Further studies have to clearify, whether this scintigraphic method can also give hints for a possible therapeutic benefit of labeled or unlabeled somatostatin analogues, according to the therapeutic use of octreotide in acromegaly. Due to the high somatostatin receptor density, meningiomas of the skull or the orbit could be differentiated from somatostatin receptor negative tumors. Therefore, in vivo receptor imaging may narrow the spectrum of differential diagnoses, especially confirming or excluding meningiomas. This may be important for planning therapeutic interventions.

References

1 Bakker W H, Albert H, Bruns C, Breeman WAP, Hofland LJ, Marbach P, Pless J, Pralet D, Stolz B, Koper JW, Lamberts SWJ, Visser TJ, Krenning EP (1991) (111-In-DTPA-d-Phe)1-octreotide, a potential radio-pharmaceutical for imaging of somatostatin receptor-positive tumors: synthesis, radiolabeling and in vitro validation. Life Sciences 49:1583-1591
2 Greenberg SM, Weiss MH, Spitz IM, Ahmadi J, Sadun A, Russel CP, Lucci L, Stevenson LL (1991) Treatment of unresectable meningiomas with the antiprogesterone agent mifepristone. J Neurosurg 74:861-866
3 Ikuyama S, Nawata H, Kato K, Karashima T, Ibayashi H, Nagkagaki H (1985) Specific somatostatin receptors on human pituitary adenoma cell membranes. J Clin Endocrinol Metab 61:666-671
4 Krenning EP, Bakker WH, Breeman WAP, Koper J W, Kooij PPM, Ausema L, Lameris JS, Reubi JC, Lamberts SWJ. Localisation of endocrine related tumors with radioiodinated analogue of somatostatin. Lancet (i) 242-245

5 Lamberts SWJ (1988) The role of somatostatin in the regulation of anterior pituitary hormone secretion and the use of its analogues in the treatment of human pituitary tumors. Endocr Rev 9:417-419
6 Lamberts SWJ, Krenning EP, Bakker WH, Breeman WAP, Kooy PM, Reubi JC (1991) Somatostatin receptor imaging in the diagnosis of pituitary and parasellar tumors. In: Melmed S, Robbins RJ (eds) Molecular and clinical advances in pituitary disorders. Blackwell Scientific Publications Boston, pp 285-294
7 Rachlin JR, Rosenblum ML (1991) Etiology and biology of meningiomas. In: Al-Mefty O (ed), Meningiomas. New York, pp 27-35
8 Reubi JC, Horisberger U, Lang W, Koper JW, Braakman R, Lamberts SWJ (1989) Coincidence of EGF receptors and somatostatin receptors in meningiomas but inverse, differentiation-dependent relationship in glial tumors. Am J Pathol 134:337-344
9 Reubi JC, Kvols L, Krenning EP, Lamberts SWJ (1990) Distribution of somatostatin receptors in normal and tumor tissue. Metabolism 39:78-81
10 Reubi JC, Landolt AM (1984) High densitiy of somatostatin receptors in pituitary tumors from acromegalic patients. J Clin Endocrinol Metab 59:1148-1151
11 Reubi JC, Maurer R (1985) Autoradiographic mapping of somatostatin receptors in the rat CNS and pituitary. Neurosciences 15:1183-1195
12 Reubi JC, Maurer R, Klijn JGM, Stefanko SZ, Foekens JA, Blaauw G, Blankenstein MA, Lamberts SWJ (1986) High incidence of somatostatin receptors in human meningiomas: biochemical characterisation. J Clin Endocrinol Metab 63:433-438
13 Reubi JC, Maurer R, Lamberts SWJ (1986) Somatostatin binding sites in human leptomeninx. Neuroscience 70:183
14 Ruenzi MW, Jaspers C, Windeck R, Benker G, Mehdorn HM, Reinhardt, Reinwein D (1989) Successful treatment of meningioma with octreotide. Lancet 1:1074

Address for correspondence:
Dr. med. K. Scheidhauer
Abteilung für Nuklearmedizin
Universitätskrankenhaus
Joseph-Stelzmann-Straße 9
D-50924 Köln, Germany

Visualization of peptide hormone receptor complexes using [¹¹¹In]octreotide in breast cancer in vivo

A. Scharl[a], U.-J. Göhring[a], K. Scheidhauer[b], K. Schomäcker[b]

[a]Departments of Obstetrics and Gynecology, [b]Department of Nuclear Medicine, University of Cologne, Cologne, Germany

Introduction

Somatostatin is a tetradecapeptide. The hormone effects are mediated via a transmembrane receptor protein and include mainly inhibition of metabolic processes (7). The expression of somatostatin receptors is preserved in certain tumors including tumors of the CNS (meningiomas, astrocytomas) and the gastrointestinal tract (APUDomas), and carcinomas of prostate and breast (2, 3, 6, 7, 9, 10). Somatostatin has been demonstrated to inhibit growth in certain tumor cell lines in vitro including human carcinomas, and in animal tumor models (4, 6, 12).

In this study, we used the somatostatin receptor as a model to evaluate the potential for imaging of peptide hormone receptors utilizing radiolabeled receptor ligands. Possible clinical applications of this technique include receptor detection in vivo, tumor localization and staging. On the other hand somatostatin receptors may be utilized as targets for site-directed radiotherapy using ligands which are tagged with high energy radionuclides.

Patients, materials, and methods

25 patients (age 43–76 years) with suspicious breast masses were studied before surgery. All masses were removed in toto and examined histologically. In case of malignancy, breast conserving therapy or Patey mastectomy including axillary lymphonodectomy level 2 were performed according to tumor stage and patients' consent.

Radiolabeling of octreotide, a somatostatin analogue, with [¹¹¹In]chloride was performed on site (Octreoscan®, Mallinckrodt Diagnostica, Fetten, The Netherlands). HPLC analyses proved radiochemical purity of [¹¹¹In]DTPA-octreotide to approximate 96%.

Patients received an intravenous bolus injection of 10 ng [¹¹¹In]octreotide ([¹¹¹In]O), which equals approximately 110 MBq (3 mCi) ¹¹¹In. Planar images of the thorax in ventral and oblique (RAO, LAO) views were scanned up to 15 minutes and 3–6 hours after injection, respectively. During the latter time interval additional SPECT (single photon emission computed tomography) was performed. We used single-head gamma cameras (planar, 128 x 128 matrix, 5 min per view) and double-head SPECT cameras (64 x 64 matrix, 64 projections of 40 sec) equiped with medium-energy, parallel-hole collimators, respectively. Peaks were set to 173 keV and 247 keV with 20% windows. Tumor localization was not known before image interpretation.

In one patient serum levels of ¹¹¹In and excretion into urine were measured for 48 hours: Venous blood was drawn at 10, 20, 30, 40, 60 minutes, 2, 3, 4, 5, 6, 10, 23, 27 and 48 hours after injection. Total urine production was collected in 4-hour fractions.

Results

Analysis of serum activity of ¹¹¹In demonstrated a short blood pool phase: 3/4 of the activity were eliminated from the blood within one hour. Five hours after injection activity in blood approximated zero. Urine excretion of [¹¹¹In]O was 78% and 98% of injected dose after 8 hours and 48 hours, respectively.

Histological diagnoses of masses were adenofibroma or mastopathy in five patients and breast cancer in 20 patients. Tumor size and nodal status is given in table I.

Positive images were seen in two patients with benign disease (1 adenofibroma, 1 mastopathy). 15 of 20 breast cancer patients yielded well defined images, which correlated favorably with the clinical localization of the masses (figure I). In five cancer patients imaging was negative (table I).

Six of 12 node-positive patients displayed axillary uptake (figure 1), whereas no axillary uptake was seen in node-negative patients. Planar scintigraphy was sufficient to detect all tumors eventually considered positive. SPECT did not improve sensitivity but provided a superior anatomical orientation and a higher tumor/background-ratio than planar imaging.

Table I. Results of [¹¹¹In]octreotide imaging in patients with breast masses with regard to histology, tumor size and nodal status.

	Benign	Carcinoma	Tumor size				Nodal status	
			ca. in situ	T1	T2	T3/4	N0	N+
Patients	5	20	1	4	8	7	8	12
Positive imaging	2[a]	15 (75%)	1	3	6	5	0	6

[a]One adenofibroma, one mastopathy

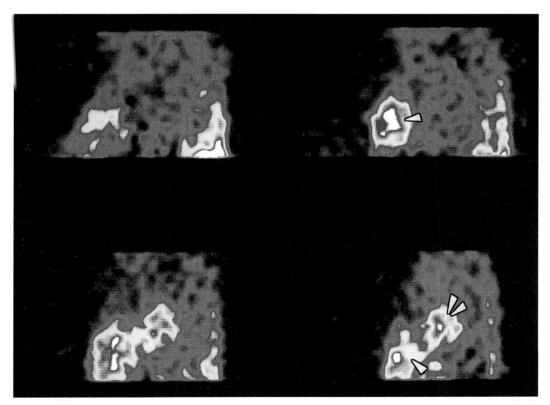

Figure 1. [¹¹¹In]octreotide images (SPECT) of a patient with T4 N+ breast cancer (coronar sections). Focal uptake in the left breast (>) and axillary region (>>).

Discussion

Our study utilizing [^{111}In]O as a prototype radioligand demonstrated that non-invasive techniques for detection in vivo of peptide hormone receptors are feasible. This receptor imaging is not based on characteristics specific for malignant tissues and consequently positive images are not restricted to carcinomas. However, it uses high affinity molecules which are specific for the presence of receptors, and therefore tests the biology of a tumor, and provides informations on selective molecular biological characteristics. Receptor imaging may eventually be of clinical use for staging and offers therapeutic guidance.

We demonstrated a short blood pool phase of [^{111}In]O and a rapid cumulative excretion via the kidneys confirming data published by *Krenning* et al. (5) and *Adrian* et al. (1). 75% of tumors investigated accumulated radioactivity sufficient for distinct and clear imaging. This is in accordance with data of *Lamberts* and colleges (6). We postulate that this sequestration of [^{111}In]O is receptor-mediated and visualizes the presence of ligand-receptor-complexes in the tumors. However, we have not yet completed to further support this notion by demonstrating somatostatin receptors in surgical specimens of the tumors. With respect to this task it is interesting that data available on receptor detection in vitro report frequencies of positive carcinomas ranging between 15 and 46% only (2, 3, 9, 10). These are considerably lower than rates achieved with imaging techniques.

Although the number of patients tested is insufficient, it is interesting that accumulation or radioactivity in the axillary region was strictly confined to patients with node metastases. More data are needed to answer the question whether positive axillary [^{111}In]O images are a reliable marker for node involvement.

At present, somatostatin and somatostatin receptors have no clinical applications in breast cancer. However, there was experimental evidence for the ability of somatostatin to block epidermal growth factor (EGF)-induced cell proliferation (8) three years prior to the first reports on the prognostic significance of EGF receptor in breast carcinoma (11). Investigations in vitro and in vivo detected somatostatin receptors in breast cancer and noted a potential prognostic significance (6). *Reubi* and *Torhorst* (10) demonstrated concordance between the expression of receptors for somatostatin and for steroid hormones in breast carcinomas. Thus they concluded the expression of somatostatin receptors to be a marker for well preserved functional differentiation. When *Foekens* and collaborators (3) analyzed 110 patients whose breast carcinomas were tested for the presence or absence of somatostatin receptors, they reported the clinical outcome to be significantly poorer when tumors tested negative for somatostatin receptors as compared to somatostatin receptor-positive carcinomas (3).

References

1. Adrian HJ, Dörr U, Bach D, Bihl H (1993) Biodistribution of 111In-pentatreotide and dosimetric considerations with respect to somatostatin receptor expressing tumor burden. Hormone Metabol Res 27:18–23
2. Fekete M, Wittliff JL, Schally AV (1989) Characteristics and distribution of receptors for [D-TRP6]-luteinizing hormone-releasing hormone, somatostatin, epidermal growth fator, and sex steroids in 500 biopsy samples of human breast cancer. J Clin Lab Anal 3:137–147
3. Foekens JA., Portengen H, van Putten WLJ, Trapman MAC, Reubi J-C, Alexieva-Figusch J, Klijn JGM (1989) Prognostic value of receptors for insulin-like growth factor 1, somatostatin, and epidermal growth factor in human breast cancer. Cancer Res 49:7002–7009
4. Haijri A, Aprahamian M, Vonderscher J, Damgé C (1989) Antitumoral effect of sandostatin in an exocrine pancreatic tumor trans-planted in the rat. Bull Cancer 76:504
5. Krenning EP, Bakker WH, Kooij PPM, Breeman WAP, Oei HY, de Jong M, Reubi J-C, Visser TJ, Bruns C, Kwekkeboom DJ, Reijs AFM, van Hagen PM, Koper JW, Lamberts SWJ (1992) Somatostatin receptor scintigraphy with Indium 111-DTPA-D-Phe-1-oc-treotide in man: metabolism, dosimetry and comparison with Iodine-123-Tyr-3-octreotide. J Nucl Med 33:652–658
6. Lamberts SWJ, Krenning EP, Reubi J-C (1991) The role of somatostatin and its analogs in the diagnosis and treatment of tumors. Endocrin reviews 12/4: 450–482
7. Lewin M (1986) Somatostatin receptors. Scand J Gastroenterol 21 (suppl 119): 42–46
8. Mascardo RN, Sherline P (1982) Somatostatin inhibits rapid centrosomal separation and cell pro-

liferation induced by epidermal growth factor. Endocrinol 111:1394
9. Reubi JC, Waser B, Foekens JA, Klijn JGM, Lamberts SWJ (1990) Somatostatin receptor incidence and distribution in breast cancer using receptor autoradiographiy: relationship to EGF receptors. Int J Cancer 46:41
10. Reubi JC, Torhorst J (1989) The relationship between somatostatin, epidermal growth factor, and steroid hormone receptors in breast cancer. Cancer 64:1254–1260
11. Sainsbury JRC, Malcolm AJ Appleton DR, Farndon JR, Harris AL (1985) Presence of epidermal growth factor receptor as an indicator for poor prognosis in patients with breast cancer. J Clin Pathol 38: 1225–1228
12. Scambia G, Panici PB, Baiocchi G et al (1988) Antiproliferative effects of somatostatin and the somatostatin analogue SMS 201-995 on three human breast cancer cell lines. J Cancer Res Clin Oncol 114: 306–308

Address for correspondence:
Priv.-Doz. Dr. med. A. Scharl
Universitätsfrauenklinik
Kerpenerstraße 34
D-50931 Köln, Germany

Detection and delineation of rhabdo- and leiomyosarcomas using ^{111}In labeled antimyosin-antibodies (Fab) as a hopeful tool in oncology

W.-G. Franke[a], S. Wiener[a], S. Weiß[a], E. Siegert[b], K. Koehler[c]

[a]Clinic and Policlinic for Nuclear Medicine, [b]Clinic for Pediatrics,
[c]Clinic and Policlinic for Radiology, Klinikum of the Technical University, Dresden, Germany

Introduction

Myosarcomas (MS) play a not insignificant role among the tumor entity of malignant soft tissue tumors. After all, rhabdomyosarcomas (RMS) predominate in the infancy (embryonal and alveolar species) except the rare pleomorphic species and amount to 20% of the soft tissue tumors and to 50% of the soft part sarcomas in childhood (3). Leiomyosarcomas (LMS), the other group of MS, occur in about 7% of all the primary soft tumors favoring the adulthood. Because of the considerable difficulties to distinguish MSs from some other types of tumors by histologic investigation alone addition of immunohistochemical specifying by evidence of desmin, vimentin, myosin and/or myoglobin possibly in a lot of cases is to value as very meaningful.

An early and comprehensive diagnosis is very important especially because of two causes:
MSs metastasize prematurely. 30–40% of RMSs show a hematogenous metastasizing prefered to lung, liver and skeleton already at the date of the initial confirmation of diagnosis. Under conditions of up-to-date therapeutic approaches an overall 5-years survival rate of more than 50% can be reached (3). The contribution from *de Jong* et al. (2) on the specific enrichment of antimyosin antibodies in RMS and in tumors with rhabdomyoblastic parts exhibited a very meaningful knowledge with regard to a new diagnostic tool in MSs. Few years later some authors confirmed the correctness of these findings by scintigraphic presentation of LMSs as well as RMSs following administration of ^{111}In labeled antimyosin antibodies (1, 4, 5, 6, 7, 8, 9).

Because the radioimmunoscintigraphy (RIS) by means of the antimyosin antibodies seems to be a promising method for tumor detection in MSs, own scintigraphic studies were accomplished in patients suffering from such malignancies.

Patients and methods

A kit ("Myoscint", formerly Centocor, Leiden, recently Mallinckrodt, the Netherlands) is used for scintigraphic studies. The murine antibody (hybridic cell line R11D10) of the subclass IgG_{2a} exists as a Fab fragment (molecular weight about 50.000 dalton) coupled with DTPA and solved in a 10 mM phosphate buffer. For a single study the patient is injected i.v. with about 80 MBq of ^{111}In labeled antibody fragment corresponding to 0.2–0.5 mg of the substances. Imaging takes place 3, 24 and 48 h after administration of the radiopharmaceutical. Planar scintigraphy and SPECT of suspicious regions are carried out in each case. For optimization of image quality a MEGP collimator and a matrix of 128 times 128 are used. The energy windows lie at 172 and 247 keV. For SPECT investigations the 360° rotation takes place divided in 64 steps taking 60 seconds for each one. The images become evaluated by visualization. Additionally, the heart / lung court ratio is calculated. Values > 1.7 were estimated as elevated. A certain quantification of intratumoral uptake was possible by calculation of a ratio count rate over the tumor/ count rate over the opposite region.

Ten patients suffering from MS were studied by antimyosin Fabs in our department until now as seen in table I. Follow-up studies were carried out in four persons. Male patients and RMSs prevailed in the case material. At all times the diagnosis was ascertained by histological examination of the primary tumor. Suspicion of metastases and/or recurrences could be confirmed or excluded in each case using up to four anatomical methods. Whereas MRT and/or XCT are used customarily, sonography and x-ray are accomplished often additionally. Because of special urgency for treatment some patients had been already submitted to therapeutic procedures when the radionuclide studies were accomplished. In some cases the study took place not before a recurrence or metastazation were supposed after a preceding treatment of the primary tumor.

Results

Side effects, adverse reactions or increase of HAMA levels never were seen even not after repetition of studies in the same patient. Follow-up observations of imagings over 3, 24 and 48 h after antimyosin administration showed frequently an intratumoral radioactivity uptake already after 3 h sufficient for tumor scintigraphy. However, the best possible scintigraphic presentation were found 48 h p.i. attributable to the optimal relation between intratumoral and background radioactivity concentration. The highest non-tumoral radionuclide uptake was seen in the later phases of radioactivity time course always in the kidneys followed by liver. Results of tumor imaging become illustrated by some case reports.

Case 1

An eight years old boy suffered from a cold in the head resistant against therapy for eight weeks. Diagnostic excision from a epipharyngeal tumor showed by histological and immunohistochemical examination an embryonal RMS. An intensive radioactivity concentration was seen by scintigraphy in the tumoral region corresponding to findings of XCT and MRT concerning the extent of the pathological process (figure 1).

Case 2

Scintigraphic images obtained from an adult man (age 52 years) may serve as an example for scintigraphic detectability of metastases and

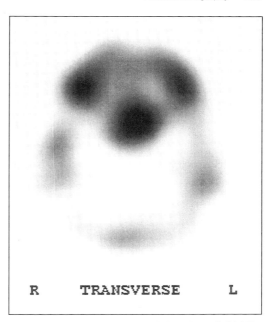

Figure 1. Scintigram after administration of 80 MBq ^{111}In labeled antimyosin Fab-fragments in an eight years old boy suffering from an embryonal RMS (for details see report on case 1).

recurrences. This patient endured the fourth relapse of a pleomorphic RMS first localized into the galea capitis. After explorative excision the diagnosis was ascertained by microscopy and immunohistochemistry detecting aktin, vimentin, and myoglobin. Scintigraphic studies (figure 2) presented areas with raised radioactivity uptake besides of the galeal region at glandula parotis and prae-auricular region also in correspondence with the morphologic changings seen by MRT.

Case 3

A tumoral mass localised submandibularily on the right side of the neck found in a four years old girl was resistant against therapy. Histological and immunohistochemical analysis of the excided tissue material showed an embryonal RMS containing desmin, vimentin and aktin. By antimyosin RIS (figure 3) the tumor could been visualized similarly extended as established by XCT. A follow-up scintigraphic study about nine month after the first one and after application of various

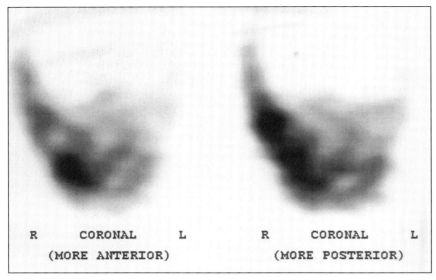

Figure 2. ^{111}In anti-myosin-Fab scintigram after the 4th recurrence (RMS) of a 52 years old man (for details see case 2).

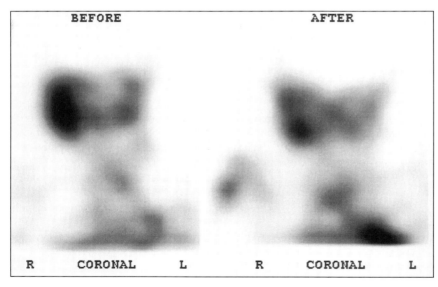

Figure 3. Scintigraphic follow-up of a four years old girl with an embryonal RMS using ^{111}In antimyosin Fab fragments (for details see case 3).

therapeutic procedures (EVAIA scheme and radiation therapy) was accomplished. Increased radioactivity uptake was still detected in the same place even if lower than before therapy. However, comparison of the ratio countrate over the tumor/countrate over the opposite region processed at both dates of study demonstrates a distinct decrease of radioactivity storage with time probably as a consequence of preceded treatment. Moreover, an increase of the heart/lung ratio was stated at the second study in the same patient.

The most important data of all patients investigated are presented more detailed in table I. As can be seen, all of MS, i.e. RMS as well as LMS and different histological and histochemical identified subgroups, primary tumors, recurrences and metastases, found by anatomical methods, were also detected by antimyosin RIS except one case of recurrent LMS. In some cases

Table I. Scintigraphic results compared with results of reference methods.

Patient	Sex	Age (years)	Histology	Histo-chemistry	Site	Scintigraphic results agreeing with reference		Reference
						primary tumor	recurrence/ metastases	
M.K.	male	8	embryonal RMSa	desmin	head, epi-pharynx	+	–	XCT, MRT x-ray
L.H.	female	4	embryonal RMS	vimentin desmin aktin	head	+	–	XCT sonography x-ray
J.L.	male	13	alveolar RMS	vimentin desmin myoglobin	head	+	–	XCT sonography x-ray
W.M.	male	52	pleomorph. RMS	aktin desmin myoglobin	head	+	head (recurr.) lymphonodi	MRT XCT x-ray
A.W.	male	5	embryonal RMS	aktin vimentin	head	+	bone lung	MRT x-ray
J.S.	male	17	alveolar RMS	desmin vimentin myoglobin	bone	–	lung bone	XCT MRT x-ray
M.I.	female	3	embryonal RMS	not investigated	foot	–	foot	XCT
S.R.	female	68	LMSb	aktin vimentin	thigh	–	thigh	XCT MRT
S.P.	male	40	LMS	aktin	thigh	–	–	XCT sonography
						scintigraphic result not agreeing with reference		
						primary tumor	recurrence/ metastases	
E.H.	male	40	LMS	not investigated	abdomen	–	–	XCT bone scan

[a] Rhabdomyosarcoma; [b] leiomyosarcoma

the tumors could been delineated more clearly than by means of MRT or other anatomical methods. Furtheron the extent of the tumoral process was often presented greater than expected from the results of the various reference methods. A distinct reduction of radioactivity was evident in two of four cases controlled by repeated scintigraphy. Cytostatic therapy protocols were taken from these patients.

Discussion

A synoptic view on the results obtained by antimyosin RIS published by some authors until now including our own contribution demonstrates very distinctly, that the great majority of MS is visualizable by antimyosin RIS. This detectability is apparently not depending from histology and histochemistry and concerns primary tumors as well as secondaries and recurrences. As prerequisites for antimyosin enrichment rhabdomyolysis and intracellular existence of myosin could been supposed. In contrary to other tumor markers the localization takes place intracellularily and not an increased but a decreased perfusion is necessary for tumor detection. It seems to be ascertained, that not an unspecific radioactivity uptake occurs (7), but a specific process of storage inwardly of the tumor cells. This supposition is supported by the results of antibody binding studies accomplished by *Reuland* (8). The author could prove, that the antimyosin antibody R11D10 can be bound specifically and very fast in cells descending from the MS cell line A 204.

Therefore, it should been noted, that antimyosin Fab fragments used in tumor scintigraphy signalize myosin containing malignant tumors. Consequently, it may be obvious on the one hand, that positive scintigramms were obtained by rhabdoid tumors and in one case of a primitive neuroectodermal tumor, and on the other hand MSs can be remained undetected by imperfect differentiation. This could be one argument for the single case with a false negative result in our patient group.

Experiences are not yet sufficient concerning the quantification of therapeutic effects although hitherto known results of follow-up studies made by *Reuland* (8) and our preliminary experiences can be interpreted in this sense. A moderate variation of the velocity of antimyosin uptake is possible, which could be related to "biological activity".

Correspondence exists relating to improvement of diagnosis in primary or secondary MRs, especially for exact destination of extent and delineation of the process as well as in case of tumor localization near kidneys or liver. Especially the intensive intratubular storage of antimyosin antibodies under normal conditions and the decrease of uptake in pathologic situations allow probably very meaningful diagnostic informations on renal disturbances after cytostatic therapy.

Finally, as seen from of other authors, in one case of our patients also an increasing of heart/lung ratio can be detected as an accessory finding. Because indicating damage of cardiac musculature these findings could be important for patients treated by cytotoxic drugs.

Conclusions

Antimyosin (Fab) antibodies seem to be a hopeful additional tool in the diagnostic program of tumors, which are suspected as myosin containing. In this sense it could be assessed as a tumor marker. The possibility of overlaying processes induced by other muscular damages, e.g. postoperative reaction, have to be taken into consideration.

Following expectations are attached to prospective application: sensitive and specific detection, localization and elimination of primary tumors, recurrences and secondaries; estimation of progress and therapeutic influence by follow-up studies; judgement of biological activity with regard to tumor grading simultaneously to proof of (therapeutically induced) toxic cardiomyopathy. Of course, a critical re-evaluation will be necessary after having greater numbers of examinations to decide on routineous diagnostic use of this method. Furthermore, methodical development for quantification of intratumoral antibody uptake is urgently necessary.

Reference

1 Cox PH, Verweij J, Pillay M et al (1988) Indium-[111] antimyosin for the detection of leiomyosarcoma and rhabdomyosarcoma. Eur J Nucl Med 14:50–522
2 De Jong ASH, van Vark M, Albus- Lutter CH E et al (1984) Myosin and myoglobulin as tumor markers in the diagnosis of rhabdomyosarcoma. A comparative study. Am J Surg Pathol 8:521–528
3 Harms D (1984) Tumoren des Kindesalters. In: Remmele W (ed) Pathologie. Vol 3, Springer, Berlin-New York, pp 613–638
4 Hoefnagel CA, de Kraker J, Voute PA, Behrendt H (1988) Tumor imaging of rhabdomyosarcoma using radiolabelled fragments of monoclonal antimyosin antibody. J Nucl Med 29(suppl):791
5 Kairemo KJ, Lehtovirta P (1990) Radioimmun- detection of uterine leiomyosarcoma with [111]In- labeled monoclonal antimyosin antibody Fab fragments. Gynecol Oncol 36:417–422
6 Kairemo KJ, Wiklund TA, Liewendahl K et al (1990) Imaging of soft-tissue sarcomas with In-[111] labeled monoclonal antimyosin Fab fragments. J Nucl Med 31:23–31
7 Kalevi JA, Kairemo MD, Wiklund TA (1990) Imaging of soft-tissue sarcomas with In-labeled monoclonal antimyosin Fab fragments. J Nucl Med 1:23–31

8 Reuland P (1992) Nuklearmedizinische Untersuchungen bei embryonalen Tumoren. Habilitationsschrift (Thesis), Tübingen
9 Weiß S, Franke WG, Wiener S (1984) Myosin-Antikörper in der Diagnostik von Rhabdo- und Leiomyosarkomen. Deutsche Gesellschaft für Nuklearmedizin, 31. Internationale Jahrestagung, Köln (abstr)

Address for correspondence:
Prof. Dr. med. W.-G. Franke
Technische Universität Dresden
Universitätsklinikum "Carl Gustav Carus"
Klinik und Poliklinik für Nuklearmedizin
Fetscherstraße 74
D-01307 Dresden, Germany

Immunoscintigraphy with the B72.3 antibody in presurgical patients with suspected colorectal cancer[1]

A. Bockisch[a], M. Mörschel[b], A. Hach[a], Anja Schmitz[a]
[a]Clinic for Nuclear Medicine, [b]Clinic for General and Abdominal Surgery,
Klinikum of the Johannes-Gutenberg-University, Mainz, Germany

Introduction

The ^{111}In labeled antibody B72.3 (OncoScint®) (3, 7) has been commercially available in Germany for the last three years. This antibody is directed against the tumor marker TAG-72 (4), which is commonly expressed in colorectal cancer. In early human studies the sensitivity for detecting tumor sites has been proven to be about 66% averaged over all sites and sizes (5). In a prospective study we investigated patients suffering from colorectal cancer with the B72.3 antibody prior to surgery in order to determine the local tumor extent and especially to detect peri-aortic and peri-iliacal lymph node metastases.

The sensitivity for detecting the primary tumor or recurrencies was 75%, the specificity 80%. Concerning (regional) lymph node metastases or distant metastases, the numbers were less favorable. The sensitivity was found to be 40% and 33%, respectively, with the specificity of app. 85%, in both cases.

Patients and methods

Thirty patients have been investigated, which included 18 men and 12 women, aged 31 to 90 years. Most patients were in the age group of 60 to 80 years. Surgery was planned because of suspicion of rectal (n = 18), sigmoid (n = 1), or colonic (n = 10) carcinoma. In one case the primary was in the gall bladder. The majority of patients investigated had primary tumors.
180 to 200 MBq ^{111}In labeled OncoScint were administered intravenously and planar whole body scintigrams were acquired after 24 or 48 hours. In addition, a second image was obtained after a delay of 48 hours (at 72 or 96 hours). At each time of investigation, in addition single photon emission computed tomograms (SPECT) were obtained of the pelvic and the abdominal regions, using a double head large field of view gamma camera (Picker Prism 2000®). A total of

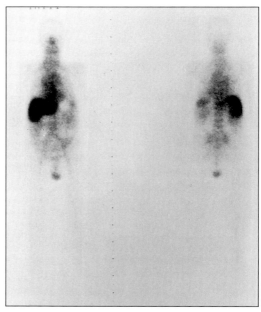

Figure 1. Typical activity distribution of the OncoScint® antibody four days after application, ventral view left, dorsal view right. There is quite high uptake in liver, spleen, and bone marrow. The blood pool is largely cleared and the unspecific activity in the urinary bladder is low.

---

[1]The paper contains parts of the thesis of *Anja Schmitz*.

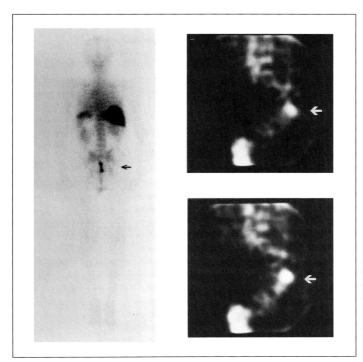

Figure 2. Typical image of a patient with rectal carcinoma. Left: Even on whole body scans (dorsal view) the tumor is clearly visible. Right: The SPECT images demonstrate the anatomical correlation to bladder and spine. Two consecutive sagittal slices of the pelvis are shown.

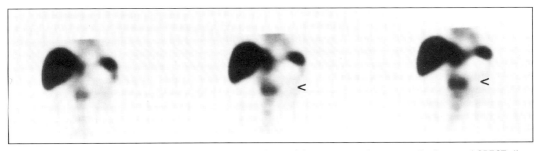

Figure 3. Extended peri-aortic lymph node metastases. A set of three consecutive prevertebral coronal SPECT slices is demonstrated, in front of the spine and slightly below the liver, lymph node metastases are clearly delineated. The serum CEA level was increasing for more than six months and was repeatedly measured (> 80 ng/ml) during the months prior to scintigraphy. Abdominal CT and sonography were negative, but a later performed 2-FDG PET scan also demonstrated pathology.

64 views every 6° were acquired, requiring a total acquisition time of 20 minutes. The scintigraphic results were compared with presurgical sonography or CT-findings, when available, and with histological data.

Figure 1 displays the typical activity distribution of the antibody four days after administration. There is moderate uptake in liver, spleen, and bone marrow. The blood pool activity has mostly cleared. There is also only low non-specific activity in the urinary bladder that might diminish the sensitivity for of rectal carcinoma detection.

Figure 2 demonstrates the typical image of a patient with rectal carcinoma. Even on whole body scans the tumor is clearly visible. The additionally acquired SPECT images demonstrate anatomical correlation to bladder and spine.

In Figure 3 multiple metastases are demonstrated. The abdominal CT was negative, but a later fluoro (^{18}F)-deoxyglucose (2-FDG) PET scan also demonstrated pathology.

Results and discussion

In 29 of the 30 patients surgery was performed. In 25 of the patients who had surgery, colorectal carcinoma was found including 23 primaries, and two local recurrencies. In 17 of those patients immunoscintigraphy was true positive, in six cases false negative. The scintigraphic finding of the last patient was unambiguous. In four patients benign histological findings were reported corresponding mostly to postsurgical fibrosis. These patients were always rated true negative by immunoscintigraphy. One presacral malignant melanoma metastasis, which showed low radiotracer uptake was the only false positive finding concerning the primary tumor site. In the remaining case scintigraphy was unambiguous.

Sixteen of the 24 patients bearing colorectal cancer were free of lymph node metastases. In 11 of those 16 cases scintigraphy was true negative, in two cases false positive and in three cases unambiguous. In three of the nine patients with lymph node metastases, immunoscintigraphy was true positive, in four cases false negative and twice unambiguous.

Distant metastases occured in three of the above mentioned patients. In one patient with intraperitoneal metastases, the scan was true positive, and one case with lung metastases was missed. In the third patient, liver metastases were missed by immunoscintigraphy, but lung metastases were reported, that could not be established with CT till now.

In the remaining 30th case surgery has not yet been performed because of the unexpectedly widespread disease that was detected by immunoscintigraphy. In spite of CEA serum levels that were rising for more than six months and were > 80 ng/ml at the time of scintigraphy, CT and sonography were negative. The 2-FDG PET scan performed after immunoscintigraphy supported the diagnosis of extended peri-aortic lymph node metastases.

The results of the present study coincide with those reported earlier (5) using the B72.3 antibody. Over all sensitivity and specificity are comparable with those of other antibodies used for routine scintigraphy (1, 2, 6). Planar imaging gave good results, which surprisingly could not be reallyimproved by SPECT. This result is in contrast

Table I. Summary of results described in detail in the text. In spite of the small number of cases, the percent values are provided for orientation purposes. Their statistical uncertainty must be considered.

Site	True pos.	True neg.	False pos.	False neg.	Unambiguous
Colorectal	17	4	1	6	1
Lymph nodes	3	11	2	4	5
Distant	1	17	2	2	2
unambiguous, counted as positive					
Colorectal	18	4	1	6	–
Lymph nodes	4	11	5	4	–
Distant	1	17	4	2	–
	sensitivity (%)	specificity (%)			
Colorectal	74	80			
Lymph nodes	43	85			
Distant	33	89			
	unambiguous, counted as positive				
Colorectal	75	80			
Lymph nodes	50	69			
Distant	33	81			

to the experience with $^{99}T_c^m$-labeled antibodies directed against colorectal carcinoma. Possible reasons are the lower blood pool activity because of later imaging times or the higher gamma photon energy of ^{111}In.

Conclusion

Immunoscintigraphy was found to be highly specific and quite sensitive for the detection of primary or recurrent colorectal carcinoma. The only false positive finding in this respect corresponded to malignancy involving the metastasis from malignant melanoma. However, in our pre-surgical patients the sensitivity for lymph node metastases was not high enough to plan the surgical strategy based on the results of immunoscintigraphy. The sensitivity for lymph node metastases was below 50% of the histologically proven metastases, but the size of the metastases was often on the millimeter scale. Nevertheless, immunoscintigraphy was able to demonstrate unsuspected tumor sites in two patients, which had been previously thoroughly investigated by morphologic imaging. According to our results, the B72.3 antibody is suitable for the use in colorectal cancer diagnosis. Its sensitivity, however, is not high enough to exclude malignant disease and the procedure therefore must be indicated thoroughly. In that case, immunoscintigraphy using the B72.3 antibody is of value as a routine clinical procedure.

References

1. Bischof-Delaloye A, Delaloye B, Buchegger F et al (1989) Clinical value of immunoscintigraphy in colorectal carcinoma patients: A prospective study. J Nucl Med 30:1646–1656
2. Bockisch A, Oehr P, Biltz H et al (1991) The clinical value of radioimmunodetection (RID) using anti melanoma antibody. Tumordiagn u Ther 12:112–116
3. Brown BA, Comeau RD, Jones PL (1987) Pharmacokinetics of the monoclonal antibody B72.3 and its fragments labeled with either 125I or 111In. Cancer Res. 47:1149–1154
4. Colcher D, Hand HP, Muti M et al (1989) A spectrum of monoclonal antibodies reactive with human mammary tumor cells. Proc Natl Acad Sci USA 78:3199–3203
5. Doerr RJ, Abdel-Nabi H, Krag D, Mitchell E (1991) Radiolabeled antibody imaging in the management of colorectal cancer. Ann Surg 214:118–124
6. Siccardi AG, Burragi GL, Callegro L et al (1989) Immunoscintigraphy of adenocarcinomas by means of radiolabelled F(ab')2 fragments of an anti-carcinoembryonic antigen monoclonal antibody: A multicenter study. Cancer Res 49:3095–3103
7. Thor A, Ouchi N, Szpak CA et al (1986) The distribution of oncofetal antigen TAG-72 defined by monoclonal antibody B72.3. Cancer Res 46:3118–3124

Address for correspondence:
Prof. Dr. med. Dr. rer. nat. A. Bockisch
Klinik für Nuklearmedizin
Johannes-Gutenberg-Universität
Langenbeckstraße 1
D-55101 Mainz, Germany

Application of anti-TPS antibodies for in vivo diagnostics and therapy

P. Oehr, U. Germer, Q. Liu
University of Bonn, Germany

Introduction

TPS is a cytokeratin 18 (1) tumor marker suitable for the in vitro detection of different kinds of cancer. The aim of our study was to investigate whether anti-TPS antibodies could be applied for the in vivo diagnostics and therapy of cancer.

Materials and methods

Antibody labeling

The anti-TPS antibodies (M 3 MAK 2/87, 1.35 mg/ml, 1 part glycerol, 1 part citrate buffer pH 7.0.) were a present from B. Björklund, SBL, Stockholm. The antibodies were separated from glycerol by PDG-6 gel column chromatography with PBS buffer at pH 7.2 and concentrated by centrifugation in Amicon-10 filters to the final volume of 0.5 ml. ^{131}I-labeling was made according to the chloramin T technique using the iodobead method of *Pierce*. Three iodobeads were incubated for 10 min with 370 MBq ^{131}I at room temperature, after which 700 µg anti-TPS antibodies in 500 µl PBS buffer (pH 7.2) were added. The incubation was stopped 12 min later by removal of the beads. The labeled antibodies were separated from the unbound ^{131}I activity by Sephadex-G-25 PD10 gel filtration in PBS buffer (pH 7.2) containing 0.01% albumin at a flow rate of 1.5 ml/min. The specific activity of the antibodies was 20–100 kBq/µg.

Intraperitoneal injections

Wistar rats were immuno-suppressed by diurnal treatment with cyclosporin A and a single whole-body x-ray irradiation of 3 Gy three days before the tumor transplantation. Under ether-anesthesia the animals were injected with 3 ml HeLa cell suspension ($3 \cdot 10^6$ cells/ml) followed by an injection of 0.5 ml antibodies. Subsequent injections of antibodies were made in different groups four and eight days after the first injection: first day 140 µg antibodies (specific activity 100 kBq/µg), fourth day 140 µg (specific activity 26 kBq/µg), eighth day 200 µg (specific activity 76 kBq/µg).

Determination of tumor weight and radioactivity uptake

Under ether-anestesia the animals were bled 22 days after the tumor implantation and perfused with saline. Organs and solid tumors were removed and weighed, and the radioactivity was measured in a scintillation well-counter. The biodistribution of the antibodies was determined using the tumor/organ index per gram tissue.

Results

Figure 1 compares the uptake of radioactivity by the tumor and organs regarding a single and repeated antibody injection after four days. Repeated application of antibodies improved the uptake of the ^{131}I activity. For all organs the tumor/tissue index for uptake of the radiolabel increased after a subsequent injection of antibodies. The smallest change was found in relation to the kidney (1.2 times), the highest in relation to the liver and muscle (4.4 and 3.9. times, respectively).

Figure 2 displays the tumor weights and their mean value obtained for four animals after three

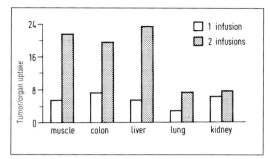

Figure 1. Effect of ^{131}I anti-TPS antibody infusions in vivo on the radiolabel uptake.

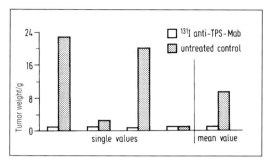

Figure 2. In vivo inhibition of tumor growth by ^{131}I anti-TPS.

repeated antibody injections in comparison with four control animals without the antibody treatment. The mean value of the tumor weight for the treated animals showed a 15-fold reduction of the tumor weight as compared to the control.

Discussion

Our study provides information on the applicability of radiolabeled antibodies for the in vivo localization of tumors and the reduction of the tumor weight by a repeated infusion of the ^{131}I-labeled anti-TPS antibodies.

The results in figure 1 indicate that there is an accumulation of the ^{131}I radiolabel 22 days after a single injection of ^{131}I anti-TPS. This uptake is normally sufficient for the in vivo tumor localization with a gamma camera. A twofold injection of radiolabeled antibodies within four days of each other leads to an increased tumor/tissue uptake index which is reflected in an improved image of the tumor as compared to the organ-background radioactivity. This increased uptake ratio is leading to a more efficient tumor treatment. The improved ratio can be explained by three different mechanisms: 1. increased availability of antigens in the tumor, 2. decreased non-specific binding of specific antibodies in the organs, 3. decreased availability of specific antigen in the organs in comparison with the tumor.

The TPS-antigen decorates the cytosceleton of HeLa cells. This means that most of the target antigen is in the cytoplasm of the tumor cells and cannot be easily reached by the antibodies. In the first mechanism we assume that the number of accessible TPS-antigen in the tumor tissue in- creased after the first antibodies injection. The antigen might have been released due to the tumor-cell destruction caused by the first injection of radiolabeled antibodies, whereas in organs which probably contain only a small number of cells with cross-reacting non-specific membrane epitopes for anti-TPS antibodies no further antigen was released. In such a case an additional injection of antibodies would mainly lead to the binding of anti-TPS antibodies at the tumor. In the second mechanism the non-specific binding sites in the organs might have been blocked after the first injection of the specific antibodies, and the uptake of radioactivity in the organs was therefore lower after the second injection. In the third mechanism some of the organs might also exhibit specific epitopes for TPS in a limited number of TPS-positive cells as compared with the tumor. In such a case the amount of destroyed cells and released antigen would have been much lower than that in the tumor which consisted of HeLa cells.

Apart from these three distinctly different mechanisms there could also be a mixed reaction which includes them all. In different experiments (data not shown) we observed a decreased background radioactivity in the organs after injection of small quantities of non-labeled specific antibodies prior to the injection of specific radiolabeled antibodies. This result is in an agreement with the hypothesis of epitope blocking in the organs after repeated injections of anti-TPS antibodies.

The improvement of the antibodies binding to the tumor has an impact on the antibody treatment. Since repeated injections enhance the accumulation of antibodies and/or radioactivity, we made a triple injection of labeled antibodies and compared the tumor weights to those from untreated animals who received only the tumor cells. Although the results in figure 2 show some variations in the tumor weight of each individual untreated animal, the trend of tumor weight reduction by treatment with radiolabeled antibodies is clearly distinguishable. This reduction of tumor weight can be explained either by a tumor cell destruction or by a growth inhibition. In the case of the tumor cell destruction there would be an agreement with the hypothesis that repeated infusions can lead to more accessible antigen for binding of radiolabeled antibodies.

Our data do not allow a conclusion of whether it was the antibody or the radioactivity which caused the observed treatment effect. It could have been been due to a combined effect of both of them. Since the antibodies were used for intraperitoneal treatment of a transplanted cell suspension, the results can only account for a successful inhibition of micrometastatic growth. With respect to the treatment of patients this finding would call for a repeated postsurgical treatment with radiolabeled antibodies which should inhibit or prevent the growth of extruded single tumor cells. Such a treatment could be implemented only within a limited period of time inasmuch as the repeated monoclonal antibody administrations might provoke formation of human anti-mouse antibodies (HAMA) which might in turn inactivate the subsequently injected antibodies. For a long term treatment it would be necessary to "humanize" the TPS-antibodies. The experiments were stopped 22 days after the beginning of the treatment. We can expect that the effect of the radiolabel on the reduction of tumor weight could be even higher after a longer waiting period (1–3 months), as is the case with the ^{131}I-treatment of the thyroid cancer. A more extended study with longer time intervals was, however, not possible due to limited availability of the antibodies.

Summary

Intraperitoneally infused ^{131}I-labeled anti-TPS antibodies accumulated in the intraperitoneally injected HeLa cells in immuno-suppressed rats. Repeated injections of ^{131}I anti-TPS antibodies increased the tumor/organ index for the uptake of the radiolabel into the tumor. Triple injection of ^{131}I-labeled anti-TPS antibodies within eight days led to a 20-fold decrease in tumor weight within 22 days as compared with the tumors in untreated animals. As a result, the multiple infusion of ^{131}I anti-TPS antibodies inhibited the micrometastatic tumor growth. The treatment of tumor cells with ^{131}I anti-TPS may lead to tumor-cell destruction which increases the number of accessible antigen-binding sites in the tumor tissue. The repeated infusion of radiolabeled anti-TPS antibodies might therefore be a promising method for the in vivo diagnostics and treatment of cancer with cytokeratin antibodies.

References

1   Oehr P, Liu Q, Jin HJ, Halim AB, El Ahmady O, Nap M, Lackner, Schultes B, Ota Y (1992) TPS: Biology and clinical value. In: Klapdor R (ed) Tumor associated antigens, oncogenes, receptors, cytokines in tumor diagnosis and therapy at the beginning of the nineties. Zuckschwerdt, München, pp 213–218

Address for correspondence:
Priv.-Doz. Dr. P. Oehr
Experimentelle Strahlenbiologie
Universitätskliniken Bonn
Sigmund-Freud-Straße 25
D-53105 Bonn, Germany

Formation of anti-idiotype antibodies and the induction of cellular immunity after in vivo administration of the monoclonal antibody OC 125

H. Richter[a], J. Reinsberg[b], U. Wagner[b], H.J. Biersack[a]
[a]Clinic for Nuclear Medicine, [b]Center for Obstetrics and Gynecology,
University of Bonn, Germany

Introduction

The murine monoclonal antibody OC125 binds to Cancer Antigen 125 (CA 125), a determinant expressed on the cell-surfaces of 80% of non-mucinous ovarian adenocarcinomas, and subsequently shed into the general circulation (1, 2). In vivo administration of OC125 is thought to offer an approach to immunotherapy of ovarian cancer by activating the immunological network postulated by *Jerne* (3). Mimicking the epitope of the CA 125-antigen and presenting it in an immunogenic environment, anti-idiotype antibodies (Ab2) of the "internal image"-type, which bind to the paratope of the OC125 (Ab1), are thought to induce anti-anti-idiotype antibodies (Ab3) reacting with the CA 125-antigen like the OC125-antibody and to activate T-cell immunity against the tumor (4, 5).

This study was designed to demonstrate the development of Ab2 after the infusion of radiolabeled OC125 F(ab)$_2$-fragments and to investigate their effect on T-cell immunity. Therefore Ab2 were determined and their specificity was characterized using inhibition assays. Furthermore the activation of the T-cell system was monitored by following the production kinetics of the soluble interleukin-2 receptor (sIL-2R) and a soluble subunit of the CD8 T-cell receptor (sCD8), two cytokines which are useful parameters for indicating T-cell activity (6–11), and correlating them to the formation of Ab2.

Materials and methods

The patient

Patients were treated with multiple infusions of ^{131}I-labeled OC125-F(ab)$_2$-fragments (1 mg each time) and the patient U.M. was chosen for further study. For this 63-years old patient, a non-metastatic, papillary carcinoma of the ovary (FIGO stage II) was diagnosed in the course of a tumor reduction in January 1988. In the first month after the surgery irradiation of the abdomen and a polychemotherapy were performed. For the next 12 month a mono-chemotherapy with treosulfan followed. In April and July 1988, ^{131}I-labeled OC125-F(ab)$_2$-fragments were infused. A recurrence of the tumor, detected in July 1991, was only treated with a third infusion of ^{131}I-labeled OC125-F(ab)$_2$-fragments. Six weeks after this infusion the recurrence was not longer detectable by computed tomography. 68 month after the surgery (in January 1988) the patient U.M. was still alive, undergoing no further therapeutical treatments.

Serum samples

Serial serum samples were taken over a period of 22 days after the third infusion. The samples were aliquoted and stored at –18 °C until use. To detect and characterize Ab2, serum samples, which were supposed to contain high Ab2-levels, were pooled.

Preparation of serum IgG

Immunoglobulin-G was purified from the pool-serum by affinity-chromatography using a Protein G Sepharose column (MabTrap G kit, Pharmacia LKB, Uppsala, Sweden) according to the instructions of the manufacturer using 0.5 ml pool-serum diluted 1:2 with the included binding buffer. The purified IgG was concentrated with Centricon-30 microcentrators (Amicon, Danvers, Massachusettes, USA).

Determination of sIL-2R and sCD8

The concentrations of sIL-2R and sCD8 were measured using the Cellfree-IL-2R and the Cell-free CD8 (both supplied from Biermann, Bad Nauheim, Germany). Both are immunometric assays, which were performed according to the instructions of the manufacturer.

Determination of Ab2

Ab2 levels were determined with the CA 125-EIA Monoclonal (Abbott, Wiesbaden-Delkenheim, Germany) and the CA 125 ELSA (CIS Isotopendiagnostik, Dreieich, Germany), respectively, according to the instructions of the manufacturers. Because these immunometric assays use OC125 as capture and detector antibody the two assays, which were original designed to determine CA 125, can also measure Ab2 directed against the OC125. Since the CA 125-EIA Monoclonal and the CA 125 ELSA cannot distinguish between CA 125 and anti-OC125-antibodies, such as Ab2, and both assay were calibrated using CA 125, the material measured with those assays was named CA 125-equivalents.

For the direct determination of Ab2, an immunological "sandwich-assay" with immobilized OC125 as capture antibody and horseradish peroxidase labeled anti-human-IgG as detector antibody was used. The assay was based on the Enzygnost-HAMA micro (Behring, Marburg, Germany) and performed according to the instructions of the manufacturer. To adapt the assay to the determination of Ab2 against the OC125 instead of unspecific murine antibodies, ^{125}I-labeled OC125 from the CA 125 RIA (Abbott, Wiesbaden-Delkenheim, Germany; radiolabeling not used for detection) was bound to the layer of anti-murine-IgG (developed in goat) coating the solid phase of the microtitration plates.

To inhibit the binding of human anti-murine antibodies (HAMA) directed against iso- and allotype determinants on the OC125, polyclonal murine IgG (Sigma, Deisenhofen, Germany) in different concentrations was added to the samples to mask these HAMA, so that only the Ab2 directed against the idiotype were bound.

Determination of CA 125

CA 125 was determined with the IM$_x$ CA 125 (Abbott, Wiesbaden-Delkenheim, Germany). The assay was performed in the IM$_x$-analyser (Abbott, Wiesbaden-Delkenheim, Germany) according to the instructions of the manufacturer. Because in this "sandwich-assay" a polyclonal anti-CA 125-antibody (developed in sheep) is used as the capture antibody and the OC125 is only employed as the detector antibody, only "real" CA 125 was measured and not anti-diotype anti-OC125-antibodies.

Inhibition of the binding of Ab2 to immobilized OC125 (inhibition assay I)

In order to characterise the specificity of Ab2, the assay used for the determination of Ab2, which was based on the Enzygnost-HAMA micro (see above), was performed in the presence of 200 µg/ml polyclonal murine IgG (Sigma, Deisenhofen, Germany) and increasing concentrations of CA 125 (Biomira, Edmonton, Alberta, Canada). In this assay (inhibition assay I) the CA 125 should inhibit the binding of "internal image"-Ab2 to the paratope of immobilized OC125 antibodies.

Inhibition of the binding of OC125 to immobilized Ab2 (inhibition assay II)

In another assay to characterize the specificity of Ab2 (inhibition assay II), CA 125 was used to inhibit the binding of radiolabeled OC125 to immobilized Ab2. First, the purified IgG of the pool-serum was diluted with phosphate buffer saline of pH 7.4 (PBS; 10 mM PO_4^{3-}, 137 mM NaCl, 2.7 mM KCl). 50 µl per well were pipetted into a Polysorb microtitration plate (Nunc, Roskilde, Denmark) and incubated over night at 2–8° C. Then the plate was decanted and blocked by incubating each well for 1 h at room temperature with 300 µl of a solution containing 5% (5 g/100 ml PBS) bovine serum albumin. After washing the microtitration plate three times with 400 µl PBS per well, 50 µl of ^{125}I-labeled OC125 (tracer from the CA 125 RIA; Abbott, Wiesbaden-Delkenheim, Germany) and 25 µl of a solution containing CA 125 and murine IgG were dispensed into each well and incubated at 2–8° C over night. For this solution, CA 125 (Biomira, Edmonton, Alberta, Canada) and polyclonal murine IgG (Sigma, Deisenhofen, Germany; 200 µg/ml final concentration) were diluted in PBS. The murine IgG should inhibit immunoreactions between HAMA and the OC125. By washing each well again three times with 400 µl of PBS this incubation was stopped. After dividing the microtitration plate, the bound activity of each well was measured for 5 min using a gamma-scintillation-counter.

Results

In the first three days after the third infusion of OC125 antibody fragments the concentrations of sIL-2R and sCD8 showed only slight fluctuations, which were followed by a strong increase by the 10th day (sIL-2R up to 5,992 U/ml and sCD8 up to 824 U/ml), indicating an activation of the T-cell system (figure 1). By the 21th day after the infusion, the concentration of sCD8 returned to a lower level, whereas the concentration of sIL-2R remained elevated. The concentrations of CA 125 equivalents (determined with the CA 125 ELSA) increased from 589 U/ml to 3,072,440 U/ml by the 10th day suggesting that Ab2 had been formed. Even by day 21 nearly 2 million units were detected.

In the pooled sera of the patient a concentration of 198,570 U/ml CA 125-equivalents was measured using the CA 125-EIA Monoclonal. The concentration of "real" CA 125 measured with the IM_x CA 125 was 29 U/ml, indicating the presence of anti-OC125-antibodies. This was confirmed by the finding, that the IgG fraction from the pool serum, purified by Protein G affinity chromato-

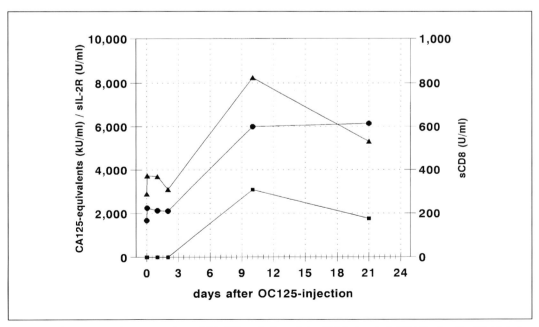

Figure 1. Time-course of concentrations of CA 125-equivalents (■), sCD8 (▲) and sIL-2R (●) after the third infusion of ^{131}I-labeled OC125-F(ab)$_2$-fragments into the patient U.M. One sample taken immediately before infusion is marked at time zero on the x-axis.

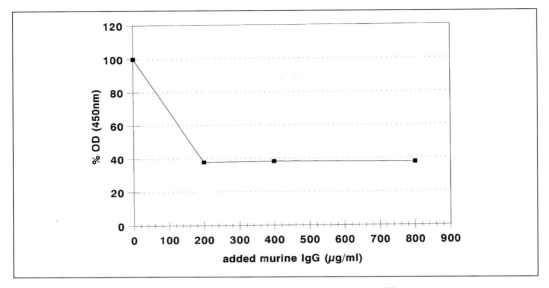

Figure 2. Inhibition of the binding of human anti-OC125-IgG to immobilized ^{125}I-labeled OC125-antibodies by polyclonal murine IgG. A dilution of the IgG purified from the pool-serum of the patient U.M. (resulting in a concentration of 4,910 U/ml CA 125-equivalents) was mixed with murine IgG in increasing concentrations (x-axis labels indicate the final concentrations) and incubated with immobilized OC125-antibodies. Bound human IgG was detected with enzyme-labeled anti-human-IgG antibodies. After the development with 3,3',5,5'-tetramethylbenzidine the optical density (OD) was read at 450 nm. The data are displayed as percent OD of the control without murine IgG.

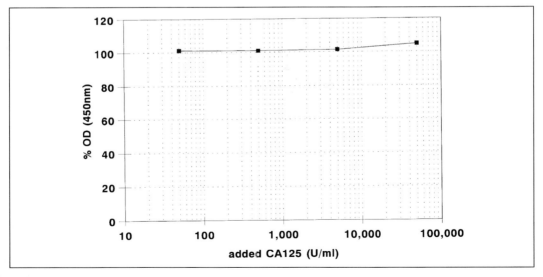

Figure 3. Inhibition of the binding of human anti-OC125-IgG to immobilized ^{125}I-labeled OC125-antibodies by CA 125 (inhibition assay I). A dilution of the IgG purified from the pool-serum of the patient U.M. (resulting in a concentration of 4,910 U/ml CA 125 -equivalents) was mixed with CA 125 in increasing concentrations (x-axis labels indicate the final concentrations) and incubated with immobilized OC125-antibodies. 200 µg/ml of polyclonal murine IgG (final concentration) were added to all samples. Bound human IgG was detected with enzyme-labeled anti-human-IgG antibodies. After the development with 3,3',5,5'-tetramethylbenzidine the optical density (OD) was read at 450 nm. The data are displayed as percent OD of the control without CA 125.

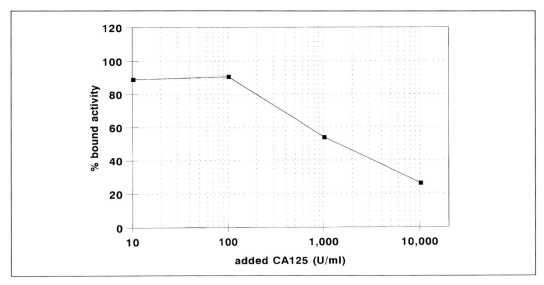

Figure 4. Inhibition of the binding of ^{125}I-labeled OC125-antibodies to immobilized human IgG by CA 125 (inhibition assay II). A dilution of the IgG purified from the pool-serum of the patient U.M. (resulting in a concentration of 1,093 U/ml CA 125-equivalents) was immobilized and then incubated with radiolabeled OC125-antibodies, which had been mixed with murine IgG (final concentration of 200 µg/ml) and CA 125 in increasing concentrations (x-axis labels indicate the final concentrations). Afterwards the bound activity was measured. The data are displayed as percent bound activity of the control without CA 125.

graphy contained 39% of the CA 125-equivalents applied to the column (38,311 U/ml of 99,285 U/ml CA 125-equivalents).

Upon mixing the IgG purified from the pool serum with murine IgG in increasing concentrations and incubating it with immobilized ^{125}I-labeled OC125 (inhibition assay I), only 62% of the binding of anti-OC125-IgG was inhibited (figure 2). This indicated, that only a portion of the anti-OC125-IgG was bound to iso- and allotype determinants on the OC125, whereas the remaining portion was bound to the idiotype of the OC125.

Adding increasing concentrations of CA 125 to the sample mixed with murine IgG (inhibition assay I) the remaining binding between Ab2 and the immobilised OC125 could not be inhibited (figure 3). The binding of ^{125}I-labeled OC125 to immobilised IgG purified from the pool serum, which was mixed with murine IgG to block the binding of the OC125 to HAMA present in the sample, was inhibited by CA 125 (inhibition-assay II) in a concentration depending manner (figure 4). This indicates, that the CA 125 and a portion of the immobilised Ab2 of patient U.M. competed for the binding to a common determinant of the OC125. In the presence of 10,000 U/ml CA 125 the binding to the immobilized Ab2 was inhibited for about 70%.

Discussion

The results confirm, that the patient U.M. developed Ab2 after the infusion of ^{131}I-labeled F(ab)$_2$-fragments of the OC125-antibody.

With the CA 125-EIA Monoclonal could be shown, that the pool serum of the patient U.M. contained high concentrations of a material binding bivalent to the OC125, and therefore reacting in a manner equivalent to CA 125. The material was not "real" CA 125, since the CA 125-equivalents could not be similary detected with the IM$_x$ CA 125. Additionally, 39% of the CA 125-equivalents were recovered in the IgG fraction of the pool-serum, confirming that a portion of the CA 125 equivalents was anti-OC125-IgG.

Patients often develop HAMA after the infusion of murine antibodies (12, 13). When investigating the specificity of our anti-OC125-IgG by means of inhibition assays, only a portion of the anti-

OC125-IgG could be masked with polyclonal murine IgG in order to inhibit its binding to the OC125. This showed that the patient U.M. developed not only antibodies directed against iso- and allotype determinants on the OC125 (HAMA) but also Ab2 impossible to be masked.

It is one characteristic of "internal image"-Ab2, that their binding to the Ab1 (OC125) can be inhibited by the antigen (CA 125). However, a definite characterization of the Ab2 developed by the patient produced mixed results. In one assay the binding of Ab2 to immobilized OC125 was not inhibited with increasing concentrations of CA 125, suggesting no formation of "internal image"-Ab2. In another type of assay the binding of Ab2 to soluble OC125 was inhibited with CA 125 in a concentration depending manner, suggesting the formation of "internal image"-Ab2.

When investigating the induction of cellular immunity, the formation of Ab2 was monitored using the concentration of CA 125-equivalents, because it has been shown above, that a portion of the CA 125-equivalents were Ab2. Increased concentrations of the sIL-2R and the sCD8 were observed simultaneously with the induction of Ab2 suggesting a correlation. This is in accordance with *Lee* et al., who showed the induction of a T-cell-immunity against a tumor after administration of Ab2 in vitro and in vivo by means of an animal model (15). Also the fact, that the recurrence being diagnosed prior to the administration of the OC125 was no longer detectable six weeks after the infusion, suggests an induction of cellular immunity by the Ab2 formed after the infusion of ^{131}I-labeled OC125-F(ab)$_2$-fragments, regardless their specificity of binding to the OC125-paratope like "internal image"-Ab2 or not.

References

1. Bast RC, Feeny M, Lazarus H, Nadler LM, Colvin RB, Knapp RC (1981) Reactivity of a monoclonal antibody with human ovarian carcinoma. J Clin Invest 68:1331–1337
2. Kabawat SE, Bast RC, Welch WR, Knapp RC, Colvin RB (1983) Immunopathologic characterization of a monoclonal antibody that recognizes common surface antigenes of human ovarian tumors of serious, endometrioid, and clear cell types. Am J Clin Pathol 79:98–104
3. Jerne NK (1974) Towards a network theory of the immune system. Ann Immunol (Inst Past) 125C: 373–389
4. Wagner U, Reinsberg J, Oehr P, Briele B, Werner A, Kerbs D, Biersack HJ (1990) Clinical courses of patients with ovarian carcinomas after induction of anti-idiotypic antibodies against a tumor-associated antigen. Tumoriagnostik Therapie 11:1–4
5. Wagner UA, Oehr PF, Reinsberg J, Schmidt SC, Schlebush HW, Schultes B, Werner A, Prietl G, Krebs D (1992) Immunotherapy of advanced ovarian carcinomas by activation of the idiotypic network. Biotechn Ther 3:81–89
6. Rubin LA, Nelson DL (1990) The soluble interleukin-2 receptor: Biology, function, and clinical application. Ann Int Med 113:619–627
7. Reske-Kunz AB, Osawa H, Josimovic-Alasevic O, Rüde E, Diamantstein T (1987) Soluble interleukin 2 receptors are released by long term-cultured insulin-specific T-cells transiently after contact with antigen. J Immunol 138:192–196
8. Tomkinson BE, Wagner DK, Nelson DL, Sullivan JL (1987) Activated lymphocytes during acute Epstein-Barr virus infection. J Immunol 139:3802–3807
9. Tomkinson BE, Brown MC, IP SH, Carrabis S, Sullivan JL (1989) Soluble CD8 during T cell activation. J Immunol 142:2230–2236
10. Fujimoto J, Stewart SJ, Levy R (1984) Immunochemical analysis of the released Leu-2 (T8) molecule. J Exp Med 160:116–124
11. Fujimoto J, Levy S, Levy R (1983) Spontaneous release of Leu-2 (T8) molecule from human T cells. J Exp Med 159:752–766
12. Schroff RW, Foon KA, Beatty SM, Oldham RK, Morgan AC (1985) Human anti-murine immunoglobulin responses in patients recieving monoclonal antibody therapy. Cancer Res 45:879–885
13. Shawler DL, Bartholomew RM, Smith LM, Dillman RO (1985) Human response to multiple injections of murine monoclonal IgG. J Immunol 135:1530–1535
14. Lee VK, Harriott TG, Kuchroo VK, Halliday WJ, Hellström I, Hellström KE (1985) Monoclonal anti-idiotypic antibodies related to a murine oncofetal bladder tumor antigen induce specific cell-mediated tumor immunity. Proc Natl Acad Sci USA 82:6286–6290

Address for correspondence:
Dipl. Biol. H. Richter
Klinik für Nuklearmedizin der
Universität Bonn
Sigmund-Freud-Straße 25
D-53127 Bonn, Germany

Biodistribution and tumor visualization with ^{111}In labeled B72.3 antibodies

Studies in nude mice bearing xenografts of human pancreatic carcinomas

A. Popp[a], M. Bahlo[a], R. Klapdor[a], D. Platz[b]

[a]Department of Medicine, [b]Department of Nuclear Medicine, University Hospital, Hamburg, Germany

Introduction

Basing on previous studies on immunoscintigraphy in nude mice bearing xenografts of human g.i. carcinomas using ^{131}I, 99mTe or ^{111}In labeled CA 19-9, anti CA 125 and anti CEA antibodies (2) and encouraged by clinical sensitivity/specificity studies with the recently introduced "tumor marker" CA 72-4 in gastric and pancreatic cancer (3) as well as by clinical immunoscintigraphy of colorectal carcinomas with the B72.3 antibody we started experimental studies to investigate the potential relevance of ^{111}In labeled B72.3 antibodies for immunoscintigraphy of tumors of the pancreas.

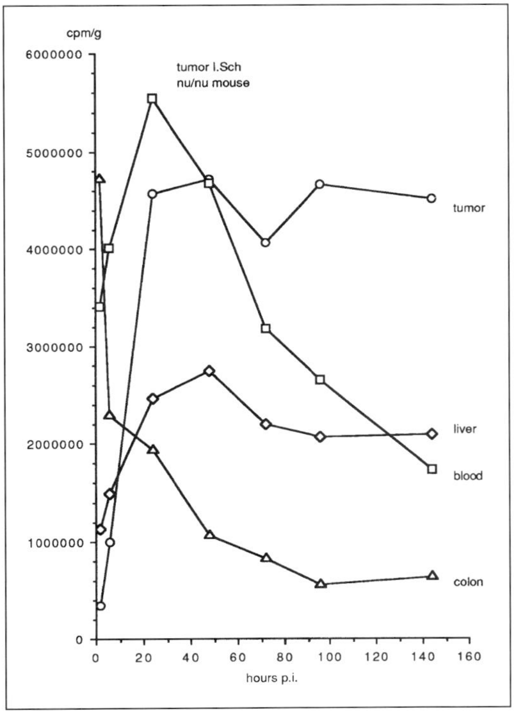

Methods

The studies were performed in nude mice, age 6–8 weeks, 30–50 g body weight, females or castrated males, bearing xenografts of human pancreatic carcinomas (n = 6), secreting CA 72-4 into the serum to a low, middle and higher extend.
We injected i.v. 100 µCi per animal of the ^{111}In labeled B72.3 antibody (CYT-103-[111]In: OncoScint CR 103) into the tail vein and measured the distribution and the tumor/blood ratios after 2, 4,

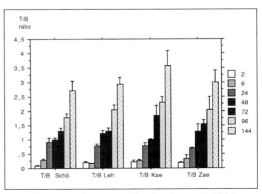

Figure 1. Uptake of the injected ^{111}In labeled B72.3 antibody by the tumor, the liver and the colon in studies in nude mice bearing the human exocrine pancreatic cancer I.Sch.

Figure 2. Increasing tumor/blood ratio up to 144 hours after i.v. injection of the ^{111}In labeled B72.3 antibody in nude mice bearing four different human pancreatic carcinomas.

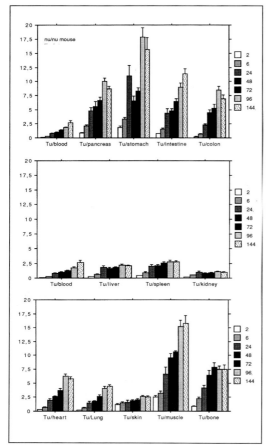

Figure 3. Tumor/blood and tumor/organ ratios in the studies on nude mice bearing the human pancreatic xenograft I.Sch. in relation to time after injection of the ^{111}In labeled antibody B72.3

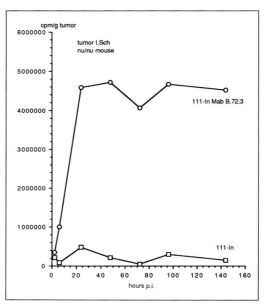

Figure 4. Evidence for a specific uptake of the injected antibody B72.3 by comparing the tumor uptake of the ^{111}In labeled antibody B 72.3 with the uptake of unconjugated ^{111}In.

6, 24, 48, 72 and 144 hours. Scintigraphy was done with Bodyscan-Kamera (Siemens). Tumor uptake, tumor/blood ratios as well as organ/blood ratios were measured and calculated as described previously. CA 72-4 serum concentrations were measured using the CA 72-4 RIA Sorin, serum CEA using the Enzymun EIA BM.

In addition the effects of a three weeks treatment with mitomycin C (2.4 mg/kg per week i.p.) and 5-fluorouracil (80 mg/kg per week i.p.) on antibody uptake by the tumor and tumor/blood ratios as well as on secretion of the tumor marker CEA were studied.

Results and discussion

In contrast to the absolute tumor uptake (figure 1) the tumor/blood ratios as well as the tumor/pancreas and tumor/stomach ratios after 144 hours increased up to 2.5–3.5 and 8–10 and 10–15, respectively (figures 2, 3), that means values significantly higher than the T/liver, T/spleen and T/kidney ratios (figure 3).

Comparative studies with injection of uncoupled ^{111}In suggest a specific tumor uptake of the injected labeled antibody (figure 4). Consequently immunoscintigraphy resulted in good visualization. Chemotherapy with mitomycin C (figures 5a–c) resulted in the three studies in a significant antitumoral effect (SD, SD, PR), chemotherapy with 5-fluorouracil only in retardation of tumor growth compared to the untreated controls (figure 5a). In general, serum levels of CEA reflected the tumor answer to therapy (figure 5b), that means progressive increase in the 5-FU treated animals, and stable course or decrease in the mitomycin C treated animals. The tumor/blood ratios and the tumor uptake of the labeled antibody were found in a similar or slightly

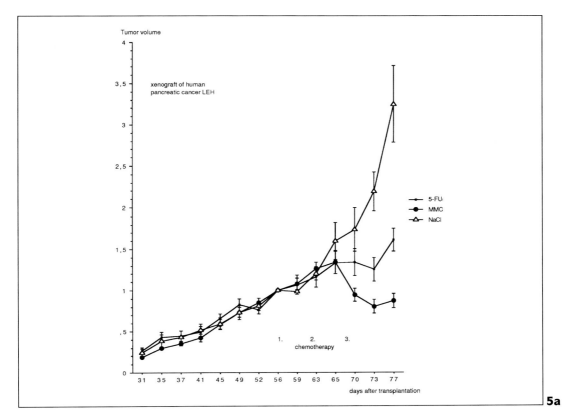

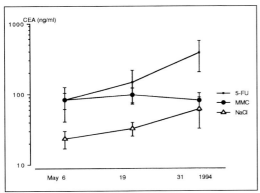

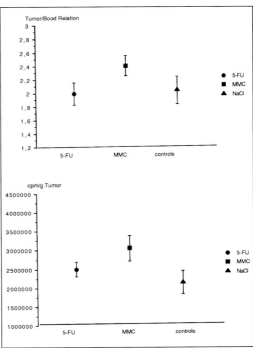

Figure 5. Effects of chemotherapy for three weeks with mitomycin C and 5-fluorouracil on the tumor volume of the xenografts of the human exocrine pancreatic carcinoma Leh, on serum CEA levels (5b) and on the tumor/blood ratios as well as on the antibody B72.3 uptake per tumor weight (5c).

elevated range compared to the control group in two of these studies (figure 5c) and slightly or significantly decreased in the third one.

Summarizing, these experimental studies suggest a specific uptake of the ^{111}In labeled B72.3 antibody by human exocrine pancreatic carcinomas, even in the case of effective chemotherapy. Clinical studies have to evaluate the potential role of this antibody for clinical immunoscintigraphy, for intraoperative scintigraphy and RIGS.

References

1. Doerr RJ, Abdel-Nabi H, Krag D, Mitchell E (1991) Radiolabelled antibody imaging in the management of colorectal cancer. Ann Surg 214:118–124
2. Klapdor R, Montz R (1989) Immunoscintigraphy of pancreatic cancer: Relevance for diagnosis and therapy. In: Chatal JF (ed) Monoclonal antibodies in immunoscintigraphy. CRC Press, Boca Raton, Florida, pp 153–163
3. Patzke B, Klapdor R, Meier-Pannwitt U, Weh P, Schreiber HW (1990) TAG 72 in comparison with CA 19-9, CEA and CA 125 in diagnosis and follow-up of stomach cancer. In: Klapdor R (ed) Recent results in tumor diagnosis and therapy. 5th Symposium on Tumor Markers, Hamburg, Zuckschwerdt, München, pp 31–36

Address for correspondence:
Prof. Dr. R. Klapdor
Medizinische Abteilung
Universitätskrankenhaus
Martinistraße 52
D-20246 Hamburg, Germany

Therapy

Intratumoral radioimmunotheraphy in glioblastomas by means of ^{131}I radiolabeled monoclonal antibodies

P. Riva[a], A. Arista[b], C. Sturiale[b], G. Franceschi[a], N. Riva[a], A. Spinelli[a],
M. Casi[a], G. Moscatelli[a], F. Campori[a], R. Gentile[a]

[a] Nuclear Medicine Department and Istituto Oncologico Romagnolo
[b] Neurosurgery Department, "M.Bufalini" Hospital, Cesena, Italy

Introduction

Brain malignant gliomas represent a major therapeutical problem in modern neurosurgery. They are tumors normally confined to the brain and very rarely give extra neural metastases. On the contrary, local recurrences with extension to other brain regions are the rule and the cause of patient death. Surgery, radiotherapy and chemotherapy are the current approaches for the therapy of glioblastomas (GBM) (1) but, in most cases are ineffective or produce transient results. The prognosis of affected patients is always poor with a median survival of 12 months; if the tumor relapses after these treatments, the patient's life expectancy is not longer than six months (2). The lack of an effective treatment led us to experiment an innovative therapeutical approach based on the use of specific murine radiolabeled monoclonal antibodies (MAbs), directly administered into the neoplastic mass (3). We choose this route of administration in order to accumulate in the neoplastic tissue the maximum amount of radiolabeled MAbs to strongly irradiate and completely destroy the tumor. Intravenous (i.v.) and intra-arterial (i.a.)(4) routes in fact, have been proven to deliver to the tumor mass a low amount of immunoconjugates, not enough for therapeutical purpose. This is mainly due to the brain blood barrier (BBB) which limits the penetration of the macromolecules in the extravascular space.

Aim of this study was the evaluation of brain and systemic toxicity following the intratumor injection of escalating doses of radiopharmaceutical, the study of MAbs biodistribution in the tumor and in the body as well as the dosimetry data. Finally, the possible effectiveness of radioimmunotherapy in this kind of very aggressive diseases, was assessed.

Materials and method

Monoclonal antibodies

We applied radioimmunotherapy (RIT) by employing singly or as a cocktail two murine MAbs (IgG$_1$): BC-2 and BC-4 (Sorin Biomedica Italy) which recognize two different epitopes on the molecul of tenascin (5). This antigen is constantly expressed in very large amounts in the stroma of many tumors and in particular in glioblastomas but not in the normal glia (6).

Isotope and labeling method

All MAbs were labeled with iodine-131 by means of iodogen method. The radiochemical purity of the compound was higher than 98%. After labeling procedures MAbs immunoreactivity was over 60%.

Dosimetry evaluation

The radiation dose which could be delivered to target neoplastic tissue and to healthy parenchymas (bone marrow, liver, kidneys) was previously calculated before RIT, by administering intratumorally a tracer dose (mg 1 of MAb and mCi 1 of ^{131}I). Serial planar and SPECT scintigraphies were performed immediately after the injection and daily thereafter for at least five days. Brain, chest and abdomen were carefully studied also with the aid of Roi method to calculate the amount of radioactivity in the tumor bed and in critical extraneural parenchymas. MAbs residence time in pathological and normal tissues was estimated. Tumor mass volume was established by CT scan or MRI. By this data and applying MIRD (7) formalism the radiation dose to tumor and to healthy major organs was in advance forecasted.

Patients

48 patients with brain glioblastoma and one with spinal cord glioblastoma were recruited to this protocol. Patients age ranged from 11 to 68 years (mean 50). They were 23 females and 26 males. By histological examination the tumors resulted six anaplastic astrocytomas (grade 3° or 4°) and 35 glioblastomas.

All patients, except one, were previously operated once or more times. 48 patients received after surgery radiotherapy and/or chemotherapy. So radioimmunotherapy was applied as 3rd or 4th line care. 41 out 49 patients are, at present, evaluable. The patients were admitted to intratumor Rit protocol: a) when immunohistochemistry examination of tumor specimen demonstrated a very high expression of tenascin antigen, b) if Karnofsky performance score was > 60% and the patient was self-sufficient, c) if the dosimetry data (calculated in vivo as above expounded) showed the possibility to deliver to the tumor a radiation dose higher than 15,000 cGy without harming normal organs.

Radioimmunotherapy protocol

Before radioimmunotherapy application the patients were pretreated with thyroid blocking agents in order to avoid or reduce free iodine-131 uptake. Antiepilectic and corticosteroid medications were given whenever necessary. MAbs were injected through plastic catheter placed in the tumor bed. At the beginning of our study we utilized a removable catheter inserted by stereotaxy, which was left in place for two or three weeks allowing one or two injections to be made. More recently we use an indwelling catheter placed in the site of the disease. The surgeon removes the primary or recurrent tumor and makes a cavity where the antibodies are injected and easier bind to their antigens on the cavity walls. Repeated injections can be safely carried out through a Rickam reservoir set under the skin. The ^{131}I doses administered were progressively increased and ranged from 15 to 58 mCi. More in particular, six patients received up to 15 mCi, nine received 16-30 mCi, 23 a dose ranging between 31 to 50 and three patients more than 50 mCi of iodine-131. The MAbs mean dose per cycle was 2.8 milligrams. Usually multiple courses of therapy are carried out to obtain a very high cumulative radiation dose (3-5 courses per patient). Ten patients underwent one cycle, 13 were submitted to two cycles, ten patients to three cycles, six to four courses and two had five radioimmunotherapy courses. RIT was always performed under strictly radioprotection rules. Patients were kept in a shielded room and daily, calculation of radioactivity was obtained.

Results

Untoward effects

No systemic, hepatic, renal and hematological adverse reactions were recorded following single or multiple intratumor injections of escalating doses of radiolabeled MAbs. Major organs like kidneys, liver or bone marrow received in fact a very low radiation dose (less than 50 cGy per cycle). In some patients we observed a low thyroid uptake of free iodine-131 with a cumulative dose of about 400 cGy to the organ without endocrinological alterations. Brain toxicity consisted only of transient post injection headache of short duration (13 pats) and seizure in one case who was bearing a bulky tumor mass with cerebral oedema.

HAMA production

In 19 cases the development of human antimouse antibodies (HAMA) (8) after one or more radioimmunotherapy did not occur. In 22 patients a slight HAMA production was demonstrated owing to the leakage of the radiopharmaceutical in the ventricules and afterwords in the blood but no allergic reactions were observed.

Dosimetry

The mean radiation dose to the tumor resulted of 39,800 cGy during the first cycle, 33,500 during the second cycle and 32,700 and 28,300 cGy in the third and fourth course, respectively. In the patients who received a fifth irradiation the mean dose resulted of 47,500 cGy. The cumulative dose was, on average, 80,000 cGy and resulted definitively higher than the radiation achievable by employing the external beam therapy.

Survival

The median survival of our group of patients was about 18 months. The objective response to RIT was evaluated according to WHO suggestions (9). In nine cases no recurrence was observed at follow-up ranging from 12 to 50 months. These patients had an excellent clinical outcome (post RIT Karnofsky score > 70%). In seven patients a partial remission was radiologically documented with consequent clinical improvement and extended survival time (9 months, range: 6–15). In nine cases we observed a stabilization of the neoplastic mass which lasted 12 months. In the remaining 16 patients tumor grew up in 4.8 months as median time (range 2–8 months) after radioimmunotherapy. The response rate (CR+PR) was 39%.

Conclusions

Present multimodality therapies for malignant glioblastomas such as surgery, radiotherapy and chemotherapy have had a relatively little impact on patients survival. The intralesional radio-immunotherapy of gliomas did not produce local or systemic toxicity and even if it resulted rather invasive, it was well tolerated by the patients. The clinical results recorded were favorable and were improved by injecting multiple doses by mean an indwelling catheter placed in the tumor mass or in the cavity after surgery. The intralesional route of administration of radiolabeled monoclonal antibodies seems to be the best method to concentrate in the tumor tissue the largest amount of radioactivity to destroy the most of glioblastoma mass. Radioimmunotherapy can be proposed in an adjuvant setting immediately after surgery and external radiotherapy and should represent a form of tumor radiation boost. The high tolerability and the sharp specificity of this treatment are important features for this purpose.

Further amelioration will be achieved by employing more energetic Beta-emitters such as Yttrium 90 (10) or Rhenium 186 (11).

Acknowledgements

This work was carried out within the National Research Council (CNR, ITALY) program: Clinical Applications of Oncology Research, subproject 8.

References

1. Chang CH, Horton J, Schoenfeld D, Salazer O, Perez-Tamay, Kramer S, Weinstein A, Nelson JS, Tsukada Y (1983) Comparison of postoperative radiotherapy and combined postoperative radiotherapy and chemotherapy in the multidisciplinary management of malignant gliomas. Cancer 52:997–1007
2. Jellinger K, Vole D, Grisold W, Weiss R, Flament H (1983) Multimodality treatment of high-grade supratentorial gliomas. In: Proc 13th Internat Chemother Congr 249:6–12
3. Riva P, Arista A, Sturiale C, Moscatelli G, Tison V, Mariani M, Seccamani E, Lazzari S, Fagioli L, Franceschi G, Sarti G, Riva N, Natali PG, Zardi L, Scassellati GA (1992) Treatment of intracranial human glioblastoma by direct intratumoral administration of ^{131}I labeled antitenascin monoclonal antibody BC-2. Int J Cancer 51:7–13
4. Epenetos AA, Courtenay-Luck N, Pickering D (1985) Antibody guided irradiation of brain glioma by arterial infusion of radioactive monoclonal antibody against epidermal growth factor receptors and blood group A antigen. Br Med J 290:1463–1466
5. Natali PG, Zardi L (1989) Tenascin: an exameric adhesive glycoprotein. Int J Cancer, suppl 4:66–68
6. Erikson HP, Lightner WA (1988) Hexabrachion protein (tenascin, cytotactin, brachionectin) in connective tissues, embryonic brain and tumors. Adv Cell Biol 2:55–90
7. Mird Pamphlet, n°11 (1975) Society of Nuclear Medicine, NY
8. Dillman RO (1990) Human antimouse and antiglobulin responses to monoclonal antibodies. Antibody Immunoconj Radiopharm 3:1–8
9. World Health Organization handbook for reporting

results of cancer treatments (1979) Offsets publication Geneva, Switzerland WHO, no 40

10. Hird V, Snook C, Kosmas B, Dhokia S, Stewart P, Mason J, Lambert C, Meares C, Epenetos A (1991) Intraperitoneal radioimmunotherapy with yttrium-90-labeled immunoconjugates. In: Epenetos A (ed) Monoclonal antibodies application in oncology. Chapman and Hall, London, pp 267–271

11. Schroff RW, Weiden PC, Appelbaun J, Fer M, Breitz H, Van derheuden J-L, Ratliff BA, Fisher D, Foisie D, Hanelin LG, Morgan Jr AC, Fritzberg AR, Abrams PG (1990) Rhenium-186 labeled antibody in patients with cancer: report of a pilot phase I study. Antibody Immunoconj Radopharmac 2:99

Address for correspondence:
Dr. P. Riva
Unita Sanitaria Locale N 39
Ospedale "Maurizio Bufalini"
Servizio Multizonale di Medicina Nucleare
Via Ghirotti
I-47023 Cesena, Italy

Fusion protein mediated tumor-selective prodrug activation

K. Bosslet, J. Czech, D. Hoffmann
Research Laboratories of Behringwerke AG, Marburg, Germany

Introduction

The major limitations of conventional chemotherapy are its lack of tumor selectivity resulting in high toxicity as well as generation of multidrug-resistant tumor cells under the influence of long-term treatment with insufficient drug concentrations at the tumor site (for review see (1)). To overcome these problems of toxicity and multidrug resistance several groups tried to develop antibody-enzyme conjugates which ideally shall activate non-toxic prodrugs to toxic drugs in high concentrations at the tumor site only (for review see (2)).

To get these site-specific activation systems working at least two or preferably three steps are needed (3). The first step includes the injection of a tumor-selective antibody-enzyme conjugate into the tumor bearing individual. After an appropriate localization phase of one or two days a second antibody directed to the enzyme is injected in order to clear the antibody-enzyme conjugate from the plasma. Thereafter a non-toxic prodrug which can be cleaved to a cytotoxic drug by the enzyme moiety of the antibody-enzyme conjugate localized at the tumor is injected.

The whole procedure as shown by studies in nude mice and by preliminary clinical trials generates superior therapeutic effects in comparison to conventional chemotherapy (3, 4). Nevertheless, the high immunogenicity of the antibody-enzyme conjugates, which consist of murine monoclonal antibodies chemically linked to xenogeneic enzymes, does not allow repetitive application of the conjugate leading to a limitation of the therapy. Furthermore, the insufficient clearance of the antibody-enzyme conjugates and the inappropriate plasma stability of the prodrug result in high concentrations of drug in the plasma. This deficiency causes a significant toxicity to non-tumorigenic tissues (4).

To reduce the problem of immunogenicity our group has generated a fusion protein consisting of a humanized CEA-specific binding region and human β-glucuronidase using recombinant DNA technology (5). Under native conditions, the fusion protein has an apparent molecular weight of > 250 kD and is composed of two heavy and two light chains. The enzyme moiety of the fusion protein is located at the carboxyterminal part of the fusion protein's heavy chains. Further characteristics of the fusion protein with respect to its specificity and avidity as well as enzymological and protein chemical properties have already been described in detail (5).

In the present study we present information concerning the pharmacokinetics, tumor and tissue distribution and metabolism of the fusion protein after i.v. injection in human tumor bearing nude mice. Furthermore, we present data on the pharmacokinetics, organ distribution, stability and toxicity of an appropriate glucuronyl-spacer-doxorubicin prodrug whose synthesis (6) and in vitro cleavability by human β-glucuronidase was described before (6, 7).

In addition, data concerning the drug concentrations in tumor tissue and normal organs after therapy with fusion protein and prodrug are shown and compared with values received using chemotherapy with doxorubicin. Finally, data concerning the therapeutic efficiency of the concept of fusion protein mediated prodrug activation (FMPA) on the growth of established human tumor xenografts in nude mice are reported.

Results

Pharmacokinetics and metabolism of fusion protein in vivo

Quantitative determination of functionally active fusion protein

After a single i.v. injection of fusion protein having an immunoreactivity of 90% and a specific enzyme activity of 12 µmol/mg x min at pH 4.5 in tumor bearing nude mice (400 µg/mouse), a selective retention of functionally active fusion protein only was observed in CEA-expressing (Mz-Sto-1, LoVo) but not in CEA-negative tumors (LXF-529). At day 7 after i.v. injection of fusion protein, 200 ng or 430 ng of functionally active fusion protein were found per gram of Mz-Sto-1 or LoVo tumors respectively, whereas fusion protein concentration in LXF-529 tumors were below the detection limit of the assay (< 1 ng/g). Thus, the in vivo specificity of fusion protein for CEA-expressing tumor is about 100 times higher than for not CEA-expressing tumors. At day 7 similar specificity ratios were also observed between fusion protein concentration in CEA-expressing tumors and plasma or normal tissues. Detectable, but minor amounts of functionally active fusion protein were observed only in the liver, gut and lung.

The absolute masses of fusion protein detected in tumor and organs 3 min after i.v. injection sum up to approximately 100% of the injected dose, if the respective tissue weights of nude mice as well as the plasma content in the removed organs is considered. The absolute masses of fusion protein detected at later times are far below 100 % and decrease continuously in the various organs.

Quantitative determination of functionally active β-glucuronidase

In addition to the analysis of functionally active fusion protein, tissues investigated in the above mentioned experiments were analyzed with respect to concentrations of non fusion protein bound, functionally active human β-glucuronidase. In plasma of fusion protein treated animals concentrations of free active β-glucuronidase were below 20 ng/ml during the observation period from 3 min to 168 h after fusion protein injection, outlining the high stability of fusion protein in plasma. In contrast, high levels of free active β-glucuronidase were detected in the livers of these animals. In this tissue a time dependent increase of free β-glucuronidase was observed with a maximum of 181–256 µg/g at 24 h after fusion protein application. Thereafter free β-glucuronidase values slowly declined to concentrations of 12–84 µg/g which were still present 168 h after fusion protein application. In opposite to the liver, concentrations of free human β-glucuronidase in other organs were found to be in the range of 1–14 µg/g and remained fairly constant during time.

Histochemical determination of β-glucuronidase

Histochemical analysis of normal tissues derived from either fusion protein treated or untreated nude mice revealed that β-glucuronidase activity was exclusively associated with intracellular organelles. The microscopically visible red spots most probably are located in lysosomes of liver and other organs. The semiquantitative histochemical procedure performed at different times shows that the intracellular β-glucuronidase activity is higher in liver parenchymal cells from nude mice treated with fusion protein than in untreated control mice in which the endogenous mouse β-glucuronidase activity is only marginally detectable. Addition of 10 mM saccharolactone, a selective competitive inhibitor of β-glucuronidases (8) completely abolishes the staining reaction. Already 3 min after fusion protein injection β-glucuronidase activity was detected in most liver parenchymal cells. Staining intensity remained constant up to 24 h and thereafter decreased to background levels till day 7.

Immunohistochemical determination of fusion protein

In addition to the histochemical studies and the quantitative data generated, a semiquantitative immunohistochemical method was applied, allowing the visualization of the fusion protein on cryopreserved tumor tissue sections in its microenvironment. Already 3 min after i.v. injection of 400 µg of fusion protein in nude mice bearing established CEA-positive Mz-Sto-1 xenograft a heterogeneous staining of certain areas in the tumor thin sections was seen. The strength of staining slightly increased up to 24 h after injection, however remaining heterogeneous. Thereafter a decrease of staining intensity was observed which, however, at day 7 is above background level.

In summary, with respect to normal organs, especially liver, the results from the quantitative analysis as well as the histochemical data suggest that the kinetics of the fusion protein concentration in normal organs parallels its concentration in plasma. However, free human β-glucuronidase activity accumulates in liver parenchymal cells. This could be explained by a preferential uptake of the fusion protein into liver parenchymal cells and cleavage to an enzymatically active protein lacking the variable region. The concentrations of functionally active fusion protein in liver 7 days after its application are very low. The fusion protein's rapid uptake and degradation, mainly in normal liver, is in contrast to its fate in the tumor in which 7 days after i.v. injection 200 - 400 ng of functionally active fusion protein can be detected per g tumor. This obvious difference in the fusion protein's fate in liver and normal organs compared to CEA-expressing malignant tissue results in the unexpectedly high specificity ratios reported above.

Furthermore, in contrast to the intracellular histochemical reactions in normal tissues, the immunohistochemical staining observed in tumor tissue was localized extracellulary. Furthermore, the semiquantitative immunohistochemical staining reactions are in agreement with the quantitative data presented above. They clearly demonstrate that the fusion protein selectively binds to CEA-positive human tumor xenografts remaining there as a functionally active molecule for at least 7 days.

Plasma stability of prodrug and in vitro cleavage

In order to take advantage of the pharmacokinetics and metabolism of the fusion protein with respect to tumor chemotherapy a prodrug (N-[4-β-glucuronyl-3-nitro-benzyloxycarbonyl]doxorubicin) has been synthesized (6, 7). The prodrug is very stable under in vitro conditions in human, rat or mouse plasma. After 50 h of incubation of the prodrug at 100 µg/ml maximally 20% of the prodrug is cleaved. Addition of 1.6 µg/ml of fusion protein to a solution of prodrug (335 µg/ml) results in a quick disappearance of prodrug due to cleavage of the glucuronide moiety. The resulting doxorubicin spacer derivative spontaneously decomposes and gives raise to generation of doxorubicin.

Based on a number of similar in vitro cleavage experiments in buffer at pH 7.2, Km and Vmax were calculated to be 1.3 mM and 0.635 nMol/min x µg at 37° C. Similar data have been previously reported for other mammalian β-glucuronidases with respect to cleavage of the synthetic substrate 4-nitrophenyl-β-glucuronide (9).

Pharmacokinetics of prodrug in disease free and tumor bearing animals

Plasma half-life of prodrug was determined after a single bolus i.v. injection of 50 mg/kg prodrug in tumor free CD-1 nu/nu mice, in CD rats and in Macaca fascicularis monkeys. Prodrug and drug concentrations were determined using reversed phase HPLC followed by data analysis with the HoeRep computer program.

In all three animal systems, pharmacokinetics of the prodrug fit into a two compartment model with an elimination half-life (t1/2β) between 0.4 and 2.6 hours and a distribution half-life (t1/2α) between 2 and 7 min. Differences between the pharmacokinetic parameters are observed between the three species especially with respect to a significantly higher AUC value for monkeys compared to rodents. For comparison distribution and elimination half-lives of doxorubicin are determined to be 2 min and 8.1 hours in rats.

After a 5 min infusion of prodrug in a therapeutic dosage (250 mg/kg) only minor amounts of doxorubicin were found in the plasma of tumor free nude mice. Depending on the evaluation time doxorubicin plasma concentration in these animals represents 0.08% to 3.2% of the corresponding plasma prodrug concentration. A similar percentage of liberation of doxorubicin from the prodrug (0.1–0.6%) was observed in Macaca fascicularis monkeys. Infusion of a maximum tolerated dose of free doxorubicin resulted in similar plasma concentrations as doxorubicin concentrations observed after prodrug infusion.

In a separate set of experiments fusion protein was injected into tumor (Mz-Sto-1) bearing nude mice followed by an infusion of prodrug (250 mg/kg) seven days later. At the same time other animals received an infusion of doxorubicin (12 mg/kg). The concentrations of doxorubicin in plasma of prodrug or doxorubicin treated animals were found to be similar to those found in plasma of non-fusion protein treated, tumor free animals. However, major differences were found with respect to doxorubicin concentrations in organ and tumor tissues. In mice treated with fusion protein and prodrug the amounts of doxorubicin in various organ tissues were found up to 5-fold lower than the amounts observed in doxorubicin treated animals. In contrast, the amount of drug present in tumor tissues was 4 to 12-fold higher for fusion protein and prodrug treated mice than in animals which received a single application of doxorubicin. Thus, these data show that treatment of tumor bearing mice with fusion protein and prodrug results in an increase of drug concentration in the target tissue (Mz-Sto-1 tumor) and a reduction of drug concentration in non-target tissues.

Maximal tolerable dose (MTD) of prodrug and drug in vivo

The MTD of prodrug and drug was determined by 5 min i.v. infusions of increasing dosages of prodrug or drug in CD-1 nu/nu mice. MTD of the drug was 12 mg/kg (0.022 mmol/kg), that of the prodrug was 1600 mg/kg (1.8 mmol/kg), if applied in doses of 800 mg/kg in 6 h intervals. Applications of a single dose larger than 800 mg/kg were not possible due to the water solubility of the prodrug (30 mg/ml). According to these data, the prodrug is at least 130-fold less toxic (wt/wt) in vivo than the drug. MTD of prodrug, if applied eight days after fusion protein application was > 1600 mg/kg as well.

Therapeutic efficacy

Based on the in vivo distribution and tumor retention data generated using the fusion protein as well as on the pharmacokinetics and in vivo prodrug activation data obtained, therapy experiments were performed. Seven days after injection of 20 mg/kg of fusion protein into nude mice bearing established CEA-expressing human tumor xenografts (tumor diameter 3–5 mm) (LoVo) 250 mg/kg of prodrug were infused. In addition, separate groups of animals were treated with prodrug alone, doxorubicin, or physiological saline.

Therapeutic efficacy was documented by monitoring tumor growth. Significant growth retardation with partial regression was obtained only in those animals receiving fusion protein and prodrug (26% T/C, day 24). Prodrug alone (68% T/C) or doxorubicin (61% T/C, day 24, respectively) had no significant antitumoral effect against this particular tumor. These superior therapeutic effects were obtained, without any obvious signs of toxicity to the animals, at 1/6 of the prodrug's MTD.

Discussion

This preclinical study demonstrates that appropriate in vivo application of a tumor selective humanized fusion protein and a non-toxic prodrug generates tumor therapeutic effects superior to conventional chemotherapy. These therapeutic effects were obtained in a human tumor xenograft model relatively resistant to doxorubicin treatment and with a single cycle of fusion protein and prodrug. Due to the presumably low immunogenicity of the fusion protein consisting of a humanized CEA-specific binding region and human β-glucuronidase (5), repetitive applications of fusion protein should be possible. Furthermore, the prodrug dose used in our therapy experiment (250 mg/kg) is only approximately 1/6 of the MTD of the prodrug. Therefore, repetitive treatment cycles probably can be applied in patients hopefully resulting in even superior therapeutic effects than those reported in our in vivo nude mouse studies.

In contrast, the application of repetitive treatment cycles does not seem to be possible without immunosuppressive therapy in systems containing mouse MAbs chemically linked to xenogenic enzymes (10). In addition, to be effective some xenogenic antibody-enzyme conjugate systems (3) need as a third component the injection of a galactosylated anti-enzyme MAb to clear the xenogenic antibody-enzyme conjugate from the plasma before prodrug injection. Such a clearing step is not needed in our system, because the fusion protein is quickly eliminated from plasma probably by internalization into parenchymal cells of the liver. Internalization is most probably mediated by mannose 6-phosphate- and galactose-receptor mediated uptake known to be a highly active internalization pathway in liver parenchymal cells. Galactosilated and mannosilated glycoproteins like human β-glucuronidase are efficiently taken up and transported to the lysosomal compartment, where enzymatic degradation occurs as observed similarly for the fusion protein (manuscript in preparation). Intracellulary, the fusion protein is cleaved to enzymatically active human β-glucuronidase lacking the CEA-binding region. During time, intracellularly accumulated human β-glucuronidase activity is slowly reduced. This efficient internalization and degradation mechanism is one of the parameters responsible for the very high ratios (100:1) of functionally active fusion protein between tumor and plasma or organs obtained at day 7 after fusion protein injection as shown in two independent kinetic studies using two different CEA-expressing human tumor xenografts.

The mechanistic intepretation suggested above is supported by the fusion protein's high stability (> 80%) during incubation for four weeks at 37° C in rodent or human plasma arguing against easily accessible plasmatic protease cleavage sites (data not shown). This finding which is in concordance with the non-detectable amounts of free human β-glucuronidase in plasma after fusion protein application supports the hypothesis that the increase of free β-glucuronidase in liver parenchymal cells is rather due to internalization of the fusion protein into the liver cells and intracellular cleavage of the fusion protein than to extracellular removal of the V-region followed by internalization of functionally active β-glucuronidase.

Despite of its high molecular weight (> 250 kD) under non-denaturing conditions and the known diffusion barriers reported for solid tumors (11) the fusion protein is able to penetrate human tumor xenograft tissues. Although the staining reaction after i.v. application of the fusion protein remains heterogeneous the amounts of functionally active fusion protein in the tumor at day seven are still suitable to activate the prodrug in vivo. Compared to standard chemotherapy using doxorubicin, the doxorubicin generated by fusion protein mediated prodrug activation results in 4–12-fold higher doxorubicin concentrations in the tumor and up to 5-fold lower doxorubicin concentrations in normal tissues. The pharmacokinetic advantage observed using the FMPA system can be explained by the high hydrophilicity of the prodrug resulting preferentially in doxorubicin liberation mainly at sites where extracellularly accessible β-glucuronidase is available. However, small amounts of doxorubicin are probably generated from the prodrug in plasma and normal tissues catalyzed by the minute amounts of accessible plasmatic and normal tissue associated glucuronidase. In contrast, the unfavorable normal tissue doxorubicin levels obtained after i.v. injection of doxorubicin are a consequence of the high lipophilicity of the drug leading to rapid tissue uptake and a concomittant decrease of plasma levels. Furthermore, the advantageous in vivo drug distribution using FMPA is only possible, because the prodrug has several favorable characteristics. First, the high in vivo tolerability (> 1600 mg/kg) of the prodrug should be emphasized resulting in an exceptionally high detoxification factor between prodrug and drug (> 130-fold). A second favorable characteristic of the prodrug is its long term plasma stability in mouse, rat and human plasma avoiding significant unspecific drug liberation. Thirdly, the in vitro prodrug activation kinetics performed in plasma shows, that addition of enzymatically active fusion protein leads to a rapid cleavage of the prodrug to the drug, with similar characteristics as observed for the activation of conventional substrates such as methylumbelliferyl β-glucuronide or 4-nitrophenyl β-glucuronide used to evaluate natural human β-glucuronidase. In contrast to the ADEPT-system (antibody directed enzyme mediated prodrug therapy) suggested by the groups of Senter (12), Meyer (13) and Bagshawe (14) using xenogenic enzymes like β-lactamase or carboxypeptidase G2 as catalytic moiety, our FMPA system uses human β-glucuronidase as a catalytic moiety. The turnover rate of our fusion protein is significantly below the activities reported for the above mentioned antibody-enzyme conjugates due to the high K_m (1.3 mM) and relatively low V_{max} (0.635 nMol/min x µg, pH 7.2) of human β-glucuronidase. This disadvantage of our fusion protein is more than compensated by its superior pharmacokinetic resulting in unusually high specificity ratios totally in agreement with the pharmacodynamic model constructed by *Yuan* et al. (15). These authors suggest, that in two step systems a significant delay between the first injection of the catalytic component and the prodrug will result in little toxicity and superior therapeutic efficacy.

Indeed, after a delay of seven days between fusion protein injection and prodrug infusion with a single dose of 250 mg/kg of prodrug, therapeutic effects in a CEA-positive human tumor xenograft system were observed which are superior to treatment with standard doxorubicin therapy. This superior efficacy of FMPA is supported by the more favorable in vivo drug distribution in the tumor as well as in normal tissues as discussed above. A comparison of our in vivo drug distribution data after FMPA with those obtained in the ADEPT-system (14) reveals that in our system a tumor selective drug deposition is observed, whereas the ADEPT-system based on antibody-carboxypeptidase G2 conjugates leads to a more systemic drug distribution. The advantageous drug distribution in our system is not only mediated by the high in vivo specificity ratio of the fusion protein but also by the high prodrug stability in plasma and its favorable pharmacokinetic characteristics. Thus, the finding that plasma AUC values were significantly higher in monkeys as compared to rodents suggests that the prodrug dose needed in human beings can presumably be reduced by a factor of 5–10. This hypothesis is based on the assumption that tumor tissue prodrug levels are influenced by the respective prodrug plasma levels and that tumor tissue prodrug levels allowing efficient catalysis are available for prolonged periods of time in monkeys and probably also in human beings compared to rodents.

Summary

The prospective low immunogenicity of our fusion protein, the high specificity ratio obtained in vivo combined with tumor selective disposition of doxorubicin after prodrug activation resulting in superior therapeutic effects, recommend our FMPA system for clinical development.

Acknowledgement

The skilful technical assistance of *Mr. H. Lind, N. Döring, R. Straub* and *Ms. C. Wetzler* is gratefully acknowledged. The authors thank *Ms. S. Lehnert* for secretarial assistance.

References

1. Ford JM, Hait WN (1990) Pharmacology of drugs that alter multidrug resistance in cancer. Pharmacol Rev 42:155–199
2. Senter PD, Wallace PM, Svensson HP, Vrudhula VM, Kerr DE, Hellström I, Hellström KE (1993) Generation of cytotoxic agents by targeted enzymes. (Review) Bioconjugate Chem 4:3–9
3. Sharma SK, Bagshawe KD, Springer CJ, Burke PJ, Rogers GT, Boden JA, Antoniw P, Melton RG, Sherwood RF (1991) Antibody directed enzyme-prodrug therapy (ADEPT): a three phase system. Disease Markers 9:225–231
4. Bagshawe KD, Sharma SK, Springer CJ, Antoniw P, Boden JA, Rogers GT, Burke P, Melton RG (1991) Antibody directed enzyme prodrug therapy (ADEPT): clinical report. Disease Markers 9 233–238
5. Bosslet K., Czech J, Lorenz P, Sedlacek HH, Schuermann M, Seemann G (1992) Molecular and functional characterisation of a fusion protein suited for tumor specific prodrug activation. Brit J Cancer 65:234–238
6. Jacquesy J-C, Gesson J-P, Monneret C, Mondon M, Renoux B, Florent J-C, Koch M, Tillequin F, Sedlacek HH, Kolar C, Gaudel G (1991) Prodrogues glycosylées, leur procédé de préparation et leurs utilisation. Demande de brevet européen, EP 0 511 917 A1
7. Adrianomenjanahary S, Koch M, Tillequin F, Michel S, Monneret C, Florent JC, Gesson JP, Jacquesy JC, Mondon M, Bosslet KN (1992) (D-glycopyranosyl)-chlorbenzyloxycarbonyl daunorubicine prodrugs and their enzymatic cleavage. Int J Carbohydrate Symp Paris, A 264, p 299
8. Lojda Z, Gossrau R, Schiebler TH (1979) Enzyme histochemistry. Springer, Berlin, p 166–167
9. Tomino S, Paigen K, Tulsiani TPP, Touster O (1975) Purification and chemical properties of mouse liver lysosomal β-glucuronidase. J Biol Chem 250: 8503–8509

10. Bagshawe KD, Sharma SK, Springer CJ, Antoniw P, Rogers GT, Burke PJ, Melton R, Sherwood R (1991) Antibody-enzyme conjugates can generate cytotoxic drugs from inactive precursors at tumor sites. Antibody Immunoconj Radiopharmac 4:915–922
11. Jain RK (1987) Transport of molecules in the tumor interstitium: a review. Cancer Res 47:3039–3051
12. Goshorn SC, Svensson HP, Kerr DE, Sommerville JE, Senter PD, Fell HP (1993) Genetic construction, expression and characterization of a single chain anti-carcinoma antibody fused to β-lactamase. Cancer Res 53:2123–2127
13. Meyer DL, Jungheim LN, Law KL, Mikolajczyk SD, Shepherd TA, Mackensen DG, Briggs SL, Starling JJ (1993) Site-specific prodrug activation by antibody-β-lactamase conjugates: Regression and long-term growth inhibition of human colon carcinoma xenografts models. Cancer Res 53:3956–3963
14. Antoniw P, Springer CJ, Bagshawe, KD, Searle F, Melton RG, Rogers GT, Burke PJ, Sherwood RF (1990) Disposition of the prodrug 4-(bis(2-chloroethyl)amino)benzoyl-L-glutamic acid and its active parent drug in mice. Brit J Cancer 62:909–914
15. Yuan F, Baxter LT, Jain RK (1991) Pharmacokinetic analysis of two-step approaches using bifunctional and enzyme-conjugated antibodies. Cancer Res 51:3119–3130

Address for correspondence:
Dr. rer. nat. K. Bosslet
Behringwerke AG
Postfach 1140
D-35001 Marburg, Germany

Immunocytological monitoring of antibody-mediated reduction of individual disseminated breast cancer cells

K. Pantel[a], G. Schlimok[b], I. Fackler-Schwalbe[b], R. Oberneder[c],
A. Hofstetter[c], H. Loibner[d], G. Riethmüller[a]

[a]Institute for Immunology, [b]Medical Clinic II, Zentralklinikum, Augsburg, [c]Department of Urology, University of Munich, Germany; [d]Sandoz Research Institute, Wien, Austria

Introduction

Over almost a decade, murine monoclonal antibodies (MAbs) to tumor-associated cell surface molecules have been tried for therapy of various types of human solid tumors (for review, see (1)). Except for a few anecdotal and transient remissions, the failure of this experimental therapy has become undeniable. Although MAbs might lack the capacity to kill tumor cells in vivo, there is ample evidence that malignant cells encased in solid parenchyma are largely inaccessible for intravenously administered macromolecules (2). Thus, instead of aiming antibody therapy at solid metastases, the present study was designed to evaluate the cytotoxic effect of systemic application of MAb BR55-2 (also called ABL 364) to the Lewis Y blood group precursor antigen on individual dispersed breast cancer cells present in bone marrow. Since these cells can now be identified by immunocytochemistry with MAbs to cytokeratins (3), which are integral components of the epithelial cytoskeleton, the attempt was undertaken to monitor their eradication by analyzing sequential bone marrow aspirates.

Material and methods

MAb ABL 364 (IgG3) to the Lewis Y carbohydrate antigen (4), was exclusively manufactured in vitro for human use and provided by Sandoz, Switzerland. Immunostaining with ABL 364 is found on a variety of malignant epithelial tumors (including breast cancer) while expression on mesenchymal neoplasms is quite rare (table I). The serum half life of ABL 364 is in the order of 50 (23–105) hours (5). The in vitro cytotoxicity against several Lewis Y+ tumor cell lines obtained with fresh serum from antibody-treated patients could be shown to be both complement dependent and antibody mediated (5).

Ten breast cancer patients with more than 20 CK+ cells per $4 \cdot 10^5$ nucleated bone marrow cells were consecutively recruited into the therapeutic study. All patients had either failed or refused current treatment modalities; three patients were staged M0, while the other seven patients displayed stage M1 disease (metastases of the bone, brain, lung, liver or skin). The treatment consisted of 6 x 100 mg ABL 364 i.v. infusions administered over two weeks on day 1, 3, 5, 8, 10, and 12; the three placebo-treated patients received HSA

Table I. Immunostaining of MAb ABL 364 on primary epithelial tumor cells.

Tumor tissue origin	Positive/total samples[a]	% of total
Breast	16/23	69.6
Pancreas	20/28	71.4
Colorectum	118/179	66.0
Stomach	6/10	60.0
Lung (SCLC + NSCLC)	26/37	70.3

[a]Based on the immunostaining (APAAP-technique) of cryostat tumor sections with MAb ABL 364

Bone marrow aspirations were performed before and on day 15 and 60 after antibody treatment. The marrow was aspirated from the iliac crest and processed by Ficoll-Hypaque density centrifigation. Following cytocentrifugation on glass slides and overnight airdrying, a total of $4 \cdot 10^5$ nucleated cells per patient were stained and screened. For immunocytochemical analysis, single epithelial tumor cells were identified with MAb CK2 (IgG1, Boehringer Mannheim, Germany) to CK component no. 18 (CK18), as previously described (3). Consecutive preparations were stained with MAb ABL 364, which does not crossreact with normal hematopoietic cells. After incubation with the respective primary antibody, the reaction was developed using the alkaline phosphatase anti-alkaline phosphatase (APAAP) technique (6).

Results

Over the past decade, several groups (including ours) have been interested in the detection of individual disseminated tumor cells in bone marrow of patients with operable primary carcinomas (1, 7). The prognostic relevance of this minimal residual tumor load has thus far been demonstrated in patients with carcinomas of the breast, lung, colorectum and stomach (8–13). Table II demonstrates the broad applicability of the immunocytochemical screening for cytokeratin expression in bone marrow, which is presently used as standard assay in our laborartory.

The specificity of our assay for detection of individual epithelial tumor cells was supported by the observation that $CK18^+$ cells were only detected in six out of 215 (2.8%) control marrows

Table II. Incidence of cytokeratin-positive tumor cells in bone marrow of patients with primary epithelial cancer (TNM-stage M0).

Tumor origin	No. of patients analyzed	No. of patients with CK18+ samples (% of total)
Lung (NSCLC)	101	26 (25.7)
Breast	116	35 (30.2)
Stomach	80	25 (31.2)
Colon/Rectum	195	53 (27.2)
Prostate	80	27 (33.8)
Kidney	76	12 (15.8)
Bladder	66	15 (22.7)
Control group[a]	215	6 (2.8)

[a]Patients with no evidence for an epithelial malignancy at the time of bone marrow analysis

Table III. Monitoring of cytokeratin-positive tumor cells in bone marrow of breast cancer patients during treatment with MAb ABL 364.

Patient/treatment	n CK18+ cells per $4 \cdot 10^5$ marrow cells		
	pre-MAb	day 15 post-MAb	day 60 post-MAb
ABL 364			
B.P.	860	28[a]	47[a]
D.G.	27	0	0
R.O.	22	10[a]	0
W.H.	114	2	12[a]
M.W.	349[a]	437[a]	n.d.
S.H.	62[a]	353[a]	950[a]
R.R.	37	12	0
Placebo			
K.U.	320	300	380
B.R.	22[a]	55[a]	192[a]
H.H.	1051[a]	900[a]	259[a]

[a]All cells in this sample were ABL 364-negative

from patients without evidence of malignant epithelial disease at the time of marrow aspiration (table II). It should be noted that all patients displayed benign epithelial tumors and that colon cancer was diagnosed ten months later in one of them, suggesting that tumor cell dissemination had already occurred before the primary tumor could be detected. Furthermore, our previous studies have shown that CK18+ cells lack coexpression of hematopoietic marker proteins such as the common leukocyte antigen CD45 (3). Thus, expression of CK18 in normal bone marrow cells, as suggested by previous investigations (14), appears to be a very rare event, at least at those levels detected by immunoenzymatic staining techniques.

The frequency of disseminated cancer cells in bone marrow is extremely low, ranging from 10^{-4} to 10^{-6}. In order to perform a meaningful monitoring of CK18+ cells, we therefore decided to select breast cancer patients who presented with more than 20 positive cells per sample of 4×10^5 marrow cells. As shown in table III, five of seven antibody-treated patients displayed a distinct reduction of CK18+ cells in bone marrow. Interestingly, CK18+ cells found on day 60 post-treatment appeared to be ABL 364-, suggesting the induction of a negative selection process. The two antibody-treated patients, who presented only with ABL 364- tumor cells, as well as those patients in the placebo-treated group, showed no significant response to the antibody infusion. As to the seven patients with overt metastases, no objective regression of metastatic lesions were documented. On the other hand, no relapses were observed in the three patients without overt metastasis (TNM-stage M0).

Except for nausea, no major adverse effects, such as anaphylactic reactions, were documented. The titers of human anti-mouse antibodies were found to be low in all ABL 364-treated patients.

Discussion

The primary aim of this study was to explore the feasabilty of monitoring individual metastatic tumor cells dispersed in bone marrow, using an immunocytochemical assay previously developed in our laborartory (3). The rationale for an antibody treatment was supported by our recent finding that individual breast tumor cells present in bone marrow rest frequently in the G_0-phase of the cell cycle (15), which limits the cytotoxic action of many chemotherapeutic agents. Furthermore, the recent evaluation of our clinical trial with the systemic application of MAb 17-1A in colorectal cancer clearly demonstrated the significant benefit of such treatment in patients without overt metastases (stage Dukes C) (16).

The number of patients treated in the present study is rather small which certainly limits the interpretation of our data. However, the validity of the observed reduction of metastatic cells is strenghtened by the lack of any measurable response in CK18+ cell numbers in patients where the tumor cells lack the targeted Lewis Y antigen. In addition, the consistent absence of a respective response in placebo-treated, control patients supports the specificity of the observed antibody-mediated responses. Masking of Lewis Y antigens by the injected antibody appears to be unlike since labeled cells were consistently absent on control slides stained with anti-murine-Ig secinary antibodies alone. The question, however, remains whether the antibody-treatment favors the selection of Lewis Y- tumor cell clones, as indicated in some patients (table III).

The strong complement dependent cytotoxicity of MAb ABL 364 may be attributed to the nature of the IgG3-isotype, which by its peculiar Fc-Fc cooperativity can act as a potent activator of the C1q complement component, when bound to the repetitive carbohydrate determinants of the cell membrane (17). It may thus circumvent the otherwise effective complement inhibitory activity of the homologous restriction factors that control various homologous complement factors (18). The engagement of natural effector mechanisms, such as complement or antibody-dependent cellular cytotoxicity (ADCC) by unmodified MAbs, may offer advantages over immunotoxins and other antibody-conjugates that carry the risk of severe adverse effects due to a considerable risk of unspecific uptake (19).

Our present therapy failed to induce a remission of overt metastatic lesions which is consistent with previous disappointing antibody trials performed on patients with advanced stage solid tumors (1). One reason for this disappointment is the fact that solid metastatic tumors inherit multifold barriers which protect them against i.v.

injected anticancer agents. These barriers include an aberrant vasculature, the basement membrane, a dense mesh of interstitial proteoglycans, intercellular tight junctions, and the high oncotic pressure within the tumor interstitium (2). Furthermore, immune effector cells and complement are readily detectable in the tumor stroma but appear to be rather rare in the epithelial parenchyma.

Thus, a strong plea can be made that antibody therapy should be more effective in the stage of minimal residual disease, in which the total tumor cell load is more limited and the dispersed neoplastic cells are more accessible. Furthermore, application of double marker analysis may help to define the phenotype of micrometastatic tumor cells in individual patients (15), thus allowing the design of individualized treatment protocols. However, because of the difficult cell retrieval at low tumor cell frequencies, the current immunocytochemical assays need to be improved. Our ongoing in-depth methodological analysis has thus far resulted in a more than 10-fold enrichment of tumor cells in bone marrow aspirates. The development of new techniques, such as the amplification of epithelial mRNA species by the polymerase chain reaction (20) or the detection of solubilized epithelial marker proteins by enzyme-linked immunoassays (7), may further increase the sensitivity of tumor cell detection.

The total number of remaining tumor cells in the patients with minimal residual disease can now be estimated to be in the range of 10^6 to 10^8 tumor cells. Considering the 10 to 100-fold reduction in tumor cell number achieved in this study, an adjuvant treatment with an appropriate antibody might therefore contribute to a considerable improvement of the clinical outcome of patients with primary breast cancer.

Acknowledgements

This work was supported by the Deutsche Krebshilfe Bonn and the Wilhelm Sander Stiftung, Neuburg, Germany. The authors thank *Gaby Barowsky*, *Simone Bayer*, and *Tanja Hoffmann* for their excellent technical work.

References

1. Riethmüller G, Johnson JP (1992) Monoclonal antibodies in the detection and therapy of micrometastatic epithelial cancers. Current Opinion in Immunology 4:647–655
2. Jain RK (1990) Physiological barriers to delivery of monoclonal antibodies and other macromolecules in tumors. Cancer Res 50:2747–5271
3. Schlimok G, Funke I, Holzmann B et al (1987) Micrometastatic cancer cells in bone marrow: in vitro detection with anti-cytokeratin and in vivo labeling with anti-17-1A monoclonal antibodies. Proc Natl Acad Sci USA 84:8672–8676
4. Steplewski Z, Blaszezyk Thurin M et al (1990) Oligosaccharide Y specific monoclonal antibody and its isotype switch variants. Hybridoma 9:201–210
5. Scholz D, Lubeck M, Loibner H et al (1991) Biological activity in the human system of isotype variants of oligosaccharide -Y-specific murine monoclonal antibodies. Cancer Immunol Immunother 33:153–157
6. Cordell JI, Falini B, Erber WN et al (1984) Immunoenzymatic labeling of monoclonal antibodies using immune complexes of alkaline phosphatase and monoclonal anti-alkaline phosphatase (APAAP-complexes). J Histochem Cytochem 32:219–229
7. Pantel K, Koprowski H, Riethmüller G (1993) Meeting report: Conference on cancer micrometastasis: Biology, methodology and clinical significance. Int J Oncol 3:1019
8. Cote RJ, Rosen PP, Lesser ML et al (1991) Prediction of early relapse in patients with operable breast cancer by detection of occult bone marrow micrometastases. J Clin Oncol 9:1749–1756
9. Diel IJ, Kaufmann M, Goemer R et al (1992) Detection of tumor cells in bone marrow of patients with primary breast cancer: A prognostic factor for distant metastasis. J Clin Oncol 10:1534–1539
10. Schlimok G, Lindemann F, Holzmann K et al (1992) Prognostic significance of disseminated tumor cells detected in bone marrow of patients with breast and colorectal cancer. Proc Am Soc Clin Oncol 11:102
11. Pantel K, Izbicki JR, Angstwurm M, Braun S, Passlick B, Karg O, Thetter O, Riethmüller G (1993) Immunocytochemical detection of bone marrow micrometastasis in operable non-small cell lung cancer. Cancer Res 53:1–5
12. Lindemann F, Schlimok G, Dirschedl P, Witte J, Riethmüller G (1992) Prognostic significance of micrometastatic tumor cells in bone marrow of colorectal cancer patients. Lancet 340:685–689
13. Schlimok G, Funke. I, Pantel K, Strobel F, Lindemann F, Witte J, Riethmüller G (1991) Micrometastatic tumor cells in bone marrow of patients

with gastric cancer: methodological aspects of detection and prognostic significance. Eur J Cancer 27:1461–1465
14. Franke W, Moll R (1987) Cytoskeletal components of lymphoid organs. Synthesis of cytokeratin 8 and 18 and desmin in subpopulation of extrafollicular reticulum cells of human lymph nodes, tonsil and spleen. Differentiation 36:145–163
15. Pantel K, Schlimok G, Braun S et al (1993) Differential expression of proliferation-associated molecules in individual micrometastatic carcinoma cells. J Natl Cancer Inst 85:1419–1424
16. Riethmüller G, Schneider-Gädicke E, Schlimok G et al (1994) Randomized trial of monoclonal antibody for adjuvant therapy of resected Dukes' C colorectal carcinoma. Lancet 343:1177–1183
17. Greenspan NS, Dacek DA, Cooper LJN (1989) Cooperative binding of two antibodies to independent antigens by an Fc-dependent mechanism. FASEB J 3:2203–2208
18. Lachmann PJ (1991) The control of homologous lysis. Immunol Today 12:312–315
19. Vitetta ES, Thorpe PE, Uhr JW (1993) Immunotoxins: magic bullets or misguided missiles? Immunol Today 14:252–259
20. Gerhard M, Juhl H, Kalthoff H et al (1994) Specific detection of carcinoembryonic antigen-expressing tumor cells in bone marrow aspirates by polymerase chain reaction. J Clin Oncol 12:725–729

Address for correspondence:
Dr. med. K. Pantel
Institut für Immunologie
Universität München
Goethestraße 31
D-80336 München, Germany

Determination and characterization of human antibodies after application of the monoclonal antibody B72.3

B. Gast, J. Reinsberg

Department of Gynecology and Obstetrics, University of Bonn, Germany

Introduction

The benefit of the treatment with monoclonal antibodies (MAb) directed against tumor associated antigens has been shown for the MAb CO17-IA in patients with colorectal carcinomas (5) and for the MAb OC125 in patients with ovarian adenocarcinomas (4). It is proposed that the applied antibodies modulate the immune system via the idiotypic network, as postulated by *Jerne* et al. (2). It is accompanied by formation of anti-idiotypic "internal image" antibodies (Ab2β) and at last by formation of anti-anti-idiotypic antibodies (Ab3) directed against the original tumor antigen. Another antibody against a tumor associated antigen is the murine MAb B72.3 which recognizes a high-molecular-weight tumor associated glycoprotein (TAG 72) expressed on 95% of ovarian adenocarcinomas (3). The aim of the present study was to demonstrate in a patient treated with B72.3 antibodies the formation of human anti-B72.3 antibodies and to examine their specificity.

Material and methods

Patients and samples

Serial serum samples were obtained routinely during follow-up of a patient with an ovarian adenocarcinoma stage I (FIGO) who had received four infusions of 1 mg B72.3 of the MAb (Eurocetus, Frankfurt, Germany). A serum sample with a high TAG 72 concentration drawn from an ovarian cancer patient not yet treated with B72.3 served as control. All samples were aliquoted and stored at −20 °C until analysis.

Removal of IgG from serum samples

Serum IgG were removed by affinity chromatography on Protein-G-Sepharose (Pharmacia, Freiburg, Germany). 1 ml of serum sample diluted 2-fold with phosphate buffer (0.02 mol/l sodium phosphate, pH 7.0) was applied to a 3 ml column equilibrated with phosphate buffer. Then the column was washed with 30 ml of phosphate buffer to elute the unadsorbed fraction. The adsorbed IgG fraction was eluted with 15 ml of elution buffer (0.1 mol/l glycine-HCL, pH 2.7). The eluate was neutralized immediatly with l.5ml of neutralizing buffer (1 mol/l tris(hydroxymethyl)-aminomethane-HCl, pH 9.0).

Determination of TAG 72

TAG 72 was determined with two different assays: Assay I (B72.3-M-K-S, Sorin Biomedica, Saluggia, Italy) is an one-step solid-phase immunometric assay involving the B72.3 antibody as both the immobilized and the labeled antibody. In an assay of that kind, anti–idiotypic anti-B72.3 antibodies can crosslink both antibodies resulting in falsely high values for TAG 72. Assay II (ELSA-CA-72-4, CIS, Gif-sur-Yvette Cedex, France) is a two-step solid-phase immunometric assay with cc49 capture antibodies; the B72.3 serves only as radiolabeled detector antibody. In this assay cross-reaction with anti–idiotypic anti-B72.3 antibodies are not to be expected. Both assays were performed according to the manufacturer's instructions.

Inhibition assays

To examine the specificity of the human anti-B72.3 IgG, inhibition assays were performed: To block binding of anti-iso/allotypic anti-B72.3 antibodies, polystyrene beats coated with B72.3 antibodies (Sorin Biomedica, Saluggia, Italy) were incubated with 0.2 ml serum diluted with Tris-buffer (0.05 mol/l tris(hydroxymethyl)-amino-methane-HCl, 0.15 mol/l NaCl, 0.001 mol/l $MgCl_2$, 0.1% Tween 20, pH 8.0) supplemented with increasing concentrations of non-specific polyclonal mouse IgG (Sigma, Deisenhofen, Germany) (20 h, 4 °C). After incubation the unbound material was removed by washing. The bound human IgG was detected by incubation with 0.2 ml alkaline phosphatase-labeled murine anti human-IgG antibodies (Sigma, Deisenhofen, Germany, diluted 1:2000 with Tris-buffer) for 4 hours at 4° C. After a further washing step the beads were incubated with 0.3 ml p-nitrophenyl phosphate (1 g/l p-nitropheny phosphate in 0.1 mol/l glycine buffer, 0.001 mol/l $MgCl_2$, 0.001 mol/l $ZnCl_2$, pH 10.4) for 10 min at room temperature. The reaction was stopped by addition of 0.75 ml 3 mol/l NaOH. The absorbence was measured at 405 nm. To inhibit the binding of antibodies directed against the paratope of the B72.3 a bovine mucin (Sigma, Deisenhofen, Germany) containing a high TAG 72 concentration was added.

Determination of human anti-idiotypic anti-B72.3 IgG

Human anti–idiotypic anti-B72.3 IgG was determined by incubating polystyrene beats coated with B72.3 antibodies with 0.2 ml serum diluted 1:50 with Tris-buffer. The sample was supplemented with 80 mg/l of non-specific polyclonal mouse IgG to block anti-iso/allotypic anti-B72.3 antibodies. Binding of human IgG was detected as described above.

Results

Figure 1 shows the relationship between the apparent TAG 72 concentrations measured with assay I and assay II, respectively, and the time of B72.3 infusions. The apparent TAG 72 concentrations measured with assay I increased from 13 U/ml before treatment up to 12,900 U/ml after the fourth infusion while the values measured with assay II only slightly increased up to 515 U/ml indicating false-positive TAG 72 values in assay I. In order to characterize the responsible interfering factors, serum IgG was removed by affinity chromatography with Protein G-Sepharose from a sample drawn after four infusions: 97% of the false-positive TAG 72-like material was bound by Protein G-Sepharose; 70% was recovered in the eluat. In contrast, 84% of the TAG 72 activity of the control sample passed through the column

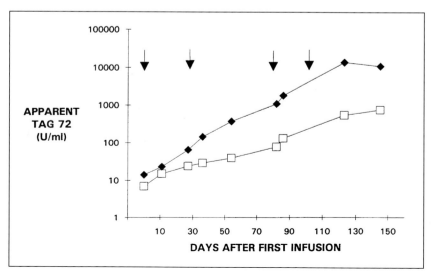

Figure 1. Time course of apparent TAG 72 concentrations measured with assay I (◆) and assay II (□) during repeated treatment with B72.3 antibodies. Arrows indicate the time of B72.3 infusions.

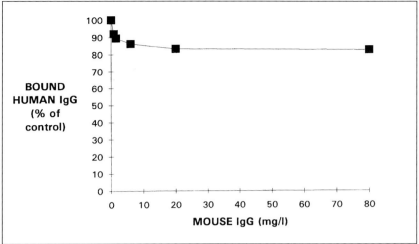

Figure 2. Inhibition of human anti-B72.3 IgG binding to B72.3 antibodies by non-specific mouse IgG. Immobilized B72.3 was incubated with serum diluted 1:300 with Tris buffer containing increasing concentrations of non-specific mouse IgG.

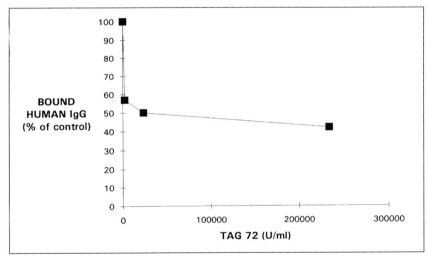

Figure 3. Inhibition of human anti–idiotypic anti-B72.3 IgG binding to B72.3 antibodies by TAG 72 antigen. Immobilized B72.3 was incubated with serum diluted 1:300 with Tris buffer containing increasing concentrations of TAG 72. Anti-iso/allotypic antibodies were blocked by addition of 80 mg/l non-specific mouse IgG.

directly, and no TAG 72 was found in the eluate. These data suggested that the false-positive results in assay I were due to human anti-idiotypic anti-B72.3 IgG. For further characterization, binding of human anti-B72.3 IgG was determined directly in the presence of increasing concentrations of non-specific polyclonal mouse IgG to inhibit binding of anti-iso/allotypic anti-B72.3 antibodies. In the presence of 20 mg/l mouse IgG binding was inhibited only slightly about 13% (figure 2). Larger amounts of mouse IgG did not further reduce binding indicating the anti-idiotypic nature of a high percentage of the newly formed anti-B72.3 antibodies. However, the anti-idiotypic portion of anti-B72.3 IgG binding, which could not be blocked by mouse IgG, was inhibited by addition of the antigen TAG 72 about 52% (figure 3). To validate that the anti-idiotypic anti-B72.3 antibodies were induced by administration of B72.3 antibodies, the relationship between the time of antibody infusions and the appearance of anti-idiotypic antibodies was examined. As shown in figure 4, after the first infusion anti-idiotypic antibody concentrations slightly increased, followed by a dramatic rise after the second infusion and a further increase after each following infusion.

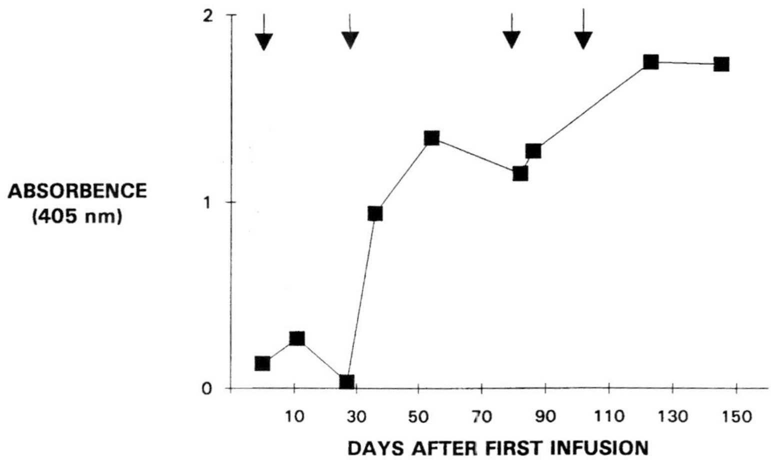

Figure 4. Time course of anti–idiotypic anti-B72.3 antibody concentration during repeated treatment with B72.3 antibodies. Anti-iso/allotypic antibodies were blocked by addition of 80 mg/l non-specific mouse IgG. Arrows indicate the time of B72.3 infusions.

Discussion

The presented results support the hypothesis that human anti–idiotypic anti-B72.3 antibodies (Ab2) are induced by treatment with the MAb B72.3, which cannot be masked by non-specific mouse IgG. Obviously, these Ab2 do not crossreact with the anti-TAG 72 MAb cc49 used in assay II but – as to be expected – interfere with the homologous assay I. According to *Bona* and *Köhler* (1) anti-idiotypic antibodies can be classified as Ab2α directed against regulatory idiotopes, Ab2γ directed against determinants near the paratope and Ab2β directed against determinants within the paratope. Ab2β and Ab2γ are antigen inhibitable but only Ab2β mimic functional and structural characteristics of the antigen. The fact, that a high percentage of Ab2 binding to MAb B72.3 was inhibited by the antigen TAG 72, suggests that a considerable portion of Ab2 binds at (Ab2β) or near to (Ab2γ) the antigen binding site of the MAb B72.3. A further discrimination of Ab2β and Ab2γ and identification of "internal image" antibodies cannot be done by means of inhibition assays.

Conclusion

The application of the monoclonal antibody B72.3 stimulates the production of antibodies directed against different determinants on the B72.3: 1. anti-iso/allotypic antibodies, which can be masked by nonspecific mouse IgG; 2. anti-idiotypic antibodies, which bind to epitopes on the B72.3 antibody not inhibited by non-specific mouse IgG but partly by the antigen TAG 72.

References

1. Bona CA, Köhler H (1984) Anti-idiotypic antibodies and internal images. Recept Biochem Methodol 14:141–149
2. Jerne NK, Roland J, Cazenave PA (1982) Recurrent idiotypes and internal images. EMBO J 1:243–247
3. Schlom J, Colcher D, Szpak CA et al (1989) A monoclonal antibody (B72.3) to adenocarcinoma of the colon and related tumors. Immun Cancer 2:63–72
4. Wagner U, Oehr P, Reinsberg J, Schmidt S, Schlebusch H, Werner A, Krebs D (1992) Immunotherapy of advanced ovarian carcinomas by the activation of the idiotypic network. Biotech Therapeutics 3:81–89
5. Wettendorf M, Iliopoulos D, Tempero M, Kay D, DeFreitas E, Koprowski H, Herlyn D (1989) Idiotypic cascades in cancer patients treated with monoclonal antibody CO17-IA. Proc Natl Acad Sci 86:3787-3791

Address for correspondence:
Dr. rer. nat. J. Reinsberg
Zentrum für Frauenheilkunde und Geburtshilfe
Universität Bonn
Sigmund-Freud-Straße 25
D-53127 Bonn, Germany

Toxicity of local continuous and cyclic, high-dose bladder perfusion with recombinant and natural interleukin-2 in advanced cancer of the urinary bladder

H. Schwaibold, Edith Huland, H. Heinzer, H. Huland

Department of Urology, University of Hamburg, Germany

Introduction

Interleukin-2 (IL-2) has a key function in proliferation and activation of immune cells (9). The benefits of IL-2 treatment for tumor regression have been demonstrated successfully (12). Systemic application, however, induces severe side effects, can be given only to patients in good condition, and often must be restricted to inpatients (3, 8). We were the first group to demonstrate that high-dose local application of IL-2 in advanced bladder carcinoma can be given without toxicity during two 5-day continuous treatment cycles (4). There is increasing evidence that IL-2 is involved in the therapeutic effects of BCG (8, 11) and other immunotherapeutic substances (1) used to prevent recurrence of superficial bladder carcinoma. However, the use of high-dose local IL-2 in patients with less advanced disease requires solid knowledge of the safety of long-term high-dose application, the development of safe equipment for outpatient treatment, and the study of cyclic and continuous application schedules.

Materials and methods

Patients

Between January 1988 and December 1989 18 out of 89 patients, referred to our hospital for advanced but not metastatic transitional-cell carcinoma of the bladder in purpose to perform radical cystectomy entered this study. Two had clinical stage T2, G2/G3 tumors, two had clinical stage T3, G3 tumors and 14 clinical stage T4, (G2/G3) tumors. T4 was assessed by bimanual examination during anesthesia and by CT scans. None of the patients was eligible for any other form of treatment – such as cystectomy, chemotherapy or radiation – because of age (12/18 patients were older than 70 years), poor performance status (9 of them had Karnofsky index below 70), increased creatinine levels (7/18) or cardiac risks (9/18). Metastatic disease was excluded by chest rays, bone scans, and computed tomographic scans of the abdomen and pelvis.

Interleukin

nIL-2 was produced from phytohemagglutinin stimulated, pooled, freshly donated human mononuclear cells. It was provided to us as a solution of 100,000 U/ml or 150,000 U/ml (Biotest Pharma GmbH/Frankfurt, FRG). In this paper all units given are Biological Response Modifier Programm Units (BRMPU). rIL-2 was produced in E. coli transfected with the gene for IL-2. The specific activity of rIL-2 was $18 \cdot 10^6$ international units (IU) per milligram (Eurocetus/Amsterdam, Netherlands). rIL-2 was not glycosylated. It was provided to us as a lyophilized powder that had to be reconstituted with 1.2 ml of sterile water per vial. According to information provided by EuroCetus/Amsterdam, Netherlands, $6 \cdot 10^6$ international units correspond to $2.3 \cdot 10^6$ BRMPU. Treatment schedule see table I.

TUR was performed 2–5 days before IL-2 perfusion started, bi-monthly in group A and before every second treatment cycle in groups B and C. In group A permanent nIL-2 perfusion was performed in a complete outpatient setting using the combination of a battery driven portable Pharmacia Deltec CADD-I pump (Pharmacia, Minnesota, USA) and a subcutaneous catheter system developed by our group for this study. In group B and C cyclic IL-2 perfusion was performed in the clinic. Continuous perfusion was through a double-line transurethral catheter. Each patient received 15 l of IL-2 solution during the five days for a total dose of $15 \cdot 10^6$ units nIL-2 (group B) or rIL-2 at an increasing dose, starting with $32.10 \cdot 10^6$ BRMPU/5 days[a] (cycle 1) up to $107.85 \cdot 10^6$ BRMPU/5 days[a] (cycle 5) (see table I). The 5-day treatment was repeated every four weeks, if possible, up to 15 times in group B and up to six times in group C. Patients with "complete remission" were offered an additional treatment cycle every 120 days for the next two years. Toxicity and response criteria were graded according to World Health Organization procedure.

Results

Side effects

No serious side effects were observed in any of the patients. Fever occured in three patients during therapy. In all three, IL-2 accidentally entered the vascular system, due two bladder wall perforation after TUR or subcutaneous IL-2 application in case of a dislocation of the needle of the pump system. Except for short-term (less than 24-hour) toxicity, systemic side effects – i.e., side effects of IL-2 – did not appear. Creatinine levels were increased in four patients, but all suffered from urinary obstruction due to bladder carcinoma and infusions were not discontinued. All other blood measures remained normal during the whole treatment period. One patient in group A (78 years old) developed signs of local contrast media hypersensitivity requiring intensive care a few hours after local intraurethral application of iodine containing radiographic contrast medium. Steroid and symptomatic therapy led to relief of symptoms within 24 h (6, 7). Uncomplicated urinary tract infections appeared a mean of 4.8 times per patient in group A, 2.2 times per patient in group B and 2.6 times per patient in group C. Only bacterial infections of the subcutaneous catheter system, seen in three patients in group A required therapy-stop. The low numbers of side effects were achieved despite extraordinarily long treatment periods (especially in group A) and high IL-2 doses (table I).

Table I. Treatment schedules.

Group	A	B	C
Therapy-mode	permanent	cyclic	cyclic
IL-2 BRMPU*	natural IL-2	natural IL-2	recombinant IL-2
Dose	100,000 U/ml	1,000 U/ml	2,140–7,140 U/ml
ml/min	0.01	2	2
Schedule	permanent infusion (24 h/day)	one cycle: 5 day continuous infusion (24 h/day), stop therapy day 6- day 28	one cycle; 5 day continuous infusion (24 h/day) stop therapy day 6- day 28
Overall-treatment period, mean (range) days	206 (81–420)	179 (162–420)	129 (112–168)
Single treatment days, mean (range)	141 (81–283)	32,2 (29–75)	23 (20–30)
Therapy cycles, mean (range)	–	7.3 (6–15)	4.8 (4–6)
Mean overall IL-2 dose, BRMPU[a] (range)	$305 \cdot 10^6$ (40–688)	$305 \cdot 10^6$ (90–870)	$432 \cdot 10^6$ (289–506)

[a] According to information provided by EuroCetus/Amsterdam, the Netherlands, $6 \cdot 10^6$ international units correspond to $2.3 \cdot 10^6$ BRMPU.

Tabel II. Results of IL-2 treatment.

Therapy-schedule	Complete remission	Stable disease	Progressive disease
Group A	1/7 (540 days)	1/7 (283 days)	5/7 ($\bar{x}$ 139; 81-217 days)
Group B	3/7 (990, 147, 152 days)	2/7 (207, 291 days)	2/7 ($\bar{x}$ 153; 150-156 days)
Group C	0/4	0/4	4/4 ($\bar{x}$ 114; 104-156 days)

Clinical results

According to the definition of complete remission, i.e. no evidence of tumor in at least six randomized biopsies taken with cystoscopy from urothelium, "complete remission" was achieved in one of seven patients in group A (initial stage T2), three of seven in group B (two patients with initial stage T4-tumors and one patient with initial stage T3-tumor), and none of four in group C (see table II). Two patients with "complete remission" still receive 5-day cycles of nIL-2 perfusion every 120 days, and no evidence of bladder carcinoma has been found on histologic examination of TUR material 540 and 990 days after the start of therapy. Another patient with complete remission underwent cystectomy because of urinary incontinence (low-capacity bladder) due to previous pelvic irradiation. Histologic examination of the cystectomy specimen did not show any remaining tumor. Stable disease was achieved in one patient in group A and two patients in group B but in no patients in group C.

Discussion

In view of the fact that IL-2 seems to play a role in BCG immunotherapy for prevention of recurrent bladder cancer (8, 11) and in view of our data that show for the first time that high-dose local continuous application of IL-2 does not induce any side effects (4), there is increasing readiness to enter a new level of IL-2 immunotherapy: Application in diseases to reduce toxicity and increase effectiveness, even if alternative therapy might be available. Our data show for the first time that even long-term (up to 420 days) and high-dose continuous application into the bladder is tolerated extremely well. Despite the long treatment period blood measures remained normal or unchanged except in patients in whom increased values could be explained by the presence of other conditions. None of the schedules and none of the substances produced toxicity if administration into the bladder was accurate. That is not due to a lack of effectiveness of the substances: When bladder perforation or needle dislocation permits systemic access of IL-2, typical side effects, such as fever and malaise occurred within a few hours. During local IL-2 administration, only uncomplicated, but frequent urinary tract infections pose problems. These infections seem not to be peculiar to IL-2 treatment, but rather result from repeated TURs and the repeated transurethral or long-term suprapubic catheterization needed for bladder perfusion. In case of implantation of a subcutaneous Port-a reservoir, there may be an increased risk of local infection requiring explantation. We recommend low-dose antibiotic prophylaxis to reduce the infection rate. Very important for the clinician is the observation that the local application of IL-2 can induce severe toxicity if local contrast medium is used for diagnostic purposes. It was not the purpose of this study to evaluate effectivity of this treatment-schedule by two reasons: 1. Remission can not be adequately defined unless cystectomy is done. 2. We used two therapeutic modalities such as local immunotherapy and repeated TURs.

With these limitations the four complete remissions are encouraging in respect to the especially bad constitution of the patients. Additionally, the duration of "complete remission" in two patients (up to 540 and 990 days) is encouraging. However, from a scientific point of view it has yet to be determined whether IL-2 or TUR is responsible for effectiveness of treatment. We have further evidence that local IL-2 application may induce local and systemic cellular immunce activation. In previous studies with much shorter treatment periods, we evaluated different local and systemic immune reactions after natural IL-2 application in the bladder. We found local and systemic cellular immune activation, e.g. an increase in IL-2 receptor-positive cells in the blood up to 17% (7). We were able to show tumor-associated eosinophilia of up to 65% (i.e., eosinophils constituting 65% of leucocytes) during IL-2 treatment, local activation of eosinophils attached to bladder tumor cells and active degranulation of eosinophils on bladder tumor cells. In the present study we could also confirm local immune reactions in the first weeks of therapy such as IL-2-receptor expression and eosinophilia. The present study shows the safety of local IL-2 bladder application even at high doses and for extremely long periods. Our data provide a basis for the safe use of IL-2 to prevent recurrent bladder carcinoma when alternative treatment schedules exist but have distinct local and potential systemic toxicity, which according to our data can be avoided with IL-2.

Acknowledgements

This work was supported by the Deutsche Forschungsgemeinschaft.

References

1. Bradley LM, Duncan DD, Tonkonogy S, Swain SL (1991) Characterization of antigen-specific CD4+ effector T cells in vivo: Immunization results in a transient population of MEL-14-, CD45 RB- helper cells that secretes interleukin 2 (IL-2), Il-3, Il-4, and interferon gamma. J Exp Med 174:547–559
2. Heinzer H, Huland H, Huland E (1990) Activated eosinophil leucocytes in interleukin-2 treated patients: Evidence for a new antitumor effector mechanism. J Cancer Res Clin Oncol (abstr) 369
3. Herr H (1987) Conservative management of muscle-infiltrating bladder cancer: Prospective experience. J Urol 138:1162–1163
4. Huland E, Huland H (1989) Local continuous high dose interleukin-2: a new therapeutic model for the treatment of advanced bladder carcinoma. Cancer Res 49:5469–5474
5. Huland E, Heinzer H, Huland H (1991) Increased toxicity to local and systemic n-Interleukin-2 (nIl-2) after iodine-containing radiographic contrast media (ICCM). J Urol 145:334
6. Huland E, Huland H (1992) Tumor associated eosinophilia in interleukin-2 treated patients: evidence of toxic eosinophil degranulation on bladder cancer cells. J Cancer Res Clin Oncol 118:463–467
7. Huland E, Huland H, Heinzer H (1992) Interleukin-2 by inhalation: Local therapy for metastatic renal cell carcinoma. J Urol 147:3443–348
8. Lee RE, Lotze MT, Skibber JM, Tucker E, Bonow RO, Ognibene FP, Carra squillo JA, Shelhamer JH, Parrillo JE, Rosenberg SA (1989) Cardiorespiratory effects of immunotherapy with interleukin-2. J Clin Oncol 7:7–20
9. Mertelsmann R, Welte K (1986) Human interleukin-2: molecular biology, physiology and clinical possibilities. Immunobiol 172:400–419
10. Sosnowski JT, De Haven JI, Abraham FM, Riggs DR, Lamm DL (1992) Sequential immunocytological evaluation of murine transitional cell carcinoma during intralesional bacillus Calmette-Guerin and interleukin-2 immunotherapy. J Urol 147:1439–1443
11. Wang MH, Flad HD, Böhle A, Chen YQ, Ulmer AJ (1991) Cellular cytoxicity of human natural killer cells and lymphokine-activated killer cells against bladder carcinoma cell lines. Immunol Lett 27:191–197
12. West WH, Tauer KW, Yannelli JR, Marshall GD, Orr DW, Thurmann GB, Oldham RK (1987) Constant-infusion recombinant interleukin-2 in adoptive immunotherapy of advanced cancer. N Engl J Med 316:898–905

Address for correspondence:
Dr. med. H. Schwaibold
Abteilung für Urologie
Universität Hamburg
Martinistraβe 52
D-20252 Hamburg, Germany

Inhalative natural interleukin-2 (IL-2) in combination with low dose systemic IL-2 and interferon-α (IFNa)

Longterm follow-up and toxicity of patients with pulmonary metastasis of renal cell carcinoma

H. Heinzer, Edith Huland, B. Falk, H. Huland

Department of Urology, Universiy of Hamburg, Germany

Introduction

Experimental models in immunotherapy with interleukin-2 (IL-2) alone (12, 14) or in combination with lymphokine-activated killer (LAK) cells (11, 12) or tumor-infiltrating lymphocytes (TILs) (3, 5, 13) have shown anti-tumor effectivity in tumor diseases. Despite promising trials using systemic immunotherapy in patients with metastic renal cell carcinoma (RCC) the overall response rate is less than 20% with a complete remission under 10%. The widely use of systemic IL-2 is limeted to severe, possible fatal side effects. Despite new application forms of systemic cytokines (1, 2, 6) sytemic IL-2 treatment is still toxic and patients at risk have to be excluded from treatment.

In a former study we have shown that local continuous IL-2 can be given in very high doses without side effects in patients with advanced bladder cancer (7) and induced local and systemic immunomodulation (8).

In patients with pulmonary metastasis of RCC we have shown that a combination of intravenous IL-2 (40% of total IL-2 dose), inhaled IL-2 (60% of total IL-2 dose) and subcutaneous interferon-a (IFN-α) has toxicity only in systemic treatment and anti-tumor effectivity while pulmonary metastases responded in 5/5 patients (9).

In this study we report the longtime follow-up of 21 patients receiving a modified therapy with inhalative natural IL-2 (90% of total IL-2 dose) in combination with low dose subcutaneous natural IL-2 (10% of IL-2 dose) and interferon-α.

Material and methods

We included 21 patients in the protocol. Five had received prior treatment as published recently (9). All patients have histologically confirmed renal cell carcinoma. All pulmonary metastases had documented progression before treatment start. Characteristics of patients are given in table I. All patients received natural human interleukin-2 provided by Biotest Pharma GmbH, Frankfurt.

Table I. Characteristics of patients receiving immunotherapy.

Patients	
Total	21
Male	15
Female	6

Age (years)	
41–50	4
51–60	9
61–70	8

Performance status[a]	
0	6
1	10
2	4
3	1

[a]According to criteria of Eastern Cooperative Oncology Group (ECOG)

Prior treatment	
Nephrectomy	19
Interferon	5
Hormone therapy	2
Surgery of metastases	4
Chemo- or radiotherapy	0

Table II. Toxicity of inhaled IL-2.

	WHO grade 0	WHO grade I	WHO grade II
Dyspnea	0	20	1
Hypotension	19	2	0
Skin	12	9	0
Nausea	3	18	0
Fever	6	15	0
Fatigue	2	19	0
Arthralgia	9	12	0
Infection	19	2	0
Allergy (contrast media)	18	1	2

Table III. Response of pulmonary metastases.

	n	Percentage	Duration (months)
Complete respone	1	5	6
Partial response	10	48	33, 24, 24[a], 24+, 18, 18, 8, 5, 4, 3
Stable disease	7	38	23, 20, 17, 12,7[a], 6,5+, 3,2+
Progressive disease	1	5	

[a]Complete surgical response

Recombinant IFN-a2b was purchased from Essex/ Schering, Munich, Germany. Treatment was performed exclusively on an outpatients basis. Inhalation of IL-2 was performed with a Salvia Lifetec nebulizer five times daily. The treatment protocol is shown in detail in figure 1. Toxicity was assessed in terms of WHO grades. Response was considered according to WHO response criteria and actual mean survival was compared to expected mean survival according to risk factors (4).

Results

Toxicity

A total of 275 months of continuous inhalation in these 21 patients has been performed (mean 14.7, range 1–33.5 months). Only grade I toxicity was observed during the whole treatment time, except that three patients had a single grade II event (bronchospasm and allergy to contrast media) (table II). No development of autoimmune diseases or interstitial lung diseases occured during longtime treatment.

Response of pulmonary metastases

In 20/21 patients pulmonary metastases responded with complete remission, partial remission or stabilization (table III).

Response of non-pulmonary metastases

Non-pulmonary metastases were present in ten patients. Partial response occured in two pleural metastases and in one abdominal lymph node metastases.

Overall tumor response (WHO critiria)

One complete response, two surgical complete responses, five partial responses, three mixed responses, seven stable diseases and three progressive diseases (table IV).

Table IV. Overall response (WHO).

	n	Percentage
Complete response	1	5
Partial response	5	24
Stable disease	7	33
Mixed response	3	14
Complete surgical response	2	10
Progressive disease	3	43

Survival

Of the 19 evaluable patients, eight are still alive. The mean expected survival was 9.4 months while so far a mean actual survival of 22.3 months has been achieved ($p < 0.001$, paired t-test).

Discussion

This is the first report of a non-toxic outpatient treatment schedule for metastatic renal cell carcinoma with high antitumor effectivity. The responses cannot be explained by patient selection alone, in as much as patients at risk were included and all patients had progressive disease before entry. Even patients with stabilization of up to 23 months had a good quality of life during treatment. The main advantage of this new combination therapy may not be to achieve better response rates with lower toxicity than traditional schedules but the fact that in nearly all patients pulmonary progress safely can be stopped. If this could be achieved even in a larger group of patients it will influence the further treatment of metastic RCC. By using mainly local cytokines applications the tools of response evaluation have to be used critically.

An unexpected finding is the extremely low toxicity of inhaled IL-2, no severe side effects occured during 275 treatment months.

Survival in our patients seems to prolonged. According to risk factors (4) patients achieved an average of more than two times their expected mean survival. IL-2 is highly effective and non toxic if local treatment is used. Toxicity and antitumor effectivity of IL-2 seem not be connected but independent from each other.

References

1. Atzpodien J, Körfer A, Franks CR et al (1990) Home therapy with recombinant interleukin 2 and interferon-α2b in advanced human malignancies. Lancet 335:1509
2. Bartsch HH, Adler M, Ringert RH et al (1990) Sequential therapy of recombinant interferon alpha (IFN-A) and recombinant interleukin 2 (IL-2) in patients with advanced renal-cell carcinoma (RCC). Proc Ann Meet Am Soc Clin Oncol 9: A 556
3. Bukowski RM, Sharfman W, Murthy S et al (1991) Clinical results and characterization of tumor-infiltrating lymphocytes with or without recombinant interleikin-2 in human metastic renal cell carcinoma. Cancer Res 51: 4199–4205
4. Elson PJ, Witte RS, Trump DL (1988) Prognostic factors for survival in patients with recurrent or metastatic renal cell carcinoma. Cancer Res 48:7310
5. Figlin R, Belldegrun A, De Kernion J (1992) Immunotherapy of patients with metastic renal cell carcinoma (RCCa) using an outpatients regimen of interleukin-2 (IL-2) and interferon-alpha (IFN) administered either alone or with in vivo primed tumor infiltrating lymphocytes (pTIL): The UCLA experience [abstract]. Proc Am Soc Clin Oncol 11:197
6. Figlin R, Citron M, Whitehead R et al (1990) Low dose continuous infusion recombinant human interleukin 2 (rhIL-2) and roferon; an active outpatient regimen for metastatic renal-cell carcinoma (RCCa). Proc Ann Meet Am Soc Clin Oncol 9: A 553
7. Huland E, Huland H (1989) Local continuous high dose interleukin 2: a new therapeutic model for the treatment of advanced bladder carcinoma. Cancer Res 49:5469
8. Huland E, Huland H (1992) Tumor-associated eosinophilia in interleukin 2-treated patients: evidence of toxic eosinophil degranulation on bladder cancer cells. J Cancer Res Clin Oncol 118:463
9. Huland E, Heinzer H, Huland H (1992) Effective non-toxic treatment of pulmonary metastases of renal cell carcinoma by inhalation of interleukin-2. J Urol 147:421A
10. Huland E, Huland H, Heinzer H (1992) Interleukin 2 by inhalation: local therapy fo metastatic renal cell carcinoma. J Urol 147: 344
11. Rosenberg SA, Lotze MT, Muul LM et al (1985) Observations on the systemic administration of autologous lymphokine-activated killer cells and recombinant interleukin 2 to patients with metastatic cancer. N Engl J Med 313:1485–1492
12. Rosenberg SA, Lotze MT, Muul LM et al (1987) A progress report on the treatment of 157 patients with advanced cancer using lymphokine activated killer cells and interleukin 2 or high dose interleukin 2 alone. N Engl J Med 316:889
13. Rosenberg SA, Spiess P, Lafreniere R (1986) A new approach to the adoptive imunotherapy of cancer with tumor-infiltrating lymphocytes. Science 223:1318
14. West WH, Tauer KW, Yannelli JR et al (1987) Constant-infusion recombinant interleukin 2 in adoptive immunotherapy of advanced cancer. New Engl J Med 316:898

Address for correspondence:
Dr. med. H. Heinzer
Abteilung für Urologie
Universitätsklinik Hamburg-Eppendorf
Martinistraße 52
D-20246 Hamburg, Germany

Intrapleural administration of interleukin-2 in malignant pleural mesothelioma

A phase I-II study

A. M. M. Eggermont[a], S. H. Goey[b], R. Slingerland[b], C. J. A. Punt[b], J. W. Gratama[c], R. Oosterom[d], R. L. H. Bolhuis[c], G. Stoter[b]

Departments of [a]Surgical Oncology, [b]Medical Oncology, [c]Immunology and [d]Clinical Chemistry, Rotterdam Cancer Institute, Rotterdam, The Netherlands

Introduction

No effective therapy for malignant pleural mesothelioma exists. It has been demonstrated in intraperitoneal tumor models that intracavitary administration of interleukin-2 (IL-2) can induce very high numbers of lymphokine activated killer cells with high antitumor activity in the peritoneal exudate (1). Intrapleural administration of IL-2 for pleural mesothelioma, a condition that tends to remain confined to the pleural cavity throughout or for most of its natural course, could therefore be considered a reasonable therapeutic approach. A recent report by *Yasumoto* and co-workers described the complete clearance of malignant cells from the pleural fluid in patients with malignant pleurisy due to lung cancer after intrapleural instillations of IL-2 (2). Based on these data a phase I-II study with intrapleural IL-2 was initiated in patients with pleural mesothelioma stage I-IIA according to the Butchart staging system (3).

Patients, materials and methods

Patients

According to Butchart's staging system (3) stage I-IIA is defined as tumor confined within the capsule of the parietal pleura, i.e. involving only ipsilateral pleura, lung, diaphragm, and external surface of the pericardium within the pleural reflection. Stage IIA is defined as mesothelioma invading chest wall or mediastinal tissues with or without lymph node involvement ipsilaterally inside the chest.

Twenty-four male patients with malignant pleural mesothelioma stage I or IIA, without prior treatment, entered the study. Their median age was 53 (range 47-71) and their median Karnofsky performance status 100% (range 90-100%). Eligibility criteria required histologically confirmed pleural mesothelioma stage I-IIA, sufficient pleural effusion to insert an intrapleural catheter, no signs of loculation on the CT scan, no prior chemo-, radio-, immunotherapy, age < 76 years, Karnofsky performance status > 80%, no cardiovascular disease, a white blood cell count > 4000/ml, a platelet count > 100,000/ml, hematocrit > 30%, serum bilirubin and creatinine levels within the institution's normal range, no active infections, no use of corticosteroids, informed consent.

Treatment

One to two weeks prior to the first administration of IL-2 a port-a-cath system was surgically inserted under general anaesthesia. The correct intrapleural position of the catheter was checked radiographically and a colloid scan was made to check for good distribution throughout the pleural effusion.

Recombinant human interleukin-2 (IL-2) (Euro-Cetus B.V., Amsterdam, the Netherlands) was administered as a continuous intrapleural infusion at a dose according to a groupwise (at least three consecutive patients) dose escalation schedule (group A: $3 \cdot 10^4$, B: $3 \cdot 10^5$, C: $3 \cdot 10^6$, D: $6 \cdot 10^6$, E: $18 \cdot 10^6$, and F: $36 \cdot 10^6$ IU/day; this is the equivalent of $5 \cdot 10^4$ up to $6 \cdot 10^6$ Cetus units) for a period of 14 days at 2 week intervals. Thereafter, patients with stable disease or better could receive up to a maximum of four maintenance cycles at the same dose and route.

Response and toxicity

Response was evaluated after two treatment cycles. Tumor response and toxicity assessment used the World Health Organization (WHO) criteria (4). Toxicity was recorded and analyzed using the WHO grading system. For toxicities not included in the WHO guidelines, a grading system was used ranging from mild (grade I) to life-threatening (grade IV).

Determination of cytokine levels

In the patients where pleural fluid could be easily obtained, this was done prior to and during the treatment with IL-2. At the same time blood samples were taken in order to be able to determine and compare intrapleural IL-2 and TNFα levels with concurrent systemic IL-2 and TNFα levels.
IL-2 was measured with a double antibody radio immunoassay which uses a polyclonal antiserum (IRE-Medgenix, Fleurus, Belgium). The detection limit is about 0.5 U/ml (3.0 IU/ml). The interassay coefficient of variation at a level of 10.4 U/ml was 6.8%. One unit in this assay corresponds with 6 IU. TNFα was measured wit a coated tube immuno radiometric assay (IRE-Medgenix, Fleurus, Belgium). The detection limit is 5 ng/l and the interassay coefficient of varation at a level of 131 ng/l was 7.2%.

Results

Tumor response

Of 24 eligible patients with pleural mesothelioma, 17 patients were fully evaluable (both for toxicity and tumor response) as they received at least one full 14 day cycle of intrapleural IL-2. Cycles were administered at two week intervals. Three patients were not evaluable at all. In two patients this was due to catheter related problems, prohibiting the delivery of IL-2 and one patient did not receive IL-2 due to the development of a broncho-oesophageal fistula in the period between the insertion of the catheter and the first administration of IL-2. Four patients at the highest dose level were not evaluable for tumor response as they were unable to finish one cycle of 14 days because of dose limiting systemic toxicity that occurred only at that dose level. At least one treatment cycle of 14 days was received by four patients at $3 \cdot 10^4$ IU/day, three patients $3 \cdot 10^5$ IU/day, three patients $3 \cdot 10^6$ IU/day, three patients $6 \cdot 10^6$ IU/day, three patients $18 \cdot 10^6$ IU/day, and 1 patient $36 \cdot 10^6$ IU/day. Patients received 1 up to 5 treatment cycles. Four patients had a partial remission of 5, 11, 20, and 30 months (table I). Five patients had stable disease lasting 4, 4, 5, 6 and 8 months, and seven patients had progressive disease. The partial remissions occurred at the three lowest dose levels (A, B, C), Therefore no dose response relationship is evident. In two patients massive infected necrosis, in one patient massive sterile necrosis of the mesothelioma occured.

Table I. Responses and time to progression.

Response (n)	Time to progression (mts)
Complete remission (0)	
Partial remission (4)	5, 11, 20, 30
Stable disease (5)	4, 4, 5, 6, 8
Progressive disease (8)	2

Toxicity and complications

Toxicity has been virtually absent in this study at all dose levels except for the highest. Toxicity is summarized in table II. All patients received their treatment in an outpatient setting except for the last five patients of the study who were started on the highest dose level of $36 \cdot 10^6$ IU/day. Only minor flu-like symptoms were observed in the patients treated at the two higher dose levels. No systemic adverse effects, especially no hypotension or other cardiovascular effects, no pulmonary complications, no renal or liver dysfunction was observed. A slight leukocytosis (10,000–12,000 cells/ml) and an eosinophilia (2000–3500 cell/ml) were seen in most patients at the higher dose levels. Complications of the

Table II. Toxicity in relation to dose level in 17 fully evaluable patients.

Dose level	Symptoms	No. patients
$3 \cdot 10^4$ IU	flu-like	0/4
$3 \cdot 10^5$ IU		0/3
$3 \cdot 10^6$ IU		0/3
$6 \cdot 10^6$ IU		1/3
$18 \cdot 10^6$ IU		3/3
$36 \cdot 10^6$ IU		1/1[a,b]
All levels	cardiovascular	0/17
All levels	pulmonary	0/17
All levels	gastrointestinal	0/17
All levels	skin rash	0/17
	biochemical	
All levels	renal	0/17
All levels	hepatic	0/17

	hematologic (cells/mm^3)	
	leukocytosis > 10,000 (n/n)	eosinophilia > 2,000 (n/n)
$3 \cdot 10^4$ IU	1/4	0/4
$3 \cdot 10^5$ IU	1/3	1/3
$3 \cdot 10^6$ IU	1/3	2/3
$6 \cdot 10^6$ IU	3/3	2/3
$18 \cdot 10^6$ IU	3/3	1/3
$36 \cdot 10^6$ IU	1/1	0/1

[a] Only one patient fully evaluable (finished one cycle). MTD was reached here as two patients had to stop treatment at this dose level before finishing the 1st cycle because of sytemic toxicity: extreme fatigue in one patient and renal failure grade III in the other patient.
[b] Two other patients had to stop before finishing 1 cycle because of an infected catheter system. All five patients at the highest dose level had fever and flu-like symptoms.

treatment consisted of infected catheter systems in four patients. At the highest dose level systemic toxicity was quite prominent and dose limiting. Only one patient managed to complete one cycle of 14 days. The four other patients were hospitalized and had to stop treatment because of dose limiting malaise. The systemic toxicity corresponded with serum IL-2 levels of up to 30 IU/ml in patients treated at the highest dose level. At these high dose levels infections of the catheter systems occurred in the majority of the patients, and the catheters had to be removed before completion of the first cycle.

Determination of cytokine levels

Intrapleural as well as serum IL-2 levels were determined. Intrapleural concentrations were very high and correlated with the administered dose of IL-2. Intrapleural levels varied from 6–110 IU/ml at the lowest dose level to as high as 66,000–192,000 IU/ml at the highest dose level. Serum IL-2 levels became measurable only at the two highest dose levels and varied from < 3 IU/ml up to 30 IU/ml. Intrapleural IL-2 levels were up to 6000 times higher than serum levels. Intrapleural TNFα levels varied greatly from 50–125 pg/ml at the lowest dose level up to 235–405 pg/ml at the highest dose level. However no clear relation with IL-2 levels or dose levels was observed as TNFα levels at the intermediate IL-2 levels varied from 292–1141 pg/ml.

Discussion

We observed in this phase I-II the toxicity and efficacy of intrapleural administration of IL-2 in patients with pleural mesothelioma significant antitumor effects in four out of 17 evaluable patients at dose levels that were not associated with systemic toxicity. Regarding the intrapleural administration of IL-2 Yasumoto and coworkers (2) demonstrated that low doses of IL-2 were allready sufficient to induce lymphokine activated killer activity in the pleural exudate and lead to the disappearance of malignant pleural effusions. These activated lymphocytes were shown to be able to kill NK cell-resistant human mesothelioma cells (5). We made similar observations in our study. Significant regionally induced LAK activity was displayed by lymphocytes collected from the pleural effusions after intrapleural administration of IL-2. No LAK activity was displayed by the peripheral lymphocytes, except at the two highest dose levels of IL-2. However, LAK activity did not correspond with IL-2 dose level, intrapleural IL-2 level or intrapleural TNFα level. In this study where IL-2 dose did not correlate with response rate, none of the parameters investigated by immunophenotyping, cytotoxicity assays and determination of cytokine levels corresponded with the outcome of therapy.
IL-2 given intrapleurally has antitumor activity against mesothelioma showing a response rate of

24% in 17 evaluable patients with this disease, known to be refractory to almost any treatment. *Boutin* and collegues recently reported similar antitumor activity with intrapleural interferon-gamma (6). We conclude on the basis of our study and the reports in the literature that intrapleural administration of cytokines should be further explored as a new mode of treatment for malignant pleural mesothelioma.

References

1. Eggermont AMM, Sugarbaker PH, Marquet RL, Jeekel J (1988) In vivo generation of lymphokine activated killer (LAK) activity by ABPP and Interleukin-2 and their antitumor effects against immunogenic and nonimmunogenic tumors in murine tumor models. Cancer Immunol Immunother 26:24–30
2. Yasumoto K, Miyazaki K, Nagashima A et al (1987) Induction of lymphokine-activated killer cells by intrapleural instillations of recombinant interleukin-2 in patients with malignant pleurisy due to lung cancer. Cancer Res 47:2184–2187
3. Butchart EG, Ashcroft T, Barnsley WC et al (1976) Pleuropneumectomy in the management of diffuse malignant mesothelioma of the pleura. Thorax 31:15–24
4. WHO Handbook for Reporting Results of Cancer Treatment (1979) Geneva, World Health Organisation
5. Manning LS, Bowman RV, Darby SB, Robinson BWS (1989) Lysis of human malignant mesothelioma cells by natural killer (NK) and lymphokine-activated killer (LAK) cells. Am Rev Respir Dis 139:1369–1374
6. Boutin C, Viallat JR, Van Zandwijk N et al (1991) Activity of intrapleural gamma-interferon in malignant mesothelioma. Cancer 67:2033–2037

Address for correspondence:
A. M. M. Eggermont, M.D., PhD
Department of Surgical Oncology
Rotterdam Cancer Institute
P.O. BOX 5201
NL-3008 AE Rotterdam, The Netherlands

High dose TNFα, gamma-interferon and melphalan in isolated limb perfusion for stage III melanoma and irresectable soft tissue sarcomas of the extremities – A highly effective regimen

A. M. M. Eggermont[a], D. Lienard[b], H. Schraffordt Koops[c],
B. B. R. Kroon[d], F. Rosenkaimer[e], F.J. Lejeune[b]

[a]Department of Surgical Oncology, Rotterdam Cancer Institute, The Netherlands,
[b]Centre Pluridisciplinaire d'Oncologie, Lausanne, Switzerland,
[c]University Hospital Groningen, Groningen, [d]Netherlands Cancer Institute, Amsterdam,
The Netherlands; [e]Boehringer Ingelheim GmbH, Ingelheim, Germany

Introduction

Tumor necrosis factor-alpha (TNFα)

TNFα is a cytokine with pleiotropic actions, with direct and indirect antitumor effects, and is an important mediator of septic shock (1). Systemic administration of TNFα in cancer patients is associated with severe toxicity and negligible antitumor effects. Phase I-II studies indicate that the maximal tolerated dose (MTD) in humans is ± 350 µg/m^2 intravenously (2). Based on data in murine tumor models one might expect a 10–50-fold higher dose to be necessary to achieve antitumor effects (3). These differences may only be overcome in the setting of isolated limb perfusions (ILP). The antitumor effects of TNFα seem to be related to endothelial activation and vascular damage resulting in hemorrhagic necrosis, which starts within 1–4 hours after the administration of TNFα (4).

Melanoma stage III (intransit metastases)

Isolated limb perfusion for stage III melanoma permits regional cytostatic concentrations 15 to 20 times higher than those reached after systemic administration. The standard drug in this setting is melphalan (L-phenyl-alaninemustard). ILP with melphalan alone produces a 40–50% complete response rate with a median duration of local tumor control for all patients treated for only six months (5). True hyperthermia (>41.5 °C) may improve response rates, but may lead to severe regional toxicity (6). The modest efficacy of ILP with melphalan alone in stage III melanoma led to the addition of high doses of tumor necrosis factor-α (TNFα). The results of the initial observations in stage III melanoma have been recently published by *Lienard* and *Lejeune* (7, 8). Interferon-gamma (IFN) is added in this schedule because of synergistic antitumor activity of IFN plus TNFα (9).

Irresectable soft tissue sarcomas of the limbs

Isolated limb perfusion for stage III melanoma permits regional cytostatic concentrations 15 to 20 times higher than those reached after systemic administration. The standard drug in this setting is melphalan (L-phenyl-alaninemustard). ILP with melphalan alone produces a 40–50% complete response rate with a median duration of local tumor control for all patients treated of only six months (5). True hyperthermia (> 41.5 °C) may improve response rates, but may lead to severe regional toxicity (6). The modest efficacy of ILP with melphalan alone in stage III melanoma led to the addition of high doses of tumor necrosis factor-α (TNFα). The results of the initial observations in stage III melanoma have been recently published by *Lienard* and *Lejeune* (7, 8). Interferon-gamma (IFN) is added in this schedule because of synergistic antitumor activity of IFN plus TNFα (9).

Irresectable soft tissue sarcomas of the limbs

Isolated limb perfusion for soft tissue sarcomas (STS) can be an attractive option to render an irresectable tumor resectable, and in some cases of a sarcoma with hematogenous metastases this technique may be used palliatively for the local alleviation of pain and to avoid ablative surgery. *Krementz* and *Muchmore* reported only six CRs and six PRs in a series of 50 ILPs in 50 STS patients (10). *Lejeune's* initial experience with TNFa in ILP for STS lead to a multicenter study (11). Here we report on the collaborative experience with high dose TNFa ILP in the first 25 patients with irresectable STS of the limb.

Material and methods

Patients

Melanoma patients: Fifty-eight patients entered the study (46 females and 12 males); median age was 64 years (range 22–84). Most patients (38) had in transit metastases only (stage IIIa), 16 patients had in transit metastases associated with regional lymph node metastases (stage IIIab) and seven patients had systemically disseminated disease (stage IV) in association with transit metastases. The majority of these patients (31) had been previously treated: 25 had been perfused with melphalan.

Sarcoma patients: Twenty five patients with irresectable STS of the leg (21) or arm (4) were treated. There were 12 males and 13 females. Median age was 58 years (range 13-78). All tumors were locally advanced and considered irresectable because of fixation to the neurovascular bundle and or bone. The tumors were all grade II-III tumors of ten different histological types.

Drugs

Recombinant human tumor necrosis factor-α (TNFα: 0.2 mg/ampoule) and recombinant human interferon-gamma (IFN: 0.2 mg or 1.5×10^6 U/ampoule) were a gift from Boehringer Ingelheim GmbH, Germany. The cytostatic drug melphalan (Alkeran) was obtained as a sterile powder (100 mg) that was dissolved aseptically using solvent and diluent provided by Burroughs Wellcome (London, England).

Treatment schedule

Patients received 0.2 mg IFN s.c. on the two days prior to the ILP. ILP consisted of a 1 1/2 hour long perfusion with 0.2 mg IFN, 2 or 3 (arm) – 4 mg (leg) TNFα, and 10 mg/l leg or 13 mg/l arm volume of melphalan at mild hyperthermia (40 °C). IFN and TNFα were injected successively as a bolus into the arterial line. Melphalan was administered 30 minutes later. The whole perfusion lasted 90 minutes. At the end of ILP, the limb was washed with at least 1l of Haemaccel and 1l of 6% dextran. Leakage of the drugs was measured with radio-iodinated human serum albumin. Dopamine was administered peroperatively and/or postoperatively in about half of the patients at 2 µg/kg/min by continuous infusion, usually for several hours up to 48 hours. Fluid loading was applied before releasing the tourniquet after the completion of washing.

Assessment of tumor response

Complete remissions (CR), partial remissions (PR), no change (NC) and progressive disease (PD) were assessed by standardized criteria. In patients who underwent a resection of residual tumor histopathological examination was performed. If the clinical response was a PR the response could only be upgraded to a CR if histology showed 100% necrosis of the tumor.

Results

Tumor response in melanoma patients

In most cases a rapid softening of the nodules was seen within the first three days after TNFα ILP, as the first sign of tumor response. Objective regression rapidly followed. There were complete remissions in 51 of 58 patients (88%) and partial remissions in seven patients (12%). Median follow-up time has been 18+ months and the median response time 14+ months.

Local recurrences have been observed in 22 out of 58 patients (38%, median 6 months). In 25 patients (43%) distant metastases developed.

Response rate and limb salvage in sarcoma patients

After a pilot study in eight patients (8, 11), following a policy of not resecting the sarcoma sometime after the perfusion, we report here on 25 consecutive patients, adhearing to the principle of resecting the sarcoma 2–4 months after the perfusion except when systemic metastases, or multiple sarcomas in the limb were present, and the goal of limb salvage had been achieved.

At a median follow-up of 14+ months (12–28+ months) our results demonstrate that long lasting complete remissions and valuable partial remissions, making irresectable tumors resectable, can be obtained. Ten patients had a CR, twelve patients a PR and three patients a minimal response. In 20 patients the previously irresectable sarcoma was resected. In 13 of the 20 resected specimens > 90–100% necrosis was seen, in five specimens > 50% necrosis. Limb salvage was achieved in 22/25 patients (88%). A local recurrence developed in three patients, which led to an amputation in two patients and a reperfusion in the other.

Regional toxicity

All patients had a perfusion reaction grade II-III (grade II: redness of the skin; grade III: blisters). In one patient grade IV toxicity was observed and in one patient there was a rapid (within 48 hours) grade V toxicity of the foot which had been previously irradiated a part of sarcoma treatment. This is similar to the toxicity observed after ILP with melphalan alone.

Systemic toxicity

All patients developed fever and chills within four hours of the ILP, treated effectively with paracetamol or indomethacine. Although most patients went through a phase of lowered blood pressure, this was easily managed (fluid, low dose dopamine). In five patients hypotension in the postoperative period was severe and prolonged but reversible. Pulmonary toxicity was severe in six patients, who developed an ARDS, that usually resolved in two days. Liver toxicity was mild, only a transient increase in liver enzymes was observed in some patients. No grade III–IV renal toxicity occurred. Transient grade II–III leukopenia and thrombocytopenia were occasionally observed but did not require interventions. Systemic toxicity has been minimal in the last 60 patients treated.

Discussion

TNFα ILP in melanoma

ILP with high dose TNFα in combination with IFN and melphalan appears very effective against melanoma intransit metastases. Both the 88% complete response rate and the duration of local tumor control of 14+ months, are quite superior to results obtained with melphalan alone. After TNFα ILP the typical acute antitumor effects of TNFα as observed in murine models are also observed in patients. Acute softening and redness of the tumor associated with a prominent inflammatory response is observed. This rapid tumor response suggests that also in humans TNFα has an important vascular mediated effect (12).

TNFα ILP in irresectable soft tissue sarcoma

ILP with high dose TNF in combination with IFN and melphalan appears extraordinarily effective against locally advanced irresectable STS. The limb salvage rate of 88% in the 25 patients described here with irresectable STS is very high. The possibly selective effects of TNFα of tumor associated vessels, can be visualized by pre- and post-ILP angiographies. These often highly vascularized tumors show a prominant "blush" of pathological tumor associated vessels. Angiography 1–2 weeks after ILP with TNFα show that all the tumor associated vessels have disappeared.

Conclusions

The results in the 83 patients described here demonstrate that typical TNF-mediated antitumor effects can be obtained in man, provided sufficiently high TNF levels can be delivered to the tumor site. Whether gamma-IFN plays an important role is unclear. An ongoing randomized phase 2 study may soon elucidate the role of IFN. High dose TNF can be administered safely in isolation perfusion provided leakage during ILP is well controlled. After the toxicity observed during the learning curve, it is now clear after > 130 perfusions, that this therapy can be administered safely without significant toxicity. TNFα may thus establish itself as an important drug in isolation perfusion for a number of tumors, in particular stage III melanoma and irresectable soft tissue sarcomas.

References

1. Carswell EA, Old LJ, Kassel RL (1975) An endotoxin induced serum factor that causes necrosis of tumors. Proc Nat Acad Sci USA 72:3666–3370
2. Spriggs DR, Sherman ML, Michie H (1988) Recombinant human tumor necrosis factor administered as a 24 h intravenous infusion. A phase I and pharmacologic study. J Natl Cancer Inst 80:1039–1044
3. Asher AL, Mule JJ, Reichert CM, Shiloni E, Rosenberg SA (1987) Studies of the antitumor efficacy of systemically administered recombinant tumor necrosis factor against several murine tumors in vivo. J Immunol 138:963-974
4. Watanabe N, Niitsu Y, Umeno H (1988) Toxic effect of TNF on tumor vasculature in mice. Cancer Res 49:2179–2183
5. Klaase JM, Kroon BBR, Van Geel AN, Van Wijk J, Franklin HR, Eggermont AMM, Hart AAM (1993) Prognostic factors for tumor response and limb recurrence free interval in patients with advanced melanoma of the limbs treated with regional isolated perfusion using melphalan. Surg Gynaec Obstet (in press)
6. Kroon BBR, Klaase JM, Van Geel AN, Eggermont AMM (1992) Application of hyperthermia in regional isolated perfusion of melanoma of the limbs. Reg Cancer Treatment 4:223–226
7. Lienard D, Ewalenko P, Delmotte J-J, Renard N, Lejeune FJ (1992) High dose tumor necrosis factor-α in combination with IFN-gamma and melphalan in isolated perfusion of the limbs for melanoma and sarcoma. J Clin Oncol 10:52–60
8. Lejeune FJ, Lienard D, Leyvraz S, Mirimanoff RO (1993) Regional therapy of melanoma. Eur J cancer 29A:606–612
9. Schiller JH, Bittner G, Storer B, Wilson JKV (1987) Synergistic antitumor effects of TNFα and gamma-IFN on human colon carcinoma cell lines. Cancer Res 47:2809–2813
10. Krementz ET, Muchmore JH (1983) Soft tissue sarcomas: Behaviour and management. Adv Surg 16:147–196
11. Eggermont AMM, Lienard D, Schraffordt Koops H, Lejeune FJ (1993). Treatment of irresectable soft tissue sarcomas of the limbs by isolation perfusion with high dose TNFα, gamma-interferon and melphalan. In: Fiers W, Buurman WA (eds) Tumor necrosis factor: molecular and cellular biology and clinical relevance. Karger, Basel, pp 239–243
12. Lejeune FJ, Lienard D, Eggermont AMM, Renard N, Gérain J (1993) Evidence for early endothelium activation, IL6 production and high systemic TNFα levels after isolation perfusion with high dose rTNFα associated with rIFN. In: Fiers W, Buurman WA (eds) Tumor necrosis factor: molecular and cellular biology and clinical relevance. Karger, Basel, pp 244–248

Address for correspondence:
A. M. M. Eggermont, M.D., PhD
Department of Surgical Oncology
Rotterdam Cancer Institute
P.O. Box 5201
NL-3008 AE Rotterdam, The Netherlands

Formation and proliferative effects of leukotrienes and lipoxins in human bone marrow cells

M. Mansour[a], L. Stenke[b], O. El-Ahmady[a], J.A. Lindgren[b]

[a]Tumor Marker Oncology Research Center, Al-Azhar University Cairo, Egypt,
[b]Department of Physiological Chemistry, Karolinska Institute, Stockholm, Sweden

Introduction

Leukotrienes are formed from arachidonic acid by the 5-lipoxygenase pathway. These compounds seem to play an important role as regulator and modulator of various physiological events in inflammation and allergy (1)

Leukotrienes may also play a role in immune function, thus LTB4 appears to act as an inducer of T-suppressor cell activity (2).

The lipoxins constitute a novel class of oxygenated arachidonic acid derivatives sharing the common structure features of conjugated tetraenes (3). Myeloid cells, including granulocytes and monocytes produce leukotrienes (LTs) from arachidonic acid.

Recent reports have indicated that the leukotrienes may have regulatory effects on cell proliferation, thus both LTB4 and LTC4 have been demonstrated to increase the in vitro growth of arterial smooth muscle (4) and airway epithelial cells (5). The leukotrienes have also been indicated to regulate myelopoiesis. Although both stimulatory and inhibitory effects have been reported (6, 7, 8), the biological significance of the lipoxins is not fully established, These compounds have been reported to possess activities such as bronchoconstriction, vasodilation, stimulation of protein kinase C and inhibition of NK cells (9).

In the present study we have investigated the synthesis of leukotrienes and lipoxins in human bone marrow cells and the effect of these compounds on human myelopoiesis.

Materials and methods

Reagents

Leukotrienes B4, C4, D4 and E4 were kind gifts from *Dr. T. Miyamato* (ONO company, Osaka, Japan). Ficoll-hypaque was supplied from pharmacia fine chemicals (Uppsala Sweden) and E. coli derived recombinant human GM-CSF from Amersham international (Amersham, UK). Bacto-Agar was from Difco Laboratories. Lipoxin A4 and Lipoxin B4 were obtained from cayman chemical Co. (Ann Anbor, MI). Ionophore A23187 was obtained from Calbiochem – Boehring. The solvents for HPLC were from Rathburn chemicals LTd (Walkerburn, Scotland).

Cell preparations

Bone marrow samples from healthy volunteers were aspirated from the iliac crest during local anesthesia, the cells were centrifuged at 900 x g for 15 min, the buffy coat layer isolated and remaining erythrocytes lysed by incubation in hypotonic ammonium chlorid. Bone marrow cells were resuspended in phosphate saline buffer containing 0.9 mM calcium (10^7 cells in 1 ml, after initial 5 min period at 37 °C, the cell suspensions were incubated for 5 min in the presence of 1 µM ionophore A23187, the incubation were terminated by addition of 5 volumes of ethanol. All samples were stored at –20 °C until analyzed.

Colony assay

The mononuclear bone marrow cells were resuspended in a mixture of Iscov's medium with 10% fetal calf serum and 0.3% agar. One ml portions of the cell suspenions containing 0.2×10^6 cells were placed in petri dishes on the top of a one ml feeder layer which contains 0.5% agar in Iscov's medium and recombinant human GM-CSF. Dose response curve from preliminary experiments demonstrated an optimal progenitor cell growth in the presence of 25 units of GM-CSF per dish. Sub-optimal concentrations of GM-CSF (12.5 units per dish) were employed. Various concentrations of leukotrienes and lipoxins were added from stock solutions in ethanol to the cell layers during plating, the final ethanol concentrations in the dishes never exceeded 0.05%, a concentration which did not affect colony growth. All cultures were incubated for ten days at 37 °C in a cell incubator with an automatically regulated fully humidified atmosphere of 5% CO_2 in air. Control dishes were made in sets of six, all other dishes in triplicates. The dishes were coded, numbered and scored blindly directly after cultivation using an inverted microscope.

The growth in test dishes was compared to that in parallel control dishes and the relative difference between mean values of sets of control and test dishes were analyzed using the two tailed student's t-test for paired samples.

Assay procedure

After removal of precipitated material by centrifugation the supernatant was evaporated and dissolved in mobile HPLC-phase, the samples were subjected to reversed-phase HPLC using Nucleosil 120-3 C18 column eluted with acetonitril/methanol/water/acetic acid (29: 19: 52: 1 v/v, pH 5.6). At a flow rate of 1 ml/min the products were identified by cochromatography with synthetic standards and UV-spectroscopy.

Results

1. Leukotriene formation in suspensions of human bone marrow cells: Human bone marrow cell suspensions readily produced leukotrienes after stimulation with ionophore A23187, the bone marrow cells synthesized mainly LTB4 (figure 1). The amounts of leukotrienes produced by these cells were similar to those produced by peripheral blood leukocytes, the capacity of human bone marrow to produce lipoxins is shown in figure 1.

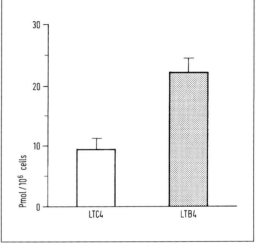

Figure 1. Leukotrienes formation by bone marrow cells from healthy donors.

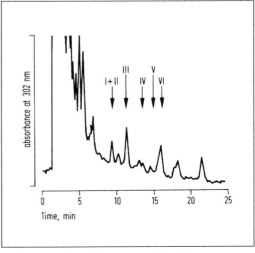

Figure 2. HPLC chromatogram of lipoxins formed by human bone marrow cell suspension. I + II: trans isomers of LXB4; III: LXB4; IV + V: trans isomers of LXA4; VI: LXA4.

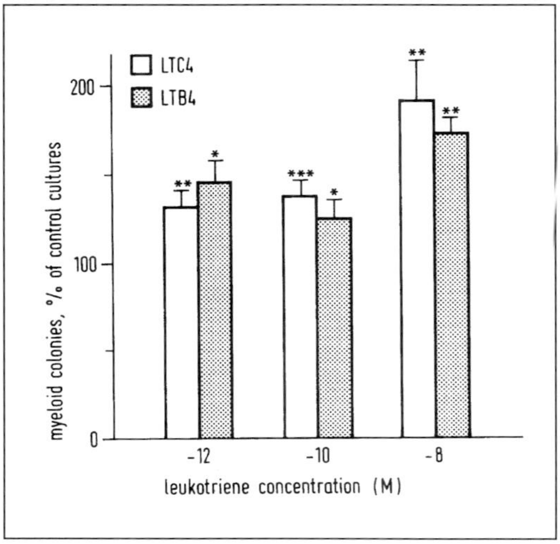

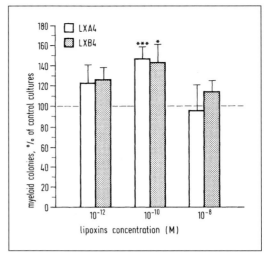

Figure 3. Stimulatory effect of LTC4 and LTB4 on bone marrow cells.

Figure 4. Effect of LXA4 and LXB4 on human bone marrow cells.

2. Effects of leukotrienes on GM-CSF induced bone marrow colony formation: Leukotrienes C4 induced a dose-dependent increase in GM-CSF induced myeloid progenitor cell growth. Maximal effects were observed at 10^{-8} M LTC4. However, addition of LTC4 10^{-10} M stimulate the growth of myeloid progenitor cells with mean increase 38 ± 9% whereas the increase at 10^{-12} M LTC4 was 32 ± 9%. In contrast, the highest and lowest concentrations of LTC4 (10^{-6} M and 10^{-14} M) failed to induce significant stimulation (figure 3). Addition of LTB4 to GM-CSF stimulated bone marrow cultures resulted in elevated colony formation, the strongest effect was observed with 10^{-8} M LTB4 which induce mean increase of 73 ± 22%. The stimulatory capacity of LTB4 was significant also at lower (concentration 25 ± 11% increase at 10^{-10} M and 46 ± 20% increase at 10^{-12} M (figure 3)).

3. Effects of lipoxins on human myeloid progenitor cell growth: The effects of lipoxins in cultures with suboptimal GM-CSF concentrations is displayed in figure 4; lipoxin A4 at 10^{-1} M increased the number of colonies with a mean increase of 47 ± 11% (M+SEM) as compared to the control dishes. The equivalent concentration of LXB4 also induced significant stimulation with mean increase of 44 ± 16%. However, addition of higher or lower concentrations (10^{-8} M and 10^{-12} M) of either LXA4 or LXB4 failed to induce significant effects on the colony formation (figure 4).

Discussion

The present investigation demonstrates that the bone marrow cell suspensions possess the capacity to produce leukotrienes and lipoxins. This indicates that also less mature cells (myeloid cells) are capable of leukotriene and lipoxin formation. This may be of interest, since it is important to study the role of leukotrienes in the regulation of human myelopoiesis.

A limited number of studies have previously addressed the question whether leukotrienes can influence the production of leukocytes in man. However, the results so far have been somewhat contradictory. Some of the proposed conclusions of the previous studies were based on only two or three experiments. In the present study, using a large number of bone marrows, we have accumulated data clearly supporting the stimulatory role for LTC4 and LTB4 in this system with the use of suboptimal concentrations of recombinant human GM-CSF which optimize the modulatory role exerted by lipoxygenase products. LTC4 was by far the most effective stimulator of myeloid progenitor cell growth. Proliferation of human myeloid progenitor cells was also stimulated by LTB4 with a similar potency like LTC4. These results are in agreement with an initial paper which reported that addition of LTB4 to human bone marrow cells induced a moderate increase in the colony formation (6). Another report disputed these results and stated that neither LTB4 nor LTC4 could potentiate the growth of human myeloid progenitor cells in the presence of colony stimulating factor (7). However, addition of dual lipoxygenase and cycloxygenase inhibitor could reduce colony formation and LTC4 or LTD4 but not LTB4 could reverse the inhibition.

The opposite effects, stimulation of myeloid cell growth by NDGA (nor dihydroguaretic acid) and inhibition by LTB4 or LTC4 have been reported (8). Another group of lipoxygenase products, the lipoxins, not only are formed from endogenous substrate in normal bone marrow but also can modulate the growth of the bone marrow derived myeloid stem cells. Highly significant synergistic effects were observed when low concentrations (10^{-10} M) of LXA4 or LXB4 were added to myeloid progenitor cells. The lipoxin induced effect appeared to be dose dependent resulting in a bell shaped dose response curve.

It was recently reported that 10^{-9} M LXB4 increased the colony formation from human peripheral mononuclear cells placed in diffusion chamber in the peritoneal cavity of mice during seven days (10).

In summary, the results demonstrate that leukotrienes and lipoxins are synthesized in the bone marrow and link these findings with potent biological effects in the same tissues.

References

1 Samuelsson B (1983) Leukotrienes: mediators of immediate hypersensitivity reactions and inflammation. Science 220:568
2 Pleszczynski M, Borgeat P, Sirosis P (1982) Leukotriene B4 induces human suppressor lymphocytes. Biochem Biophys Res Commun 198:1531
3 Serhan N, Hamberg M, Samuelsson B (1984) Lipoxins: Novel series of biologically active compounds formed from arachidonic acid in human leukocytes. Proc Natl Acad Sci USA 81:5335
4 Palmberg L, Lindgren JA, Thyberg I, Claesson HE (1991) On the mechanism of induction of DNA synthesis in cultured arterial smooth muscle cells by leukotrienes: Possible role of prostaglandin endoperoxide synthase products and platelets derived growth factor. J Cell Sci 98 141–149
5 Leikauf G, Claesson HE, Doupnik C, Hybbinette S, Grafstrom R (1989) Cysteinyl leukotrienes enhance growth of airway epithelial cells. Am J Physiol 259:255-261
6 Claesson H, Dahlberg N, Gahrton G (1985) Stimulation of human myelopoiesis by leukotriene B4. Biochem Biophys Res Commun 131:579–585
7 Miller AM, Wiener RS, Ziboh VA (1986) Evidence for the role leukotriene C4 and D4 as essential intermediates in CSF stimulated human myeloid colony formation. Exp Hematol 14:760–764
8 Estrov Z, Halperin DS, Coceani F, Freedman MH (1988) Modulation of human bone marrow hematopoiesis by leukotrienes in vitro. Br J Hematol 69:321
9 Samuelsson B, Dahlèn SE, Lindgren JÅ, Rouzer CA, Serhan CN (1987) Leukotrienes and lipoxins: structures, biosynthesis and biological effects. Science 237:1171–1176
10 Popov GK, Nekrasov AS, Khshivo AL, Pochinskii AG, Lankin VZ, Vikhert AM (1989) Bull Exp Biol Med 107:93–95

Address for correspondence:
Prof. O. EL-Ahmady
Tumor Marker Oncology Research Center
Al-Azhar University
2 Roshdy Street, Safeer Square
ET-Heliopolis, Cairo, Egypt

Immediate adjuvant hormonal therapy and radiotherapy following radical prostatectomy for stage D1 adenocarcinoma of the prostate

T. Wiegel[a], M. Baumann[a], M. Bressel[b], H. Arps[c]

[a] Department of Radiotherapy, University Hospital Hamburg-Eppendorf, [b] Department of Urology, General Hospital Hamburg-Harburg, [c] Institute of Pathology, General Hospital Fulda, Germany

Introduction

Although for most urologists radical prostatectomy is the treatment of choice for patients with localized adenocarcinoma of the prostate, there is a greater controversy for patients with stage D1 (lymph node metastases) tumors (6, 10).
Treatment options include observation, hormonal therapy, radical surgery with or without adjuvant irradiation and irradiation with or without hormonal therapy (6, 8, 10, 12). Adjuvant radiotherapy aims to reduce local recurrence, as it is stated that patients with local recurrence following radical prostatectomy have a worse prognosis, which leads to death (11). As pelvic lymph node dissection (PLND) aims to reduce lymph node metastases to a microscopic residual tumor, radiotherapy of the pelvic lymphatics has a curative intent. We investigated the outcome of 30 patients treated with adjuvant radiotherapy following radical prostatectomy and hormonal treatment at the Department of Radiotherapy at the University Hospital Hamburg-Eppendorf.

Material and methods

Patients

From 1975 to 1991 83 patients with pathological stage D1 adenocarcinoma of the prostate (evidence of pelvic lymph node metastases) with a mean age of 64.6 years (range: 52-78 years) underwent radiotherapy with curative intent at the University Hospital Hamburg-Eppendorf. Thirty of these 82 patients had a radical prostatectomy and received radiotherapy as adjuvant treatment. After examining the number of involved lymph nodes, seven patients had one microscopically positive node. The remaining 23 patients had one or more gross positive nodes. In detail, six patients had one macroscopically positive node, six patients had two nodes and eleven patients had more than two positive nodes. The grading was done based on the recommendations of the German grade of malignancy (4). All 30 patients exhibited moderate or poor tumor differentiation. Date of evaluation was 6/1991. Table I gives detailed information concerning patient characteristics.

Table I. Patient characteristics.

No. of patients (total 82 with stage D1)	30
Mean age	5.1
Median follow-up (months)	53.4
German grade of malignancy	
Ia–IIa	–
IIb–IIIb	30
Pathological stage (UICC 1987)	
pT2	2
pT3	26
pT4	2
Number of positive lymph nodes	
1 (microscopic)	7
1	6
2	6
> 2	11

Urological treatment

All patients underwent radical retropubic prostatectomy as was previously described (2). In all cases, a staging lymphadenectomy was performed, which was comprised of bilateral samples from four lymphatic vessel areas (arteria iliaca communis, a. iliaca interna, a. iliaca externa and fossa obturatoria). Urological treatment was carried out in all cases with an orchiectomy in addition to medication with Androcur.

Radiotherapy

Patients were either treated with 42 MV photons from a betatron, 16 MV photons from a linear accelerator or with Co60 (1/30) in a previous treatment. Five patients underwent a boost with 14 MV fast neutrons. Radiation therapy was initiated, usually two or three months after the operation, in order to allow sphincter function to consolidate.

The pelvic field area included the prostate, periprostatic tissue and pelvic lymph nodes up to the promontorium. All fields were subjected to daily treatment. The pelvic lymphatics were usually treated with a four field-box (AP/PA and lateral) to deliver 4,000–5,000 cGy (median: 4,000 cGy). In 25 patients, this was followed by a boost of 1,000 to 2,500 cGy with photons through reduced fields to complete 6,000-7,000 cGy (median: 6,500 cGy) to the prostate or the prostatic bed. In five patients, this boost was carried out using 14 MV fast neutrons to deliver 400-600 cGy. Boost treatment was done usually by a four field-box technique (AP/PA and lateral) or with 120° bilateral arcs. Daily dose consisted of 200 cGy for the pelvic portals and reduced fields of five fractions per week for the prostatic bed.

Follow-up

Continued observation of all patients varied from 3 to 183 months after radiotherapy (median: 53.4 months). The follow-up examinations routinely included complete history, physical examination including rectal palpation, chest x-ray, an annual bone scintigraphy, serological determination of prostatic acid phosphatase and prostate-specific antigen levels (PSA). PSA determination has only been part of the follow-up since 1987. These investigations were done earlier in cases where pathological findings or subjective complaints occured. A verifying histological investigation was performed if, after rectal palpation, a local recurrence was suspected. Tumor progress was implicated by the continuous increase in PSA levels over a period of six months, although no signs of local relapse or metastases occured.

Statistical analysis

For all patients, survivals from the beginning of radiotherapy to death regardless of course or detection of any progression (local and systemic), were estimated by the Kaplan-Meier method (5). Patients, who did not die from prostatic carcinoma were handled as censored observation. Differences were considered significant, when p-values of less than 0.05 were obtained.

Results

Overall survival

With a median follow-up of 53.4 months, six out of 30 patients (20%) died. Prostate cancer was the cause of death for three patients (10%). The 5- and 10-year-survival occured in 95% and 53% of the patients, respectively (figure 1). No significant differences were seen in patients treated with fast neutrons or photons.

Disease free survival (DFS)

Four out of thirty patients (15%) developed metastases. One patient developed a local recurrence along with bone metastases. The median time to progression was 23 months after the initiation of treatment. The 5- and 10-year-DFS was 78% in both cases (figure 1). No significant differences were found between patients who were treated with fast neutrons and those treated with photons.

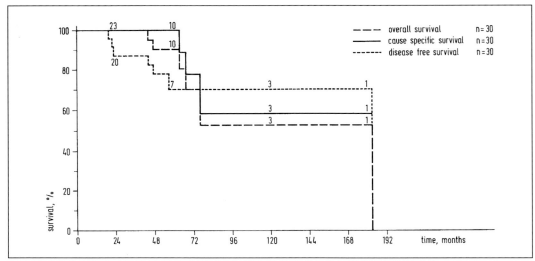

Figure 1. Overall survival, cause specific survival and disease free survival of all treated patients.

Local control

Local control was exhibited in 96% of the patients for 3 years and in 88% for both five and ten years. One local recurrence appeared 28 months after beginning treatment. Another recurrence developed in a patient after 57 months.

Side effects

A mild proctitis or cystitis (grade 1/2 RTOG) appeared in a total of 13 patients. Major complications occurred in four patients: two patients had a severe proctitis which made a colostomy necessary and a severe cystitis (grade 3 RTOG) was observed in two other patients. All major complications were seen in patients who had received a total dose of 70 Gy.

Discussion

Many investigators have demonstrated an increase of local control in patients with adjuvant radiotherapy following radical prostatectomy with extent of tumor beyond the prostatic gland (pathological stage C) (3, 8, 10). Because there are no results of randomized trials available, only a few investigators were able to demonstrate a beneficial effect on survival and disease free survival (8).

Only two of our patients had pathological stage pT2 tumors (tumor confined to the gland). Twenty-six patients had pT3 and two patients had pT4 tumors. With a median follow-up period of 53.4 months, two patients (7%) developed a local recurrence. These findings are comparable with the results from other investigations, where the incidence of recurrence ranged from 0–10% (3, 10).

The effect of radiotherapy in stage D1 prostate cancer remains uncertain. Some authors report long term survivors with definitive radiotherapy with an overall survival for 5 and 10 years occurring in 76% and 33%, respectively (6). In our patients who had received the combined treatment, the overall survival for 5 and 10 years was 95% and 33%, respectively. In the work done by Morgan in the Mayo Clinic, 85 out of 93 patients with stage D1 disease underwent an adjuvant treatment, which was hormonal in most cases. The 5-year overall survival was 78%, 10 year survival was not noted (7).

At this time, it is not exactly clear how much influence the extent of nodal disease has on the prognosis. Some authors found a better prognosis for patients, when one microscopically or gross lymph node was involved (1, 11, 12). In these investigations, seven patients had one microscopically positive node and six patients had one gross positive node, which comprised 41% of the patients. In 37% of the Mayo-Clinic patients, on the other hand, one positive node appeared (7). In another report of this clinic, 266 patients with stage D1 carcinoma showed a survival rate of 84% (±3%) and 62% (±5%) for 5 and 10 years, respectively (11).

Reported side effects of definitive and adjuvant radiotherapy have varied from insignificant to severe permanent disabilities. Following definitive radio-therapy, severe side effects (grade 3 and 4 RTOG) occur in up to 5% (1, 6). In the case of adjuvant irradiation, some investigators have demonstrated increased rates of side effects (3, 10). In four out of 30 patients severe complications occured. These included two cases of grade 3 for the bladder and in two cases of grade four for the rectum, which made a colostomy necessary. All four patients underwent adjuvant irradiation with a total dose of 70 Gy. On account of good results, but at the same time considering the high grade of toxicity, adjuvant radiotherapy was limited to 62 Gy (10).

In conclusion, the results support a combined treatment in patients with stage D1 adenocarcinoma of the prostate, but it was noted that an increase in the rate of severe side effects occured, which also has been found by other investigators (3). Therefore, the total dose to the prostate for adjuvant irradiation was reduced to 62 Gy, as severe side effects occured only in patients who had received 70 Gy to the prostate area. For the pelvic lymphatics we apply 50 Gy, as this is necessary for patients with microscopic metastatic disease. Although it is impossible to differentiate between the effect of hormonal therapy and radiotherapy, these results are to be considered hopeful, but further investigations in the form of randomized trials are required in the future.

References

1. Anscher MS, Prosnitz LR (1992) Prognostic significance of extent of nodal involvement in stage D1 prostate cancer treated with radiotherapy. Urol 39:39–43
2. Bressel M (1990) Radical prostatectomy-indication, surgical technique, results. Akt Urol Supl I:115–119
3. Gibbons RP et al (1986) Adjuvant radiotherapy following radical prostatectomy: results and complications. J Urol 135:135–142
4. Helpap B, Böcking A, Dohm G, Faul P, Kastendieck H, Leistenschneider W, Müller HA (1985) Klassifikation, histologisches und zytologisches Grading sowie Regressionsgrading des Prostatakarzinoms. Pathologe 6:3–7
5. Kaplan EL, Meier P (1958) Nonparametric estimation from incomplete observations. J Amer Stat Ass 53:457–462
6. Lawton CA, Cox JD, Glisch C, Murray KJ, Byhardt RW, Wilson JF (1992) Is long-term survival possible with external beam irradiation for stage D1 adenocarcinoma of the prostate? Cancer 69:2761–2766
7. Morgan WR, Bergstrahl EJ, Zincke H (1993) Long-term evaluation of radical prostatectomy as treatment for clinical stage C (T3) prostate cancer. Urol 41:116–120
8. Stein A, de Kernion JB, Dorey F, Smith RB (1992) Adjuvant radiotherapy in patients post-radical prostatectomy with tumor extending through capsule or positive seminal vesicles. Urol 39:59–63
9. Wiegel T, Bressel M, Arps H, Hübener KH (1992) Radiotherapy of local recurrence following radical prostatectomy. Strahlenther Oncol 168:351–355
10. Wiegel T, Bressel M, Baumann M, Schwarz R, Hübener KH (1993) Adjuvant radiotherapy following radical prostatectomy – acute and late toxicity. Strahlenther Oncol 169:152–158
11. Zincke H (1989) Extended experience with surgical treatment of stage D1 adenocarcinoma of prostate. Suppl Urol 33:27–35
12. Zincke H (1990) Combined surgery and immediate adjuvant hormonell treatment for stage D1 adenocarcinoma of the prostate: Mayo Clinic experience. Semin Urol 8:175–183

Address for correspondence:
Dr. med. T. Wiegel
Abteilung für Radiotherapie
Universitätsklinikum Benjamin Franklin
Hindenburgdamm 30
D-12200 Berlin, Germany

Three-dimensional treatment planning for radiotherapy of prostate cancer: Technique und acute toxicity

T. Wiegel[a], R. Schmidt[a], P. Steiner[b], H. Arps[c], B. Göckel-Beining[d]

[a]Department of Radiotherapy, [b]Department of Diagnostic Radiology, University Hospital Hamburg-Eppendorf, [c]Institute of Pathology, General Hospital Fulda, [d]Department of Surgery, St. Rochus-Hospital, Steinheim, Germany

Introduction

Treatment options for stage A-C prostate cancer include radical prostatectomy and definitive radiotherapy, both with or without hormonal manipulation with nearly equivalent results (1, 3, 13). Radical prostatectomy is the therapy of choice for most urologists, but there is no proven advantage in survival compared with definitive radiotherapy for stage A–C (3). The problem of radiotherapy is the rate of late side effects for doses greater than 65 Gy as normally used for stage C prostate cancer. Between 65 and 70 Gy, the rate of severe late side effects increases strongly (5).

The 3-dimensional treatment planning offers the possibilty of a reduction of acute and late normal tissue damage. Using the "beams eye view" and irregulary shaped fields it is possible to reduce the treated volume and the dose of the organs at risk, in case of prostate cancer the bladder and the rectum (2, 8, 11, 12).

Based on a prospective, non-randomized clinical trial we demonstrate the technique and acute toxicity of 26 patients, who were treated using 3-dimensional treatment planning for prostate cancer between 1991 and 1993 at the Department of Radiotherapy, University Hospital Hamburg-Eppendorf.

Material and methods

Patients

From 6/91 to 11/92 26 patients with adenocarcinoma of the prostate underwent 3-dimensional planned radiotherapy with curative intent (for detailed information see table I). In 12 cases only a PE was performed, in seven patients a radical prostatectomy, in three patients a TURP and four patients had a local recurrence following radical prostatectomy. 15 out of 26 patients also had an additional hormonal treatment.

Staging

Staging was done according to the American Joint Cancer Comittee classification and the UICC

Table I. Caracteristics (number) of patients and tumor diseases.

Median age	64
Range	56–84
Karnofski stage 100	26
Stage	
adjuvant radiotherapy	7
pT2 pN0 - R1	1
pT3 pN0	6
stage B2	2
stage C	5
macroscopical tumor	19
T2 N0	4
T3 N0	7
T4 N0	1
T3/4 Nx M1	3
local recurrence following rad. prostatectomy	4
stage B2	4
stage C	8
stage D2	3
German grade of malignancy	
GIa-IIa	11
GIIb-IIIb	15

staging system (1987). Grading was done based on the recommandations of the German grade of malignancy (4).

Radiotherapy

For all patients a three-dimensional treatment-planning was performed using irregular coplanar fields. 17 patients had an irradiation of the prostate and the seminal vesicles including a security margin of 15 mm as previously published (12). Using a 4-field-box technique (figure 2) or 5 fixed fields (figure 1) a total dose of 62 Gy or 70 Gy with a single dose of 2 Gy was given. Nine out of 26 patients had also an irradiation of the pelvic lymphatics up to a total of 50 Gy using a 3-dimensional planned 4-field-box technique (for detailed information see table II).

Table II. Overview of all treatment groups, single dose 2.0 Gy.

No. of patients	Pelvic lymphatics	Prostate
3	–	62 Gy
14	–	70 Gy
4	50 Gy	62 Gy
5	50 Gy	70 Gy
Total 26		

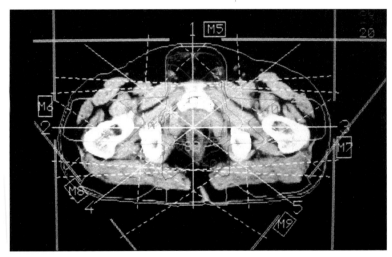

Figure 1. 3-Dimensional treatment plan with 5 fixed fields.

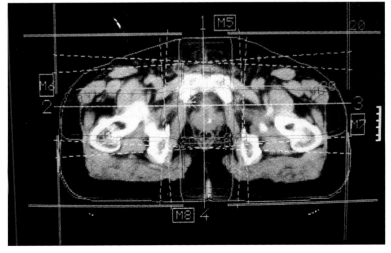

Figure 2. 3-Dimensional treatment plan with 4 fixed fields (4-field-box).

Acute toxicity

Classification of acute side effects was done using the RTOG-score for acute side effects (grade I/II milde, grade III/IV severe). Patients were seen weekly at the time of treatment and later on every 12 weeks. Side effects were scored for rectum, urinary bladder and the skin. The follow-up examinations routinely included complete history, physical examination including rectal palpation, chest x-ray, an annual bone scintigraphy, serological determination of prostatic acid phosphatase and prostate-specific antigen levels (PSA).

Results

All together 17 out of 26 patients (65%) developed one or more acute side effects. 11 out of 26 patients (44%) (i.e. 9 grade I and two grade II) showed side effects for the skin. Six patients (22%) had only grade I toxicity for the urinary bladder whereas eight out of 26 patients (30%) (i.e. seven grade I and one grade II) had these for the rectum. One patient had a mild proctitis and stopped therapy for personal reasons at 36 Gy. In all cases the side effects disappeared within six weeks after the end of treatment.

Discussion

There are two different ways using 3-dimensional treatment planning in general. On the one hand 3-dimensional treatment planning demonstrates a chance to decrease side effects (6). On the other hand it seems possible to raise up the dosage without higher rates of normal tissue damage (7). Several investigators calculated, that 3-dimensional planning for radiotherapy of prostate cancer can reduce the involved volume of the rectum for about 14% and 19% (range: 9.5–36%) and for about 14% and 28% (range: 9–46%) for the urinary bladder (9, 12). For this reason different clinical trials were opened to investigate this possible advantage of 3-d planning in decreasing the acute and late side effects (7, 10). *Soffen* reported results of a prospective non-randomized trial. 26 patients underwent a conformal, 3-d planned radiotherapy of the prostate up to 68 Gy (range: 64-68 Gy). The acute side effects were compared to a group of 20 2-d planned patients with equivalent doses and treated volumes. The rate of patients with an interruption of radiotherapy or higher grade of acute side effects was significantly higher for 2-d treated patients (9).

These findings are similar to ours. 65% of our patients had grade I of acute toxicity with a dose of 62 Gy or 70 Gy. Only three out of 26 patients had grade II RTOG side effects.

Sandler et al. demonstrated the first results of 20 patients with stage C prostate cancer using a 3-dimensional planned dose escaltion. Irradiation field included the prostate, the seminal vesicles, the locoregional lymphatics and a surrounding margin of 2 cm. This volume was irradiated up to 44–50 Gy and then reduced fields for the primary up to 74–80 Gy. With a median follow-up of 19 months three patients had grade I or II side effects for the rectum (rectal bleeding). Side effects for the bladder were not seen (7). Taking the short follow-up into consideration, this rate of side effects is extremly low.

In summary we conclude, that 3-dimensional treatment planning for radiotherapy of prostate cancer is practicable and the rate of acute side effects seems to be the same or smaller than for 2-dimensional planned therapy. More important, it seems to be a hopeful way reducing late side effects especially for the rectum and the bladder. On the other hand it seems possible to raise up the dosage aiming higher local control rates for patients with stage C without higher rates of long term side effects as demonstrated by *Sandler*.

References

1. Bressel M (1990) Radical prostatectomy-indication surgical technique, results. Akt Urol Supl I:115– 119
2. Gademann N, Schlegel W, Buerkelbach J, Laier C, Behrens S, Brieger S, Wannenmacher M (1993) Dreidimensionale Bestrahlungsplanung. Untersuchungen zur klinischen Integration. Strahlenther Onkol 169:159–167
3. Hanks GE (1988) Radical prostatectomy or radiation therapy for early prostate cancer: two roads to the same end. Cancer 61:2153–2160
4. Helpap B, Böcking A, Dohm G, Faul P, Kastendieck H, Leistenschneider W, Müller HA (1985) Klassifikation, histologisches und zytologisches Grading sowie Regressionsgrading des Prostatakarzinoms. Pathologe 6:3–7

5 Lawton CA, Won M, Pilepich MV, Asbell SO, Shipley WU, Hanks GE, Cox JD, Perez CA (1991) Long term treatment sequelae following external beam irradiation for adenocarcinoma of the prostate: analysis of RTOG studies 75-06 and 77-06. Int J Radiat Oncol Biol Phys 21:935–939

6 Low N, Vijayakumar S, Rosenberg I, Rubin S, Virudachalam R, Spelbring D, ChenGT (1990) Beams eye view based prostate treatment planning: is it useful? Int J Radiat. Oncol Biol Phys 19:759–768

7 Sandler HM, Perez-Tamayo C, Ten Haken RK, Lichter AS (1992) Dose escalation for stage C (T3) prostate cancer: minimal rectal toxicity observed using conformal therapy. Radiother Oncol 23:53–54

8 Schmidt R, Schiemann T, Riemer M, Höhne KH, Hübener KH (1992) 3-D visualization of photon treatment plans. Z Med Phys 2:158–164

9 Soffen EM, Hanks GE, Hwang CC, Chu JC (1991) Conformal static field therapy for low volume low grade prostate cancer with rigid immobilization. Int J Radiat Oncol Biol Phys 20:141–146

10 Soffen EM, Hanks GE, Hunt MA, Epstein BE (1992) Conformal static field radiation therapy treatment of early prostate cancer versus non-conformal techniques: a reduction in acute morbidity. Int J Radiat Oncol Biol Phys 24:485–488

11 Ten Haken RK, Perez-Tamayo C, Tesser RJ, McShan DL, Fraass BA, Lichter AS (1989) Boost treatment of the prostate using shaped fixed fields. Int J Radiat Oncol Biol Phys 16:193–200

12 Wiegel T, Schmidt R, Krüll A, Schwarz R, Sommer K, Hübener KH (1992) Advantage of three-dimensional treatment planning for localized radiotherapy of early stage prostatic cancer. Strahlenther Onkol 168:692–697

13 Wiegel T, Schmidt R, Baumann M, Schwarz R, Huebener KH (1993) Adjuvant radiation therapy following radical prostatectomy. Strahlenther Oncol 169:152–158

Address for correspondence:
Dr. med. T. Wiegel
Universitätsklinikum Benjamin Franklin
Abteilung Strahlentherapie
Hindenburgdamm 30
D-12200 Berlin, Germany

Para-aortic radiation treatment in FIGO stage III ovarian carcinomas – A sensible complementary approach in connection with cytotoxic drugs?

U. M. Carl[a], J. Bahnsen[a], G. Fröschle[b], T. Wiegel[c]

University Hospital Hamburg-Eppendorf; Hamburg, Germany
[a]Department of Gynecological Radiology, [b]Department of General Surgery,
[c]Department of Radiation Therapy, University of Düsseldorf, Germany

Introduction

In general the outcome of treatment in gynecological cancers can be improved considerably when the target of second order is treated initially together with the target of first order (figure 1) (3, 4). Once metastases become clinically apparent the amount of needed radiation dose will exceed the threshold of high toxicity. Thus para-aortic metastases govern the prognosis. It has been demonstrated by many authors, that already early stages of gynecological cancers can have a high rate of para-aortic nodal involvement (table I). Apart from peritoneal spread early para-aortic involvement is a major problem of FIGO stage III ovarian cancers. In former times the radiotherapeutic approach consisted mainly of an open beam irradiation (6) or a whole abdominal irradiation (13, 20) basically not exceeding the total dose of 25–30 Gy. This dose cannot be understood to be sufficient in order to sterilize a considerable rate of tumors nor can it treat macroscopically involved para-aortic lymph nodes sufficiently. But higher doses in such large treated volumes were linked to an increased rate of side effects especially in patients who had first been operated on (9, 15, 18).

With the application of intraperitoneal (IP) chemotherapy treatment results of advanced ovarian cancers have been improved considerably within the last decade. Speyer et al. (17) found the best results of IP carboplatin in patients with microscopical disease. Obviously the combination with other treatment modalities such as radiotherapy might further improve the outcome (19). In patients with macroscopical para-aortic lymph node involvement the low toxicity rate of platin containing treatment schedules permits and urges an additional treatment, such as radiotherapy. Most of the radiation techniques for treating the para-aortics have been demonstrated to be linked with a number of problems (3). The biaxial-four-

Table I. Many authors that have found gynecological tumors turn to show an early spread to the para-aortic lymph nodes

Author	Stage						
	Ib	IIa	IIb	IIIa	IIIb	IVa	IVb
Ballon (1981)	23.0	19.0	19.0	–	17.0	–	–
Berman (1984)	5.0	12.0	16.7	33.3	24.9	12.5	100
Chen[a] (1983)	18.2	20.0		41.9		66.7	
Fletcher (1972)	3.3	10.3	20.0	17.4	8.0	–	–
Hughes (1980)	4.3	8.5	24.4	20.0	24.4	50.0	28.5
Lagasse (1980)	5.6	18.2	32.8	–	31.1	33.3	–
Podczaski (1990)	8/10	3/3	9/12	–	8/11	–	–
Carl (1992)	28.0	10.0		67.6		60.0	

[a]Ovarian carcinomas

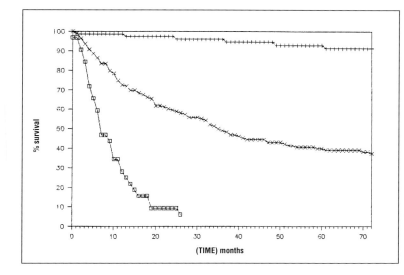

Figure 1. Crude survival of patients (n = 173) with gynecological cancers. Either para-aortic irradiation was part of the initial treatment (x) when lymph node involvement was proven lymphographically (n = 141) or when recurring para-aortic disease became clinically apparent (n = 32, □). The results of the latter were poor. For comparison survival data of age-matched healthy women were plotted (+).

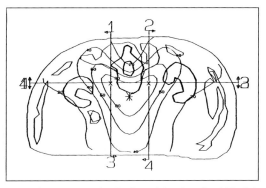

Figure 2. The dose distribution of the described biaxial-foursegmental-rotating-field-technique on a cobalt-unit as described elsewhere (3, 8). The dose to the maximum was 50 Gy, not exceeding 20 Gy in the kidneys.

segmental-rotating-field-technique has been described to be a valid method. A small rate of side effects was seen while the survival probability was improved (3) for cervical cancers. The presented retrospective analysis is concerned with results after FIGO stage III ovarian cancers.

Patients and methods

From 1965 to 1986 33 patients with ovarian carcinomas received a radiation treatment of the primary side as well as a consecutive para-aortic irradiation in the Department of Gynecologic Radiology, University Hospital, Hamburg. 13 patients presented with FIGO stage III tumors. Fractionated radiotherapy with total doses of 50 to 60 Gy to the small pelvis and up to a maximum dose (100%) of 50 Gy to the para-aortic lymph nodes were administered. Irradiation was performed using a biaxial-foursegmental-rotating-field-technique on a cobalt-unit as described elsewhere (3, 8). The dose distribution is shown in figure 2. Kaplan-Meyer analysis (11) has been applied to all data. Data have then been compared to the FIGO Annual Report (14).

Results

Figure 3 shows the survival data of patients (n = 13) with ovarian carcinomas Figo stage III who received a para-aortic radiation treatment. The 5-year survival rate of 38% is better than described in the Annual Report (14). The results are poor in eight patients in any initial stage but with clinical recurring para-aortic disease. So far 173 patients with various gynecological cancers were treated using the described RT-method. Only three cases of ureter stenosis and two cases of small bowel complications were documented.

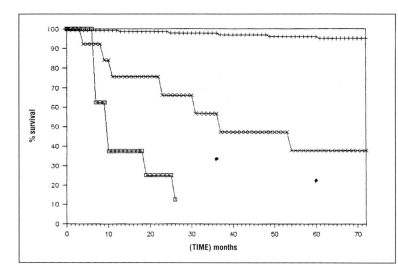

Figure 3. In ovarian carcinomas FIGO stage III initial radiotherapy of the para-aortic region improves survival considerably even in 13 patients with lymphographically proven involvement of the para-aortic lymph nodes (x). 3- and 5-year survival rates taken from the 21. Annual Report (14) (♦) are below our own data. The prognosis of clinically para-aortic recurring disease is poor (□). For comparison survival data of matched healthy women were plotted (+).

Discussion

The 5-year survival rate in FIGO stage III ovarian carcinomas has been improved considerably within the last decade while it has remained relatively constant for stages I and II. Due to extensive disease in stage IV the 5-year survival rate has always been poor (14). By radiation treatment of the primary site as well as the para-aortic lymph nodes the presented results appear to be promising, but those are based on small patient numbers. Despite of that alterations in the treatment modalities have constantly improved the therapeutic outcome for FIGO stage III ovarian carcinomas. The major success might be due to cytotoxic drugs (13, 17). Still, a sole chemotherapy cannot cope with residual tumors (> 2 cm). The adjuvant radiation method we offer is limited to the para-aortics. We found an acceptable rate of side-effects (3). Therefore we would like to suggest, that the described method could be a sensible adjuvant approach in order to overcome the problem of macroscopic (residual) para-aortic disease. Any clinical trial should also include the role of radiotherapy.

References

1 Ballon SC, Berman ML, Lagasse LD, Petrilli ES, Castalado TW (1981) Survival after extraperitoneal pelvic and para-aortic lymphadenectomy and radiation therapy in cervical carcinoma. Obstet Gynaecol 57:90–95
2 Berman ML, Keys H, Creasman W, DiSaia P, Bundy B, Blessing J (1984) Survival and patterns of recurrence in cervical cancer metastatic to periaortic lymph nodes. Gynaecol Oncol 19:8–16
3 Carl UM, Bahnsen J, Rapp W, (1992) Radiation therapy of para-aortic lymph nodes in gynecologic cancers: techniques, results and complications. Strahlenther Onkol 168:383–389
4 Carl UM, Bahnsen J, Wiegel Th (1993) Radiation-therapy of para-aortic lymph nodes in cancer of the uterine cervix. Acta Oncologica 32:63–67
5 Chen SS, Lee L (1983) Incidence of para-aortic and pelvic lymph node metastases in epithelial carcinoma of the ovary. Gynaecol Oncol 16:95–100
6 Delclos L, Dembo AJ (1980) Ovaries. In: Fletcher GH (ed) Textbook of Radiotherapy. Lea and Febinger, Philadelphia, 3rd ed, pp 834–851
7 Fletcher GH, Rutledge FN (1972) Extended field technique in the management of the cancers of the uterine cervix. Am J Radiol 114:116–122
8 Frischbier HJ, Karl B (1970) Zur Telekobalt-bestrahlung der aortalen Lymphknoten. Strahlentherapie 140:32–36
9 Hamberger, AD and Fletcher, GH (1982) Is surgical evaluation of the para-aortic nodes prior to irradiation of benefit in carcinoma of the cervix? Int J Radiat Oncol Biol Phys 8:151–153
10 Hughes RR, Brewington KC, Hanjani P, Photopulos G, Dick D, Votava C, Noran M, Coleman S (1980) Extended field irradiation for cervical cancer based on surgical staging. Gynaecol Oncol 9:153-158

11. Kaplan EL, Meier P (1958) Nonparametric estimation from incomplete observations. J Am Stat Assoc 53:457–481
12. Lagasse LD, Creasmen WT, Shingleton HM, Ford JH, Blessing JA (1980) Results and complications of operative staging in cervical cancer: experience of the Gynecologic Oncology Group. Gynaecol Oncol 9:90–98
13. Lindner H, Willich H, Atzinger A (1990) Primary adjuvant whole abdominal irradiation in ovarian carcinoma. Int J Radiat Oncol Biol Phys 19:13–18
14. Pettersson F (ed) (1991) 20 Annual Report on the results of treatment in gynecological cancer. 21. Volume. Statements of results obtained in patients treated in 1982 to 1990, inclusive 3- and 5-year survival up to 1990. Int J Gynaecol Obstet 36
15. Piver MS, JJ Barlow (1973) Para-aortic lymphadenectomy, aortic node biopsy, and aortic lymphangiography in staging patients with advanced cervical cancer. Cancer 32:367–370
16. Podczaski E, Stryker JA, Kaminski P, Ndubisi B, Larson J, DeGeest K, Sorosky J, Mortel R (1990) Extended-field therapy for carcinoma of the cervix. Cancer 66:251–258
17. Speyer JL, Beller U, Colombo N, Sorich J, Wernz JC, Hochster H, Green M, Porges R, Muggia FM, Canetta R, Beckmann M (1990) Intraperitoneal carboplatin favorable results in women with minimal residual ovarian cancer after cisplatin therapy. J Clin Onc 8:1335–1341
18. Tewfik HH, Buchsbaum HJ, Latourette HB, Lifshitz SG, Tewfik FA (1982) Para-aortic lymph node irradiation in carcinoma of the cervix after exploratory laparatomy and biopsy-proven positive aortic nodes. Int J Radiat Oncol Biol Phys 8:13–18
19. Wang CC, Nelson JH, Shimm DS (1988) In: Wang, CC (ed) Clinical radiation oncology. PSG Publishing Company, Littleton, Massachusetts, pp 317–320
20. Wang CC (1988) In: Wang CC (ed) Clinical radiation oncology. PSG Publishing Company, Littleton, Massachusetts, pp 440–444

Address for correspondence:
Dr. med. U. M. Carl
Klinik für Strahlentherapie
Universität Düsseldorf
Moorenstraße 5
D-40225 Düsseldorf, Germany

Local tumor control in patients with advanced stages of squamous cell carcinomas of the oral cavity: Interstitial brachytherapy with iridium-192

R. E. Friedrich[a], A. Krüll[b], D. Hellner[a], K. Plambeck[a], R. Schwarz[b]

[a]Department of Oral and Maxillofacial Surgery, [b]Department of Radiotherapy, Eppendorf University Hospital, University of Hamburg, Germany

Introduction

In the treatment of oral squamous cell carcinomas (OSCC) ablative surgery and additionally a percutaneous irradiation are used (2, 3, 4, 5). Despite curative intended therapy, however, in some patients local recurrences are occuring in already irradiated areas. In these cases an additional percutaneous irradiation often is limited or not applicable. Due to an easy access a local brachytherapy (interstitial afterloading technique) can be applied in tumors of the oral cavity (1, 6).

Material and methods

Over a period of four years 34 patients with OSCC were treated by an interstitial high dose rate afterloading therapy.
Equipment: Gammamed 12i, Sauerwein, Germany; source: iridium-192; half time: 74.2 days; initial radioactivity: 10 Curie.
Application: 1 to 3 fractions, interval = 7 days, 10 to 30 Gy (n = 20 (20 Gy), 8 (30 Gy), 5 (10 Gy), 1 (15 Gy)). In patients with a primary OSCC an additional brachytherapy was applied only in cases with a residual malignant tumor intended for curative ablative surgery.
Handling: translucent plastic cannulas with a trocar were used.
Patients (females: males = 15:19, age: 38–89 (mean: 62) years) with an advanced stage of their disease at the time of the first diagnosis were treated (n = 3 (T_1), 9 (T_2), 6 (T_3), 16 (T_4), 5 (N_0), 11 (N_1), 15 (N_2), 2 (N_3), 1 (N_X), 32 (M_0), 2 (M_X). 22 of 30 patients were already percutaneously irradiated (60.0–75.6 Gy) and in seven patients only ablative surgery had been performed. The indications for brachytherapy are summarized in table I. The effects of brachytherapy were estimated clinically and morphologically.

Results

A complete remission of the tumor was found in 11 (32%) patients. The devitalization of the OSCC was proven by morphological investigations in ten cases. A partial remission was found in 16 patients (47%), a "no change" in two (5.8%) and a progress of the tumor growth despite brachytherapy in five (14%).
Concerning follow-up in 23 of 34 patients an ablative surgery was carried out. In these cases the results of follow-up are based on radiotherapeutical and surgical treatments. The total rate of local tumor control after six months is 58% decreasing to 44% after one year (figure 1). Ten patients are still alive without recurrences of an OSCC (29.4%) and three are alive with recurrences. Due to the malignant diasease 14 patients

Table I. Indications for high-dose rate afterloading therapy of 34 patients with oral squamous cell carcinomas (OSCC).

Residual tumor after percutaneous irradiation	14
Residual tumor after surgery	1
Progress of tumor growth during irradiation	5
Progress after surgery and percut. irradiation	1
Recurrence after surgery and percut. irradiation	4
Recurrence after irradiation	3
Palliative intended (reduced general conditions)	4
Second OSCC after surgery and percut. irradiation	2

died (41.2%) and five died intercurrently (one with a known recurrence). One patient deceased with an unknown cause of death and one was lost for follow-up. The total survival rate of the patients is 82% after six months and 53% after one year (figure 2).

Discussion

Due to the available equipment a high-dose-rate afterloading technique and an iridium-192 source is used in weekly fractions.

Calculating the benefits of the technique in patients with OSCC best results are achieved in cases with a complete remission. Eight of eleven patients are still alive without a detectable tumor, three deceased intercurrently. It is remarkable that we could correlate the clinical impression of a shrinking ulcer to the lack of morphological signs of vital tumor cells in a lot of cases.

Summarizing our experiences, interstitial brachytherapy can be applied as a local tumor boost after percutaneous irradiation in patients with local recurrences of an OSCC and in patients with a second malignant tumor of the head and neck

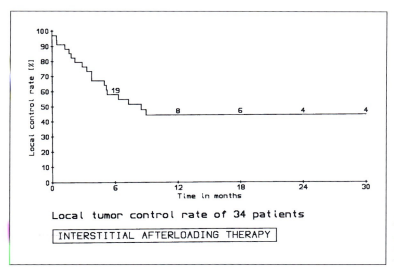

Figure 1. Local tumor control in patients with OSCC treated by high-dose rate afterloading therapy and surgery.

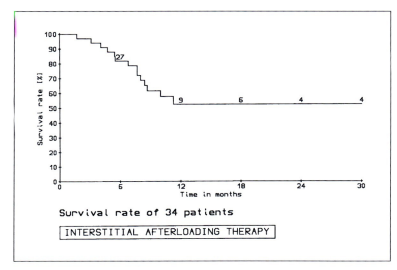

Figure 2. Survival rate in patients with OSCC treated by high-dose rate afterloading therapy and surgery.

region which already had been irradiated. Patients with large tumors and an advanced stage of their disease will gain some benefit by this treatment but any effect regarding their survival time is doubtful. A partial remission can be achieved improving the patient's quality of life for a limited period of time in many cases.

References

1. Declos L (1984) Interstitial irradiation techniques. In: Levitt SH, Tapley N du V (eds) Technological basis of radiation therapy. Practical clinical applications. Lea, Febiger, Philadelphia, pp 55–84
2. Freeman SB, Hamaker RC, Singer MI, Pugh P, Garrett P (1990) Intraoperative radiotherapy of head and neck cancer. Arch Otolaryngol Head Neck Surg 116:165–168
3. Frommhold W, Hübener KH (1986) Computertomographie in der Strahlentherapie. Thieme, Stuttgart
4. Gundlach KKH, Schmelzle R, Hübener KH (1992) Hat die praeoperative Bestrahlung des Mundhöhlenkarzinoms Vorteile gebracht? In: Schwenzer N (Hrsg) Therapie des Mundhöhlenkarzinoms. Fortschr Kiefer- Gesichts-Chir 37:21–22
5. Nilles A, Stoll P, Frommhold DH, Schilli W (1993) Intraoperative Radiotherapie (IORT) bei Kopf-Hals-Tumoren. Dtsch Z Mund Kiefer Gesichts Chir 17:28–31
6. Vaeth JM (1978) Renaissance of interstitial brachytherapy. Frontiers of radiation therapy andoncoloy. Vol 12, Karger, Basel

Address for correspondence:
Dr. med. Dr. med. dent. R. E. Friedrich
Klinik für Mund-, Kiefer- und Gesichtschirurgie
Universitätskrankenhaus Eppendorf
Martinistraße 52
D-20246 Hamburg, Germany

A caseous-tuberculoid reaction in lymph node metastases following radiochemotherapy of undifferentiated nasopharyngeal carcinoma

R. E. Friedrich[a], K. Donath[b], D. Hellner[a]

[a]Department of Oral and Maxillofacial Surgery, [b]Department of Oral Pathology, Eppendorf University Hospital, University of Hamburg, Germany

Introduction

Undifferentiated nasopharyngeal carcinomas (UCNT) are highly proliferative carcinomas not endemic in Western Europe. The first clinical manifestations often are tumors of the neck indicating an advanced stage of the neoplastic disease (6). UCNT are radiosensitive (2, 8) and sensitive to chemotherapeutics (3). The residual findings in lymph nodes after radiochemotherapy of resection specimens, e.g. lymph nodes of the neck, might be difficult to estimate (6).

Case report

A 14 years old boy of White Russia was referred to the department of oral and maxillofacial surgery for resection of tumor recurrence in a histologically proven UCNT (figure 1). First symptoms of the disease (swelling of the left side of neck) occurred a few weeks before diagnosis. Poor clinical data of the patient were available: 5 1/2 months before two cycles of chemotherapy were applied (1. cycle: 10 mg vinblastin, 3800 mg cyclophosphamid, 270 mg prednisolon for a week; 2. cycle 10 mg rosevin, 3600 mg cyclophosphamid, 345 mg prednisolon (three weeks later) leading to an unchanged state of the disease. Then a local and regional percutaneous irradiation of the nasopharynx and lymph nodes of the neck (total: 44 Gy, single dose: 2 Gy, duration: 20 days) was added. About three month later again swelling of the tumor of the left neck was noticed and the patient was submitted for surgical therapy. A restaging of the patient revealed multiple enlarged lymph nodes of the neck (CCT, ultrasound) and by panendoscopy no local tumor recurrence was detectable neither by clinical inspection nor by histological investigation of tissue samples. Then a neck dissection was carried out and multiple enlarged lymph nodes were found in the situs (figure 2). The patient recovered quickly. Surprisingly, the morphological investigation of lymph nodes demonstrated two of them with central caseation necrosis, epitheloid cell granulomas and a few Langhans cells (figure 3). In none of the lymph nodes (total: 6) a carcinoma was found. In follow-up repeated clinical and serological investigations excluded a tuberculosis in this patient. One year later the patient was still alive and in our restaging no tumor recurrence was found.

Discussion

In malignant tumors, especially in lymph node metastases, tuberculoid lesions might occur mimicking Morbus Boeck like lesions. Due to a similar appearance the lesions are known as "sarcoid-like lesions" (5). The tuberculoid reactions are characterized by groups of epitheloid cells and sometimes complete "tubercle" might be found. Usually caseation of tumors is missing (7). A caseous and tuberculoid-like alteration in carcinomas without any tbc-related etiology was rarely reported (1, 4) but was recurrently found in lymphoepithelial carcinomas (7): in lymph node metastases of lymphoepithelial carcinomas (n = 155) were found epitheloid cells in 17.8% and caseation necrosis in 8.5%. Caseous-tuberculoid reaction in 40 lymph nodes, with or without metastasis, was found in eleven patients. The

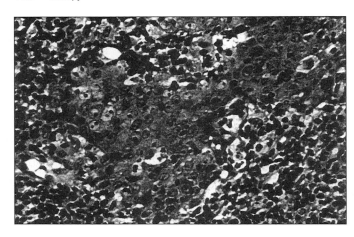

Figure 1. Undifferentiated carcinoma, nasopharynx. (HE, magnification x 67).

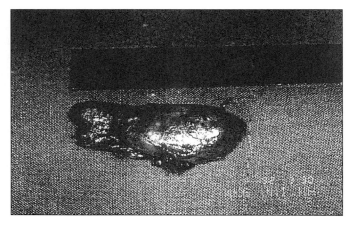

Figure 2. Lymph node of the left neck in a patient with a known UNCT after radiochemotherapy (largest diameter 15 mm).

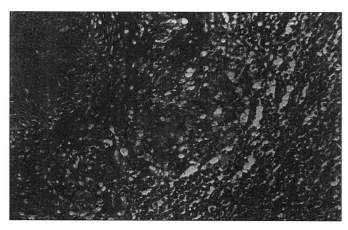

Figure 3. Lymph node. Central caseation necrosis (left), epitheloid granuloma and Langhans cells (center). (EvG, magnification x 67).

association of epitheloid cells and caseation was restricted to lymph nodes with carcinoma metastasis in this study. Mycobacterium tuberculosis was not found in any of the lymph nodes. Tuberculoid lesions, with or without caseation necrosis, and marked eosinophilia and plasmacytosis are highly characteristic for lymph node metastases of lymphoepithelial carcinomas (6), presently termed UCNT (9).

In one case of the reported study the diagnosis of UCNT was delayed for years due to a misdiagnosis as tbc-based on the finding of caseous-tuberculoid necrosis in lymph nodes (6). A caseous-tuberculoid reaction in lymph nodes is proposed to be fairly specific for UCNT. In addition, in non-keratinizing carcinomas after irradiation of lymph node metastases the same phenomenom was occasionally reported (7).

The finding of a caseous necrosis with epitheloid cell granulomas strongly suggests a regression of regional lymph node metastases in a young boy with a known UCNT explored after radiochemotherapy. Although curative irradiation of UCNT was reported a careful follow-up of patients with UCNT is recommended.

References

1 Birnmeyer G (1967) Epitheloidzellige Reaktionen im Halslymphknotenbereich und ihre ätiologische Deutung. Z Laryngol Rhinol 46:357–361
2 Ho JHC, Lau WH, Fong M, Chan CL, Au GKH (1981) Treatment of nasopharyngeal carcinoma (NPC). In: Grundmann E, Krueger GRF, Ablashi DV (eds) Nasopharyngeal Carcinoma. Fischer, Stuttgart, New York, pp 279–286
3 Huang AT, Cole TB, Fishburn RI, Baughn SG, Lucas VS (1981) Chemotherapy for nasopharyngeal carcinoma. In: Grundmann E, Krueger GFR, Ablashi DV (eds) Nasopharyngeal carcinoma. Fischer, Stuttgart, New York, pp 263–268
4 Krische K (1913) Kombination von Krebs und Tuberkulose in metastatisch erkrankten Drüsen. Frankfurt Z Path 12:63–79
5 Lennert K (1961) Lymphknoten. Diagnostik in Schnitt und Ausstrich. Bandteil A: Cytologie und Lymphadenitis. In: Henke, Lubarsch, Roessle, Uehlinger (Hrsg) Handbuch der speziellen pathologischen Anatomie und Histologie. Bd. I/3A, Springer, Berlin, Göttingen, Heidelberg
6 Lennert K, Kaiserling E, Mazzanti T (1978) Diagnosis and differential diagnosis of lymphoepithelial carcinoma in lymph nodes: Histological, cytological and electron-microscopic findings. In: de-Thé G, Ito Y, Davis W (eds) Nasopharyngeal carcinoma: etiology and control. WHO, IARC Scientific Publications No. 20, Lyon, pp 51–64
7 Rennke H, Lennert K (1973) Käsig-tuberkuloide Reaktionen bei Lymphknotenmetastasen lymphoepithelialer Carcinome (Schmincke-Tumoren). Virchows Arch (A) 358:241–247
8 Sack H (1981) Radiation therapy of nasopharyngeal cancer. In: Grundmann E, Krueger GFR, Ablashi DC (eds) Nasopharyngeal carcinoma. Fischer, Stuttgart, New York, pp 273–277
9 Shanmugaratnam K, Sobin LH (1991) Histological typing of tumors of the upper aerodigestive tract and ear. Springer, Berlin pp 32–33

Address for correspondence:
Dr. med. Dr. med. dent. R. E. Friedrich
Klinik für Mund-, Kiefer- und Gesichtschirurgie
(Nordwestdeutsche Kieferklinik)
Martinistraße 52
D-20246 Hamburg, Germany

Longterm continuous release and bioactivity of interleukin-2 depot preparations in human tumor bearing nude mice

B. Falk, Edith Huland, D. Hübner, H. Huland

Department of Urology, University of Hamburg, Germany

Introduction

Our group has shown that continuous local high-dose interleukin-2 (IL-2) application in patients with transitional cell carcinoma (TCC) of the bladder and in patients with pulmonary metastases of renal cell carcinoma (RCC) is not toxic but highly effective against tumor. To extend the possibilities of local tumor treatment either for animal or in vitro experimentation or for clinical use in patients we developed depot preparations releasing cytokines for continuous application at tumor sites.

Material and methods

Depot construction consisting of a carrier substance ethylene-vinyl-acetat-copolymer (ELVAX) plus 25% w/v human serum albumine (HSA) and either natural interleukin-2 (IL-2 depot containing $5 \cdot 10^5$ BRMP U IL-2) or natural interferon-a (IFN-a depot containing $3 \cdot 10^5$ U IFN-α) were prepared, sterile and suitable for in vivo use. We developed a model using nude mice subcutaneously transplanted with human tumors and placed depot preparations locally to the tumor to confirm the in vivo longterm biological activity of these depot preparations by the activity of IL-2 to trigger precursor cells in nude mice.

Four different human tumors (2 RCC, 2 TCC) were used. Tumor bearing mice of each tumor were devided into 5 groups of 6–8 mice with different treatment: Control (no treatment), HSA depot (no cytokine), IL-2 depot, IFN-α depot and IFN-α plus IL-2 depot preparations. 3–6 weeks after tumor transplantation and only after proven in vivo tumor growth these depot preparations were implanted subcutaneously directly at the tumor site.

Results

Reduction of tumor growth could be achieved for 3-4 weeks after depot implantation proving in vivo long term biological activity of interleukin-2 in Elvax depot preparations. Tumor size was significantly reduced in the IL-2 depot and IFN-a plus IL-2 depot treated groups compared to the other groups. After that period tumors startet to grow again and the growth rate was comparable to the rate before treatment. No complete tumor remission was achieved in any of the tumors and IFN-α alone did not show considerable influence on tumor growth.

Conclusions

We have shown that the nude mouse is a highly valuable model to test biological activity and release time of IL-2 depot preparations in vivo. Evidence for biological activity of depots in vivo is a promising step to extend our concept of an innovative and effective way of immuno therapy: the local continuous high dose IL-2 application in cancer patients.

References

1. Queseda JR, Swanson DA, Trindade A, Gutterman JU (1983) Renal carcinoma: Antitumor effects of leucocytes interferon. Cancer Res 43:940–947
2. Lotze MT, Chang AE, Seipp CA, Simpson C, Vetto J, Rosenberg SA (1986) High-dose recombinant interleukin-2 in the treatment of patients with cancer. JAMA 256:3117–3124
3. Rosenberg SA, Lotze MT, Muul LM, Chang AE, Avis FP, Leitman S, Lineham WM, Robertson CN, Lee RE, Rubin JT, Seipp CA, Simpson CG, White DE (1987)

A progress report on the treatment of 157 patients with a advanced cancer using lymphokine activated killer cells and interleukin-2 alone. N Engl J Med 316:889–897
4. Hosokawa M, Morikawa K, Okada F, Kobayashi H (1986) An enhaced therapeutic effect in the treatment of rat transplanted tumors by mixing interleukin 2 in a Pluric gel, a sustained-released vehicle. In: Urushizaki I, Aoki T, Tsubura E (eds) Host defence mechanisms against cancer. Excerpta Medica, Amsterdam, pp 26–35
5. Wagner H, Hardt C, Heeg K, Rollinghoff M, Pfitzenmaier K (1980) T-cell-derived helper factor allows in vivo induction of cytotoxic T-cells in (nu/nu) mice. Nature 284:278–289
6. Bubenik J, Kieler J, Tromholt V, Indrova M, Lotzova E (1986) Recombinant interleukin-2 inhibits growth of human tumor xenografts in congenitally athymic mice. Immol Lett 14:325–330
7. Huland E, Huland H (1988) Local continous high dose interleukin 2: A new therapeutic model for the treatment of advanced bladder carcinoma. Cancer Res 49:5469–5474
8. Huland E, Huland H, Heinzer H (1992) Interleukin 2 by inhalation: Local therapy for metastatic renal cell carcinoma. J Urol 147:344–348

Address for correspondence:
Dr. med. B. Falk
Abteilung für Urologie
Universitätskrankenhaus
Martinistraße 52
D-20246 Hamburg, Germany

Successful labeling of the murine monoclonal anti-EGF-receptor-antibody MAb 425 with technetium-99m

First experimental results

S. Adams, R.P. Baum, H.G. Schnürch, M. Stegmüller, H.G. Bender, G. Hör

Department of Nuclear Medicine and Department of Gynecologic Oncology,
University Medical Center, Frankfurt/Main, Germany

Introduction

The epidermal growth factor (EGF) is a polypeptide of 53 amino acids with a molecular weight of approximately 6000 kD (1). This factor interacts with specific cell surface receptors and stimulates the proliferation and differentiation of target cells in vitro and in vivo (2). The epidermal growth factor receptor (EGF-R) is a transmembrane mitogenic glycoprotein with a molecular weight of 170 kD (3). The EGF-R represents the product of the c-erbB protooncogene (4). Many kinds of tumors such as thyroid carcinoma, gastric cancer, non-neuronal brain tumors and squamous cell carcinomas have been reported to express enhanced EGF-R levels (5). The expression of high levels of EGF-R in malignant tissues also correlates with poor differentiation and depth of invasion (6, 7, 8). In experimental animal studies the iodine-131 labeled monoclonal antibody MAb 425 (directed against the external domain of the EGF receptor) was used for radioimmunodetection of human glioma xenografts in nude mice (9). The iodine-125 labeled MAb 425 was used successfully for antibody-guided therapy of EGF-R positive human brain gliomas (10, 11). Soo et al. (12) used an In-111 labeled antibody (EGF-R1) to image patients with squamous cell carcinoma of the head and neck. The radionuclides used up to now have many disadvantages for radioimmunoscintigraphy (unfavorable energy, inadequate half-life, costs, and availability). Technetium-99m (Tc-99m) is an optimal radionuclide for scintigraphic imaging (physical energy peak 140 keV, half-life 6 hours). Our interdisciplinary group was the first to use Tc-99m labeled MAb 425 for the localization of EGF receptors in cervical cancer and squamous cell carcinomas of the head and neck (13). The aim of the present investigation was to study the biokinetics and biodistribution of the Tc-99m labeled murine IgG 2a monoclonal antibody MAb 425 in athymic nude mice, xenotransplanted with EGF-R positive cervical carcinomas: A high dose saturation of EGF-receptors ("blocking experiment") was performed to find out how long the receptors were blocked after a single injection of 2.5 mg of cold MAb 425. In order to get further information on the binding kinetics of MAb 425 in vivo, a "saturation experiment" was carried out to determine the minimal dose of cold (unlabeled) MAb 425 required for blockade of EGF-R positive cervix carcinoma xenotransplants.

Material and methods

Antibody

MAb 425 binds to the external domain of the epidermal growth factor receptor and was first characterized by *Murthy* et al. 1987 (4). We received the antibody (EMD 55900) for research purposes from Merck Darmstadt, Germany.

Radiolabeling MAb 425

The 2-component instant labeling kit (based on a modified Schwarz Technique) consisted of two vials, one with 1 mg lyophilized MAb 425, 2 mg natrium phospate buffer and 4 mg D(+)-trehalose and another vial containing the tin component (2.7 mg PTP, 0.12 mg Zn-II-Cl x H_2O and 0.2 mg

NaCl). The labeling efficiency after addition of up to 1.1 GBq (30 mCi) technetium-99m was controlled by HPLC, gel filtration and by thin layer chromatography using methylethylketone as runnning medium. Labeling time (incubation) was ten minutes. Purity check by HPLC resulted in > 96% of the monoclonal antibody in monomer form containing more than 96% of the Tc-99m activity. The immunoreactivity of MAb 425 labeled with Tc-99m was more than 85%.

Xenotransplants

Tumor pieces from EGF-R positive cervical carcinomas from patients of the Department of Gynecologic Oncology, Frankfurt University Medical Center were transplanted bilaterally to athymic nude mice (25 to 30 g) and grown to a weight of 200 to 600 mg (14).

High-dose saturation of EGF receptors ("Blocking experiment")

The xenotransplanted nude mice were given injections of 2.5 mg unlabeled (cold) MAb 425 intraperitoneally (i.p.) at day 0 (D0). 20 µg of MAb 425 labeled with 20 MBq Tc-99m were then injected at daily intervals up to six weeks. Immunoscintigraphy of the xenotransplanted nude mice was performed 24 to 36 hours post injection (p.i.), and then at daily intervals by gamma camera imaging (acquisition time 1 hour, 256 x 256 matrix, high resolution low energy collimator, Sopha Medical Gamma Camera) and region of interest (ROI) analysis was performed for measuring the activity (counts per pixel) in the whole body, in the tumor and in representative organs. After immunoscintigraphy, the mice were dissected. Tumors and organs were weighed and measured in a gamma counter detecting the specific activity/gram. From these results, tumor-to-non-tumor (T/NT) ratios were calculated.

Titration of saturation dose ("Saturation experiment")

Between 3.75 µg and 2 mg of cold (unlabeled) MAb 425 were injected in different nude mice carrying bilateral EGF-R positive cervix carcinoma xenografts. After 24 hours, the nude mice were sacrified and immuniscintigraphy was performed. After immunoscintigraphy, the tumors were weighed and measured in a gamma counter.

Results

High-dose saturation of EGF-receptors ("Blocking experiment")

After a single intraperitoneal injection of 2.5 mg of cold (unlabeled) MAb 425, the uptake of Tc-99m labeled MAb 425 in the EGF-R positive cervix carcinomas was blocked for about six days as calculated from the T/NT ratios (see figure 1 and table I) and as also demonstrated by immunoscintigraphy. Seven days after injection of cold MAb 425, there was an increasing uptake of the Tc-99m labeled MAb 425 in the growing cervical tumors.

Titration of saturation dose ("Saturation experiment")

After injection of different doses of unlabeled MAb 425 (between 3.75 µg and 2 mg), the tumor to-non-tumor ratios revealed that doses of 250 to 2000 µg of cold MAb 425 resulted in blockade of tumor uptake of 20 µg of the technetium-99m labeled antibody (see figure 2). Doses between 3.75 and 30 µg were not effective in blocking tumor uptake.

Discussion

EGF is a powerful mitogen for a wide variety of benign and malignant cells and increases tumor growth by an acceleration of cellular division (15). The mature EGF-receptor is a glycoprotein with intrinsic tyrosin-specific kinase activity that has been sequenced and is present on a wide range of normal epithelial tissues and malignant tumors. The expression of EGF receptors on different malignant tissues shows a direct correlation with poor differentiation (6, 7, 8). In breast cancer there is an inverse correlation of EGF-R expression and the expression of oestrogen recep-

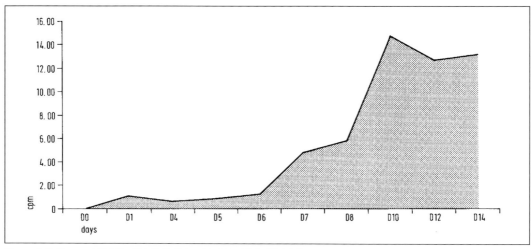

Figure 1. 2.5 mg cold MAb 425 (D0), 20 µg Tc-99m MAb 425 daily.

Table I. 2.5 mg MAb 425 (cold preload at D0), 20 µg Tc-99m MAb 425 daily i.p.

Day pi	Tumor cts	Muscle cts	Tumor/muscle cts	% cts Tumor/whole body
D0				
D1	977	879	1.11	0.78
D4	358	559	0.64	0.71
D5	431	497	0.87	0.79
D6	969	788	1.23	0.8
D7	11048	2300	4.8	3.4
D8	18349	3168	5.49	4.27
D10	20983	1427	14.7	10.83
D12	17472	1380	12.66	6.57
D14	13340	1012	13.88	8.17

tors (8). *Schnürch* et al. (14) demonstrated that breast and cervical tumors with high EGF-R expression showed significant tumor growth inhibition after treatment with MAb 425, whereas tumors with low or unmeasurable EGF-R levels remained unchanged in their growth pattern. In our study, we demonstrated that the epidermal growth factor receptors in tumors were blocked for about six days after a single injection of 2.5 mg of cold MAb 425. *Senekowitsch* et al. (16) demonstrated an increasing tumor uptake of iodine-125 labeled MAb 425 until nine days p.i. in breast and colon carcinoma xenografts in nude mice after intraperitoneal injection. In our studies, doses between 3.75 and 30 µg of cold MAb 425 caused no blockade of the EGF-receptors and no saturation effect, whereas doses of more than 250 µg blocked the EGF-R. The iodine-125 labeled MAb 425 was used successfully for antibody-guided therapy of human brain gliomas (17, 18). The biokinetic data obtained from our

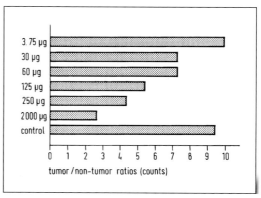

Figure 2. Saturation experiment.

investigations in the nude mice model, may be important for radio- or immunotherapy using cold or radiolabeled MAb 425 for treatment of advanced EGF-R positive tumors. MAb 425 might be useful for immunodiagnostic and immunotherapeutic purposes but more pharmacokinetic or pharmacodynamic studies in humans are still desirable.

References

1. Conteas C, Desai TK, Arlow FA (1988) Relationship of hormones and growth factors to colon cancer. Gastroenterol Clin 17:761
2. Rakowicz-Szulczynska EA, Otwiaska D et al (1989) Epidermal Growth Factor (EGF) and monoclonal antibody to cell surface EGF-receptor bind to the same chromatin receptor. Arch Biochem Biophys 268:456-464
3. De Wit PEJ, Moretti S et al (1992) Increasing epidermal growth factor receptor expression in human melanocytic tumor progression. J Invest Dermatol 99:168-173
4. Murthy U, Basu A et al (1987) Binding of an antagonistic monoclonal antibody to an intact and fragmented EGF-receptor polypeptide. Arch Biochem Biophys 252:549-560
5. Rodeck U, Herlyn M et al (1987) Tumor growth modulation by a monoclonal antibody to the epidermal growth factor receptor: immunologically mediated and effector-cell independent effects. Cancer Res 47:3692-3696
6. Real FX, Rettig WJ et al (1986) Expression of epidermal growth factor receptor in human cultured cells and tissues: relationship to cell lineage and stage of differentiation. Cancer Res 46:4726-4731
7. Mueller BM, Romerdahl CA et al (1986) Suppression of spontaneous melanoma metastasis in SCID mice with an antibody to the epidermal growth factor receptor. Cancer Res 51:2193-2198
8. Malkowicz SB, Rodeck U et al (1991) Inhibition of human TCC metastases by an anti epidermal growth factor receptor monoclonal antibody (MAb 425) in an orthotopic nude mice model. J Urol 227A:145
9. Takahashi H, Herlyn D et al (1987) Radioimmunodetection of human glioma xenografts by monoclonal antibody to epidernal growth factor receptor. Cancer Res 47:3847-3850
10. Brady LW, Miyamoto C, Woo DV et al (1991) Malignant astrocytomas treated with iodine-125 labeled monoclonal antibody 425 against epidermal growth factor receptor: a phase II trial. Int J Rad Oncol Biol Phys 22:225-230
11. Faillot T, Magdalenat H et al (1991) A Phase I study of the anti-EGF-R monoclonal antibody 425 in patients with malignant gliomas. Neurology 41 (suppl 1):383
12. Soo KC, Ward M et al (1987) Radioimmunoscintigraphy of squamous carcinomas of the head and neck. Head Neck Surg 9:349-352
13. Baum RP, Adams S, Schwarz A et al (1992) Successful labeling of anti EGF-R MAb 425 with Tc-99m: First experimental and clinical results in squamous cell carcinomas. Work in Progress, EANM Congress, Lissabon, Portugal, August 22-26
14. Schnürch HG, Beckmann MW (1992) Growth inhibition of human female genital and breast cancer tissues transplanted in nude mice by a monoclonal antibody (MAb 425) directed against the epidermal growth factor receptor (EGF-R). In: Kalpdor R (ed) Tumor-associated antigens, oncogenes, receptors cytokines in tumor diagnosis and therapy at the beginning of the nineties. Zuckschwerdt, München, pp36
15. Sinletary SE, Baker FL et al (1987) Biological effect of epidermal growth factor on the in vitro growth of human tumors. Cancer Res 47:403-406
16. Senekowitsch R, Reidl G et al (1990) In vivo binding of I-125-EGF and anti-EGF-receptor MAb 425 to human tumor xenografts depending on the EGF-receptor density. J Cancer Res Clin Oncol 116 (suppl 1):384
17. Bender H, Takahashi H et al (1992) Immunotherapy of human glioma xenografts with unlabeled, I-131, or I-125 labeled monoclonal antibody 425 to epidermal growth factor receptor. Cancer Res 52:121-126
18. Capone PM, Papsidero LD et al (1984) Relationship between antigen density and immunotherapeutic response elicited by monoclonal antibodies against solid tumors. JNCI 72:400

Address for correspondence:
Dr. med. S. Adams
Klinik und Poliklinik für Nuklearmedizin
Johann-Wolfgang-Goethe-Universität
Theodor-Stern-Kai 7
D-60590 Frankfurt, Germany

Anti-EGF-receptor MAb 425 has a growth-inhibiting influence on tumor cells and leads to a differentiation of multicell tumor spheroids

J. Nußbaumer, B. Gunsenheimer, J. Haunschild, K. Steiner, Reingard Senekowitsch

Nuklearmedizinische Klinik und Poliklinik, Technische Universität, Munich, Germany

Introduction

One important problem of cancer research is the understanding of the cellular processes, which control cell growth and proliferation. Growth factors and their receptors play an important role in the growth regulation of various normal and malignant cells.

The epidermal growth factor receptor is a transmembrane glycoprotein on the surface of many human cells. An increased EGF receptor expression on malignant tissue and cell lines has been described for tumors of diverse tissue origin. Binding of EGF to the receptor triggers multiple biological responses in the target cell, such as phosphorylation of the receptor, stimulation of DNA synthesis and cell proliferation. Substances binding to the EGF receptor, as different monoclonal antibodies, could play an important role in tumor therapy by blocking the stimulating effects of EGF-binding.

The aim of these studies was to investigate the influence of MAb 425 and its (Fab)$_2$- or Fab-fragment on growth inhibition of tumor cells.

Material and methods

For our studies the A431 cell line, a squamous cell carcinoma of the vulva, respectively the SW707 cell line, an adenocarcinoma of the colon, were used.

With a displacement assay on viable tumor cells the ability of MAb 425 or its fragments to block receptor binding of EGF was investigated. A431 cells were incubated at 4 °C for 1.5 h with MAb 425 or its fragments at different concentrations. Afterwards, I-125-EGF was added to the reaction volume and incubated for another 1.5 h at 4 °C.

By means of repeated centrifugation and washing, the cell-bound radioactivity was separated from the free radioactivity. The amount of I-125-EGF bound to the EGF-receptor was measured in a gamma-counter. This parameter represents a marker for the EGF-receptors which aren't occupied by MAb 425 or its fragments.

To assess the vitality and the proliferation capacity of A431 cells, a clonogenic assay in soft agar technique was carried out. The tumor cells were incubated for ten days at 37 °C, 5% CO_2 under humid conditions in glas capillaries. Their medium contained 0.3% agar and different concentrations of MAb 425 or its fragments, ranging from 0.1 to 100 pmol/ml. After incubation, the agar solution was transferred to microscopy glasses and colonies were measured and counted. As criterion for colony formation, the number of tumor cell colonies with a diameter more than 50 μm was taken.

The effect of MAb 425 on spheroid growth was tested by means of a spheroid proliferation assay. A431 multi-tumor cell spheroids were cultivated in agarose coated 96-well-plates for 22 days. Their culture media contained different concentrations of MAb 425 (0.1 to 100 pmol/ml). Every two days the spheroid volume was measured and the growth curve was made out.

Penetration studies, on A431 multi-tumor cell spheroids with MAb 425 and its fragments, were made by using autoradiographic technique. Spheroids with a diameter more than 300 μm were incubated by gentle mixing for 1, 2 and 24 h in culture medium containing 2.5 to 270 nmol/l of I-125 labeled MAb 425 or its fragments. After incubation and washing, the spheroids were embedded in mounting medium on cutting blocks and frozen down to –30 °C. 10 μm sections were cut in a cryostat, and the sections sealed in contact with x-ray film for eight days.

SW707 spheroids with a diameter about 500 μm were cut in histological sections after incubation with MAb 425 or its fragments for ten days. These sections were stained with HE and afterwards checked through for any histological changes in comparison to the untreated control spheroids.

Human tumor xenografts were established by subcutaneous inoculation of athymic mice with $5 \cdot 10^6$ A431 cells. Mice bearing tumors with a weight of 500 to 800 mg were intravenously injected with 185 kBq of I-125-MAb 425 or I-125 labeled fragments. The biodistribution data were obtained by killing and dissecting the animals in groups of 6 mice at 1, 2, 6, 9 and 15 days after injection of the intact MAb or at 6, 24 and 48 h after injection of the fragments. Different tissues were removed, weighed and the radioactivity measured in a gamma-counter. The results were expressed as percent injected dose per gramm of tissue.

Results

The results of the displacement assay show, that the intact antibody MAb 425 and the (Fab)$_2$-fragment as well as the small Fab-fragment can completely displace I-125-EGF from its receptor (figure 1). The intact antibody and its fragments have different affinities to the EGF-receptor. Therefore, a ten-fold concentration of the Fab-fragment is necessary for complete displacement of EGF compared to the intact MAb 425.

The evaluation of the clonogenic assay shows, that MAb 425 and its fragments can suppress the forming of tumor cell colonies (figure 2). The higher the antibody concentration, the better the inhibitory effect. At a concentration of 100 pmol MAb 425/ml medium there was not any colony formation. The colony inhibiting effect of the (Fab)$_2$-fragment was comparable to MAb 425. The small Fab-fragment could reduce the number of colonies to approximately 50% compared to the untreated control group.

The growth curves of the A431-spheroids revealed, that MAb 425 reduces the volume of the spheroids to approximately 50% at antibody concentrations of 100 pmol/ml. Lower antibody concentrations (0.1 to 10 pmol/ml) had no effect on spheroid growth compared to the control group (figure 3).

The autoradiographic studies on A431-spheroids demonstrated that the intact MAb 425 could hardly penetrate the spheroid. MAb 425 was mainly localized on the spheroid's circumference. In contrast, both antibody fragments showed a far more homogenous distribution in the whole spheroid.

The histological sections of SW707 spheroids treated with MAb 425 or its (Fab)$_2$-fragment showed a higher grade of differentiation compared to the untreated spheroids. The tissue

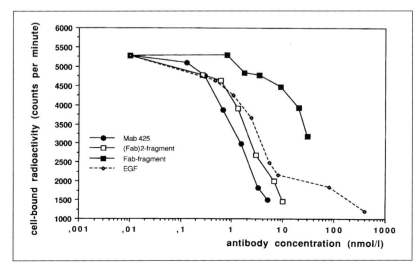

Figure 1. Displacement assay with EGF, MAb 425, (Fab)$_2$- and Fab-fragment on viable tumor cells.

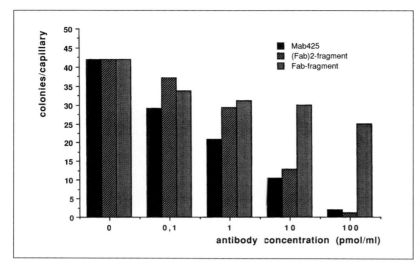

Figure 2. Clonogenic assay of A431 cells during incubation with different concentrations of MAb425 or the (Fab)$_2$- and Fab-fragments.

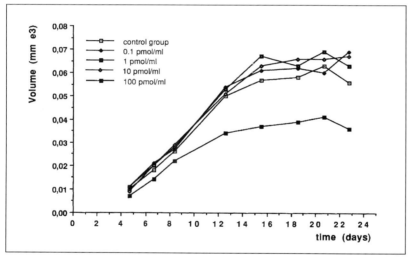

Figure 3. Spheroid proliferation assay with A431 cells during incubation with Mab425 in different concentrations.

looked like colon epithelium and the nucleus-cytoplasmic-relation was shifted to the cytoplasma. The spheroids exhibited structures of intestinal epithelium similar to the original tissue. The cells were arranged like along a basilemma.

The results of the in vivo experiments on athymic mice show a high and rapid uptake of the (Fab)$_2$-fragment in the tumor with 23 %/g at 24 p.i., leading to tumor-blood-ratios of 15 at 24 h and 55 at 48 h p.i. (table I). 48 hours after injection the intact MAb 425 and the (Fab)$_2$-fragment obtained similar concentrations. The small Fab-fragment achieved the lowest tumor uptake and was cleared from the blood very rapidly. Comparing the tumor-blood-ratios, the (Fab)$_2$-fragment shows the most favorable constellation with high tumor uptake and low concentrations in the blood.

Conclusions

The results show, that both the MAb 425 and its fragments can completely inhibit EGF-binding. We demonstrated that MAb 425 and its fragments can inhibit tumor cell proliferation, as shown by the clonogenic assay and the spheroid proliferation assay. Furthermore MAb 425 causes redifferentiation of SW707 cells.

Table I. Concentration of MAb 425 and its fragments in the tumor and blood (% injected dose/g tissue) and tumor-blood-ratios (T/B).

	Time	Tumor	Blood	T/B
MAb 425	1 d	14.3	20.1	0.7
	2 d	14.6	19.1	0.8
	6 d	15.4	10.9	1.4
	9 d	15.8	8.6	1.8
	15 d	11.9	4.5	2.6
(Fab)$_2$-fragment	6 h	19.4	16.2	1.2
	24 h	23.0	1.5	15.2
	48 h	16.1	0.3	55.5
Fab-fragment	6 h	3.7	1.4	2.7
	24 h	1.5	0.1	15.0
	48 h	1.1	0.05	22.0

The antibody penetration studies showed a good permeability into the spheroid for the (Fab)$_2$- and the Fab-fragment, but the intact MAb 425 was mainly localized in the spheroid's circumference.
The results of the biodistribution experiments favor the (Fab)$_2$-fragment.

References

1. Ennis BW, Lippmann ME, Dickson RR (1991) The EGF receptor system as a target for antitumor therapy. Cancer Invest 9:553–562
2. Carpenter G (1987) Receptors for epidermal growth factor and other polypeptide mitogens. Ann Rev Biochem 56:881–914
3. Masui H, Kawamoto T, Sato JD, Wolf B, Sato G, Mendelsohn J (1984) Growth inhibition of human tumor cells in athymic mice by anti-epidermal growth factor receptor monoclonal antibodies. Cancer Res 44:1002–1007
4. Defize LHK, Mummery CL, Moolenaar WH, de Laat SW (1987) Anti-receptor antibodies in the study of EGF-receptor interaction. Cell Differ 20:87–102
5. Langmuir VK, Mendonca HL, Woo DV (1992) Comparisons between two monoclonal antibodies that bind to the same antigen but have different affinities: uptake kinetics and I-125-antibody therapy efficacy in multicell spheroids. Cancer Res 52: 4728–4734
6. Langmuir VK, Mendonca HL (1992) The role of radionuclide distribution in the efficacy of I-131-labeled antibody as modeled in multicell spheroids. Antibody, Immunoconj Radiopharmac Vol 5, no 3
7. Jain RK (1990) Physiological barriers to delivery of monoclonal antibodies and other macromolecules in tumor. Cancer Res 50:814–819

Address for correspondence:
Prof. Dr. Dr. Reingard Senekowitsch
Nuklearmedizinische Klinik
Technische Universität München
Ismaninger Straße 22
D-81675 München, Germany

Evidence of a growth inhibition effect of high levels of recombinant human erythropoietins on sarcoma cell lines in vitro

R. E. Friedrich[a], P. Mestmacher[a], D. Hellner[a], H. Arps[b]

[a]Department of Oral and Maxillofacial Surgery, Eppendorf University Hospital, University of Hamburg, [b]Institute of Pathology, Municipal Hospital, Fulda, Germany

Introduction

Previous investigations of the influence of human recombinant erythropoietins (rhE) proved a lack of tumor cell growth stimulating activity in human tumor specimens including cell cultures of different solid malignant tumors in the majority of tissues (2, 3, 10). In previous investigations in individual cell lines we noted a mild anti-proliferative activity of the drug which seems to be without therapeutic relevance (4). In pilot studies of successfull treatment of tumor associated anemias in men the dosage of rhE was elevated to about 150 to 450 U/kg body weight (bw) (end stage renal failure: 25 to 75 U/kg bw), particularily applied in patients with malignant myelomas and low-grade non-Hodgkin's lymphomas (8, review: 7). In patients with refractory anemia due to a myelodysplastic syndrome rhE (i.v. ≤ 450 U/ml, sc 10,000 U/ml) were applied leading to an elevation of reticulocytes count (6). On the other hand production of erythropoietin has been reported for various tumor cell lines in vitro at least in subsets of leukemias (9, 11) and there are clinical data about an aberrant synthesis and release of erythropoietin in cancer patients, particularily in renal cell cancer (12). So far there are just a few studies of rhEs effects on solid malignant tumors and there is none published concerning high levels of this drug in vitro. In a second series of cell culture studies of erythropoietin we compared the effects of high concentrations of two rhE products on the growth of sarcoma cell lines.

Material and methods

To establish further information about the action of rhE we applied very high concentrations of two commercially available rhEs (Recormon™, Boehringer Mannheim GmbH, Mannheim; Erypo™, Cilag GmbH, Sulzbach/Ts., Germany) on sarcoma cell lines in the monolayer proliferation assay. For toxicity testing the in vitro concentrations were calculated for both rhEs identically (K_1 =50 U/ml, K_2 = 200 U/ml, K_3 = 1000 U/ml). The details of the test are presented elsewhere (1) and are identical to the procedures presented in this volume (5). The cell cultures used are listed in table I. The incubations were done three-fold.

Results

After incubation of the sarcomas with Recormon™ in five cell lines a linear degression of relative tumor growth was found. Although two liposarcomas initially were stimulated up to

Table I. Sarcoma cell lines tested in the monolayer proliferation assay against high concentrations of human recombinant erythropoietins (rhE).

89/148	Rhabdomyosarcoma
87/266	Rhabdomyosarcoma
89/063	Schwannoma
86/324	Schwannoma
87/214	Liposarcoma
86/197	Liposarcoma
87/072	Fibrosarcoma
89/096	Fibrosarcoma

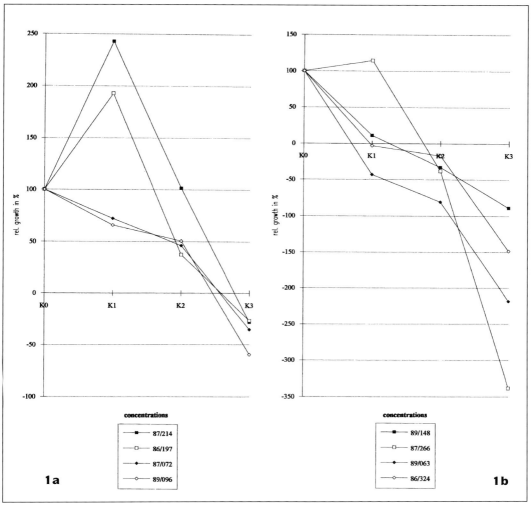

Figure 1a and b. Dose/response curves of sarcoma cell lines after incubation with recombinant human erythropoietin (Recormon™).

almost 200% and 250%, resp. (K_1), at higher levels of rhE these tumors were inhibited, too. At K_3-levels no tumor cell growth was detectable. After incubation of the sarcomas with Erypo™ at the K_1-levels a reduction of cell growth was measured in four lines (< 0–80% relative growth). The two sarcomas stimulated after incubation of rhE (Recormon™, 50 U/ml) were not affected or mildly stimulated after incubation with Erypo™ but cell growth was stimulated in a rhabdomyosarcoma (K_2, > 200%). Comparing relative cell-growth after application of Erypo™ of K_2 and K_3 levels, in all lines there was a degression found. A total or almost total inhibition of the growth of sarcoma cell lines at K_3-levels was found in five cases. The results are summarized in figures 1 and 2.

Discussion

In a previous study an inhibition of tumor cell growth by rhE was found in 5 of 53 tumor cell lines in a soft agar cloning system. In four of five cases this effect was found in the highest rhE dose applied (400 U/ml) (2). Neither stimulation nor inhibition occured in the majority of cell lines. Two soft tissue sarcomas were stimulated in a non-dose-dependent manner (0.4 U/ml, 40 U/ml).

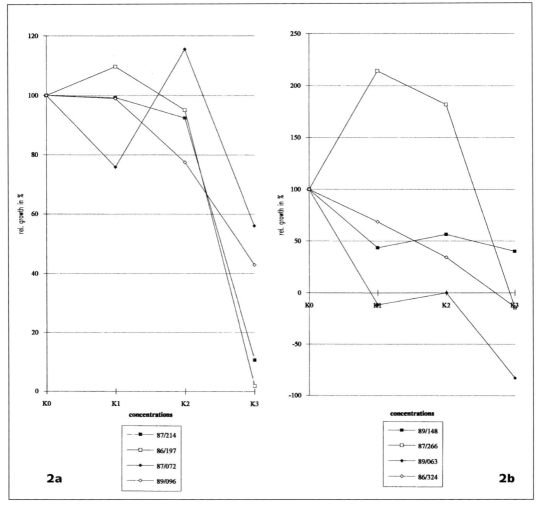

Figure 2a and b. Dose/response curves of sarcoma cell lines after incubation with recombinant human erythropoietin (Erypo 4000™).

No tumor cell growth stimulating effect was found in 53 cell lines at the highest levels (400 U/ml). Comparing these results and our findings occasionally a stimulation of sarcoma cell lines after incubation of rhE, which is not dose dependent, has to be taken into account in lower levels of the drug as far as in vitro data are concerned. Very high levels of the drug in both formulations act cytotoxic on sarcoma cell lines in vitro. Differences of cytotoxic activity of both the rhEs commercially available might be due to differences of the biological properties of the charges used. It is concluded erythropoietin to be cytotoxic to sarcoma cell lines in vitro at high levels so far not used for clinical application in cancer patients.

References

1 Arps H (1988) Maligne humane Tumoren in der Zellkultur. Habilitationsschrift, Universität Hamburg
2 Bauer E, Danhauser-Riedl S, De Riese W, Raab HR Sandner S, Meyer HJ, Neukam D, Hanauske U Freund M, Poliwoda H, Rastetter J, Hanauske AF (1992) Effects of recombinant human erythropoietin on clonogenic growth of primary human tumor specimens in vitro. Onkol 15:254–258

3 Berdel WE, Oberberg D, Reufi B, Thiel E (1991) Studies on the role of recombinant human erythropoietin in the growth regulation of human non hematopoietic tumor cells in vitro. Ann Hematol 63:5-8

4 Friedrich RE, Arps H (1993) Zur Wirkung von humanem rekombinanten Erythropoietin (rHu-EPO) auf Zellen solider maligner Tumoren in vitro. Dtsch Z Mund Kiefer Gesichts Chir (im Druck)

5 Friedrich RE, Mestmacher P, Hellner D, Arps H (1994) Lack of tumor cell growth stimulating activity of human recombinant erythropoietins (Erypo 4000™, Recormon 1000™) on sarcoma cell lines in vitro (this volume)

6 Ganser A, Seipelt G, Hoelzer D (1991) The role of GM-CSF, G-CSF, Interleukin-3, and erythropoietin in myelodysplastic syndrome. Am J Clin Oncol (CCT) 14 (Suppl 1):S34-S39

7 Heinrichs H, Oster W (1991) Zur Therapie der Anämie bei malignen Erkrankungen. Die gelben Hefte XXXI:172-179

8 Ludwig H, Fritz E, Kotzmann H, Hoecker P, Gisslinger H, Barnas U (1990) Erythropoietin treatment in anemia associated with multiple myeloma. N Engl J Med 322:1693-1699

9 Motoji T, Hoshino S, Ueda M, Takanashi M, Masuda M, Nakayama K, Oshimi K, Mizoguchi H (1990) Enhanced growth of clonogenic cells from acute myeloblastic leukemia by erythropoietin. Br J Haematol 75:60-67

10 Mundt D, Berger MR, Bode G (1992) Effect of erythropoietin on a human melanoma cell line in vitro (RHEPO) and in vivo (RMEPO). J Cancer Res Clin Oncol 118 R54 (Suppl) Abstr No MI.16.05

11 Salem M, Delwel R, Mahmoud LA, Clark S, Elbasousy EM, Lowenberg B (1989) Maturation of human acute myeloid leukemia in vitro: the response to five recombinant haematopoietic factors in a serum-free system. Br J Haematol 71:363-270

12 Sytkowski AJ, Bicknell KA, Smith GM, Garcia JF (1984) Secretion of erythropoietin-like activity by clones of human renal carcinoma cell line GKA. Cancer Res 44:51-55

Address for correspondence:
Dr. med. Dr. med. dent. R. E. Friedrich
Klinik für Mund-, Kiefer- und Gesichtschirurgie
(Nordwestdeutsche Kieferklinik)
Universitätskrankenhaus Eppendorf
Martinistraße 52
D-20246 Hamburg, Germany

Tumor cell growth stimulation by stable PGE$_1$ and PGI$_2$ derivatives on human sarcoma cell lines in vitro

R. E. Friedrich[a], P. Mestmacher[a], D. Hellner[a], A. Reymann[b], H. Arps[c]

[a]Oral and Maxillofacial Surgery, [b]Institute of Pharmacology, Eppendorf University Hospital, University of Hamburg, [c]Institute of Pathology, Municipial Hospital, Fulda, Germany

Introduction

After the establishment of microvascular surgery techniques a lot of donation areas of (osteo-)myocutaneous flaps have come into the focus of practice of reconstructive surgery of head and neck, especially for the therapy of patients which are suffering from malignant diseases of this region (12, 17). However, due to the fact that the majority of patients are of an age where chronic degenerative vascular diseases are prevalent, e. g. atherosclerosis, thrombosis of the microvascular anastomoses or other parts of the prepared vessels might happen and necrobiosis or at least damage of the superficial and marginal layers of the autograft is threatening. Routinely applied heparin, neither local during microvascular surgery nor systemical by intravenous infusion is no guarantee for avoiding thrombosis in the selected vessels. So there is a basic surgical interest in managing the perioperative vulnerability of the new vascular supply.

The knowledges about physiological and pharmacological properties of the products of the arachidonic acid have rapidly increased (for review: 6, 9, 13). Some of the cyclooxygenase products are potent antagonists of blood clotting and effective vasodilators (PGE$_1$, PGI$_2$) and recently stable derivatives of these substances have become available for therapy or scientific investigations (2, 16). The application of prostacyclin seems to avoid thrombus formation in intimectomized/arteriotomized small arteries (15) and there are promising reports of a benefit of applying the prostacyclin-analogue to futures for the prevention of postoperative arterial and venous thrombosis in the rat (4, 11). However, up to the knowledge of the authors there are no published data of in vitro studies available elucidating the question of a stimulation of tumor growth of sarcoma cell lines by PGI$_2$ and PGE$_1$ derivatives designed for clinical therapy and so the drugs were investigated in the monolayer proliferation assay (1).

Material and methods

Nine cell lines of histogenetically different soft tissue sarcomas (table I) were tested against varying concentrations of PGE$_1$ and PGI$_2$ derivates (ranging from 21.3 pg/ml to 7.1 ng/ml for PGE$_1$ (MW 354.49) (K$_1$ = 200.2 pmol/l, K$_2$ = 2.002 µmol/l, 20.02 µmol/l) and from 0.75 pg/ml to 250 pg/ml for PGI$_2$ (MW 347) (K$_1$ = 7.21 pmol/l, K$_2$ = 72.04 pmol/l, K$_3$ = 720.46 pmol/l resp.) in the monolayer proliferation assay. The PGE$_1$ derivative is the active agent of a commercially available drug (Prostavasin™). The stable PGI$_2$ derivative (Iloprost™) was kindly supplied by Schering AG, Berlin. For a single concentration the preparations for all sarcomas were done three-fold. K$_2$ is the estimated value for a human

Table I. Sarcoma cell lines tested in the monolayer proliferation assay against varying concentrations of PGE$_1$ and PGI$_2$ derivatives.

86/197	Liposarcoma
87/015	MFH
87/072	Fibrosarcoma
87/214	Liposarcoma
87/266	Rhabdomyosarcoma
87/324	Schwannoma
89/063	Schwannoma
89/096	Fibrosarcoma
89/148	Rhabdomyosarcoma

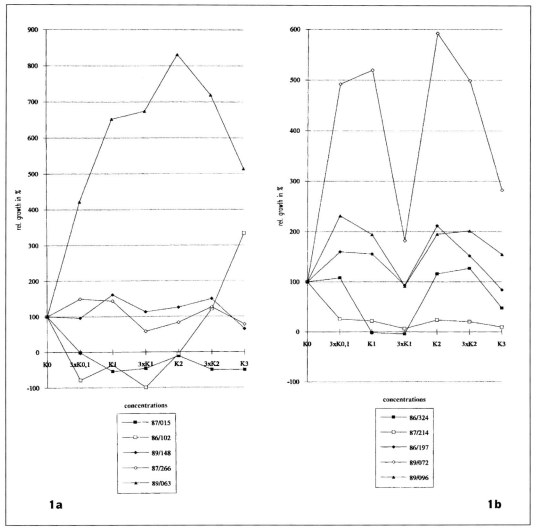

Figure 1a and b. Action of stable derivatives of PGI$_2$ on sarcoma cell lines in vitro: to improve the clearness of the dose/response relations the data are presented in splitted diagrams. For details see text.

individual weighing 70 kg (clinical application: PGI$_2$ = 5 µg/kg/min and PGE$_2$ = 0.1–0.6 ng/kg/min).

Results

Tumor cell lines showed individual reactions to the substances applied. While rhabdomyosarcomas and liposarcomas demonstrated only slight stimulative effects up to a two-fold, a fibrosarcoma and a malignant schwannoma were stimulated up to 500% and 800% growth, respectively. Correlating the effects of both the prostaglandin derivates the substances did not show substantial differences in their growth stimulating effects (figure 2).

Discussion

The cell growth of the majority of cell lines investigated were not or only moderately altered by the application of the prostaglandin derivatives. Surprisingly, two of the cell lines were

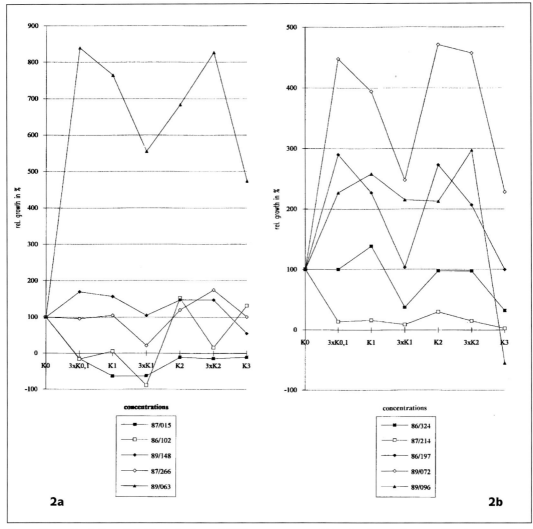

Figure 2a and b. Action of stable derivatives of PGE_1 on sarcoma cell lines in vitro: to improve the clearness of the dose/response relation the data are presented in splitted diagrams. For details see text.

stimulated by both prostaglandin derivatives in the monolayer proliferation assay (89/063 and 89/072 resp.). In general it would have been expected that prostaglandins and their derivatives were of no effect on tumor cell proliferation. Due to their antithrombogenic properties the antimetastatic effects of these substances are well known (7). Antimetastatic effects of a drug are no guarantee for similar effects on tumor cell growth stimulation. *Ellis* et al. (5) reported of a differential role of PGE_1 on tumor metastasis in Lewis Lung carcinoma in the nude mouse. The substances acted as a promotor in artificial metastases (i.v. infusion of carcinoma cells during constant PGE_1 infusions) in contrast to its antimetastatic effect in animals with primary LLC (5). PGI_2 was found to have an antimetastatic activity on hepatic metastases from a human pancreatic adenocarcinoma in the nude mouse (17) and due to platelet/tumor cell interaction Iloprost™ and prostacyclin have an antimetastatic effect in other experimental studies (3, 8). In an experimental study several prostaglandins were evaluated regarding the effects on protein and glycoprotein synthesis and secretion. PGE_2 and 16,16-dimethyl-PGE_2 enhanced the incorporation of the amino sugar into cellular compartments and secreted acid insoluble macromolecules in a concentration dependent manner. On the other hand, Iloprost™ was found to be ineffective in stimulating pig gastric mucosa cells in this model (10). Prostaglandins (i.e., $PGF2\alpha$, PGE_1, PGE_2), thromboxane B_2 and fatty acids plasma levels were not altered by doxorubicin application in rats up to nine weeks after application (14) supporting the hypothesis that endogenous prostaglandin synthesis hardly is altered in normal cells during chemotherapy. Up to now the available data concerning the drug safety of PGE_1 and PGI_2 derivatives with regard to the lack of tumor cell growth stimulation are limited. It is concluded that although clinical benefit in microvascular surgery might be reached by using platelet aggregation inhibitors caution is warranted to control patients for individual tumor stimulating effects when these drugs are used at least in cases with a prolonged perioperative application of these anti-aggregatory substances.

References

1. Arps H (1988) Maligne humane Tumoren in der Zellkultur, Habilitationsschrift, University, Hamburg
2. Chan PS, Cervoni P (1986) Prostaglandins, prostacyclin and thromboxane in cardiovascular diseases. Drug Dev Res 7:341–359
3. Costantini V, Fuschiottii P, Allegruci M, Agnelli G, Nenci GG, Fioretti MC (1988) Platelet tumor cell interaction: effect of prostacyclin and asynthetic analogon on metastasis formation. Cancer Chemother Pharmacol 22:289–293
4. Eddy CA, Laufe LE, Dunn RL, Gibson JW (1986) The use of prostacyclin analogue-containing suture for the prevention of postoperative venous thrombosis in the rat. Plast Reconstr Surg 78:504–510
5. Ellis LM, Copeland EM, Bland KI, Sitren HS (1990) Differential role of prostaglandin E1 on tumor metastases. J Surg Res 48:333–336
6. Friedrich RE (1986) Quantitative Messungen erythematöser Hautveränderungen an Menschen nach epidermaler Applikation des Prostazyklinderivates Iloprost™ (ZK36374). Med Diss (Thesis), Free University, Berlin
7. Gastpar H (1982) Die Beeinflussung der Metastasierung durch Gerinnungsmechanismen. In: Schmähl D (Hrsg) Krebsmetastasen. Thieme, Stuttgart, pp118–128
8. Giraldi T, Sava G, Perissin L, Zorzet S, Piccini P, Rapozzi V (1988) Antimetastatic activity of the prostacyclin analog iloprost in the mouse. Pharmacol Res Commun 20 (suppl):182
9. Gryglewski RJ (1987) The impact of prostacyclin studies on the development of its stable analogues. In: Gryglewski RJ, Stock G (ed) Prostacycline and its stable analogue iloprost. Springer, Berlin, pp 3–16
10. Heim HK, Oestmann A, Sewing KF (1990) Stimulation of glycoprotein and protein synthesis in isolated gastric mucosal cells by prostaglandins. Gut 31:412–416
11. Kort WJ, De Kam J, Westbroek DL (1987) Peroperative topical administration of ZK 36374 (iloprost) acts favourably on patency of small artery anastomoses in rats. Microsurgery 8:17–21
12. Manktelkow T (1986) Microvascular Reconstruction. Springer, Berlin
13. Moncada S, Higgs A (1987) Prostaglandins in the pathogenesis and prevention of vascular disease. Med Clin North Am 1:141–145
14. Robinson TW, Giri SN (1987) Effects of chronic administration of doxorubicin on plasma levels of prostaglandins, thromboxane B2, and fatty acids in rats. Cancer Chemother Pharmacol 19:213–220
15. Salemark L, Wieslander JB, Dougan P, Arnljots B (1991) Infusion of prostacyclin reduces in vivo thrombus formation following arteriotomy/intimectomy in small arteries. An experimental study in the rabbit. Eur J Plast Surg 14:89–93
16. Schwalke MA, Tzanakakis GN, Vezeridis MP (1990) Effects of prostacyclin on hepatic metastases from human pancreatic cancer in the nude mouse. J Surg Res 49:164–167
17. Schillinger E, Krais TH, Lehmann M, Stock G (1986) Iloprost. In: Scriabine A (ed) New cardiovascular drugs. Raven Press, New York, pp 209–231
18. Seidenberg B, Rosenak SS, Hurwitt ES, Som ML (1959) Immediate reconstruction of the cervical esophagus by means of revascularized isolated jejunal loop. Ann Surg 149:162–171

Address for correspondence:
Dr. med. Dr. med. dent. R. E. Friedrich
Klinik für Mund-, Kiefer- und Gesichtschirurgie
Universitätskrankenhaus Eppendorf
Martinistraße 52
D-20246 Hamburg, Germany

Lack of tumor cell growth stimulating activity of recombinant human erythropoietins (Erypo 4000™, Recormon 1000™) on sarcoma cell lines in vitro

R. E. Friedrich[a], P. Mestmacher[a], D. Hellner[a], H. Arps[b]

[a] Department of Oral and Maxillofacial Surgery, Eppendorf University Hospital, University of Hamburg, [b] Institute of Pathology, Municipial Hospital, Fulda, Germany

Introduction

Human recombinant erythropoietin (rhE) is a hormone successfully applied in patients with anemia in end stage renal failure and there are promising data concerning the benefit of patients with tumor associated anemias treated with rhE. Indeed, in tumor associated anemias a decrease of erythropoietin was found (6) and the recovery of reticulocyte count is associated with an increase of rhE-substitution in cancer patients (5). However, a tumor cell stimulating activity of this hormone can not entirely be ruled out and there are reports of a rhE related stimulation of leukoblastic cells in vitro (7). Recent in vitro studies confirmed a lack of tumor growth stimulating activity of rhE in a soft agar cloning system, particularily in colorectal and renal cancer but a non-dose-dependent stimulation of soft cell sarcomas by rhE has been reported. Interestingly, the levels of tumor growth stimulating activity of rhE on sarcoma cell lines was in the range of therapeutical application (2). So the dose response of a panel of sarcoma cell lines incubated with rhEs in therapeutical levels was investigated.

Material and methods

The effects of two rhEs (Erypo 4000™, Recormon 1000™) on eight human sarcoma cell lines were investigated in the monolayer proliferation assay (1). In clinical applications (end stage renal failure) according to different data of the literature the dosages are about 3 x 15 U/kg body weight (bw) up to 3 x 200 U/kg bw (5, 6). For this in vitro test for both the rhEs a range of concentration was chosen (10–40–200/kg bw; e.g.: 10 U/kg bw, in a patient with 70 kg bw = 700 U/14.000 ml extracellular body fluid = 0.05 U/ml = 50mU/ml for in vitro application). The cell lines used are presented in table I. A cell growth of up to 100% is calculated to be within the statistical range.

Results

In Erypo™ the K_1 levels did not interfere with the proliferation of sarcoma cells in the monolayer proliferation assay in four lines but another four lines demonstrated a mild inhibitory effect. In K_2 and K_3 levels all cell lines which demonstrated a decrease of tumor cell growth at K_1 levels were again inhibited. In one cell line the inhibition was not dose dependent (89/148).
In Recormon™ in five cell lines even at K_1 levels demonstrated an inhibition of tumor cell growth (< 0% cell growth). Theses cell lines showed an almost identical reaction as it was to be seen in Erypo™ application. Two cell lines again were not altered by Recormon™ application. Comparing the concentrations applied at K_2 levels to the K_1 levels in seven of eight cell lines additionally a

Table I. Sarcoma cell lines tested in the monolayer proliferation assay against varying concentrations of human recombinant erythropoietins (rhE).

89/148	Rhabdomyosarcoma
87/266	Rhabdomyosarcoma
89/063	Schwannoma
86/324	Schwannoma
87/214	Liposarcoma
86/197	Liposarcoma
87/072	Fibrosarcoma
89/096	Fibrosarcoma

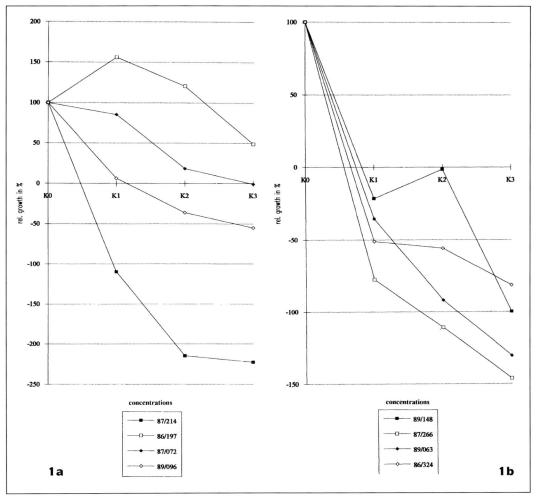

Figure 1a and b. Dose/response curves of sarcoma cell lines after incubation with recombinant human erythropoietin (Recormon™).

relative inhibitory effect could be demonstrated. In K_3 levels the relative cell growth of sarcoma cell lines in all but one is ≤ 0% (figure 1 and 2).

Discussion

The application of rhE in patients with tumor associated anemias needs confirmation of drug safety concerning a lack of tumor cell growth stimulating activity. Calculating in vitro concentrations of rhE related to levels which are desirable in vivo for therapeutic reasons we could not find any tumor cell growth stimulating activity in sarcoma cell lines. These results are confirmed by other reports (2, 3). Although we could find a growth inhibitory effect of both the erythropoietin drugs this antiproliferative activity seems to be without therapeutic relevance. Based on data of the in vitro analysis a tumor stimulating activity of this hormone on sarcomas therefore is unlikely. On the other hand pharmacological properties of a drug have to be distinguished from effects which can be measured at physiological levels (4).

References

1 Arps H (1988) Maligne humane Tumoren in der Zellkultur. Habilitationsschrift, University Hamburg

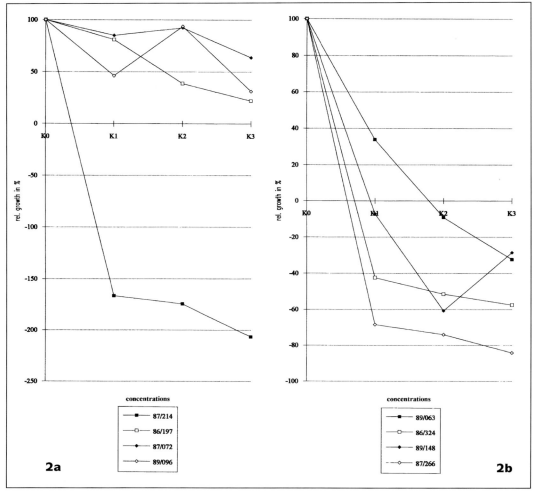

Figure 2a and b. Dose/response curves of sarcoma cell lines after incubation with recombinant human erythropoietin (Erypo™).

2. Bauer E, Danhauser-Riedl S, De Riese W, Raab HR, Sandner S, Meyer HJ, Neukam D, Hanauske U, Freund M, Poliwoda H, Rastetter J, Hanauske AR (1992) Effects of recombinant human erythropoietin on clonogenic growth of primary human tumor specimens in vitro. Onkologie 15:254–258

3. Berdel WE, Oberberg D, Reufi B, Thiel E (1991) Studies on the role of recombinant human erythropoietin in the growth regulation of human non hematopoietic tumor cells in vitro. Ann Hematol 63:5–8

4. Friedrich RE, Mestmacher P, Hellner D, Arps H (1994) Evidence of a growth inhibition effect of high levels of recombinant human erythropoietins on sarcoma cell lines in vitro (this volume)

5. Ludwig H, Fritz E, Kotzmann H, Hoecker P, Gisslinger H, Barnas U (1990) Erythropoietin treatment in anemia associated with multiple myeloma. N Engl J Med 322:1693–1699

6. Miller CB, Jones RJ, Piantadosi S, Abeloff MD, Spivar JL (1990) Decreased erythropoietin response in patients with anemia of cancer. N Engl J Med 322:1689–92

7. Motoji T, Hoshino S, Ueda M, Takanashi M, Masuda M, Nakayama K, Oshimi, Mizoguchi H (1990) Enhanced growth of clonogenic cells from acute myeloblastic leukemia by erythropoietin. Br J Haematol 75:60–67

Address for correspondence:
Dr. med. Dr. med. dent. R. E. Friedrich
Klinik für Mund-, Kiefer- und Gesichtschirurgie
Universitätskrankenhaus Eppendorf
Martinistraße 52
D-20246 Hamburg, Germany

In vitro studies to assess the response of human adenocarcinoma cell spheroids to radiotherapy using fluorodeoxyglucose and thymidine

J. Mattes, K. Matzen, Regine Truckenbrodt, Reingard Senekowitsch
Clinic for Nuclear Medicine and Policlinic, Technical University, Munich, Germany

Introduction

Neoplastic tissue is characterized by an increased uptake of glucose due to the increased metabolic demand of tumor tissue.
Fluorodeoxyglucose (FDG) a glucose analogue has been reported to accumulate in many kinds of malignant tumors as shown by F-18-FDG and positron emission tomography (PET).
It was reported (1, 4) using FDG in an experimental murine cancer model, that metabolic alterations of tumor cells precede morphologic alteration as depicted by a change in tumor size. In addition the response of cancers to irradiation or chemotherapy can be more precisely assessed by using FDG, thymidine and amino acids (2).
The aim of this in vitro study was to investigate the effects of irradiation on the glucose and thymidine metabolism of SW 707 cells, a human colon carcinoma cell line, which has been grown as multicellular tumor spheroids. Tumor cell spheroids are cultured cancer cells in the form of three-dimensional multicell model that simulate micrometastases or intravascular microregions of larger tumors.
Furthermore a clonogenic assay after irradiation was carried out as a measure of proliferative capacity in irradiated and control spheroids.
The final question was whether there is a possibility to determine non-invasively significant changes in tumor physiology and metabolism early after therapy as a predictor of long term therapy response.

Materials and methods

Spheroids were cultured by the liquid overlay technique, i.e. by seeding suspended SW 707 cells in agarose-coated wells of a culture dish with 96 wells allowing the cells to aggregate into small cell clusters.
The culture medium used was RPMI 1640 with L-glutamine (2 mM), 10% FKS, penicillin (100 units/ml) and streptomycin (100 mg/ml) without glucose.
On day 6 of their growth spheroids were irradiated with 6 Gy. Afterwards 15 irradiated spheroids with comparable diameter (microscopic control) as well as 15 untreated spheroids (control) were transferred individually into a well of a culture plate containing incubation medium with 37 kBq/ml C-14-FDG or H3-thymidine at 1, 4, 8, 24 and 48 h after irradiation.
The spheroids were incubated at 37 °C for 1 h, subsequently washed in PBS and the intracellular activity was measured in a liquid scintillation counter. The number of viable cells of the spheroids was determined by the MTT-test, a measure of the activity of mitochondrial dehydrogenases in viable cells.
The proliferation capacity of irradiated and control spheroids was assessed after disintegration by using a clonogenic assay. The proliferation capacity of the irradiated cells was expressed in % of the control.

Results

1 h after irradiation a considerable decrease in glucose uptake per viable cell of irradiated spheroids by 40% of the control was determined. This decrease was followed by a quick increase in FDG-uptake after 4 (to 149%) and 8 h (to 183% of control). 24 and 48 h after irradiation the glucose uptake per viable cell was below control (44 and 39%) (figure 1).

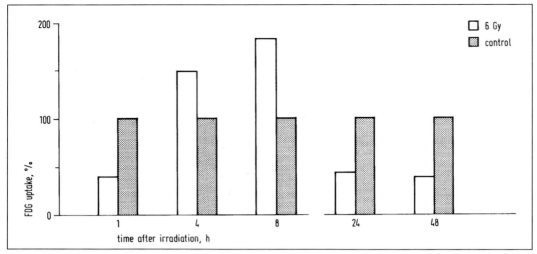

Figure 1. C14-FDG-uptake per viable cell at different time points after irradiation with 6 Gy in comparison to C14-FDG-uptake of control spheroids per viable cell (control=100%).

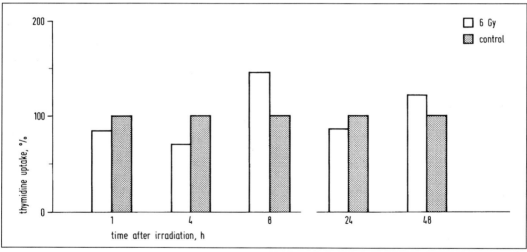

Figure 2. H3-thymidine-uptake per viable cell at different time points after irradiation with 6 Gy in comparison to H3-thymidine-uptake of control spheroids per viable cell (control =100%).

The thymidine uptake of viable cells after irradiation was less than for the control during the first four hours. 8 h after irradiation a distinct increase in thymidine uptake to 145% of that of the control was found. 24 h after irradiation the thymidine uptake decreased again but was followed by an increase to 121% of the control at 48 h (figure 2). The clonogenic assay resulted in a proliferative capacity of the irradiated cells of 4% of control 1 h after irradiation. At 48 h an increase to 21% of the control was determined (figure 3).

The histology of the spheroid sections did not reveal any differences between the irradiated and control spheroids considering the individual cells till 48 h after irradiation.

Discussion

It has been reported that FDG accumulates in many kinds of human malignant tumors. *Minn* et al. (6) compared the changes of FDG uptake and

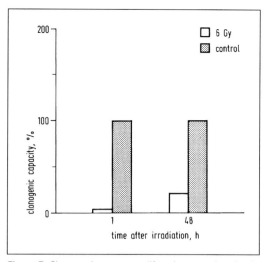

Figure 3. Clonogenic assay: proliferative capacity of cells of irradiated spheroids 1 h and 48 h after irradiation with 6 Gy in comparision to control spheroids (control = 100%).

tumor size by therapy in patients with head and neck tumors and found that decreases in FDG uptake in clinical responders were more prominent than those in non-responders. *Ichiya* et al. (4) noted that FDG uptake before therapy was higher in the relapse group than that in the non-relapse group.

Lesions with no change of tumor size by conventional morphologic examinations are usually thought to have undergone ineffective therapy. *Ichiya* et al. (4) described in his study one lesion which had no change in tumor size but showed a prominent decrease in FDG uptake after therapy. This result indicates the possible use of FDG to predict prognosis in the no change group. In vitro studies of *Higashi* et al. (3) showed that the changes in the proliferation index and H-3-thymidine uptake is highest during lag phase of cell growth and declines rapidly through the exponentional phase. So the proliferative rate is highest before the exponential growth. This correlates with our results that show an increase of thymidine uptake before the recovery of the proliferative capacity after radiotherapy.

Higashi et al. (3) found a smaller variation in FDG uptake during the cell growth cycle, and the changes in FDG uptake were not clearly related to the changes in proliferative activity. Further a direct correlation of the FDG uptake per total number of cells was described.

In our study we could not find a strong relation between FDG uptake and the number of viable cells. Changes in FDG uptake seem to be a very variable indicator of the actual metabolic situation of tumor cells but do not correlate directly with the number of cells.

FDG is a sensitive substance for the evaluation of early effects after radiotherapy but it is difficult to make a prediction about a long term therapy response.

In contrast, H3-thymidine uptake appears to be more suited as an indicator of the proliferative capacity of tumor cells. It seems that using some metabolic substances as FDG, thymidine and amino acids together allows a more precise evaluation about a long term tumor response to therapy.

Conclusion

The presented studies submitted show that already at an early stage after beginning of a therapy changes in metabolism can be assessed with radioactive metabolic tracers. Further investigations are required to have more generally valid findings concerning early tumor effects after a therapy as a prediction for long term therapy response.

References

1. Abe Y, Matsuzawa T, Fujiwara T et al (1986) Assessment of radiotherapeutic effects on experimental tumors using F-18-fluoro-2-deoxy-D-glucose. Eur J Nucl Med 12:325–328
2. Haberkorn U, Strauss LG, Dimitrakopoulou A et al (1991) PET studies of fluorodeoxyglucose metabolism in patients with recurrent colorectal tumors receiving radiotherapy. J Nucl Med 3:1485–1490
3. Higashi K, Clavo A, Wahl RL (1993) In vitro assessment of 2-fluoro-2-deoxy-D-glucose, L-methionine and thymidine as agents to monitor the early response of a human adeno-carcinoma cell line to radiotherapy. J Nucl Med 34:773–779
4. Ichiya J, Kuwabara Y, Otska M et al (1991) Assessment of response to cancer therapy using fluorine-18-fluorodeoxy-glucose and positron emission tomography. J Nucl Med 32:1655–1660

5. Kubota K, Ishiwata K, Kubota R et al (1991) Tracer feasibility for monitoring tumor radiotherapy: a quadruple tracer study with fluorodeoxyuridine, L-(methyl-C-14)-methionine, (6-H-3-) thymidine, and gallium-67. J Nucl Med 32:2118–2123
6. Minn H, Paul R, Ahonen A (1988) Evaluation of treatment response to radiotherapy in head and neck cancer with fluorine-18-fluorodeoxyglucose. J Nucl Med 29:1521–1525

Address for correspondence:
Prof. Dr. Dr. Reingard Senekowitsch
Nuklearmedizinische Klinik und Poliklinik
Klinikum rechts der Isar
Technische Universität München
Ismaninger Straße 22
D-81675 München, Germany

Autoradiographical studies to evaluate C14-FDG uptake by human tumor cell spheroids as response to radiotherapy

K. Matzen, J. Mattes, Regine Truckenbrodt, Reingard Senekowitsch
Clinic for Nuclear Medicine and Policlinic, Technical University, Munich, Germany

Introduction

One of the characteristics of malignant tumors is an increased glucose uptake due to a higher metabolic demand of neoplastic tissue. With autoradiographical studies the change in uptake of the glucose analogue C14-FDG in tumor cell spheroids after irradiation was investigated and compared with the uptake by unirradiated control spheroids.

The results of the autoradiographical studies were set in relation to the number of viable cells which was determined by the MTT-test that measures cell viability by the activity of mitochondrial dehydrogenases.

The in vitro autoradiography should demonstrate the ability of tomographic procedures as positron emission tomography (PET) using F18-FDG to predict the response of tumor treatment from early alterations of the tumor metabolism.

Material and methods

Autoradiography

Spheroids of SW 707 cells, a human adenocarcinoma cell line were grown as three-dimensional multicellular tumor cell spheroids by the liquid overlay technique. On day 6 of their growth the spheroids were irradiated with 6 Gy. Irradiated and control spheroids were incubated for 1 h at 37 °C in incubation medium containing C14-FDG (37 kBq/ml). Then the spheroids were washed twice in PBS and embedded in Methylan and frozen to –26 °C. 10 mm sections were cut in a cryostat, and the sections sealed in contact with x-ray film for five days.

MTT-test

The MTT-test measures the activity of the mitochondrial dehydrogenases of viable cells. The yellow 3-(4,5-dimethylthiazol-2-yl)-2,5-diphenyl-tetrazolium bromide (MTT) penetrates into spheroids and is taken up by the tumor cells. The ring of the tetrazolium molecule is broken up by the mitochondrial dehydrogenases, resulting in the water insoluble dark-blue formazan.

The test is an indicator for the viability of the cells. The calibration curve allows to relate the MTT-extinction value to a defined number of viable cells. Six different cell concentrations in 50 ml incubation medium were prepared for the calibration curve. After an incubation time of 4 h in MTT-solution and the addition of DMSO (dimethylsulfoxide) the optical density was measured photometrically at 490 nm (figure 1). The same procedure was applied to spheroids after their mechanical disaggregation.

Results

The evaluation of the MTT-viability-test proved that 1 h after irradiation the number of the viable cells of irradiated spheroids was decreased by about 25% compared to control spheroids from 2608 to 2008 (figure 2).

24 h and 48 h after irradiation the number of viable cells in the control spheroids increased according to the growth curve to 3417 and 3565 cells per spheroid. The amount of viable cells in the irradiated spheroids remained unchanged during the same time interval with approximately 2200 viable cells (figure 2).

The autoradiographic sections of spheroids 1 h after irradiation with 6 Gy showed a clear

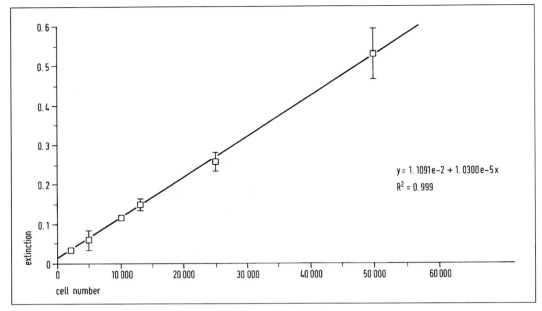

Figure 1. MTT-calibration-curve.

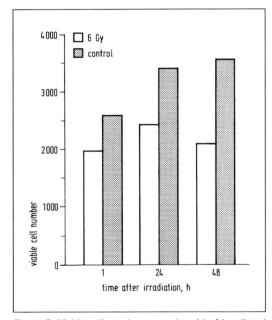

Figure 2. Viable cell number per spheroid of irradiated and control spheroids calculated from the MTT calibration curve.

reduction in FDG-accumulation in comparison with untreated control spheroids. 1.5 h after irradiation, however, the spheroids demonstrated an increase in FDG uptake. The further autoradiographical examinations 24 h and 48 h after irradiation indicate a decrease of FDG uptake compared to the control.

Discussion and conclusion

The irradiated spheroids with a lower number of viable cells are characterisized by an increase in FDG-uptake after irradiation. In comparison untreated control spheroids with a higher number of viable cells showed a lower FDG-uptake than the irradiated spheroids. A possibility to explain the time-dependent uptake of FDG in spheroids after irradiation can be seen as a result of repair mechanisms. How far membrane effects after irradiation are responsible for the variability of FDG uptake of spheroids has to be clarified by further studies. The exact evaluation of the variable FDG uptake of spheroids after irradiation allows a non-invasive prediction of an early response of tumors to radio- or chemotherapy preceding morphological changes.

References

1. Hoekstra OS, Ossenkoppele GJ, Golding R et al (1993) Early treatment response in malignant lymphoma, as determined by planar fluorine-18-fluorodeoxyglucose scintigraphy. J Nucl Med 34:1706–1710
2. Ichiya Y, Kuwabara Y, Otsuka M et al (1991) Assessment of response to cancer therapy using fluorine-18-fluorodeoxyglucose and positron emission tomography. J Nucl Med 32:1655–1660
3. Kubota R, Yamada S, Kubota K et al (1992) Intratumoral distribution of fluorine-18-fluorodeoxyglucose in vivo: high accumulation in macrophages and granulation tissues studied by microautoradiography. J Nucl Med 33:1972–1980
4. Lindholm P, Leskinen-Kallio S, Minn H et al (1993) Comparison of fluorine-18-fluorodeoxyglucose and carbon-11-methionine in head and neck cancer. J Nucl Med 34:1711–1716
5. Minn H, Paul R (1992) Cancer treatment monitoring with fluorine-18-2-fluoro-2-deoxy-D-glucose and positron emission tomography: frustration or future. Eur J Nucl Med 19:921–924

Address for correspondence:
Prof. Dr. Dr. Reingard Senekowitsch
Nuklearmedizinische Klinik und Poliklinik
Klinikum rechts der Isar
Technische Universität München
Ismaninger Straße 22
D-81675 München, Germany

Workshop 1

10 Years CA 19-9 and CA 125

CA 19-9 and CA 125 –
10 Years Hamburg Symposia on Tumor Markers

R. Klapdor
Medical Department, University of Hamburg, Germany

The clinical introduction of the new tumor associated antigens CA 125 and CA 19-9 in 1983, defined by monoclonal antibodies and determined by assay systems using monoclonal antibodies, opened a new area in the field of tumor diagnosis and therapy.

Monoclonal antibodies could be expected as a new and promizing tool to improve serological diagnosis as well as the results of immunoscintigraphy and immunotherapy, by detection and clinical introduction of new and highly sensitive and specific tumor makers or tumor associated substances and by providing the clinicians with monoclonal antibodies in amounts necessary to develop clinically relevant methods of immunoscintigraphy and immunotherapy.

The 15 presentations given at the 1st Hamburg Symposium on Tumor Markers in 1983 confirmed the results published by *del Villano* et al. and *Bast* et al. in 1983 in that way that since CA 19-9 and CA 125 represent the tumor markers of choice for exocrine pancreatic and ovarian cancer respectively, with sensitivities between 80–90% at time of primary diagnosis using cut-offs based on a 95% specificity. However, they did also confirm, that both markers could not fullfill the criteria of so-called ideal markers: they do not allow early diagnosis or screening for early cancers in the asymptomatic population and they do not fulfill the criteria of organ and /or tumor specificity.

As a consequence, the introduction of these new markers was followed by evaluation of their clinical relevance in serological diagnosis and immunohistology. At the same time several groups startet to evaluate the potential clinical relevance of immunoscintigraphy and immunotherapy using monoclonal antibodies directed against these antigens. In contrast to trials with anti-CA 19-9 antibodies immunoscintigraphy and immunotherapy with anti-CA 125 antibodies still represent an actual and interesting theme.

In correlation to the increasing number of newly detected tumor associated antigens and the increasing interest in tumor marker determinations in the following years we find an increasing number of assay systems introduced by manufacturers with a trend from RIA/IRMA assays to non-RIA assays like EIA or LIA and with the trend from manual to semi- or automized tests.

These trends again reinforced increasing efforts concerning quality control and standardization since the beginning of the nineties and trials to handle effectively problems like hook effects or HAMA interference.

The Hamburg Tumor Marker Symposia 1–6 as well as the actual 7th Symposium reflect these developments and trends during the past decade (1–6).

The number of presentations did increase from 15 in 1983 to about 40, 60, 110 up to about 120 in 1991. The actual 7th Symposium comprises more than 250 oral or poster presentations in main sessions, workshops or within the Satellite Symposium. The number of participants increased from about 20 in 1983 to more than 400 in 1991. Since 1986 the offical languages of the Sympsosia are German and English. The themes extended from serological diagnosis with CA 19-9 and CA 125 antigens in 1983 to immunohistochemical studies, various aspects of immunoscintigraphy and immunotherapy, newer fields of tumor diagnosis like oncogenes, cytokines and receptors and actually gene technology as well as e.g. to new disease entities, like immunodeficient syndromes.

Standardization and quality control are main themes since 1989, automation since 1991. The working group Standardization and Quality Control under the Auspices of the Hamburg Symposia on Tumor Markers was founded in 1991. The actual 7th Symposium on Tumor Markers includes the 6th Meeting of this international "European" standardization working group.

The submitted abstracts of the Hamburg Symposia have been published in Abstract books, the final presentations mainly as original papers in Proceedings of increasing volumes, from 261 pages in 1984 to 788 pages in 1991 and more than 850 pages in the Proceedings of the 7th Hamburg Symposium on Tumor Markers in 1993 (1–6).

The presentations of the workshop "10 Years CA 19-9 and CA 125" will focus your attention to some of these developments during the past decade on the following pages of these Proceedings.

References

1. New Tumour Associated Antigens – Two years clinical experience with monoclonal antibodies. 2nd Sympsoium on tumor markers, Hamburg. Greten H, Klapdor R (eds) Georg Thieme, Stuttgart-New York, 1986, 261 pages
   This volume includes the abstracts of the 1st Hamburg Symposium on Tumor Markers (pp 238–261)
2. Clinical Relevance of New Monoclonal Antibodies. 3rd Symposium on tumour markers, Hamburg. Greten H, Klapdor R (eds) Georg Thieme, Stuttgart, New York, 1986, 455 pages
3. New Tumour Markers and their Monoclonal Antibodies – Actual clinical relevance for diagnosis and therapy of solid tumors. 4th Symposium on tumour markers, Hamburg. Klapdor R (ed) Georg Thieme, Stuttgart, New York, 1987, 592 pages
4. Recent Results in Tumor Diagnosis and Therapy. Satellite Symposium: Cancer of the pancreas-state and trends in diagnosis and therapy. 5th Symposium on tumor markers, Hamburg. Klapdor R (ed) Zuckschwerdt, München, Bern, Wien, San Francisco, 1990, 642 pages
5. Tumor Associated Antigens, Oncogenes, Receptors, Cytokines in Tumor Diagnosis and Therapy at the Beginning of the Nineties. Satellite Symposium: Cancer of the breast-state and trends in diagnosis and therapy. 6th Symposium on tumor markers, Hamburg. Klapdor R (ed) Zuckschwerdt, Bern, Wien, San Francisco, 1992, 788 pages
6. Current Tumor Diagnosis: Applications – Clinical Relevance – Research – Trends. Satellite Symposium: Cancer of the lung-state and trends in diagnosis and therapy. 7th Symposium on tumor markers, Hamburg. Klapdor R (ed) Zuckschwerdt, München, Bern, Wien, San Francisco, 1993, 642 pages

Address for correspondence:
Prof. Dr. R. Klapdor
Medizinische Abteilung
Universitätskrankenhaus
Martinistraβe 52
D-20246 Hamburg, Germany

10 years experience of CA 19-9 in patients with pancreatic cancer

C. Haglund, J. Lundin, P. J. Roberts
Fourth Department of Surgery, Helsinki University Central Hospital, Helsinki, Finland

Introduction

CA 19-9 was first described in 1979 by *Koprowski* et al. and the CA 19-9 assay in 1983 by *Del Villano* et al. CA 19-9 is defined by monoclonal antibody 1116 NS 19-9 (19-9 antibody), reacting with sialosyl-fucosyl-lactotetraose, i.e. sialylated Lewis[a] blood group antigen (8, 11). Although the CA 19-9 assay is based on a monoclonal antibody raised against a colorectal carcinoma cell line, it was soon shown to be at its best in the diagnosis of pancreatic cancer and proved to be superior to CEA (4, 7, 13). During the ten years that CA 19-9 has been available for clinical use it has gained a position as reference marker for pancreatic cancer. In this short review, we report our experience on CA 19-9 in the diagnosis and follow-up of patients with pancreatic cancer.

Results

CA 19-9 in the primary diagnosis of pancreatic cancer

Preoperative serum samples from 248 consecutive patients with verified pancreatic cancer were analyzed. Patients were classified according to the UICC TNM-classification: 55 patients had stage I disease, 82 patients stage II–III disease and 111 patients stage IV disease. Most of the patients with stage II–III disease underwent a palliative operation. In these operations, local lymph nodes were not always removed adequately to allow differentiation between stages II and III. Therefore, patients with stage II and III tumors, representing locally spread, non-resectable disease, were combined for analysis.

The serum CA 19-9 concentration was higher than 37 U/ml in 201 out of 248 patients with pancreatic cancer (81%) (figure 1, table I, II). The median value was 575 U/ml, mean 18 422 U/ml, and range < 6.2 – 1 858 900 U/ml. Of these patients, 90 (36%) had a level higher than 1400 U/ml, which was the highest value of the benign group. CA 19-9 was elevated in 37 out of 55 patients with stage I disease (67%), in 71 out of 82 patients with stage II–III disease (67%) and in 93 out of 111 patients with stage IV disease (84%). The CA 19-9 level was significantly higher in stage II–III ($p = < 0.05$) and in stage IV patients ($p = < 0.001$) than in patients with stage I disease. The difference between stage II–III and stage IV patients was not significant ($p = 0.067$). The CA 19-9 level in all stages of pancreatic cancer was significantly higher than in patients with benign diseases ($p = < 0.0001$).

CA 19-9 in benign diseases

The results of cancer patients were compared with a control group, consisting of 238 patients with benign diseases that might cause symptoms and signs similar to those of pancreatic cancer. Benign pancreatic disease was found in 81 patients: 51 patients with acute pancreatitis and 30 with chronic pancreatitis. The 117 patients with benign biliary tract diseases included 60 patients with stones in the common bile duct, 42 patients with gall bladder stones and 15 with acute cholecystitis. Variable degree of cholestasis was seen in 69% of patients with common bile duct stones. Benign liver diseases were seen in 40 patients.

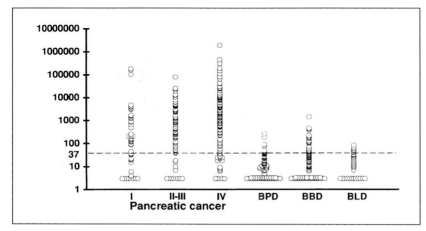

Figure 1. Serum CA 19-9 concentrations in patients with pancreatic cancer, and with benign pancreatic (BPD), biliary (BBD) and liver (BLD) diseases. The cut-off value for the CA 19-9 test is marked with a dashed line.

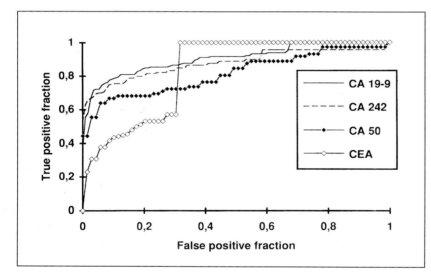

Figure 2. ROC curves for CA 19-9, CA 242, CA 50 and CEA. The true positive fraction was calculated from patients with pancreatic cancer and the false positive fraction from patients with benign pancreatic, biliary and liver diseases.

Table I. Serum CA 19-9 in patients with pancreatic cancer, and patients with benign pancreatic, biliary and liver diseases.

	No.	CA 19-9 > 37 U/ml
Pancreatic cancer	248	81%
stage I	55	67%
stage II–III	82	87%
stage IV	111	84%
Benign diseases	238	21%
benign pancreatic diseases	81	15%
benign biliary diseases	117	26%
benign liver diseases	40	20%

Table II. Assay parameters of the CA 19-9 assay in pancreatic cancer, using the recommended cut-off level and cut-off levels representing the 90% and 95% specificity levels. The specificity was calculated from patients with benign pancreatic, biliary and liver diseases.

Assay parameter	CA 19-9 >37 U/ml	CA 19-9 >72 U/ml	CA 19-9 >170 U/ml
Sensitivity	81%	76%	66%
Specificity	79%	90%	95%
Positive predictive value	80%	89%	93%
Negative predictive value	80%	89%	93%

The serum concentration of CA 19-9 was increased above the cut-off level of 37 U/ml in 50 out of 238 patients with benign diseases of the pancreas, biliary tract and liver (21%; median 12.5 U/ml; mean 40 U/ml; range < 6.2–1400 U/ml) (figure 1, table I, II). The CA 19-9 level was elevated in 30 out of 117 patients with benign biliary diseases (26%) and in eight patients with benign liver disease (20%). In benign pancreatic diseases CA 19-9 was elevated in five patients with chronic and seven patients with acute pancreatitis (15%).

Comparison of CA 19-9 with CEA, CA 50 and CA 242

The CEA level was available in 207 patients with pancreatic cancer and in 130 patients with benign diseases. Using linear regression there was no correlation between CA 19-9 and CEA ($r^2 = 0.197$). The sensitivity of CA 19-9 (81% > 37 U/ml) was clearly higher than that of CEA (46% > 5 ng/ml). This has also been shown previously (4, 13). CA 50 is closely related to CA 19-9 (9). The CA 50 antibody like the CA 19-9 antibody reacts with sialylated Lewis[a] (12). CA 242 is a novel tumor marker, also closely related to CA 19-9 (10). The antigenic detrminant of this new marker is still not defined. Receiver operating characteristic (ROC) curve analysis showed almost identical curves for CA 19-9 and CA 242, whereas CA 19-9 was superior to both CA 50 and CEA (figure 2). Only some patients with advanced disease had an elevated CEA level, but a normal CA 19-9 level. There was no advantage of combining CA 19-9 and CEA, which has also been shown previously (4). Neither was there any advantage of combining CA 19-9 with CA 50 or CA 242 (5, 6).

CA 19-9 in jaundiced patients

Patients with benign disease and an elevated serum bilirubin level (> 20 μmol/l) had significantly higher mean serum CA 19-9 concentration than patients with a normal bilirubin level ($p < 0.05$). In cancer patients, the difference between patients with elevated versus normal bilirubin level was not significant in any stage group. CA 19-9: stage I, $p = 0.78$; stage II–III, $p = 0.13$; stage IV, $p = 0.10$.

Using linear regression there was no correlation between the serum levels of tumor markers CA 19-9 and serum bilirubin ($r^2 = 0.11$) and alkaline phosphatase ($r^2 = 0.07$).

CA 19-9 in postoperative monitoring of radically operated patients with pancreatic cancer

We have used CA 19-9 in postoperative monitoring of patients with pancreatic cancer operated for cure. Out of 23 analyzed patients, 15 patients had verified recurrence. In ten out of 15 patients the CA 19-9 value began to increase 3–13 months (mean 7 months) before appearance of other signs of recurrence. In three patients, the CA 19-9 level increased by the time of detection of recurrence, and in one patient the CA 19-9 level slightly increased one month after detection of recurrence. One patient had no CA 19-9 detectable in serum either pre- or postoperatively. Postoperative monitoring of 33 pancreatic cancer patients treated by palliative surgery plus chemotherapy showed a good correlation between the serum level of CA 19-9 and status of the disease, evaluated by radiological methods.

The prognostic value of preoperative serum levels of CA 19-9 in pancreatic cancer

The prognostic value of preoperative serum levels of CA 19-9 was evaluated in 128 patients with pancreatic cancer. The survival of patients whose tumor marker value was below 370 U/ml was significantly longer than those with a preoperative CA 19-9 level higher than 370 U/ml. When patients were classified according to stage, a significant difference in survival was found only in stage II–III patients. The results are described in detail in this book by *Lundin* et al.

Discussion

In our series, CA 19-9 showed an overall sensitivity of 81% for pancreatic cancer. The highest serum levels of CA 19-9 were found in patients with non-resectable disease, which can rather easily be diagnosed also by other clinical, radiological and laboratory investigations. In stage I disease, when surgical treatment with curative intent is possible, 67% of the patients had an elevated CA 19-9 level (> 37 U/ml). If seven patients with resectable stage II–III tumors were included, 69% of patients with resectable disease had an elevated CA 19-9 level.

Because of high correlation of the test results there was no advantage of combining CA 19-9 with CA 242 or CA 50. No correlation was seen between CA 19-9 and CEA. However, a combination of CA 19-9 and CEA increased the sensitivity only by 4%. The majority of patients with elevated CEA and normal CA 19-9 had disseminated disease.

The highest frequency of false positive CA 19-9 levels has been described in patients with extrahepatic jaundice (4, 7, 8, 13), and this was confirmed in this patient series. The highest CA 19-9 serum concentrations in benign diseases have been described in patients with cholangitis (1). In the present study, one patient with a CA 19-9 value of 1400 U/ml had cholangitis. In an unpublished series of patients with cholangitis 13 out of 15 patients with cholangitis had an elevated CA 19-9 serum concentration (*Haglund* et al., unpublished data).

At the time of diagnosis, most patients with pancreatic cancer show extrahepatic cholestasis with elevated serum levels of bilirubin and alkaline phosphatase. It seems obvious that cholestasis contributes to elevated marker levels in these patients. In stage II–IV cancer patients, the mean values of CA 19-9 appeared higher in jaundiced than in non-jaundiced patients, although the difference was not significant. In clinical practice, biliary decompression has been found to reduce the CA 19-9 levels to a variable degree (*Haglund* et al., data not shown). In spite of the higher frequency of elevated marker levels in cancer patients with cholestasis, there was no clear-cut correlation between the serum levels of CA 19-9 in malignant or benign diseases and the serum levels of bilirubin or alkaline phosphatase. This may be explained by the fact that a minority of tumors do not express CA 19-9 (3), and these patients have a normal serum level even though they might be jaundiced. On the other hand, some patients show strong tissue expression and high serum concentration of CA 19-9 without obstruction of the common bile duct.

Preoperatively, chronic pancreatitis can sometimes be very difficult to differentiate from pancreatic cancer. In these patients tumor markers might be helpful. Five out of 20 patients with chronic pancreatitis had an elevated CA 19-9 level (17%). The highest value found in chronic pancreatitis was 265 U/ml. Hence, a clearly elevated tumor marker level strongly indicated malignant disease. On the other hand, 62% of patients with stage I tumors and 39% of patients with stage II–III tumors had a CA 19-9 serum level below 265 U/ml.

Preliminary results indicate that CA 19-9 is a simple and sensitive way of monitoring the postoperative course of patients with pancreatic cancer. In many patients, it gives a lead time of several months before detection of recurrence by other means. Also in patients with a normal preoperative value, the serum concentration of CA 19-9 may increase before or at the time of recurrence.

In conclusion, CA 19-9 has in many studies and in clinical practice been shown to be a useful complement to other methods in the diagnosis of symptomatic patients with pancreatic cancer and in monitoring patients after surgery for cure. An elevated tumor marker level may lead to an intensified search for primary pancreatic cancer or recurrent disease respectively.

References

1. Albert MB, Steinberg WM, Henry IP (1988) Elevated serum levels of tumor marker CA 19-9 in acute cholangitis. Digest Dis Sci 33:1223–1225
2. del Villano BC, Brennan S, Brock P, Bucher C, Liu V, McLure M, Rake B, Westrick B, Schoemaker H, Zurawski VR (1983) Radioimmunometric assay for a monoclonal antibody-defined tumor marker, CA-19-9. Clin Chem 29:549–552
3. Haglund C, Lindgren J, Roberts PJ, Nordling S (1986) Gastrointestinal cancer-associated antigen CA 19-9 in histological specimens of pancreatic tumors and pancreatitis. Br J Cancer 53:189–195
4. Haglund C, Roberts PJ, Kuusela P, Scheinin TM, Mäkelä O, Jalanko H (1986) Evaluation of CA 19-9 as a serum tumor marker in pancreatic cancer. Br J cancer 53:197–202
5. Haglund C, Kuusela P, Jalanko H, Roberts PJ (1987) Serum CA 50 as a tumor marker in pancreatic

cancer: A comparison with CA 19-9. Int J Cancer 39:477–481
6. Haglund C, Lundin J, Kuusela P, Roberts PJ (1994) CA 242, a new tumor marker for pancreatic cancer: A comparison with CA 19-9, CA 50 and CEA. Br J Cancer 70:487–492
7. Jalanko H, Kuusela P, Roberts P, Sipponen P, Haglund C, Mäkelä O (1984) Comparison of a new tumor marker, CA 19-9™, with alpha-fetoprotein and carcinoembryonic antigen in patients with upper gastointestinal diseases. J Clin Pathol 37:218–222
8. Koprowski H, Steplewski Z, Mitchell K, Herlyn M, Herlyn D, Fulner P (1979) Colorectal carcinoma antigens detected by hybridoma antibodies. Somat Cell Genet 5:957–972
9. Lindholm L, Holmgren J, Svennerholm L, Fredman P, Nilsson O, Persson B, Myrvold H, Lagergård T (1983) Monoclonal antibodies against gastrointestinal tumor-associated antigens isolated as monosialogangliosides. Inst Arch Allergy Appl Immun 71:178–181
10. Lindholm L, Johansson C, Jansson E-L, Hallberg C, Nilsson O (1985) An immunometric assay (IRMA) for the CA 50 antigen. In: Holmgren J (ed) Tumor marker antigens. Studentlitteratur, Lund, pp 122–133
11. Magnani JL, Nilsson B, Brockhaus M, Zopf D, Steplewski Z, Koprowski H, Ginsburg V (1982) A monoclonal antibody-defined antigen associated with gastrointestinal cancer is a ganglioside containing sialylated lacto-n-fucopentaose II. J Biol Chem 257:14365–14369
12. Månsson JE, Fredman P, Nilsson O, Lindholm L, Holmgren J, Svennerholm L (1985) Chemical structure of carcinoma ganglioside antigens defined by monoclonal antibody C-50 and some allied gangliosides of human pancreatic adenocarcinoma. Biochim Biophys Acta 834:110–117
13. Steinberg WM, Gelfand R, Anderson KK, Glenn, J, Kurzman SH, Sindelar WF, Toskes PP (1986) Comparison of the sensitivity and specificity of the CA 19-9 and carcinoembryonic antigen assays in detecting cancer of the pancreas. Gastroenterol 90:343

Address for correspondence:
C. Haglund, M.D.
4th Department of Surgery
Helsinki University Central Hospital
Kasarmikatu 11-13
SF-00130 Helsinki 13, Finland

The occurrence of the carbohydrate antigen 19-9 in the organism of man[1]

J. Makovitzky

Department of Pathology, Martin-Luther-University, Halle-Wittenberg, Germany

General remarks

Since the introduction of the hybridoma-technique (11) a great number of new tumor-associated antigens have been found on the surface of the cells and in the serum of the tumor patients. First of these tumor-associated antigens is the carbohydrate antigen 19-9 (CA 19-9). CA 19-9 antigen has been isolated and characterized as the oligosaccharide sialylated lacto-N-fucopentaose II, which is related to Lewis blood group substance (sialylated Lewis[a]) (1, 2, 3, 9, 10, 12). In the first time it has gained great clinical importance for the diagnosis of gastrointestinal tumors, later for differential diagnosis and follow-up of human exocrine pancreatic carcinoma (5, 6, 8). High levels of the CA 19-9 in the serum of patients with benign diseases such as acute and chronic pancreatitis in some of the cases contradict the tumor specifity of this antigen. The immunohistochemical proof of the CA 19-9 in the normal (healthy) tissue of the fetus and adult contradicts the fact, too. One could demonstrate CA 19-9-epitopes immunohistochemically in the fetal large and small intestine, stomach, pancreas and liver. In the adult one could prove CA 19-9 immunohistochemically in the following organs and their malign tumors: glandula submandibularis, glandula parotis, glandula thyreoidea, lung, breast, gastrointestinal tract, liver (biliary ducts-carcinoma) exocrine pancreas, ovary, endometrium, prostatic gland and vesicula seminalis (4, 13, 14, 15, 17, 18). However, *Uhlenbruck* et al. have detected a CA 19-9 positivity in human saliva, gastric juice, meconium, pancreatic secretion, amniotic fluid, urine, seminal plasma, ovarian cyst fluid and post-colostral milk (21, 22). That means CA 19-9 is neither tumor- nor organ specific. In the clinical practice exists however a high diagnostic sensitivity for the following tumors: exocrine pancreas-, colorectal carcinoma, carcinoma of the stomach and bile ducts (5, 6, 8, 13).

Own examinations

We have tested the glycoprotein nature of the carbohydrate antigen CA 19-9 by sialidase digestion and chemical desialylation, i.e. acid and alkaline hydrolysis.
According to this reaction we have found in examined tissues a CA 19-9 negative immunohistochemical reaction with anti CA 19-9, thus proving the glycoprotein nature of this antigen in our routinely fixed paraffin-embedded material (14, 15). We detected a discontinuous and sometimes weak positivity in the small, medium and large branches of the pancreatic duct from autopsy-material of individuals aged between four days and 80 years and two fetal pancreatic glands (at 29 and 31 weeks gestation). Based on these examinations CA 19-9 is an oncofetal antigen. The monoclonal antibody defined CA 19-9 is specific for human tissue, it does not show any reactions with pancreas or any other tissue of the rat. Futhermore we could confirm the examinations from various authors (5, 6, 8, 17, 18) on different normal and tumor tissue.

---

[1] Dedicated to *Professor Dr. Sabine von Kleist* (Freiburg i. Br., FRG) on the occasion of her 60th birthday.

CA 19-9 reaction in pancreatic tissue

Normal pancreas

Fetal and adult ductal epithelial cells were labeled with anti-CA 19-9 in membrane bound pattern.

Chronic pancreatitis

In chronic pancreatitis the reaction pattern did not differ from that in normal pancreas.

Exocrine pancreatic carcinoma

The CA 19-9 (and CA-50) antigens exhibited a change in cellular expression pattern between well differentiated (G1) carcinomas on one side, and moderately to poor differentiated (G2/G3) carcinomas on the other; their antigen localization was predominantly membrane-bound in G1, and more cytoplasmatic in G2/G3 carcinomas. Lewis[a] and Lewis[b] negative individuals did not show a positive reaction with CA 19-9. Because anti-CA 19-9 binds in chronic pancreatitis as well as in pancreatic carcinoma, and the difference between them is merely quantitative, the presence of CA 19-9 epitopes and the binding of anti-CA 19-9 to them does not allow discrimination between benign and malignant processes in the pancreas.
The reaction is of greater intensity in chronic pancreatitis, whilst in carcinoma of the exocrine pancreas a massive expression is found, which corresponds to the elevated serum value. Thus the tissue reaction is not appropriate in the discrimination of chronic pancreatitis from pancreas carcinoma and the possibility of demonstrating a transition from chronic pancreatitis to pancreas carcinoma cannot be fulfilled.
The antigen CA 19-9 was the starting point for the clinical and immunhistochemical use from the Lewis blood group family and CA-50 (7, 16, 19, 20, 22).

References

1 Arends JW, Verstynen C, Bosman T, Hilgers J, Steplewski Z (1983) Distribution of monoclonal antibody-defined monoganglioside in normal and cancerous human tissues: An immunoperoxidase study. Hybridoma 2:219–229
2 Ernst C, Atkinson B, Wysocka M (1984) Monoclonal antibody localization of A and B isoantigens in normal and malignant fixed human tissues. Am J Pathol 117:451–456
3 Del Villano BC, Brenan S, Brock P, Bucher C, Liu V, McClure M, Rake B, Space S, Westrick B, Schoemaker H, Zurawski VR Jr (1983) Radio-immunometric assay for a monoclonal antibody-defined tumour marker CA 19-9. Clin Chem 29:549–552
4 Göhring UJ, Scharl A, Crombach G, Vierbuchen M, Göttert Th (1992) CA 19-9: A differentation marker for adenocarcinomas of the Müllerian Duct. In: Klapdor R (ed) Recent results in tumor diagnosis and therapy. 5th Symposium on Tumor Markers. Zuckschwerdt, München, Bern, Wien, San Francisco, pp 362–365
5 Haglund C, Lindgren J, Roberts PJ, Nordlings S (1986) Tissue expression of the tumor marker CA 50 in benign and malignant pancreatic lesions. A comparison with CA 19-9. Int J Cancer 38:841–846
6 Haglund C, Lindgren J, Roberts PJ, Nordling S (1986) Gastrointestinal cancer associated antigen CA 19-9 in histological specimens of pancreatic tumours and pancreatitis. Brit J Cancer 53:189–195
7 Hanisch FG, Auerbach B, Bosslet K, Kolbe K, Karsten U, Nakahara Y, Ogawa T, Uhlenbruck G. Monoclonal antibody BW494 a blood group Lewis a/type 1 chain-related antigen on carcinoma-associated mucins. Hoppe Seyler's Z Physiol Chem (in press)
8 Jalanko H, Kuusela P, Roberts P, Sipponen P, Haglund C, Mäkelä O (1984) Comparison of a new tumour marker CA 19-9 TM, with alfa-fetoprotein and carcinoembyonic antigen in patients with upper gastrointestinal diseases. J Clin Path 37:218–222
9 Koprowski H, Steplewski Z, Mitchell K, Herlyn M, Herlyn D, Fuhrer P (1979) Colorectal carcinoma antigens detected by hybridoma antibodies. Somatic Cell Mol Genet 5:957–972
10 Koprowski H, Steplewski Z, Herylin M, Sears HF (1981) Specific antigen in serum of patients with colon carcinoma. Science 212:53–55
11 Köhler G, Milstein C (1975) Continuous cultures of fused cells secreting antibody of predefined specificity. Nature 256:495–497
12 Magnani JL, Nilsson B, Brockhaus M, Zopf D, Steplewski Z, Koprowski H, Ginsburg V (1982) A monoclonal antibody-defined antigen associated with gastrointestinal cancer is a ganglioside containing sialylated lacto-N-fucopentaose II. J Biol Chem 257:14365-14369.
13 Magnani JL, Steplewski Z, Koprowski H, Ginsburg V (1983) A gastrointestinal and pancreatic cancer-

associated antigen in human sera detected by monoclonal antibodies is a mucin. Fed Proc 42:2096

14. Makovitzky J (1986) The distribution and localization of the monoclonal antibody-defined antigen 19-9 (CA 19-9) in chronic pancreatitis and pancreatic carcinoma. Virchows Arch (Cell Pathol) 51:535–544

15. Makovitzky J (1987) The localization and distribution of the carbohydrate antigen 19-9 (CA 19-9) in chronic pancreatitis and pancreatic carcinoma. In: Klapdor R (ed) New tumour markers and their monoclonal antibodies:actual clinical relevance for diagnosis and therapy of solid tumours. 4th Symposium on tumour markers. Thieme, Stuttgart, pp 359–364

16. Mollicone R, Bara J, Le Pendu J, Oriol R (1985) Immunohistologic pattern of type 1 (Le a, Le b) and type 2 (X, Y H) blood group-related antigens in the human pyloric and duodenal mucosae. Lab Invest: 53:219-227

17. Prantl F (1987) Expression des tumorassoziierten Antigens CA 19-9 in benignen und malignen Tumoren der Glandula parotis. Tumor Diagnostik Therapie 8:64–68

18. Prantl F, Johannes A (1986) Vorkommen und Verteilung des tumorassoziierten Antigens CA 19-9 in der Glandula submandibularis des Menschen. Tumor Diagnostik Therapie 7:171–174

19. Schwenk J, Makovitzky J (1989) Comparative study on the expression of the blood groups antigens Le a, Le b, Le x, Le y and the carbohydrate antigens CA 19-9 and CA-50 in chronic pancreatitis and pancreatic carcinoma. Virchows Arch A (Pathol Anat) 414:465–476

20. Schwenk J, Makovitzky J (1990) The occurence of carbohydrate antigens CA 19-9, CA-50) in chronic pancreatitis and pancreatic carcinoma. Acta Histochem Suppl XXXVIII, pp 183–187

21. Uhlenbruck G, van Meensel-Maene U, Hanisch FG, Dienst C (1984) Unexpected occurence of the CA 19-9 tumor marker in normal human seminal plasma. Hoppe Seyler's Z Physiol Chem 365:613–617

22. Uhlenbruck G, Höller U, Heising J, van Mil A, Dienst C (1985) Sialylated Le a blood group substances detected by the monoclonal antibody CA 19-9 in human seminal plasma and other organs. Urol Res 13:223–226

Address for correspondence:
Prof. Dr. med. J. Makovitzky
Institut für Pathologie
Martin-Luther-Universität
Magdeburger Strasse 14
D-06097 Halle/Saale, Germany

10 years experience with the tumor marker CA 125 in ovarian cancer

A critical review

W. Meier[a], Petra Stieber[b], L. Baumgartner[a], U. Hasholzner[b], A. Fateh-Moghadam†[b]

[a]Department of Obstetrics and Gynecology, Department of [b]Clinical Chemistry, Klinikum Großhadern, Ludwig-Maximilians-University, Munich, Germany

Introduction

CA 125 is an antigenic determinant expressed by epithelial ovarian tumors and other tissues of Müllerian origin (1, 19). The function of CA 125 is still unknown and information about the nature of this antigen is limited (19). Serum levels can be measured with a radioimmunoassay by means of the monoclonal antibody OC 125, which was first described by *Bast* (2, 3). Despite of an excellent correlation with the course of disease, CA 125 – measurable in the serum by various immunoassays today – has not yet been well established in therapy decisions. After measuring CA 125 serum levels over a period of more than ten years, a critical review about its further role in the treatment of ovarian cancer is necessary.

CA 125 in primary therapy

A lot of studies have demonstrated a high sensitivity of pre-operative CA 125 levels especially in serous cystadenocarcinomas of the ovary (2, 3, 5, 7, 9, 11, 12, 13, 21, 22, 23, 28, 32, 36). Using an upper limit of 35 U/ml serum levels were elevated in about 97% of the cystadenocarcinomas and in about 87% of all ovarian carcinomas. Also in 65% of the mucinous carcinomas elevated CA 125 levels could be demonstrated (5, 7, 22). On the other hand, elevated values can be found in other malignancies and even in benign gynecological disease, i.e. endometriosis, benign ovarian tumors and pregnancy (2, 20, 22, 28).

There is general agreement that CA 125 levels are related to the stage and histology of the ovarian tumor, only a few investigators found a significant correlation between the grade of tumor and CA 125 levels (7, 29). Consequences cannot be drawn of this results, because in several cases high CA 125 levels are accompanied by low stage malignancy and low levels can be found even in stage IV tumors.

Until now no correlation between pre-operative CA 125 levels and disease outcome could be demonstrated. Only patients with levels below 65 U/ml showed a better prognosis than patients with more than 65 U/ml (8, 25). But these findings are consistent with the relation to stage of disease and pre-operative levels. Patients with early-stage disease rarely have high CA 125 levels and are known to have an optimal prognosis. On the other side the majority of ovarian malignancies are disseminated at the time of first diagnosis, associated with elevated CA 125 values and have a very poor outcome. Postoperative CA 125 values reflect the tumor burden after primary surgery and cannot be used as independent prognostic factors.

Although ovarian cancer patients respond to a variety of chemotherapeutic agents, there are still many who have a poor outlook. An early predictor of good or bad responders would be useful so that treatment decisions could be made earlier than in the current clinical practice after six cycles of chemotherapy. Therefore the prognostic significance of CA 125 half-life (6, 14, 16, 18, 24, 26, 34) and the rate of fall of CA 125 post-operatively was investigated in 220 of our own ovarian cancer patients. Former studies by *van der Burg* 1988 (34) are lacking of a very low number of investigated patients.

CA 125 half-life for individual cases was calculated with the formula first described by *van der Burg* 1988 (34):

$T1/2 = dT/_2 \log(CA1/CA2)$.

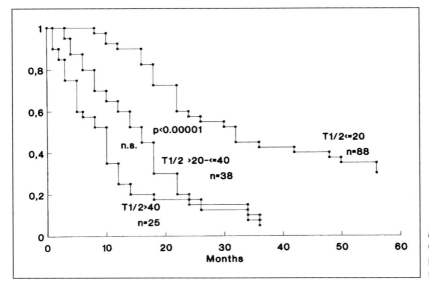

Figure 1. Survival and CA 125 half-life in patients with stage III und IV disease.

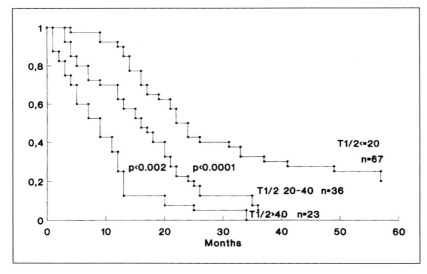

Figure 2. Survival and CA 125 half-life in patients with residual tumor after primary surgery.

CA1 is the pre-therapeutic value, CA2 the first normal CA 125 value or the lowest CA 125 value, if CA 125 did not normalize within three months after start of therapy, and dT is the time in days between CA1 and CA2. The patients were grouped as having half-life values less or more than 20 days. In addition, patients with serum CA 125 half-life of more than 20 days were grouped as having intermediate values between 20 and 40 days and highest values above 40 days. CA 125 half-life increased with tumor stage, showing 22% of the patients with stage I and 58% of patients with stage IV disease as having elevated half-life values. CA 125 half-life was also depending on residual tumor size after primary surgery. 26% of the patients with macroscopically free disease showed elevated values, compared with 51% of elevated half-life values in patients with residual tumor of more than 2 cm. No correlation could be found between elevated values and tumor grade.

Considering only patients with FIGO stage III and IV, median survival was significantly greater (p < 0.00001) in patients with the shorter CA 125 half-life. Median survival in this group was 42 months compared with only 15 months in the group with half-life values above 20 days (figure 1). No difference was seen between patients with intermediate half-life and patients with values of more then 40 days. Time to progression also achieved statistical significance (p < 0.00001) between the main groups with values lower and higher than 20 days.

Concerning the prognostic outcome, patients with residual tumor after primary surgery are of special interest. Even in this worst prognostic group serum CA 125 half-life can distinguish significantly different groups (figure 2). Patients with short half-life show a median survival of 34 months compared with only 14 months in patients with long half-life values. Discriminating patients with high half-life values in the intermediate group and in a group with more than 40 days, significant differences in median survival between all groups can be demonstrated. Median survival in the intermediate group was 17 months compared with 9 months in the long half-life group (p < 0.002). Time to progression achieved statistically is also significant (p < 0.002).

Taking 20 days as prognostic limit of CA 125 half-life in patients with residual disease after primary surgery, positive predictive value concerning death within two years was 81% with a negative predictive value of 57%. If the prognostic limit is calculated as 40 days, positive predictive value was 91 % with a negative predictive value of 46%. After confirming the prognostic importance of CA 125 half-life even for patients with residual disease after primary surgery, treatment modifications in primary therapy are possible at an earlier stage. Especially in patients with long CA 125 half-life values a reduction of toxicity by avoidance of ineffective chemotherapy can be achieved. On the other hand treatment modifications could include changes to other drugs or giving increased doses of the original drug if this is possible. Using the CA 125 half-life it should also be possible to adapt treatment of individual patients so that therapy that will not be of long-term benefit is modified as soon as possible.

CA 125 in recurrent disease

Complete surgical cure is not a realistic goal in the majority of epithelial ovarian cancer patients (10, 15, 17, 27, 30, 31, 33, 35). Although most patients respond to first line chemotherapy, the relapse rate is high. At the time of clinical diagnosis, recurrent tumor is likely to be widespread and difficult to treat.

A great number of studies have reported on the correlation between the course of disease and CA 125 serum levels (4, 5, 12, 22, 25, 29). Rising CA 125 levels are a stronger predictor of progressive disease than a falling CA 125 is of

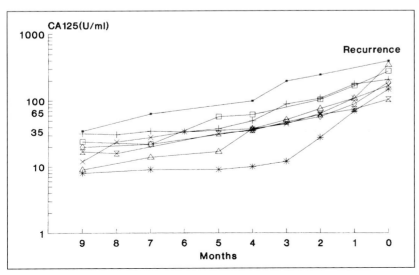

Figure 3. CA 125 lead time in eight patients with recurrent ovarian cancer.

partial or complete remission. In more than 90% of recurrences CA 125 serum levels are elevated several months before clinical occurence of the disease, with a median lead time of 3.6 months (figure 3). In our patients with CA 125 determinations during follow-up we calculated a sensitivity of 92% and a specificity of 89% for detecting recurrent disease. Because of a lower specificity than 100% therapeutic consequences have not yet been drawn from a persistently rising CA 125 level. On the other hand no study has addressed the question of whether earlier detection of recurrent disease by CA 125 monitoring is translated into an improved outlook for the patient. Prospective trials are urgently necessary. In order to get a 100% specificity for detecting recurrence in ovarian cancer patients we graphically determined the grade of increase of CA 125 by regression curves. In 52 patients with recurrence mean grade of CA 125 increase was 75 U/ml/month compared with 4 U/ml/month in 55 patients in clinical remission. Looking at the different ranges of increase, there is no patient in clinical remission with a grade of CA 125 increase of more than 25 U/ml/month. Taking 25 U/ml/month as the upper limit of normal in grade of CA 125 increase, we can achieve a 100% specificity in detecting partially occult recurrences.

The grade of CA 125 increase, first described in this review, can help to improve therapy results in recurrent ovarian cancer patients. We must learn to accept grade of CA 125 increase values of more than 25 U/ml/month as a reliable predictor of recurrence. If elevated CA 125 values can be confirmed after a period of four weeks, grade of CA 125 increase has to be calculated and further diagnostic tools, even as explorative laparotomy, have to be initiated immediately. Only by consequent utilization of these results, therapy in recurrent ovarian cancer can be started at an earlier stage and can help to improve the usually poor outcome in these patients.

Conclusion

In accordance to these results concerning the prognostic importance of CA 125 half-life and the grade of CA 125 increase, an individualized therapy in ovarian cancer patients is possible at an early stage of the course of primary or recurrent disease. The time has come to utilize the full weight of CA 125 data to make treatment decisions rather than to wait for the reappearance of bulky disease.

References

1. Bast RC, Feeney M, Lazarus H, Nadler LM, Colvin RB, Knapp RC (1981) Reactivity of a monoclonal antibody with human ovarian carcinoma. J Clin Invest 68:1331–1337
2. Bast RC, Klug TL, St.John E, Jenison E, Niloff JM, Lazarus H, Berkowitz RS, Leavitt T, Griffiths T, Parker L, Zurawski VR (1983) A radioimmunoassay using a monoclonal antibody to monitor the course of epithelial ovarian cancer. N Engl J Med 309:883–887
3. Bast RC, Klug TL, Schaetzl E, Lavin P, Niloff JM, Greber TF, Zurawski VR, Knapp RC (1984) Monitoring human ovarian carcinoma with a combination of CA 125, CA 19-9 and carcinoembryonic antigen. Am J Obstet Gynecol 149:553–559
4. Berek JS, Knapp RC, Malkasian GD et al (1986) CA 125 serum levels correlated with second-look operations among ovarian cancer patients. Obstet Gynecol 67:685
5. Brioschi PA, Irion O, Bischof C, Bader, M, Forni M, Krauer F (1987) Serum CA 125 in epithelial ovarian cancer. A longitudinal study. Br J Obstet Gynaecol 94:196–201
6. Buller RE, Berman ML, Bloss JD, Manetta A, DiSaia PJ (1991) CA 125 regression: A model for epithelial ovarian cancer response. Am J Obstet Gynaecol 165:360–367
7. Crombach G, Zippel HH, Würz H (1985) Erfahrungen mit CA 125, einem Tumormarker für maligne epitheliale Ovarialtumoren. Geburtsh u Frauenheilk 45:205–212
8. Cruickshank DJ, Fullerton WT, Klopper A (1987) The clinical significance of pre-operative serum CA125 in ovarian cancer. Br J Obstet Gynaecol 94:692–695
9. Daunter, B (1990) Tumor markers in gynecologic oncology. Gynecol Oncol 39:1–15
10. Einzig AI, Wiernik PH, Sasloff J, Runowicz CD, Goldberg GL (1992) Phase II study and long-term follow-up of patients treated with taxol for advanced ovarian adenocarcinoma. J Clin Oncol 10:1748–1753
11. Fioretti P, Gadducci A, Ferdeghini M, Prontera C, Malagnino, G, Facchini V, Mariani G, Bianchi R (1992) The concomitant determination of different serum tumor markers in epithelial ovarian cancer: Relevance for monitoring the response to chemotherapy and follow-up of patients. Gynecol Oncol 44:155–160

12. Fish RG, Shelley MD, Maughan T. Rocker I, Adams M (1987) The clinical value of serum CA 125 levels in ovarian cancer patients receiving platinum therapy. Eur J Cancer Clin Oncol 23:831–835
13. Gallion HH, Hunter JE, van Nagell JR, Averette HE et al (1992) The prognostic implications of low serum CA 125 levels prior to the second-look operation for stage III and IV epithelial ovarian cancer. Gynecol Oncol 46:29–32
14. Hawkins RE, Roberts K, Wiltshaw E. Mundy J, Fryatt IJ, McCready VR (1989) The prognostic significance of the half-life of serum CA 125 in patients responding to chemotherapy for epithelial ovarian carcinoma. Br J Obstet Gynaecol 96:1395–1399
15. Heintz AP, Hacker NF, Berek JS et al (1986) Cytoreductive surgery in ovarian carcinoma: Feasibility and morbidity. Obstet Gynecol 67:783–788
16. Hogberg T, Kagedal B (1990) Serum half-life of the tumor marker CA125 during induction chemotherapy as a prognostic indicator for survival in ovarian carcinoma. Acta Obstet Gynecol Scand 69:423–429
17. Hoskins WJ, Rubin SC, Dulaney E, Chapman D, Almadrones L (1989) Influence of secondary cytoreduction at the time of second-look laparotomy on the survival of patients with epithelial ovarian carcinoma. Gynecol Oncol 34:365–371
18. Hunter VJ, Daly L, Helms M, Soper JT, Berchuck A, Clarke-Pearson DL, Bast RC jr (1990) The prognostic significance of CA 125 half-life in patients with ovarian cancer who have received primary chemotherapy after surgical cytoreduction. Am J Obstet Gynecol 163:1164–1167
19. Kawabat SE, Bast RC, Welch WR, Knapp RC, Colvin RB (1983) Immunopathologic characterization of a monoclonal antibody that recognizes carcinoma surface antigens of human ovarian tumors of serous, endometrioid and clear cell types. Am J Clin Pathol 79:98–104
20. Klug TL, Bast RC, Niloff JM, Knapp RC, Zurawski,VR (1984) Monoclonal antibody immunoradiometric assay for an antigenic determinant (CA 125) associated with human epithelial ovarian carcinoma. Cancer Res 44:1048–1053
21. Kreienberg R (1986) Möglichkeiten und Grenzen der Tumormarkeruntersuchungen in der Nachsorge bei Ovarialkarzinom-Patientinnen. Gynäkologe 19:178–185
22. Meier W, Stieber P, Fateh-Moghadam A, Eiermann W, Hepp H (1987) CA 125 in gynecological malignancies. Eur J Cancer Clin Oncol 23:713–717
23. Meier W, Stieber P, Eiermann W, Schneider A, Fateh-Moghadam A, Hepp H (1989) Serum levels of CA 125 and histological findings at second-look laparotomy in ovarian carcinoma. Gynecol Oncol 35:44–46
24. Meier W, Stieber P, Fateh-Moghadam A, Eiermann W, Hepp H (1992) Prognostische Bedeutung der CA 125-Halbwertszeit für den weiteren Krankheitsverlauf beim Ovarialkarzinom. Geburtsh u Frauenheilk 52:526–532
25. Möbus V, Kreienberg R, Crombach G, Würz H, Caffier H, Kaesemann H, Hoffmann FJ, Schmid-Rhode P, Sturm G, Kaufmann M (1988) Evaluation of CA 125 as prognostic and predictive factor in ovarian cancer. J Tumor Marker Oncol 3:251–258
26. Mogensen O (1992) Prognostic value of CA 125 in advanced ovarian cancer. Gynecol Oncol 44:207–212
27. Morris M, Gershenson DM, Wharton JT, Copeland LJ, Edwards CL, Stringer CA (1989) Secondary cytoreductive surgery for recurrent epithelial ovarian cancer. Gynecol Oncol 34:334–338
28. Niloff JM, Knapp RC, Schaetzl E et al (1984) CA 125 antigen levels in obstetric and gynecologic patients. Am J Obstet Gynecol 151:703–707
29. Niloff JM, Knapp RC, Lavin PT et al (1986) The CA 125 assay as a predictor of clinical recurrence in epithelial ovarian cancer. Am J Obstet Gynecol 155:56–60
30. Omura G, Blessing JA, Ehrlich CE (1987) A randomized trial of cyclophosphamide and doxorubicin with or without cisplatin in advanced ovarian carcinoma. Cancer 56:1725–1728
31. Pfleiderer A (1991) Tumoren des Eierstocks. In: Bender HG (Hrsg) Gynäkologische Onkologie. Thieme, Stuttgart, New York
32. Podczaski E, Whitney C, Manetta A, Larson JE, Kirk J, Stevens CW, Lyter J, Mortel R (1990) Use of CA 125 to monitor patients with ovarian epithelial carcinomas. Gynecol Oncol 33:193
33. Umbach G. (1984) Review of tumor markers for ovarian cancer. Med Hypotheses 13:329–339
34. van der Burg MEL, Lammers FB, van Putten WJL, Stoter G (1988) Ovarian Cancer: The prognostic value of the serum half-life of CA 125 during induction chemotherapy. Gynecol Oncol 30:307–312
35. Wharton J, Edwards C (1984) Cytoreductive surgery for common epithelial tumors of the ovary. Clin Obstet Gynecol 10:235–239
36. Zurawski VR, Knapp RC, Einhorn N, Kenemans P, Mortel R, Ohmi K, Bast RC, Ritts RE, Malkasian GD (1987) An initial analysis of preoperative serum CA125 levels in patients with early stage ovarian carcinoma. Gynecol Oncol 30:7–14

Address for correspondence:
Dr. med. W. Meier
Abteilung für Geburtshilfe und Gynäkologie
Klinikum Großhadern
Ludwig-Maximilians-Universität
Marchioninistraße 15
D-81377 München, Germany

Current status of immunoscintigraphy after ten years of clinical experience

J. F. Chatal, P. Peltier, A. Chetanneau, I. Resche

Nuclear Medicine Division, Centre René Gauducheau, Nantes, France

Introduction

The clinical evaluation of immunoscintigraphy over the last ten years has indicated the advantages, sometimes determinant, of this new imaging method in oncology as well as its methodological limitations. During this decade, technological advances have been rapid concerning the characteristics of the immunospecific radiopharmaceutical agent and, to a lesser degree, the performance of detection equipment. Clinical results have defined the anatomical localizations for which immunoscintigraphy is of significant value compared to other imaging techniques as well as the clinical indications in which it can play a useful role in therapeutic strategy.

After ten years of experience, and in the context of biotechnological developments, it is feasible to consider the future methodological and clinical prospects for immunoscintigraphy specifically from the viewpoint of cost and the benefit to the patient. This analytic approach can be illustrated by the application of immunoscintigraphy in targeting CA 125 antigen associated with ovarian carcinomas.

Technological developments

Radioimmunoconjugates: Whole antibodies have been replaced by fragments, the tumor uptake kinetics of F(ab')2 fragments being more suitable to the longer physical half-life of indium-111, and the rapid tumor kinetics of Fab' fragments to the shorter physical half-life of technetium-99m.
Iodine-131 has been replaced by indium-I11 or technetium-99m, and sometimes by iodine-123.
The chemical labeling of technetium-99m was initially difficult but has been facilitated by the development of simple, rapid and relatively stable direct labeling techniques.
Instrumentation: The technical performances of the gamma cameras used for scintigraphic detection have been improved, particularly in SPECT mode. However, these technical advances in detection have been of less importance than the improvement of radioimmunoconjugate characteristics.

Clinical results

It has been clearly established that immunoscintigraphy is the most efficient imaging technique for detection of abdominopelvic recurrences of adenocarcinomas, particularly ovarian ones (1). In 20 to 30% of cases, it is the only imaging method to visualize occult recurrences, and such early visualization, guided by a rise in the serum concentration of CA 125 marker in the case of ovarian cancer, enables the surgeon to perform total macroscopic resection of the recurrence (2).
Immunoscintigraphy is generally less efficient for other anatomical sites, particularly lung and bone for which computed tomography and bone scan provide clearly superior results.
The indications of immunoscintigraphy have also been defined. It is useful in determining the spread of certain types of carcinoma, particularly small-cell lung cancer, non-Hodgkin's lymphoma and cancer of the prostate for which it can detect lymph node invasion in the pelvis. It is especially useful in the detection of early recurrences of colorectal and ovarian carcinomas and can lead to effective surgical resection. Finally, it is useful before undertaking radioimmunotherapy, particularly for non-Hodgkin's lymphoma, in order to

select the cases in which clear scintigraphic imaging is predictive of good radioimmunotherapeutic results (3).

Future prospects

There are two main drawbacks of immunoscintigraphy at the present time, which unquestionably limit its clinical development. First, the immunogenicity of the murine antibodies used until now often prevents the repetition of examinations. Secondly, tumor to non-tumor ratios are often inadequate to obtain easily interpretable images. It is frequently necessary to resort to the SPECT mode, which can raise problems for physicians lacking the experience required to interpret the images. Moreover, immunoscintigraphy is not accepted by clinicians in the case of cancers for which no effective therapeutic alternative is available. It is thus essential to provide a clear definition of the future indications of this imaging method.

Methodological prospects: One very active research area in the biotechnological field is the synthesis of peptides which mimick the peptide sequences of antibody hypervariable regions corresponding to the sites of antigenic recognition. It will be possible to label these non-immunogenic peptides with technetium-99m and inject them repeatedly. Their rapid kinetics will allow visualization of tumor targets within the first hours after injection.

It will also be possible to use humanized or human antibodies or their fragments characterized by a reduced immogenicity allowing repeated injections. Finally, two-step targeting techniques will provide a very significant increase in tumor to non-tumor ratios and thus allow clear visualization of tumor targets on whole-body images. Many of these techniques are currently being developed through the use of bifunctional immunoconjugates (4), the avidin-biotin system, the DNA-DNA system or the enzyme-enzyme inhibitor system. The most promising application of these two-step techniques is for radioimmunotherapy.

Clinical prospects: In addition to solely iconographic factors independent of the clinical situation, it is advisable to consider the indications in which immunoscintigraphy can be truly beneficial for the patient within the context of therapeutic strategy.

As radioimmunotherapy of epithelial tumors is only feasible for curative purposes when there are microscopic residues, it is essential to visualize such recurrences early by immunoscinitigraphy in order to achieve optimal surgical tumor reduction. Such is the case for ovarian cancer in which immunoscintigraphic visualization of a recurrence guided by a rise in CA 125 serum concentration often allows complete and therefore optimal tumor resection. Intraperitoneal radioimmunotherapy can then be effective on the microscopic residual disease by delivering potentially tumoricidal doses greater than 100 Gy (5).

It may be concluded that the potential advantages and limitations of immunoscintigraphy have been defined within the last 10 years. During the next decade, it is likely that this imaging technique will be used in close association with the development of radioimmunotherapy.

References

1. Peltier P, Dutin JP, Chatal JF et al (1993) Bayesian analysis of indium-111-labeled OC125 immunoscintigraphy in the diagnostic strategy of ovarian carcinoma recurrence. Diagn Oncol 3:21–24
2. Peltier P, Dutin JP, Chatal JF et al (1993) Usefulness of imaging ovarian cancer recurrence with In-111-labeled monoclonal antibody (OC125) specific for CA 125 antigen. Ann Oncol 4:307 311
3. Press OW, Eary JF, Appelbaum FR et al (1993) Radiolabeled antibody therapy of B-cell lymphoma with autologous bone marrow support. N Engl J Med 329:1219–1224
4. Le Doussal JM, Chetanneau A, Gruaz-Guyon A et al (1993) Bispecific monoclonal antibody-mediated targeting of an indium-111-labeled DTPA dimer to primary colorectal tumors: phamacokinetics, biodistribution, scintigraphy and immune response. J Nucl Med 34:1662–1671
5. Bardies M, Thedrez P, Gestin JF et al (1992) Use of multicell spheroids of ovarian carcinoma as an intraperitoneal radio immunotherapy model: uptake, retention kinetics and dosimetric evaluation. Int J Cancer 50:984–991

Address for correspondence:
Prof. Dr. J. F. Chatal
Laboratoire de Recherche, INSERM U.211
Institute de Biologie – CHR
9, Quai Moncousu
F-44035 Nantes Cédex 01, France

Achievements, failings and promises of radioimmunotherapy

K. N. Syrigos, A. A. Epenetos

Department of Clinical Oncology, Royal Postgraduate Medical School, Hammersmith Hospital, London, UK

Introduction

The management of cancer by exploiting properties distinguishing neoplastic and normal cells has always been an attractive concept. Hybridoma technology and the resulting tumor-associated monoclonal antibodies (MoAb) offered new prospects on that strategy, expecting to decrease the side effects, by increasing the specificity of tumor localization. Some of the applications of MoAb to oncology include immunohistochemistry, radioimmunodetection and immunotherapy with "naked" MoAbs, or MoAbs conjugated with a toxic agent such as drugs, toxins, enzymes and isotopes (1).

The use of MoAbs as carriers of high activity radionuclides for the treatment of malignant diseases (radioimmunotherapy, RIT) spurred an unprecedented effort in oncology and nuclear medicine research, with the main field of interest being the surgically inaccessible tumors, the recurrences and the distant metastases. The MoAb-isotope conjugate, after binding to the target cell and delivering a lethal radiation dose, could offer the advantage of killing many untargeted cells through "crossfire irradiation" (2). This distribution of the cytotoxic activity by the radiolabeled MoAb could, in theory, be the solution to the considerable problem of tumor heterogeneity in antigen expression. Unfortunately, but not surprisingly, the clinical application of the above model proved to be rather more complicated.

The radioimmunoconjugate

The choice of the most effective radionuclide has been the issue of intensive study. The ideal isotope should have decay compatible with the carrier MoAb's biological half-life in the human body. 131I, one of the earliest used isotopes for the treatment of thyroid malignancies, is the first and commonest applied in radioimmunotherapy studies, not only because of its availability and moderate cost, but also because of the easy technique of protein halogenation. Unfortunately, the emission of unwanted y-radiation, its β-particles of low energy and the potential decrease of its biological half-life in the tumor area by tissue dehalogenases (3, 4), made it less than ideal and led to the use of other radionuclides for RIT, such as the ^{90}Y, ^{153}Sm, ^{166}Rh, ^{168}Rh, ^{111}At, ^{32}P, ^{199}Au and ^{212}Bi. Some of the isotope selection criteria include 1. the physical data of the radionuclide: half-life, type of energy produced. Dosimetry studies on artificial models indicate that for tumors diameter bigger than 1 cm high energy beta-emitters are more effective, while for smaller tumors medium energy beta-emitters should be prefered; unfortunately one cannot expect all malignant nodules to be of uniform size in vivo (5, 6); 2. the rate of particulate radiation to gamma-ray energy, 3. the specific activity of the isotope per amount of MoAb's (MBq/mg), which mainly depends on the method of radiolabeling, 4. the availability and cost of the isotope, the convenience and efficiency of the labelling technique, the stability of the conjugate (7) and 5. the tumor radiosensitivity.

Table I. Examples of isotopes with potential value in RIT.

Isotope	Decay mode	Half-life
Rhenium-186	beta	3.5 days
Yttrium-90	beta	2.5 days
Iodine-131	beta	8 days
Iodine-125	electron capture	60 days

The choice of the antibody to be radiolabeled greatly depends on the tumor antigenic expression and the accessibility, the macro- and microdistribution, the kinetics and the in vivo stability of the MoAb. When an antibody is injected into the blood stream only 0.007%–0.01% of it finally targets to the tumor. The rest of it, passing through the body compartments (vascular network, organs and body fluid) is catabolised and excreted. Furthermore, some MoAbs bind to tumor antigen present in normal organs, such as the liver. Other factors interfering with MoAb targeting include the antigen size, density, location and accessibility (8). The perfect MoAb-isotope combination should have pharmacokinetics, physical half-lives and emission matched to achieve the biggest therapeutic ratio. As stability of the radioconjugate is of great importance, efforts have been made to improve the labeling techniques and chelator efficiency. For example, for isotopes such as ^{90}Y, previously used chaletor DTPA (diethylene-triamine-pentaacetic acid) has been replaced by new chelators, such as DOTA (2-p-nitrobenzyl – 1, 4, 7, 10- tetraazocylododecane – N, N', N", N'''-tetracetic acid), CITC ((s)-4-[2,3 bis [bis (carboxymethyl) amino] propyl]-phenyl-isothyocyanate of DTPA) and TETA (6-p-nitrobenzyl-1,4,8,11-tetraazocyclotetradecane-N, N', N", N'''-tetraacetic acid), which provide more stability in vivo and allow the administration of the amount to be calculated with accuracy (9, 10, 11).

Systemic radioimmunotherapy

Promising results have been obtained in the treatment of lymphomas and chronic lymphocytic leukemia using MoAb given intravenously (12). These malignancies offer good access to antibodies, in contrast to epithelial solid tumors where poor access is a limiting factor. The inner parts of the tumor often have relatively impaired blood flow compared to the surface area and, as the tumor's blood supply is from the surface inwards, the MoAbs have poor access to the core of the tumor. MoAbs' penetration of the tumor is made even more difficult by the tumor's lack of lymph vessels. In addition, because of the impaired blood flow, the deeper parts of large tumors are less oxygenated and therefore less radiosensitive. The result of all the above is that these parts not only receive less amount of radiolabeled MoAb, but also the radiation delivered is less effective. Preclinical animal studies have suggested that the greater quantity of the antibody administered the deeper the penetration. Increasing the amount of MoAb administered, more radioconjugate is delivered to the tumor, but there is a concomitant increase of deposition in normal tissues, because only a very small percentage of it finally reaches the tumor. It has been estimated that only 1% of the radioactivity administered binds to the tumor, while 30% is excreted and 69% binds normal tissue. Non-specific binding, mainly by the reticuloendothelial tissue and selective accumulation in critical organs, such as the bone marrow, the liver and the spleen, worsen the therapeutic ratio. In fact, bone marrow is the dose limiting organ. Bone marrow toxicity appears principally as thrombocytopenia, arising 4–6 weeks after treatment, but leukopenia has also been described. The extent of hematologic toxicity is dose dependent and more severe in patients being compromised by previous chemotherapy or radiotherapy. Other side effects described after RIT include oesophagitis, diarrhoea and symptoms of allergic reaction against the murine MoAb administered.

The response of the host immune system to the repeated administration of murine protein and the development of human anti-mouse immunoglobulin antibodies (HAMA) is one of the most commonly encountered problems of RIT (13, 14). The clinical manifestations include serum sickness, fever, dyspnea, urticaria and hypotension. HAMA reactions usually occurs two to three weeks after initial administration and usually are unrelated to dose and rate of administration. HAMA responses can intervene with therapy through the impairment of targeting and the enhancemant of the MoAb clearance. Genetic engineering may overcome the HAMA reactions. The production of human and chimeric antibodies, composed of the Fc region of a human IgG immunoglobulin and parts of variable region of a murine globulin, are probably less immunogenic than murine antibodies, although the repeated use of humanised antibodies can lead to anti-isotype and anti-idiotype antibodies. An other alternative for reducing HAMA is the development of small antibody fragments such as the Fab and F(ab)2, single chain antibodies, single domain antibodies and antibody derived oligopeptides (15, 16).

Many innovative approaches are also being developed to resolve the already described poor permeability of the tumor and the non-specific binding. Methods to increase the tumor permeability and consequent MoAb uptake include inducing tumor inflammation, the use of vascular dilators and of external irradiation (17, 18). Another approach is to target structures vital for the survival of the tumor instead of individual tumor cells. As vessels are the main source of nutrients for neoplastic cells, efforts have been made to use MoAbs raised against the tumor vascular endothelium (19).

A novel and rather promising approach is the introduction of bifunctional or bispecific antibodies based on a two- or three- stages administration. An example of this approach is the tumor-associated antibody firstly administered intravenously, without the radionuclide but being conjugated with avidin or streptavidin (modified MoAb). It binds the tumor, where it can remain for a long period. The unbound MoAb is eventually removed from the circulation. This is succeeded by the administration of radiolabeled biotin (second step). The extremely high affinity of biotin for streptavidin (Kd = 10–15 M) leads to enhanced tumor uptake of the radioconjugate while its small molecular size ensures its fast clearance from the circulation via the kidneys. The unconjugated radiolabeled biotin will be cleared quickly by the kidneys and the remaining radioactivity will be mainly tumor bound (20, 21, 22).

Regional radioimmunotherapy

Since access to the tumor site may be a limiting factor in the targeting of solid tumors, other routes of administration, except the systemic one, have been considered for the regional delivery of the radiocongugate. The intraperitoneal route for ovarian carcinoma, the intrathecal for meningeal carcinomatosis, the intravesical for superficial bladder carcinoma and intratumoral routes of administration have been tried at preclinical and clinical levels.

Intraperitoneal RIT as salvage treatment for patients with ovarian cancer has been reported with the use of the MoAbs HMFG1, HMFG2, AUA1, and H17E2. The MoAbs were labeled with ^{131}I or ^{90}Y and injected through a peritoneal dialysis catheter into the peritoneal cavity under local anesthetic and after any ascites had been drained off. When ^{131}I is used, the patient is given potassium iodate or iodide for two days before and for one month after therapy to protect the thyroid gland. The effective dose is thought to be above 150 mCi (23, 24, 25) Side effects described include myelosuppression, abdominal pain, fever and diarrhea.

After intraperitoneal injection, 80% of the given radioactivity is found as free iodine in the urine. Urinary excretion results in reduction of normal tissue irradiation, while a frequent bladder emptying and a high fluid intake are required to decrease absorbion by the bladder wall. RIT for ovarian cancer, using ^{90}Y labeled antibodies, has provided responses in patients with small-volume disease and is currently being evaluated in phase III clinical trials (26).

Intravesical administration of chemo- or immunotherapeutic agents is currently used to reduce the recurrence rate in superficial bladder carcinoma. Recently, the possibility of the intravesical administration of radiolabeled MoAb has been investigated. Biodistribution data showed selective uptake of antibody by tumor cells, with minimal uptake by normal urothelium and no circulating radioactivity in the patients' serum resulting in lack of systemic toxicity (27, 28).

Malignant glioma, a fatal rapidly progressive disease, despite the improvements in neurosurgical and adjuvant therapeutic modalities, has also been the subject of RIT trials. The MoAbs UJ13A, ERIC-1 and MUC 2-63 labeled with ^{111}In, ^{90}Y, or ^{131}I have been administered systematically, intrathecally, or intratumorly. The intratumoral administration of the radioimmunoconjugate has proved to be without systemic and with acceptable acute central nervous toxicity (raised intracranial pressure and brain oedema readily responded to steroids). Although the RIT efficacy needs further evaluation, early results are encouraging (29, 30).

Conclusions

Therapy with radiolabeled MoAbs has an excellent potential for establishing itself as an important part of the treatment of human malignancies. Clinical data presented in this and other studies suggest an encouraging outlook. Regional delivery of the radioimmunocongugate is promising, but further clinical trials are needed to accurately evaluate this approach. The production of chimaeric or human antibodies and of immunoreactive fragments or peptides, as well as the introduction of two- and three- step pretargeting techniques may solve many of the present problems of RIT and lead to its more widespread applications.

References

1. Goldenberg DM (1993) Monoclonal antibodies in cancer detection and therapy. Am J Med 94:297
2. Britton KE, Mather SJ, Granowska M (1991) Radiolabeled monoclonal antibodies in oncology. III. Radioimmunotherapy. Nuclear Medicine Communications 12:333
3. Leichner PK, Klein JL, Garrison JB (1981) Dosimetry of ^{131}I labeled anti-ferritin in hepatoma. A model for radioimmunoglobulin dosimetry. Int J Radiat Oncol Biol Phys 7:323
4. Buchsbaum D, Randall B, Hanna D et al (1985) Comparison of the distribution and fate of monoclonal antibodies labeled with ^{131}I or ^{111}In. Eur J Nucl Med 10:398
5. Humm JL (1986) Dosimetric aspects of radiolabeled antibodies for tumor therapy. J Nucl Med 27:1491
6. Howell RW, Rao DV, Sastry KS (1989) Macroscopic dosimetry for radioimmunotherapy: Non uniform activity distributions in solid tumors. Med Phys 16(1):66
7. Mausner LF, Srivastava SC (1993) Selection of radionuclides for radioimmunotherapy. Med Phys 20(2):503
8. Epenetos AA, Snook D, Durbin H et al (1986) Limitations of radiolabeled monoclonal antibodies for localisation of human neoplasms. Cancer Res 46:3183
9. Moi MK, DeNardo SJ, Meares CF (1990) Stable bifunctional chelates of metals used in radiotherapy. Cancer Res 50:789
10. Cole WC, DeNardo SJ, Meares CF et al (1987) Comparative serum stability of radiochelates for antibody radiopharmaceuticals. J Nucl Med 28:83
11. Snook DE, Rowlinson G, Meares C, Epenetos AA (1992) Indium-111 and ytrium 90 labeled macrocyclic chelating agents. In: Epenetos AA (ed) Monoclonal antibodies. Applications in clinical oncology. Chapman and Hall, London, pp 155–164
12. DeNardo GL, DeNardo SJ, O'Grady LF et al (1990) Fractionated radioimmunotherapy of B-cell malignancies with ^{131}Y-Lym-1. Cancer Res 50: 1014–1016
13. Schroff RW, Foon KA, Beatty SM et al (1985) Human anti-murine immunoglobulin responses in patients receiving monoclonal antibody therapy. Cancer Res 45:879
14. Courtenay-Luck NS, Epenetos AA, Larche M et al (1986) Development of primary and secondary immune responses to mouse monoclonal antibodies used in the diagnosis and therapy of malignant neoplasms. Cancer Res 46:6489
15. Neuberger MS, Williams GT, Fox RO (1984) Recombinant antibodies possessing novel effector functions. Nature 312:604
16. LoBuglio AF, Wheeler RH, Trang J et al (1989) Mouse/human chimaeric monoclonal antibody in man: Kinetics and immune response. Proc Natl Acad Sci USA 86:4220
17. Evans ML, Graham MM, Mahler PA, Rasey JS (1986) Changes in vascular permeability following thorax irradiation in rat. Radiat Res 107:262
18. Krishnan L, Krishnan EC, Jewell WR (1988) Immediate effect of irradiation on microvasculature. Int J Radiat Oncol Biol Phys 15:147
19. Burrows FJ, Thorpe PE (1993) Eradication of large solid tumors in mice with an immunotoxin directed against tumor vasculature. Proc Natl Acad Sci USA 90:8996
20. Paganelli G, Malcovati M, Fazio F (1991) Monoclonal antibody pretargeting techniques for tumor localization: the avidin-biotin system. Nucl Med Comm 12:211
21. Paganelli G, Magnani P, Zito F et al (1991) Tree-step monoclonal antibody tumor targeting in CEA-positive patients. Cancer Res 51:5960
22. Bosslet K, Steinstraesser A, Hermentin P et al (1991) Generation of bispecific monoclonal antibodies for two-phase radioimmunotherapy. Br J Cancer 63:6816
23. Stewart JS, Hird V, Sullivan M, Epenetos AA (1989) Intraperitoneal radioimmunotherapy for ovarian cancer. Br J Obst Gyn 86:529
24. Epenetos AA, Munro AJ, Stewart S et al (1987) Antibody-guided irradiation of ovarian cancer with intraperitoneally administered radiolabeled monoclonal antibodies. J Clin Oncol 5:1890
25. Ward BG, Mather SJ, Hawkins LA et al (1987) Localisation of radioiodine conjugated to monoclonal antibody HMFG2 in human ovarian carcinoma: assessment of intravenous and intraperitoneal ratios of administration. Cancer Res 47:4719

26 Hird V, Maraveyas A, Snook D et al (1993) Adjuvant therapy of ovarian cancer with radioactive monoclonal antibody. Br J Cancer Aug 68 (2):403–6
27 Bamias A, Keane P, Krausz T et al (1991) Intravesical administration of radiolabeled antitumor monoclonal antibodies in bladder carcinoma. Cancer Res 51:724.
28 Bamias A, Bowles MJ, Krausz T et al (1993) Intravesical administration of Indium 111 labeled monoclonal antibodiy in superficial bladder carcinoma. Int J Cancer 54(6):899
29 Westlin JE, Snook D, Nilsson S et al (1993) Intravenous and intratumoral therapy of patients with malignant gliomas with 90-yttrium-labeled monoclonal antibody MUC 2-63. In: Epenetos AA (ed) Monoclonal antibodies. Applications in clinical oncology. Chapman and Hall, London, pp 17
30 Riva P, Arista A, Sturiale C et al: Treatment of intracranial human glioblastoma by direct intratumoral administration of 131I-labeled anti-tenascin monoclonal antibody BC2.

Address for correspondence:
Dr. A. A. Epenetos
Department of Clinical Oncology
I.C.R.F. Oncology Unit
Royal Postgraduate Medical School
Hammersmith Hospital
Du Cane Road
London W12 OHS, UK

Monoclonal antibody B 43.13 for immunoscintigraphy and immunotherapy of ovarian cancer

A. A. Noujaim[a], R. P. Baum[b], T. R. Sykes[a], R. Madiyalakan[a], C. J. Sykes[a], A. Hertel[b], A. Nielsen[b], G. Hör[b]

[a]Biomira Research Inc., University of Alberta, Edmonton, Alberta, Canada;
[b]Johann Wolfgang Goethe Universitätsklinikum, Frankfurt/Main, Germany

Introduction

The mucin-like molecule CA 125 has been the most thoroughly studied serum marker for ovarian cancer (1). Monoclonal antibodies generated against this marker have been effectively used for 1. monitoring the disease in patients, 2. the early prediction of treatment outcome, and 3. for the identification of tumor status after completion of therapy (2). The monoclonal antibody (MAb) B43.13 has been previously reported to specifically recognize the CA 125 antigen (3, 4, 5) in serum of ovarian cancer patients with bulky disease. It has also been identified to be of particular utility in the management of patients with metastatic adenocarcinoma of unknown primary origin (4). We are now reporting on the potential use of a Tc-99m radiolabeled form of the antibody for the in vivo detection and therapy of ovarian cancer.

Materials and methods

Monoclonal antibody (MAb) B43.13

The monoclonal antibody (MAb) B43.13 (IgG1, kappa isotype) was developed and provided to us by Biomira Inc. (Edmonton, Alberta) in a purified form from murine ascites. It was supplied as a sterile, pyrogen-free, virus-free solution (3–5 mg/ml) in 50 mM phosphate buffered saline (PBS) at a pH of 7.4. The protein concentration in the solution was determined by absorbance at 280 nm.

Tissue specificity of MAb-B43.13

Tumors and histologically normal adult human tissues were obtained from surgical pathology and autopsy specimens. Fresh tissues were embedded in OCT compound in cryomolds, frozen, and stored at –70 °C until needed. MAb-B43.13 was diluted in PBS containing 2% bovine serum albumin and purified mouse IgG1 diluted in a similar buffer, was used as the negative control. Biotinylated horse anti-mouse IgG was used as the secondary antibody with avidin-biotin-peroxidase complexes and DAB as the staining reagent.

Preparation of the radiolabeled kit

MAb-B43.13 was formulated for this study as a kit allowing for facile labeling with Tc-99m pertechnetate solution. The preparation was provided to us as a sterile, pyrogen free solution containing 2 mg of functionalized antibody ready for radiolabeling. Immediately prior to use, the vials were thawed at room temperature and a sterile solution of up 40 mCi of Tc-99m pertechnetate was added to the vials. In our most recent experiments, we have used a photo-activated product prepared as previously described (6).

Quality control

To ascertain the purity of the administered radiolabeled antibody, we have performed a number of quality-control steps to satisfy ourselves as to the biochemical, radiochemical and immunochemical integrity of the preparation. In addition to the previously mentioned MAb protein determination, SDS-PAGE electrophoretic analysis under reducing conditions was performed. The sample were further subjected to isoelectric focusing analysis and size-exclusion HPLC analysis. In

Table I. MAb-B43.13 specific human tumor reactivity.

Tumor type tested	Frozen tissue positive/total tested	Fixed tissue positive/total tested
Astrocytoma	0/2	0
Bladder carcinoma	0/3	0
Breast carcinoma		
intraductal	1/8	0
infiltrating cells	0/3	0
Colon carcinoma	0/10	0
Gastric carcinoma	0/1	–
Larynx carcinoma		
squamous	0/1	–
Lung carcinoma		
adenosquamous	1/3	0–2+
small cell	0/3	0
squamous	1/3	0–2+
Lymphoma	0/3	0
Melanoma	0/3	0
Prostate carcinoma	0/5	0
Renal carcinoma	0/3	0
Sarcoma	0/3	0
Ovarian Tumors		
serous tumors		
adenoma	2/2	1/3
borderline	3/3	5/5
primary carcinoma	4/4	4/6
metastatic carcinoma	1/1	1/1
endometrioid tumors		
primary	2/2	4/5
metastatic	1/1	2/2
mucinous tumors		
adenoma	3/3	0/5
borderline	1/1	0/1
primary carcinoma	2/2	0/2
metastatic carcinoma	1/1	N/A
ovarian cysts		
endometriotic	2/3	0/3
corpus luteum	1/2	0/3
para-ovarian	1/1	0/1

addition to the previously mentioned immunohistochemical staining of ovarian cancer tissue sections with the injectable preparation we have used both a CaOV3 cell line bioassay as well as an inhibition radioimmunoassay to ensure that no significant loss of immunoreactivity has taken place prior to usage. The radiochemical assessment of Tc-99m MAb-B43.13 was performed with a variety of standard techniques such as silica gel thin layer chromatography and size exclusion HPLC using continuous flow NaI(T1) radiation detection and in-line UV detection to monitor and quantitate the various elution peaks. On-site radiochemical analysis using ITLC-SG and a methanol saline (85:15) mobile phase demonstrated that the labeling efficiency was always > 95%.

Animal biodistribution studies

Biodistribution studies of intravenously administered MAb-B43.13, radiolabeled with either Tc-99m or In-111-DTPA, have been conducted. These studies were carried out in both non-tumor

Table II. Biodistribution of Tc-99m MAb-B43.13 in non-tumor bearing balb/c mice and OVCar 3 tumor-bearing Balb/c (nu/nu) mice and In-111-DTPA MAb-B43.13 in and OVCar 3 tumor-bearing Balb/c (nu/nu) mice.

Tissue	Non-tumor bearing Balb/c mice				
	Tc-99m MAb-B43.13				
	0.1 h (n = 4)	1.0 h (n = 4)	3.0 h (n = 4)	6.0 h (n = 4)	24.0 h (n = 4)
Blood	35.0 ± 3.2	28.4 ± 2.0	19.3 ± 1.2	17.5 ± 2.5	9.6 ± 0.9
Lungs	12.7 ± 2.1	9.1 ± 1.5	7.2 ± 0.8	7.1 ± 0.9	4.5 ± 0.5
Heart	8.6 ± 1.4	7.4 ± 0.3	6.8 ± 0.6	6.2 ± 0.5	3.2 ± 0.4
Stomach	1.2 ± 0.1	1.3 ± 0.4	1.3 ± 0.4	0.9 ± 0.2	0.7 ± 0.2
Small intestine	1.0 ± 0.1	3.4 ± 0.3	2.7 ± 0.6	1.8 ± 0.3	1.1 ± 0.2
Liver	15.1 ± 1.9	13.3 ± 1.3	9.3 ± 0.5	8.9 ± 1.0	4.8 ± 0.3
Spleen	6.6 ± 0.6	6.7 ± 0.5	5.1 ± 0.5	5.1 ± 0.8	3.3 ± 0.5
Kidneys	11.2 ± 1.5	12.4 ± 1.0	9.9 ± 0.8	9.0 ± 1.0	5.3 ± 0.3
Bone (femur)	n. d.	n. d.	n. d.	n. d.	n. d.
Tumor	n. a.	n. a.	n. a.	n. a.	n. a.

n. d. = not determined; n. a. = not available

Tissue	OVCar 3 tumor bearing Balb/c (nu/nu) mice			
	Tc-99m-MAb-B43.13	In-111-DTPA-MAb-B43.13		
	24 h (n = 3)	24 h (n = 3)	72 h (n = 4)	20 h (n = 3)
Blood	11.1 ± 1.7	11.4 ± 3.1	5.5 ± 1.0	6.2 ± 1.6
Lungs	5.2 ± 1.2	5.6 ± 1.4	3.9 ± 0.5	4.7 ± 1.0
Heart	5.2 ± 1.0	3.9 ± 3.1	3.2 ± 0.3	3.8 ± 0.7
Stomach	0.7 ± 0.2	0.9 ± 0.1	0.9 ± 0.2	1.0 ± 0.2
Small intestine	1.1 ± 0.1	2.4 ± 0.6	2.4 ± 0.2	2.2 ± 0.3
Liver	6.0 ± 1.3	6.6 ± 0.3	6.0 ± 0.3	7.4 ± 0.2
Spleen	4.0 ± 1.1	5.7 ± 1.7	5.7 ± 0.7	8.6 ± 0.8
Kidneys	6.7 ± 1.3	14.5 ± 3.8	11.7 ± 0.4	14.6 ± 2.1
Bone (femur)	1.7 ± 0.8	2.5 ± 0.7	2.4 ± 0.3	3.3 ± 0.5
Tumor	7.2 ± 1.4	14.0 ± 1.3	15.0 ± 3.9	15.5 ± 1.4

Table III. Immunoscintigraphic results with Tc-99m MAb-B43.13 by anatomic region.

Disease sites identified by RIS	No. of lesions detected	No. of new lesions detected	New lesions	FN/FP
Peritoneal carcinosis	12	9	7	–
Lymph node metastases	10	8	5	–
Liver metastases	6	5	2	–
Local recurrence	5	3	3	–
Primary	1	1	–	–
Other		0	–	-1
Negative	3	–	–	1
Sum	35	26	17	2

bearing Balb/c (normal) mice and OVCar-3 tumor-bearing Balb/c (nu/nu) mice. Pretreated MAb-B43.13 was radiolabeled with Tc-99m to a specific activity of 20 mCi/mg. Animals were injected via the tail vein with approximately 20 µCi of Tc-99m labeled antibody solution containing 20 µg of protein. DTPA-derivatized MAb-B43.13 was radiolabeled with In-111 to a specific activity of 2 mCi/mg. Animals were injected via the tail vein with approximately 20 µCi of In-111 labeled antibody solution containing 10 µg of protein. The animals were euthanized at selected time intervals and the various organs were removed, blotted to remove adhering blood and weighed. The dose standards as well as the selected organs were counted in a multisample NaI(T1) gamma spectrometer to less than 1% counting error.

Clinical studies

For radioimmunoscintigraphy, a single injection of 2 mg of MAb-B43.13 radiolabeled with 40 mCi of Tc-99m was injected intravenously. Images were obtained immediately after injection and at 6 hours and 24 hours. For therapeutic trials, Tc-99m MAb-B43.13 was administered repeatedly and some patients received more than ten injections over a period of several years. The CA 125, HAMA and Ab2 levels were monitored at various time intervals throughout this period.

Results and discussion

MAb-B43.13

Initial screening and selection identified a large number of MAbs that reacted with the CA 125 antigen. Of these, two MAbs (MAb-B43.13 and MAb B27.1) were selected on the basis of their high affinity for CA 125 and their ability to function in a sandwich immunoassay format to detect serum CA 125. The affinity for CA 125 was measured against both CA 125 expressing ovarian carcinoma cells in vitro and CA 125 antigen-coated beads. These two MAbs are currently formatted in a two-step immunoradiometric assay for CA 125 determination (TruQuant® OV™ - Biomira Inc.). Thus, the assays for serum CA 125 were conducted without significant interference from Ab2 HAMA production after injection of MAb-B43.13. MAb-B43.13 is of the IgG$_1$ kappa isotype and has an affinity of approximately 1 x 10^{10} M^{-1} (K_a) towards the CA 125 antigen. This SP2/0 derived hybridoma is a good producer of the antibody in both cell culture and murine ascitic fluid. The sequences of the antigen combining sites of the heavy and light chains of B43.13 have been determined by genetic engineering techniques.

Tissue specificity of MAb-B43.13

MAb-B43.13 was tested for cross reactivity by immunohistochemical procedures employing the avidin-biotin-peroxidase system of staining of fresh frozen as well as paraffin-embedded tissue. A series of benign and malignant ovarian tumors were shown to stain positive with MAb-B43.13 (table I). A variety of normal human tissues (data not shown) as well as malignancies of non-ovarian origin (table I) were also tested to establish the reactivity spectrum of MAb-B43.13.

Serous and endometrioid tumors, whether malignant or benign, stained positive in 100% of frozen tissue samples (13/13) and in 77% of formalin-fixed paraffin-embedded tumors (17/22) (table I). Borderline malignancies and well-differentiated carcinomas had typical staining of apical cytoplasm and/or extracellular material. Poorly-differentiated carcinomas showed cytoplasmic staining. Mucinous tumors were positive on frozen sections (7/7) and negative on formalin-fixed tissue (0/8). A variety of normal tissues as well as malignancies of non-ovarian origin were negative. MAb-B43.13 does not show any significant cross-reactivity with selected human organs and tissues. In particular, the MAb was not reactive with brain, heart and lung tissues. With the exception of weakly positive reactions with the collecting tubules, most elements of the kidney were also negative. Hepatocytes in the liver exhibited weak staining with MAb-B43.13. Results of testing of other normal tissues showed that MAb-B43.13 was not reactive with connective, nervous and lymphatic tissue. Also, most types of epithelia were not stained by MAb-B43.13. The pattern of reactivity of MAb-B43.13 with normal tissues was specifically limited to organs of common Müllerian

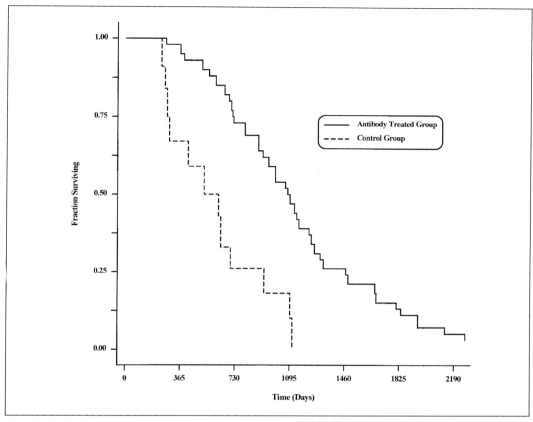

Figure 1. Survival curves for ovarian carcinoma patients, FIGO stage III. Control group treated post operatively with conventional chemotherapy (either cis-platinum/treosulfan or cis-platinum/cyclophosphamide, n = 39). Antibody treated group received MAb-B43.13 post operatively in addition to chemotherapy (n = 39).

origin (on a scale of 0 to 4+, reactivity with endocervical, endometrial, oviductal epithelium is 1+ to 2+). This is interpreted to mean that CA 125 antigen is present in small amounts on normal epithelia of the female reproductive system. MAb-B43.13 showed reactivity with some samples of normal breast acini. The limited study of non-ovarian malignancies shows that the MAb also reacts with about 20% of breast carcinoma samples. Other tumors tested did not stain with MAb-B43.13.

Animal biodistribution studies

The biodistribution pattern of Tc-99m MAb-B43.13 after intravenous injection in normal mice reflects the biological behavior of the MAb and its metabolites (table II). At early time points the blood accounts for a considerable portion of the dose with clearance half-lives of about 2.5 and 24 hours. The major organs responsible for uptake of the radiotracer are the liver and kidneys, which are also sites for the metabolism and excretion of the radiolabeled MAb and its metabolites. Most organs exhibited a rapid uptake phase followed by a clearance phase. The lack of significant stomach (table II), salivary or thyroid gland (data not shown) accumulation is indicative of an absence of free pertechnetate in the preparation or formed during metabolism. The whole body elimination in mice followed a biphasic pattern with estimated biological half-lives of 3 and 37 hours. Approximately 50% of the dose remains in the body at 24 hours.

The biodistribution pattern of Tc-99m MAb-B43.13 in tumor-bearing mice (table II) is remarkably similar to that in the normal mice. In addition, this data also indicates that the tumor has considerable uptake of the radiotracer at 24 hours. The biodistribution pattern of the In-111-DTPA MAb-B43.13 is also similar to Tc-99m in the tumor-bearing mice (table II) with the noted exception of kidney, bone and tumor. This is attributable mainly to the nature of the In-111 radioisotope and its known clearance mechanisms from the body and again indicates that the tumor is accumulating the radiotracer over time.

Clinical studies

Imaging results from a single dose level of 2 mg of Tc-99m MAb-B43.13 were obtained at various time intervals up to 24 hours post-injection. The images were read unblinded to the patient's disease status and clinical history. The lesions detected by immunoscintigraphy were compared with lesions detected by other techniques (clinical, CT, MRI, US, surgery). The results were used to calculate the imaging efficacy. Human anti-mouse antibody (HAMA-anti-isotype) levels were monitored for each patient. Additionally, Ab2 levels (anti-idiotype) were measured to determine the extent of anti-idiotype response as a function of time.

To date, over 150 patients in several centres have been injected with MAb-B43.13 for the scintigraphic detection of ovarian carcinoma. The clinical results of the first 20 patients studied have been reported by *Baum* et al. (7, 8) as shown in table III. In 12 patients peritoneal carcinomatosis was detected by immunoscintigraphy, nine of these cases were previously unknown and of these, seven have now been confirmed on follow-up (surgery, CT, US or MRI). Lymph node metastases were seen in ten patients, eight of which were previously unknown and five of which have been subsequently confirmed. Liver metastases were seen as "hot" lesions in six patients, five of which were previously unknown, two of which have subsequently been confirmed. Local recurrence was demonstrated in five patients, three of which were previously unknown, but subsequently confirmed. In total, 35 lesions were demonstrated with immunoscintigraphy using Tc-99m MAb-B43.13, 26 of which were unknown prior to scanning. Analysis has revealed two false negative results. HAMA was demonstrated in approximately 50% of patients following a single administration of Tc-99m MAb-B43.13.

The use of murine monoclonal antibodies (MAb) such as MAb-B43.13 for diagnostic imaging has, however, yielded some unexpected and provocative results. One well-known biologic effect of murine MAb directed against human tumor antigens has been the generation of an antibody response against the mouse protein in the host (9, 10, 11). The generation of human anti-mouse antibodies (HAMA) is seen often after exposure to murine MAb such as those used in radioimmunoscintigraphy (RIS). These antibodies in turn result in another generation of antibody production. These host antibodies are anti-idiotypic, that is they match the most specific region of the mouse protein, that area that matches the tumor marker as expressed on the tumor itself. By the »anti-idiotypic cascade« the host develops humoral immunity to her ovarian tumor. This strategy therefore acts much like a vaccine, inducing the host to produce circulating immunoglobulins directed against cancer-specific proteins, and may also augment cell-mediated immunity and delayed-type hypersensitivity (12, 13). RIS may therefore not only be diagnostic, but may also confer an unexpected survival advantage to ovarian cancer patients (14, 15). The rationale for studying this approach as therapy comes from several reports in the literature attributing a significant survival to patients with refractory tumors exposed to diagnostic radiolabeled MAb (9, 14, 16, 17).

We have recently retrospectively analyzed data from 61 patients (FIGO stage III and IV, recurrent disease) who were given Tc-99m MAb-B43.13. These patients were given up to ten injections in an effort to induce host anti-idiotypic antibody response. This group of patients was compared to a large group that had been studied prospectively as controls in another study. Cases were matched according to stage, grade, residual tumor after debulking surgery, first line agents, number of cycles of previous chemotherapy and outcome after first line therapy. Kaplan-Meier survival analysis reveals a statistically significant survival advantage to treatment with the antibody ($p < 0.03$) (figure 1 – stage III data only). In 218 administrations, seven mild to moderate acute hypersensitivity reactions (3%) which responded to standard measures were the only observed toxicities. These most encouraging results lead us to believe that some antibodies, while administered in small diagnostic doses, may indeed carry an unintended, beneficial pharmacologic action. The role of circulating antigens, and further complexation with either administered Ab1 (such as MAb-B43.13) or any endogenously produced Ab3 (resulting from the anti-idiotypic cascade) must be re-examined. This may indeed explain, at least partially, the immune response and therapeutic effect observed after MAb-B43.13 administration.

Acknowledgements

The authors would like to thank *Ms. Trudy Chimko, Mr. Thomas Woo, Ms. Birgit Schultes, Dr. Ze Peng and Professor Detlev Behnke* for their expert technical assistance with this project.

References

1. Einhorn N, Sjovall K, Knapp RC, Schoenfeld DA, Hall P, Eklund G, Scully RE, Bast RC Jr, Zurawski VR (1992) Specificity of serum CA 125 radioimmunoassay for early detection of ovarian cancer: A prospective study. Obst Gynecol 80:14–18
2. Kenemaus P, Yedema CA, Bon GG, von Mensdorff-Pouilly S (1993) CA 125 in gynecological pathology – a review. Europ J Obst Gynecol Reprod Biol 49:115–124
3. Jensen JL, MacLean GD, Suresh MR, Almeida A, Jette D, Lloyd S, Bodnar D, Krantz M, Longenecker BM (1991) Possible utility of serum determinations of CA 125 and CA 27.29 in breast cancer management. Int J Biol Markers 6:1–6
4. Capstick V, MacLean GD, Suresh MR, Bodnar D, Lloyd S, Shepert L, Longenecker BM, Krantz M (1991) Clinical evaluation of a new two-site assay for CA 125 antigen. Int J Biol Markers 6:129–135
5. Krantz MJ, MacLean GD, Longenecker BM, Suresh MR (1988) A radioimmunoassay for CA 125 employing two new monoclonal antibodies. UCLA Symposia on Molecular and Cellular Biology. Keystone, Colorado, April 23–30
6. Sykes TR, Woo TK, Qi P, Baum RP, Noujaim AA (1993) Direct labelling of monoclonal antibodies with technetium-99m by a novel photoactivation process. J Nucl Med 5:100
7. Hertel A, Baum RP, Niesen A, Noujaim AA (1992) A new Tc-99m-labelled monoclonal antibody (B43.13) against CA 125 for early detection of ovarian cancer recurrences – First Clinical Results. J Nucl Med 33:904
8. Baum RP, Hertel A, Baew-Christow T, Noujaim AA, Hör G (1991) A novel Tc-99m-labelled monoclonal antibody against CA 125 (B43.13) for radioimmunodetection of ovarian cancer – initial results. Europ J Nucl Med 18:535
9. Baum RP, Noujaim AA, Nanci A, Moebus V, Hertel A, Niesen, A, Donnerstag B, Sykes T, Boniface G, Hör G (1993) Clinical course of ovarian cancer patients under repeated stimulation of HAMA using MAb OC 125 and MAb-B43.13. Hybridoma 12: 583
10. Baum RP, Niesen A, Hertel A, Nanci A, Hess H, Donnerstag B, Sykes TR, Sykes CJ, Suresh, MR, Noujaim AA, Hör G (1994) Activating anti-idiotype human anti-mouse antibodies for immunotherapy of ovarian carcinoma. Cancer Suppl 73:1121–1125
11. Donnerstag B, Baum RP, Oltrogge JB, Hertel A, Hör G (1994) A preliminary study on the functional analysis of peripheral blood lymphocytes from ovarian cancer patients developing HAMA after immunoscintigraphy. Int J Biol Markers 9:115–120
12. Fagerberg J, Frödin J-E, Ragnhammar P, Steinitz M, Wigzell, H, Mellstedt H (1994) Induction of an immune network cascade in cancer patients treated with monoclonal antibodies (Ab1). II. Is induction of anti-idiotype reactive T-cells (T3) of importance for tumor response to MAb therapy? Cancer Immunol Immunother 38:149–159
13. Wagner UA, Oehr PF, Reinsberg J et al (1992) Immunotherapy of advanced ovarian carcinomas by activation of the idiotypic network. Biotech Ther 3:81–9
14. Barrada M, Pateisky N, Schember M et al (1994) Influence of immunoscintigraphy using monoclonal antibodies on survival of ovarian cancer patients. (personal communication)
15. Roitt IM, Brostoff J, Male DK (1985) Regulation of the immune response. In: Roitt IM (ed) Immunology, St. Louis, Mosby
16. Cheung N-K, Cheung I, Canete A et al (1994) Antibody response to murine anti-GD2 monoclonal antibodies: Correlation with patient survival. Cancer Res 54:2223–2228
17. Fagerberg J, Frödin J-E, Wigzell H, Mellstedt H (1993) Induction of an immune network cascade in cancer patients treated with monoclonal antibodies (Ab1). Cancer Immunol Immunother 37:264–270

Address for correspondence:
Prof. Dr. A. A. Noujaim
Biomira Research Inc.
1134 Dentistry-Pharmacy Bldg.
University of Alberta
CDN-Edmonton, AB T6G 2N8, Canada

Evolution of CT and MRI in oncologic diagnosis and their current value

K. Sommer, W. Crone-Münzebrock
Department of Diagnostic Radiology,
University Hospital Hamburg-Eppendorf, Hamburg, Germany

The evolution of radiological diagnostic modalities has been dramatic, especially in the field of oncology. This is even more true for computerized tomography (CT) and – more recently – magnetic resonance imaging (MRI), a technology highly depend on modern data processing which has been improved in an unprecedented way during the last decade.

The following short review was written in an attempt to summarize both the history and the current status in this field with its possible implications for the future.

Cormack (1) started his first experiments for CT as early as 1964 which eventually resulted in the legendary EMI-scanner prototype in London 1972. This first generation of scanners could only acquire one slice at a time with a scanning time of not less than 4.5 minutes with an additional 1.5 minutes of reconstruction time. The gantry was barely large enough to position the head of the patient which had to be placed inside a water bag. The second generation of scanners already reduced scanning time for a single slice to 18 seconds and the gantry was wide enough to accomodate the body of the patient. In 1975, the third generation of CTs worked with scanning times of four seconds per scan employing a matrix of 256 pixels. Cormack and Hounsfield (2) both received the Nobel prize for their work in 1979. The fourth generation of scanners was introduced in 1980 with scanning times as low as 0.75 seconds and a matrix of 512 pixels. Finally, and most recently so far, in the beginning of the nineties 1024 pixel matrix was beginning to become standard equipment and features such as 3-dimensional reconstruction algorithms and spiral CT were introduced.

The evolution of MRI leads even further back to 1946, when first experiments of magnetic resonance were conducted at Harvard university. It took another twenty years, until in 1967 magnetic resonance signals could be received from a living animal by Jackson. In 1972, Lauterbur (3) published a 2-D proton image of a test sample and in 1974 of a live animal. The first 2-D image of the human brain was obtained in 1978 (4) and, finally, in 1980 the first prototypes of MR-scanners were constructed. In 1983, the first systems were commercially available including simple motion reduction techniques such as cardiac triggering or respiratory gating. Gadolinium-DTPA was introduced as MRI contrast agent. In 1984 the number of worldwide installed MR-systems was 147, including the first low field machines. New, time-saving data-acquisition modes such as 3-D scans were introduced. In 1991, already more than 5500 systems were in use worldwide. The most recent developments include new coil systems, surface and intracorporal, ultrafast imaging sequences and new modalities such as MRI-angiography.

In prostatic carcinoma, MRI employing conventional surface coils can find tumors down to a size of 7–8 mm, with intrarectal coil systems the minimum size is approximately 3 mm. Transrectal sonography can differentiate lesions as small as 5 mm. CT can only detect tumors extending into the surrounding tissues. Specifities (T-stage) are 67–83% (sonography), 83–89% (MRI surface coils) and > 90% (MRI intrarectal coil). For lymph node staging, sensitivity ranges from 7–50% (CT) to 50–54% (MRI) and specifity ranges from 70–96% (CT) to 100% (MRI). Transrectal sonography is – apart from the clinical examination – ideal as primary diagnostic measure whereas MRI can especially evaluate invasion of the neurovascular bundle or of the seminal vesicles. Diagnostic problems in MRI pose patients after radio- or antiandrogen therapy, because tumor tissue can not be differentiated from post-therapeutic fibrotic changes.

In breast cancer, there are three major types of examination: mammography, sonography and MRI. Mammography can detect microcalcifications even smaller than 0.5 mm, the lowest detectable size of other lesions depends largely upon their configuration and topography, existence of scar tissue and multiple other factors. In MRI, the smallest detectable lesions are 5 mm, when utilizing new sequences providing ultra-thin slices even as small as 2 mm. The results for sensititivity and specifity in MRI are highly controversial. Sensitivity ranges from 65-98%, specifity from 68-98% but the negative predictive value has been shown to be as high as 99.5%. One series could show evidence of disease in 70/400 patients with previous negative or equivocal mammographies (5). The primary radiologic diagnostic procedure should doubtlessly be mammography and sonography. The current opinions about indications for MRI differ somewhat, nevertheless it can be safely stated that patients after partial mastectomy suspected of local recurrence profit. Other possible indications seem to be discrepant or equivocal results in clinically supicious cases after mammography and sonography as well as the preoperative exclusion of multicentric carcinoma.

Pancreatic cancer has been investigated by a wide variety of radiologic procedures including percutaneous and endoluminal sonography, endoscopic retrograde cholangiopancreatography (ERCP), CT and MRI. In general, detection of lesions is more probable and earlier in the course of the disease when the duct system is obstructed and thus widened. Approximate smallest detectable lesion sizes vary considerably: doubtlessly, endosonography (> 5-15 mm) and ERCP (when duct system is obstructed, even by smalles lesions) are among the most sophisticated procedures available. Percutaneous sonography (> 2 cm), CT (> 1.5-2 cm) and MRI (> 2-3 cm) detect only considerably larger lesions, but are also much more susceptible to inter-patient variants such as body weight, peristalsis and intestinal air-content. Specifity is probably highest for ERCP (> 88%) and endosonography (70-84%). CT (38-77%), MRI (60-81%), and percutaneous sonography (50-72%) are somewhat lower, but needle aspiration biopsy (60-95%) can possibly enhance their performance. Diagnostic problems, especially in MRI, can be insidious: There is no peroral contrast medium (yet) to differentiate intestinal loops from pancreatic tissue, and respiratory, peristaltic and aortic pulsational artifacts can make diagnosis extremely difficult. On top of that, microcalcifications cannot be detected, since calcium produces no signal whatsoever in MRI. Both CT and MRI have considerable problems differentiating pancreatitis from carcinoma, and the detection of peritoneal carcinosis in an early stage is nearly impossible. Nonetheless, sonography, CT and ERCP are the methods of choice for the radiologic detection of pancreatic cancer. MRI can possibly be beneficial in cases of vessel encasement, detection of liver metastasis and in patients with a history of previous allergy to iodine or patients undergoing treatment for thyroid cancer by radioactive iodine.

The specifities for the detection of colorectal cancer by CT (70-88%) or MRI (70-85% for rectal cancer) are almost equal. Hepatic metastasis in this disease can be diagnosed fairly safely by CT (78%), sonography (80%) or MRI (80%). Problems in this entity include low spatial resolution, peristalsis and no oral contrast medium for MRI and in CT, the differential diagnosis of intestinal contents versus tumor and the differentiation of local recurrence from presacral fibrosis in rectal cancer. CT should be employed for lymph node staging, detection of liver metastasis and larger primary tumors. MRI is best when trying to differentiate presacral fibrosis from local recurrence in rectal cancer. In the pelvic region, sagittal and coronal planes provide additional information. Patients with a history of previous allergy to iodine or patients undergoing treatment for thyroid cancer by radioactive iodine profit as well from MRI using Gadolinium-DTPA.

Hepatocellular carcinoma (HCC) can be detected by MRI with a specifity of 75% (lesions < 1 cm) or 85% (< 2 cm). CT (75%) or portal CT (75%) provide equal specifity, sonography somewhat less (69%). Sensitivity is probably highest with digital subtraction angiography (DSA, 67-95%), portal CT (75-87%) and sonography (73-94%). CT by itself is less sensitive (72-77% over all), especially in early disease (< 2 cm: 44%). MRI has an intermediate sensitivity of 70-75%. Diagnostic problems pose diffuse and multicentric HCC as well as perivascular tumor growth.

In conclusion, three major ideas for the presence and future of radiologic diagnosis in oncology seem evident. 1. The history of the development of radiologic tools shows, that reducing the distance between the detection device and the organ system in question has largely contributed to an increase in spatial resolution and thus in sensitivity and specifity. Or, from a different point of view, the size of the smallest detectable lesion has been reduced in this process. 2. There will always be a lowest detectable tumor size in radiology, depending on the biology and physics involved. Small singular disease as well as diffuse disease will therefore continue to be at risk of not being detected. This obviates the need for other diagnostic tools, such as tumor markers. 3. The multiplicity of radiologic types of examinations, the constant evolution of new modalities and the consecutive shift of indications and detection probabilities demand an ever increasing interdisciplinary approach of radiologists and clinicians, especially in the light of the recent explosion in health care costs.

References

1. Cormack AM (1964) Representation of a function by its line integrals with some radiological applications, II. J App Phys 35:2908–2913
2. Hounsfield GN (1973) Computerized transverse axial scanning (tomography): Part I: Description of system. Br J Radiol (1973) 46:1016–1022
3. Lauterbur WS (1973) Image formation by induced local interactions: examples employing nuclear magnetic. Nature 243:190
4. Hinshaw WS, Bottomley PA, Holland GN et al (1977) Radiographic thin section imaging of the human brain by nuclear magnetic resonance imaging. Nature 270:722
5. Kaiser WA (1991) Magnetic resonance mammography. Medica Mundi 36:168–182

Address for correspondence:
Dr. med. K. Sommer
Abteilung für diagnostische Radiologie
Universitätskrankenhaus
Martinistraβe 52
D-20246 Hamburg, Germany

Workshop 2

Gene Technology in Diagnosis and Therapy

Recombinant DNA technology: Diagnostic and therapeutic aspects

H. E. Blum

Department of Medicine, University Hospital Zurich, Zurich, Switzerland

Molecular biology and recombinant DNA technology are of increasing significance for diagnosis, therapy and prevention of human diseases. In the following we will briefly discuss the principle of recombinant DNA technology and its applications in clinical medicine.

Principle of recombinant DNA technology

Recombinant DNA technology is centered on the in vitro manipulation of deoxyribonucleic acid (DNA). DNA carries the genetic information of all living organisms. In humans it is mainly localized in the cell nucleus where it is structurally organized in 46 chromosomes (2 x 23 chromosomes, 2 x 22 autosomes and 2 x 1 sex chromosome). In chromosomes DNA sequences are arranged as structural units with protein encoding function, termed genes. The human genome carries about 130,000 genes, for most of which a function has not been identified as of now. For biological activity, genes are expressed resulting in protein synthesis: A DNA sequence is transcribed into a complementary messenger RNA (mRNA) sequence which in turn is translated into an amino acid sequence (protein). Since the mRNA sequence is complementary to the DNA sequence and each amino acid is, via the genetic code, encoded by a defined triplet of three bases (codon), the DNA sequence defines the amino acid sequence and thereby the protein (1–4).

Recombinant DNA technology allows the cloning of DNA fragments or genes and their expression in vitro. For conventional cloning, the DNA sequences of interest are recombined via a ligase with a vector to form the recombinant DNA molecule (figure 1). The most frequently used vectors are bacterial plasmids which are self-replicating circular DNA molecules that usually carry an antibiotic resistance gene (e.g., ampicillin resistence gene encoding a beta-lactamase). The recombinant DNA molecule, consisting of the

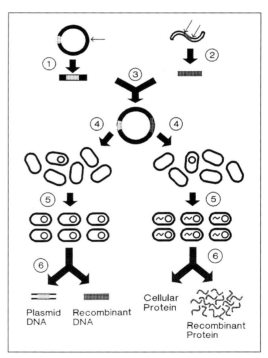

Figure 1. Principle of recombinant DNA technology: DNA multiplication (left) and protein synthesis (right): (1) linearization of vector; (2) preparation of DNA fragment or gene; (3) Ligation of vector and DNA fragment to form recombinant DNA molecule; (4) introduction of recombinant DNA molecule into bacteria (transformation); (5) selection of bacteria in the presence of an antibiotic and DNA multiplication or gene expression protein synthesis; (6) isolation of the recombinant products: cloned DNA or recombinant protein.

Table I. Molecular detection of infectious, genetic and malignant diseases.

1. Bacteria
   Bordetella, Legionella, M. leprae, M. tuberculosis, Mycoplasma, Chlamydia, N. gonorrhoeae, N. meningitidis, Treponema, Hemophilus, Helicobacter, Salmonella, Shigella, Borrelia, enterotox. E. coli, Tropheryma whippelii

2. Viruses
   Adenoviruses, Cytomegalovirus, Epstein-Barr Virus
   Hepatitis A-E viruses
   Herpes simplex viruses
   Human T-cell-leukemia virus 1 und 2
   Human immunodeficiency virus 1 und 2
   Human papilloma viruses

3. Parasites
   Plasmodia, Entamoeba histolytica, Giardia lamblia
   Pneumocystis carinii, Toxoplasma gondii

4. Fungi
   Candida albicans, Coccidioides immitis, Cryptococcus neoformans

5. Hemoglobinopathies
   Sickle cell anemia, Beta-thalassemias

6. Metabolic and other diseases
   Alpha-1-antitrypsin deficiency,
   Lesch-Nyhan-syndrome
   Xeroderma pigmentosum,
   Duchenne muscular dystrophy
   Cystic fibrosis, Hemophilia A or B

7. Malignant Diseases
   Retinoblastoma
   Leukemias, Lymphoma, Burkitt's lymphoma, Nasopharyngeal carcinoma, Cervical cancer, Liver cancer

Table II. Recombinant proteins in clinical practice.

Human insulin (1982)
Growth hormone (1985)
Hepatitis B vaccine (1986)
Interferon alpha (1986)
Tissue plasminogen activator (1987)
Erythropoietin (1988)
Interferon gamma (1989)
Interleukin-2 (1989)
Granulocyte colony stimulating factor (G-CSF; 1991)
Granulocyte macrophage colony stimulating factor (GM-CSF; 1991)
Factor VIII (1993)

Table III. Concepts of gene therapy.

Disease	Gene Therapy
Classic monogenic diseases	gene replacement
Complex genetic diseases	gene augmentation
Acquired genetic diseases	block of gene expression

antibiotic resistance gene carrying plasmid and the DNA fragment of interest (e. g., insulin gene), is then transferred into an appropriate cell, in most cases bacteria (e. g., E. coli strains). In the presence of ampicillin, the bacteria containing the recombinant DNA molecule are selected and allow the multiplication of the recombinant DNA molecule (insulin gene) or its expression (insulin). The result of these in vitro manipulations is either the multiplication of the DNA fragment (cloned DNA) figure 1, left)) or protein synthesis (recombinant protein, figure 1, right).

Conventional cloning by transformation of appropriate cells with recombinant DNA constructs has been revolutionized by the polymerase chain reaction (PCR) amplification which allows cell-free DNA or RNA cloning in vitro (5, 6).

Clinical applications of recombinant DNA technology

The products of recombinant DNA technology are cloned DNA and recombinant proteins (figure 1). Recombinant proteins are of increasing significance for the diagnosis, therapy and prevention of human diseases. Some of the recombinant proteins have already been successfully introduced into clinical practice (table I!).

Cloned DNA, together with PCR amplification, is used as molecular probe for the early and specific detection of known infectious, inherited and malignant diseases by molecular hybridization analyses (table I). In addition, such molecular hybridization analyses for the first time permit an understanding of the molecular basis of inherited and malignant diseases which in turn allows the early identification of patients at risk. Impressive recent examples for the successful clinical application of molecular techniques are the identification of the agent causing Whipple's disease (7), the early non-invasive detection of individuals at risk for familial adenomatous polyposis (8) or colorectal cancer (9).

Table IV. Monogenic diseases.

Defective gene	Disease
Adenosine deaminase	severe combined immunodeficiency
Alpha-1-antitrypsin	emphysema, liver cirrhosis
Argininosuccinate synthetase	citrullinemia
CD-18	leucocyte adhesion deficiency
Cystic fibrosis transmembrane regulator	cystic fibrosis
Factor VIII	hemophilia A
Factor IX	hemophilia B
Alpha-L-fucosidase	fucosidosis
Glucocerebrosidase	M. Gaucher
Beta-glucuronidase	mucopolysaccharidosis type VII
Beta-globin	thalassemia
Beta-globin	sickle cell anemia
Alpha-L-iduronidase	mucopolysaccharidosis type I
LDL-receptor	familial hypercholesterinemia
Ornithin transcarbamylase	hyperammonemia
Purine nucleoside phosphorylase	severe combined immunodeficiency
Sphingomyelinase	Niemann-Pick disease

Apart from diagnostic aspects and the clinical use of recombinant proteins for therapy and prophylaxis, gene therapy is being evaluated for the treatment or prevention of human diseases. Conceptually, gene therapy can follow three strategies (10, 11), depending on the nature of the genetic disease (table III):

1. Gene replacement. For classical genetic diseases, following the rules of Mendelian inheritance, the missing or defective gene is replaced by introduction of the respective normal gene into appropriate cells (table IV). An example is the replacement of the adenosine deaminase (ADA) gene in patients with ADA deficiency and consecutive severe immunodeficiency (figure 2).

2. Gene augmentation. For complex genetic diseases, such as cardiovascular diseases, hypertension, rheumatic diseases or malignancies, the introduction of a gene with a new function is a strategy with substantial promise. An example is the ex vivo introduction of a cytokine gene (interleukin-2 [Il-2] or tumor necrosis factor [TNF]) into tumor infiltrating lymphocytes (TIL) and reinfusion after in vitro expansion of the genetically engineered cells with consecutive destruction of tumor cells by the local production of Il-2 or TNF in the face of low systemic toxicity (figure 3).

3. Block of gene expression. For acquired genetic diseases, such as infectious and malignant diseases, a block of gene expression by oligonucleotides holds substantial promise. Conceptually, there are several strategies: block of transcription by binding of transcription factors or triple helix formation, destruction of mRNA by ribozymes or block of mRNA translation by antisense oligonucleotides as well as protein inactivation by protein-protein or potein-nucleic acid interactions. A well-studied strategy is the use of antisense oligonucleotides to arrest mRNA translation (figure 4) in the treatment of infectious (12–16) or malignant diseases (17).

While many issues central to the clinical application of gene therapy remain to be resolved (gene targeting and delivery, gene integration and expression, specificity of gene suppression and others), molecular biology clearly has become an integral part of both basic medical research and clinical medicine.

References

1. Watson JD, Gilman M, Witkowski J, Zoller M (1992) Recombinant DNA. 2nd Edition. Scientific American Books, W. H. Freeman and Company, New York
2. Sambrook J, Fritsch E F, Maniatis T (1989) Molecular Cloning. A Laboratory Manual. Cold Spring Harbor Press, Cold Spring Harbor
3. Knippers R, Philippsen P, Schäfer KP, Fanning E (1990) Molekulare Genetik. Georg Thieme Verlag, Stuttgart, New York

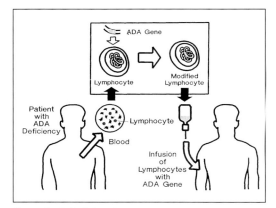

Figure 2. Principle of gene replacement therapy: ex vivo introduction of adenosine deaminase (ADA) gene for therapy of severe combined immunodeficiency.

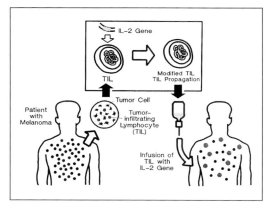

Figure 3. Principle of gene augmentation therapy: ex vivo introduction of interleukin-2 (IL-2) gene for therapy of malignant melanoma.

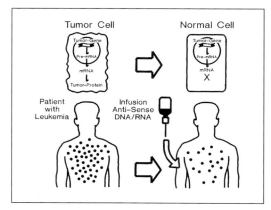

Figure 4. Principle of block of gene expression: antisense strategy in acquired genetic diseases.

4. Darnell J, Lodish H, Baltimore D (1990) Molecular Cell Biology. 2nd Edition. Scientific American Books, W. H. Freeman and Company, New York
5. Erlich HA (1989) PCR Technology. Principles and applications for DNA amplification. Stockton Press, New York, London, Tokyo, Melbourne, Hong Kong
6. Innis MA, Gelfand DH, Sninsky JJ, White TJ (1990) PCR protocols. A guide to methods and applications. Academic Press, San Diego, New York, Boston, London, Sydney, Tokyo, Toronto
7. Relman DA, Schmidt TM, Richard P, MacDermott P, Falkow S (1992) Identification of the uncultured bacillus of Whipple's disease. N Engl J Med 327: 293–301
8. Powell SM, Petersen GM, Krush AJ, Booker S, Jen J, Giardiello FM, Hamilton SR, Vogelstein B, Kienzler KW (1982-1987, 1993) Molecular diagnosis of familial adenomatous polyposis. N Engl J Med 329
9. Sidransky D, Tokino T, Hamilton SR, Kinzler KW, Levin B, Frost P, Vogelstein B (1992) Identification of ras oncogene mutations in the stool of patients with curable colorectal tumors. Science 256:102–105
10. Anderson WF (1992) Human gene therapy. Science 256:808–813
11. Morgan RA, Anderson WF (1993) Human gene therapy. Annu Rev Biochem 62:191–217
12. Blum HE, Galun E, von Weizsäcker F, Wands JR (1991) Inhibition of hepatitis B virus by antisense oligodeoxynucleotides. Lancet 337:1230
13. Offensperger W-B, Offensperger S, Walter E, Teubner K, Igloi G, Blum HE, Gerok W (1993) In vivo inhibition of duck hepatitis B virus replication and gene expression by phosphorothioate modified antisense oligodeoxynucleotides. EMBO J 12:1257–1262
14. Wu GY, Wu CH (1992) Specific inhibition of hepatitis B viral gene expression by targeted antisense oligonucleotides. J Biol Chem 267:12436–12439
15. Chatter JS, Johnson PR, Wong KK (1992) Dual-target inhibition of HIV-1 in vitro by means of an adeno-associated antisense vector. Science 258:1485–1488
16. Calabretta B (1991) Inhibition of proto-oncogene expression by antisense oligodeoxynucleotides: biological and therapeutic implications. Cancer Res 51:4505–4510

Address for correspondence:
Prof. Dr. H. E. Blum
Department für Innere Medizin
Medizinische Klinik B
Universitätsspital
Rämistraße 100
CH-8091 Zürich, Switzerland

Applications of the polymerase chain reaction to tumor analysis and diagnosis

R. Shipman
Molecular Oncology, University Hospital Research Center (ZLF), Basel, Switzerland

The development and refinement of methods used in molecular biology and molecular genetics have had profound effects on medical research. Of the many techniques used routinely in molecular biology, the polymerase chain reaction (PCR) likely represents the most substantial advance in molecular technology since the introduction of DNA cloning and sequencing. The specificity and sensitivity of PCR permits the analysis of target sequences in the DNA of fixed tissue blocks and sections, archival tissue sections, cells present in urine or stool, single human hairs, single sperm or oocytes, cells from pre-implantation embryos and archeological specimens such as amber-embedded insects, ancient mummies or dinosaur bones. In the medical sciences, PCR has been used primarily as an analytical or diagnostic method. In this sense, PCR has been employed in screening protocols to establish "carrier" status, and to provide evidence of asymptomatic or residual disease. PCR has also been used to establish causal relationships between viral infection and cancer, oncogene expression and cancer, and the linkage of specific alleles with genetic disorders. In myeloproliferative disorders, PCR has been used to monitor the re-emergence of malignant clones in remission patients or bone marrow transplant patients. In human hereditary disease syndromes, the linkage of a specific allele with disease allows PCR to be employed as a means of determining genotype and therefore verifying "carrier" status. As such, PCR has the potential to be both a diagnostic and prognostic method.

A brief list of some of the applications of PCR to medical science is given in table I. The use of PCR in these various areas of research relies entirely on the previous demonstration of a link between a particular disease and the altered expression or genetic alteration of a particular "marker gene".

In tumor analysis, PCR can be used to determine the spectrum and type of genetic alterations that occur during tumor formation and progression. If a significant correlation can be established between a specific genetic alteration and tumor development, the utility of this genetic alteration for tumor diagnosis can be evaluated.

Tumor analysis and diagnosis using PCR require certain prerequisites, the most important of which are listed below.

1. For analytical PCR, the tumor sample should be primarily tumor cells or tissue (minimal normal cell or tissue "contamination").

2. For analytical PCR, the genetic alteration tested should occur preferentially in the tumor cell population (present at low levels or in a minority of normal cells).

3. For diagnostic PCR, the genetic alteration used to detect the presence of tumor cells should occur exclusively in all tumor cells.

The problems with sample acquisition, handling and processing also play a determinative role in the success of both analytical and diagnostic PCR. Depending on the source material used for a particular PCR application (genomic DNA, total RNA, mRNA, cDNA), the manner in which the sample is prepared will influence the ability to amplify the specific PCR product. In addition, the techniques used for detection, quantitation or sequencing of the PCR product will be influenced by the sample preparation.

Similar sampling and technical problems plague the analysis of tumor material using immunohistochemical (IHC) approaches. IHC can be used to detect the expression of a "tumor-associated marker" on abnormal cells in a tissue sample and as such has the potential to be both an analytic and diagnostic method. A comparison of IHC and PCR in the analysis of tumor samples is shown in table II.

Table I. Applications of PCR in medical science.

Virology	infectious disease diagnosis	
	AIDS, TB, hepatitis, pediatric diseases	
Molecular genetics	hereditary disease diagnosis (carrier genotype?)	
	prenatal diagnosis (fetal genotype)	
	HLA polymorphism disease susceptibility	
	disease syndromes and susceptibility loci	
	(fragile X, myotonic dystrophy, CF, WT, RB)	
Molecular oncology	allelic loss analysis	RFLP-/AFLP-PCR
	expression studies	RT-PCR and quantitation
	mutation analysis	exon-specific PCR and sequencing
	linkage analysis	microsatellite PCR
	disease locus mapping	microsatellite PCR
	disease locus isolation	PCR analysis of human genomic
		DNA-YAC and -cosmid libraries
Cancer biology	oncogene/tumor suppressor gene expression	
	colon, bladder, lung	(p53, ras, FAP, WT1)
	breast, ovary	(p53, ras, BRCA1)
	leukemia	(p53, ras, bcr-abl, PML, WT1)
Tumor biology	"oncofetal" gene expression	(AFP, CEA, CALLA, CAMAL)
	cytokine/growth factor expression	
	cytokine/growth factor receptor expression	
	angiogenic factor expression	(FGFs, EGF, PDGF)
	matrix factor expression	(TGF)
	metastasis	(CD44)

The ability to use PCR for tumor analysis is due mainly to the nature of the sample. Usually, the cell or tissue sample consists primarily of tumor cells and the genetic alteration is expected to be present in all the tumor cells. The ability to detect gene deletion, mutation or expression in tumor samples by PCR is a direct result of normal cells constituting a minority of the total cell or tissue sample. The contribution, if any, of the normal cells to the PCR signal is thus minimised and is unlikely to prevent the detection of the desired genetic alteration.

This stands in contrast to the use of PCR for tumor diagnosis. In this instance, PCR is used to detect a genetic alteration in a population of cells that may constitute < 1% of the total sample. The contribution of normal cells to the PCR signal is therefore overwhelming and will most likely prevent the detection of the genetic alteration. Consequently, the application of PCR to tumor diagnosis requires that the genetic alteration exists exclusively in the tumor cells. Providing such a "tumor-specific" alteration exists, the detection of the few "tumor" cells present in a cell or tissue sample should be possible.

To describe or summarise the many and varied applications of PCR to medical science over the last few years is a daunting prospect. Reciting a catalogue of the diseases to which PCR analysis has been applied and how the PCR protocol differs from one application to the next is not likely to be particularly informative or interesting. The application of PCR to specific research areas has already been addressed in a number of comprehensive reviews (1–5).

Rather than reviewing PCR reviews, I would prefer to illustrate the application of PCR to the molecular analysis of clinical samples in which the status of particular genes and genetic loci are examined in a group of cancer patients. This approach will hopefully indicate when and where PCR can be applied, how PCR can most effectively be used, what information PCR can provide and whether PCR analysis is appropriate.

In our hypothetical cancer patient group, the availability of matched normal tissue (N) and

Table II. Comparison of immunohistochemical and PCR methods for the examination of tumor samples.

| Immunohistochemical methods |
| --- |//

Advantages:
1. Diagnosis can be made on the basis of the presence and identification of abnormal cells.
2. Proportion of normal cells and tumor cells can be determined.
3. Pattern of expression of specific cellular markers on tumor cells versus normal cells can be determined.
4. Correlation of cellular marker expression with tumor status (TMN parameters).
5. Cellular marker expression can be used to monitor residual or recurrent disease.

Disadvantages:
1. Sampling problems (do normal cells also express marker?).
2. Disease is usually "advanced" before diagnosis is possible.
3. Sensitivity and cross-reactivity problems preclude early diagnosis or detection of rare tumor cells.
4. Detection of the genetic alteration is dependent on gene expression.

Polymerase chain reaction

Advantages:
1. Sensitivity and specificity for the gene or genetic alteration.
2. Sensitivity permits identification of rare tumor cells.
3. Can also be used to monitor residual or recurrent disease.
4. Detection of genetic alteration is independent of gene expression.

Disadvantages:
1. Sampling problems (do normal cells constitute a significant proportion of the cell sample?).
2. Analytical PCR requires homogenous tumor and normal cell samples to permit the discrimination of genetic alterations between the two sample populations.
3. Diagnostic PCR requires unique genetic alterations in the tumor cell population to permit the detection of rare tumor cells in a "normal" cell sample.

tumor tissue (T) is assumed. The next logical and perhaps most critical step is deciding what genetic alteration(s) to examine. This decision will dictate how the PCR primers are chosen, what methods of sample collection and preparation will be followed and whether quantitation of the PCR product will be necessary.

As a starting point, we will want to determine the status of particular genetic loci in N and T genomic DNA before we proceed to the analysis of specific gene expression in these same samples. In this instance, the genes in question are known (cDNA and/or genomic DNA sequence, tissue expression pattern, altered expression or mutation in cancer), have been localised to specific chromosomal sub-regions, contain characteristic mutations which affect gene expression or function and have been associated with particular diseases.

In this sense, we know what to expect and want to demonstrate that the altered nature of this gene(s) is relevant to the development or progression of the disease being studied. The general approach and PCR methods employed are shown in table III and figure 1.

PCR analysis of allelic loss on specific chromosomes is accomplished using primers specific for polymorphic repetitive DNA sequences located at specific chromosomal loci (figure 1: VNTR or microsatellite PCR). By using genomic DNA isolated from normal and tumor tissue of the same patient, the loss of "VNTR alleles" for specific genetic loci in the tumor tissue can be determined. Depending on the chromosomal region chosen, the allelic loss analysis can proceed fairly quickly from the examination of gross chromosomal and chromosomal sub-region deletions to the detailed analysis of gene deletion and mutation. Such analyses require microsatellite sequence primers located within the region identified in the initial deletion analysis. Such microsatellite primers are being identified and assigned to specific chromosomal regions by a number of laboratories worldwide and are available through Généthon or Research Genetics. This analysis allows us to assess whether allelic loss is

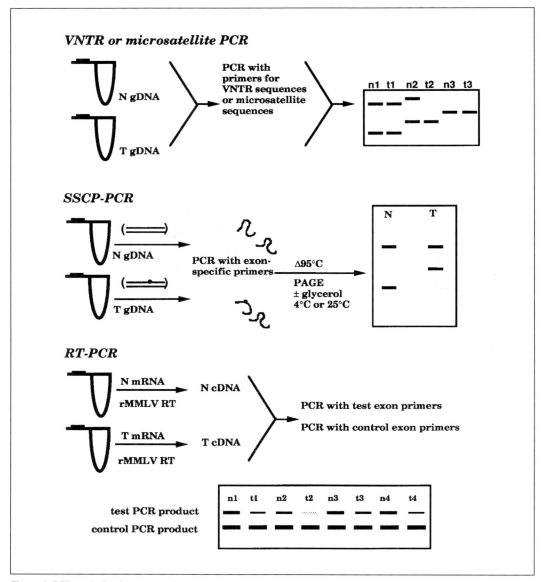

Figure 1. PCR analysis of normal and tumor issue.

a frequent, non-random event at a particular chromosomal locus in our study group and, if so, whether further analysis of known genes located within the deleted region is likely to be informative. Non-random allelic loss analysis generally provides a reasonable "jumping-off" point for a number of PCR-based analyses. If genes known to harbour specific mutations (affecting gene expression or function) are located within the deleted chromosomal region, then exon-specific PCR followed by direct sequencing or SSCP is the standard methodology for "mutation analysis" (figure 1: SSCP-PCR). Another analytical approach relies on the differential expression of a particular gene in normal versus tumor tissue. cDNA is synthesized from total RNA, isolated from the normal and tumor source tissues, using recombinant Mouse Moloney Leukemia Virus Reverse

Table III. PCR-based approach to the analysis of paired samples of tumor and normal tissue.

1. Analysis of allelic loss at specific chromosomal loci (> 500 kb)
    homozygous or hemizygous deletion of specific chromosomal regions
        normal tissue DNA compared to tumor tissue DNA
        Variable Number Tandem Repeat or microsatellite PCR (6–8)
        Restriction Fragment Length Polymorphism-PCR (9–12)
        Arbitrary Fragment Length Polymorphism-PCR (13)

2. Analysis of known genes within the "deleted" region (< 300 kb)
    translocation, inversion or duplication, aberrant gene splicing,
    expansion of repetitive inter- or intragenic sequences
        normal tissue DNA compared to tumor tissue DNA
        Variable Number Tandem Repeat or microsatellite PCR

3. Analysis of gene expression (< 10 kb)
    point mutations in exons or introns (expression?), truncations (creation of stop codon in exon),
    abnormal mRNA (mutation of splice donor or acceptor site), mutated gene expressed (wild-type activity?)
        normal tissue DNA compared to tumor tissue DNA
        exon-specific PCR followed by either direct sequencing or
        Single Strand Conformation Polymorphism PCR (14–16)
        normal tissue mRNA compared to tumor tissue mRNA
        Reverse Transcription-PCR for specific gene or genes (17–19)
        quantitative RT-PCR to assess the relative level of gene expression in the tissue samples (20–24)

4. Correlation with tumor status
    statistical correlation between immunohistochemistry, molecular analyses and TMN parameters

Transcriptase (rMMLV RT). This cDNA is then used in a PCR with exon-specific primers for the "test" gene and primers specific for a ubiquitously-expressed "control" gene (β-actin, glyceraldehyde-3-phosphate dehydrogenase (GAPDH), hypoxanthine-phospho-ribosyl transferase (HPRT), β2-microglobulin). When the samples are analysed on agarose gels, the "test" signal can be normalised to the "control" signal to give a "relative level of expression" for the "test" gene in normal versus tumor tissue (figure1; RT-PCR). RT-PCR or "semi-quantitative PCR" has been used to examine the differential expression of a number of defined genes and due to its specificity and sensitivity is particularly suited for the analysis of small amounts of tissue (25–27). If the molecular basis of the differential expression is known, this genetic alteration can be examined by coupling the RT-PCR with SSCP-PCR or PCR-based direct sequencing.

The application of PCR to tumor diagnosis has less to do with the PCR method and more to do with the nature of the genetic alteration itself. For tumor diagnosis by PCR, the genetic alteration examined must occur exclusively in all the tumor cells to permit the detection of the rare tumor cells in an overwhelming excess of normal cells. The best candidates for such exclusive genetic alterations are the specific chromosomal translocations that occur in various myeloproliferative or lymphoproliferative disorders (table IV).

The ability to detect rare abnormal cells harbouring characteristic chromosomal translocations in peripheral blood samples has been demonstrated in a number of studies (28–30). The ability to use PCR-based analysis to monitor residual disease or predict disease progression has also been established (31–33). The limitation of tumor diagnosis by PCR lies with the genetic alteration itself. Most of these "specific" alterations occur only in a proportion of the patients at disease presentation. Providing a panel of such "specific" alterations exists for each disease, it should be possible to design diagnostic PCR procedures to detect all the possible genetic alterations for a particular disease. The ability to detect such genetic alterations at the single cell level and thereby monitor residual disease or impending relapse indicates the value of PCR in the clinical setting. The early detection of malignant cells by

Table IV. Chromosomal breakpoints in myeloproliferative or lymphoproliferative disorders.

Translocation	Gene (Locus)	Disease
t(1:19)	PBX1(1q):E2A (19p)	acute pre-B cell leukemia
t(14:18)	IgH(14q):BCL2(18)	follicular lymphoma
t14:19)	IgH(14q):BCL3(19q)	B-CLL
t(3:14)	BCL6(3q):IgH(14q)	diffuse large-cell lymphoma
t(5:14)	IL3(5q):IgH(14q)	B-ALL
t(9:22)	cABL(9q):BCR(22q)	CML and AML
t(6:9)	CAN(6p):DEK(9q)	AML
t(15:17)	PML(15q):RARa(17q)	APML
t(11:17)	PLZF(11q):RARa(17q)	APML
t(8:14)	cMYC	Burkitt's lymphoma
t(8:22)	cMYC	Burkitt's lymphoma
t(8:14)	cMYC	T-ALL
t(2:8)	cMYC	B-ALL
t(7:19)	LYL1	T-ALL
t(1:14)	TAL1	T-ALL
t(7:9)	TAL2	T-ALL
t(11:14)	Rhom1	T-ALL
t(11:14)	Rhom2	T-ALL
t(7:11)	Rhom2	T-ALL
t(10:14)	HOX11	T-ALL
t(7:10)	HOX11	T-ALL
t(7:9)	TAN1	T-ALL

PCR and the subsequent initiation of treatment should improve the clinical outcome of these diseases.

References

1. White TJ Arnheim N, Erlich HA (1989) The polymerase reaction.Trends Genet 5:185–189
2. Eisenstein BI (1990) The polymerase chain reaction: A new method of using molecular genetics for medical diagnosis. New Engl J Med 322:178–183
3. Erlich HA, Gelfand D, Sninsky JJ (1991) Recent advances in the polymerase chain reaction. Science 252:1643–1651
4. Persing DH (1991) Polymerase chain reaction: Trenches to benches. J Clin Micro 29:1281–1285
5. Grompe M (1993) The rapid detection of unknown mutations in nucleic acids. Nature Genet 5:111–117
6. Nakamura Y, Leppert M, O'Connell P, Wolff R, Holm T, Culver M, Martin C, Fujimoto E, Hoff M, Kumlin E, White R (1987) Variable number of tandem repeat (VNTR) markers for human gene mapping. Science 235:1616–1622
7. Kasai K, Nakamura Y, White R (1990) Amplification of a variable number of tandem repeats (VNTR) locus (pMCT118) by the polymerase chain reaction (PCR) and its application to forensic science. J Forensic Sci 35:1196–1200
8. Budowle B, Giusti AM, Waye JS, Baechtel FS, Fourney RM, Adams PE, Presley LA, Deadman HA, Monson KL (1991) Fixed-bin analysis for statistical evaluation of continuous distributions of allelic data from VNTR loci for use in forensic comparisons. Am J Hum Genet 48:841–855
9. Horn GT, Richards B, Klinger KW (1989) Amplification of a highly polymorphic VNTR segment by the polymerase chain reaction. Nucl Acids Res 17:2140
10. Batanian JR, Ledbetter SA, Wolff RK, Nakamura Y, White R, Dobnyns WB, Ledbetter DH (1990) Rapid diagnosis of Miller-Dieker syndrome and isolated lissencephaly sequence by the polymerase chain reaction. Hum Genet 85:555–559
11. Budowle B, Chakraborty R, Giusti AM, Eisenberg AJ, Allen RC (1991) Analysis of the VNTR locus DS180 by PCR followed by high resolution PAGE. Am J Hum Genet 48:137–144
12. Sajantila A, Puomilahti S, Johnsson V, Ehnholm C (1992) Amplification of reproducible allele markers for amplified fragment length polymorphism analysis. BioTechniques 12:16–22
13. Williams JGK, Kubelic AR, Livak KJ, Rafalski JA, Tingey SV (1990) DNA polymorphisms amplified by

arbitrary primers are useful as genetic markers. Nucl Acids Res 18:6531–6535
14. Orita M, Iwahana H, Kanazawa H, Hayashi K, Sekiya T (1989) Detection of polymorphisms of human DNA by gel electrophoresis as single-stand conformation polymorphisms. Proc Natl Acad Sci USA 86:2766–2770
15. Orita M, Suzuki Y, Sekiya T, Hayashi K (1989) Rapid and sensitive detection of point mutations using the polymerase chain reaction. Genomics 5:874–879
16. Michaud J, Brody LC, Steel G, Fontaine G, Martin LS, Valle D, Mitchell G (1992) Strand-separating conformational polymorphism analysis: Efficacy of detection of point mutations in the human ornithine δ-aminotransferase gene. Genomics 13:389–394
17. Doherty PJ, Huesca-Contreas M, Dosch HM, Pan S (1989) Rapid amplification of complementary DNA from small amounts of unfractionated RNA. Anal Biochem 177:7–10
18. Brenner CA, Tam AW, Nelson PA, Engleman EG, Suzuki N, Fry KE, Larric JW (1989) Message amplification phenotyping (MAPPing): A techinque to simultaneously measure mRNAs from small numbers of cells. BioTechniques 7:1096–1103
19. Dallman MJ, Montgomery RA, Larsen CP, Wanders A, Wells AF (1991) Cytokine gene expression: Analysis using northern blotting, polymerase chain reaction and in situ hybridisation. Immunol Rev 119:163–179
20. Wang AM, Doyle MV, Mark DF (1989) Quantitation of mRNA by the polymerase chain reaction. Proc Natl Acad Sci USA 86:9717–9721
21. Noonan KE, Beck C, Holzmayer TA, Chin JE, Wunder JS, Andrulis IL, Gazdar AF, Willman CL, Griffith B, Von Hoff DD, Ronsison IB (1990) Quantitative analysis of MDR1 (multidrug resistance) gene expression in human tumours by polymerase chain reaction. Proc Natl Acad Sci USA 87:7160–7164
22. Wages JM, Dolenga L, Fowler AK (1993) Electrochimiluminescent detection and quantitation of PCR-amplified DNA. Amplifications 10:1–6
23. Katz ED, DiCesare JL, Picozza E, Anderson MS (1993) General aspects of PCR quantitation. Amplifications 10:7–8
24. Van Houten B, Chandrasekhar D, Huang W (1993) Mapping DNA lesions at the gene level using quantitative PCR methodology. Amplifications 10:10–17
25. Rappolee D, Mark D, Banda MJ, Werb Z (1988) Wound macrophages express TGF-α and other growth factors in vivo: Analysis by mRNA phenotyping. Science 241:708–712
26. Chelly J, Kaplan JC, Maire P, Gautron S, Kahn A (1988) Transcription of the dystrophin gene in human muscle and non-muscle tissues. Nature 333:858–860
27. Thompson JD, Brodsky I, Yunis JJ (1992) Molecular quantification of residual disease in chronic myelogenous leukemia after bone marrow transplantation. Blood 79:1629–1635
28. Dobrovic A, Trainor KJ, Morley AA (1988) Detection of the molecular abnormality in chronic myeloid leukemia by use of the polymerase chain reaction. Blood 72:2063–2065
29. Hermans A, Selleri L, Gow J, Grosveld GC (1988) Absence of alternative splicing in bcr-abl mRNA in chronic myeloid leukemia cell lines. Blood 72:2066–2069
30. Kawasaki ES, Clark SS, Coyne MY, Smith SD, Champlin R, Witte ON, McCormick FP (1988) Diagnosis of chronic myeloid and acute lymphocytic leukemias by detection of leukemia-specific mRNA sequences amplified in vitro. Proc Natl Acad Sci USA 85:5698–5701
31. Hughes TP, Morgan GJ, Martiat P, Goldman M (1991) Detection of residual leukemia after bone marrow transplant for chronic myeloid leukemia: Role of polymerase chain reaction in predicting relapse. Blood 77:874–878
32. Lion T, Haas OA, Harbott J, Bannier E, Ritterbach J, Jankovic M, Fink FM, Stojimirovic A, Hermann J, Riehm HJ, Lampert F, Ritter J, Koch H, Gadner H (1992) The translocation t(1;22)(p13;q13) is a non-random marker specifically associated with acute megakaryocytic leukemia in young children. Blood 79:3325–3330
33. Lion T, Henn T, Gaiger A, Kalhs P, Gadner H (1993) Early detection of relapse after bone marrow transplantation in patients with chronic myelogenous leukemia. Lancet 341:275–276

Address for correspondence:
Dr. R. Shipman
Molekulare Onkologie
Forschungszentrum (ZLF)
Universitätskrankenhaus
Hebelstraße 20
CH-4031 Basel, Switzerland

Adjuvant therapy with recombinant CSFs in patients with solid tumors

J. Frisch[a], G. Schulz[a], J. Nemunaitis[b], W. P. Steward[c], J. Verweij[d],
W. Brugger[d], L. Kanz[d], R. Mertelsmann[e]

[a]Behringwerke AG, Marburg, [b]Baylor Medical Centre, Dallas, [c]Beatson Oncolgy Centre, Western Infirmary, Glasgow, [d]Rotterdam Cancer Institute Daniel den Hoed Kliniek, [e]University of Freiburg, Department of Hematology and Oncology, Freiburg, Germany

Introduction

Colony stimulating factors (CSFs) are gaining increasing importance since recombinant gene technology allows that they are produced in sufficient amounts for therapeutic doses in humans. CSFs play a major role as promoting factors in hematopoiesis. They determine together with various interleukins the process of differentiation from a pluripotent hematopoietic stem cell into specific cell lineages, e.g. granulopoiesis, myelopoiesis, megakaryopoiesis and erythropoiesis. Due to their proliferative activity in hematopoiesis the therapeutic use of CSFs is nowadays established in disorders with cytopenia, especially in those induced by oncological cytotoxic regimen.

The use of recombinant human granulocyte-macrophage colony stimulating factor (rh GM-CSF) after autologous bone marrow transplantation is well established since a large placebo-controlled study in patients with lymphoid malignancies showed that significantly earlier engraftment with rh GM-CSF directly translates into clinical benefit such as a six days shorter hospitalization period and a shorter duration of intravenous antibiotic therapy in GM-CSF treated patients (1). Apart from autologous bone marrow transplantation recently the first double blind placebo-controlled trial using rh GM-CSF after standard chemotherapy of acute myeloid leukemia (AML) demonstrated a significant reduction of infectious complications and thus decreasing the early treatment related mortality in AML induction therapy leading to a significant prolongation of the median survival of rh GM-CSF treated patients (2). Two approaches are now followed for further evaluation of the therapeutic use of CSFs: the search for more effective cytokine combinations and the efforts to intensify chemotherapy by adjuvant CSF therapy. Data referring to rh GM-CSF and interleukin-3 (IL-3) in either of these fields are presented in the following.

Cytokine combination

In a phase I study the megakaryopoietic action of rh IL-3 was recently identified. The sequential administration of rh IL-3 and rh GM-CSF was shown to induce increase of neutrophils as well as platelets (3). Thus the therapeutic advantage of the rh IL-3/rh GM-CSF combination was evaluated after a standard chemotherapy combination of etoposide, ifosfamide and cisplatin (VIP).

36 patients with advanced malignancies were treated with etoposide (VP16) 500 mg/m^2, ifosfamide 4 g/m^2 and cisplatin 50 mg/m^2 followed by the sequential administration of rh IL-3 (day 1 to 5, 250 µg/m^2 subcutaneously) and rh GM-CSF (day 6 to 15, 250 µg/m^2 subcutaneously). Control patients either received rh GM-CSF alone (for 15 days) after VIP chemotherapy or received VIP without any hematopoietic growth factor (4).

The 36 patients received a total of 50 chemotherapeutic treatment cycles. The allocation to control group (without growth factors), to rh GM-CSF alone or the sequential cytokine combination of rh IL-3/rh GM-CSF is listed in table I. These three treatment groups were balanced with respect to baseline characteristics. In addition patients were categorized according to their chemotherapeutic pretreatment status: One

Table I. IL-3 and GM-CSF following VIP chemotherapy.

Patient characteristics	Control	GM-CSF	IL-3 and GM-CSF
No. of patients	11	13	12
No. of cycles	13	17	20
Sex			
male	54	71	65
female	46	29	35
Median age (years)	52	51	50
range	37–64	21–64	21–68
Performance status (% of group)			
ECOG0	31	35	35
ECOG 1–2	69	65	65
Pretreatment status (no. of cycles)			
no.	7	6	6
mild-moderate	6	6	7
intensive	0	5	7

Table II. IL-3 and GM-CSF following VIP chemotherapy. Duration of neutropenia after VIP chemotherapy with or without hematopoietic growth factors. Data are indicated as median days of neutropenia. Ranges are indicated in parentheses.

Neutrophils ($\times 10^9/l$)	Control (IF = 13)	GM-CSF (n = 17)	p	IL-3/GM-CSF (n = 20)	p
< 1.0	10 (6–12)	5 (0–10)	< 0.005	5 (1–13)	< 0.01
< 0.5	8 (1–10)	3 (0–10)	< 0.01	4 (0–11)	< 0.01
< 0.1	3 (0–5)	0 (0–5)	< 0.02	1 (0–11)	< 0.05

group had no prior chemotherapy before entering the trial, one group was classified as having received mild to moderate cytotoxic pretreatment (less than six chemotherapy cycles and/or irradiation to less than 20% of their bone marrow) and a third subgroup having received intensive cytotoxic pretreatment (more than six chemotherapy cycles and/or irradiation to more than 20% of bone marrow) (table I). Rh GM-CSF as well as the sequential cytokine combination rh IL-3 plus rh GM-CSF was able to significantly reduce the duration of neutropenia after VIP chemotherapy in comparison to the control group without growth factors after VIP table II). The recovery times for platelets after standard chemotherapy are usually uneffected by rh GM-CSF therapy. In this trial the overall duration of thrombocytopenia was identical in all three treatment groups. As 64% of the patients did not show platelet counts less than $50 \cdot 10^9/l$ it is considered that the application of IL-3 in patients with less severe thrombocytopenia has no marked impact on platelet recovery time.

However, one third of the patients had a platelet nadir less than $50 \cdot 10^9/l$ and all these patients had been intensively pretreated with chemotherapy. In these patients the platelet recovery was accelerated after rh IL-3/rh GM-CSF combination compared to rh GM-CSF alone (figure 1). Control data without growth factor treatment in intensively pretreated patients cannot be presented. Because of ethical considerations all patients of this subgroup received adjuvant cytokine therapy after VIP.

The toxicity of the cytokine combination was mainly consisting of mild fever, headache, bone pain, arthralgia and myalgia. The most frequent event was fever observed in 14 cycles, two thirds

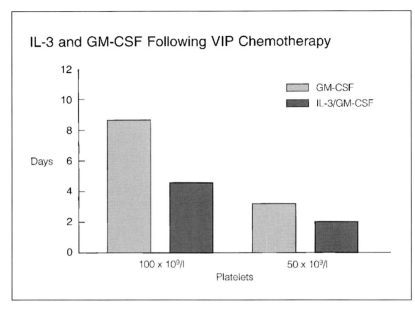

Figure 1. Median duration of thrombocytopenia in intensively pretreated patients. Median days of less than $100 \cdot 10^9/l$ or less than $50 \cdot 10^9/l$ platelets after VIP chemotherapy followed by either rh GM-CSF alone squential rh IL-3/rh GM-CSF (4).

WHO grade I, one third WHO grade II. Local erythema in a mild degree was observed in three cycles and only once the occurrence of dyspnoea (WHO grade III) was reported. No hypotension or signs of fluid retention and formation of effusions was seen.

Our results indicate that the sequential administration of IL-3 and GM-CSF seems to enhance platelet recovery only in patients who experienced grade III to IV thrombocytopenia after VIP chemotherapy. Especially in patients with severe thrombocytopenia a stimulatory effect on megakaryopoiesis would be most valuable and the sequential administration of IL-3 and GM-CSF might offer for the first time a therapeutic means to improve platelet recovery. The tolerability of the cytokine combination was as good as the single therapy with rh GM-CSF alone and in this respect our results are considered to be the basis for further evaluation of cytokine combinations including perhaps other CSFs with megakaryocytic activity like IL-6 or IL-II. The search for cytokine combinations providing advantages over the single adjuvant cytokine therapy has just begun and will most probably lead to a more effective supportive therapy in the future.

Dose intensification by rh GM-CSF

Maximal success of treatment has not been achieved even in chemotherapy sensitive tumors, because hematotoxicity is limiting further dose intensification. As rh GM-CSF may overcome this limitation the question whether tumor response may be improved is investigated in a series of clinical studies including patients with soft tissue sarcomas and small cell lung cancer.

Doxorubicin and ifosfamide are the most active substances to treat soft tissue sarcomas. A phase II study was conducted with the European Organization for Research and Treatment of Cancer (EORTC) Soft Tissue Sarcoma Group to test the feasibility of administering a regimen of high dose doxorubicin in combination with ifosfamide by support of rh GM-CSF.

104 patients with advanced soft tissue sarcoma were entered into the trial. 70 patients had metastatic disease only and 34 patients had local recurrence and metastases. Median age was 49 years (range 20 to 73) and all patients had a good performance status (WHO grade 0 or I, only two patients grade II). Patients received doxorubicin 75 mg/m^2 as an intravenous bolus injection followed immediately by ifosfamide 5 g/m^2 as a 24 hour infusion together with uroprotection of

Mesna. 24 hours after the end of ifosfamide infusion rh GM-CSF was commenced at a total daily dose of 250 µg/m². Rh GM-CSF was administered up to 14 days but discontinued earlier if neutrophil counts were grater than $10 \cdot 10^9/l$. Six chemotherapeutic courses were administered at 3 week intervals (5).

Throughout all six chemotherapeutic cycles the median leucocyte nadir was found to be greater than $1.0 \cdot 10^9/l$ even in later cycles. However, the median platelet nadir decreased continuously throughout the six chemotherapeutic cycles (table III). The chemotherapeutic courses could be administered every 21 days (median length), only 23% to a maximum of 39% of patients per cycle had to be delayed. High dose chemotherapy could be administered as planned: the median dose of doxorubicin was 75 mg/m², median dose of ifosfamide was 5 g/m² throughout all six courses. In each course in less than 5% patients, a dose reduction had to be realized. In summary this trial demonstrated that the high dose doxorubicin plus ifosfamide regimen could be administered by the additional application of rh GM-CSF (250 mg/m²/d) with a hematotoxicity being comparable to lower chemotherapeutic doses without growth factor. The response rate in this study was 45% and thus the highest so far seen by this cooperative multinational group for treatment of advanced soft tissue sarcomas. Previous trials with high dose doxorubicin alone or with a combination of ifosfamide, and standard doxorubicin without GM-CSF demonstrated lower overall response rates (table IV). The response rate found in this trial may indicate that the dose increase achieved by support of rh GM-CSF may finally achieve more favorable tumor response rates. This has to be proven in a controlled and randomized study which is currently running.

Another randomized double blind placebo-controlled trial in patients with small cell lung cancer of favorable prognosis is currently conducted in a European study group comprising 17 oncological centres. The question in this trial is whether the chemotherapeutic dose can be increased by shortening of the length of chemotherapeutic cycles. Patients receive a chemotherapy combination of ifosfamide (5 g/m² as 24 hour infusion given on day 1), carboplatin (300 mg/m² i.v. on day 1 and 3), etoposide (120 mg/m² i.v. on day 1 and 2, 240 mg/m² p.o. on day 3) with midcourse vincristine (0.5 mg/m² i.v. on day 14). On day 4 rh GM-CSF therapy (or placebo) is commenced at a dose of 250 µg/m² subcutaneously for a maximum of 14 days. Patients are randomized to either one arm with a constant administration of each ICE chemotherapy every 28 days or to the second arm with intensified chemotherapy where each course is started as soon as hematological recovery has occured (WBC $> 3 \cdot 10^9/l$ and platelets $> 100 \cdot 10^9/l$). Preliminary data of 142 patients of this ongoing trial indicate that in the

Table III. High dose doxorubicin/ifosfamide + rhu GM-CSF in soft tissue sarcoma (EORTC 62883). Hematoxicity per cycle (median nadir (range) $\cdot 10^9/l$).

	n	WBC	Platelets
Cycle 1	51	1.0 (0.2–3.9)	122 (20–344)
Cycle 2	47	1.8 (0.1–9.4)	78 (14–412)
Cycle 3	39	1.0 (0.0–7.1)	29 (4–215)
Cycle 4	33	1.1 (0.2–4.1)	32 (4–173)
Cycle 5	22	1.2 (0.1–6.0)	35 (5–282)
Cycle 6	17	1.1 (0.2–5.3)	37 (7–98)

Table IV. Tumor response in EORTC soft tissue sarcoma trials using chemotherapy with or without rh GM–CSF.

Chemotherapy	No. of evaluable patients	Tumor response (%)			
		CR	PR	NC	PD
Doxorubicin (75.0 mg/m²)	83	7 → 25 ← 18		45	30
Doxorubicin (50.0 mg/m²) + ifosfamide (5.0 g/m²)	175	9 → 35 ← 26		47	18
Doxorubicin (75.0 mg/m²) + ifosfamide (5.0 g/m²) + rh GM-CSF (250 µg/m²/day)	104	10 → 45 ← 35		35	20

intensified arm a median cycle length of 21 days throughout all cycles compared to 28 days in the fixed arm can be achieved. Overall the dose intensity could be increased by a median of 30% in the intensified arm and the preliminary data seem to indicate a more favorable complete response rate by this intensified dose.

Conclusions

It has been a major breakthrough to get CSFs from the laboratory to the patients. Clinical use of cytokines such as G-CSF, GM-CSF and Erythropoietin is meanwhile standard in oncology departments to prevent or shorten time of severe neutropenia or anemia. Since hematopoiesis involves the interaction of a variety of CSFs and as those actions are overlapping, additive or synergistic, the development of those cytokines is complex. It is unlikely that a single factor provides sufficient treatment for complex hematopoietic disorders regardless of whether they are due to endogenous or exogenous causes. Further clinical research will have three major goals:
1. to optimize combinations of CSFs in order to improve efficacy and to diminish toxicity;
2. to prove that clinical use of CSFs allows more intensive chemotherapy resulting in a higher rate of tumor remission and a better longterm survival of cancer patients;
3. to characterize and produce new CSFs like a megakaryocyte-CSF.

Acknowledgement

The authors thank *A. Immel* and *C. Prinz* for typing the manuscript.

Reference

1. Nemunaitis J, Rabinowe S, Singer J, Bierman P, Vose J, Freedman A, Onetto N, Gillis S, Oette D, Gold M, Buckner C, Hansen J, Ritz J, Appelbaum F, Armitage J, Nadler L (1991) Recombinant granulocyte-macrophage colony-stimulating factor after autologous bone marrow transplantation for lymphoid cancer. N Engl J Med 324:1773–1778
2. Rowe J, Andersen J, Mazza J, Paietta E, Bennett J, Hayes A, Oette D, Wiernik P (1993) Phase III randomized placebo-controlled study of granulocyte-macrophage colony-stimmulating factor (GM-CSF) in adult patients (55–70 years) with acute myelogenous leukemia (AML). A study of the eastern cooperative oncology group (ECOG). Blood 82 (suppl 1):329a
3. Ganser A, Lindemann A, Ottmann O, Seipelt G, Hess U, Geissler G, Kanz L, Frisch J, Schulz G, Herrmann F, Mertelsmann R, Hölzer D (1992) Sequential in vivo treatment with two recombinant human hematopoietic growth factors (Interleukin-3 and granulocyte-macrophage colony-stimulating factor) as a new therapeutic modality to stimulate hematopoiesis: Results of a phase I study. Blood 79:2583–2591
4. Brugger W, Frisch J, Schulz G, Pressler K, Mertelsmann R, Kanz L (1992) Sequential administration of interleukin-3 and granulocyte-macrophage colony-stimulating factor following standard-dose combination chemotherapy with etoposide, ifosfamide and cisplatin. J Clin Oncol 10:1452–1459
5. Steward W, Verweij J, Somers R, Spooner D, Kerbrat P, Clavel M, Crowther D, Rouesse J, Tursz T, Tueni E, van Oosterom A, Warwick J, Greifenberg B, Thomas D, van Glabbeke M (1993) Granulocyte-macrophage colony-stimulating factor allows safe escalation of dose-intensity of chemotherapy in metastatic adult soft tissue sarcomas: A study of the European organization for research and treatment of cancer soft tissue and bone sarcoma group. J Clin Oncol 11:15–21

Address for correspondence:
Prof. Dr. med. G. Schulz
Behringwerke AG
Postfach 1140
D-35001 Marburg, Germany

Modification of local and systemic host response by topical cytokine application in malignant disease

Experimental and clinical experiences

Edith Huland, H. Heinzer, B. Falk, H. Schwaibold, D. Hübner, H. Huland
Department of Urology, University of Hamburg, Hamburg, Germany

Cytokines were shown to have potent antitumor-activity in preclinical and clinical studies. Especially interleukin 2 (IL-2) and interferons are promising in this respect. However, systemic cytokine treatment in general induces toxic systemic effects preventing long-term treatment which seems to be neccessary for complete tumor eradication. In addition cytokines are small molecules, cleared rapidly by glomerular filtration leading to short half-life in serum and uneconomical use of such expensive and rare substances. Topical injection of interferon in melanoma, colorectal carcinoma, Kaposi´s sarcoma and other malignancies have been reported to induce effective antitumor responses. Our group has therefore evaluated in a multistep approach the toxicities and therapeutic possibilities of local continuous IL-2 application in localized and systemic tumor diseases. In a first step we have proven that high dose local continuous IL-2 perfusion in human bladders of patients with advanced transitional cell carcinoma does not induce local or systemic toxicity, even when applied for months. In five patients with T4 N0 M0 transitional cell carcinoma of the bladder we used continuous IL-2 perfusion of the bladder (1000 U BRMP/ml, 2 ml/min, 24 h/day) for 5 days/cycle. None of our patients showed any evidence of side effects. Before treatment no Il- 2 receptor positive cells were found in urine, after treatment a distinct increase in IL-2 receptor positive cells occured not only in urine but also in peripheral blood. One patient had a complete histologically proven remission of his tumor (1). In urinary sediment eosinophils were attached to the tumor cells and according to staining with specific monoclonal antibodies actively secreted eosinophil granules on these tumor cells locally (2). In a second step the inhalatory application of IL-2 in patients with pulmonary metastatic renal cell carcinoma was shown to be a non-toxic and highly effective support to patients treated with low dose systemic cytokines. Treatment duration is possible and effective for up to three years now, toxicity of treatment was low with no evidence for pulmonary damage. Treatment can be combined with i.v. or subcutaneous additional cytokine therapy (3, 4, 5) or in patients with high risk factors not allowing systemic treatment without additional systemic cytokine treatment with antitumor effect (6). With addtional low dose systemic cytokine pulmonary metastases responded in one patient completely (six months) in nine patients partially (33, 24, 24, 21+ ,18, 18, 8, 5, 4 months) and were stabilized in eight patients in a total of 18 patients.

In a further step we developed depot preparations containing IL-2 and INF a which release cytokines continuously for more than four weeks and are sterile and suitable for in vivo use. This depot systems have been proved to induce effective antitumor responses in nude mice transplanted with human tumor tissue, when the depots were located directly at the tumor site. IL-2 can induce immune responses in the nude mouse. Longterm in vivo bioactivity of released IL-2 from depot preparations was proven with this model.

We conclude that local cytokine treatment is not toxic and highly effective. The development of pharmaceutically acceptable depot preparations will enable us to make use of these advantages in advanced and systemic tumor diseases.

References

1. Huland E, Huland H (1989) Local continuous high dose interleukin 2: a new therapeutic model for the treatment of advanced bladder carcinoma. Cancer Res 49: 5469–5474
2. Huland E, Huland H (1992) Tumor-associated eosinophilia in interleukin-2-treated patients: evidence of toxic eosinophil degranulation on bladder cancer cells. J Cancer Res Clin Oncol 118:463–467
3. Huland E, Heinzer H, Huland H (1994) Inhaled interleukin-2 in combination with low dose systemic interleukin-2 and interferon-a in patients with pulmonary metastatic-renal cell carcinoma: effectiveness and toxicity of mainly local treatment. J Cancer Res Clin Oncol 120:221–228
4. Heinzer H, Huland E, Huland H (1993) Lokale Immuntherapie urologischer Tumoren – ein neues Therapiekonzept in der Applikation von Cytokinen. Urologie Nephrologie 5:240–249
5. Huland E, Huland H, Heinzer H (1992) Interleukin 2 by inhalation: Local therapy for metastatic renal-cell carcinoma. J Urol 147:344–348
6. Aulitzky WE, Kessler M, Wilhelm M, Huland E, Thews C, Peschel C, Huber C, Lorenz J (1993) Aerosolized natural interleukin-2 for treatment of advanced malignancy: Results of a phase I trial. Ann. Hematol 66 Suppl II : A 109
7. Heinzer et al (this volume)
8. Falk et al (this volume)

Address for correspondence:
Dr. med. Edith Huland
Abteilung für Urologie
Universität Hamburg
Martinistraβe 52
D-20252 Hamburg, Germany

Workshop 3

Immunosuppression, -deficiency (Transplantation/AIDS) and Cancer

De novo cancers in renal transplant recipients

R. Brunkhorst, H. Lang, M. Behrendt, U. Frei
Center for Internal Medicine and Dermatology, Hannover, Germany

Introduction

In 1969 Mc Khann and Penn et al. (7, 11) reported an association between cancer and immunosuppression in renal allograft patients. The reported incidence of cancer in renal transplant patients under use of cyclosporine (which represented the basic immunsuppressive drug in the recent years) ranges from 1 to 16% at various centers (1, 2, 9, 10) . This great variation is due to methodological reasons: Only short observation times were covered and in some studies the numbers of patients without malignancies were not reported; the populations were heterogenous with different immunosuppressive regimens and different ethnic and geographic background. Frequently a comparison to a non-transplanted control population is lacking. Therefore the present study was performed in the homogenous population of renal allograft recipients of a single transplant center treated by a well defined immunosuppressive regimen; as control served the data of a regional cancer registry.

Patients and methods

Between May 1981 (when cyclosporin A was introduced) and the end of 1991 a total of 1620 grafts were performed at our institution, 1352 of them were first transplants. Last date of follow-up was July 1992. 966 transplants were performed in male, 654 in female recipients. Total observation time was 6015 patient years (3510 in male and 2504 in female patients). Mean age of the recipients at time of transplant was 39.5 years (median 41.9, range 1–73 years; mean of males 40.2, of females 38.4 years). 89.1% of the patients received cadaver kidneys, the remaining received grafts from living related donors. Grafts were allocated according to Eurotransplant exchange criteria. More than 60% of the grafts were shipped from elsewhere for optimal HLA-matching.

The control data were taken from the cancer registry of the Saarland (german federal state of 1 million inhabitants) (12) .

All patients were controlled at the outpatient clinic in close cooperation with the referring nephrologists. A screening programm for detection of tumors and skin malignancies was carried out at least twice per year.

Prophylactic immunosuppression consisted of prednisolone 1 mg/kg/bodyweight (BW)/day initially which was tapered down to 0.1 mg/kg BW/day after three months to a final maintenance dose of 5 to 7.5 mg/day. Cyclosporine was administered at 10 mg/kg/day postoperatively and subsequently adjusted to RIA whole blood trough levels. Until 1984 the initial dose was 14 mg/kg/BW/day. Levels of 400–800 ng/ml until 1984 and 300–600 ng/ml until 1988 measured by the polyclonal RIA were tolerated. Thereafter the therapeutic range was 100–150 ng/ml measured by the more specific monoclonal assay (RIA). In addition 19.8% of the male and 13.8% of the female patients received azathioprine (2 mg/kg/day) for some periods because of initial non-function or cyclosporine toxicity. Rejection treatment consisted of 500 mg methylprednisolone boluses daily for 3–5 days, in steroid resistant rejections (7% of all patients) poly- or monoclonal antilymphocytic sera were administered.

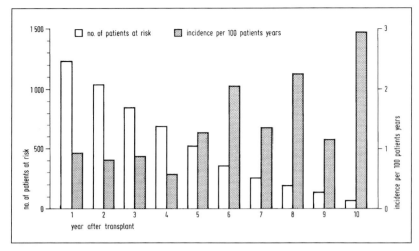

Figure 1. Annual incidence of malignancies per 100 patient years.

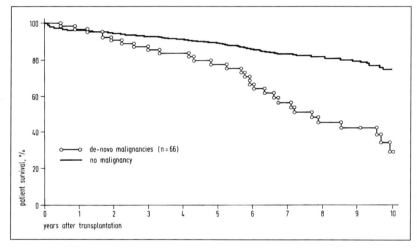

Figure 2. Patient survival after kidney transplantation compared for patients with or without malignant disease.

Results

Incidence of de-novo malignancies: Development of a de novo malignant disorder was observed in 66 patients (40 males and 26 females). Mean age of the recipients developing a malignancy was 48.8 years (males 48.2, females 49.8 years) at the time of transplant. Mean age at the time when the cancer was diagnosed was 52.9 years (males 52.1, females 54.2 years). The incidence for development of a malignant disease is given in figure 1. The figure shows that the incidence was less than 1/100 patient years until year four after renal transplantation. In the following years the incidence rose to numbers between 1.3 and 2.9 cases per 100 patient years.

Sites of malignancies: 18 out 66 malignancies detected were skin cancers, two of them malignant melenomas, five lymphomas were observed, one of them Hodgkin's lymphoma (8). None of these patients had ever received poly- or monoclonal antibodies. Time of development ranged ranged between 8 and 128 months after transplant. The remaining malignancies consisted of solid tumors of different sites resembling the distribution in a non-transplanted population except for urotheliomas which were found in eight cases. Original disease in seven of them was analgesic nephropathy.

Risk estimation: The ratio between expected and observed de novo malignanies was calculated for al age groups in five year intervals comparing the

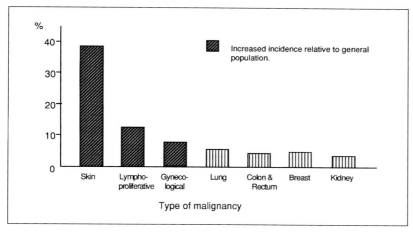

Figure 3. Distribution of the most common malignancies occurring in organ transplant recipients (from (9)).

study population with a cancer registry. For 2504 observed patient years in the female population the expected number of malignancies was 7.3 compared to 26 observed cases in our population, which means a 3.5 fold increased risk in female kidney transplant recipients. In 3510 patient years observed in males the expected number was 13.3, compared to an observed number of 40 malignancies what resembles a 3-fold increase. The difference was significant for males and females ($p < 0.01$, x-square test). When the cumulative risk to develop a de novo malignancy was calculated by life table analysis, the risk after TEN years was 13.5%.

Survival: The development of a malignant disorder after kidney transplantation affected the patient survival significantly when the patient survival curve for affected and non-affected patients was compared by life table analysis (figure 2).

Discussion

Several theories have been proposed for the increased incidence of cancer in immune deficient individuals, including impaired immune surveillance mechanisms (5), chronic antigenic stimulation (3), reactivation of latent oncogenic viruses (6, 13), and direct oncogenic effects of immunosuppressive drugs (9–11). These pathogenetic mechanisms increase the risk for skin and lip cancer (4, 14), lymphoproliferative disease in heart transplant patients and renal transplant recipients (15, 16) and for gynecological neoplasms (10) compared to the general population (see figure 3). Unfortunately most studies only give the percentage of affected patients out of the total transplant population irrespective of the time of exposure to risk. Furthermore the mode of immunosuppression and the racial and geographic background varied and were reported inadequately in most studies. The present study analyzed a population homogenous with respect to selection criteria, mode of immunosuppression and ethnic and geographic background. Compared to a regional cancer registry the risk to develop de novo malignancy was increased 3.0–3.5-fold for males and females. This is in agreement with the report of *Walz* et al. from another german center using a comparable immunosuppressive regimen (17). Under the limited immunosuppression with steroids and cyclosporine and the cautious use of antibodies no excess numbers of malignancies ocurred during the first years after transplantation. However, our data suggest an increasing incidence of cancer with time of exposure irrespective of age. The cumulative risk to develop a malignancy within ten years is 13.5% under our renal transplant conditions. Development of malignancy after kidney transplantation worsened markedly survival in affected patients. In summary, development of malignant tumors remains a serious long term problem in patients after kidney transplantation even under cautious immunosuppressive regimens and in regions without increased risk for skin cancer.

References

1. Birkeland SA (1983) Malignant tumors in renal transplant recipients. Cancer 51:1571–1575
2. Cockburn I (1987) Cancers after renal transplantation. Transplant Proc 19:1804–1808
3. Gleichmann E, Gleichmann H, Schwartz RS, Weinblatt A, Armstrong MYK (1975) Immunologic induction of malignant lymphoma: Identification of donor and host tumors in the graft versus host model. J Natl Cancer Inst 54:107–116
4. Gruber SA, Skjei KL, Sothern RB (1991) Skin tumors in renal transplant patients. Transplant Proc 23:1104–1110
5. Klein G, Klein E (1977) Immune surveillance against virus-induced tumors and nonrejectability of spontaneous tumors: Contrasting consequences of host versus tumor evolution. Proc Natl Acad Sci 74:2121–2125
6. Matas AJ, Simmons RL, Najarian JS (1975) Chronic antigenic stimulation, herpes virus infection, and cancer in transplant recipients. Lancet 1:1277–1279
7. Mc Khann CF (1969) Primary malignancy in patients undergoing immunosuppression for renal transplantation. Transplantation 8:209–212
8. Oldhafer K, Bunzendahl H, Frei U (1989) Hodgkin's lymphoma in a renal transplant patient. Am J Med 47:218–219
9. Penn I (1988) Development of new tumors after transplantation. In: Cerilli GJ (ed) Organ transplantation and replacement. Lippincott, Philadelphia, pp 612–620
10. Penn I (1989) Risk of cancer in the transplant patient. In: Flye M W (ed) Principles of organ transplantation. Saunders, Philadelphia, pp 254–261
11. Penn I, Hammond W, Brettschneider L, Starzl T (1969) Malignant lymphomas in transplantation patients. Transplant Proc 1:106–112
12. Sonderhefte Statistisches Amt des Saarlandes. Tumorstatistik (1989) 166:30–45
13. Saemundsen AK, Klein G, Cleary M, Warnke R (1982) Epstein Barr virus carrying lymphoma in cardiac transplant recipients. Lancet 2:158
14. Sheil AGR, Disney APS, Mathew TH (1991) Cancer development in renal transplant patients. Transplant Proc 23:1111–1115
15. Starzl TE, Nalesnik MA, Porter KA (1984) Reversibility of lymphomas and lymphoproliferative lesions developing under cyclosporine – steroid therapy. Lancet 1:583–587
16. Swinnen LJ, Constanzo-Nordin MR, Fisher SG (1990) Lymphomas under cyclosporine – steroid therapy after heart transplantation. N Engl J Med 323:1723-1726
17. Walz MK, Albrecht KH, Niebel W, Eigler W (1992) De novo Malignome unter medikamentöser Immunsuppression. Dtsch med Wschr 117:927–931

Address for correspondence:
Priv.-Doz. Dr. R. Brunkhorst
Zentrum für Innere Medizin und Dermatologie
Abteilung Nephrologie
Postfach 610180
D-30625 Hannover, Germany

Limiting factors of liver transplantation in patients with liver tumors

X. Rogiers, T. E. Langwieler, M. Malagó, R. Kuhlencordt,
W. T. Knoefel, L. Fischer, M. Sterneck, C. E. Broelsch

Abteilung Allgemeinchirurgie, Universitäts-Krankenhaus Eppendorf, Hamburg, Germany

In the seventies, liver transplantation has developed to a routine operation. It was hoped that this kind of procedure could also be used as a radical operation for treatment of hepatic tumors. Potential indications can be devided in two groups: tumors that were previously not resectable because they occured in cirrhotic livers and tumors in normal livers that are so big or badly located that they could not be resected without vital damage to the remaining liver.

Since these early times, many patients with liver tumors have been treated with liver transplantation. Several single cases with longterm survival have been reported. Looking closer at the published data from Pittsburgh, Chicago, Hannover etc., however, one finds that good results are not the rule.

In a consecutive series at the University of Chicago which we studied one can see that the earlier results of liver transplantations in tumor patients are extremely good and even clearly better than those of cirrhotic patients. One month survival rate was 95%. By looking at longer survival times, however, the results are very bad (25%). Results in patients with a fibrolamellar hepatocellular carcinoma or a hepatocellular carcinoma smaller than 5 cm were clearly better. But also in this group the results published by the university of Pittsburgh are clearly worse than those of patients without malignoma (46% and 68% respective three year survival rates).

An especially bad group is composed by the cholangiocellular carcinomas. In our view, with very few exceptions, this kind of carcinoma should be considered as a contraindication for liver transplantation.

The bad results of liver transplantation for tumors are also illustrated in table II, where we looked at the patients transplanted for tumors in Germany in 1991 that were reported to the European Liver Transplant Registry (ELTR).

The conclusion is clear, that liver transplantation for tumors is certainly not an efficient use of the few available organs for transplantation. Still it is at least problematic to refuse transplantation to these patients as a small chance of longer survival.

Therefore, in our view, liver transplantation for liver malignomas still has to be possible, although in very selected cases and only in the frame of controlled studies.

In order to reduce the impact of such a transplantation on the organ pool, split liver transplantation should be considered in these patients. Split liver transplantation, in which the liver is

Table I. Liver transplants at the university of Chicago (4).

	Tumor	Cirrhosis
Operating time	7 ± 3 h	11 ± 3 h
Blood loss	0.8 ± 1 units	3.4 ± 4 units
ICU stay	3 ± 2 days	7 ± 9 days
Hospital stay	15 ± days	35 ± 20 days
1 Month survival	95%	90%
1 Year survival	26%	72%

Table II. Patients transplanted for tumor in Germany in 1991 (ELTR data).

	Tumor patients	Actuarial survival time (01.01.1993)
All	48 (12.5%)	23 (48%)
Liver transplant centers with < 40 LTx/year	27 (20%)	13 (41%)

divided in two, using the left lateral liver lobe for a child and the right liver for an adult has shown clearly worse results in the early experience (Chicago). One has to say to this that many of these patients where in acute hepatic failure and were transplanted as high urgently patients, carrying a higher peri-operative risk.

The increasing surgical expierence with reduced-sized livers and living related liver transplantation, however, should allow to improve the management of technical complications. In addition, tumor patients have the advantage of being technically easier than cirrhotic patients. The good coagulation of these patients increases the risk of bleeding from the cut section of the reduced liver. As a disadvantage one can see that, in order to bridge the radically resected liver hilum, vascular interponates may be nessesary.

The most recent experiences with the split liver transplantation in Europe provides hope that, in elective conditions, results of split liver transplantation may be equal to those of "full-size" liver transplantation.

Conclusion

Specific indications for liver transplantation in patients with tumors still remain a matter of debate. In the context of the existing organ shortage and the ethical considerations mentioned above, it is essential that such transplants are performed in the context of a controlled study.

An improvement of the number of organs could be achieved by the use of split liver transplantation for this indication. Because of the good pre-operative blood coagulation and electivity of the procedure tumor patients may be especially suitable for this kind of procedure.

References

1. Funovics JM, Fritsch A, Herbst F, Piza F, Mühlbacher F, Längle F, Iwatsuki S, Gordon RD, Shaw BW, Starzl TE (1985) Role of liver transplantation in cancer therapy. Ann Surg 202 (4):401–407
2. Pichlmayr R, Ringe B, Lauchart W, Neuhaus P (1988) Approach to primary liver cancer. Recent Results in Cancer Research 110:65-73
3. Pichlmayr R, Ringe B, Lauchart W, Bechstein WO, Gubernatis G, Wagner E (1988) Radical resection and liver grafting as the two main components of surgical strategy in the treatment of proximal bile duct cancer. World J Surg 12:68–77
4. Rouch DA, Emond JC, Thistlethwaite JR, Brolesch CE (1989) Liver transplantation for hepatic malignancy. In: Lygidakis NS, Tytga GNS (eds) Hepatobiliary and pancreatic malignancies. Thieme, Stuttgart, pp 248–253
5. Schemper M (1988) Primary hepatic cancer – The role of limited resection (?) and total hepatic resection with orthotopic liver replacement. Hepatogastroenterol 35:316–320
6. Wolff H, Sperling P (1986) Die chirurgische Therapie des Leberkarzinoms. Zentrbl Chir 111:3–15
7. Yokoyama I, Todo S, Iwatsuki S, Starzl TE (1990) Liver transplantation in the treatment of primary liver cancer. Hepatogastroenterol 37:188–193

Address for correspondence:
Dr. med. X. Rogiers
Universitätskrankenhaus Eppendorf
Abteilung für Allgemeine Chirurgie
Lebertransplantation
Martinistraße 52
D-20246 Hamburg, Germany

Determination of tumor markers after heart transplantation

H. Nägele[a], R. Klapdor[b], M. Bahlo[b], P. Kalmar, W. Rödiger[b]
[a]Department of Thoracic and Cardiovascular Surgery,
[b]Department of Internal Medicine, University Hospital, Hamburg, Germany

Introduction

Immunosuppressive therapy after transplantation of solid organs is discussed as a decisive factor for the 100fold incidence of carcinomas and the 40fold risk for non-Hodgkin's lymphomas in these patients (8, 11). In various studies incidence of cutaneous tumors and lymphomas is reported between 1 and 16%.

In these transplanted patients there is reported a relevant association between lymphoproliferative diseases and an induction treatment with OKT3- (16) and anti-thymocyte globulin (10). In our experience, during the time period 1984-1994, six (7.5%) of our 81 transplanted patients (mean age 49 ± 12 years) developed a malignoma (mean age 49 years) (see table I). According to Kaplan-Meier statistics the risk for developing cancer amounts to 30% about seven years post-Tx (figure 1). All these patients died from tumor disease in spite of various treatment trials and in spite of encouraging reports on treatment results after heart transplantation (14, 15).

Simultaneous determination of sensitive tumor markers in addition to clinical investigation and imaging methods might improve an earlier and more specific tumor diagnosis in these high risk patients (2). On the other hand transplantation and post-transplantation treatment or rejection may influence the serum concentrations of various tumor markers (2, 3, 12, 18).

Therefore we started a prospective study to evaluate the potential value of tumor marker determinations in our collective of patients with heart transplantation.

Methods

At the University of Hamburg heart transplantation is followed by rATG (Fresenius) induction therapy in the first postoperative week in combination with cyclosporin A and decreasing doses of methylprednisolon. Chronic immunosuppression comprises triple therapy with cyclosporin A (levels between 100 and 140 ng/ml), azathioprin (50–100 mg/die) and 4–8 mg methylprednisolon.

Up to now, the tumor markers CA 125 (Enzymun EIA BM), CA 19-9 (Cobas® Core EIA Roche) CEA (Enzymun EIA BM), TAG 72 (IRMA Sorin), TPA cyk (ELISA medac) and TPS (IRMA Beki) were determined in three months intervals in all 47 patients admitted to the hospital for follow-up

Table I. Tumor diseases after heart transplantation (Hamburg).

Patient	Age at HTx	Years after Tx	Tumor	Death (days after tumor diagnosis)
W.H.	32	4.3	hypopharynx ca.	288
K.P.	41	6.5	small cell lung ca.	7
B.U.	53	3.7	MALT-lymphoma	217
L.F.	54	6.0	liposarcoma	41
K.F.	54	2.9	Burkitt lymphoma	18
E.E.	62	4.0	squamous cell lung ca.	176
Mean	49.3	4.5		124

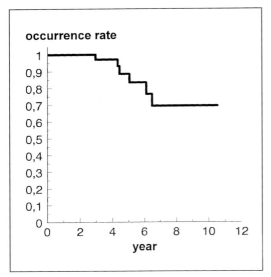

Figure 1. Occurrence of malignancies (n = 6) in Htx patients (Hamburg, n = 81 patients 1984–1994) (Kaplan-Meier-analysis).

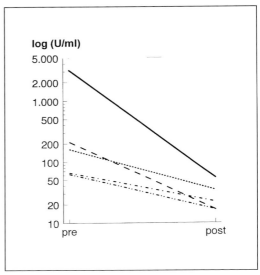

Figure 3. Course of the pre- and post Htx serum concentrations of CA 125 in 5 consecutive patients.

after heart transplantation over a time period of 13 months. In addition, the markers were determined in 34 patients admitted for HTx because of terminal heart insufficiency to study the effects of effective heart transplantation on the serum levels (blood samples were taken 1–8 weeks before transplantation and about three months after stabilization of clinical situation after Tx).

The statistical analyses were done using the SPSS 6.0 for Windows (U-test according to *Mann-Whitney*).

Results

Comparison of pre- and postoperative determinations

Considering CA 125 we found a significant difference between the pre- and the postoperative serum concentrations (277 ± 649 and 53 ± 166 U/ml, p = 0.026) (figure 2). Some typical examples are shown in figure 3. For the other markers measured we did not find a significant difference (CA 19-9 35 ± 56 versus 28 ± 33 U/ml, CEA 2.9 ± 1.7 versus 2.7 ± 1.5 ng/ml, TAG 72-4 3.2 ± 0.4 versus 3.3 ± 1.4 U/ml, TPAcyk 0.85 ± 0.8 versus 0.89 ± 1.3 and TPS 118 ± 114 versus 97 ± 83 U/l) (figures 4a–e).

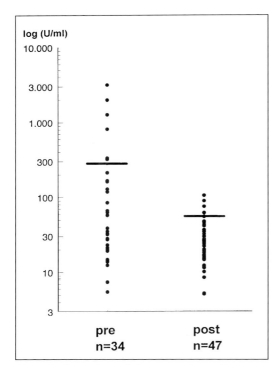

Figure 2. Comparison of the pre- and post Htx serum concentrations of CA 125 (p = 0.026).

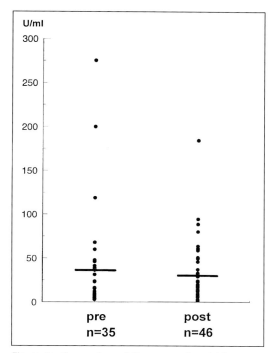

Figure 4a. Comparison of the pre- and post Htx serum concentrations of CA 19-9.

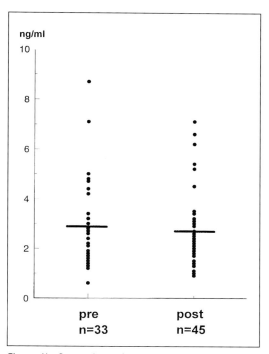

Figure 4b. Comparison of the pre- and post Htx serum concentrations of CEA.

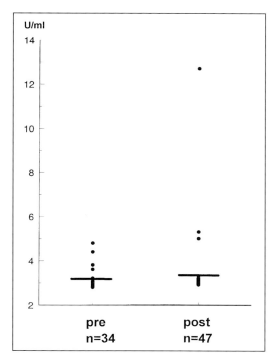

Figure 4c. Comparison of the pre- and post Htx serum concentrations of CA 72-4.

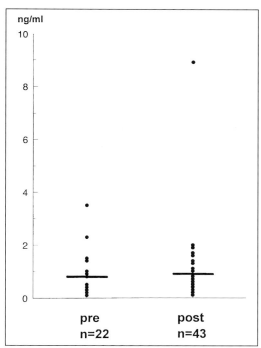

Figure 4d. Comparison of the pre- and post serum concentration of TPAcyk.

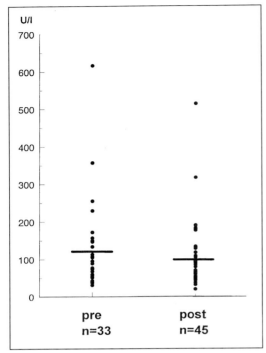

Figure 4e. Comparison of the pre- and post Htx serum concentrations of TPS.

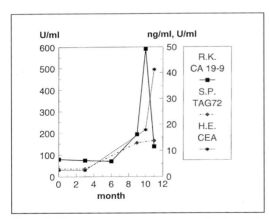

Figure 5. Time course of tumor markers in three Htx patients without overt malignancies.

Patients with histologically verified tumors

The results of two patients with proven tumors at time of tumor marker determination are shown in table II.

Patients with increase of single tumor markers

Three patients showed as suspicious increase of a single tumor marker without evidence for malignoma in endoscopy, sonography or CT, clinical investigation and x-ray examination. Furthermore, in patient R.K. we did not find increased levels for bilirubin or transaminases, however, a spontaneous decrease of CA 19-9 in the further follow-up. All three patients did not show signs of rejection and no signs of liver or kidney disfunction.

Discussion

Patients after organ transplantation represent a high risk group for the development of malignant tumor diseases. Consequently, regular tumor marker determinations might be of clinical relevance. However, actually there are mainly two limitations:
1. We do not have a relevant tumor marker available for non-Hodgkin's lymphomas the tumors with the highest incidence after organ transplantation. On the other hand, in order to "screen" for the various tumors we would need a spectrum of tumor markers, such as CA 125 for ovarian cancer, CA 19-9 for pancreatic, CEA for colorectal, CA 72-4 for stomach, CA 15-3 for breast, CYFRA 21-1 for lung and TPA e.g. for proliferating epithelial tumors. In males PSA should be added for detection of prostate cancer. In our patient with the squameous cell lung cancer

Table II. Tumor marker serum concentrations in two patients with proven malignomas (K.P. metastasized SCLC, E.E. squameous cell lung cancer).

Patient	CA 125 U/ml	CA 19-9 U/ml	CEA ng/ml	TAG72-4 U/ml	TPAcyk ng/ml	TPS U/l	SCC U/ml	NSE ng/ml
K.P.	1162	2390	1016	3	15	3175	–	–
E.E.	29	25	1.8	3	2.8	274	25	14.4

e.g. the SCC determination was the first sign of tumor disease.

2. In patients before and after organ transplantation there are some unspecific effects on serum concentrations of tumor markers. Our data suggest an increase of CA 125 serum levels in patients suffering from cardial insufficiency. Probably the "tumor marker" CA 125 may correlate with the degree of cardial insufficiency. Recently there was reported the usefulness of serum CA 125 measurement for monitoring pericardial effusion (13).

Hepatitis and liver cirrhosis may induce elevated CA 19-9 serum concentrations (4). Rejection after liver transplantation may induce transient increases of CA 19-9 (12). Transient increases of various tumor markers are reported after kidney transplantation (18). The significant increase of serum CA 19-9 in our patient has probably to be explained by bile stone passage. Actually, we do not have an explanation for the increase of CEA and TAG 72 in the other two patients.

However, further prospective studies have to evaluate the definitive role of repetitive tumor marker determinations in transplanted patients.

References

1. Björklund B, Björklund V (1957) Antigenicity of pooled human malignant normal tissues by cyto-immunological technique: Presence of an insoluble heatlabile tumor antigen. Int Arch Allergy 10:209–223
2. Brandt M, Hirt SW, Walluscheck K, Sievers HH, Haverich A (1994) Einsatz von Tumormarkern zur Diagnostik und Verlaufskontrolle von malignen Tumoren nach Herztransplantation. Abstr No 59, 23. Jahrestagung der dt. Ges. f. THG-Chirurgie, p 69
3. Cases A, Filella X, Molina R, Ballesta AM, Lopez-Pedret J, Revert L (1991) Tumor markers in chronic renal failure and hemodialysis patient. Nephron 57:183–186
4. Collazos J (1992) Clinical and laboratory evaluation of CA 19-9 in cirrhotic patients. Eur J Med 1(4):215–8
5. Couteil JP, McGoldrick JP, Wallwork J, English TAH (1990) Malignant tumors after heart transplantation. J Heart Transplant 9:622–6
6. Haglund C, Roberts PJ, Kuusela P, Scheinin TM, Mäkelä O, Jalanko H (1986) Evaluation of CA 19-9 as a serum tumor marker in pancreatic cancer. Br J Cancer 53:197–202
7. Johnston WW et al (1986) Use of a monoclonal antibody (B72.3) as an immunocytochemical adjunct to diagnosis of adenocarcinoma in human effusions. Cancer Res 45:850
8. McLeod AM, Gatto GD (1988) Cancer after transplantation. Br Med J 297:4–5
9. Nägele H, Döring V, Kalmar P, Rödiger W, Stubbe HM (1994) Zehn Jahre Herztransplantation im Universitäts-Krankenhaus Eppendorf. Hamb Ärzteblatt 48:71–75
10. Opelz G, Henderson R (1993) Incidence of non-Hodgkin lymphoma in kidney and heart transplant recipients. The Lancet 342:1514–1516
11. Penn I (1981) Depressed immunity and the development of cancer. Clin Exp Immunol 46:459–75
12. Sameshima Y, Chia D, Terasaki PI, Imagawa DK, Busut RW (1992) Appearance of the tumor marker CA 19-9 in liver transplant patients during rejection episodes. Transplantation 53:580–582
13. Seo T, Ikeda Y, Onaka H, Hayashi T, Kawaguchi K, Kotake C, Toda Kobayashi K (1993) Usefulness of serum CA 125 measurement monitoring pericardial effusion. Jpn Circ J 57(6):489–94
14. Stauch C, Fischer B, Bernhard A (1993) Malignancies after heart transplantation. Onkologie 338–343
15. Swinnen LJ, Costanzo-Nordin MR, Fisher SG (1990) Increased incidence of lymphoproliferative disorder after immunosuppression with the monoclonal antibody OKT3 in cardias transplant recipient. N Engl J Med 323:1723–8
16. Wiebe K, Wahlers Th, Hirt SW Schäfers HJ, Fieguth HG, Jurmann M, Hausen B, Gräter T, Borst HG (1994) Prävalenz, Verlauf und Behandlung maligner Erkrankungen nach Herzplantation unter Dreifach-Immunsuppression. Abstr No 60, 23. Jahrestagung der dt. Ges. f. THG-Chirurgie, p 69
17. Wood WG, Werner A (1984) CEA, TPA and CA 125 levels in different patient groups with benign and malignant disease. Ärztl Lab 30:309–315
18. Wood WG, Steinhoff J, Kessler AC (1993) Anomalous marker concentrations in renal transplant patients. Eur J Biochem 31:75–82

Address for correspondence:
Dr. med. H. Nägele
Abteilung für Thorax-Herz-Gefäßchirurgie
Universitätskrankenhaus Eppendorf
Martinistraße 52
D-20246 Hamburg, Germany

Serum level of tumor necrosis factor receptor p55 and p75 in patients with kidney transplantations

H. Gallati[a], I. Pracht[a], A. Bock[b], G. Thiel[b]

[a]F. Hoffmann-La Roche, [b]Nephorologie, Kantonsspital, Basel, Switzerland

Introduction

Recently, naturally occuring inhibitors of tumor necrosis factor (TNF) activity have been found in the urine of normal individuals and febrile patients (1–4), as well as in the serum of patients with renal insufficiency (5). This host mediators, originally termed TNF binding proteins, have subsequently been identified as the soluble extracellular domains of the respective 55 and 75 kD membrane-bound TNF receptors (TNFR). The expression and the serum concentration of the soluble TNF receptors (sTNFR 55 and sTNFR 75) have already been demonstrated to correlate with a state of immunoactivation. The correlation of the sTNFRs levels with acute clinical events in the post transplant course strengthens the hypothesis that the sTNFRs can be regarded as markers for the acute rejections of the allograft.

The aim of this study was the determination of the sTNFRs level during a few weeks after kidney transplantation. It was studied whether TNFRs levels indicate graft rejection or if the TNFRs level could even be used as an early diagnostic indicator for graft rejection and if the nature of the rejection could be diagnosed.

Patients and methods

Of the 71 kidney transplanted patients (28 males and 43 females with a mean age of 52 years, range 17–71 years) blood was drawn every second or third day. The plasma was stored at –25 °C until analyzed. Ten patients received a living kidney, 59 received a first allograft. 28 patients were treated with the anti-lymphocytic substance ATG, 31 patients with OKT3. In addition, both groups received azathriopin, prednison and cyclosporin for immune-suppression. Graft rejections were treated during three days with 0.5 g of methylprednisolon. The criteria for the diagnosis of a graft rejection were: results of biopsy, increase of plasma creatinine, urine volume and improvement of the kidney function after therapy. The sTNFRs levels were not taken into account.

sTNFRs-assays

Concentrations of sTNFR 55 and sTNFR 75 were measured with an enzyme-linked immunological and biological binding assay (ELIBA): Samples and sTNFRs standards were added together with recombinant human TNF-a-peroxidase conjugate to the well of a microtiter plate precoated with non-neutralising monoclonal (mouse) antibodies to sTNFRs (clone htr 20 for the sTNFR 55 and clone utr 4 for the sTNFR 75). After this immunological and biological reaction, the unbound material was removed by a washing step and the quantity of peroxidase bound to the microtiter plate was measured enzymatically. The resulting color intensity was determined photometrically. It was directly propotional to the sTNFRs concentrations in the sample. The detection limit was about 100 pg/ml sTNFRs.

Results

The normal values for sTNFRs in urine are the following:
Men (n = 25; age 18–65 years): 4.0 ng/ml for sTNFR 55 and 8.3 ng/ml for sTNFRs 75. Females (n = 25, age 18–65 years): 1.8 ng/ml for sTNFR 55 and 4.1 ng/ml for sTNFRs 75. The serum levels

of sTNFRs (normal levels for sTNFR 55 are 1 ng/ml and for sTNFRs 75 are 3 ng/ml) increase with progressive kidney insufficiency (5) and they can reach values of 20 to 80 ng/ml for patients undergoing kidney dialysis. These values do not significantly change during dialysis. sTNRF levels decrease after a kidney transplantation to a degree that depends on the ability of the new organ to function. The normal sTNFRs values are never reached (figure 1). If the function of the new organ is incapacitated due to an infection, immunological graft rejection or nephrotoxicity caused by medication, the serum levels of sTNFRs increase. After the reversal of these incapacitations the serum levels decrease (figure 2). If it is not possible to stop the graft rejection, the sTNFRs remain high or continue to increase (figure 3). In all 71 cases that were investigated the sTNFRs levels were in parallel with the creatinine levels (figure 2).

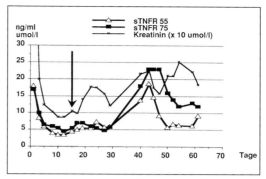

Figure 2. Patient no. 689: sTNFR and creatine levels during 61 days following kidney transplantation. On day 15 (↓) an acute graft rejection occured.

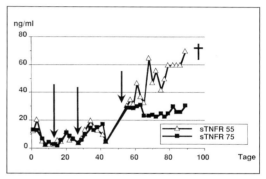

Figure 3. Patient no. 650: sTNFR levels during 90 days following kidney transplantation (↓), the third one could not be kept under control and the patient died as a result of that.

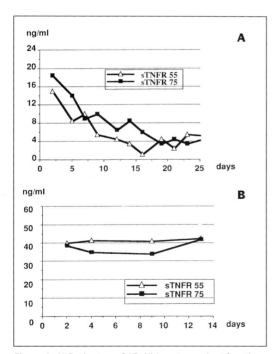

Figure 1. A) Patient no. 643: Kidney transplant functions without any problem during the observation period. sTNFR levels return to normal. B) Patient no. 641: Kidney transplant does not function and has to be removed 14 days after. Accordingly the sTNFR levels remain high.

Discussion

The immune competent cells continuously produce sTNFRs which are enzymatically shed from the cell membrane. It is not known whether or how the sTNFRs concentration in blood is regulated. From the data presently known it can be assumed that the sTNFRs are removed continually and exclusively through the kidneys. Therefore, kidney malfunctions will always lead to increased sTNFRs levels as well as increased creatinine levels. For kidney dialysis patients the levels are extremely high. While creatinine can be removed from the blood through dialysis, the sTNFRs remain. It is not yet known whether the dialysis patients synthesize less sTNFRs or if sTNFRs are metabolized via an alternative path and are in this way eliminated from the blood. If the kidney function is returned to normal either by medication or by kidney transplantation, the removal of sTNFRs and of creatinine from the blood is guaranteed and the blood levels of these analytes decrease to normal levels.

Rejection of the implanted kidney and decrease in kidney function as a consequence of the rejection are reflected in an increase of the sTNFRs and the creatinine levels in the blood. The immunological rejection of the kidney provokes an additional increase of the sTNFRs levels, but it is low compared to the increase caused by kidney failure. The data from this study clearly shows that the determination of sTNFRs can be used like creatinine as diagnostic parameter of an acute graft rejection and for the control of treatment of kidney rejection in patients that underwent kidney transplantation. However, sTNFRs are no early indicators for graft rejection and they do not answer the question if the rejection is due to immunological reasons. Further studies are needed to determine, if and how sTNFRs can be of use for the surveillance of patients that received other organs.

References

1. Seckinger P, Isaaz S, Dayer J-M (1988) A human inhibitor of tumor necrosis factor a. J Exp Med 167: 1511–1516
2. Peetre C, Thysell H, Grubb A, Olsson I (1988) A tumor necrosis factor binding protein is present in human biological fluids. Eur J Haematol 41:414–419
3. Olsson I, Lantz M, Nilsson E et al (1989) Isolation and characterisation of a tumor necrosis factor binding protein from urin. Eur J Haematol 42: 270–275
4. Seckinger P, Isaaz S, Dayer J-M (1989) Purification and biologic characterization of a specific tumor necrosis factor a inhibitor. J Biol Chem 264:11966–11973
5. Brockhaus M, Bar-Khayim Y, Gurwicz S, Frensdorff A, Hara N (1992) Plasma tumor necrosis factor-soluble receptors in chronic renal failure. Kidney Int 42:663–667

Address for correspondence:
Dr. H. Gallati
F. Hoffmann-La Roche
Pharmaceutical Research
CH-4002 Basel, Switzerland

Genetic variability of HIV – A new HIV subtype from Cameroon

H.-P. Hauser[a], L. Gürtler[b], S. Knapp[a], J. Eberle[b], A. von Brunn[b], L. Kaptue[c]

[a]Behringwerke AG, Marburg, [b]Max-von-Pettenkofer-Institute, München, Germany,
[c]Centre Hospitalier Universitaire, Youndé, Cameroon

In 1991 a new HIV strain (MVP-5180) was isolated from a Cameroonian AIDS patient. By cocultivation, the virus could be adapted to several human T-cell lines (HUT78, MT-2, Jurkat and C8166) and to the monocytic U937 line. DNA from MVP-5180 infected cells could not be amplified by using conventional pairs of primers for PCR detection of HIV. In addition its reverse transcriptase showed a reduced molecular weight. Most of German, Ivorian and Malawian anti-HIV1 sera reacted faintly or moderately with the env-proteins in a MVP-5180-immunoblot, whereas some Cameroonian sera reacted strongly. Together these data indicated that the MVP-5180 genome shows pronounced structural differences compared to known HIV strains (1).

Since variants of the rapidly mutating HIV might be of diagnostic relevance, we were interested in characterizing the new isolate on a molecular level. We established novel PCR conditions (using the primers sk168 AGC AGC AGG AAG CAC TAT GG and envb GAG TTT TCC AGA GCA ACC CC) which allowed us to amplify part of the glycoprotein gp41 of MVP-5180. In this region, which is important for HIV serodiagnosis, we found a very low homology to other published HIV sequences. We then isolated total DNA of MVP-5180 infected HUT78 cells, fragmented it randomly by partial Sau3A digestion and cloned the 12 kb to 20 kb fraction of DNA-fragments into the bacteriophage lambda "DASHTM". The subsequent screening of this genomic library by hybridizing the radioactively labeled PCR-fragment sk168-envb led to the cloning of 99% of the total genome of MVP-5180.

Sequencing the whole viral genome enabled us to determine the relationship of MVP-5180 to other members of the HIV family. The genomic organization of MVP-5180 (ltr, gag, pol, vif, vpr, vpu, tat, env, nef, ltr) was like that of other members of the HIV1 family. Homology comparisons (table I) and a pedigree analysis (exemplified for the env protein in figure 1 showed that MVP-5180 is closer related to HIV1 than to HIV2. Within the highly divergent and highly immunogenic V3-loop most variants of HIV1 show a conserved "crown" consisting of the aminoacids GPGR, whereas MVP-5180 shows the novel sequence GPMR or GPLR. Together with another Cameroonian strain, ANT70 (2), MVP-5180 represents a novel subtype within the HIV1 family which has been designated subtype O (3).

Table I. Comparison of the sequence of MVP-5180 with the consensus sequences of HIV1 and HIV2 and with the partially published sequence from ANT-70 (2).

Gene	HIV2-Consensus	HIV1-Consensus	ANT70
ltr	51%	67%	82%
gag	62%	70%	
pol	66%	74%	
env	49%	53%	

MVP-5180 represents the most divergent and probably the most ancient HIV1 subtyp characterized so far. Such a divergent strain might be difficult to detect by using conventional assays. To address this question we initiated a study in Cameroon which will give us more information about the prevalence of this virus and of its diagnostic relevance. Using the sequence information MVP-5180 provides, it is well conceivable, that even more divergent HIV1 variants will be detected.

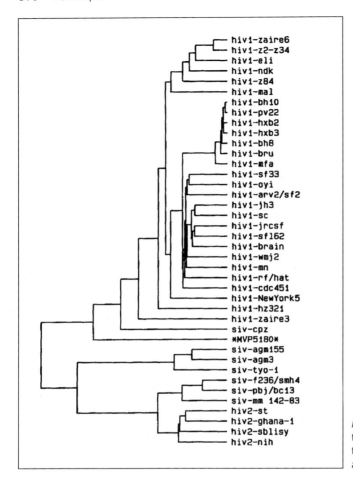

Figure 1. Pedigree analysis comparing the env protein of MVP-5180 by using the PILEUP programm of the GCG DNA analysis package.

References

1. Gürtler LG, Hauser H-P, Eberle J, von Brunn A, Knapp S, Zekeng L, Tsague JM, Kaptue L (1994) Characterisation of a new and ancient subtype of the Human Immunodeficiency Virus (HIV-1), MVP-5180 from Cameroon. J Virol (in press)
2. De Leys R, Vanderbroght B, Haesfelde MV, Heyndrickx I, von Geel A, Wauters C, Bernaerts R, Saman E, Nijs P, Willems B, Taelman H, van der Groen G, Piot P, Tersmette T, Huisman JG, von Heuverswyn H (1990) Isolation and partial characterisation of an unusual human immuno-dificiency retrovirus from two persons of West-Central African origin. J Virol 64:1207-1216
3. Los Alamos HIV Sequence Data Base, August 1993

Address for correspondence:
Dr. H.-P. Hauser
Behringwerke AG
Mikrobiologische Diagnostik
Postfach 1140
D-35001 Marburg, Germany

Immunological phenomenons and problems after organ transplantation

B. H. Markus

Clinic for General Surgery, Johann Wolfgang Goethe-University, Frankfurt/Main, Germany

Introduction

Organ transplantation, especially liver transplantation offers many immunologically interesting features. With now many thousand organ transplants performed worldwide the understanding of the basic immunological characteristics is rapidly advancing. Liver transplants are the most difficult transplants to be performed and perhaps the immunologically most interesting ones. For end stage liver diseases transplantation offers a much superior survival to conventional treatment options (1).

Immunobiology of liver transplantation

Liver transplants are more resistant to rejection and apparently can protect other organs transplanted shortly thereafter against the deleterious effects of humoral rejection (2). Lymphopoietic chimerism has been reported in liver transplant recipients as a significant mechanism for long lasting survival. Current studies are therefore evaluating the effect of combined bone marrow and liver transplants. In addition HLA matching seems to have a "dualistic effect" on the outcome of liver transplantation with mismatching being responsible for rejection and matching responsible for the role of other e.g. HLA restricted underlying immune mechanisms (3). CMV hepatitis is now in part attributed to better HLA matching.

Factors influencing the immunological course

Underlying mechanisms for the original liver disease can be non-immunological (perhaps biliary atresia), immunologically mediated (e.g. autoimmune disease, infections) and in addition HLA-associated. Currently our understanding for these disease mechanisms is only very limited and therefore it is difficult to understand, how these mechanisms react in a new environment with the diseased liver removed, another liver with another HLA-type being sewn in, and various immunosuppressive and other drugs started. Disease mechanisms e.g. of cytotoxic lymphocytes, which are by nature at least in part restricted by HLA-antigens will most likely function differently with the new organ in place. So survival after transplantation might also depend on whether former disease mechanisms will still be active, but perhaps disguised by immunosuppressive effects. The presentation of alternative proteins as there are e.g. foreign proteins (viral, bacterial, soluble donor HLA antigens), other self proteins as well as stress proteins (so called heat shock proteins) might induce under such extreme conditions additional immune effector mechanisms which we just start to discover now.

Immunosuppressive drugs function by different mechanisms. On the one hand there are T-cell depleting drugs as e.g. anti-T-cell-globulin, anti-lymphocyte-globulin or OKT3, a monoclonal antibody against the CD3 receptor, which are used during the early postoperative days for induction immunosuppression or later for steroid resistant rejection. On the other hand the drugs used mainly for long term immunosuppression as there are Ciclosporin, Azathioprin and newly FK506 are acting by suppressing T-cell functions. So each drug alters the immunological course after transplantation by its own nature and in relation to various other factors.

Furthermore the recipients macro- and micro-environment with ischemic damage to tissue, infections and local cytokine production, all leading in part to antigen upregulation, affects all other immunological systems.

Clinical relevance

In liver transplants some clinical states are of major importance. The differentiation between acute rejection, chronic rejection and recurrent disease mechanisms is long being debated. Some groups e.g. claim to see a substantial number of recurrent primary biliary cirrhosis after liver transplants, while other investigators point out, that these alleged features are also important in the development of chronic rejection. Chronic rejection per se is still ill defined and the underlying mechanisms, as there are cellular and humoral mechanisms, not yet clearly established. Acute rejection at least, most often in the early weeks after transplant, seems to be mainly mediated by specific cellular rejection mechanisms. However, all of the above mentioned factors might play a role in the development of the clinically apparent conditions. In order to develop more specific anti-rejection drugs or to induce disease free tolerance we further need to achieve a better understanding of the basic immunological mechanisms after transplantation.

Liver transplantation for primary or secondary tumors

The role of liver transplantation as a clinical alternative for primary hepatic malignancies and metastatic tumors still needs to be better defined. Survival analysis in patients who received a liver graft for primary or secondary tumors show excellent survival within the first few months with a steady decline thereafter. Survival at later time intervals is significantly reduced in these patients than in the patient group receiving a transplant for non-malignant indications. Tumor recurrence is in most of these patients the reason for death with recurrence often noted first in the transplanted liver.

Primary tumors: Earlier studies have suggested that certain tumors as e.g. the fibrolamellar tumor have a better prognosis. Unfortunately these results could not be substantiated in more recent and larger analyses. While in recent years patients with primary malignancies of the liver were refered to transplantation when tumors were too large or to widespread to be resectable, many of them died because of early recurrence. Since studies on hepatic resection of smaller hepatic tumors have also demonstrated a fairly high recurrence rate, it is suggested today to preferentially transplant those patients having smaller hepatic tumors with only few intrahepatic nodules, given the excellent results of these patients with low recurrence rate in long term follow-up studies.

Secondary tumors: Transplantation for metastatic tumors to the liver needs further evaluation. Neuroendocrine tumors are believed to carry a better prognosis. Nevertheless we experienced tumor recurrence in all of our three patients surviving the perioperative period despite of an extensive upper abdominal cluster resection and an excellent liver graft function. Liver transplanta-

Table I. Factors influencing the immunological course after liver transplantation.

Disease mechanisms	non-immunological	immunological mediated	HLA-associated
Donor/recipient HLA matching	match	partial match	mismatch
Alternative protein presentation	foreign proteins (viral, bacterial, soluble donor HLA antigens)	self proteins	stress protein (heat shock proteins)
Recipient macroenviroment	regular	ischemic damage	infection
Recipient macroenviroment	regular	increased cytokine production	
Immunosuppression	T-cell depleting (ATG,ALG,OKT3)	T-cell suppressive (CsA, Azathioprin, FK506)	

tion for colorectal metastasis carries an even greater risk of tumor recurrence. Still these procedures might be justified under individual circumstances. In addition there might be a role of transplantation as a palliative procedure, unfortunately putting heavy constraints on the limited number of available donor organs and the health care system.

Chemotherapy and chemoembolization: Pre-, peri- and post-operative chemotherapy as well as pre-operative chemoembolization is currently used by various centers to reduce tumor recurrence after transplantation and to overcome the long waiting period. With various regimens under evaluation, leading in part to some better patient selection for transplantation, this strategy offers some hope for future developments. The effect of post-transplant immunosuppression on tumor growth and cell proliferation is not yet clearly established. This effect seems to be different for each immunosuppressive drug. The most often seen development of B-cell lymphomas is in addition related to an Eppstein Barr virus infection. Modern strategies to reduce immunosuppression as much as tolerable will help to minimize this problem.

Conclusion

While organ transplantation and especially liver transplantation offers some very unique insights into immunological mechanisms, we still need a more profound understanding in order to develop better immunosuppressive drugs or to induce disease free tolerance.

References

1. Markus BH, Dickson ER, Grambsch PM, Fleming TR, Mazzaferro V, Klintmalm GBG, Wiesner RH, Van Thiel DH, Starzl TE (1989) Efficacy of liver transplantation in patients with primary biliary cirrhosis. N Engl J Med 320:1709-1713
2. Fung JJ, Griffin M, Duquesnoy RJ, Shaw BW, Starzl TE (1987) Successful sequential liver-kidney transplantation in a patient with preformed lymphocytotoxic antibodies. Transplant Proc 19:767
3. Markus BH, Duquesnoy RJ, Gordon RD, Fung JJ, Vanek M, Klintmalm G, Bryan C, Van Thiel D, Starzl TE (1988) Histocompatibility and liver transplant outcome: Does HLA exert a dualistic effect? Transplantation 46:372-377

Address for correspondence:
Dr. med. B. H. Markus
Klinik für Allgemeinchirurgie
Johann Wolfgang Goethe Universität
Theodor-Stern-Kai 7
D-60590 Frankfurt am Main, Germany

Satellite Symposium

Cancer of the Lung – State and Trends in Diagnosis and Therapy

Histopathologic diagnosis of lung cancer – Classification, problems, pitfalls

M. Amthor

Institute of Pathology, Diaconate Hospital, Rotenburg/W., Germany

Classification

Carcinoma of the lung is a common tumor; it is the most common malignant tumor in males, in females it ranks on the fourth place (5). Thus, every physician is confronted with lung carcinoma, every histopathologist must be able to diagnose and type it. Other tumors of the lung are, with the exception of malignant mesothelioma, much rarer and do not play that role in the daily diagnostic work. Therefore it seems to be justified to discuss the classification mainly under the topic of malignant epithelial tumors, group C of the WHO nomenclature.

Diagnosis means coordination to a system of classification, also called "typing". This statement may seem to be commonplace, but it is important to point out that we are dealing with a taxonomic problem, being a function of diverse factors mainly such as the aim of the classification and the method based on (1). From a suitable classification we expect (12):

1. that the individual entities exclude each other (no overlaps, no "grey zones"),
2. that the sum of all entities represents all features of the group, it must be possible to classify every tumor according the taxonomy adopted;
3. that the classification is of biological and therapeutic relevance (WHO: "to show biological consistency, in that tumors similarly typed would have the same important biological properties in common").

Because carcinoma of the lung is a common tumor we also can expect:

1. that the method the taxonomic system is based on is sufficiently simple to be used in a histopathologic routine laboratory (*Hoepker* and *Luellig* 1987, p. 57 (12) for the problem of reclassification of routine diagnoses by a second pathologist),
2. that the entities formulated in that way can be diagnosed with sufficient ease and security (*Hirsch* et al. 1982 (10)) for the problem of insufficient agreement in case of terminological haziness; they found an inter-observer agreement of 90% with small cell lung carcinoma but only of 54% if subtyping of small cell carcinomas was requested),
3. that authority and acceptance of the applied taxonomic system makes a general communication of diagnoses possible.

The Veterans Administration Lung Cancer Therapy Study Group (VAL-Group) had set up the basis for the WHO-classification of lung tumors which first appeared 1967. It was the first of the so called "blue books", designed to standardize the nomenclature of tumors world wide. This WHO-classification now is available in its second edition (1981). In addition the Working Party of Lung Cancer (WP-L) and the Lung Cancer Study Group (LCSG) have to be mentioned (for review see 8, 12). The second edition of the WHO-classification of lung tumors has changes in terminology and substance as well. A new spindle-celled subtype of squamous cell carcinoma, further changes in the group of small cell carcinoma with the introduction of combined small cell carcinomas, and the classification of solid tumors with mucin as adenocarcinoma have to be mentioned. Important is also the fact that the carcinoid is no longer classified as adenoma. The classification of the WHO is a compromise trying to fulfil the above mentioned postulates. The classification is almost exclusively based on the histopathologic standard procedure, the H/E-staining. Only for adenocarcinomas a mucin reaction is needed, for the diagnosis of the carcinoid a reaction for argyrophilia is recommended (Grimelius-reaction) but not optional. Immunohistochemical techniques are not the basis of this classification.

Problems

Problems derive from different reasons:
1. from classification of a) multiform carcinomas (tumors of different differentiation), b) combination tumors (tumors with compartments of different types or subtypes), c) composition tumors (tumors with epithelial and non-epithelial components).
2. The classification of the WHO is based exclusively on light microscopy and almost exclusively on H/E-stain. By use of electron microscope *Auerbach* et al. (1) have found a mis-interpretation in about one third of the cases. According to *Hoepker* and *Luellig* (12) a reduction of mis-interpretation could already be achieved if combination tumors and multiform tumors could be mentioned as subentities. Against this, however, stands the WHO recommendation to classify those tumors under the main type.
3. The general problem of the large cell carcinoma. This type comprises under application of conventional histological methods a "waste basket" (8). The application of more sophisticated methods probably would dissolve that type at least partly.
4. The whole group of neuroendocrine tumors has experienced new knowledge by immunohistochemical methods (3, 6, 16, 9, 13, 14, 18, 25). New entities have been formulated like the neuroendocrine large cell carcinoma (22). Here the WHO classification of 1981 needs revision.
5. This causes an increasing loss of the mentioned aim, i.e. a uniform, semantic unequivocal and communicable nomenclature.

Pitfalls

Pitfalls or mis-interpretations can have different causes:
1. the classification (difficulties in interpretation of given definitions, lack of general application, overlaps of types, obsolete),
2. the technique of biopsy. Especially centrally situated tumors are diagnosed in biopsies. This implies the possibility of misinterpretation (8, 11, 24). Also combination tumors and composition tumors may not be biopsied in sufficient amount to be diagnosed correctly (7). Thus statistics of the distribution of different types are different if based on biopsies or based on surgical/autopsy material. In biopsy material also peripheral tumors such as adenocarcinomas are under-represented. Actually they are increasing as a group (2).
3. The impossibility to distinguish between primary and metastasis in many cases, which applies especially to adenocarcinomas. Metastases can grow like bronchioloalveolar carcinomas, metastases can also grow as endobronchial tumors (15, 17, 19, 23),
4. the lack of experience of the histopathologist with a given problem such as artefacts, lymphocytic infiltration versus small cell carcinoma and squamous metaplasia versus squamous carcinoma (5).

Conclusions

1. A classification of lung tumors should be qualified to diagnose at least the common neoplasms accordingly as base of therapeutic procedures.
2. For this (i.e. for routine purposes) a limited panel of stains and immunohistochemical methods should be defined and sufficient.
3. Every classification means a compromise between realisation of all scientific knowledge and reality of daily work pathology, between communicability and scientific progress. Every classification will be obsolete from a scientific standpoint when finally generally adopted.
4. Still, a classification as formulated in the blue books of the WHO "Histopathological Typing and Tumors" seems to be the only realistic way to achieve a practicable, therapeutically relevant, semantic uniform and communicable histopathological diagnostic systems.
5. Pitfalls, mis-interpretations, can be reduced by optimal techniques, clinicopathological communication, personal experience and a good classification, but they cannot be avoided completely.

References

1. Auerbach O, Trasca JM, Parks VR, Charter HW (1982) A comparison of World Health Organisation (WHO) classification of lung tumours. Cancer 50:2079–2088
2. Auerbach O, Garfinkel L (1991) The changing pattern of lung carcinoma. Cancer 68:1973–1977
3. Barbareschi M, Detassis C, Dalla Palma Parrigoni GL (1991) Atypical bronchial carcinoids lack S-100 positive sustentacular cells (letter). Pathol Res Pract 187:856
4. Becker N, Frenzel-Beyme R, Wagner G (1994) Krebsatlas der Bundesrepublik Deutschland (Atlas of cancer mortality in the Federal Republic of Germany). Springer, Berlin, Heidelberg,
5. Chandraratnam EA, Henderson DW, Meredieth DJ, Jain S (1987) Regenerative atypical squamous metaplasia in fibreoptic bronchial biopsy sites – a lesion liable to misinterpretation as carcinoma on rebiopsy: report of 5 cases. Pathol 19:419–424
6. Christen B, Trojanowski JQ, Pietra GG (1987) Immunohistochemical demonstration of phosphorylated forms of human neurofilament subunits in human pulmonary carcinoids. Hum Pathol 18:997–1001
7. Churg A. (1988) Tumors of the lung. In: Thurlbeck (eds) Pathology of the lung. Thieme, Stuttgart
8. Hammar SP (1987) Common neoplasms. In: Dail DH, Hammar SP (eds) Pulmonary pathology. Springer, New York, pp 727–845
9. Hasleton PS, Al-Saffar N (1989). The histological spectrum of bronchial carcinoid tumors. Appl Pathol 7:205–218
10. Hirsch FR, Metthews MJ, Yesner R (1982) Histopathological classification of small cell carcinoma of lung. Cancer 50:1360–1366
11. Homna K, Mishina M, Watanabe Y (1988) Polypoid endobronchial extension from invasive thymoma. Virch Arch A 413:469–474
12. Hoepker WW, Luellig H (1987) Lungenkarzinom, Resektion, Morphologie und Prognose. Springer, Berlin
13. Kominoth P, Roth J, Lackie PM, Bitter-Suermann D, Heitz PU (1991) Polyeystic acid of the neural cell adhesion molecule distinguishes small cell carcinoma from carcinoids. Am J Pathol 139:297–304
14. Lauweryns JM, Godderis P (1975) Neuroepithelial bodies in the human child and the adult lung. Am Rev Respir Dis 111:469
15. Lee DW, Ro JY, Sahin AA, Ayala AG (1990) Mucinous adenocarcinoma of the prostate with endobronchial metastasis. Am J Clin Pathol 94:641–645
16. El-Nagar AK, Ballance W, Karim FW, Ordonez NG, McLemore D, Giacco GG, Batsakis JG (1991) Typical and atypical bronchopulmonary carcinoids. A clinicopathologic flow cytometric study. Am J Clin Pathol 95:828–834
17. Rosenblatt MB, Lisa JR, Collier F (1967) Primary and metastatic broncho-alveolar carcinoma. Dis Chest 52:147–152
18. Said JW, Vimadalal S, Nash G, Shintaku IP, Heusser RC, Sassoon AF, Lloyd RV (1985) Immunoreactivite neuron-specific enolase, bombesin, and chromogranin as markers for neuroendocrine lung tumors. Hum Pathol 16:236–240
19. Schrijver M, Havenith MG, Hupperets PS, Greve LH, Wouters EF (1987) Endobronchial non-Hodgkin lymphoma: report of two cases. Respiration 52:228–231
20. The World Health Organisation: Histological typing of lung tumors. 2nd ed. Geneva 1981
21. Torre M, Barberis M, Barbiere B, Bonacina E, Belloni P (1989) Resp Med 83:305–308
22. Travis WD, Linnoila R Ilona, Tsakos Maria G, Hitchcock ChL, Cutler GB, Niemann Lynette, Chrousos G, Pass H, Doppman J (1991) Neuroendocrine tumors of the lung with proposed criteria for large-cell neuroendocrine carcinoma. Am J Surg Pathol 15:529–553
23. Umcki S (1990) Multiple endobronchial metastases due to renal carcinoma and laser therapy (letter, comment) Chest 98:778–779
24. Vanmaele L, Noppen M, Frecourt N, Impens N, Welch B, Schandevijl W (1990) European Respir J 3:927–929
25. Warren WH, Faber LP, Gould VE (1989). Neuroendocrine neoplasms of the lung. A clinicopathologic update. J Thoracic Cardiovasc Surg 98:321–332

Address for correspondence:
Prof. Dr. med. M. Amthor
Pathologisches Institut
Diakoniekrankenhaus
Postfach
D-27342 Rotenburg/Wümme, Germany

Clinical staging of primary lung cancer

P. Steiner
Department of Radiology,
University Hospital, Hamburg, Germany

Introduction

The appropriate staging of a patient with lung cancer has been the subject of continuing debate since the introduction of cross-sectional body imaging in the 1970s. The debate has been stimulated by the observation that approximately 40% to 50% of patients with lung cancer are found to be unresectable at the time of exploratory thoracotomy. The preoperative recognition of the reasons for unresectability of primary lung cancers are the following:

a) extrathoracic metastatic disease;
b) intrathoracic malignant pleural effusion, invasion of critical mediastinal structures, contralateral mediastinal lymph node involvement.

It would seem reasonable to assume that current methods of imaging should demonstrate the intrathoracic reasons for non-resectability, providing pathologic confirmation support these findings. Experience has shown, through multiple patient trials, that our current imaging techniques lack the sensitivity and specificity to confidently catalogue lung cancer patients preoperatively into those who have resectable and non-resectable disease. These data and appropriate recommendations for the selective application of cross-sectional imaging techniques will be reviewed and recommendations made.

The staging of the patient with lung cancer is based on the TNM classification, a system now in worldwide use. For the patient with lung cancer, this TNM system was revised in 1988 and made consistent with similar systems which existed throughout the world (7).

Imaging technologies used in staging the patient with lung cancer

Routine chest radiographs

The routine chest radiograph is an extremely useful tool in staging, as well as the way in which most primary lung cancers are initially detected. This examination should be performed with high kilovoltage (120 to 130 kVp) postero-anterior and lateral projections. Much of the T-staging criteria can be extracted from the plain film, including the size of the primary lesion, its location, any lobar or segmental atelectasis, the presence of a pleural effusion, and abnormalities of the hilum or mediastinum suggesting lymph node enlargement. The chest radiograph is insensitive to small moderate-sized lymph nodes involved with metastatic disease. Mediastinal invasion by direct extension from a centrally located primary lung cancer can not be detected by plain films. The size and location of the primary tumor correlates with the prevalence of mediastinal lymph node involvement. The larger and more central primary lung cancers have a much higher prevalence of mediastinal lymph node involvement and should be the subject of extensive presurgical staging procedures. The small, peripheral lesions have a significantly lower prevalence of mediastinal lymph node involvement, and if the plain chest radiographs show no evidence of mediastinal abnormalities, many thoracic surgeons proceed directly to thoracotomy in these instances. Arguments against this practice are based on the lack of sensitivity of routine chest radiographs in the assessment of mediastinal lymph node involvement. When the mediastinum is abnormal on chest radiographs, suggesting nodal spread, it is quite specific for involvement secondary to the primary lung cancer. Thoracic surgeons tend to approach the staging of the patient with primary lung cancer based on routine/plain film findings or abnormalities. If the patient presents with a peripheral, small (less than 3 cm) lesion with a normal mediastinal contour on plain films, no further radiographic work-up or mediastinal exploration will be performed prior to exploratory thoracotomy. Thoracic surgeons generally use plain film abnormalities to justify the need for cross-sectional imaging (2).

Justification can also be made for using routine radiographic abnormalities to eliminate the need for cross-sectional imaging techniques when contour abnormalities suggest an underlying mediastinal mass lesion. In these instances, a case can be made to proceed directly with biopsy confirmation of the abnormality within the mediastinum (7).

In most centers, CT is used to validate the plain film abnormalities or further characterize those questions found on plain films. The lack of specificity of those findings on plain films justifies this additional cost.

Sophisticated imaging procedures used for staging

Computed tomography (CT)

CT staging of the thorax for the patient with primary lung cancer is the dominant imaging modality in use today. The technique utilized for CT staging employs 10 mm continuous sections from lung apex through the upper abdomen to include the adrenals. Todays "state of the art" CT-modality represents the use of the so called spiral-mode or volume scanning in which the whole thorax is scanned in a single breath-hold time during which the patient is transported continuously through the CT-gantry while the x-ray tube performs a continuous rotation (6, 11). Contrast enhancement is necessary to separate the vascular structures from lymph nodes, particularly in the hilum.

All patients undergoing cross-sectional imaging for staging should have that examination include the upper abdomen, especially the adrenal. Approximately 10% to 12% of patients with primary lung cancers will have enlarged adrenal glands requiring biopsy prior to thoracotomy as the majority of these lesions will be found to be benign (10). Similarly, all enlarged mediastinal lymph nodes must be confirmed histologically before they are assumed to be involved by metastatic cancer. The operator may vary sensitivity and specificity of CT in the evaluation of mediastinal lymph node enlargement based on the threshold size selected for defining abnormally enlarged lymph nodes (7). The inherently superior resolution of CT especially in the combination with contrast enhancement of the hilar vascular structures makes the detection of individual lymph nodes easier than with magnetic resonance (MR). CT is therefore recommended as the standard for cross-sectional imaging used in staging the patient with lung cancer.

Magnetic resonance (MR)

MR imaging provides additional staging information to the CT evaluation of patients with Pancoast's or superior sulcus tumors, as well as with primary lung cancers that are centrally located for detection of mediastinal invasion. MR imaging is superior to CT in the assessment of mediastinal penetration and critical organ invasion. CT and MR imaging both have disappointing accuracy in the assessment of chest wall invasion; however, MR imaging may have a slight advantage over CT (5).

Lymph node detection

The fundamental basis for the application of cross-sectional imaging techniques in staging the patient with lung cancer relate to detection of enlarged lymph nodes or invasion of critical structures, which would preclude surgical resection. The recognition of abnormal lymph nodes is based solely on size criteria, and at least for the foreseeable future, imaging will not be able to provide any tissue-specific characteristic signals to suggest metastatic disease.

The numerous conflicting reports that have appeared in the literature summarizing the results of cross-sectional imaging in staging the patient with lung cancer reflect this dependence on lymph node size, geographic variations that relate to the prevalence of non-neoplastic lymph node involvement, the accuracy of the local "gold standard" (the thoroughness by which node sampling has occured in study populations), the population characteristics of the primary cancers, and the state of evolution of imaging technology. Based on a 15 mm size threshold separating the normal and abnormal lymph node, sensitivity will vary between 61% and 88%. Specificities will vary from 89% to as high as 98%, with accuracies varying from 81% to 92% (7). The Radiologic Diagnostic Oncology Group trials reported the accuracy of CT in distinguishing N0-N1 from N2-N3 disease as 65%, with a 69% specificity and a 52% sensitivity. MR performed slightly below that CT standard, with an accuracy of 61%, specificity 64% and sensitivity 48%.

The gold standard, mediastinoscopy and open thoracotomy, is not without fault. In one report, 33% of patients with primary lung cancers who had undergone a negative mediastinoscopy were subsequently found to have mediastinal lymph node metastatic disease at open thoracotomy (7). To reduce this inaccuracy, coordination between the radiologist and clinician performing the mediastinoscopy needs to occur to identify the blind areas of various mediastinal exploration techniques. For example, the usual transcervical mediastinal exploration limits access to the anterior mediastinum, aorticopulmonary window region, and posterior mediastinum (7).

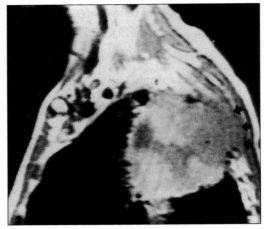

Figure 1. T1-weighted MRI image demonstrating signs of chest wall invasion on MRI. Large mass locally invading the chest wall (arrows).

T-classification

Unfortunately, neither CT nor MR imaging have sufficient accuracy to be used confidently as predictors of chest wall invasion (13). In one study, chest wall pain was a more accurate predictor of invasion than cross-sectional imaging. Nonetheless, cross-sectional imaging techniques will help in planning the surgical procedure if specific criteria for mediastinal penetration/invasion are used and the limitation of the techniques appreciated. Chest wall invasion should not be reported without evidence of either bone destruction or tumor penetration through the thoracic cage (figure 1). Less dependable criteria for invasion include the area of tumor contact with the chest wall and loss of fat plane on MR imaging (figure 2). Mapping of the area of involvement will enable the surgeon to more appropriately plan for an anticipated chest wall resection at the time of thoracotomy (9). A recent article reviewed the controversial topic of imaging and chest wall invasion. The authors found T1-weighted MR images provided the most accurate information (MR sensitivity of 89%, accuracy of 88% compared with CT with 45% and 68%, respectively). Gadolinium enhancement was not found to be helpful (8).

Mediastinal invasion is more accurately assessed with MR imaging than CT. The ability to image the vascular compartment, esophagus, trachea, and cardiac structures are more easily performed with the multiple imaging planes afforded with MR imaging (figure 3).

With superior sulcus or Pancoast's tumors, both CT and MR imaging should be used as they provide complimentary staging information. CT will allow one to evaluate the bony and nodal compartments of the chest wall structures more accurately and MR imaging, the soft tissue elements, including the neurovascular bundle. This is a critical step in the evaluation of these patients, as most centers now favor preoperative radiation therapy followed by surgical resection for Pancoast's tumors, with an improved overall survival approaching 25% at five years (4).

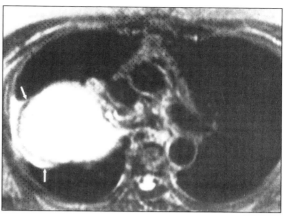

Figure 2. A) Coronal T1-weighted scan demonstrates large tumor in the right upper lobe with extensive chest wall contact. However, the pleura and the subpleural fat layer appear undistorted. B) T2-weighted axial scan through the lower tumor portion shows band of high signal intensity surrounding the tumor laterally and extending to the chest wall. Surgery confirmed reactive pleural thickening extending into the minor fissure (arrows). No tumor invasion of chest wall was seen.

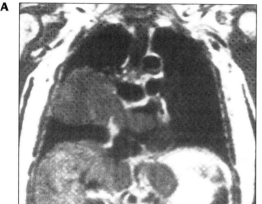
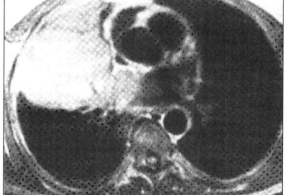

Figure 3. Lung cancer with intracardiac invasion. Coronal (A) and axial (B) T1-weighted images demonstrate a large mass in the right lung invading the left atrium via the right superior pulmonary vein. Note the large tumor thrombus within the left atrium.

M-classification

Extrathoracic staging of the patient with primary lung cancer should be reserved for the patient with a small cell anaplastic lung cancer or the individual who has symptoms suggesting extrathoracic metastatic disease. In the absence of symptoms, extrathoracic staging can not be justified for the patient with a non-small cell anaplastic lung cancer. A possible exception to this statement is the patient with an adenocarcinoma primary in the lung who has a greater incidence of developing metastatic brain disease within the first three to four months following initial detection, suggesting a role for preoperative MR image scanning of the brain (1).

Radionuclide studies have been applied to the staging process for years. The most common radioisotope used has been gallium. Although the majority of primary lung cancers tend to be gallium-avid, a number of adenocarcinomas tend not to be visible. In addition, seperation of the gallium-avid central lesions and contiguous mediastinal involvement is often difficult if not impossible with radionuclide scanning (3). Recently, positron emission tomography using fluorodeoxyglucose has been shown to be more accurate than CT in staging the mediastinum of patients with primary lung cancer. These preliminary results are reported from a small number of patients and must be proved in subsequent clinical trials (12).

Imaging algorithms for lung cancer staging

Table I lists three possible algorithms in common usage for staging the patient with primary lung cancer. Most radiologists advocate the application of cross-sectional imaging, usually CT, for all patients with primary lung cancer. The majority of thoracic surgeons on the other hand, selectively use cross-sectional imaging procedures based on clinical, histological, and chest radiographic features. Radiologists involved in staging the patient with lung cancer should be familiar both with the limitations and applications of cross-sectional imaging, as well as the needs and the treatment and follow-up of patients with primary lung cancers. In an effort to illustrate the problem, three possible approaches to the application of imaging in staging the patient with lung cancer will be presented.

Physicians should select the appropriate imaging algorithm from table I appropriate to the clinical problem, the surgical philosophy within one's own institution and the needs of the individual patient. In my opinion, cross-sectional imaging can not be justified in staging all patients with primary lung cancer. The inherent inaccuracy of the techniques induce unnecessary interventional procedures to explore the detected abnormalities and add further to the cost and morbidity of the patient work-up. The majority of thoracic surgeons in practice tend to base the decision to request cross-sectional imaging on plain film abnormalities, a problematic approach (table II). This concept tends to ignore the lack of sensitivity of the routine chest radiograph in the detection of involved mediastinal lymph nodes.

The selective use of cross-sectional imaging, based on clinical and histological criteria, combined with chest radiographic abnormalities,

Table I. Imaging algorithms for lung cancer staging.

I. Chest radiographs and CT for all patients

II. Chest radiographs as a guide for selective CT/MR imaging staging

III. Use of selective CT/MR imaging based upon clinical, histological, and chest radiographic criteria

Table II. Chest radiographs as a guide for selective CT staging.

I. Small (< 3 cm) peripheral primary; normal hilum and mediastinum on chest radiograph:
No need for CT staging

II. Large (> 3 cm) primary and/or central location and/or contact with pleural surface and/or lobar atelectasis:
Perform CT and/or MR imaging staging

III. Abnormal hilum or mediastinum on chest radiograph suggesting nodal disease:
Perform CT for staging

Table III. Selective use of cross-sectional imaging based on clinical and histological criteria.

I. Marginal surgical candidate-added risk for surgery:
Perform CT staging

II. Symptomatic (weight loss or extrathoracic symptoms suggesting metastatic disease) patient:
Perform CT and extrathoracic staging

III. Small cell anaplastic lung cancer:
Perform CT and extrathoracic staging

IV. Adenocarcinoma-primary lung cancer:
Perform CT staging and MR imaging brain scan

seems to represent a logic compromise. Often, the clinically marginal surgical candidate needs to be explored more completely to obviate the additional morbidity imposed by exploratory thoracotomy. One could therefore justify the added expense of cross-sectional imaging to detect criteria more accurately that would make the patient unresectable (table III).

The symptomatic patient, usually the lung cancer patient with significant weight loss at the time of initial presentation, exhibits the most ominous symptom suggesting a poor outcome and prognosis. Individuals with significant weight loss should also be evaluated for the possibility of more extensive disease, both within the thorax and in extrathoracic symptoms suggesting metastatic disease should also be worked up with appropriate imaging techniques prior to attempted resection of primary lung cancer.

The patient with a small cell anaplastic lung cancer generally is considered for extrathoracic staging of the brain, liver, and skeleton. These procedures provide the clinician with a baseline to assess the tumor burden and follow the patient subsequently to treatment. As mentioned previously, it has been suggested that the patient with a primary adenocarcinoma of the lung undergo MR imaging evaluation of the brain, as they seem to be at higher risk for specific metastatic involvement of that compartment.

References

1. Armstrong JD, Bragg DG (1986) Thoracic neoplasms: Imaging requirements for diagnosis and staging. In: Bragg DG, Rubin P, Youker JE (eds) Oncologic imaging. Pergramon Press, Elmsford, NY
2. Epstein DM, Stephenson LW, Geften WB et al (1986) Value of CT in the preoperative assessment of primary lung cancer: A survey of thoracic surgeons. Radiol 161:423-427
3. Friedmann PJ, Feigin DS, Liston SE et al (1987) Sensitivity of chest radiography, computed tomography and gallium scanning to metastases of lung carcinoma. Cancer 54:1300-1306
4. Heelan RT, Demas BE, Caravelli JF et al (1989) Superior sulcus tumors: CT and MRI imaging. Radiol 170:637-641
5. Heelan RT (1992) Primary lung cancer RDOG trials: MRI versus CT. Categorial course on imaging of cancers. Scottsdale, Arizona, American College of Radiology
6. Kalender WA, Seißler W, Klotz E, Vock P (1990) Spiral volumetric CT with single-breathhold technique, continuous transport and continuous scanner rotation. Radiol 176:181-183
7. Klein JS, Webb WR (1991) The radiologic staging of lung cancer. J Thorac Imaging 7:29-47
8. Padovani B, Mouroux J, Seksik L et al (1993) Chest wall invasion by bronchogenic carcinoma: Evaluation with MR imaging. Radiol 187:33-38
9. Ratto GB, Piacenza G, Frola C et al (1992) Chest wall involvement by lung cancer: Computed tomographic detection and results of operation. Ann Thorac Surg 51:182-188
10. Sandler MA, Pearlberg JL, Madrazo BL et al (1982) Computed tomographic evaluation of the adrenal gland and the preoperative assessment of bronchogenic carcinoma. Radiol 145:733-736
11. Vock P, Soceck M, Daepp M, Kalendar WA (1990) Lung: Spiral volumetric CT with single-breath-hold technique. Radiol 176:864-867
12. Wahl RL, Quint LE, Orringer M et al (1992) Staging non-small cell lung cancer in the mediastinum: Comparison of FDG-PET, CT and hybrid "anatometabolic" fusion images with pathology. Radiol 185:324
13. Webb WR, Gatsonis C, Zerhouni EA et al (1991) CT and MR imaging in staging non-small cell bronchogenic carcinoma: Report of the radiologic diagnostic oncology group. Radiol 178:705-713

Address for correspondence:
Dr. med. P. Steiner
Radiologische Klinik und Strahleninstitut
Universitätskrankenhaus
Martinistraße 52
D-20246 Hamburg, Germany

Tumor markers in lung cancer

Petra Stieber[a], H. Dienemann[b], Ute Hasholzner[a], A. Zimmermann[b], Karin Hofmann[a], A. Fateh-Moghadam†[a]

[a]Institut for Clinical Chemistry, [b]Surgical Clinic and Policlinic,
Klinikum Großhadern, Ludwig-Maximilians-University, Munich, Germany

Introduction

In industrialized countries, lung cancer is the most common cancer in men and is climbing quickly toward the same incidence in women. In the European Community (EC) lung cancer accounts for 29% of all cancer deaths, and 21% of all cancers among men. The increasing mortality rate from lung cancer is occuring at a time when death rates from other leading causes of cancer are either leveling off (breast cancer) or starting to decrease (colorectal cancer). In contrast to other frequent solid tumors, adequate follow-up care and control of efficiency of therapy existed up to now only for small cell lung cancer (SCLC). The clinical significance of the determination of neuron specific enolase (NSE) as the marker of choice in this histological type of lung cancer is well known and documented since many years (1, 8). In contrary, a detection of a change in the tumor behavior of non-small cell lung carcinomas (NSCLC) with the help of established tumor-associated antigens such as carcinoembryonic antigen (CEA), squamous cell carcinoma antigen (SCC) and many other markers was not yet satisfactory. Therefore many efforts have been made to develop a useful serum marker for the monitoring of these tumors. The important part of cytokeratins and other intermediate filaments like vimentin and desmin in histopathology for the classification of tumors was well known since a long time (3, 5). Some years ago it became evident that in contrast to cytokeratins themselves fragments of intermediate filaments are soluble in serum and can be detected by aid of monoclonal antibodies. As cytokeratin 19 is particularly abundant in carcinoma of the lung a test system called CYFRA 21-1 combining two monoclonal antibodies directed specifically against this cytokeratin was developed (4). At the same time it became evident that also TPA detects fragments of cytokeratins (8, 18 and to a small degree 19) as well as TPS does (mainly cytokeratin 18, to a small degree 8 and 19). In meanwhile many investigations CYFRA 21-1 proved to be a kind of "pan-marker" in lung cancer, especially in non-small cell lung carcinomas (NSCLC) and herewith in squamous cell carcinomas of the lung (7, 9, 10, 13, 14, 15, 16). As all these serological markers are neither organ nor tumor specific they can not be suitable for screening purposes in asymptomatic patients or early stages of tumor disease. But those few markers with a satisfying ability of discrimination between benign and malignant diseases (in this case of the lung) can represent an important tool in diagnosis, follow-up care and control of efficiency of therapy of lung cancer patients.

Specificity and cut-off values

Corresponding to the high incidence of lung cancer there is almost no tumor associated antigen described in the literature which has not been investigated in its clinical relevance for this kind of tumor. The problem is that a fair comparison of all these data is not possible as single values with corresponding clinical background are seldom shown in publications and many different cut-off values served as basis for the calculation of sensitivities and specificities. As none of the so called tumor-associated antigens is tumor specific and only very few are organ specific like PSA, it is evident that every marker will be more or less "true" positive also in lung cancer. The question is to find out which of the markers at the moment available possesses the best profile of specificity

Table I. Cut off-values of the most frequently described tumor markers in lung cancer at a specificity of 95% versus healthy persons and benign diseases of the lung.

Marker	Healthy (n = 99)	Benign lung deseases (n = 84)
CYFRA 21-1 (ng/ml)	1.8	2.1
TPA (U/l)	133	131
TPS (U/l)	97	237
TPA-CYK (ng/ml)	0.6	2.1
CEA (ng/ml)	2.3	7.4
SCC (ng/ml)	1.3	2.4
NSE (ng/ml)	9.8	18.0
CASA (U/ml)	3.1	10.6
NCAM (U/ml)	12.0	13.6
Chromogranin (ng/ml)	10.3	14.7
CA 19-9 (U/ml)	35	39
CA 72-4 (U/ml)	4.0	7.0
CA 50[a] (U/ml)	?	52
CA 242[a] (U/ml)	ca. 20.0	?

[a] Results taken from the literature

and sensitivity in lung cancer. Therefore we choose benign pulmonary diseases as clinically relevant control group and furthermore we fixed specificity versus this reference group at 95%. The resulting cut-off values were taken as basis for the calculations of sensitivities of the different markers in lung cancer. In table I it becomes evident, that for some markers the cut-off values are rather similar for healthy persons and benign diseases of the lung, whereas for others like for example for CEA, TPS and CASA there is a great discrepancy between the values of the two reference groups. The sometimes extremely high difference in sensitivities between some publications and our results are due to cut-off values which have been taken into account for the investigations.

Small cell lung carcinoma (SCLC)

Neuron-specific enolase (NSE) is the tumor marker of choice for small-cell lung carcinoma, both for diagnosis and for monitoring of therapeutic response (table II). Histological diagnosis is of great importance for a sensible therapeutic approach to this type of tumor. However, given that unfavorable location of the tumor results in bronchoscopy and bronchial lavage failing to establish a histological diagnosis in 10 to 20% of patients, NSE can sometimes provide evidence of the presence of a small cell lung carcinoma. Investigating the NSE as a diagnostic tool in lung tumors of unknown origine and dignity we found (figure 1) that in 5% of the patients with benign disorders of the lung NSE was > 12 ng/ml and < 20 ng/ml. Lung metastases from other solid tumors showed in general rather low NSE-concentrations but in 2% of the patients values

Table II. Sensitivities (%) for different types of lung cancer of the markers mentioned in table I at a specificity of 95% versus benign lung diseases.

Marker	All	SCLC	NSCLC	Squamous	Adeno-	Large cell
NSE	19	55	5	5	3	9
CYFRA 21-1	61	52	64	79	54	60
CEA	29	18	33	25	41	27
TPA	51	52	50	62	40	41
TPS	22	32	17	18	16	18
TPA-cyk	15	20	10	11	6	17
SCC	18	6	19	38	5	
CASA	16	37	11	14	8	6
NCAM	22	30	4	3	6	
Chromogranin A	24	27	20	31	19	14
CA 19-9	16	26	14	13	20	22
CA 72-4	15	2	18	13	25	10
CA 50[a]	12					
CA 242[a]			29			

[a] Results taken from the literature

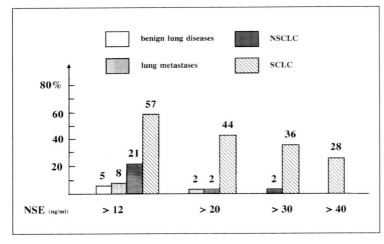

Figure 1. Differential diagnosis of lung tumors of unknown dignity by neuron specific enolase: NSE (%) in various benign and malignant diseases of the lung.

could reach 30 ng/ml. All the NSE values higher than 30 ng/ml were due to primary carcinomas of the lung, but in 2% of these patients also non-small cell lung carcinomas proved to have NSE values up to 40 ng/ml. But all NSE results > 40 ng/ml were due to small cell lung carcinomas. The combined determination of NSE and CYFRA 21-1 showed significant additive sensitivities higher than those reached in former times by combining NSE and CEA, and can therefore be recommended in SCLC.

Non-small cell lung carcinomas (NSCLC)

In non-small cell lung carcinomas CYFRA 21-1 proved to be the marker of choice. At 95% specificity versus benign diseases of the lung CYFRA 21-1 has with 64% a considerably higher number of tue positive test results than established markers like CEA (33%), TPA (50%), TPS (17%) and all the other antigens investigated (table II). In squamous cell carcinomas of the lung this leading position of CYFRA 21-1 becomes with 79% sensitivity even more evident (CEA: 25%, TPA: 62%, TPS: 18%, SCC:38%). Also in adenocarcinomas CYFRA 21-1 is with 54% true positive results superior to CEA (41%) and TPA (40%), but as has been described before (10, 16) the combined determination of CYFRA 21-1 and CEA can be recommended until one of these two markers becomes clearly positive. In large cell carcinomas CYFRA 21-1 (60%) is significantly superior to CEA (27%) and the other markers but following our experiences in routine laboratory diagnosis there might be some cases were only CEA becomes positive; therefore we recommend

Table III. Tumor marker determinations in lung cancer in routine laboratory diagnosis at time of primary diagnosis and for follow-up care and therapy monitoring.

Histology	Before therapy	Follow-up control
Unknown	CYFRA 21-1, NSE, CEA	post surgery: following the result of histology; without surgery: following the result of tumor markers
Adeno-	CYFRA21-1 and CEA	CYFRA 21-1 and/or CEA
Squamous cell	CYFRA 21-1	CYFRA 21-1
Small cell	NSE and CYFRA 21-1	NSE and CYFRA 21-1
Large cell	CYFRA 21-1 and CEA	CYFRA 21-1 and/or CEA

also for this histological type of lung cancer the combined determination of CYFRA 21-1 and CEA (table III).

Follow-up care

Besides the aid in differential diagnosis in lung tumors of unknown dignity the main indication for tumor marker determinations in lung cancer is of course the control of efficiency of therapy and the postoperative follow-up care. Tumor marker kinetics, not individual values, are critical in this respect. For most of the tumor markers in various carcinomas the speed of postoperative decrease of the corresponding tumor marker serves as a first sign of prognosis. Basic condition is a significantly elevated tumor marker value at time of primary diagnosis. Decreasing values after primary surgery corresponding to the half-life period (2-3 days for CEA and SCC, several hours for CYFRA 21-1 and NSE) is a first sign of curative resection and therefore of good prognosis, so assay of tumor marker levels therefore constitutes an important non-invasive method of monitoring the course of the disease. Tumor marker values which are decreasing slowly and perhaps even not moving down to the reference range can be a sign of non curative surgery (tumor rest).

During follow-up care an increase of tumor marker values (even within the reference range) can be the first sign of recurrent disease. This increase can be more than six months earlier than the detection of progressive disease by medical imaging or clinical manifestation (lead time).

Depending on its rapidity, a secondary rise in tumor marker concentration following postoperative normalization is strongly suggestive either of local recurrence or of distant metastasis. One example for the potential value of relevant tumor markers for the control of efficiency of therapy and follow-up care of lung carcinomas is demonstrated in figure 2. The cut-off values are fixed at a specificity of 95% versus benign diseases of the lung. For the follow-up presentation the tumor marker values are divided by these cut-offs. Figure 2 represents the graphical follow-up of a 70 year old man suffering from an adenocarcinoma of the lung (T2 N2 Mo G3). At time of primary diagnosis only CYFRA 21-1 showed a slight elevation (5.1 ng/ml). After surgery this value decreases to 1.3 ng/ml. At the first date of post-examination there was clinically and by medical imaging (chest x-ray) no evidence of disease. CYFRA 21-1 had significantly increased up to 6.1 ng/ml. Three months later progressive disease was confirmed by sceleton scintigraphy and computed tomography of the chest (detection of multiple bone metastases). At this time CYFRA 21-1 was 82.0 ng/ml, a serum concentration which corresponds in most cases to distant metastases.

Conclusions

Following the results from the literature and our own findings there are at the moment three serological markers which are helpful in monitoring

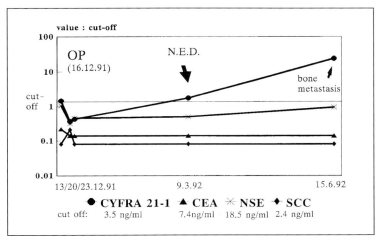

Figure 2. Follow-up of lung cancer, pT2 pN2 MO pG3 adenocarcinoma.

the disease of lung cancer patients: NSE, CYFRA 21-1 and CEA. Depending on the histological type of the tumor these marker show a significant better profile of specificity and sensitivity than the other parameters do.

Our recommendation for the use of tumor markers in routine laboratory work to support diagnosis, follow-up care and control of efficiency of therapy in lung cancer patients is summarized in table III. As "marker-negative" large primary tumors or distant metastases are unlikely to become marker-positive subsequently or after therapy, regular checks of tumor marker levels make little sense in such cases. In the case of marker-negative small tumors, by contrast, regular checks are worth-while, as progression may well lead to expression of the antigen. If during follow-up care one of the two markers used becomes significantly positive the single determination of this "leading" marker is enough for further control of efficiency of therapy.

In summary, patients suffering from lung cancer, can benefit from assay and correct interpretation of tumor marker levels in the following circumstances.

1. Aid in differential diagnosis between NSCLC and SCLC: as histological diagnosis is of great importance for a sensible therapeutic approach to small cell lung carcinomas and bronchial lavage is sometimes failing to establish histological diagnosis, NSE can sometimes provide evidence of a small cell lung carcinoma (figure 1).

2. Determining the prognosis at time of primary diagnosis can sometimes be helpful for therapeutical decisions. CYFRA 21-1 proved to possess a good prognostic tool at time of primary diagnosis (9).

3. Checking the effectiveness of therapy: the change of tumor marker concentration can indicate at an early stage whether the patient is likely to benefit from continuation of therapy (like chemotherapy or radiotherapy in lung cancer) or whether – in the case of continuously rising marker concentrations – a change in therapeutic approach is required or whether therapy can be dispensed with altogether. Tumor marker assay makes no sense in untreatable tumor patients.

4. Identification of residual tumor: after surgery the markers should decrease following their half life period (CYFRA 21-1 and NSE: several hours, CEA: 2-3 days) to the reference range, which would be a typical sign for complete removal of the tumor. Failure of tumor marker levels to fall adequately or at all after therapy is suggestive either of incomplete removal of tumor or of the presence of multiple tumors. Such a finding therefore has therapeutic and prognostic implications.

5. Monitoring of the course of the disease: the use of tumor markers to monitor the course of disease not uncommonly permits identification of metastatic spread and/or recurrent disease six months or more before these become clinically manifest. The rapidity of rises in tumor marker levels generally also permits conclusions as to the nature of the progression or metastatic spread that is taking place. Changes in tumor marker levels can sometimes also help in selection of the optimal time for the performance of further detailed investigations. Our recent results indicate that if CYFRA 21-1 is positive pretherapeutically and decreases to the reference range after surgery, further investigations involving invasive – or expensive – techniques are rendered unnecessary as long as CYFRA 21-1 is investigated in short intervals and shows stable kinetics and no sign of increase. Conversely, where the level of CYFRA 21-1 is rising and knowing that the disease is progressing would have therapeutic consequences, such investigations are indicated.

As seen from the above, correct use of tumor markers in lung cancer can bring benefit to patients and can even help to reduce costs. Uncritical use of them like monitoring untreatable tumor patients, on the other hand, can greatly increase costs and can cause severe psychological trauma to patients. Failure to correctly evaluate results obtained with tumor markers can even lead to mistaken medical decisions.

References

1 Akoun G, Scarna H, Milleron B, Benichou M, Herman D (1987) Serum neuron-specific enolase. A marker for disease extent and response to therapy for small cell lung cancer. Chest:39–43

2 Bergmann B, Brezicka F, Engström C (1992) Clinical utility of serum assays of neuron specific enolase, carcinoembryonic antigen and CA-50 antigen in the diagnostic evaluation of lung cancer patients. Eur J Cancer 29:198–202

3. Broers JL, Ramaekers FC, Rot MK, Oostendorp T, Huysmans A, van Muijen GN (1988) Cytokeratins in different types of human lung cancer as monitored by chain-specific monoclonal antibodies.Cancer Res 48 (11):3221–3229
4. Bodenmüller H, Banauch D, Ofenloch B, Jaworek D, Dessauer (1992) Technical evaluation of a new automated tumor marker assay: the Enzymun-Test CYFRA 21-1. In: Klapdor R (ed) Tumor associated antigens, oncogenes, receptors, cytokines in tumor diagnosis and therapy at the beginning of the nineties. Zuckschwerdt, München, pp 137–138
5. Debus E, Moll R, Franke WW, Weber K, Osborn M (1984) Immunohistochemical distinction of human carcinomas by cytokeratin typing with monoclonal antibodies. A J Pathol 114(1):121–130
6. Devine P, McGuckin M, Ramm L, Ward B, Pee D, Long S (1993) Serum mucin antigens CASA and MSA in tumors of the breast, ovary, lung, pancreas, bladder, colon and prostate. Cancer 72, 6:2007–2015
7. Dienemann H, Stieber P, Zimmermann A, Hoffmann H, Müller C, Banauch D (1994) Tumor-marker CYFRA 21-1 in non small cell lung cancer (NSCLC): Role for detection of recurrence. Lung Cancer 11, suppl 1:46
8. Ebert W, Hug G, Stabrey A, Bülzebruck H, Drings P (1989) Evaluation of tumormarkers NSE and CEA for the diagnosis and follow-up of small cell lung cancer. Ärztl Lab 35:1–10
9. Ebert W, Leichtweis B, Schapöler B, Muley Th (1993) The new tumor marker CYFRA is superior to SCC antigen and CEA in the primary diagnosis of lung cancer.Tumor Diagn Ther 14:91–99
10. Ebert W, Dienemann H, Fateh-Moghadam A, Scheulen M, Konietzko N, Schleich T, Bombardieri E (1994): Cytokeratin 19 fragment CYFRA 21-1 compared with carcinoembryonic antigen, squamous cell carcinoma antigen and NSE in lung cancer. Eur J Clin Chem Clin Biochem 32:189–199
11. Fischbach W, Ring G (1988) SCC-Antigen: Ein sensitiver und spezifischer Tumormarker für Plattenepithelkarzinome? Dtsch med Wochenschr 113:289–293
12. Klapdor R (1992) Arbeitsgruppe Qualitätskontrolle und Standardisierung von Tumormarkertests im Rahmen der Hamburger Symposien über Tumormarker. Tumordiagn u Ther 5, XIX–XXII
13. Stieber P, Hasholzner U, Bodenmüller H, Nagel D, Sunder-Plassmann L, Dienemann H, Meier W, Fateh-Moghadam A (1993) CYFRA 21-1 – a new marker in lung cancer. Cancer, 72, 3:707-713
14. Stieber P, Müller Ch, Hasholzner U, Dienemann H, Fiebig M, Fateh-Moghadam A (1993) CYFRA 21-1 – Ein neuer Marker beim Bronchialkarzinom. Lab med 17: 7-8/93, 328–332
15. Stieber P, Bodenmüller H, Banauch D, Hasholzner U, Dessauer A, Ofenloch-Hänle B, Jaworek D, Fateh-Moghadam A (1993) Cytokeratin 19 fragments: A new marker for non-small-cell-lung cancer. Clin Biochem 26:301–304
16. Stieber P, Dienemann H, Hasholzner U, Müller Ch, Poley S, Hofmann K, Fateh-Moghadam A (1993) Comparison of cytokeratin fragment 19 (CYFRA 21-1), tissue polypeptide antigen (TPA) and tissue polypeptide specific antigen (TPS) as tumor markers in lung cancer. Eur J Clin Chem Clin Biochem 31, 10:689–694

Address for correspondence:
Dr. med. Petra Stieber
Institut für Klinische Chemie
Klinikum Großhadern
Marchioninistraße 15
D-81366 München, Germany

Stage related surgery of bronchial carcinoma

J. Schirren, S. Trainer, W. Richter, P. Schneider, H. Bülzebruck, I. Vogt-Moykopf

Thorax-Clinic, Heidelberg-Rohrbach, Germany

For patients with NSCLC not presenting with metastasis the primary operation provides the best chance of cure. This therapeutic concept encloses the TNM categories Tl-T3, N0-N2, M0 (UICC Stage I to IIIa). But a resection, however, is only feasible in 30% of all patients with NSCLC. Size and location of the lesion are decisive for the extent of the surgical intervention. Standard procedures are lobectomy, organ-sparing operations (sleeve resections of the bronchial tree or the lung vessels) and pneumonectomy. Because of the problematic lymphatic drainage, segmental resections are carried out only in patients with poor ventilatory capacity or other severe risk factors. Pneumonectomy often can be avoided by organ-sparing operations with equally complete surgical remission. These procedures improve postoperative life quality and the preconditions for any necessary chemo- or radiation therapy.

Organ-sparing operations are lobectomies combined with a defect resection of the main bronchus. Additional segmental resection of pulmonary vessels is possible. The severed bronchial and vascuclar structures are anastomosed end to end. In most challenging cases lobe transposition and/or the extracorporeal resection with autotransplantation of healthy parts of the lung are requested. For patients with reduced lung function these methods allow a radical oncologic operation, where pneumonectomy would be impossible. Also some adjuvant chemotherapies are not possible after pneumonectomy, because the obligatory extensive infusion therapy would cause a volume overload.

Wedge and segmental resections

Wedge and segmental resections principally are not performed in young patients with good ventilatory function for the reason of insufficient radicality due to lymphatic drainage (3). These procedures are left up to patients with severe cardio-respiratory failure.

Extended resections

These operations are modifications of standard procedures which are combined with additional resections of adjacent structures or organs (f.e. pericardium, left atrium, recurrent nerve, phrenic nerve, chestwall, diaphragm, trachea, esophagus, v. cava). Also in tumors encroaching on the mediastinum extended resections may be useful, if a complete excision can be achieved. Even infiltration of the carina or the distal trachea (T4) can be managed by use of these techniques. In this case a pneumonectomy with resection of the carina is performed en bloc. The airway is reconstructed by end to end anastomosis between trachea and opposite main-bronchus. This technique enables a long time survival for locally advanced stages. Thus tumor invasion of adjacent structures (T3/4) is not necessarily a contraindication for a surgical treatment. These cases of extensive tumor growth require an individual decision for every patient. Often the question of operability can only be answered after thoracotomy. Encouraging reasons for an extended resection are the absence of effective therapeutic alternatives, young age and lack of other risk factors. A circumscribed invasion of parietal pleura or chestwall can be resected with the same radical intent as strictly intrapulmonary lesions. The resulting defects are sufficiently covered by synthetic patches (Marlex mesh®, Gore-Tex®). Also half of the pericardium can be resected without significant increase of risk. The replacement of the excised pericardium is usually performed with Gore-Tex® (Surgical membrane).

Table I. Radiological versus postoperative T-stage (primary tumor, n = 1404).

	pT 1	2	3	4	Total
T1	111	66	2	3	182
T2	75	579	48	51	753
T3	1	98	92	48	239
T4	4	78	48	100	230
Total	191	821	190	202	1404

Correctly staged: 63%   T1 correctly staged: 61%
Overstaged: 22%   T2 correctly staged: 77%
Understaged: 15%   T3 correctly staged: 38%
                        T4 correctly staged: 43%

Table II. Radiological versus postoperative N-stage (lymph nodes, n = 1404).

	pN 1	2	3	4	Total
N0	318	102	88	12	520
N1	126	153	88	17	384
N2	94	155	181	36	466
N3	4	5	13	12	34
Total	542	415	370	77	1404

Correctly staged: 47%   N0 correctly staged: 61%
Overstaged: 28%   N1 correctly staged: 40%
Understaged: 25%   N2 correctly staged: 39%
                        N3 correctly staged: 35%

The pancoast carcinomas represent a special group of T3/4 tumors. The surgical procedure consists of upper lobectomy, resection of the first and probably more ribs, mobilization of axillary nervous plexus and vessels and, if necessary, prosthetic vascular reconstruction. The operation is combined with pre- and postoperative radiation. Remaining tumor (R1/2) demands, if possible, an implantation of "afterloading" tubes or intraoperative radiation therapy.

Systematic lymph node dissection

A correct TNM staging and stage related surgical procedure requires a systematic mediastinal lymph node dissection (table I). The preoperative assessment of mediastinal lymph nodes with CT-scan is very uncertain. The involvement of N2-lymph nodes could be predicted correctly only in 38%. The main problem in this context is, that enlargement of lymph nodes can be caused by other reasons than metastatic invasion. The combination of CT-scan and mediastinoscopy does not improve the preoperative sensitivity. The small, harmless appearing T1-tumor is combined with mediastinal lymph node metastasis in 19–20% (4). The aim of the lymph node dissection is the discovery of hidden N2/N3 disease and the complete resection of it. In case of metastatic invasion, the operation must be followed by a postoperative mediastinal radiation therapy.

The regular lymphatic drainage direction in the mediastinum is caudal, cranial or to the contralateral thoracic cavity. The metastatic spread does not respect the topographic order of the lymph nodes. A "skipping" within this drainage system has been described. For this reason an affection of mediastinal lymph nodes despite of free broncho-pulmonal or hilar lymph nodes is possible (4). The complete removal of all regional mediastinal lymph node metastasis requires a systematic mediastinal lymph node resection, including the contralateral positions. This procedure is more difficult, when it has to be performed by a left posterolateral thoracotomy compared to a right one. But mobilization of the aortic arch together with the subclavian artery faciliates the same radical dissection as from the right side. In our experience the postoperative morbidity is not increased by this additional procedure.

The dissection of tumor free lymph nodes provides a security distance, which is an established principle of primary tumor resection. So lymph node dissection, as far as possible into healthy lymph node regions is an important requirement for a real R0-resection (TNM-Atlas, 1989).

Therapy of distant metastasis

Stage IV is characterized by distant metastasis. This means a generalization of the disease, which normally is a contraindication for a surgical intervention. Nevertheless there are situations, where resections of isolated metastasis (e.g. in the liver, suprarenal gland or brain) provided a prolongation of lifetime. A solitary pulmonary metastasis, ipsi- or contralateral, can be resected together with the primary tumor in one operation. The

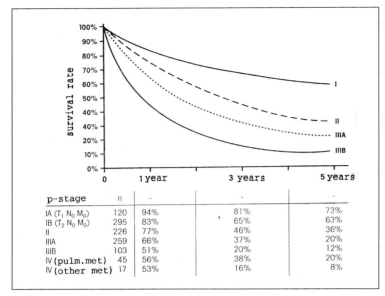

Figure 1. Prognosis according to p-stage and radical resection.

simultaneous removal of abdominal or retroperitoneal metastasis can be performed by a transdiaphragmatic approach or by combining a median sternotomy with a laparotomy. It must be emphasized that the postoperative staging often differs significantly from the preoperative assessment. For example supposed suprarenal metastasis turn out to be adenoma or supposed liver metastasis might really show themselves as hemangiomas. All types of coin lesions can simulate lung metastasis.

The problem, to undertake a resection of stage IV bronchial carcinoma is an individual decision. Possible risks and expected benefit must be assessed in an interdisciplinary manner for every single patient.

References

1. Bülzebruck H, Bop R, Drings P, Bauer E, Krysa S, Probst G, van Kaick G, Müller KM, Vogt-Moykopf I (1992) New aspects in the staging of lung cancer, Cancer 70:1102–1110
2. Schildberg FW, Sunder-Plassmann L (1990) Chirurgische Therapie des Bronchialkarzinoms. Chirurg 61: 558–564
3. Junker K, Müller KM (1989) Metastasierungsmuster beim Bronchialkarzinom. Z Herz-Thorax-Gefäßchir 3:189-194
4. Schirren J, Cuenoud PF, Bülzebruck H, Krysa S (1992) N2-surgery in bronchial carcinoma. Gen Thorac Surg 1: 32–41
5. Martini N, Bains MS, Kaiser IR, Burt ME, Pomerantz AH (1988) Surgical treatment of non-small cell carcinoma of the lung. The Memorial Sloan Kettering Experience. In: Hoogstraten B, Adis BJ, Hansen HH, Martini N, Spiro SG (eds) Lung tumors (VICC – Current treatment of cancer) Springer, Berlin Heidelberg New York, pp 111
6. Seely JM, Mayo I, Müller R, Müller N (1993) T1-lung-cancer: Prevalence of mediastinal nodal metastases and diagnostic accuracy of CT. Radiology 136:129
7. Maasen W (1985) Staging issues problems: Accuracy of mediastinoscopy. In: Delarve NC, Eschapasse H (eds) lung cancer (International trends in general thoracic surgery. Vol I) Sanders, Philadelphia London Toronto, pp 42
8. Shields TW (1993) Surgical therapy for carcinoma of the lung. Clin Chest Med 14:121–147

Address for correspondence:
Dr. med. J. Schirren
Thoraxklinik Heidelberg-Rohrbach
Amalienstraße 5
D-69126 Heidelberg, Germany

Chemotherapeutic treatment of bronchial carcinoma

Marlene Heckmayr, U. Gatzemeier
Department of Thoracic Oncology, Hamburg-Großhansdorf, Germany

Introduction

Bronchial carcinomas are often inoperable at the time of diagnosis. Without treatment the median survival time is about 2-3 months and the 5-year survival rate is about 8% (1). With chemotherapeutic treatment it is possible to prolong the overall survival time and to improve the 5-year survival rate (2). Because of different chemotherapeutic sensitivities it is important to distinguish between small cell and non-small cell carcinomas of the lung.

Small cell carcinomas

20-25% of all bronchial carcinomas are small cell carcinomas. In small cell bronchial carcinomas combination chemotherapy is the first line therapy. The prognosis of these tumors depends on the factors listed in table I.

Table I. Prognostic factors of small cell carcinomas.

Tumor stage
Performance index
Weight loss
Sex
Serum-LDH
Tumor response

Platin derivatives, Vinca alkaloids, alkylating agents, etoposide and adriamycin are the most effective cytostatic drugs in small cell lung cancer. With combination chemotherapy the following remission rates and survival times are available (table II).

Under cisplatin containing- regimens remission rate and median survival time improved in comparison to adriamycin with cyclophosphamide and vincristine (ACO). In the last six years we have treated all of our patients with the combination-chemotherapy carboplatin-etoposide and vincristine (CEV)

The median survival time (months) for all patients is 10.5, for LD/ED 13.0/9.0. The 1-year survival time for all is 41.7%, for LD/ED 51.7%/9.0%. The 3-year survival time for all is 19.1%, for LD/ED 29.1/8.6%

Following chemotherapy local recurrences at the site of the primary tumor occured in 22.8% and distant metastases in 31.4% of all cases. Primary tumor and distant metastases could be observed in 45.7%, cerebral metastases in 48.5%, liver metastases in 17.1% and bone metastases in 14.3%. Thoracic radiotherapy following complete remissions under chemotherapy moderately improves the 3-year survival time (5.4%) in limited diease. The optimal schedules of radiotherapy to chemotherapy – concurrent, alternating or sequential – is without influence on remission rate or survival time.

Table II. SCLC combination-chemotherapy results.

	Remission rate (%)	Median survival time (months)	3-Year survival (%)
Limited diseases	70-90	14-20	10-30
Extensive diseases	40-70	9-12	0-10

That means, that in small cell bronchial carcinomas combination chemotherapy is the first line therapy. For 10 to 15% of the patients with limited disease the chemotherapy will be curative. Therefore the treatment should be as aggressive as possible. Platin containing chemotherapy improved in comparison to ACO.

In patients with good performance index more aggressive chemotherapy is indicated under curative intention.

Less agressive therapy under palliative intention is indicated in elderly patients or patients with bad performance index.

Non-small cell carcinoma

There are 40.000 newly diagnosed cases of non-small cell carcinomas every year in Germany. At the time of diagnosis 65% of all non-small cell carcinoms are inoperable. In advanced carcinomas the chemotherapy is always only palliative. There is no standard chemotherapy regimen. The cytostatic substances used should have little side-effects to secure quality of life. The most effective substances in non-small cell bronchial carcinomas today are: ifosphamide, cisplatin, mitomycin-C, vindesine, etoposide and carboplatin. The preferable combinations used are cisplatin/etoposide, cisplatin/vindesine and mitomycin-C/vindesine. With these regimens remission rates between 30 and 50% depending on stage of disease are achieved. The median survival time is between six and eight months.

A meta-analysis of seven studies with over 700 patients in the last years around the world could have demonstrated the superiority of cytostatic therapy compared to supportive care therapy alone in non-small cell lung cancer (figure 1). There was a modest survival advantage with chemotherapy (figure 2)

In the last years several new cytotoxic substances were developed like irinotecan (a topoisomerase-derivative), paclitaxel (taxol), vinorelbin (a Vinca alkaloid), edatrexat (a methotrexat-analogue), gemcitabine (a synthetic Vinca alkaloide). The remission rates are about 20–30%, the side effects are different. Recently extensive experience with preoperative chemotherapy for locally advanced non-small cell lung cancer has been reported. It appears that 60–73% of the patients may be respected to response to one of a number of preoperative regimens. For example: Under MIC-chemotherapy the median survival time prolonged from 6 to 18 months with only a less reduced resection rate from 84 to 77 % (5).

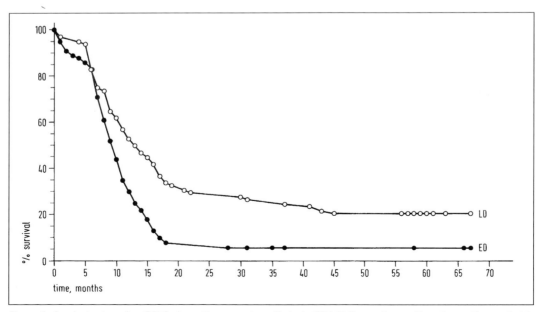

Figure 1. Survival rates after SCLC chemotherapy; phase II study CEV. Unil now the median observation period is 61.5 months, the 5-year survival rates are 21% (LD) and 7% (ED.) (● = ED, ○ = LD; p = 0.02)

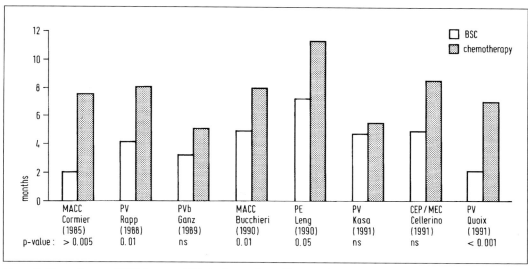

Figure 2. Chemotherapy (NSCLC versus BSC studies, review of literature).

That means, for non-small cell lung cancer there is no standard chemotherapy. Chemotherapy in non-small cell bronchial carcinoma is always only palliative. Prognostic factors are more important than chemotherapy protocols. Under chemotherapy prolongation of survival time is possible. The cytostatic substances should have little side-effects to secure quality of life.

References

1. Skarin A (1991) Bronchial carcinomas. Data without therapy. NSCLC, Cancer Medicine, Boston, p 24
2. Gatzemeier U (1990) Chemotherapie der Bronchialkarzinome. Hamburger Ärzteblatt 44:175–181
3. Gatzemeier U et al (1992) Carboplatin/etposide/vincristine therapy in small cell lung cancer. Oncol 49:25–33
4. Souquet PJ et al (1993) Polychemotherapy in advanced non small cell lung cancer: a meta-analysis. Lancet 342:19–21
5. Rosell R et al (1992) Neoadjuvant chemotherapy of advanced non-small cell lung cancer. Proc ASCO, abstr 954

Address for correspondence:
Dr. med. Marlene Heckmayr
Abteilung für Thorax-Onkologie
Krankenhaus Großhansdorf
Wöhrendamm 80
D-22927 Großhansdorf, Germany

Radiotherapy for lung cancer

*Karin Koch, I. Broll, W. Frank, H. Hartmann, D. Kaiser,
D. Krumhaar, R. Loddenkemper, W. Matthiessen, H. Neusetzer*
Department of Radiation Therapy, Klinikum Ernst von Bergmann, Potsdam, Germany

Introduction

Radiotherapy for non-small cell lung cancer is a definitive therapy for patients with inoperable lung cancer because of technical or medical reasons with curative or mostly palliative intentions.
Preoperative irradiation is recommended only in patients with Pancoast's tumors. Postoperative irradiation is indicated in patients with hilar or mediastinal lymph node metastasis or positive surgical margins.
Small cell lung cancer is sensitive to many chemotherapeutic agents. Additonal thoracic irradiation enhances control of the primary tumor and locoregional lymph node metastasis. The significance of prophylactic brain irradiation is not definitively determined.
Good and symptomatic improvement is observed as a result of radiation therapy in patients suffering from superior vena cava syndrome, poststenotic complications as pneumonia and atelectasis, locoregional recurrences, brain, bone and sometimes suprarenal and liver metastases.

Interdisciplinary cooperation

To integrate the various disciplines and provide better care for patients it is important for the radiation therapist to cooperate closely with specialists in the other disciplines in management of the patients.
Weekly tumor conferences for treatment planning and assessment of the course of the disease of every individual patient are realized in the cooperation between the Lung Clinic Heckeshorn and the Radiotherapy Department of University Hospital Rudolf Virchow in Berlin.

Patients

We report our results on treatment of 1234 lung cancer patients (949 men (77%) and 285 women (23%)) within five years. Mean (median) age amount to 65.7 (68.5) years, 73% of the patients were elder than 60 years.
The histological classification showed 3% squamous cell caricinoma, 21% small cell carcinoma, 20% large cell carcinoma, 15% adenocarcinoma, 8% carcinomas without classification and 4% without histological classification.
Stage distribution was typical for lung cancer with 8% stage I, 11% stage II, 39% stage III, 26% stage IV and 16% not classified.

Treatment modalities

Irradiations as only treatment modality were carried out in 54% of the patients, combined treatment modalities with surgery in 21%, with chemotherapy in 15%, with surgery and chemotherapy in 3%, other therapies in 7%.
All patients were treated at accelerators. Most treatment plans are calculated by computer based on individual CT to minimize radiation exposure of the lung parenchyma and other critical normal tissues.
Numerous non-randomized and randomized studies have been published on the results of radiation therapy with various fractionation schedules. Most clinical results have been obtained with single daily doses of 1.8 to 2.5 Gray and total doses ranglng from 40 to 65 Gray. Dose escalation up to 79.2 Gray is possible with hyperfractionation. Based on the results of the RTOG studies it is concluded, that higher total doses result in a greater proportion of complete

response, higher intrathoracic tumor control and a better survival up to three years.

On the other hand we have to consider the natural history of lung cancer with a high incidence of metastases and low probability of long-term survival. So, altered fractionation including different regimes of hypofractionation are justified. The reality of clinical practice is that most patients suffer from advanced diseases at presentation and have symptoms, which can be treated effectively by radiation therapy with or without influencing the prognosis.

Our patients received once a week irradiations with single doses of 4 to 5 Gray, total doses (10–60 Gray) varied depending on the aim of treatment. The tolerance is better than with conventional fractionation, remission rates are similar.

Results and survival

The remission rates inside the irradiated volume come to 21% complete remission, 32% partial remission, 16% minor response, no change 14%, progression 3% and not evaluable 14%. (The survival of the patients is shown in figures 1 to 6.) All datas are summarized from clinical practice without any selection criteria and include also all the patients with unfavorable prognosis, who received only symptomatic radiotherapy.

Toxicity results

The most frequently sequelae following lung irradiation are pneumonits and pulmonary fibrosis. In our patients mild reactions appeared in 9%, moderate in 7%, severe in 1% and life-threatening in 0.1%. Esophagitis appeared in less than 1%. No thoracic spinal cord radiation myelopathy was observed.

Brachytherapy

Indications for use of endoluminal brachytherapy in lung cancer are stenosis of the trachea or of the main or lobe bronchi caused by endobronchial tumor growth. We have ten years experience in endobronchial high dose rate afterloading therapy with iridium-192.

Patients

469 patients suffering from lung cancer with central endobronchial stenosis were evaluated.

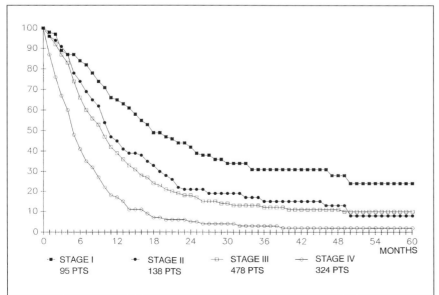

Figure 1. Stage depending overall survival (%) of the entire radiotherapy group.

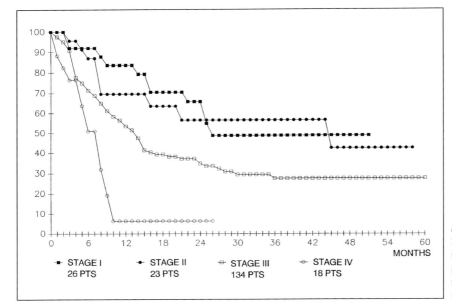

Figure 2. Stage depending survival (%) of patients with surgery and radiation therapy.

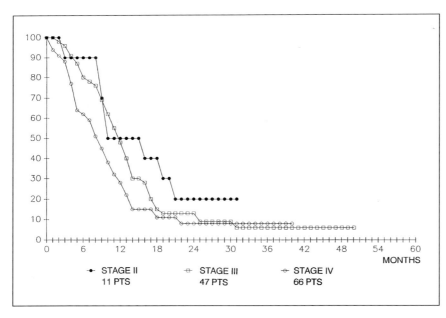

Figure 3. Stage depending survival (%) of patients with small cell lung cancer.

The mean age of 378 males and 91 females was 63 years. The tumor stage was usually advanced with 56% T3- and T4-tumors, 91% positive lymphnodes and 27% distant metastases. The most frequent histology was squamous cell carcinoma in 66%.

Treatment modalities

A total of 1526 HDR afterloading applications were administered to the 469 patients. A prescribed dose of 15 Gray for a single application was calculated at a distance of 5 mm from the

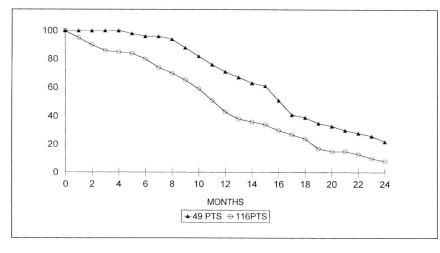

Figure 4.
Survival (%) of 49 patients with small cell lung cancer and adjuvant brain irradiation and 116 patients with SCLC and brain metastases and irradiation (non-randomized).

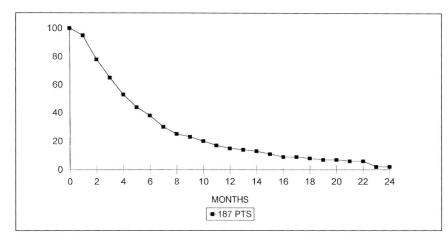

Figure 5.
Survival (%) of patients after diagnosis of brain metastasis (histological classifications) and brain irradiation (≤ 30 Gray).

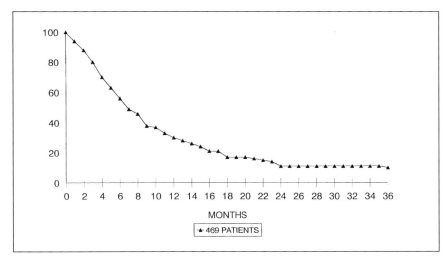

Figure 6.
Survival of patients after high dose rate afterloading therapy including the patients with recurrences.

source axis. More than half of the patients received three of four applications at two week intervals.

Because of advanced disease combined treatment modalities were mostly required. In the case of complete or severe stenosis a channel was first created with a laser for immediate restoration of the respiratory system and to permit the placement of the afterloading applicator. This occurred in 28% of the patients. Whereas the laser is capable of eliminating the endobronchial tumor growth immediately, the HDR afterloading technique offers the possibility of also dealing with peribronchial tumor growth without endangering the bronchial wall. HDR afterloading brachytherapy improves and prolongs the effect of the laser.

67% of the patients received simultaneous external beam irradiation. The total doses varied, the decision was individual to each patient depending on the extent of disease. Therapy planning was frequently palliativ, but it should be noted that high radiation doses are possible in a combined modality treatment.

The most successful therapeutic combination included surgery. This patient subgroup consisted of 6%. Preoperative afterloading therapy has to destroy tumor in the area of resection. A possibility of postoperative brachytherapy is an endangered bronchus stump if tumor cells were microscopically seen in or near the resection area. Assessments of the course of disease of 17 patients up to 85 months are encouraging.

Combined treatment with chemotherapy is indicated only in a few patients, in our series 2%. However, brachytherapy can be useful in some patients with atelectasis or pneumonia. When central stenosis and its complications improves, chemotherapy is to be started.

Results and survival

The overall response rate of our series of 469 patients is 69%, additional 7% showed a minor response. 30% of the patients received HDR afterloading because of recurrences and the response rate of this subgroup was 63%. 31% of the patients suffered from atelectasis and/or pneumonia, improvement was shown in 78%.

The overall survival (< 1–85 months) after HDR afterloading therapy of the entire patient population including those with recurrent disease after HDR afterloading is shown in figure 6.

Conclusions

Radiotherapy should be employed within the framework of the overall treatment concept for lung cancer. It presents an excellent possibility for palliative treatment, but it can also be used with curative intention.

The decision for radiotherapy has to be reflected not only in regard to survival, which is usually short, but also in regard to the symptoms and quality of life. Radiotherapy in patients with lung cancer should be tolerated well and offers the chance of improvement of the course of disease.

Address for correspondence:
Priv.-Doz. Dr. med. Karin Koch
Klinikum Ernst von Bergmann
Klinik für Strahlentherapie
Charlottenstaße 72
D-14467 Potsdam, Germany

Intrapleural administration of cytokines for malignant pleural effusions

A. M. M. Eggermont[a], G. Stoter[b]

Departments of [a]Surgical Oncology and [b]Medical Oncology, Rotterdam Cancer Institute, Rotterdam, The Netherlands

Introduction

Malignant pleural effusions are an important cause of morbidity in patients with advanced cancer. By definition, a malignant pleural effusion implies the presence of malignant cells in the pleural cavity. Although this may be caused by direct extension of a cancer into the pleural space, it is usually due to metastatic seeding onto the visceral or parietal pleural surface. Often free floating viable tumor cells in the pleural effusion are not demonstrable. In those cases where an exudative effusion is found with repeatedly negative cytology prognosis is equally poor, as is illustrated in the staging system for lung cancer (1). Almost two-thirds of all malignant pleural effusions are caused by lung and breast cancer (2). Most patients with a malignant pleural effusion have dyspnea, cough, pain and a sense of heaviness in the chest. Morbidity is significant and successful treatment may require a combination of modalities.

General treatment principles

Not always will one consider drainage followed by pleurodesis as the procedure of choice. For pleural effusions due to cancers likely to be highly sensitive to systemic chemotherapy as small cell lung cancer of lymphoma such a therapy is the treatment of choice. In breast cancer one may consider simple tube drainage followed by a course of systemic chemotherapy. In most other situations, however, one is confronted to chemo-insensitive cancers such as pancreatic cancer. Here tube drainage followed by pleurodesis is indicated. Many reports in the literature suggest that production of chest tube drainage should be less than 100 ml/24 h if a good result is to be expected from pleurodesis.

Traditional sclerosing and chemotherapeutic agents

Talc powder and tetracyclin are the agents most commonly used for pleurodesis. Both can induce a painful local inflammatory reaction, but high success rates of 96% for talc powder and of 70% for tetracyclin have been reported in the literature (3). Various cytostatic drugs have been used over the years. Some of these, e.g. nitrogen mustard and quinacrine are not used any more because resorption to the systemic compartment and concurrent toxicity. Bleomycin may be most commonly used (84% response rate) in spite of a recent poor result (30% response rate) in a trial where patients were randomised to be treated either with tetracyclin (53% response rate) or bleomycin (30% response rate) (4). Agents that have gained some recent popularity are cisplatin (49% response rate) and mitoxantrone (80% response rate) (5–7).

Unspecific immunostimulants

Bacterial preparations such as Corynebacterium parvum (C. parvum), Nocardia cell wall sceleton (N-CWS) and the streptococcal preparation OK-432, have been administered intrapleurally with comperable success. Response rates of 66–92% for C. parvum (8–9), 46% for N-CWS (10) and 40–88% for OK-432 (11–12) have been reported.

Table I. Intrapleural administration of interferons.

Dose	Patients	Response (%)	Reference
Interferon-α			
$2 \cdot 10^6$	8/14	57	Tercelj (13)
$1-10 \cdot 10^6$	5/9	55	Markowitz (14)
$7-7.5 \cdot 10^6$	14/40	70	Goldman (15)
$3-5 \cdot 10^6$	0/20	0	Davis (16)
Interferon-β			
$5-20 \cdot 10^6$	11/29	38	Rosso (17)
$5-15 \cdot 10^6$	2/22	9	Cascinu (18)
Interferon			
$2-40 \cdot 10^6$	6/19	31	Boutin (19)

Table II. Intrapleural administration of interleukin-2.

Dose	Patients	Response (%)	Reference
low	9/11	82	Yasumoto (20)
low	21/35	60	Yasumoto (21)
up to $24 \cdot 10^6$	6/25	22	Viallat (22)
Mesothelioma			
up to $36 \cdot 10^6$	4/17	23	Eggermont, 1993

Cytokines

Recombinant cytokines have been examined for their activity in the treatment of malignant pleural effusions in a number of trials over the last eight years.

The interferons

Various doses of interferon-a (IFNα), IFNβ and IFN have been evaluated both for their effect on malignant pleural effusions and on pleural tumors such as mesothelioma. The studies reported in the literature are summarized in table I. Striking differences in efficay are reported. For IFNα three studies (13–15) showed response rates from 55–70%, in contrast to Davis and coworkers (16) who did not register any responses in 20 patients treated. The same disparity is observed between the two studies performed in Italy with intrapleural IFNβ at similar doses (17–18). Boutin's study with IFNγ shows good antitumor activity of this agent, especially against pleural mesothelioma (19).

Interleukin-2

Yasumoto and coworkers reported as early as 1987 on the intrapleural application of Il-2 (20). They reported the disappearance of malignant pleural effusions in > 80% of the patients after intrapleural instillation of very low doses of IL-2. An updated report in 1991 on 35 patients showed a significant drop in response rate to about 60% (21). Viallat and colleques found a much lower response rate of 22% in a phase I dose escalation study (22).

The Rotterdam Mesothelioma Study

In Rotterdam we performed a phase I-II study in maligant pleural mesothelioma patients. This study was aimed to determine the MTD of intrapleural administration of IL-2 and to obtain an impression of the potential antitumor effects in these patients with bulky pleural tumor masses. In total 24 patients were treated. One to two weeks prior to the first administration of IL-2 a port-a-cath system was surgically inserted under general anesthesia. The correct intrapleural position of the catheter was checked radiographically and a colloid scan was made to check for good distribution throughout the pleural effusion. Twenty-four patients received recombinant human interleukin-2 (IL-2) (EuroCetus B.V., Amsterdam, the Netherlands) administered as a continuous intrapleural infusion at a dose according to a groupwise (at least three consecutive patients) dose escalation schedule (Group A: $3 \cdot 10^4$, B: $3 \cdot 10^5$, C: $3 \cdot 10^6$, D: $6 \cdot 10^6$, E: $18 \cdot 10^6$, and F: $36 \cdot 10^6$ IU/day; this is the equivalent of $5 \cdot 10^4$ up to $6 \cdot 10^6$ Cetus Units) for a period of 14 days at two week intervals. Thereafter, patients with stable disease or better could receive up to a maximum of four maintenance cycles at the same dose and route.

Tumor response: Of 24 eligible patients with pleural mesothelioma, 17 patients were fully evaluable (both for toxicity and tumor response) as they received at least one full 14 day cycle of intrapleural IL-2. At least one treatment cycle of 14 days was received by four patients at $3 \cdot 10^4$ IU/day, three patients $3 \cdot 10^5$ IU/day, three patients $3 \cdot 10^6$ IU/day, three patients $6 \cdot 10^6$ IU/day, three patients $18 \cdot 10^6$ IU/day, and one patient $36 \cdot 10^6$ IU/day. Patients received one up to five treatment cycles. Four patients had a partial remission of 5, 11, 20, and 30 months. Five patients had stable disease lasting 4, 4, 5, 6 and 8 months, and seven patients had progressive disease. The partial remissions occurred at the three lowest dose levels. Therefore no dose response relationship is evident. In two patients massive infected necrosis, in one patient sterile necrosis of the mesothelioma occured.

Toxicity and complications: Toxicity has been virtually absent in this study at all dose levels except for the highest. All patients received their treatment in an outpatient setting except for the last five patients of the study who were started on the highest dose level of $36 \cdot 10^6$ IU/day. Only minor flu-like symptoms were observed in the patients treated at the two higher dose levels. No systemic adverse effects, especially no hypotension or other cardiovascular effects, no pulmonary complications, no renal or liver dysfunction was observed. A slight leukocytosis (10,000–12,000 cells/ml) and an eosinophilia (2000–3500 cell/ml) were seen in most patients at the higher dose levels. Complications of the treatment consisted of infected catheter systems in four patients. At the highest dose level systemic toxicity was quite prominent and dose limiting. Only one patient managed to complete one cycle of 14 days. The four other patients were hospitalized and had to stop treatment because of dose limiting malaise. The systemic toxicity corresponded with serum IL-2 levels of up to 30 IU/ml in patients treated at the highest dose level. At these high dose levels infections of the catheter systems occured in the majority of the patients, and the catheters had to be removed before completion of the first cycle.

Conclusion: IL-2 given intrapleurally has antitumor activity against mesothelioma giving a response rate of 24% in 17 evaluable patients with this disease, known to be refractory to almost any treatment. Boutin and collegues recently reported similar antitumor activity with intrapleural IFN (19). We conclude on the basis of our study and the reports in the literature that intrapleural administration of cytokines should be further explored as a new mode of treatment for malignant pleural mesothelioma.

Tumor necrosis factor-α

The intrapleural administration of TNFα has been tested in few studies. Taguchi (23) and Karck (24) reported on very small numbers of patients. TNFα however was effective in almost all those patients (three out of four patients and five out of six patients).

In Rotterdam we embarked upon a phase I-II study with TNFa (Boehringer Ingelheim, GmbH) in pleural mesothelioma patients. One of the first three patients suffered from very rapid pleural effusion formation and needed tapping more than once a week of > 2 liters. This patients pleural effusion production came to a halt after six intrapleural instillations of low doses of TNFα.

Conclusion

Although the initial results are modest some good anti-effusion and antitumor effects have been observed after intrapleural administration of cytokines. Thus cytokines may play a role both in the treatment of malignant pleural effusions as in the treatment of pleural mesothelioma.

References

1. Mountain CF (1986) An international staging system for lung cancer. Chest 89:225–235 (suppl)
2. Hausheer FH, Yarbro JW (1985) Diagnosis and treatment of malignant pleural effusions. Sem Oncol 12:54–75
3. Ruckdeschel JC (1988) Management of malignant pleural effusion: An Overview. Sem Oncol (Suppl 3) 15:24–28
4. Ruckdeschel JC, Moores D, Lee YC, Einhorn LH, Mandelbaum I, Koeller J, Weiss GR, Losada M, Keller JH (1991) Intrapleural therapy for malignant pleural effusions. A randomized comparison of bleomycin and tetracycline. Chest 100:1483–84
5. Rusch VW, Figlin R, Godwin D, Piantadosi S (1991) Intrapleural cisplatin and cytarabine in the management of malignant pleural effusions: a Lung Cancer Group trial. J Clin Oncol 9:313–319
6. Feuilhade F, Brun B, Calitchi E, Otzmeguine Y, Haddad E, Le-Bourgeois JP, Pierquin B (1989) Efficacy and toxicity of intrapleural mitoxantrone: a propos of 18 cases of pleural metastases of breast cancer. Bull Cancer Paris 76:361–365
7. Torsten U, Opri F, Weitzel H (1992) Local therapy of malignant pleural effusion with mitoxantrone. Anticancer Drugs 3:17–18
8. McLeod DT, Calverley PM, Millar JW, Horne NW (1985) Further experience of Corynebacterium parvum in malignant pleural effusion. Thorax 40:515–518
9. Casali A, Gionfra T, Rinaldi M, Tonachella R, Tropea F, Venturo I, De Martino C, Curcio CG (1988) Treatment of malignant pleural effusions with intracavitary Corynebacterium parvum. Cancer 62:806–811
10. Fukuoka M, Takada M, Tamai S, Negoro S, Matsui K, Ryu S, Sakai N, Sakaguchi K (1984) Local application of anticancer drugs for the treatment of malignant pleural and pericardial effusion. Gan To Kagaku Ryoho 11:1543–1549
11. Luh KT, Yang PC, Kuo SH, Chang DB, Yu CJ, Lee LN (1992) Comparison of OK-432 and mitomycin C pleurodesis for malignant pleural effusion caused by lung cancer. A randomized trial. Cancer 69:674–679
12. Kan N, Kodama H, Hori T, Takenaka A, Yasumura T, Kato H, Ogawa H, Ohsumi K, Kuda N, Mukaihara S (1992) Intrapleural treatment of breast cancer patients with pleural effusions. Gan-To-Kagaku-Ryoho 19:1632–1635
13. Tercelj-Zorman M, Mermolja M, Jereb M, Oman M, soos E, Petric-Grabnar G, Jereb B (1991) Human leukocyte interferon alpha (HLI-a) for treatment of pleural effusion caused by non small cell lung cancer. Acta Oncologica 30:963–965
14. Markowitz A, Thielvoldt D, Yeomans A et al (1992) Beneficial effects of intracavitary interferon-α2b (IFN): a phase I study of patients with ascites or pleural effusion. Proc Am Assoc Clin Oncol 11:258 (abstract)
15. Goldman CA, Skinnider LF, Maksymiuk AW (1993) Interferon instillation for malignant pleural effusions. Ann Oncol 4:141–145
16. Davis M, Williford S, Muss HB, White DR, Cooper MR, Jackson DV, Barrett R (1992) A phase I-II study of recombinant intrapleural alpha interferon in malignant pleural effusions. Am J Clin Oncol 15:328–330
17. Rosso R, Rinaldi R, Salvati F et al (1988) Intrapleural natural beta-interferon in the treatment of malignant pleural effusions. Oncology 45:253–256
18. Cascinu S, Isidori PP, Fedeli A, Fedeli SL, Raspugli M, Rossi A, Ugolini M, Catalano G (1991) Experience with intrapleural natural beta interferon in the treatment of malignant pleural effusions. Tumori 77:237–238
19. Boutin C, Viallat JR, Van Zandwijk N et al (1991) Activity of intrapleural gamma-interferon in malignant mesothelioma. Cancer 67:2033–2037
20. Yasumoto K, Miyazaki K, Nagashima A et al (1987) Induction of lymphokine-activated killer cells by intrapleural instillations of recombinant interleukin-2 in patients with malignant pleurisy due to lung cancer. Cancer Res 47:2184–2187
21. Yasumoto K, Ogura T (1991) Intrapleural application of recombinant interleukin-2 in patients with malignant pleurisy due to lung cancer: a multi-institutional cooperative study. Biother 3:345–349
22. Viallat JR, Boutin C, Rey F, Astoul P, Farisse P, Brandely M (1992) Intrapleural immunotherapy with escalating doses of interleukin-2 in metastatic pleural effusions. Cancer 71:4067–4071
23. Taguchi T (1987) Recombinant human Tumor Necrosis Factor (rHu-TNF) phase I and early phase II study. Proc Am Soc Clin Oncol 6:233 (abstract)
24. Karck U, Meerpohl HG, Pfleiderer A et al (1990) TNF therapy of ascites and pleural effusions due to gynaecological carcinomas. J Cancer Res Clin Oncol 116:326 (abstr)

Address for correspondence:
A. M. M. Eggermont, MD
Department of Surgical Oncology
Rotterdam Cancer Institute
P.O. BOX 5201
NL-3008 AE Rotterdam, The Netherlands

Sponsors

of the 7th Symposium on Tumor Markers, Hamburg,
and the Satellite Symposium "Cancer of the Lung"

Abbott GmbH, Diagnostica, Wiesbaden-Delkenheim
ASTA MEDICA, Frankfurt am Main
Behring AG, Marburg
Biermann GmbH Diagnostica
Boehringer Mannheim
Bristol-Myers, München
Byk-Sangtec Diagnostica GmbH, Dietzenbach
Ciba Corning Diagnostics GmbH, Fernwald
Dianova, Hamburg
Glaxo GmbH, Hamburg
Hoffmann La Roche, Basel
Isotopen Diagnostik CIS GmbH, Dreieich
medac, Hamburg
Rhone-Poulenc Rorer, Köln
Schering AG, Berlin
Serva Feinbiochemica GmbH, Heidelberg
Sorin Biomedica, Düsseldorf